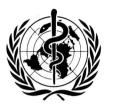

World Health Organization Classification of Tumours

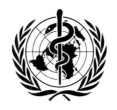

WHO   OMS

International Agency for Research on Cancer (IARC)

Revised 4th Edition

WHO Classification of Tumours of the Central Nervous System

Edited by

David N. Louis

Hiroko Ohgaki

Otmar D. Wiestler

Webster K. Cavenee

International Agency for Research on Cancer

Lyon, 2016

World Health Organization Classification of Tumours

Series Editors	Fred T. Bosman, MD PhD
	Elaine S. Jaffe, MD
	Sunil R. Lakhani, MD FRCPath
	Hiroko Ohgaki, PhD

WHO Classification of Tumours of the Central Nervous System
Revised 4th Edition

Editors	David N. Louis, MD
	Hiroko Ohgaki, PhD
	Otmar D. Wiestler, MD
	Webster K. Cavenee, PhD

Senior Advisors	David W. Ellison, MD PhD
	Dominique Figarella-Branger, MD
	Arie Perry, MD
	Guido Reifenberger, MD
	Andreas von Deimling, MD

| Project Coordinator | Paul Kleihues, MD |

| Project Assistant | Asiedua Asante |

| Technical Editor | Jessica Cox |

| Database | Kees Kleihues-van Tol |

| Layout | Stefanie Brottrager |

| Printed by | Maestro |
| | 38330 Saint-Ismier, France |

Publisher	International Agency for
	Research on Cancer (IARC)
	69372 Lyon Cedex 08, France

This volume was produced with support from and in collaboration with the

German Cancer Research Center

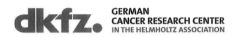

The WHO Classification of Tumours of the Central Nervous System
presented in this book reflects the views of a Working Group that convened for a
Consensus and Editorial Meeting at the German Cancer Research Center,
Heidelberg, 21–24 June 2015.

Members of the Working Group are indicated
in the list of contributors on pages 342–348.

Published by the International Agency for Research on Cancer (IARC)
150 Cours Albert Thomas, 69372 Lyon Cedex 08, France

© International Agency for Research on Cancer, 2016

Distributed by
WHO Press, World Health Organization, 20 Avenue Appia, 1211 Geneva 27, Switzerland
Tel.: +41 22 791 3264; Fax: +41 22 791 4857; email: bookorders@who.int

Second print run (5000 copies)

Format for bibliographic citations:
David N. Louis, Hiroko Ohgaki, Otmar D. Wiestler, Webster K. Cavenee (Eds):
WHO Classification of Tumours of the Central Nervous System (Revised 4th edition).
IARC: Lyon 2016.

IARC Library Cataloguing in Publication Data

WHO classification of tumours of the central nervous system / edited by David N. Louis, Hiroko Ohgaki, Otmar D. Wiestler,
Webster K. Cavenee. – Revised 4th edition.

(World Health Organization classification of tumours)

1. Central Nervous System Neoplasms – genetics
2. Central Nervous System Neoplasms – pathology
I. Louis David N

ISBN 978-92-832-4492-9   (NLM Classification: WJ 160)

Contents

WHO classification of tumours of the central nervous system

Diffuse astrocytic and oligodendroglial tumours

Diffuse astrocytoma, IDH-mutant	9400/3
Gemistocytic astrocytoma, IDH-mutant	9411/3
Diffuse astrocytoma, IDH-wildtype	*9400/3*
Diffuse astrocytoma, NOS	9400/3
Anaplastic astrocytoma, IDH-mutant	9401/3
Anaplastic astrocytoma, IDH-wildtype	*9401/3*
Anaplastic astrocytoma, NOS	9401/3
Glioblastoma, IDH-wildtype	9440/3
Giant cell glioblastoma	9441/3
Gliosarcoma	9442/3
Epithelioid glioblastoma	*9440/3*
Glioblastoma, IDH-mutant	9445/3*
Glioblastoma, NOS	9440/3
Diffuse midline glioma, H3 K27M–mutant	9385/3*
Oligodendroglioma, IDH-mutant and	
1p/19q-codeleted	9450/3
Oligodendroglioma, NOS	9450/3
Anaplastic oligodendroglioma, IDH-mutant	
and 1p/19q-codeleted	9451/3
Anaplastic oligodendroglioma, NOS	*9451/3*
Oligoastrocytoma, NOS	*9382/3*
Anaplastic oligoastrocytoma, NOS	*9382/3*

Other astrocytic tumours

Pilocytic astrocytoma	9421/1
Pilomyxoid astrocytoma	9425/3
Subependymal giant cell astrocytoma	9384/1
Pleomorphic xanthoastrocytoma	9424/3
Anaplastic pleomorphic xanthoastrocytoma	9424/3

Ependymal tumours

Subependymoma	9383/1
Myxopapillary ependymoma	9394/1
Ependymoma	9391/3
Papillary ependymoma	9393/3
Clear cell ependymoma	9391/3
Tanycytic ependymoma	9391/3
Ependymoma, *RELA* fusion–positive	9396/3*
Anaplastic ependymoma	9392/3

Other gliomas

Chordoid glioma of the third ventricle	9444/1
Angiocentric glioma	9431/1
Astroblastoma	9430/3

Choroid plexus tumours

Choroid plexus papilloma	9390/0
Atypical choroid plexus papilloma	9390/1
Choroid plexus carcinoma	9390/3

Neuronal and mixed neuronal–glial tumours

Dysembryoplastic neuroepithelial tumour	9413/0
Gangliocytoma	9492/0
Ganglioglioma	9505/1
Anaplastic ganglioglioma	9505/3
Dysplastic cerebellar gangliocytoma	
(Lhermitte–Duclos disease)	9493/0
Desmoplastic infantile astrocytoma and	
ganglioglioma	9412/1
Papillary glioneuronal tumour	9509/1
Rosette-forming glioneuronal tumour	9509/1
Diffuse leptomeningeal glioneuronal tumour	
Central neurocytoma	9506/1
Extraventricular neurocytoma	9506/1
Cerebellar liponeurocytoma	9506/1
Paraganglioma	8693/1

Tumours of the pineal region

Pineocytoma	9361/1
Pineal parenchymal tumour of intermediate	
differentiation	9362/3
Pineoblastoma	9362/3
Papillary tumour of the pineal region	9395/3

Embryonal tumours

Medulloblastomas, genetically defined	
Medulloblastoma, WNT-activated	9475/3*
Medulloblastoma, SHH-activated and	
TP53-mutant	9476/3*
Medulloblastoma, SHH-activated and	
TP53-wildtype	9471/3
Medulloblastoma, non-WNT/non-SHH	9477/3*
Medulloblastoma, group 3	
Medulloblastoma, group 4	
Medulloblastomas, histologically defined	
Medulloblastoma, classic	9470/3
Medulloblastoma, desmoplastic/nodular	9471/3
Medulloblastoma with extensive nodularity	9471/3
Medulloblastoma, large cell / anaplastic	9474/3
Medulloblastoma, NOS	9470/3
Embryonal tumour with multilayered rosettes,	
C19MC-altered	9478/3*
Embryonal tumour with multilayered	
rosettes, NOS	*9478/3*
Medulloepithelioma	9501/3
CNS neuroblastoma	9500/3
CNS ganglioneuroblastoma	9490/3
CNS embryonal tumour, NOS	9473/3
Atypical teratoid/rhabdoid tumour	9508/3
CNS embryonal tumour with rhabdoid features	*9508/3*

Tumours of the cranial and paraspinal nerves

Schwannoma	9560/0
Cellular schwannoma	9560/0
Plexiform schwannoma	9560/0

Melanotic schwannoma	9560/1
Neurofibroma	9540/0
Atypical neurofibroma	9540/0
Plexiform neurofibroma	9550/0
Perineurioma	9571/0
Hybrid nerve sheath tumours	
Malignant peripheral nerve sheath tumour	9540/3
Epithelioid MPNST	9540/3
MPNST with perineurial differentiation	9540/3

Meningiomas

Meningioma	9530/0
Meningothelial meningioma	9531/0
Fibrous meningioma	9532/0
Transitional meningioma	9537/0
Psammomatous meningioma	9533/0
Angiomatous meningioma	9534/0
Microcystic meningioma	9530/0
Secretory meningioma	9530/0
Lymphoplasmacyte-rich meningioma	9530/0
Metaplastic meningioma	9530/0
Chordoid meningioma	9538/1
Clear cell meningioma	9538/1
Atypical meningioma	9539/1
Papillary meningioma	9538/3
Rhabdoid meningioma	9538/3
Anaplastic (malignant) meningioma	9530/3

Mesenchymal, non-meningothelial tumours

Solitary fibrous tumour / haemangiopericytoma**	
Grade 1	8815/0
Grade 2	8815/1
Grade 3	8815/3
Haemangioblastoma	9161/1
Haemangioma	9120/0
Epithelioid haemangioendothelioma	9133/3
Angiosarcoma	9120/3
Kaposi sarcoma	9140/3
Ewing sarcoma / PNET	9364/3
Lipoma	8850/0
Angiolipoma	8861/0
Hibernoma	8880/0
Liposarcoma	8850/3
Desmoid-type fibromatosis	8821/1
Myofibroblastoma	8825/0
Inflammatory myofibroblastic tumour	8825/1
Benign fibrous histiocytoma	8830/0
Fibrosarcoma	8810/3
Undifferentiated pleomorphic sarcoma / malignant fibrous histiocytoma	8802/3
Leiomyoma	8890/0
Leiomyosarcoma	8890/3
Rhabdomyoma	8900/0
Rhabdomyosarcoma	8900/3
Chondroma	9220/0
Chondrosarcoma	9220/3
Osteoma	9180/0

Osteochondroma	9210/0
Osteosarcoma	9180/3

Melanocytic tumours

Meningeal melanocytosis	8728/0
Meningeal melanocytoma	8728/1
Meningeal melanoma	8720/3
Meningeal melanomatosis	8728/3

Lymphomas

Diffuse large B-cell lymphoma of the CNS	9680/3
Immunodeficiency-associated CNS lymphomas	
AIDS-related diffuse large B-cell lymphoma	
EBV-positive diffuse large B-cell lymphoma, NOS	
Lymphomatoid granulomatosis	9766/1
Intravascular large B-cell lymphoma	9712/3
Low-grade B-cell lymphomas of the CNS	
T-cell and NK/T-cell lymphomas of the CNS	
Anaplastic large cell lymphoma, ALK-positive	9714/3
Anaplastic large cell lymphoma, ALK-negative	9702/3
MALT lymphoma of the dura	9699/3

Histiocytic tumours

Langerhans cell histiocytosis	9751/3
Erdheim–Chester disease	9750/1
Rosai–Dorfman disease	
Juvenile xanthogranuloma	
Histiocytic sarcoma	9755/3

Germ cell tumours

Germinoma	9064/3
Embryonal carcinoma	9070/3
Yolk sac tumour	9071/3
Choriocarcinoma	9100/3
Teratoma	9080/1
Mature teratoma	9080/0
Immature teratoma	9080/3
Teratoma with malignant transformation	9084/3
Mixed germ cell tumour	9085/3

Tumours of the sellar region

Craniopharyngioma	9350/1
Adamantinomatous craniopharyngioma	9351/1
Papillary craniopharyngioma	9352/1
Granular cell tumour of the sellar region	9582/0
Pituicytoma	9432/1
Spindle cell oncocytoma	8290/0

Metastatic tumours

The morphology codes are from the International Classification of Diseases for Oncology (ICD-O) {742A}. Behaviour is coded /0 for benign tumours; /1 for unspecified, borderline, or uncertain behaviour; /2 for carcinoma in situ and grade III intraepithelial neoplasia; and /3 for malignant tumours. The classification is modified from the previous WHO classification, taking into account changes in our understanding of these lesions.
*These new codes were approved by the IARC/WHO Committee for ICD-O.
Italics: Provisional tumour entities. **Grading according to the 2013 *WHO Classification of Tumours of Soft Tissue and Bone*.

WHO classification and grading of tumours of the central nervous system

Louis D.N.

Combined histological–molecular classification

For nearly a century, the classification of brain tumours has been based on concepts of histogenesis, hinging on the idea that tumours can be classified according to their microscopic similarities with putative cells of origin and their developmental differentiation states. These histological similarities have been characterized primarily on the basis of the light microscopic appearance of H&E-stained sections, the immunohistochemical expression of proteins, and the electron microscopic assessment of ultrastructural features. The 2000 and 2007 WHO classifications considered histological features along with the rapidly increasing knowledge of the genetic changes that underlie the tumorigenesis of CNS tumours. Many of the canonical genetic alterations had been identified by the time the 2007 WHO classification was published, but at the time the consensus opinion was that such changes could not yet be used to define neoplasms; instead, genetic status served as supplementary information within the framework of diagnostic categories established by standard, histology-based means. In contrast, the present update (the 2016 classification) breaks with this nearly century-old tradition and incorporates well-established molecular parameters into the classification of diffuse gliomas.

Changing the classification to include diagnostic categories that depend on genotype may create certain challenges with respect to testing and reporting. These challenges include the availability and choice of genotyping and surrogate genotyping assays, the approaches that may need to be taken by centres without genotyping (or surrogate genotyping) capabilities, and the actual formats used to report these integrated diagnoses {1535}. However, an important consideration for the 2016 WHO classification was that the implementation of combined phenotypic–genotypic diagnostics in some large centres and the increasing availability of immunohistochemical surrogates for molecular genetic alterations suggest that such challenges will be readily overcome in the near future {2105}. Many of the genetic parameters included in the 2016 WHO classification can be assessed using immunohistochemistry or FISH, but it is recognized that some centres may not have the ability to carry out molecular analyses and that some molecular results may not be conclusive. With this in mind, an NOS diagnostic designation has been included in the 2016 WHO classification wherever such issues may apply. The NOS designation indicates that there is insufficient information to assign a more specific code. In this context, the NOS category includes both tumours that have not been tested for the genetic parameter(s) and tumours that have been tested but did not show the diagnostic genetic alterations. In other words, the NOS designation does not refer to a specific entity; instead, it designates the lesions that cannot be classified into any of the more precisely defined groups.

Definitions, disease summaries, and commentaries

Each entity-specific section in the 2016 WHO classification begins with a short disease definition that describes the essential diagnostic criteria. This initial definition is followed by a description of characteristic associated findings; for example, although a delicate branching vasculature and calcospherites are not essential for the diagnosis of oligodendroglioma, they are highly characteristic. The diagnostic criteria and characteristic features are then followed by the rest of the disease summary, in which other notable clinical, pathological, and molecular findings are described. Finally, for some entities, there is also additional commentary that provides information on classification, clarifying the nature of the genetic parameters to be evaluated and providing genotyping information on possibly overlapping histological entities. The classification does not specify the type of testing required to establish whether a genetic finding is present, leaving that to individual practitioners and institutions, but the commentary sections do clarify the implication of certain genetic features; for example, in what situations IDH status can be designated as wildtype.

Histological grading

Histological grading is a means of predicting the biological behaviour of a neoplasm. In the clinical setting, tumour grade is a key factor influencing the choice of therapies. Since its first publication in 1979, the *WHO classification of tumours of the central nervous system* has included a grading scheme that essentially constitutes a malignancy scale (ranging across a wide variety of neoplasms) rather than a strict histological grading system {1290,1291,2878}. WHO grading is widely used, and it has incorporated or largely replaced other previously published grading systems for brain tumours. Although grading is not a requirement for the application of the WHO classification for some tumours, including gliomas and meningiomas, numerical WHO grades are useful additions to the diagnoses. The WHO Working Group responsible for this update of the 4th edition has expanded the classification to include additional entities; however, since the number of cases of some of these newly defined entities is limited, the assignment of grades to such entities is still provisional, pending publication of additional data and long-term follow-up.

Histological grading across tumour entities

Grade I lesions are generally tumours with low proliferative potential and the possibility of cure after surgical resection alone. Grade II lesions are usually infiltrative in nature and often recur, despite having low levels of proliferative activity. Some grade II entities tend to progress to higher grades of malignancy; for example, grade II diffuse astrocytoma tends to transform to grade III anaplastic astrocytoma and glioblastoma. The grade III designation is applied to lesions with clear histological evidence of malignancy, including nuclear atypia and sometimes brisk mitotic activity. In most settings, patients with grade III tumours receive radiation and/or chemotherapy. The grade IV designation is applied to cytologically malignant, mitotically active, necrosis-prone neoplasms that are often associated with rapid pre- and postoperative disease evolution and fatal outcome. Glioblastoma and most embryonal neoplasms are examples of grade IV lesions. Widespread infiltration of surrounding tissue and a propensity for craniospinal dissemination characterize many grade IV neoplasms, although these features are not essential.

Histological grading within tumour entities

To date, the WHO classifications of CNS tumours have assigned grades as described above (i.e. across tumour entities). For the first time, the 2016 WHO classification has also adopted the principle of grading within a tumour entity,

which is the more common practice in non–nervous system tumours. Specifically, this principle is applied to solitary fibrous tumour / haemangiopericytoma, for which three different grades can be assigned within the same tumour designation. It is anticipated that the greater flexibility afforded by grading within tumour entities may be an advantage for future WHO classifications of brain tumours.

Tumour grade as a prognostic factor

WHO grade is based on histological features and is one component of a set of criteria used to predict response to therapy and outcome {1535}. Other criteria include clinical findings (e.g. patient age, performance status, and tumour location), radiological features (e.g. contrast enhancement), extent of surgical resection, proliferation index values, and genetic alterations. Genetic profile has become increasingly important because some genetic changes (e.g. IDH mutation in diffuse gliomas) have been found to have important prognostic

implications. For each tumour entity, the combination of these parameters contributes to an overall estimate of prognosis. Patients with WHO grade II tumours typically survive for > 5 years, and those with grade III tumours survive for 2–3 years. For patients with WHO grade IV tumours, prognosis depends heavily on whether effective treatment regimens are available. Most glioblastoma patients, and in particular elderly patients, succumb to the disease within a year. For those with other grade IV neoplasms, the outlook may be considerably better. For example, grade IV cerebellar medulloblastomas and germ cell tumours such as germinomas are rapidly fatal if left untreated, but state-of-the-art radiation and chemotherapy result in 5-year survival rates exceeding 60% and 80%, respectively. For some tumour types, the presence of certain genetic alterations can shift prognostic estimates markedly within the same grade, in some cases outweighing the prognostic strength of grade itself {952, 1535,2105}.

WHO grades of select CNS tumours

Diffuse astrocytic and oligodendroglial tumours	
Diffuse astrocytoma, IDH-mutant	II
Anaplastic astrocytoma, IDH-mutant	III
Glioblastoma, IDH-wildtype	IV
Glioblastoma, IDH-mutant	IV
Diffuse midline glioma, H3 K27M–mutant	IV
Oligodendroglioma, IDH-mutant and 1p/19q-codeleted	II
Anaplastic oligodendroglioma, IDH-mutant and 1p/19q-codeleted	III
Other astrocytic tumours	
Pilocytic astrocytoma	I
Subependymal giant cell astrocytoma	I
Pleomorphic xanthoastrocytoma	II
Anaplastic pleomorphic xanthoastrocytoma	III
Ependymal tumours	
Subependymoma	I
Myxopapillary ependymoma	I
Ependymoma	II
Ependymoma, *RELA* fusion–positive	II or III
Anaplastic ependymoma	III
Other gliomas	
Angiocentric glioma	I
Chordoid glioma of third ventricle	II
Choroid plexus tumours	
Choroid plexus papilloma	I
Atypical choroid plexus papilloma	II
Choroid plexus carcinoma	III
Neuronal and mixed neuronal–glial tumours	
Dysembryoplastic neuroepithelial tumour	I
Gangliocytoma	I
Ganglioglioma	I
Anaplastic ganglioglioma	III
Dysplastic gangliocytoma of cerebellum (Lhermitte–Duclos)	I

Desmoplastic infantile astrocytoma and ganglioglioma	I
Papillary glioneuronal tumour	I
Rosette-forming glioneuronal tumour	I
Central neurocytoma	II
Extraventricular neurocytoma	II
Cerebellar liponeurocytoma	II
Tumours of the pineal region	
Pineocytoma	I
Pineal parenchymal tumour of intermediate differentiation	II or III
Pineoblastoma	IV
Papillary tumour of the pineal region	II or III
Embryonal tumours	
Medulloblastoma (all subtypes)	IV
Embryonal tumour with multilayered rosettes, C19MC-altered	IV
Medulloepithelioma	IV
CNS embryonal tumour, NOS	IV
Atypical teratoid/rhabdoid tumour	IV
CNS embryonal tumour with rhabdoid features	IV
Tumours of the cranial and paraspinal nerves	
Schwannoma	I
Neurofibroma	I
Perineurioma	I
Malignant peripheral nerve sheath tumour (MPNST)	II, III or IV
Meningiomas	
Meningioma	I
Atypical meningioma	II
Anaplastic (malignant) meningioma	III
Mesenchymal, non-meningothelial tumours	
Solitary fibrous tumour / haemangiopericytoma	I, II or III
Haemangioblastoma	I
Tumours of the sellar region	
Craniopharyngioma	I
Granular cell tumour	I
Pituicytoma	I
Spindle cell oncocytoma	I

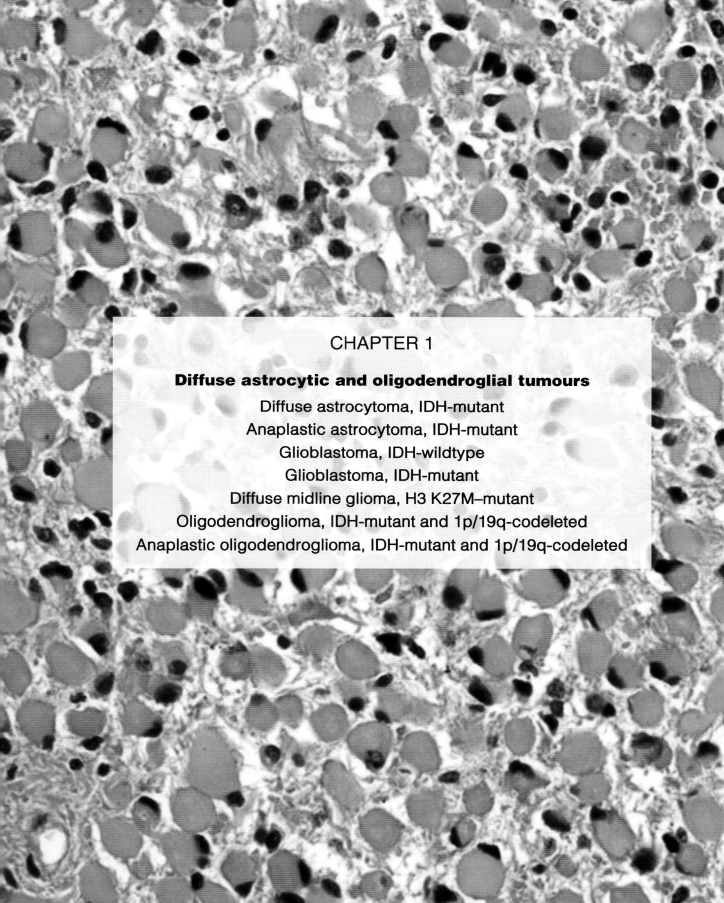

CHAPTER 1

Diffuse astrocytic and oligodendroglial tumours

Diffuse astrocytoma, IDH-mutant

Anaplastic astrocytoma, IDH-mutant

Glioblastoma, IDH-wildtype

Glioblastoma, IDH-mutant

Diffuse midline glioma, H3 K27M–mutant

Oligodendroglioma, IDH-mutant and 1p/19q-codeleted

Anaplastic oligodendroglioma, IDH-mutant and 1p/19q-codeleted

Diffuse astrocytic and oligodendroglial tumours – Introduction

Louis D.N.
von Deimling A.
Cavenee W.K.

This 2016 update of the 2007 WHO classification incorporates well-established molecular parameters into the classification of diffuse gliomas, and this nosological shift has impacted the classification in several ways. Most notably, whereas all astrocytic tumours were previously grouped together, now all diffuse gliomas (whether astrocytic or not) are grouped together, on the basis of not only their growth pattern and behaviours, but more pointedly of their shared *IDH1* and *IDH2* genetic status. From a pathogenetic point of view, this provides a dynamic classification based on both phenotype and genotype; from a prognostic point of view, it groups tumours that share similar prognostic markers; and from the eventual therapeutic point of view, it will presumably guide the treatment of biologically similar entities.

In this new classification, the diffuse glioma category includes the WHO grade II and III astrocytic tumours, the grade II and III oligodendrogliomas, the rare grade II and III oligoastrocytomas, the grade IV glioblastomas, and the related diffuse gliomas (e.g. those of childhood). This approach more sharply separates astrocytomas that have a more circumscribed growth pattern, lack IDH gene alterations, and sometimes have *BRAF* mutations (i.e. pilocytic astrocytoma, pleomorphic xanthoastrocytoma, and subependymal giant cell astrocytoma) from diffuse gliomas. In other words, diffuse astrocytoma and oligodendroglioma are now nosologically more similar than are diffuse astrocytoma and pilocytic astrocytoma; the family trees have been redrawn.

Similarly, paediatric diffuse gliomas were previously grouped together with their overall (generally adult) counterparts, despite known differences in behaviour between paediatric and adult gliomas with similar histological appearances. More recent information on the distinct underlying genetic abnormalities in paediatric diffuse gliomas has since prompted the separation of some of these entities from histologically similar adult tumours – with

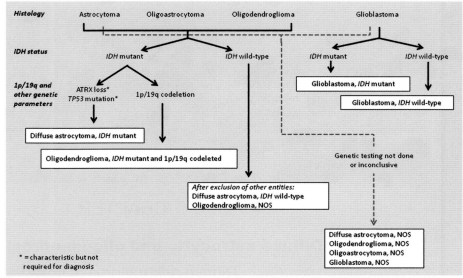

Fig. 1.01 Diffuse gliomas: from histology, IDH status, and other genetic parameters to WHO diagnosis.

a reasonably narrowly defined group of tumours characterized by K27M mutations in histone H3 genes, a diffuse growth pattern, and midline location: the newly defined H3 K27M–mutant diffuse midline glioma.

The use of integrated phenotypic and genotypic parameters in the 2016 WHO classification provides an increased level of objectivity. This will presumably yield more homogeneous and narrowly defined diagnostic entities than in prior classifications, which in turn should lead to better correlations with prognosis and treatment response. It will also result in potentially larger groups of tumours that do not fit into any of the more narrowly defined entities – groups that themselves will be more homogeneous and therefore more amenable to subsequent study and improved classification.

One compelling example of this improved objectivity relates to the diagnosis of oligoastrocytoma – a difficult-to-define category of tumours that has been subject to high interobserver variability in diagnosis, with some centres diagnosing these lesions frequently and others only rarely. The use of both genotype and phenotype in diagnosing these tumours results in essentially all of them being

placed into categories biologically compatible with either astrocytoma or oligodendroglioma {2220,2751}, with only rare cases having histological and molecular features of both {1067,2754}. As a result, the more common diagnoses of astrocytoma and oligodendroglioma both become more homogeneously defined, as does the very uncommon diagnosis of oligoastrocytoma.

The above example of classifying astrocytomas, oligodendrogliomas, and oligoastrocytomas raises the question of whether classification can proceed on the basis of genotype alone, i.e. without histology. At this point in time, it is not possible; in the classification process, a diagnosis of diffuse glioma (rather than some other tumour type) must first be established histologically in order for the nosological and clinical significance of specific genetic changes to be understood in the appropriate context. Another reason phenotype remains essential is that some individual tumours do not meet the more narrowly defined genotypic criteria; for example, a phenotypically classic diffuse astrocytoma that lacks the signature genetic characteristics of *IDH1/IDH2* and *ATRX* mutation. However, it is possible that future WHO classifications of diffuse gliomas, in the setting of deeper and broader genomic capabilities, will require less histological evaluation – perhaps only an initial diagnosis of diffuse glioma. For the time being, the current WHO classification is predicated on the concept of combined phenotypic and genotypic classification, and on the generation of so-called integrated diagnoses {1535}.

It is important to acknowledge that changing the classification to include diagnostic categories that depend on genotype may create certain challenges with respect to testing and reporting, which have been discussed elsewhere {1535}. These challenges include the availability and choice of genotyping and surrogate genotyping assays, the approaches that may need to be taken by centres without genotyping (or surrogate genotyping) capabilities, and the actual formats used to report these integrated diagnoses {1535}. However, the implementation of combined phenotypic–genotypic diagnostics in some large centres {2105} and the increasing availability of immunohistochemical surrogates for molecular genetic alterations suggest that such challenges will be readily overcome in the near future {2510A}.

Histological grading of diffuse astrocytic tumours

In neuro-oncology, histological grading has been most systematically evaluated and successfully applied to diffusely infiltrative astrocytic tumours, although recent studies suggest that molecular parameters may provide powerful

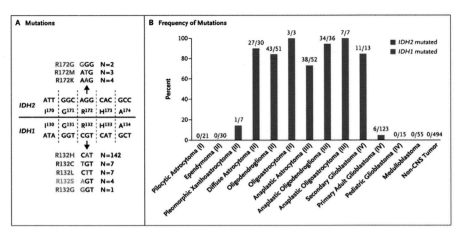

Fig. 1.02 *IDH1* and *IDH2* mutations in human gliomas, histologically diagnosed according to the 2007 WHO classification. Reprinted from Yan H et al. {2810}.

prognostic information in addition to that provided by histological grade. Nevertheless, in the 2016 WHO classification, diffuse astrocytomas are graded using a three-tiered system similar to the Ringertz system {2130}, the St. Anne–Mayo system {533}, and the previously published WHO schemes {1293,1534}. According to the WHO's current histological definition, tumours with cytological atypia alone (i.e. diffuse astrocytomas) are considered grade II, those that also show anaplasia and mitotic activity (i.e. anaplastic astrocytomas) are considered WHO grade III, and tumours that additionally show microvascular proliferation and/or necrosis are grade IV. Atypia is defined as variation in nuclear shape or size with accompanying hyperchromasia. Mitoses must be unequivocal, but no special significance is accorded to their number

or morphology. The finding of a solitary mitosis in an ample specimen is not sufficient proof of WHO grade III behaviour, but the separation of grade II tumours from grade III tumours may be facilitated by determination of the Ki-67 proliferation index {1056}. Microvascular proliferation is defined as apparent multilayering of endothelium (rather than simple hypervascularity) or glomeruloid vasculature. Necrosis may be of any type; perinecrotic palisading need not be present. Simple apposition of cellular zones with intervening pallor suggestive of incipient necrosis is insufficient. The aforementioned criteria make their appearance in a predictable sequence: atypia is followed in turn by mitotic activity, then increased cellularity, and finally microvascular proliferation and/or necrosis.

Diffuse astrocytoma, IDH-mutant

von Deimling A.
Huse J.T.
Yan H.
Brat D.J.
Reifenberger G.
Ohgaki H.
Kleihues P.
Berger M.S.
Weller M.
Nakazato Y.
Burger P.C.
Ellison D.W.
Louis D.N.

Definition

A diffusely infiltrating astrocytoma with a mutation in either the IDH1 *or* IDH2 *gene.* IDH-mutant diffuse astrocytoma typically features moderately pleomorphic cells and is characterized by a high degree of cellular differentiation and slow growth. The diagnosis is supported by the presence of *ATRX* and *TP53* mutation. The presence of a component morphologically resembling oligodendroglioma is compatible with this diagnosis in the absence of 1p/19q codeletion. This tumour most commonly affects young adults and occurs throughout the CNS, but is preferentially located in the frontal lobes {2428}. Diffuse astrocytomas have an intrinsic capacity for malignant progression to IDH-mutant anaplastic astrocytoma and eventually to IDH-mutant glioblastoma.

ICD-O code   9400/3

Grading

Diffuse astrocytoma corresponds histologically to WHO grade II.

Synonyms

Low-grade astrocytoma (discouraged); fibrillary astrocytoma (no longer recommended)

Epidemiology

Incidence

Tumour registries have not distinguished diffuse astrocytomas on the basis of IDH mutation status. However, because most cases carry an IDH mutation, the available data reflect this genetically defined tumour entity to some extent. Diffuse astrocytomas account for approximately 11–15% of all astrocytic brain tumours {1862,1863}. Annual incidence rates have been estimated at 0.55 and 0.75 new cases per 100 000 population {1862, 1863,2797}.
Some reports suggest that the incidence of astrocytomas in children has slightly increased in recent decades in several Scandinavian countries and North America {989,1015,2471}. There is a male predominance, with a male-to-female ratio of 1.3:1 {1863}.

Age distribution

The median and mean ages of patients with IDH-mutant diffuse astrocytoma are in the mid-30s. According to one study of adult patients only, the median age of patients with IDH-mutant diffuse astrocytoma is 36 years, and the mean age is 38 years. These values are similar to

those for IDH-mutant anaplastic astrocytoma {2103}.

Localization

IDH-mutant diffuse astrocytomas can be located in any region of the CNS, but most commonly develop supratentorially in the frontal lobes {2428}. This is similar to the preferential localization of IDH-mutant and 1p/19q-codeleted oligodendroglioma {1418,2871} and supports the hypothesis that these gliomas develop from a distinct population of precursor cells {1830}.

Clinical features

Seizures are a common presenting symptom; however, subtle abnormalities such as speech difficulties, changes in sensation or vision, and some form of motor change may be present earlier. Symptom onset is rarely abrupt, and some tumours are diagnosed incidentally {2390,2511}. With frontal lobe tumours, changes in behaviour or personality may be the presenting feature. Such changes may be present for months before diagnosis.

Imaging

Like clinical features, the results of neuroimaging studies can be extremely variable. On CT, diffuse astrocytomas most often present as poorly defined, homogeneous masses of low density, without contrast enhancement. However, calcification and cystic change may be present early in the evolution of the tumour. MRI studies usually show T1-hypodensity and T2-hyperintensity, with enlargement of the areas involved early in the evolution of the tumour. Gadolinium enhancement is not common in low-grade diffuse astrocytomas, but tends to appear during tumour progression.

Macroscopy

Because of their infiltrative nature, these tumours usually show blurring of the gross anatomical boundaries. There is enlargement and distortion (but not destruction) of the invaded anatomical structures (e.g. the cortex and the compact myelinated

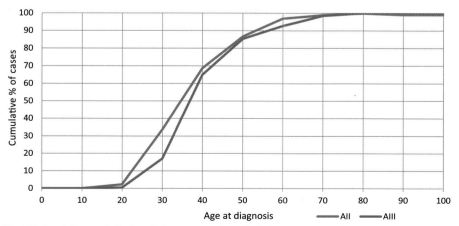

Fig. 1.03 Cumulative age distribution of astrocytomas at diagnosis, both sexes. Based on 613 cases of IDH-mutant diffuse astrocytoma (AII) and 674 cases of IDH-mutant anaplastic astrocytoma (AIII). Note that in this aggregate of patients, despite the difference in grade, the age distribution is similar, with a mean age of 35 years for AII and 37 years for AIII. This corresponds to similar data published by Reuss DE et al. {2103}, showing that IDH-mutant AII and AIII astrocytomas differ little with respect to age at diagnosis and survival in adult patients. Includes data from Reuss DE et al. {2103}.

pathways). Local mass lesions may be present in either grey or white matter, but they have indistinct boundaries, and changes such as smaller or larger cysts, granular areas, and zones of firmness or softening may be seen. Cystic change most commonly presents as a focal spongy area, with multiple cysts of various sizes. Extensive microcyst formation may cause a gelatinous appearance. Occasionally, a single large cyst filled with clear fluid is present. Tumours with prominent gemistocytes sometimes have single, large, smooth-walled cysts. Focal calcification may also be present, and a more diffuse grittiness may be observed. Extension into contralateral structures, particularly in the frontal lobes, is rarely observed.

Microscopy

Diffuse astrocytoma is composed of well-differentiated fibrillary astrocytes in a background of a loosely structured, often microcystic tumour matrix. Fibrillary astrocytoma is the classic type of diffuse astrocytoma and is no longer listed as a variant {1533}.

The cellularity is moderately increased compared with that of normal brain, and nuclear atypia is a characteristic feature. Mitotic activity is generally absent, but a single mitosis does not justify the diagnosis of anaplastic astrocytoma unless observed in a small biopsy or in the setting of obvious nuclear anaplasia. The presence of necrosis or microvascular proliferation is incompatible with the diagnosis of diffuse astrocytoma. Phenotypically, neoplastic astrocytes may vary considerably with respect to their size, the prominence and disposition of cell processes, and the abundance of cytoplasmic glial

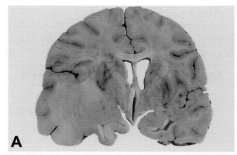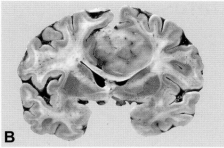

Fig. 1.04 A Large diffuse astrocytoma occupying the left temporal lobe, with extension to the Sylvian fissure. Note the homogeneous surface and the enlargement of local anatomical structures. **B** Large diffuse astrocytoma originating from the pericallosal cortex of the right hemisphere. The tumour extends into the interhemispheric fissure and shifts the midline towards the left hemisphere. Macroscopically, this lesion is well delineated and still shows structures resembling cortical architecture.

filaments. The pattern may vary markedly in different regions of the neoplasm. Histological recognition of neoplastic astrocytes using H&E staining on sectioned material depends mainly on nuclear characteristics. The normal astrocytic nucleus is oval to elongated, but on sectioning, occasional round cross-sections are seen. The nucleus is typically vesicular, with intermediate-sized masses of chromatin and often with a distinct nucleolus. Normal human astrocytes show no H&E-stainable cytoplasm that is distinct from the background neuropil. Reactive astrocytes are defined by enlarged nuclei and the presence of stainable, defined cytoplasm, culminating in the gemistocyte, which has a mass of eosinophilic cytoplasm, often an eccentric nucleus, and cytoplasm that extends into fine processes.

Differential diagnosis

The major entity in the differential diagnosis is reactive astrocytosis. Because most IDH-mutant diffuse astrocytomas have R132H mutations, immunohistochemistry

for R132H-mutant IDH1 (sometimes in combination with p53 immunohistochemistry and rarely with assessment for trisomy 7) is a powerful means to distinguish neoplastic from reactive astrocytes {347}. In other situations, however, the differential diagnosis can be challenging and may rely on standard histological differences. Diffuse astrocytoma contains astrocytes that are increased in number and usually in size, but are otherwise difficult to distinguish on an individual basis from normal or reactive cells. In minor degrees of anaplasia, it is the number of astrocytes and (most commonly) the uniformity of their morphology that is most helpful in recognizing their neoplastic nature. Reactive astrocytes are rarely all in the same stage of reactivity at the same time, so reactions reveal mixtures of astrocytes; some with enlarged nuclei, others with varying amounts of cytoplasm, most often on a somewhat rarefied background. In diffuse astrocytoma, almost all of the nuclei look identical, and the background is of at least normal density or shows increased numbers of cellular processes. Microcystic

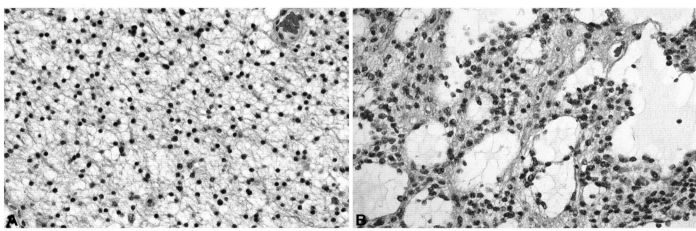

Fig. 1.05 Diffuse astrocytoma. **A** Moderately cellular tumour composed of uniform neoplastic fibrillary astrocytic cells. **B** Extensive microcyst formation.

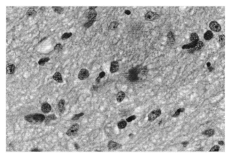

Fig. 1.06 Diffuse astrocytoma. Low cellularity and nuclear atypia.

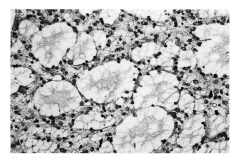

Fig. 1.07 Diffuse astrocytoma with extensive mucoid degeneration and cobweb-like architecture. This pattern was previously designated protoplasmic astrocytoma.

change may be present, but most cells look like one another, without the admixture of gemistocytes more often seen in reactions to injury. Pre-existing cell types (e.g. neurons) are often entrapped.

Intraoperative diagnosis
The smear/squash technique is often used during stereotaxic biopsies and yields similar findings, although this method is highly unreliable for estimating cellularity. Many histological features are exaggerated and amplified (e.g. nuclear folds, abnormal chromatin pattern, and astrocytic processes). The presence of many round to oval nuclei with smooth chromatin can indicate the presence of an apparent oligodendroglial component or (if the nuclei are less prominent) background white matter. Histologically, there may be significant variation between tumours and within the same lesion.

Growth fraction
The growth fraction as determined by the Ki-67 proliferation index is usually < 4%. The gemistocytic neoplastic astrocytes show a significantly lower rate of proliferation than does the intermingled small-cell component {1046,1372,1377,1847, 2706,2812}. However, microdissection

reveals identical *TP53* mutations in both gemistocytes and non-gemistocytic tumour cells {2094}. Although it has been reported that the gemistocytic variant may be particularly prone to progression to anaplastic astrocytoma and glioblastoma {1377,2204,2273}, this does not justify a general classification as anaplastic astrocytoma {320,2273}, nor is this impression based on current molecular characterization, in particular knowledge of IDH mutation status.

Immunophenotype
Diffuse astrocytomas reliably express GFAP, although to various degrees and not in all tumour cells. In particular, small round cells with scanty cytoplasm and processes tend not to label avidly for GFAP. In these cases, immunopositivity may be restricted to a small perinuclear rim and to admixed neoplastic cell processes in the fibrillary tumour background {1292}. Vimentin is typically immunopositive as well, with a labelling pattern approximating that of GFAP {995}. The signature molecular characteristics of diffuse astrocytoma (see *Genetic profile*) can often be demonstrated immunohistochemically. For example, expression of R132H-mutant IDH1 (the *IDH1* R132H mutation accounts for about 90% of all glioma-associated IDH mutations) can be detected using a mutation-specific antibody {360}. In mutant tumours, all neoplastic cells typically exhibit some degree of cytoplasmic (stronger) and nuclear (weaker) labelling, provided the staining preparation used is technically adequate {359}. For this reason, R132H-mutant IDH1 immunohistochemistry has become an invaluable diagnostic adjunct, not only in the molecular stratification of diffuse glioma, but also in the

distinction of true neoplasia from reactive gliosis {347,359}. Strong nuclear p53 expression is also frequently observed, consistent with the high incidence of *TP53* mutations in diffuse astrocytoma {915}. However, the use of p53 immunopositivity to reflect *TP53* mutation is not entirely sensitive or specific {1530,1771}. In contrast, ATRX expression is almost invariably lost in the setting of *ATRX* mutations, which also feature prominently in diffuse astrocytoma (see *Genetic profile*) {361,1160,1215,2105}. ATRX typically demonstrates strong nuclear expression in normal, unmutated tissue; therefore, retention of immunolabelling in non-neoplastic vasculature and admixed neuronal, glial, and microglial elements serves as a necessary internal control for the accurate interpretation of a negative ATRX immunostaining pattern. Finally, consistent with its inapparent mitotic activity, diffuse astrocytoma nearly always has a Ki-67 proliferation index of < 4% {492,1137,1223,2059}.

Cell of origin
The available evidence suggests that IDH-mutant and 1p/19q-codeleted oligodendrogliomas, IDH-mutant diffuse

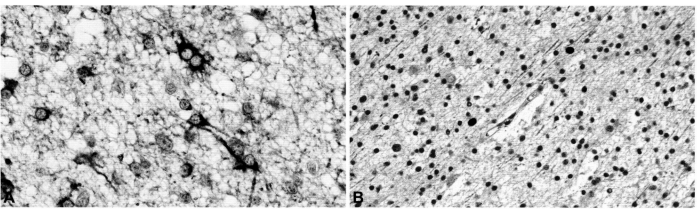

Fig. 1.08 Diffuse astrocytoma. **A** Cytoplasm and cell processes show a variable extent of GFAP immunoreactivity. **B** The Ki-67 proliferation index is low.

astrocytomas, IDH-mutant anaplastic astrocytomas, and IDH-mutant glioblastomas develop from a distinct population of precursor cells that differ from the precursor cells of IDH-wildtype glioblastoma {870,1830}.

Genetic profile
Diffuse gliomas of WHO grades II and III, including diffuse astrocytoma, are nearly all characterized by mutations in IDH genes: either *IDH1* or *IDH2* {118,953, 1895,2810}. Diffuse gliomas that occur in adults and that do not harbour IDH mutation, regardless of their WHO grade, tend to exhibit more aggressive clinical behaviour {870,2238}.

Glioma-associated *IDH1* and *IDH2* mutations impart a gain-of-function phenotype to the respective metabolic enzymes IDH1 and IDH2, which overproduce the oncometabolite 2-hydroxyglutarate {523}. The physiological consequences of 2-hydroxyglutarate overproduction are widespread, including profound effects on cellular epigenomic states and gene regulation. Specifically, IDH mutations induce G-CIMP, by which widespread hypermethylation in gene promoter regions silences the expression of several important cellular differentiation factors {1540, 2589}. In this way, IDH mutation and G-CIMP are thought to maintain glioma cells of origin in stem cell–like physiological states inherently more prone to self-renewal and tumorigenesis. In particular, it appears that IDH mutations promote glioma formation by disrupting chromosomal topology and allowing aberrant chromosomal regulatory interactions that induce oncogene expression, including glioma oncogenes such as *PDGFRA* {713A}. Consistent with this concept, IDH mutations seem to be among the first genetic alterations that occur in WHO grade II diffuse glioma {2709}. *MGMT* promoter methylation was reported in about 50% of diffuse astrocytomas in the pre-IDH era, but this proportion may be higher among IDH-mutant diffuse astrocytomas and does not correlate consistently with G-CIMP {1753,2589}.

The vast majority of IDH-mutant diffuse astrocytomas, as well as the WHO grade III anaplastic astrocytomas and grade IV glioblastomas that evolve from them, also harbour class-defining loss-of-function mutations in *TP53* and *ATRX* {1160,1215,1834,2092,2704}. *ATRX* encodes an essential chromatin-binding protein, and its deficiency has been associated with epigenomic dysregulation and telomere dysfunction {473}. In particular, *ATRX* mutations seem to induce an abnormal telomere maintenance mechanism known as alternative lengthening of telomeres {977}. *ATRX* mutations and alternative lengthening of telomeres are mutually exclusive with activating mutations in the *TERT* gene, which encodes the catalytic component of telomerase. Interestingly, *TERT* mutations are found in the vast majority of oligodendrogliomas and most IDH-wildtype glioblastomas {349,622,1270}. Distinct telomere maintenance mechanisms, mediated by either activated telomerase or alternative lengthening of telomeres, seem to be required for the pathogenesis of all diffuse gliomas.

ATRX deficiency has also been associated with generalized genomic instability, which can induce p53-dependent cell death in some contexts {488}. Therefore, *TP53* mutations in diffuse astrocytoma may enable tumour cell survival in the setting of ATRX loss. The genomic instability of IDH-mutant diffuse astrocytomas is reflected in characteristic DNA copy number abnormalities, which include low-level amplification events involving the oncogenes *MYC* and *CCND2* in mutually exclusive subsets {349}. Copy number events typically associated with IDH-wildtype glioblastoma, such as *EGFR* amplification and homozygous *CDKN2A* deletion, are rarely encountered, emphasizing the biological differences between IDH-mutant and IDH-wildtype astrocytomas {349,622,870}. On the basis of expression profiling, multiple diffuse astrocytoma subclasses have been designated, stratified by IDH mutation status as well as neuroglial lineage markers {349,870}. The transcriptional profiles of diffuse astrocytomas indicate distinct cells of origin in addition to specific genomic features.

Genetic susceptibility
Diffuse astrocytoma can occur in patients with inherited *TP53* germline mutations / Li–Fraumeni syndrome (see *Li–Fraumeni syndrome*, p. 310), although affected family members more frequently develop anaplastic astrocytoma and glioblastoma. Lower-grade astrocytoma has been diagnosed in patients with inherited Ollier-type multiple enchondromatosis, which also predisposes patients to chondrosarcoma {734,1027}.

Prognosis and predictive factors

Clinical prognostic factors
In the pre-IDH era, the median survival time was reported to be in the range of 6–8 years, with marked individual variation. The total length of disease is influenced mainly by the dynamics of malignant progression, which had been reported to occur after a median time of 4–5 years {254,1826,1834}. The European Organisation for Research and Treatment of Cancer (EORTC) trials 22844 and 22845 showed that patient age ≥ 40 years, astrocytoma histology, largest tumour diameter ≥ 6 cm, tumour crossing the midline, and neurological deficits prior to surgery were associated with inferior outcome {1975}. However, these prognostic estimates must be re-evaluated in the context of IDH mutation status; one study that included 683 IDH-mutant diffuse astrocytoma cases from three series showed a median survival of 10.9 years {2103}.

Proliferation
Low to absent proliferation rates as estimated by mitotic count or the Ki-67 proliferation index have traditionally been considered a diagnostic criterion for grading a diffuse astrocytoma as WHO grade II. Among histologically diagnosed diffuse astrocytomas, the level of proliferation has not been associated with outcome.

Histopathological factors
Gemistocytic astrocytoma has been associated with early progression and inferior outcome {1834}, but data on larger contemporary patient cohorts with known IDH mutation status are lacking. Other histological factors associated with outcome have not yet been identified.

Genetic alterations
IDH1/2 mutations distinguish astrocytomas with a more favourable course from IDH-wildtype tumours, which have a less favourable course {951}. Among IDH-wildtype tumours, a genotype of 7q gain and 10q loss is associated with a particularly poor outcome {2731}. However, as noted earlier (see *Clinical prognostic factors*), a study that included 683 IDH-mutant diffuse astrocytomas from three series reported a median survival of

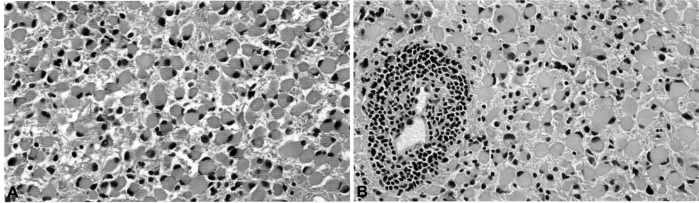

Fig. 1.09 Gemistocytic astrocytoma. **A** Tumour cells have abundant eosinophilic cytoplasm, with nuclei displaced to the periphery. **B** Perivascular lymphocytic infiltrates are common.

10.9 years. IDH mutations may be useful as a predictive biomarker when IDH-targeted therapies such as small-molecule inhibitors {2685} or vaccines {2301} become available. Comprehensive genotyping studies have shown correlations between IDH mutation status and other molecular parameters; in particular, there are strong associations between IDH mutation and TP53 mutation (present in 94% of cases) and ATRX inactivation (present in 86% of cases) {349}.

Mutant IDH catalyses the formation of 2-hydroxyglutarate, which could potentially be monitored by MR spectroscopy {449} or in body fluids {358}. However, the clinical value of these approaches has yet to be validated.

Gemistocytic astrocytoma, IDH-mutant

Definition
A variant of IDH-mutant diffuse astrocytoma characterized by the presence of a conspicuous (though variable) proportion of gemistocytic neoplastic astrocytes (gemistocytes).

For a diagnosis of gemistocytic astrocytoma, gemistocytes should constitute more than approximately 20% of all tumour cells. The presence of occasional gemistocytes in a diffuse astrocytoma does not justify the diagnosis {1533}. Reports have suggested that gemistocytic astrocytoma may progress more rapidly than standard diffuse astrocytoma to anaplastic astrocytoma and secondary glioblastoma, but these reports are from the pre-IDH era and it remains unclear whether IDH-mutant gemistocytic astrocytomas have an increased tendency for anaplastic progression {319,1533}.

ICD-O code   9411/3

Grading
IDH-mutant gemistocytic astrocytoma corresponds histologically to WHO grade II.

Epidemiology
Gemistocytic astrocytomas account for approximately 10% of all WHO grade II diffuse astrocytomas {981}. The mean reported patient age at diagnosis is 40 years {2703}, the median age is 42 years {1377}, and the male-to-female ratio is 2:1 {2703}.

Localization
Gemistocytic astrocytomas can develop in any region of the CNS, but they most commonly develop in the frontal and temporal lobes.

Macroscopy
Macroscopically, gemistocytic astrocytomas are not substantially different from other low-grade diffuse gliomas. They are often characterized by expansion of the infiltrated brain areas without clear delineation of the neoplasm. The involved areas may show greyish discolouration, granularity, firmer or softer consistency, and microcystic change {1533}.

Microscopy
The histopathological hallmark of gemistocytic astrocytoma is the presence of a conspicuous proportion of gemistocytic neoplastic astrocytes. Gemistocytes should account for more than approximately 20% of all tumour cells; the presence of occasional gemistocytes in a diffuse astrocytoma does not justify the diagnosis of gemistocytic astrocytoma. The mean proportion of gemistocytes is approximately 35% {2703}. The cut-off point of 20% is somewhat arbitrary, but a useful

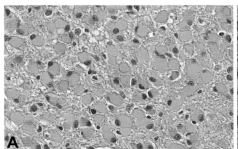
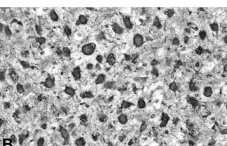
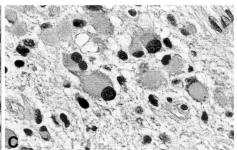

Fig. 1.10 Gemistocytic astrocytoma. **A** Tumour cells have enlarged, glassy, eosinophilic cytoplasm and eccentric nuclei. **B** Immunostaining shows a marked and consistent accumulation of GFAP in the cytoplasm of neoplastic gemistocytes. Interspersed are small tumour cells with little cytoplasm; proliferation is largely restricted to this inconspicuous cell population. **C** p53 accumulation is present in nuclei of small and gemistocytic tumour cells.

Paediatric diffuse astrocytoma

Although the histopathology of paediatric diffuse astrocytoma resembles that of adult diffuse astrocytoma, there are many important distinctions between the disease in children and in adults.

Clinicopathological aspects

The annual incidence of paediatric diffuse astrocytoma (defined by patient age < 20 years at diagnosis) is 0.27 cases per 100 000 population; lower than that of adult diffuse astrocytoma, which is 0.58 per 100 000 {1863}. Most paediatric diffuse astrocytoma are located in the cerebral hemispheres, but a significant proportion present in the thalamus, which is an unusual site for adult diffuse astrocytoma. Anaplastic progression occurs in approximately 75% of adult lesions, but is rare in paediatric tumours {284}.

Genetic aspects

Diffuse astrocytomas in children and adults have distinct genetic profiles. However, diffuse astrocytomas with genetically defined so-called adult-type disease can present in adolescents, and so-called paediatric-type disease can present in young adults. Paediatric diffuse astrocytomas are characterized mainly by alterations in *MYB* and *BRAF*. Amplification or rearrangements of *MYB* are detected in approximately 25% of paediatric diffuse astrocytomas {2518, 2855}. Rearrangements of *MYBL1* have also been described {2068}. Other paediatric diffuse astrocytomas harbour *BRAF* V600E mutations, *FGFR1* alterations, or *KRAS* mutations {2855}. Rare paediatric diffuse astrocytomas contain the H3 K27M mutation usually found in paediatric high-grade gliomas {2855}. The mutations in *IDH1*, *IDH2*, *TP53*, and *ATRX* that are frequently found in adult diffuse astrocytomas are not present in the paediatric tumours {2443}.

remains to be determined whether the prognosis of IDH-mutant gemistocytic astrocytoma differs significantly from that of IDH-mutant diffuse astrocytoma.

....

Diffuse astrocytoma, IDH-wildtype

Definition

A diffusely infiltrating astrocytoma without mutations in the IDH genes.

IDH-wildtype diffuse astrocytoma is rare. Most gliomas with a histological appearance resembling that of diffuse astrocytoma but without IDH mutation can be reclassified in adults as other tumours with additional genetic analyses. Tumours that conform to this diagnosis most likely constitute a variety of entities, and can therefore follow a broad range of clinical courses. Thus, IDH-wildtype diffuse astrocytoma is considered a provisional entity.

Gliomatosis cerebri growth pattern

Like other diffuse gliomas, diffuse astrocytoma can manifest at initial clinical presentation with a gliomatosis cerebri pattern of extensive involvement of the CNS, with the affected area ranging from most of one cerebral hemisphere (three lobes or more) to both cerebral hemispheres with additional involvement of the deep grey matter structures, brain stem, cerebellum, and spinal cord. See *Anaplastic astrocytoma, IDH-wildtype* (p. 27) for additional detail.

....

Diffuse astrocytoma, NOS

Definition

A tumour with morphological features of diffuse astrocytoma, but in which IDH mutation status has not been not fully assessed.

Full assessment of IDH mutation status in diffuse astrocytomas involves sequence analysis for *IDH1* codon 132 and *IDH2* codon 172 mutations in cases that are immunohistochemically negative for the *IDH1* R132H mutation.

ICD-O code   9400/3

criterion in borderline cases {1377,2556}. The gemistocytes are characterized by plump, glassy, eosinophilic cell bodies of angular shape. Stout, randomly oriented processes form a coarse fibrillary network. These processes are often useful in distinguishing the tumour cells from the minigemistocytes found in oligodendroglioma. Gemistocytic neoplastic astrocytes consistently express GFAP in their perikarya and cell processes. The nuclei are usually eccentric, with small, distinct nucleoli and densely clumped chromatin. Perivascular lymphocyte cuffing is frequent {322}. Electron microscopy confirms the presence of abundant, compact glial filaments in the cytoplasm and in cell processes. Enlarged mitochondria have also been noted {609}.

Proliferation

The gemistocytic neoplastic astrocytes show a significantly lower rate of proliferation than in the intermingled small-cell component {1046,1372,1377,2706}. However, microdissection has revealed identical *TP53* mutations in both gemistocytes and non-gemistocytic tumour cells {2094}.

Immunophenotype

The cytoplasm of neoplastic gemistocytes is filled with GFAP, causing displacement of nuclei to the periphery of the cell body. Expression of p53 protein is also frequently seen in gemistocytes {2706}.

Genetic profile

Gemistocytic astrocytoma is a variant of IDH-mutant diffuse astrocytoma. Reports have noted that gemistocytic astrocytomas are characterized by a particularly high frequency of *TP53* mutations, which are present in > 80% of all cases {1834, 2703}, and likely in nearly all cases of IDH-mutant gemistocytic astrocytoma. The fact that *TP53* mutations are present in both gemistocytes and non-gemistocytic tumour cells indicates that the gemistocytes are neoplastic and not reactive in nature {2094}. This interpretation is also supported by immunoreactivity to mutant IDH1 protein {359}.

Prognosis and predictive factors

Gemistocytic astrocytomas have been reported to undergo progression to anaplastic (gemistocytic) astrocytoma and IDH-mutant glioblastoma more commonly than do other diffuse astrocytomas {1377,1834,1929,1930}. However, these data pertain to histologically diagnosed gemistocytic astrocytomas irrespective of the presence of an IDH mutation. It

Anaplastic astrocytoma, IDH-mutant

von Deimling A.
Huse J.T.
Yan H.
Brat D.J.
Ohgaki H.
Kleihues P.

Berger M.S.
Weller M.
Burger P.C.
Ellison D.W.
Rosenblum M.K.
Reifenberger G.

Paulus W.
Wesseling P.
Aldape K.D.
Louis D.N.

Definition

A diffusely infiltrating astrocytoma with focal or dispersed anaplasia, significant proliferative activity, and a mutation in either the IDH1 *or* IDH2 *gene.*

Anaplastic astrocytomas can arise from lower-grade diffuse astrocytomas, but are more commonly diagnosed without indication of a less-malignant precursor lesion. The presence of a component morphologically resembling oligodendroglioma is compatible with this diagnosis in the absence of 1p/19q codeletion. Anaplastic astrocytomas have an intrinsic tendency for malignant progression to IDH-mutant glioblastoma.

ICD-O code   9401/3

Grading

IDH-mutant anaplastic astrocytoma corresponds histologically to WHO grade III. Some retrospective studies have shown that, in the setting of current therapy, IDH-mutant anaplastic astrocytomas may follow clinical courses only somewhat worse than those of IDH-mutant diffuse astrocytomas (WHO grade II) {870,2103,2464}, but this was not found in other studies {1268}. Although IDH-mutant anaplastic astrocytoma is assigned a WHO grade of III based on histological appearance, grading algorithms for distinguishing between IDH-mutant anaplastic astrocytoma and IDH-mutant diffuse astrocytoma may need to be refined.

Synonym

High-grade astrocytoma (discouraged)

Epidemiology

The peak incidence of IDH-mutant anaplastic astrocytoma occurs at a mean patient age of 38 years {2103}. However, until the discovery of IDH mutation as a molecular marker, the diagnosis of anaplastic astrocytoma was based only on histological evidence {1823,1827}. Hospital-based data from the University of Zurich in the pre-IDH era showed a mean patient age at diagnosis of approximately 45 years, with a male-to-female ratio of 1.6:1. In one population-based study, the mean patient age at biopsy was 46 years {1826}. Population-based registry data from the USA for the period 2007–2011 show an annual incidence of 0.37 cases per 100 000 population, a male-to-female ratio of 1.39:1, and median patient age at diagnosis of 53 years {1863}. In a study that incorporated IDH mutation data and included 562 IDH-mutant anaplastic astrocytomas, the median patient age at presentation was 36 years and the mean age 38 years, similar to that for IDH-mutant WHO grade II diffuse astrocytoma {2103}.

Localization

IDH-mutant anaplastic astrocytomas can develop in any region of the CNS but most frequently occur in the cerebrum. These tumours, like other IDH-mutant diffuse gliomas (including oligodendrogliomas, diffuse astrocytomas, and IDH-mutant glioblastomas), are preferentially located in the frontal lobe.

Clinical features

The symptoms are similar to those of WHO grade II diffuse astrocytoma. In some patients with a history of a diffuse WHO grade II astrocytoma, there are increasing neurological deficits, seizures, and signs of intracranial pressure (depending on the location of the tumour, the degree of oedema, and the mass effect surrounding the lesion). Patients with anaplastic astrocytoma commonly present after a history of a few months, with no evidence of a preceding WHO grade II astrocytoma.

Imaging

IDH-mutant anaplastic astrocytoma presents as a poorly defined mass of low density. Unlike in WHO grade II diffuse astrocytomas, partial contrast enhancement is usually observed, but the central necrosis with ring enhancement typical of glioblastomas is absent. More rapid tumour growth with development of peritumoural oedema can lead to mass shifts and increased intracranial pressure.

Spread

Like other diffuse gliomas, anaplastic astrocytomas are generally characterized by diffuse infiltrative growth in the brain {463}. Occasionally, leptomeningeal spread is evident {1059}.

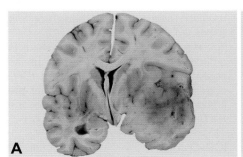
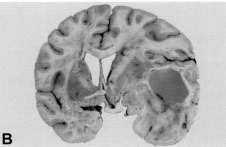
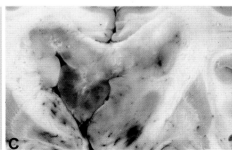

Fig. 1.11 A Anaplastic astrocytoma in the right frontotemporal region. Note the ill-defined borders with the adjacent brain structures and focal cysts. **B** Frontotemporal anaplastic astrocytoma containing a large cyst but no macroscopically discernible necrosis. **C** Anaplastic astrocytoma with diffuse, bilateral infiltration of the corpus callosum, the caudate nucleus, and the fornices. The fornices are grossly enlarged and show petechial haemorrhages.

Macroscopy

Like WHO grade II diffuse astrocytoma, anaplastic astrocytomas tend to infiltrate the surrounding brain without causing frank tissue destruction. This often leads to a marked enlargement of invaded structures, such as adjacent gyri and basal ganglia. On cut surface, the higher cellularity of the anaplastic astrocytoma results in a discernible tumour mass, which in some cases is distinguished more clearly from the surrounding brain structures than is seen in WHO grade II diffuse astrocytomas. Macroscopic cysts are uncommon, but there are often areas of granularity, opacity, and soft consistency. It is often difficult to grossly distinguish between a WHO grade III anaplastic astrocytoma and a WHO grade II diffuse astrocytoma.

Microscopy

The principal histopathological features are those of a diffusely infiltrating astrocytoma with increased mitotic activity compared with the WHO grade II equivalent, usually accompanied by distinct nuclear atypia and high cellularity. Mitotic activity should be evaluated in the context of sample size. In small specimens, such as those obtained at stereotactic biopsy, a single mitosis suggests significant proliferative activity; in such cases, Ki-67 labelling may be helpful. In large resection specimens, a few mitoses are not sufficient for WHO grade III designation {826}. Regional or diffuse hypercellularity is an important diagnostic criterion; but even in the setting of low cellularity, the diagnosis is still appropriate if there is significant mitotic activity. With progressive anaplasia, nuclear morphology becomes more atypical, with increasing variation in nuclear size, shape, coarseness, and dispersion of chromatin and increasing nucleolar prominence and quantity. Additional signs of anaplasia include multinucleated tumour cells and abnormal mitoses, but these are not obligatory for WHO grade III. By definition, microvascular proliferation (multilayered vessels) and necrosis are absent.

Proliferation

Unlike WHO grade II diffuse astrocytoma, anaplastic astrocytoma displays mitotic activity. The growth fraction as determined by the Ki-67 proliferation index is usually in the range of 5–10%, but can overlap with values for low-grade diffuse

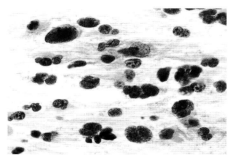

Fig. 1.12 Anaplastic astrocytoma. Smear preparations show various degrees of nuclear atypia.

astrocytoma at one end of the range and with glioblastoma at the other {492,1137, 1223,2059}. The index may vary considerably, however, even within a single tumour.

Immunophenotype

In general, the immunohistochemical features of anaplastic astrocytoma recapitulate those of WHO grade II diffuse astrocytoma, consistent with their shared histogenetic and molecular foundations. IDH-mutant anaplastic astrocytomas are typically positive for GFAP and frequently exhibit strong and diffuse nuclear expression of p53. The majority express R132H-mutant IDH1 (reflecting their underlying IDH mutation status) and display negative immunostaining for nuclear ATRX.

Cell of origin

The cell of origin is unknown. The fact that diffuse WHO grade II and III astrocytomas, IDH-mutant glioblastomas, and oligodendrogliomas all carry an IDH mutation suggests that they may share a cell of origin different from those of IDH-wildtype glioblastomas and pilocytic

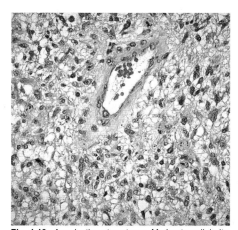

Fig. 1.13 Anaplastic astrocytoma. Moderate cellularity, marked nuclear atypia, and mitoses.

astrocytomas (i.e. gliomas that lack IDH mutations) {953}.

Genetic profile

The molecular features of anaplastic astrocytoma largely recapitulate those of WHO grade II IDH-mutant diffuse astrocytoma. By definition, mutations in *IDH1* or *IDH2* are present in all tumours, and *TP53* and *ATRX* alterations are found in the majority of tumours {118,953,1160, 1215,1834,1895,2092,2704,2810}.

Robust molecular correlates of anaplastic progression within diffuse astrocytoma lineages have yet to be established, because the biological distinctions between IDH-mutant and IDH-wildtype tumours have emerged only recently. However, compared with WHO grade II IDH-mutant astrocytomas, WHO grade III tumours have higher frequencies of chromosome arm 9p and 19q losses {349,1269}.

Prognosis and predictive factors

Clinical prognostic factors

Historically, median survival has been in the range of 3–5 years, but with marked differences in cases with older patient age and low performance status, both of which are associated with inferior outcome {2740}. In the era of subtyping anaplastic astrocytomas by IDH mutation status, survival estimates now vary more widely (see *Genetic alterations*). The extent of surgical resection at diagnosis also seems to impact outcome {2740}.

Proliferation

Proliferative activity, as estimated by mitotic count or the Ki-67 proliferation index, is not prognostic for anaplastic astrocytomas.

Histopathological factors

Histological factors are not associated with outcome of anaplastic astrocytoma, but they have not yet been carefully evaluated within the context of IDH-mutant anaplastic astrocytoma.

Genetic alterations

IDH1/2 mutations are associated with better outcome, whereas IDH-wildtype anaplastic astrocytoma has an outcome similar to that of IDH-wildtype glioblastoma {952}. A study that included 562 IDH-mutant anaplastic astrocytomas from three series showed a median survival of 9.3 years {2103}. *EGFR* amplification

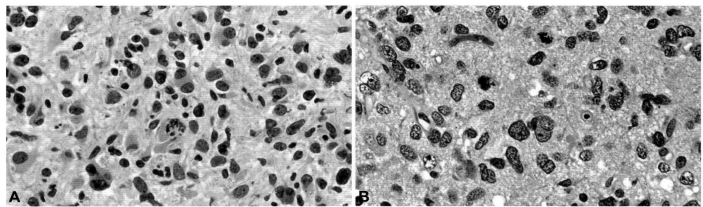

Fig. 1.14 Anaplastic astrocytoma. **A** Marked nuclear pleomorphism. Note the atypical mitosis in the centre. **B** Hypercellularity and hyperchromatic, irregular, so-called naked nuclei appearing within a fibrillary background. Two mitotic figures are present.

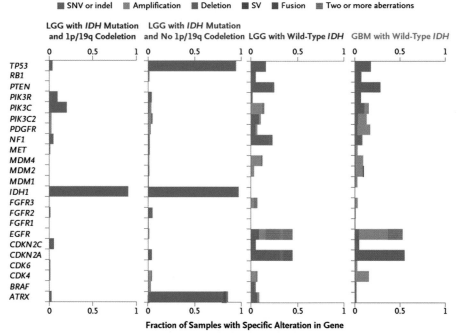

Fig. 1.15 IDH-mutant anaplastic astrocytoma. **A** Well-delineated focus with higher cellularity, mitotic activity, and a lack of GFAP expression (left). Such foci are encountered in anaplastic astrocytomas and glioblastomas and may represent new clones resulting from the acquisition of additional genetic alterations, indicating progression to a higher grade of dedifferentiation and malignancy {750}. **B** GFAP immunoreactivity. **C** Immunoreactivity for the proliferation marker MIB1, including a cell in mitosis.

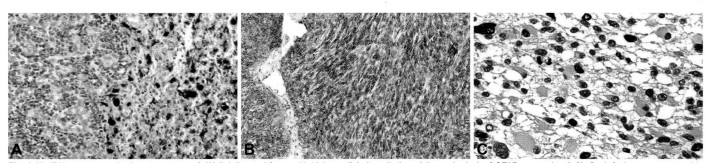

and a genotype of 7q gain and 10q loss have been associated with worse outcome. IDH mutations may be useful as a predictive biomarker when IDH-targeted therapies such as small-molecule inhibitors {2685} or vaccines {2301} become available.

Mutant IDH catalyses the formation of 2-hydroxyglutarate, which could potentially be monitored by MR spectroscopy {449} or in body fluids {358}. However, the clinical value of these approaches has yet to be validated.

Fig. 1.16 Mutations in 'lower-grade' (i.e. WHO grade II and III) gliomas (LGGs), detected in The Cancer Genome Atlas (TCGA) series {349}. Note that the mutational pattern in LGG with wildtype IDH is similar to that of glioblastoma (GBM) with wildtype IDH. LGGs with IDH mutation are divided into oligodendroglial tumours with 1p/19q codeletion and astrocytic tumours with frequent *TP53* and *ATRX* mutations but no 1p/19q codeletion. SNV, single nucleotide variant; SV, structural variant. Reprinted from: Brat DJ et al., Cancer Genome Atlas Research Network {349}.

Anaplastic astrocytoma, IDH-wildtype

Definition

A diffusely infiltrating astrocytoma with focal or dispersed anaplasia and significant proliferative activity but without mutations in the IDH genes.

IDH-wildtype anaplastic astrocytoma is uncommon and accounts for about 20% of all anaplastic astrocytomas. Nonetheless, histologically defined anaplastic astrocytomas have the highest incidence of wildtype *IDH1* and *IDH2* among the WHO grade II and III diffuse glioma variants {1269,2810}. Most gliomas with a histological appearance resembling that of anaplastic astrocytoma but without IDH mutation share molecular features with IDH-wildtype glioblastoma, and sometimes with H3 K27M–mutant gliomas if located preferentially in midline locations. Tumours in this category are more clinically aggressive than are IDH-mutant anaplastic astrocytomas and may follow a clinical course more similar to that of glioblastoma.

Grading

IDH-wildtype anaplastic astrocytoma corresponds histologically to WHO grade III.

Gliomatosis cerebri growth pattern

Like other diffuse gliomas, anaplastic astrocytoma can manifest at initial clinical presentation with a gliomatosis cerebri pattern of extensive involvement of the CNS, with the affected area ranging from most of one cerebral hemisphere (three lobes or more) to both cerebral hemispheres with additional involvement of the deep grey matter structures, brain stem, cerebellum, and spinal cord. A similar extensive, diffuse involvement of the deep grey matter structures (i.e. basal ganglia and thalamus), brain stem, cerebellum, and spinal cord can also be seen in the absence of cerebral cortical involvement. Gliomatosis was once thought to be a distinct nosological entity, but is now considered to be a pattern of exceptionally widespread involvement of the neuraxis. It can be seen in any of the diffuse glioma subtypes, but is most common in anaplastic astrocytoma. There are no unique molecular signatures that distinguish gliomatosis from the well-characterized subtypes of diffuse glioma, but IDH mutations seem to be restricted to tumours with distinct solid tumour components {2313}.

Anaplastic astrocytoma, NOS

Definition

A tumour with morphological features of anaplastic astrocytoma, but in which IDH mutation status has not been fully assessed.

Full assessment of IDH mutation status in anaplastic astrocytomas involves sequence analysis for *IDH1* codon 132 and *IDH2* codon 172 mutations in cases that are immunohistochemically negative for the *IDH1* R132H mutation.

ICD-O code   9401/3

Grading

Anaplastic astrocytoma, NOS, corresponds histologically to WHO grade III.

Glioblastoma, IDH-wildtype

Louis D.N.   Brat D.J.   Ohgaki H.   Stupp R.
Suvà M.L.   Biernat W.   Cavenee W.K.   Hawkins C.
Burger P.C.   Bigner D.D.   Wick W.   Verhaak R.G.W.
Perry A.   Nakazato Y.   Barnholtz-Sloan J. Ellison D.W.
Kleihues P.   Plate K.H.   Rosenblum M.K.   von Deimling A.
Aldape K.D.   Giangaspero F.   Hegi M.

Definition

A high-grade glioma with predominantly astrocytic differentiation; featuring nuclear atypia, cellular pleomorphism (in most cases), mitotic activity, and typically a diffuse growth pattern, as well as microvascular proliferation and/or necrosis; and which lacks mutations in the IDH genes.

IDH-wildtype glioblastoma is the most common and most malignant astrocytic glioma, accounting for about 90% of all glioblastomas and typically affecting adults, with a mean patient age at diagnosis of 62 years and a male-to-female ratio of about 1.35:1. As the synonymous designation "IDH-wildtype primary glioblastoma" indicates, this glioblastoma typically arises de novo, with no recognizable lower-grade precursor lesion. A preferentially supratentorial location is characteristic. The tumour diffusely infiltrates adjacent and distant brain structures.

ICD-O code   9440/3

Grading

Glioblastoma and its variants correspond histologically to WHO grade IV. However, in the setting of current therapy, IDH-mutant glioblastomas may follow a clinical course that is less aggressive than is typical of WHO grade IV tumours.

Synonym

Primary glioblastoma, IDH-wildtype

Epidemiology

Incidence

Glioblastoma is the most frequent malignant brain tumour in adults, accounting for approximately 15% of all intracranial neoplasms and approximately 45–50% of all primary malignant brain tumours {1826,1863}. In most European and North American countries and in Australia, the annual incidence is about 3–4 cases per 100 000 population {1863}, whereas the incidence is relatively low in eastern Asia, with 0.59 cases per 100 000 population per year in the Republic of Korea, for

Genetic parameters

The genetic alterations typical of IDH-wildtype glioblastoma include *TERT* promoter mutations (present in ~80% of cases), homozygous deletion of *CDKN2A/CDKN2B* (~60%), loss of chromosomes 10p (~50%) and 10q (~70%), *EGFR* alterations (i.e. mutation, rearrangement, altered splicing, and/or amplification; ~55%), *PTEN* mutations/deletion (~40%), *TP53* mutations (25–30%), and PI3K mutations (~25%) {277,1830}.

The prognosis of IDH-wildtype glioblastoma with current therapies is poor. Determining *MGMT* promoter methylation status provides information in these tumours on response to alkylating and methylating chemotherapies.

Ideally, the designation "IDH-wildtype" should be applied to a glioblastoma when both R132H-mutant IDH1 immunohistochemistry and subsequent *IDH1/2* sequencing reveal wildtype sequences at *IDH1* codon 132 and *IDH2* codon 172. However, in some situations it may, for practical purposes, be sufficient to rely on negative R132H-mutant IDH1 immunohistochemistry alone, most notably in older patients with a histologically classic glioblastoma that is not in a midline location (unless an H3 K27M mutation has also been excluded) and with no history of a pre-existing lower-grade glioma. Although it is not possible to establish an exact patient age cut-off point, one algorithm has suggested that, in the setting of negative R132H-mutant IDH1 immunohistochemistry in a glioblastoma from a patient without prior lower-grade glioma, the probability of an alternative IDH mutation is < 6% in a 50-year-old patient and decreases to < 1% in patients aged > 54 years {425}. The designation "IDH-wildtype" can therefore be safely applied in this setting, even in the absence of IDH sequencing. However, in younger patients, certain findings more strongly suggest the need for IDH sequencing before designating a tumour as IDH-wildtype. These include a history of a lower-grade glioma and the absence of nuclear ATRX expression (particularly if p53 immunohistochemistry shows strong and diffuse nuclear positivity and in the absence of staining for K27M-mutant H3.3). In such a setting, if IDH sequencing cannot be performed, a diagnosis of glioblastoma, NOS, should be rendered, with a note stating that R132H-mutant IDH1 immunohistochemistry was negative.

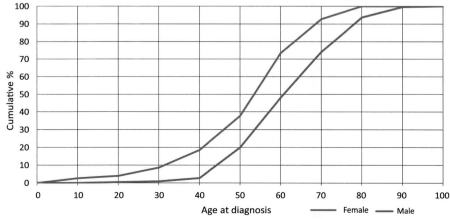

Fig. 1.17 Cumulative age distribution of patients with IDH-wildtype glioblastoma. There is a tendency for an earlier manifestation in women. Based on 371 cases from Nobusawa S et al. {1797}.

example {1861}. The annual incidence of glioblastoma in the USA, adjusted to the United States Standard Population, is 3.19 cases per 100 000 population {1863}. The corresponding rate in a population-based study in Switzerland (adjusted to the European Standard Population) was 3.55 cases per 100 000 population {1826}. Significantly lower rates have been reported in Asian and African countries, but this may be due in large part to underascertainment.

Age and sex distribution
Glioblastoma can manifest in patients of any age, but preferentially affects older adults, with peak incidence occurring in patients aged 55–85 years. Glioblastoma is the second most common type of intracranial neoplasm in adults aged ≥ 55 years {1863}. Glioblastomas are rare in individuals aged < 40 years. In the USA, the median age of patients with glioblastoma is 64.0 years, and the annual incidence rate in the 0–19 years age group, adjusted to the United States Standard Population, is 0.14 new cases per 100 000 population. The median patient age at diagnosis of IDH-wildtype glioblastomas is 62 years. The male-to-female ratio for glioblastoma is 1.60:1 in the USA {1863} and 1.28:1 in Switzerland {1825}.

Etiology
A very small proportion of glioblastomas are inherited as part of specific Mendelian syndromes (see *Genetic susceptibility*, p. 42) {1861}, but the etiology of most glioblastomas remains unknown.

A series of environmental and genetic factors have been studied as potential causes of glioblastoma. To date, these investigations have yielded inconclusive or negative results, including results on the potential influence of non-ionizing radiation (e.g. from mobile phones) and occupational exposures. The only validated risk factor associations are an increased risk after ionizing radiation to the head and neck and a decreased risk among individuals with a history of allergies and/ or atopic disease(s) {1861}. Genome-wide association studies have identified some specific heritable risk variants associated with glioblastoma (see *Genetic susceptibility*, p. 42). As our understanding of the heterogeneity of glioblastoma increases with the use of genomic technologies, our ability to discover and validate glioblastoma subtype-specific risk factors will probably improve.

Localization
Glioblastoma is most often centred in the subcortical white matter and deeper grey matter of the cerebral hemispheres. In a series of 987 glioblastomas from the University Hospital Zurich, the most frequently affected sites were the temporal lobe (affected in 31% of cases), the parietal lobe (in 24%), the frontal lobe (in 23%), and the occipital lobe (in 16%). Similar location trends are seen in the USA {1863}. Whereas primary, IDH-wildtype glioblastomas have a widespread anatomical distribution, secondary, IDH-mutant glioblastomas have a striking predilection for the frontal lobe, particularly in the region surrounding the

rostral lateral ventricles {1417}. In general, tumour infiltration extends into the adjacent cortex and through the corpus callosum into the contralateral hemisphere. Glioblastoma of the basal ganglia and thalamus is common, especially in children. Glioblastoma of the brain stem is uncommon and most often affects children {595} (see also *Diffuse midline glioma, H3 K27M–mutant*, p. 57). The cerebellum and spinal cord are rare sites.

Clinical features
Glioblastomas develop rapidly. The symptoms depend largely on the tumour location, primarily manifesting as focal neurological deficits (e.g. hemiparesis and aphasia) and tumour-associated oedema with increase in intracranial pressure. As many as half of all patients are diagnosed after an inaugural seizure. Other common symptoms are behavioural and neurocognitive changes, nausea and vomiting, and occasionally severe pulsating headaches {557,2640,2733}. In a study of 677 patients with IDH-wildtype glioblastoma, the time from first symptoms to diagnosis was < 3 months in 68% of cases and < 6 months in 84% {1827}. In patients with a significantly longer duration of symptoms, the possibility of an IDH-mutant glioblastoma that has evolved from a lower-grade astrocytoma should be considered.

Imaging
Glioblastomas are irregularly shaped and have a ring-shaped zone of contrast enhancement around a dark, central area of necrosis. They may extend widely

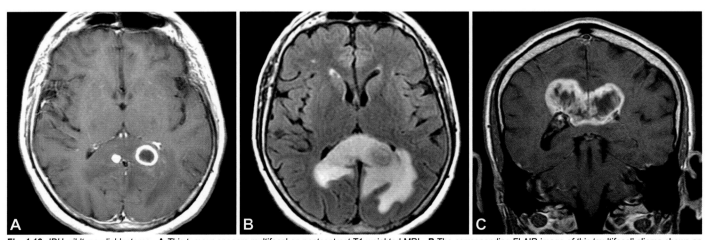

Fig. 1.18 IDH-wildtype glioblastoma. **A** This tumour appears multifocal on postcontrast T1-weighted MRI. **B** The corresponding FLAIR image of this 'multifocal' glioma shows an abnormal signal connecting the seemingly separate foci of contrast enhancement. **C** This postcontrast T1-weighted image shows the typical features of a 'butterfly glioblastoma' with extensive involvement of the corpus callosum leading to bihemispheric spread.

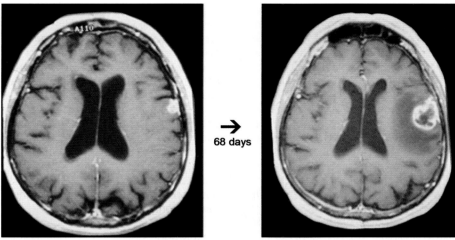

Fig. 1.19 Rare case in which the rapid development of a primary glioblastoma, IDH-wildtype, could be followed by neuroimaging. After a seizure, the 79-year-old man was hospitalized and MRI showed a small cortical lesion of 1 cm in diameter. Only 2 months later, the patient presented with a full-blown glioblastoma with ring enhancement, central necrosis, and perifocal oedema {1533,1822}.

into adjacent lobes, the opposite hemisphere, and the brain stem. In the setting of a ring-enhancing mass, biopsies showing high-grade astrocytoma but not demonstrating frank histological features of glioblastoma should be suspected to have been inadequately sampled.

Spread

Infiltrative spread is a defining feature of all diffuse gliomas, but glioblastoma is particularly notorious for its rapid invasion of neighbouring brain structures {316}. Infiltration occurs most readily along white matter tracts, but can also involve cortical and deep grey structures. When infiltration extends through the corpus callosum, with subsequent growth in the contralateral hemisphere, the result can be a bilateral, symmetrical lesion (so-called butterfly glioma). Similarly, rapid spread is observed along white matter tracts of the internal capsule, fornix, anterior commissure, and optic radiation.

Other infiltrative patterns give rise to secondary structures of Scherer, including perineuronal satellitosis, perivascular aggregation, and subpial spread {2838}. Infiltrative cells are located both inside and outside of the contrast-enhancing rim of glioblastoma and generally create a gradient of decreasing cell density with increasing distance from the tumour centre. Individual infiltrating tumour cells can be histologically identified several centimetres from the tumour epicentre, both in regions that are T2-hyperintense on MRI and in regions that appear uninvolved. These infiltrating cells are the most likely source of local recurrence after initial therapy, because they escape surgical resection, do not receive the highest dose of radiotherapy, and involve regions with an intact blood–brain barrier (which diminishes chemotherapeutic bioavailability) {834}. Interestingly, a pattern of increased infiltration has been observed in a subset of patients with glioblastoma

treated with antiangiogenic therapies, presumably due to vascular normalization {542}.

Gliomatosis cerebri growth pattern
Like other diffuse gliomas, glioblastoma can manifest at initial clinical presentation with a gliomatosis cerebri pattern of extensive involvement of the CNS, with the affected area ranging from most of one cerebral hemisphere (three lobes or more) to both cerebral hemispheres with additional involvement of the deep grey matter structures, brain stem, cerebellum, and spinal cord. See *Anaplastic astrocytoma, IDH-wildtype* (p. 27) for additional detail.

Metastasis
Despite its rapid, infiltrative growth, glioblastoma does not commonly extend into the subarachnoid space or spread through the cerebrospinal fluid, although this may be more frequent in children {90, 880} Similarly, penetration of the dura, venous sinus, and bone is exceptional {812,2002}. Although extension within and along perivascular spaces is typical, invasion of the vessel lumen is not a frequent histological finding. Extracranial metastasis of glioblastoma is uncommon in patients without previous surgical intervention, but has been documented in patients who have undergone interstitial therapies and in patients with ventricular shunts {935,1546,2676}. More recently, circulating tumour cells have been found in the blood of some patients with glioblastoma, suggesting that immune mechanisms or inhospitable environments of distant organs suppress metastatic implantation and growth {2454}. The finding that immunosuppressed recipients of organ transplants from donors with glioblastoma have developed glioblastoma in their transplanted organ suggests that the immune system normally suppresses the metastatic potential of circulating tumour cells {1161}.

Mechanisms of invasion
Mechanisms that promote the invasive properties of glioblastoma cells include those involved with cell motility, cell–matrix and cell–cell interactions, and remodelling of the extracellular matrix, as well as microenvironmental influences {160, 573}. Tumour cells produce migration-enhancing extracellular matrix components and secrete proteolytic enzymes

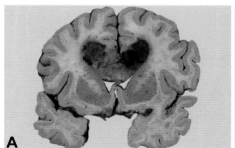
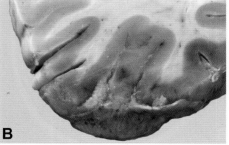

Fig. 1.20 A Glioblastoma with bilateral, symmetrical invasion of the corpus callosum and adjacent white matter of the cerebral hemispheres (butterfly glioblastoma). **B** Unusual case of a glioblastoma with focal infiltration of the cerebral cortex and the adjacent subarachnoid space, macroscopically presenting as greyish thickening of the meninges.

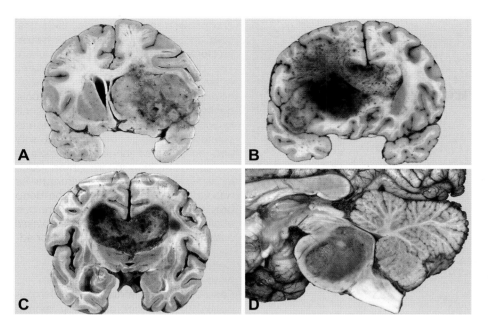

Fig. 1.21 A Glioblastoma of the right frontotemporal region with infiltration of the basal ganglia, compression of the right lateral ventricle, and midline shift towards the contralateral (left) cerebral hemisphere. **B** Large, diffusely infiltrating glioblastoma of the left frontal lobe with typical coloration: whitish-grey tumour tissue in the periphery, yellow areas of necrosis, and extensive haemorrhage. Note the extension through the corpus callosum into the right hemisphere. **C** Symmetrical glioblastoma infiltrating the lateral ventricles and adjacent brain structures. **D** Large glioblastoma of the brain stem (pons), causing compression of the fourth ventricle. This location is typical of H3 K27M–mutant diffuse midline gliomas.

that permit invasion, including the matrix metalloproteinases MMP2 and MMP9, uPA and its receptor uPAR, and cathepsins. Gliomas also express a variety of integrin receptors that mediate interactions with molecules in the extracellular space and lead to alterations of the cellular cytoskeleton and activation of intracellular signalling networks such as the AKT, mTOR, and MAPK pathways. Many growth factors expressed in glioblastoma, such as hepatocyte growth factor, fibroblast growth factor, epidermal growth factor, and VEGF, also stimulate migration by activation of corresponding receptor tyrosine kinases and downstream mediators that more directly promote migration, including FAK and the Rho family GTPases Rac, RhoA, and CDC42. In *EGFR*-amplified glioblastomas, cells with amplification are preferentially located at the infiltrating edges, suggesting a role in peripheral expansion {2385}. The overall mass migration of glioblastoma is radially outward, away from central necrosis and associated severe hypoxia, with rates substantially greater than those of pre-necrotic gliomas {2170,2467}. Hypoxia promotes invasion through the activation of HIF1 and other hypoxia-inducible transcription factors, due to both pro-

angiogenic mechanisms and direct effects that enhance glioma cell migration {1239,2840}. Hypoxic tumour cells display elevated expression of extracellular matrix components and intracellular proteins associated with cell motility {264,2170}. Activation of a pro-migration transcriptional programme seems to be associated with a decrease in proliferation, which may have therapeutic consequences {834,835}.

Multifocal glioblastoma
Although multifocality is not unusual when defined radiologically, the incidence of truly multiple, independent gliomas occurring outside the setting of inherited neoplastic syndromes is unknown. Even careful postmortem studies on whole-brain sections do not always reveal a connection between apparently multifocal gliomas, because the cells infiltrating along myelinated pathways are often small, polar, and largely undifferentiated. One careful histological analysis {143} concluded that 2.4% of glioblastomas are truly multiple independent tumours, a value similar to that reported by others (2.3%) {2204}. A postmortem study found that 7.5% of gliomas (including oligodendrogliomas) are multiple independent

tumours and that in approximately 3% of these, the tumour foci differ in histological appearance {128}. True multifocal glioblastomas are most likely polyclonal if they occur infratentorially and supratentorially (i.e. outside easily accessible routes such as the cerebrospinal fluid pathways or the median commissures) {2228}. By definition, multiple independently arising gliomas must be of polyclonal origin, and their existence can only be proven by application of molecular markers, which in informative cases enable the distinction between tumours of common or independent origin {175,197,1359}.

Macroscopy

Despite the short duration of symptoms in many cases, glioblastomas are often surprisingly large at the time of presentation, and can occupy much of a lobe. The lesions are usually unilateral, but those in the brain stem and corpus callosum can be bilaterally symmetrical. Supratentorial bilateral extension occurs as a result of growth along myelinated structures, in particular across the corpus callosum and the commissures. Most glioblastomas of the cerebral hemispheres are clearly intraparenchymal with an epicentre in the white matter. Infrequently, they are largely superficial and in contact with the leptomeninges and dura and may be interpreted by the neuroradiologist or surgeon as metastatic carcinoma, or as an extra-axial lesion such as meningioma. Cortical infiltration may produce a preserved gyriform rim of thickened grey cortex overlying a necrotic zone in the white matter.
Glioblastomas are poorly delineated; the cut surface is variable in colour, with peripheral greyish tumour masses and central areas of yellowish necrosis from myelin breakdown. The peripheral hypercellular zone presents macroscopically

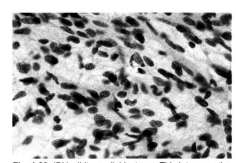

Fig. 1.22 IDH-wildtype glioblastoma. This intraoperative smear preparation shows small, elongated bipolar cells, a characteristic component of glioblastomas {1956}.

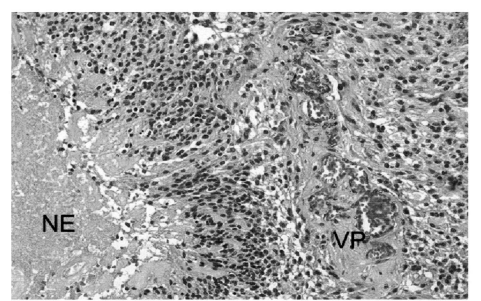

Fig. 1.23 Diagnostic hallmarks of IDH-wildtype glioblastoma. A focus of ischaemic necrosis (NE) is surrounded by palisading tumour cells and hyalinized vascular proliferation (VP).

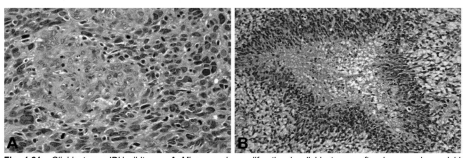

Fig. 1.24 Glioblastoma, IDH-wildtype. **A** Microvascular proliferation in glioblastomas often have a glomeruloid appearance. **B** Palisading necrosis is characterized by irregular zones of necrosis surrounded by dense accumulations of tumour cells.

The presence of highly anaplastic glial cells, mitotic activity, and microvascular proliferation and/or necrosis is required. The distribution of these key features within the tumour is variable, but large necrotic areas usually occupy the tumour centre, whereas viable tumour cells tend to accumulate in the periphery. The circumferential region of high cellularity and abnormal vessels corresponds to the contrast-enhancing ring seen radiologically, and is an appropriate target for needle biopsy. Microvascular proliferation is seen throughout the lesion, but is usually most marked around necrotic foci and in the peripheral zone of infiltration.

Cellular composition and histological patterns

Few human neoplasms are as heterogeneous in composition as glioblastoma. Poorly differentiated, fusiform, round, or pleomorphic cells may prevail, but better-differentiated neoplastic astrocytes are usually discernible, at least focally {317}. This is particularly true of glioblastomas resulting from the progression of WHO grade II diffuse astrocytomas, but these are typically IDH-mutant glioblastomas. The transition between areas that still have recognizable astrocytic differentiation and highly anaplastic cells may be either continuous or abrupt. In the case of gemistocytic lesions, anaplastic tumour cells may be diffusely mixed with the differentiated gemistocytes. An abrupt change in morphology may reflect the emergence of a new tumour clone through the acquisition of one or more additional genetic alterations (see *Primitive neuronal cells and glioblastoma with a primitive neuronal component*, below) {750}. Cellular pleomorphism includes the formation of small, undifferentiated, lipidized, granular, and giant cells. There are also often areas where bipolar, fusiform cells form intersecting bundles, and fascicles prevail. The accumulation of highly polymorphic tumour cells with well-delineated plasma membranes and a lack of cell processes may mimic metastatic carcinoma or melanoma.

Several cellular morphologies appear commonly in glioblastomas. Some glioblastomas have well-recognized patterns that are characterized by a great predominance of a particular cell type. These morphologies are discussed in the following subsections, along with the corresponding glioblastoma patterns that

as a soft, grey to pink rim or a grey band of tumour tissue. However, necrotic tissue may also border adjacent brain structures without an intermediate zone of macroscopically detectable tumour tissue. The central necrosis can occupy as much as 80% of the total tumour mass. Glioblastomas are typically stippled with red and brown foci of recent and remote haemorrhage. Extensive haemorrhages can occur and cause stroke-like symptoms, which are sometimes the first clinical sign of the tumour. Macroscopic cysts, when present, contain a turbid fluid and constitute liquefied necrotic tumour tissue, in contrast to the well-delineated retention cysts present in WHO grade II diffuse astrocytomas.

Microscopy

Glioblastoma is typically a highly cellular glioma, usually composed of poorly differentiated, sometimes pleomorphic tumour cells with nuclear atypia and brisk mitotic activity. Prominent microvascular proliferation and/or necrosis is an essential diagnostic feature.

As the outdated term 'glioblastoma multiforme' suggests, the histopathology of this tumour is extremely variable. Some lesions show a high degree of cellular and nuclear polymorphism with numerous multinucleated giant cells; others are highly cellular but relatively monomorphic. The astrocytic nature of the neoplasms is easily identifiable (at least focally) in some tumours, but difficult to recognize in tumours that are poorly differentiated. The regional heterogeneity of glioblastoma is remarkable, making histopathological diagnosis difficult on specimens obtained by stereotaxic needle biopsies {317}.

The diagnosis of glioblastoma is often based on the identification of the tissue pattern rather than of specific cell types.

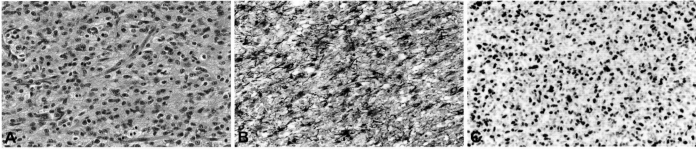

Fig. 1.25 Small cell glioblastoma. **A** Central portion of an *EGFR*-amplified, IDH-wildtype, 1p/19q-intact small cell glioblastoma showing a highly cellular monomorphic population of small tumour cells with frequent mitoses despite only mild nuclear atypia. **B** Delicate processes are evident on a GFAP immunostain. **C** The Ki-67 labelling index is very high.

can be established if a particular cellular morphology predominates. Because most of these glioblastoma patterns are found in IDH-wildtype glioblastomas, they are discussed here, but it is recognized that some of these variants (e.g. gemistocytic astrocytomas progressing to glioblastoma) are more characteristic of IDH-mutant glioblastoma.

Small cells and small cell glioblastoma
This subtype features a predominance of highly monomorphic small, round to slightly elongated, hyperchromatic nuclei with minimal discernible cytoplasm, little nuclear atypia, and (often) brisk mitotic activity. In the zone of infiltration, tumour cells can be difficult to identify as neoplastic, given their small size and bland cytology. GFAP immunoreactivity variably highlights delicate processes, and the Ki-67 proliferation index is typically high. Due to their nuclear regularity, clear haloes, microcalcifications, and chicken wire–like microvasculature, these tumours overlap with anaplastic oligodendroglioma {1937}. But unlike oligodendrogliomas, small cell glioblastomas frequently have *EGFR* amplification (present in ~70% of cases) and chromosome 10 losses (in > 95%). As in other primary glioblastomas in general, IDH mutations are absent {1183,1937}. In one series, mutations of *TP53* were found to be slightly less common in this subtype, but the difference did not reach statistical significance {1031}. The clinical behaviour of the small-cell subtype is similar to that of other primary glioblastomas in general, with a median survival time of 11 months in one series {1937}. In the same series, about a third of the cases presented as non-enhancing or minimally enhancing masses with no evidence of microvascular proliferation or necrosis on histology. However, follow-up imaging 2–3 months later often showed ring enhancement, and survival times were shorter for these cases (median: 6 months), suggesting that these cases constitute early presentations of WHO grade IV glioblastoma rather than WHO grade III anaplastic astrocytoma {1937}.

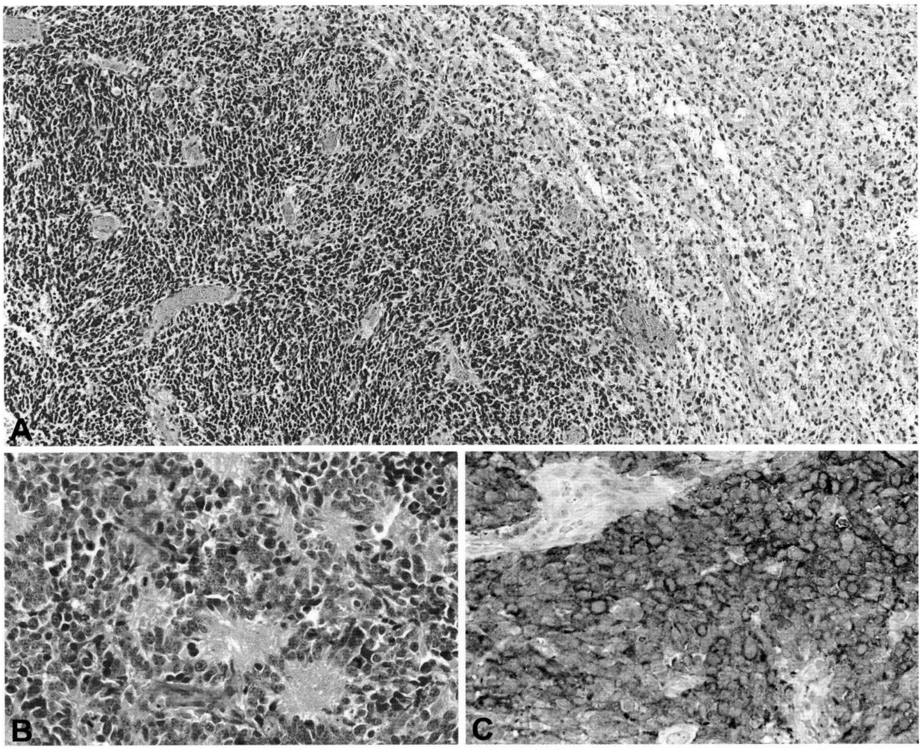

Primitive neuronal cells and glioblastoma with a primitive neuronal component
This subtype constitutes an otherwise classic diffuse glioma with one or more solid-looking primitive nodules showing neuronal differentiation. The glioma component is typically astrocytic, although rare primitive neuronal foci have also been reported in oligodendrogliomas {1946}. The primitive foci are sharply demarcated from the adjacent glioma and display markedly increased cellularity and a high nuclear-to-cytoplasmic ratio and mitosis-karyorrhexis index. More variable features include Homer Wright rosettes, cell wrapping, and anaplastic cytology similar to that of medulloblastoma or other CNS embryonal neoplasms. Additional primitive neuronal features include immunoreactivity for neuronal markers such as synaptophysin, reduction or loss of GFAP expression, and a markedly elevated Ki-67 proliferation index compared with adjacent foci of glioma. This subtype

Fig. 1.26 Glioblastoma with a primitive neuronal component. **A** Diffuse astrocytoma component on the right and primitive neuronal component on the left. **B** Homer Wright rosettes within the primitive neuronal component of a glioblastoma. **C** Strong synaptophysin positivity in the primitive cells.

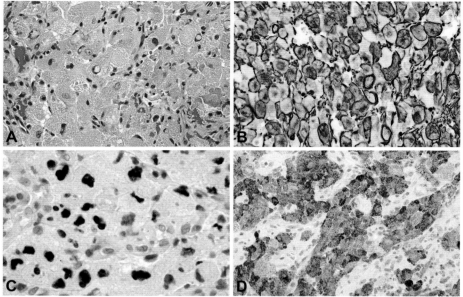

Fig. 1.27 Granular cell glioblastoma. **A** Eosinophilic cytoplasm reminiscent of a granular cell tumour of the pituitary, but with cytologically more atypical cells. **B** GFAP immunoreactivity. **C** The strong nuclear OLIG2 immunoreactivity helps to establish its glial lineage. **D** In contrast to most glioblastomas, the granular cell variant often shows immunoreactivity for EMA.

presents either de novo or during progression from a known diffuse glioma. In both settings, the survival time and genetic background are similar to those of glioblastoma in general {1946}. However, this subtype is distinctive in its high rate (30–40%) of cerebrospinal fluid dissemination and frequency (~40%) of *MYCN* or *MYC* gene amplification. *MYC* amplification is found only in the primitive-appearing nodules, and it is likely that such alterations drive the primitive-appearing clonal transformation at least in part, given that a similar phenotype has been observed in N-myc–driven murine forebrain tumours {2468}. In some cases, either new 10q losses or expanded regions of 10q loss are also found in the primitive neuronal focus {750}. Evidence that some examples of this subtype are secondary glioblastomas includes the history of a lower-grade precursor in some

patients, the typically strong and extensive tumoural p53 immunoreactivity, and the presence of *IDH1* R132H mutations in 15–20% of cases {1183,2394}.

Oligodendroglioma components
Occasional glioblastomas contain foci that resemble oligodendroglioma. These areas are variable in size and frequency, and individual pathologists' thresholds for identifying oligodendroglioma features vary. Two large studies of malignant gliomas suggest that necrosis is associated with a significantly worse prognosis in the setting of anaplastic glioma with both oligodendroglial and astrocytic components {1667,2617}; patients whose tumours had necrosis had a substantially shorter median overall survival than did patients whose tumours did not. Such tumours were classified as glioblastomas with an oligodendroglial component, and

they may have a better prognosis than standard glioblastoma {975,1031,1360}. More recent studies suggest that this is a heterogeneous tumour group, and that some cases are *IDH1*- or *IDH2*-mutant glioblastomas. The current WHO classification does not consider glioblastoma with an oligodendroglioma component to be a distinct diagnostic entity; with genetic analysis, it should be possible to classify such tumours as IDH-wildtype glioblastoma (in particular the small-cell variant, given the morphological overlap with oligodendroglial cells), IDH-mutant glioblastoma, or IDH-mutant and 1p/19q-codeleted anaplastic oligodendroglioma.

Gemistocytes and gemistocytic astrocytic neoplasms
Gemistocytes are cells with copious, glassy, non-fibrillary cytoplasm that displaces the dark, angulated nucleus to the periphery of the cell. Processes radiate from the cytoplasm, but are stubby and not long-reaching. GFAP staining is largely confined to the periphery of the cell, with the central hyaline organelle-rich zone remaining largely unstained. Perivascular lymphocytes frequently populate gemistocytic regions, but often avoid other regions in the same neoplasm. When present in large numbers, particularly in a patient known to have a pre-existing glioma (e.g. an IDH-mutant gemistocytic astrocytoma), these cells may constitute a lower-grade precursor lesion within a secondary IDH-mutant glioblastoma. Better-differentiated areas can sometimes be identified radiologically as non–contrast-enhancing peripheral regions, and in whole-brain sections, as WHO grade II to III astrocytomas clearly distinct from foci of glioblastoma {317,2266}. Immunohistochemical studies have emphasized the low proliferation rate of the neoplastic gemistocyte itself, despite the reported tendency of WHO grade II or III gemistocytic astrocytoma lesions to progress more rapidly to glioblastoma than non-gemistocytic counterparts of the same grade {2706}. The proliferating component presents as a population of cells with larger hyperchromatic nuclei and scant cytoplasm {2706}.

Multinucleated giant cells
Large, multinucleated tumour cells are often considered a hallmark of glioblastomas and occur with a spectrum of increasing size and pleomorphism.

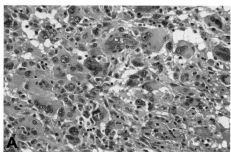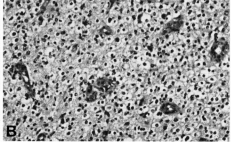

Fig. 1.28 Glioblastoma, IDH-wildtype. **A** High degree of anaplasia with multinucleated giant cells. **B** Focal oligodendroglioma-like component.

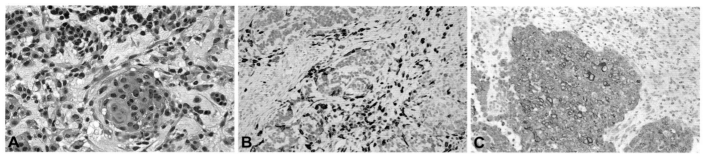

Fig. 1.29 Glioblastoma with epithelial metaplasia. **A** In addition to adenoid cytology, this glioblastoma features occasional squamous morules, indicative of true epithelial metaplasia. **B** Loss of GFAP expression within foci of epithelial metaplasia. **C** Focal squamous cell metaplasia characterized by marked cytokeratin expression.

Although common, the presence of multi-nucleated giant cells is neither an obligatory feature nor associated with a more aggressive clinical course {315}. Despite their appearance, these cells are considered a type of regressive change. If multinucleated giant cells dominate the histopathological picture, the designation of giant cell glioblastoma is justified (see *Giant cell glioblastoma*, p. 46).

Granular cells and granular cell astrocytoma/glioblastoma

Large cells with a granular, periodic acid–Schiff–positive cytoplasm may be scattered within glioblastoma. In rare cases, they dominate and create the impression of a morphologically similar but unrelated granular cell tumour of the pituitary stalk {569,948}. In the cerebral hemispheres, transitional forms between granular cells and neoplastic astrocytes can be identified in some cases, but in others it is difficult to identify any conventional astrocytoma component. Although larger and more coarsely granular, the tumour cells also resemble macrophages. Especially in the context of perivascular chronic inflammation, the tumour cells may be misinterpreted as a macrophage-rich

lesion such as demyelinating disease. Given their lysosomal content, granular tumour cells may be immunoreactive for macrophage markers such CD68, but not for specific markers such as CD163. Occasional cells may have peripheral immunopositivity for GFAP, but most cells are negative {271,793}. Some diffuse astrocytic tumours feature extensive granular cell change and have been termed "granular cell astrocytoma" or "granular cell glioblastoma". These lesions have a distinct histological appearance and are typically characterized by aggressive glioblastoma-like clinical behaviour {271}, even when the histology otherwise suggests only a WHO grade II or III designation; one review of 59 reported cases found median survival times of 11 months for WHO grade II cases and 9 months for WHO grade III–IV cases {2283}.

Lipidized cells and heavily lipidized glioblastoma

Cells with foamy cytoplasm are another feature occasionally observed in glioblastoma. The rare lesions in which they predominate have been designated malignant gliomas with heavily lipidized (foamy) tumour cells {1247,1253,2180,

2506}. The lipidized cells may be grossly enlarged {811}. If such a lesion is superficially located in a young patient, the diagnosis of pleomorphic xanthoastrocytoma should be considered, particularly if the xanthomatous cells are surrounded by basement membranes staining positively for reticulin and accompanied by eosinophilic granular bodies {1248}. Other lipid-rich lesions have epithelioid cytological features {2180}. Lobules of juxtaposed fully lipidized (i.e. not foamy) cells can simulate adipose tissue.

Metaplasia and gliosarcoma

In general, 'metaplasia' refers to the acquisition by a differentiated cell of morphological features typical of another differentiated cell type. However, the term is also used to designate aberrant differentiation in neoplasms. In glioblastoma, this is exemplified by foci displaying features of squamous epithelial cells (i.e. epithelial whorls with keratin pearls and cytokeratin expression) {320,1734}.

Occasionally, glioblastomas contain foci with glandular and ribbon-like epithelial structures {2180}. These elements have a large oval nucleus, prominent nucleolus, and round well-defined cytoplasm.

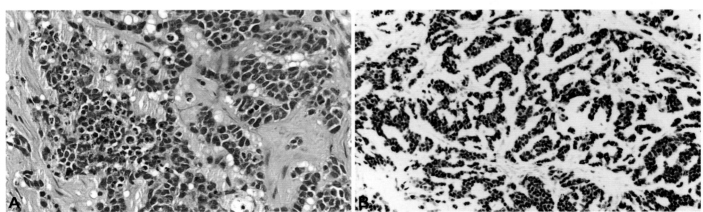

Fig. 1.30 Adenoid glioblastoma. **A** Adenocarcinoma-like cytology with small epithelioid cells arranged in nests and rows set within a mucin-rich stroma. **B** Despite the carcinoma-like appearance, the glial histogenesis of this adenoid glioblastoma is supported by strong nuclear expression of OLIG2.

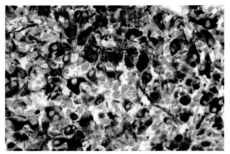

Fig. 1.31 IDH-wildtype glioblastoma. GFAP immunohisto-chemistry typically labels only some cells in glioblastoma, highlighting the tumour cell bodies and processes.

They are also referred to as adenoid glioblastomas. Expression of GFAP in these areas may be diminished, and replaced by expression of epithelial markers. Small cells with even more epithelial features and cohesiveness are less common {1250}. When there is an extensive mesenchymal component, in particular a spindle cell sarcoma–like component, a diagnosis of gliosarcoma should be considered. A mucinous background and a mesenchymal component (gliosarcoma) are not uncommon in metaplastic glioblastomas. Adenoid and squamous epithelial metaplasia are more common in gliosarcoma than in ordinary glioblastoma {1250,1734}. This is similarly true

for the formation of bone and cartilage, which predominates in gliosarcoma and in a variety of childhood CNS neoplasms {1608}.

Secondary structures
The migratory capacity of glioblastoma cells within the CNS becomes readily apparent when they reach a border that constitutes a barrier: tumour cells line up and accumulate in the subpial zone of the cortex, in the subependymal region, and around neurons (so-called satellitosis) and blood vessels. These patterns, called secondary structures {2267}, result from the interaction of glioma cells with host brain structures, and are highly diagnostic of an infiltrating glioma. Secondary structures may also be present in other highly infiltrative gliomas, such as oligodendroglioma {2266,2267}. This concept also extends to the adaptation of tumour cells to myelinated pathways, which often acquire a fusiform, polar shape as a result. Identifying neoplastic astrocytes in the perifocal zone of oedema and at more distant sites can be challenging for pathologists, in particular when dealing with stereotaxic biopsies {535}. Small cell glioblastomas pose a particular problem in this regard.

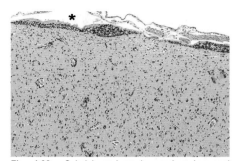

Fig. 1.32 Subpial, perivascular, and perineuronal accumulation of glioblastoma cells. Asterisk indicates uninvolved subarachnoid space.

One feature of many glioblastomas, especially the small-cell variant, is extensive involvement of the cerebral cortex. Secondary structures and most of the apparently multifocal glioblastomas arise essentially as a result of the pathways of migration of glioma cells in the CNS {1440}. The subependymal region may also be diffusely infiltrated, especially in the terminal stages of disease.

Proliferation
Proliferative activity is usually prominent, with detectable mitoses in nearly every case. Atypical mitoses are frequently present. However, there is great intertumoural and intratumoural variation in mitotic activity. The growth fraction as determined by the Ki-67 proliferation index can thus show great regional variation. Typical values are 15–20%, but some tumours have a proliferation index of > 50% focally. Rare tumours have a low proliferation index despite other histological features of malignancy. Tumours with small, undifferentiated, fusiform cells often show marked proliferative activity, in contrast to tumours composed of neoplastic gemistocytes, which typically have a lesser degree of proliferation {2706}. Despite the wide range in the proliferation index observed in glioblastoma, an association between proliferation index and clinical outcome has not been demonstrated {1715}.

Microvascular proliferation and angiogenesis
The presence of microvascular proliferation is a histopathological hallmark of glioblastoma. On light microscopy, microvascular proliferation typically presents as so-called glomeruloid tufts of multilayered mitotically active endothelial cells together with smooth muscle cells / pericytes {920,1741,2734}. Another (less

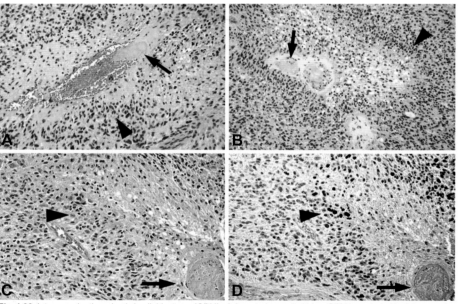

Fig. 1.33 Intravascular thrombosis in glioblastoma (GBM). **A** A central vessel within a GBM is occluded by intravascular thrombus (arrow). The vessel is dilated proximal to the occlusion and surrounded by delicate fibrillarity and scattered apoptotic cells, most likely representing the initial stages of palisade formation (arrowhead). **B** As the palisading front of tumour cells (arrowhead) enlarges around a central thrombosed vessel (arrow), perivascular necrosis becomes more prominent. **C** H&E staining of a GBM demonstrates intravascular thrombosis occluding and distending a vessel (arrow) within the centre of a palisade (arrowhead). **D** Immunohistochemistry for HIF1A of a serial tissue section shows increased nuclear staining in palisades, indicating an adaptive response to hypoxia (arrowhead). Reprinted from Rong Y et al. {2170}.

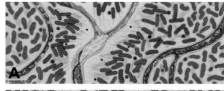

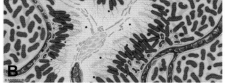

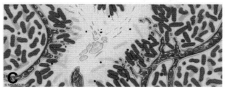

Fig. 1.34 Potential mechanism of palisade formation. **A** Endothelial injury and the expression of procoagulant factors result in intravascular thrombosis and increasing perivascular hypoxia (light blue). Tumour cells begin to migrate away, creating a peripherally moving wave of palisading cells. **B** The zone of hypoxia and central necrosis expands. Hypoxic tumour cells of palisades secrete proangiogenic factors (VEGF, IL8). **C** Microvascular proliferation in regions adjacent to central hypoxia causes an accelerated outward migration of tumour cells towards a new vasculature. Illustration © 2005 Mica Duran. Adapted from Rong Y et al. {2170}.

common) form is hypertrophic proliferating endothelial cells within medium-sized vessels. Microvascular proliferation of the glomeruloid type is most commonly located in the vicinity of necrosis and is directionally oriented to it, reflecting the response to vasostimulatory factors released from the ischaemic tumour cells. Vascular thrombosis is common and may be apparent to the neurosurgeon as so-called black veins. It may play a role in the pathogenesis of ischaemic tumour necrosis {2170}. The hyperplastic endothelial cells (which are positive for CD31 and CD34, negative for SMA, and positive for VEGFR2) are surrounded by basal lamina and an incomplete layer of pericytes (which are negative for CD31 and CD34, positive for SMA, and positive for PDGFRB) {2264}. Morphologically inconspicuous vessels have a Ki-67 proliferation index of 2–4%, whereas proliferating tumour vessels have an index of > 10% {2702}.

Glioblastomas are among the most vascularized of all human tumours. Vascularization occurs through several mechanisms, including vessel cooption (adoption of pre-existing vessels by migrating tumour cells {708,1559}), classic angiogenesis (sprouting of capillaries from pre-existing vessels by endothelial cell proliferation/migration), and vasculogenesis (homing of bone marrow–derived cells that support vessel growth in a paracrine manner {6,708,1559}). Intussusception and cancer stem cell–derived vasculogenesis have also been described {944,1127, 1989}. Hypoxia is a major driving force of glioblastoma angiogenesis {6} and leads to intracellular stabilization of the master regulator HIF1A. HIF1A accumulation leads to transcriptional activation of > 100 hypoxia-regulated genes encoding proteins that control angiogenesis (e.g. VEGFA, angiopoietins, erythropoietin, and IL8), cellular metabolism (e.g. carbonic anhydrase and lactate dehydrogenase), survival/apoptosis (e.g. BNIP), and migration (e.g. hepatocyte growth factor receptor, CXCR4, and ACKR3). VEGFA seems to be the most important mediator of glioma-associated vascular functions; it is primarily produced by perinecrotic palisading cells as a consequence of cellular stress such as hypoxia and hypoglycaemia {1239,1988,2357}. VEGFA is regulated by transcription factors, oncogenes, tumour suppressor genes, cytokines, and certain hormones. VEGFA induces tumour angiogenesis, increases vascular permeability (oedema), and regulates homing of bone marrow–derived cells {6}. Therapeutic blocking of VEGFA by monoclonal antibodies, used for the treatment of recurrent glioblastoma {1998}, seems to target primarily small, immature vessels and lead to vascular normalization accompanied by improved perfusion and oxygenation {2398}. Other signalling pathways important for glioblastoma angiogenesis include angiopoietin/Tie2 receptor signalling, IL8/IL8R signalling, platelet-derived growth factor (PDGF) / PDGF receptor signalling, WNT/beta-catenin signalling, Eph/ephrin signalling, and transforming growth factor beta signalling. Pericytes / smooth muscle cells and perivascular bone marrow–derived cells (in addition to endothelial cells) also participate in the vascular remodelling processes typically observed in glioblastoma.

Necrosis

Tumour necrosis is a fundamental feature of glioblastoma, and its presence is one of the strongest predictors of aggressive behaviour among diffuse astrocytic tumours {315,1031,2079}. Presenting on neuroimaging as a hypodense core within a contrast-enhancing rim, necrosis constitutes areas of non-viable tumour tissue that can range from extremely small to accounting for > 80% of the total tumour mass. Higher proportions of necrosis on MRI have been associated with shorter survival, and the extent of necrosis is also related to the tumour's transcriptional profile {904,1969}. Grossly, necrosis presents as a yellow or white granular coagulum. Microscopically, glioma cells in various stages of degeneration are seen within necrobiotic debris, together with faded contours of large, dilated necrotic tumour vessels. Occasionally, preserved tumour vessels with a corona of viable tumour cells can be seen within extensive areas of necrosis.

A second form of necrosis that is a histological hallmark of glioblastoma is the

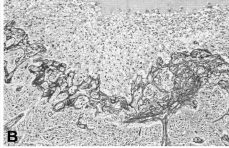

Fig. 1.35 Extensive coagulative ischaemic necrosis (right). Note several large thrombosed tumour vessels.

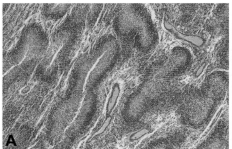

Fig. 1.36 A Longitudinal cut of perinecrotic palisades, presenting as long, serpiginous pattern. **B** Reticulin stain of a perinecrotic garland of proliferated tumour vessels.

palisading form (historically called the pseudopalisading form), which consists of multiple, small, irregularly shaped band-like or serpiginous foci surrounded by radially oriented, densely packed glioma cells {2170}. The outdated term "pseudopalisading" implied that the tumour cells did not truly aggregate around necrosis, but only created this impression, because they were believed to be a rim of hypercellular tumour cells that remained after central degeneration of a highly proliferative clone. However, this is likely not actually the case, given that the palisading cells have lower rates of proliferation than adjacent glioma cells and the central area of smaller palisading structures often consists of a fine fibrillary network without viable or necrotic glioma cells {264,1847,2170}. Palisading cells are hypoxic and strongly express HIF1A and other hypoxia-inducible transcription factors {2841,2861}. Downstream hypoxic upregulation of VEGF, IL8, and other proangiogenic factors is responsible for the microvascular proliferation that occurs immediately adjacent to palisading cells, providing a biological link between the histological hallmarks of necrosis and microvascular hyperplasia in glioblastoma {1989,2170}. The initiating necrogenic events have yet to be firmly established, but vascular cooption by neoplastic cells has been hypothesized to induce vascular regression through endothelial angiopoetin-2 expression {708,1030}. It has been speculated that microscopic vaso-occlusion and intravascular thrombosis may initiate or propagate the development of hypoxia and necrosis, given that thrombi are present near regions of necrosis in nearly all glioblastomas (but not in lower-grade, non-necrotic astrocytomas) and are often observed within or emerging from palisades {264,2529}. In this proposed sequence, hypoxia-induced cell migration away from central hypoxia establishes the palisading structures, which subsequently develop into increasingly larger regions of central necrosis and continue to expand radially outward {2170}.

Apoptosis
Apoptosis, the programmed death of individual cells, is a cell-intrinsic process characterized by nuclear fragmentation and condensation, with packaging of apoptotic bodies within an intact membrane. The process is initiated through the release of mitochondrial factors or by death receptor ligation by members of the tumour necrosis factor family, including TNFSF10/TNFRSF10B and TNFSF6/TNFRSF6 {943,1872}. The higher levels of apoptosis seen in palisading cells surrounding necrosis may be due to increased expression or ligation of death receptors {264,2485}. TNFSF10 induces apoptosis in glioblastoma by binding to TNFRSF10B and ultimately activating caspase-8 {943}. Levels of both TNFRSF6 and TNFSF6 are higher in astrocytomas than in normal brain and correlate with tumour grade {2485, 2563}. Most TNFRSF6 expression in glioblastoma is within palisading cells; physical interactions between tumour cells expressing TNFRSF6 and TNFSF6 may promote apoptosis. In malignant gliomas, the overall levels of cell death due to apoptosis are low (compared with coagulative necrosis), and apoptotic rates do not correlate with prognosis {1663,2272}.

Inflammation
The number of inflammatory cells in glioblastomas varies. Notable perivascular lymphocyte cuffing occurs in a minority of glioblastomas, most typically in areas with a homogeneous gemistocytic component. Inflammatory cells are scant if present at all in small cell glioblastomas. The inflammatory cells have been characterized primarily as CD8+ T lymphocytes, with CD4+ lymphocytes present in smaller numbers {227,2184} and with B lymphocytes detectable in < 10% of cases {2184}. Extensive CD8+ T-cell infiltrates may be more common in the tumours of long-term glioblastoma survivors {2813}. Microglia and histiocytes are also present in glioblastomas {1494, 2162}, although lipid-laden histiocytes are uncommon in untreated glioblastomas.

Immunophenotype
Glioblastomas often express GFAP, but the degree of reactivity differs markedly between cases; for example, gemistocytic areas are frequently strongly positive, whereas primitive cellular components are often negative. The gliomatous component of gliosarcoma may show expression of GFAP, as opposed to absent or meagre focal expression in the sarcomatous component, which may express alpha-1-antitrypsin, alpha-1-antichymotrypsin, actin, and EMA. S100 protein is also typically expressed in glioblastomas. In poorly differentiated tumours, the expression of OLIG2 may be of diagnostic utility, being strongly positive far more commonly in astrocytomas and oligodendrogliomas than in ependymomas and non-glial tumours {1101,1865}. The expression of cytokeratins is determined by the class of these intermediate filaments and antibodies used, some of which may indicate cross-reactivity with GFAP; keratin positivity is most often detected with the keratin antibody cocktail AE1/AE3, in contrast to the lack of positivity for many other keratins {2535}. Nestin is frequently expressed in glioblastoma and can be diagnostically useful to distinguish glioblastoma from other high-grade gliomas {88}.
Glioblastomas with missense *TP53* mutations show strong and diffuse immunohistochemical overexpression of p53 {2496}, with such overexpression evident in 21–53% of cases {276,1443,2007, 2455}. This may facilitate discrimination between neoplastic astrocytes and those in reactive gliosis in treated cases of glioblastoma {268}. Detection of WT1 expression, which is sometimes present in both low-grade and high-grade gliomas, may serve a similar purpose {2281}. EGFR expression occurs in about 40–98% of glioblastomas and correlates (to some extent) with the presence of gene amplification {198,678,1023,1443}. EGFRvIII expression is less common (occurring in 27–33% of cases) {198,678}. Tumours harbouring H3 K27M mutations (see *Diffuse midline glioma, H3 K27M-mutant*, p. 57) can be detected using an antibody specific for K27M-mutant H3, which can be useful in distinguishing these neoplasms from other astrocytic tumours {2644}. Some glioblastomas (i.e. IDH-mutant glioblastomas) express R132H-mutant IDH1, but the presence of R132H-mutant IDH1 expression is not compatible with a diagnosis of IDH-wildtype glioblastoma.

Cell of origin
The cellular origin of glioblastoma remains unknown. The expression of markers of differentiated astrocytes by glioblastoma cells has long been considered to indicate the dedifferentiation of the cells after transformation. More recently, the cellular, biochemical, and genetic heterogeneity that typify glioblastoma, together with the distinct clinical responses of histologically similar tumours, has led

to the hypothesis that the tumours arise from the malignant transformation of either a bipotential precursor cell {1794} or an even more primordial cell: the neural stem cell {1616}. This interpretation is supported by the coincident anatomical position in the subventricular zone of the brain of dividing cells with stem cell–like properties and the development of glioblastoma. Moreover, cells with stem cell–like properties have been isolated from glioblastoma tumours and cell lines and can be produced by the expression of a set of developmental transcription factors in glioblastoma cells {2461}. These cells, called brain tumour stem cells, are only a minor subpopulation, but they have the capacity of self-renewal, express markers of developmental regulation, and are tumorigenic in animals. Therefore, brain tumour stem cells may be the descendants of neural stem cells that had unrepaired DNA damage leading to mutations in cancer genes or that were subject to an environmental carcinogenic insult {1112,1756,2230,2365,2650}. Either of these initiating events could seed a tumour, given the unlimited growth potential of the neoplastic cells.

Genetic profile

Genetics

Malignant transformation of neuroepithelial cells is a multistep process driven by the sequential acquisition of genetic and epigenetic alterations. Of the astrocytic neoplasms, glioblastoma contains the greatest number of genetic changes. The following sections focus on so-called primary IDH-wildtype glioblastoma, which differs in its genetic profile from so-called secondary IDH-mutant glioblastoma (see *Glioblastoma, IDH-mutant*, p. 52). Many of the genetic alterations that are characteristic of IDH-wildtype glioblastomas are also present in the majority of WHO grade II and III IDH-wildtype gliomas, suggesting that these various grades of IDH-wildtype tumours constitute a continuum of disease and further reinforcing the necessity of distinguishing IDH-wildtype from IDH-mutant diffuse gliomas {349}.

Cytogenetics and numerical chromosome alterations

The most common chromosomal imbalances are gain of 7 and loss of 9, 10, and 13 [http://www.progenetix.net/I94403].

Table 1.01 Genetic profile of IDH-wildtype glioblastomas

Gene	Change	% of tumours	References
TERT	Mutation	72–90%	{622,1268,1270}
EGFR	Amplification	35–45%	{350,1823,1895}
CDKN2A	Deletion	35–50%	{350,1823,1895}
TP53	Mutation	28–35%	{350,1823,1895}
PTEN	Mutation	25–35%	{350,1823,1895}
NFKB1A	Deletion	25%	{273A}
NF1	Mutation	15–18%	{350,1895}
PIC3CA	Mutation	5–15%	{350,1288A,1895}
PDGFRA	Amplification	13%	{350}
PTPRD	Mutation	12%	{350}
RB1	Mutation	8–12%	{350}
PIK3R1	Mutation	8%	{1895}
MDM2	Mutation	5–15%	{350,2848A}
MDM4	Amplification	7%	{350}
MET	Amplification	4%	{350}
IDH1	Mutation	0%	{1797}
IDH2	Mutation	0%	{2810}

Chromosome 7p gain in combination with 10q loss is the most frequent genetic alteration in glioblastoma {1079,2072}. This combination is associated with EGFR amplification. Allelic loss of the chromosomal region containing the PTEN gene occurs in 75–95% of glioblastomas, whereas PTEN mutations are present in 30–44% of cases. Not only is loss of 10q the most frequent genetic alteration, but it also typically co-presents with any of the other genetic alterations. Another lesion frequently observed in glioblastoma is the combined gain of 19 and 20 {277}.

Epidermal growth factor receptor

EGFR is the most frequently amplified gene in glioblastomas {764} and is associated with overexpression; 70–90% of glioblastomas with EGFR overexpression show EGFR amplification {198, 2562}. EGFR amplification occurs in approximately 40% of primary glioblastomas {277,627,1823,2780} but rarely in secondary glioblastomas {1823,2705}. Amplification of the EGFR gene is often associated with gene truncations, most commonly truncation of the gene encoding EGFRvIII {2753}, which is present in 20–50% of glioblastomas with EGFR amplification {198,277,2306,2446}. The protein is structurally and functionally similar to v-erbB and is constitutively activated in a ligand-independent manner {458}.

Various truncations of EGFR can occur within the same tumour {732,1906}.

Receptor tyrosine kinase / PI3K / PTEN / AKT / mTOR pathway

Alterations in receptor tyrosine kinase signalling pathways occur in nearly 90% of glioblastomas {350}. In addition to EGFR alterations, alternate routes to mediate aberrant receptor tyrosine kinase signalling include PDGFRA amplification (present in 15% of cases), MET amplification (in 5%) and (in rare cases) the fusion protein FGFR1-TACC1 or FGFR3-TACC3 {2364,2645}. Amplification of the PDGFRA gene is often associated with gene truncations, the most common of which is an in-frame deletion of exons 8 and 9 (PDGFRAΔ8,9) {1869}. EGFR, PDGFRA, and MET amplifications and truncations can occur in different cells in the same tumour, which could pose a problem for targeted therapies {2385}. Mutations and amplifications in PI3K genes (e.g. PIK3CA and PIK3R1) are infrequent in glioblastomas (occurring in < 10% of cases) {350,1309,1692,1720}. The PTEN gene is involved in cell proliferation, tumour cell migration, and tumour cell invasion, and is mutated in 15–40% of glioblastomas, almost exclusively in primary glioblastomas {277,2562}. The mutation pattern suggests that PTEN truncation at any site and PTEN missense mutations in the region homologous to tensin/auxilin and dual-specificity phosphatases are associated with a malignant phenotype. Mutations in the *NF1* gene are present in approximately 20% of glioblastomas {350}.

p53/MDM2/p14ARF pathway

Alterations in the p53 pathway occur in nearly 90% of glioblastomas {350}. *TP53* mutations are more often genetic hallmarks of clinicopathologically defined secondary glioblastomas and, in almost all cases, are already present in precursor lower-grade or anaplastic astrocytomas {2705}. They are significantly less common in clinicopathologically defined primary glioblastomas (present in ~25% of cases) {1823}. G:C→A:T transitions at CpG sites are most common {1823}.

Amplification of *MDM2* or overexpression of MDM2 is an alternative mechanism for escaping p53-regulated control of cell proliferation. Amplification is observed in < 10% of glioblastomas without *TP53* mutations {2084}. Overexpression of MDM2 has been observed in > 50% of primary but only 11% of secondary glioblastomas {199}.

The *CDKN2A* locus gives rise to several splice variants encoding distinct proteins (CDKN2A and p14ARF) with tumour-suppressing function. The p14ARF protein binds directly to MDM2 and inhibits MDM2-mediated p53 degradation. Loss of p14ARF expression is frequent in glioblastomas (occurring in 76% of cases), and correlates with homozygous deletion or promoter methylation of the *CDKN2A* gene {1752}.

CDKN2A / CDK4 / retinoblastoma protein pathway

Alterations in the retinoblastoma protein pathway occur in nearly 80% of all glioblastomas {350}. In glioblastomas, *CDKN2A* deletion and *RB1* alterations are mutually exclusive {2594}. The *CDKN2A* locus encodes the CDK4 inhibitor CDKN2A as well as the alternate reading frame protein p14ARF. Inactivation of genes in this pathway is common in both primary and secondary glioblastomas {200,1752}. The *CDK4* gene is amplified in approximately 15% of all high-grade gliomas {1789,2086}, particularly in those without *CDKN2A* homozygous deletion {1789}. These homozygous deletions also involve the nearby *CDKN2B* gene on 9p {2397}. *RB1* mutations are

rare {993}, and gene promoter methylation correlated with loss of *RB1* expression is more common in secondary glioblastomas (occurring in 43% of cases) than in primary glioblastomas (occurring in 14% of cases) {1755}.

TERT promoter mutations

The promoter region of *TERT* contains two hotspots for point mutations, with most glioblastomas (~80% in one study) carrying these mutations {1270}. Within IDH-wildtype adult diffuse gliomas, *TERT* promoter mutations are inversely correlated with *TP53* mutations {1801}. They are frequent in *IDH1*-wildtype glioblastomas but rare in secondary (*IDH1*-mutant) glioblastomas and astrocytomas. *TERT* mutations are also frequent in oligodendrogliomas. *TERT* promoter mutations lead to the recruitment of multimeric GA-binding protein (GABP) transcription factor specifically to the mutant promoter, leading to aberrant TERT expression {159A}. In *IDH1*-mutant glioblastomas and astrocytomas, telomere maintenance preferentially uses the alternative lengthening of telomeres pathway, which is activated by mutations in the *ATRX* gene (see *Epigenetics, chromatin, and promoter methylation*).

IDH mutations

Mutations of the *IDH1* and *IDH2* genes, which encode IDH1 and IDH2 {1895}, are frequent in diffuse astrocytomas, anaplastic astrocytomas, oligodendrogliomas, anaplastic oligodendrogliomas, oligoastrocytomas, and anaplastic oligoastrocytomas (occurring in > 70% of cases) {2810}. These mutations are present in nearly all glioblastomas that have progressed from astrocytomas (i.e. clinicopathologically defined secondary glioblastomas), but they are exceptional in primary glioblastomas and absent in pilocytic astrocytomas {118,277,2709, 2810}. A clinically primary glioblastoma with an *IDH1* mutation may be misclassified and may actually constitute an asymptomatic lower-grade glioma that has progressed and has only become symptomatic as a secondary glioblastoma {1797}. Thus, *IDH1* mutations constitute a reliable molecular signature of a separate group of glioblastomas that may be synonymous with the secondary type {1797}. Notably, the presence of *IDH1* mutation is incompatible with the diagnosis of IDH-wildtype glioblastoma. See

Genetic parameters (p. 28) for discussion of the steps necessary to designate a glioblastoma as IDH-wildtype.

Chromatin-related genes

Mutations in chromatin-remodelling genes are common in glioblastomas. Paediatric high-grade gliomas also bear signature mutations directly affecting the histone gene *H3F3A* and less commonly *HIST1H3B/C*. These histone genes have two mutation hotspots, in codons K27 and G34, with K27 mutations more often found in midline, i.e. brain stem, thalamus, and spinal cord tumours (see *Diffuse midline glioma, H3 K27M–mutant*, p. 57) and G34 alterations in hemispheric lesions {1263,2444}. In paediatric high-grade gliomas, H3 mutations are associated with mutations in its chaperone *ATRX* and are inversely related to IDH mutations. *ATRX* mutations also occur in adult astrocytomas and glioblastomas {277}, particularly in those with IDH mutations {1160,2304,2792}.

Epigenetics, chromatin, and promoter methylation

The interplay between epigenetic regulation and gliomagenesis has several modalities. Epigenetic modifiers can be bona fide oncogenes or tumour suppressors that are directly affected by gain- or loss-of-function genetic mutations, resulting in the disruption of epigenetic regulatory processes by affecting histone modifications, DNA methylation, and chromatin remodelling {2462}. In one study, nearly half of the 291 IDH-wildtype glioblastoma samples subjected to whole-exome sequencing harboured one or more non-synonymous mutations affecting chromatin organization {277}. Even in the absence of direct genetic alterations, epigenetic modifiers can modulate gene expression to directly regulate glioma-relevant processes such as glioma stem cell programmes, senescence, genome stability, and invasion {2443,2461}.

One of the key functions of chromatin regulation is to maintain inactive portions of the genome in repressive chromatin structures with a compact organization refractory to regulatory activity. Canonical repressive states include classic heterochromatin marked by H3K27me3, a mark deposited by PRC2 and its catalytic subunit, EZH2. EZH2 is overexpressed in IDH-wildtype glioblastoma and various other cancer types, presumably contributing to the silencing of key tumour suppressor genes {556}. Loss of function of EZH2 can also promote cancer in a context-dependent manner. Although loss-of-function mutations of *EZH2* in IDH-wildtype glioblastoma are rare (occurring in < 1% of cases), studies have strongly implicated an inhibition of its enzymatic activity through a mutation of H3 genes in paediatric glioblastoma {277, 2304,2791}. Apparently, a fine-tuning of PRC2 activity must be maintained, with both gain and loss of activity linked to gliomagenesis. Mutations in *ATRX*, which encodes a chromatin remodeller that deposits H3.3 in pericentromeric and subtelomeric regions, were observed in 13 of 291 IDH-wildtype glioblastomas {277}. *ATRX* mutations are observed in about 60–70% of IDH-mutant gliomas and in about 30% of paediatric glioblastomas {1160,2304,2792}.

Within chromatin, both genes and regulatory elements are associated with characteristic chromatin modifications. Actively transcribed gene bodies are marked by H3K36me3, a mark deposited by the methyltransferase SETD2. Rare mutations in *SETD2* occur in about 2% of IDH-wildtype glioblastoma and are more common in paediatric and IDH-mutant gliomas {277,722}. Enhancers and promoters are marked by histone acetylation and H3K4 methylation. The methylation mark is catalysed by complexes that contain the mixed-lineage leukaemia (MLL) homologues. Missense mutations in *KMT2B*, *KMT2C*, and *KMT2D* have been detected in some cases (2–3%) of IDH-wildtype glioblastoma. Histone deacetylases (*HDAC2* and *HDAC9*) and a range of histone demethylases (e.g. *KDM4D*, *KDM5A/B/C*, and *KDM6A/B*) are also infrequently mutated in IDH-wildtype glioblastoma, broadly affecting chromatin activity. Both histone and DNA demethylases are inhibited by the IDH mutations, suggesting that different classes of gliomas use different modalities to inactivate key epigenetic regulators {2443}.

In addition to chromatin regulation, epigenetic gene silencing by DNA methylation of their promoters is a common mechanism of inactivating genes or noncoding RNAs with tumour suppressing functions {2010}. The *MGMT* gene is the most commonly methylated gene across tumour types {462} and encodes a DNA repair protein. It specifically removes

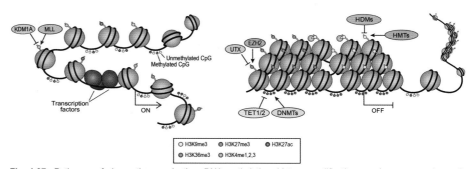

Active chromatin   **Repressive chromatin**

Fig. 1.37 Pathways of chromatin organization. DNA methylation, histone modifications, and numerous chromatin regulators determine the global structure of chromatin and are frequently altered in glioblastoma. Active chromatin (left) is globally accessible for transcriptional regulation. Repressive chromatin (right) sequesters portions of the genome, is enriched for characteristic histone modifications, and is refractory to regulatory activity. DNMTs, DNA methyltransferases; HDMs, histone demethylases; HMTs, histone methyltransferases; MLL, mixed-lineage leukaemia protein; UTX, histone demethylase UTX (also called KDM6A). Adapted from Suvà ML et al. {2462}.

promutagenic alkyl groups from the O6 position of guanine in DNA, thereby blunting the treatment effects of alkylating agents {653,798}. *MGMT* promoter methylation is common in glioblastoma (present in 40–50% of cases) {277,654, 982}, with the percentage varying depending on the assay used {2051}. It is predictive of benefit from therapy with alkylating agents such as temozolomide in patients with glioblastoma {982,1577, 2742}. A higher frequency of *MGMT* promoter methylation (> 75%) is associated with glioblastomas that have G-CIMP, which is characteristic of IDH-mutant gliomas {105,277,1830}. Distinct DNA methylation subclasses (three of which are linked with specific mutations) have been identified, which is suggestive of diverse developmental and pathogenetic/pathoepigenetic origins {277,2444}. Mutations in *IDH1* have been causally linked with G-CIMP and longer survival {1810, 2589}. Two methylation subtypes are related to hotspot mutations in H3 genes (H3 K27 and H3 G34), which are most prevalent in paediatric glioblastomas {2105,2444}. *H3F3A* G34 is associated with a CpG hypomethylator phenotype {2444}. Cancer-relevant pathways (e.g. the WNT pathway) that contribute to malignant behaviour and resistance to therapy are frequently deregulated by aberrant promoter methylation of genes encoding inhibitory factors {914,1425}.

Expression profiles
Gene expression patterns can be used to distinguish glioblastoma from

pilocytic astrocytoma {2124}, anaplastic astrocytoma {765}, and oligodendroglioma {765}; primary glioblastoma from secondary glioblastoma {2580}; and IDH-mutant glioma from IDH-wildtype glioma, across grades and histology {277,870, 1810,2444}. Unsupervised analysis of expression profiles can be used to cluster glioma into groups that correlate with histology and grade {886,1812} and may be a better predictor of patient outcome {645}. A commonly used gene expression–based classification of glioblastoma defines proneural, neural, classic, and mesenchymal subtypes, which correlate with genomic alterations including *TP53* mutation, *EGFR* mutation/amplification, and *NF1* deletion/mutation {2645}. However, individual cells characteristic of different subtypes can be found within the same glioblastoma {1906}.

Genotype–phenotype correlations
Most cases (> 90%) are glioblastomas that develop rapidly and de novo (so-called primary glioblastoma), with no known less-malignant precursor lesion, often in middle-aged or elderly patients (as opposed to the so-called secondary glioblastomas that have *IDH1* mutations; see *Glioblastoma, IDH-mutant*, p. 52). Glioblastomas in which multinucleated giant cells constitute > 5% of the tumour are associated with frequent *TP53* mutations but infrequent *EGFR* amplification {1931}, whereas small cell glioblastomas often have *EGFR* amplification {318}. In younger patients, high-grade gliomas (including glioblastomas) of the brain

Paediatric high-grade diffuse astrocytic tumours

Paediatric high-grade diffuse astrocytic tumours (WHO grade III/IV) should be considered, for therapeutic purposes, as a single category encompassing both paediatric glioblastoma and paediatric anaplastic astrocytoma. This approach is supported by our understanding of these childhood tumours' similar genetic profiles and clinical courses. Although the histopathologies of paediatric high-grade astrocytomas overlap with those of their adult counterparts, the two groups have distinct genetic alterations {2304,2444,2792}. Unlike adult glioblastomas, paediatric high-grade diffuse astrocytic tumours frequently arise in the midline of the neuraxis, commonly in the pons (as diffuse pontine glioma) or the thalamus and rarely in the spinal cord or cerebellum. These diffuse midline gliomas share genetic alterations and are discussed separately (see *Diffuse midline glioma, H3 K27M–mutant*, p. 57). Distinct from these tumours and from their adult counterparts are the cerebral hemispheric high-grade diffuse astrocytic tumours of childhood.

Clinicopathological aspects

The annual incidence of paediatric glioblastoma (defined by patient age < 20 years at diagnosis) is 0.14 cases per 100 000 population; lower than that of adult glioblastoma, which is approximately 4 per 100 000 {282,1863}. Most diffuse WHO grade II astrocytomas presenting in adults eventually progress to high-grade astrocytomas (anaplastic astrocytoma or glioblastoma). In contrast, nearly all paediatric high-grade diffuse astrocytic tumours arise de novo, rarely deriving from a WHO grade II astrocytoma.

Genetic aspects

Recurrent mutations in paediatric high-grade diffuse astrocytic tumours involve genes coding for proteins involved in chromatin and transcription regulation, or the receptor tyrosine kinase / RAS / MAPK and/or retinoblastoma protein / p53 pathways. Many of these genes are also mutated in the equivalent adult tumours, but some alterations are particularly associated with paediatric or adult disease. H3 variant (H3.1/H3.3) K27M mutations are found exclusively in diffuse midline gliomas, whereas H3.3 G34R or (rarely) G34V mutations are found exclusively in tumours of the cerebral hemispheres {2443,2792}, which are more frequently seen in teenagers and young adults. In contrast, hemispheric glioblastomas in infants harbour NTRK fusions in approximately 40% of cases, and histone mutations have not been reported. Other commonly altered genes in hemispheric high-grade astrocytomas of childhood are *TP53* (present in 30–50% of cases), *ATRX* (in ~25%), *SETD2* (in ~15%), *CDKN2A* (deletion; in ~30%), and *PDGFRA* (amplification and/or mutation; in ~30%) {2792}. In contrast, IDH mutations, *TERT* promoter mutations, and *EGFR* mutations/amplifications are rare. Several hereditary tumour syndromes predispose paediatric patients to diffuse astrocytic tumours, including Li–Fraumeni syndrome (associated with *TP53*), neurofibromatosis type 1, and constitutional mismatch repair deficiency.

Table 1.02 Frequent genetic alterations in diffuse astrocytic tumours: paediatric versus adult disease

Gene class	Paediatric
Histone protein variants	H3F3A K27M[1] H3F3A G34R/V[2] HIST1H3B K27M
Histone modification	SETD2[2]
Growth factor	ACVR1[3]
Cell signalling	BRAF V600E[2] PDGFRA mutation/ amplification
Gene class	**Adult**
Cell signalling	EGFR mutation/amplification
Telomere maintenance	TERT promoter mutation
Intermediate metabolism	IDH1 R132H
Phosphatase	PTEN mutation / biallelic deletion
Specific chromosome copy number alteration	Gain of chromosome 7 and loss of chromosome 10

[1]In tumours of midline (mutation in ~80% of diffuse intrinsic pontine gliomas), thalamus, and spinal cord.
[2]In tumours of cerebral hemispheres.
[3]In diffuse intrinsic pontine gliomas only (~20%).
[4]Both alternative lengthening of telomeres and telomerase re-expression reported.

stem and thalamus often harbour mutations in histone genes, particularly K27M mutations in H3.3 and H3.1 {1263,2444} (see *Diffuse midline glioma, H3 K27M–mutant*, p. 57). Rare glioblastomas or lower-grade astrocytic neoplasms have been reported with focal losses of SMARCB1 expression, often with monosomy 22 and epithelioid or rhabdoid cytology {1013, 1299}; these can be called SMARCB1-deficient glioblastoma. Epithelioid glioblastomas often have *BRAF* V600E mutations. Overall, glioblastomas in children have a genetic profile distinct from that of glioblastomas in adult patients; the differences between adult- and paediatric-type glioblastomas are discussed separately (see the box *Paediatric high-grade diffuse astrocytic tumours*).

Genetic susceptibility

Glioblastomas sometimes occur in more than one member of a family. This is most often the case within the setting of inherited tumour syndromes such as Turcot syndrome (in particular Turcot syndrome type 1, which is characterized by non-polyposis colorectal carcinoma), Li–Fraumeni syndrome, and neurofibromatosis type 1, as well as less common syndromes such as Ollier-type multiple enchondromatosis {734}. In rare cases, patients with L-2-hydroxyglutaric aciduria have developed malignant brain tumours, including glioblastoma {928}. Five independent genome-wide association studies have identified eight specific heritable risk variants in seven genes (*TERT, EGFR, CCDC26, CDKN2B, PHLDB1, TP53*, and *RTEL1*) associated with an increased risk of glioma {1861}.

Prognosis and predictive factors

Glioblastoma is an almost invariably fatal disease, with most patients dying within 15–18 months after diagnosis, and < 5% of patients alive after 5 years {596}. Even in clinical trials with somewhat more favourable patient selection, the 5-year survival rates do not exceed 10% {2442}. Younger age (< 50 years) and complete macroscopic tumour resection are associated with longer survival; on a molecular level, tumours associated with longer survival often exhibit two favourable molecular aberrations: *MGMT* promoter methylation {2088,2442} and/or IDH mutation {950}.

Table 1.03 IDH-wildtype glioblastoma: genetic susceptibility

Syndrome	Gene	Chromosome	OMIM
Li–Fraumeni*	TP53	17p13.1	151623
L-2-hydroxyglutaric aciduria	L2HGDH	14q21.3	236792
Turcot	MLH1, PMS2, MSH2, MSH6	3p21.3, 7p22, 2p22-p21, 2p16	276300
Neurofibromatosis type 1	NF1	7q12	162200
Ollier/Maffucci	PTHR1	3p21-22	166000

*Glioblastomas associated with Li–Fraumeni syndrome are IDH-mutant.

Age

A prospective series {2728} and numerous clinical trials {439,837,838,2442} have shown that younger patients with glioblastoma (those aged < 50 years at diagnosis) have a substantially better prognosis. In one large population-based study, patient age was a significant prognostic factor; the correlation persisted through all of the age groups in a linear manner {1823}. Because elderly patients have an inferior prognosis overall, distinct and de-escalated treatment strategies favouring a short therapeutic course and the best quality of life possible are commonly proposed to patients aged > 65–70 years. However, there is no prospectively validated age cut-off for clinical decisions. Although the frequency of MGMT promoter methylation (see Genetic alterations and biomarkers) is stable across the various age groups, recent research has identified molecular profiles associated with paediatric glioblastoma, younger patient age, and secondary glioblastoma, and these profiles may suggest novel therapeutic targets {2444,2728}.

Histopathology

In general, histopathological features do not confer significant prognostic information, but in some studies, giant cell glioblastoma (see Giant cell glioblastoma, p. 46) has been noted to have a somewhat better prognosis than ordinary glioblastoma {1356,1853}.

Greater extent of necrosis is associated with shorter survival {126,315,1031}. The presence of necrosis in a high-grade oligoastrocytic neoplasm confers a prognosis consistent with a WHO grade IV designation {1667}, but whether the presence of oligodendroglial features in a glioblastoma has prognostic value relative to other glioblastomas remains uncertain, with some studies showing a positive association {85,1667} and others having negative results {983}. It is likely that these uncertainties will be clarified by molecular-based classifications of such tumours.

Genetic alterations and biomarkers

MGMT promoter methylation is a strong predictive marker for the efficacy of and response to alkylating and methylating chemotherapy agents in glioblastoma {982,2729,2741,2742,2480}. More than 90% of long-term surviving patients with glioblastoma have a methylated MGMT promoter {2442}, versus only 35% of the general population of patients with glioblastoma {2441}. IDH1 and IDH2 mutations are positive prognostic factors and are closely associated with secondary glioblastoma {2810} (see Glioblastoma, IDH-mutant, p. 52). There is no consistent correlation between EGFR amplification and survival, regardless of patient age at clinical manifestation {1823}. Allelic loss of 10q was associated with shorter survival in one study {1823}; however, the presence of PTEN mutations is not clearly associated with prognosis {1823,2289, 2374,2728}.

Mechanisms of treatment response and resistance

Glioblastoma is highly resistant to therapy, with only modest survival increases achieved in a minority of patients, even after aggressive surgical resection, external beam radiation therapy, and maximum tolerated doses of chemotherapy with agents such as temozolomide or nitrosoureas, including in conjunction with blood stem cell transplantation or use of transgenic haematopoietic stem cells {8}. Over the past several decades, hundreds of clinical trials have achieved only limited therapeutic success; responders have been very rare and trial designs have limited the lessons learned from the failed approaches, including those of targeted therapies. The therapeutic resistance is due to a variety of factors, including: (1) uncertain drug delivery because of partial blood–brain barrier preservation and high interstitial pressure in the tumour tissue; (2) invasive properties of glioblastoma cells that enable them to spread distantly within the CNS and remain behind an intact blood–brain barrier; (3) retention of DNA repair machinery that abrogates the effectiveness of chemotherapy and radiotherapy; (4) intratumoural heterogeneity and genomic instability resulting in clonal populations of resistant cells, making it necessary to identify the driving events on an ongoing basis; (5) the presence of a population of tumour-initiating or stem cell–like cells that may harbour resistance mechanisms distinct from those of the majority of bulk tumour cells and that may contribute to cellular heterogeneity; and (6) secondary oncogenic changes induced by tumour progression.

Besides MGMT promoter methylation, there are no predictive biomarkers {2743} that facilitate the tailoring of primary {982, 2741,2742} or secondary {2480,2729} therapies, and MGMT promoter methylation is only identified in less than half of all patients using current assays {2441, 2743}. Cellular responses to DNA damage involve distinct DNA repair pathways, such as mismatch repair and base excision repair. Mismatch repair is critical for mediating the cytotoxic effect of 6-O-methylguanine. The mismatch repair pathway consists of several proteins (i.e. MLH1, PMS2, MSH2, MSH3, and MSH6) and corrects errors in DNA base pairing that occur during DNA replication. Defects in this system arise in the setting of alkylating chemotherapy and may result in resistance to such therapy {342, 2826}, potentially by causing tolerance of the mispairing of 6-O-methylguanine with thymine {2244}, but also through chemotherapy-induced mutagenesis {1167}. Temozolomide treatment of WHO grade II gliomas induces a hypermutational state and causes driver mutations in the retinoblastoma protein and AKT/mTOR pathways {2627}. In one small series, 5 of 6 hypermutated tumours showed de novo mutations in mismatch repair genes {2627}.

Molecular abnormalities in glioblastoma also provide specific mechanisms of resistance and susceptibility to therapy. Some of the signature genetic alterations in glioblastoma (e.g. mutations in PTEN, TP53, EGFR, NF1, RB1, PIK3CA, PIK3R1, and IDH1) may be related to resistance

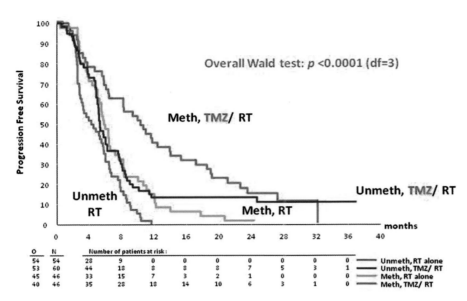

Fig. 1.38 *MGMT* promoter methylation (meth) and progression-free survival in glioblastoma patients randomized to treatment with radiotherapy (RT) alone or radiotherapy plus temozolomide (TMZ). Reprinted from Hegi ME et al. {982}.

{350,1895}. Inactivation of the p53 pathway leads to defects in apoptosis and cell cycle arrest. Mutations of the retinoblastoma protein pathway in glioblastomas result in failure of appropriate cell cycle arrest. Point mutations of the RAS genes in glioblastoma are rare, but the RAS pathway is secondarily activated through insulin-like growth factor receptor, EGFR, and PDGF receptor signalling. Downstream events such as silencing of the *NF1* tumour suppressor gene can also activate the RAS pathway, causing uncontrolled cellular proliferation. Similarly, the PI3K pathway can be activated by abnormal IGF1, epidermal growth factor, or PDGF signalling, or downstream by abnormalities in the *PTEN* gene {891, 2432}. These redundant signalling pathway abnormalities suggest that a single, specific, small-molecule signalling-pathway inhibitor could only be effective in treating glioblastoma if it targeted a downstream and driving factor. Determining such an effect may be difficult, without orthotopic patient-derived models or clinical data available to develop tightly constructed controls. For example, the assumption that testing individual glioblastoma biopsies for EGFRvIII and PTEN {1634} could potentially enable the identification of patients responsive to the EGFR kinase inhibitors is complicated by the fact that this signature characterizes a poor prognostic subgroup that currently lacks therapeutic implication {2614}. This suggests that more intensive

analyses encompassing the full genome, epigenome, and transcriptome, or even the proteome and metabolome, possibly at the single-cell level {1906}, will be necessary to identify driving changes that are accessible to targeted therapeutic approaches.

Recently, a population of glioma-initiating, potentially neural stem cell–like glioma cells has been identified in glioblastoma {122,780,2365}. These cells are highly tumorigenic in immunosuppressed mice, inducing intracranial tumours with a much smaller cellular inoculum than do non–stem cell–like glioma cells from glioblastomas. The intracranial tumours induced by these stem cell–like glioma cells have the morphological hallmarks of glioblastoma. They respond to treatment with bevacizumab (a neutralizing antibody to VEGF), and the same humanized VEGF-neutralizing antibody has achieved a 60–65% response rate in a phase II trial in recurrent glioblastomas {2671}. One of the mechanisms of radiation resistance, activation of the DNA checkpoint response, may exist preferentially in the stem cell–like glioma cell population {122}. BMP4 causes a significant reduction of stem–like precursor cells of human glioblastoma and abolishes their tumour-initiating capacities in vivo.

Given the marked vascularity of glioblastomas, antiangiogenic agents such as bevacizumab and cediranib are now widely used for the treatment of these tumours. On scans, notable responses

may be seen (in particular, decreases in enhancement and oedema). These changes reflect the effect of the agents on the tumour vasculature and may benefit patients symptomatically, but antiangiogenic agents have not clearly been shown to improve survival {141,1543}. By normalizing the tumour vasculature to some extent, antiangiogenic agents may also facilitate perfusion and oxidation of tumours.

Cellular immunotherapy / tumour vaccine approaches were initiated decades ago, but to date have had little effect on the survival of patients with glioblastoma. However, recent vaccine/immunotherapy treatment of glioblastoma may be more promising; for example, against targets such as cytomegalovirus, the poliovirus receptor, and EGFRvIII. It is also possible that combining vaccine approaches with the checkpoint inhibitors discussed below could increase efficacy. The glioblastoma microenvironment shows profound alterations compared with the normal brain microenvironment. Blood–brain barrier leakage, hypoxia, acidosis, accumulation of soluble mediators, and attraction of stromal cells from the peripheral circulation markedly alter the immunobiology of gliomas {415}. One compelling explanation is that a pool of particularly resistant and slow-proliferating cells called glioma-initiating cells, perhaps located in a perivascular or hypoxic niche, may act as a source for repopulation of the bulk tumour, thus complicating immunotherapeutic approaches. Glioma-initiating cells have been investigated with respect to their immunosuppressive potential and as a potential target for immunotherapy, given that they have antigenic properties that are different from those of bulk tumour cells {423}. Molecular mechanisms of immunosuppression involve transforming growth factor beta, STAT3, PDL1 (which is expressed by many cancer cells and binds to its receptor PD1 to suppress T-cell proliferation and IL2 production {385}), and CD276 {1469}. In addition, CTLA4, an immunoglobulin similar to the costimulatory protein CD28 that is expressed preferentially on helper T cells, transduces inhibitor signals upon engagement of the costimulatory receptors CD80 and CD86, which are expressed on antigen-presenting cells {2681}. The kynurenine pathway may also be involved in altering the immunobiology within gliomas; for

1. Cross-Resistance

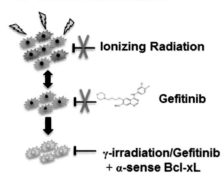

- ⊣ Ionizing Radiation
- ⊣ Gefitinib
- ⊣ γ-irradiation/Gefitinib + α-sense Bcl-xL

2. Tumor Heterogeneity

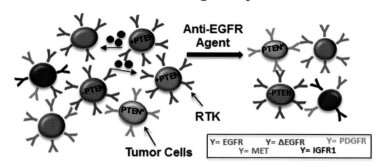

Anti-EGFR Agent

RTK

Tumor Cells

Y= EGFR	Y= ΔEGFR	Y= PDGFR
Y= MET	Y= IGFR1	

3. Cancer Stem Cell Resistance

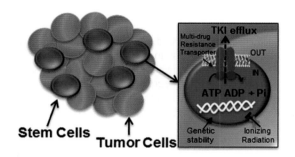

Stem Cells   Tumor Cells

TKI efflux
Multi-drug Resistance Transporter
OUT
IN
ATP ADP + Pi
Genetic stability   Ionizing Radiation

4. Tumor Microenvironment

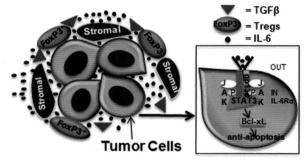

▼ = TGFβ
FoxP3 = Tregs
• = IL-6

Stromal
FoxP3
Tumor Cells

OUT
J A K   P A STAT3 K   IN IL-6Rα
Bcl-xL
anti-apoptosis

Fig. 1.39 Malignant glioma and therapeutic resistance. Glioblastomas are adept at evading inhibition of EGFR receptor function through several possible mechanisms. (**1**) Brain tumour cells that are intractable to DNA damage–induced apoptosis may also tolerate apoptotic cues driven by TKI-mediated inhibition of EGFR. Combinatorial therapy using inhibitors of anti-apoptotic activity may overcome this cross-resistance. (**2**) Intratumoural diversity within glioblastomas may drive resistance to single agent–based anti-EGFR therapy due to: RTK co-activation, *PTEN* deletion/mutations, and tumour cell–tumour cell interactions via secreted molecules. PTEN* denotes mutation. (**3**) Efflux of EGFR TKIs and increased genetic stability may lead to the maintenance of cancer stem cell populations and tumour relapse. (**4**) Enhanced immunosuppression mediated by circulating growth factors, cytokines, and suppressor T cells can antagonize the systemic immune responses generated by anti-EGFR immunotherapies. Additionally, circulating IL6 in the tumour microenvironment can facilitate resistance intracellularly via activation of the JAK/STAT3/Bcl-xL pathway. Reprinted from Taylor TE et al. {2526A}.

example, tryptophan is catabolized by key rate-limiting dioxygenases, chiefly indoleamine 2,3-dioxygenase, creating an immunosuppressive milieu due to depletion of tryptophan and accumulation of immunosuppressive tryptophan catabolites such as kynurenine {11}.

Giant cell glioblastoma

Ohgaki H.
Kleihues P.
Plate K.H.
Nakazato Y.
Bigner D.D.

Definition

A rare histological variant of IDH-wildtype glioblastoma, histologically characterized by bizarre, multinucleated giant cells and an occasionally abundant reticulin network. Despite the high degree of anaplasia, giant cell glioblastoma is often more circumscribed and has a somewhat better prognosis than ordinary glioblastoma {1356, 1853}. The genetic profile differs from that of IDH-wildtype glioblastoma in the high frequency of *TP53* mutations {1932} and in AURKB expression {2533}, whereas *EGFR* amplification is rare.

ICD-O code   9441/3

Grading

Giant cell glioblastoma corresponds histologically to WHO grade IV.

Epidemiology

Giant cell glioblastomas account for < 1% of all glioblastomas {1853}, but may be more common in paediatric populations {1356}. Giant cell glioblastoma develops in younger patients than does ordinary glioblastoma, with an age distribution covering a wider range, including children {1226, 1356,1658,1931}. In a study of 16 430 glioblastomas in the SEER database of the United States National Cancer Institute, the mean age of patients with giant cell glioblastoma (n = 171) was 51 years, significantly younger than that of patients with glioblastoma (62 years) {1356}. Similarly, in a SEER-based study of 69 935 glioblastomas, the mean age of patients with giant

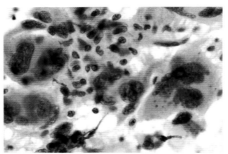

Fig. 1.41 Giant cell glioblastoma. The multinucleated giant cells are easily recognizable in the smear preparation {1956}.

cell glioblastoma (n = 592) was 54.5 years {1853}. The male-to-female ratio is 1.1–1.5:1 {1356,1533,1853}.

Localization

The localization of giant cell glioblastoma is similar to that of IDH-wildtype glioblastoma {1356,1853}.

Clinical features

Giant cell glioblastomas develop de novo after a short preoperative history and without clinical or radiological evidence of a less-malignant precursor lesion. The symptoms are similar to those of IDH-wildtype glioblastoma.

Imaging

Giant cell glioblastomas are distinctive because of their circumscription. They are

often located subcortically in the temporal and parietal lobes. On CT and MRI, they can mimic a metastasis.

Macroscopy

Due to its high connective tissue content, giant cell glioblastoma may have the gross appearance of a firm, well-circumscribed mass, which can be mistaken for a metastasis or (when attached to the dura) a meningioma. Lesions less rich in connective tissue may have features more typical of glioblastoma {1533}.

Microscopy

Giant cell glioblastoma is histologically characterized by numerous multinucleated giant cells, small fusiform syncytial cells, and a reticulin network {1584}. The giant cells are often extremely bizarre, can be as large as 0.5 mm in diameter, and can contain anywhere from a few nuclei to > 20. Giant cells are often angulated, may contain prominent nucleoli, and on occasion contain cytoplasmic inclusions. Both palisading and large ischaemic necroses are observed. Atypical mitoses are frequent, but the overall proliferation rate is similar to that of ordinary glioblastomas. A typical, (although variable) feature is the perivascular accumulation of tumour cells with the formation of a pseudorosette-like pattern {1533}. Occasionally, perivascular lymphocyte cuffing is observed. Microvascular proliferation is not common.

Immunophenotype

GFAP expression is consistently present, but the level of expression is highly variable. *TP53* mutation is present in > 80% of all cases, and these tumours typically show marked nuclear accumulation of p53

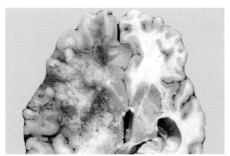

Fig. 1.40 Giant cell glioblastoma. The cut surface shows a multinodular lesion with necrosis and haemosiderin deposits.

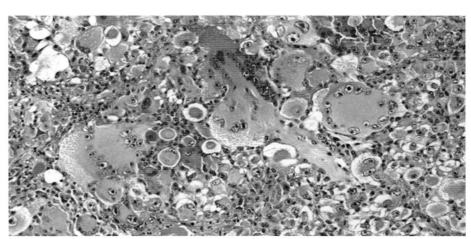

Fig. 1.42 Multinucleated cells in giant cell glioblastoma. The number of nuclei ranges from a few to > 20.

protein {1233,1931}. Neuronal markers are virtually all negative, unlike in pleomorphic xanthoastrocytoma {1597}.

Genetic profile

Giant cell glioblastomas do not carry IDH mutations and are therefore considered variants of IDH-wildtype glioblastoma. They are further characterized by frequent mutations in *TP53* (occurring in 75–90% of cases) and *PTEN* (in 33%), but typically lack *EGFR* amplification/overexpression and homozygous *CDKN2A* deletion {1596,1658,1931,1932}.

These attributes indicate that giant cell glioblastoma has a hybrid profile, sharing with IDH-wildtype glioblastoma a short clinical history, the absence of a less-malignant precursor lesion, and frequent *PTEN* mutations. Like IDH-mutant glioblastoma, which typically develops through progression from a lower-grade astrocytoma, giant cell glioblastoma has a high frequency of *TP53* mutations {1932}. The level of AURKB expression at the mRNA and protein levels is significantly higher in giant cell glioblastomas than in ordinary glioblastomas, and ectopic overexpression of aurora kinase B induces a significant increase in the proportion of multinucleated giant cells in *TP53*-mutant U373-MG (but not *TP53*-wildtype U87-MG) malignant glioma cells {2533}.

Prognosis and predictive factors

Most giant cell glioblastomas have a poor prognosis, but the clinical outcome

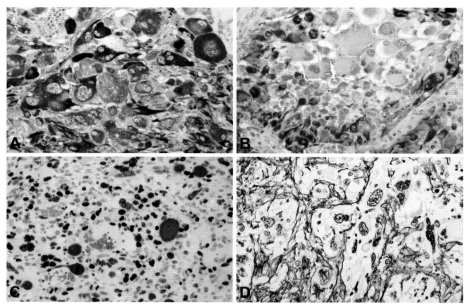

Fig. 1.43 Giant cell glioblastoma. **A** Most of the tumour cells show strong reactivity for nestin. **B** The expression of GFAP is highly variable. In this case, smaller GFAP-expressing tumour cells form a corona around GFAP-negative multinucleated giant cells. **C** High Ki-67/MIB1 proliferation index. The proliferation rate of smaller tumour cells is particularly high, whereas multinucleated giant cells are often quiescent. **D** Prominent reticulin fibre deposition.

is somewhat better than that of ordinary glioblastoma {323,1060,1356,1820,1853, 2347}. A study of 16 430 glioblastomas in the SEER database found that the median survival time of patients with giant cell glioblastoma was 11 months, significantly longer than that of patients with ordinary glioblastoma (8 months) {1356}. The overall 5-year survival rate among patients with giant cell glioblastoma was > 10%, significantly higher than that of patients

with ordinary glioblastoma (3.4%) {1356}. Similarly, a study of 67 509 glioblastomas in the USA National Cancer Data Base found that patients with giant cell glioblastoma (n = 592) had a median overall survival of 13.5 months, versus 9.8 and 8.8 months for patients with ordinary glioblastoma and gliosarcoma, respectively {1853}.

Table 1.04 Genetic profiles of histologically defined glioblastoma (GBM) variants; adapted from Oh JE et al. {1819}

	Primary GBM (IDH-wildtype)	Gliosarcoma	Giant cell GBM	Secondary GBM (IDH-mutant)
Age at GBM diagnosis	59 years	56 years	44 years	43 years
Male-to-female ratio	1.4	1.4	1.6	1.0
Length of clinical history	3.9 months	3.0 months	1.6 months	15.2 months
IDH1/2 mutation	0%	0%	5%	100%
PTEN mutation	24%	41%	33%	5%
ATRX expression loss	0%	0%	19%	100%
TERT mutation	72%	83%	25%	26%
TP53 mutation	23%	25%	84%	74%
Loss of 19q	4%	18%	42%	32%
EGFR amplification	42%	5%	6%	4%
Light blue, typical for IDH-wildtype GBMs; yellow, typical for IDH-mutant GBMs. Giant cell GBM shares characteristics with both GBM types.				

Gliosarcoma

Burger P.C.
Giangaspero F.
Ohgaki H.
Biernat W.

Definition

A variant of IDH-wildtype glioblastoma, characterized by a biphasic tissue pattern with alternating areas displaying glial and mesenchymal differentiation.

Gliosarcoma principally affects adults. The entity was originally defined as a glioblastoma in which the sarcomatous component was the consequence of malignant transformation of proliferating tumour vessels {682}, but there is cytogenetic and molecular evidence for a monoclonal origin of both the glial and mesenchymal components. Although usually associated with classic (astrocytic) glioblastoma, gliosarcomas can also arise in ependymoma (ependymosarcoma) {2153} and oligodendroglioma (oligosarcoma) {2152}. Gliosarcomas can present de novo or appear during the post-treatment phase of glioblastoma. The prognosis is poor. Occasional cases disseminate systemically and/or penetrate the skull.

ICD-O code   9442/3

Grading

Gliosarcoma corresponds histologically to WHO grade IV.

Epidemiology

Gliosarcomas account for approximately 2% of all glioblastomas {779}, although higher frequencies (as high as 8%) have also been reported {1713,2242}. The age distribution is similar to that of glioblastoma overall, with preferential manifestation in patients aged 40–60 years (mean age: 52 years). Rare cases occur in children {1228}. Males are more frequently affected, with a male-to-female ratio of 1.8:1.

Localization

Gliosarcomas are usually located in the cerebral hemispheres, involving the temporal, frontal, parietal, and occipital lobes in decreasing order of frequency. Rarely, gliosarcoma occurs in the posterior fossa {1774,1793}, lateral ventricles {2243}, or spinal cord {370}. Like standard glioblastomas, some gliosarcomas are multifocal {1881}.

Clinical features

The clinical profile of gliosarcoma is the same as that of IDH-wildtype glioblastoma, with symptoms of short duration that reflect the location of the tumour and increased intracranial pressure. Gliosarcomas can appear at the time of initial presentation of glioblastoma, but many occur during the post-treatment course of the disease {939}.

Imaging

In cases with a predominant sarcomatous component, the tumour presents as a well-demarcated hyperdense mass with homogeneous contrast enhancement, and may mimic meningioma {2166,2466}. In cases with a predominant gliomatous component, the radiological features are similar to those of glioblastomas.

Spread

Like in ordinary glioblastoma, the infiltrative growth of this variant is generally restricted to the brain parenchyma. Invasion of the subarachnoid space is uncommon. Haematogenous spread with extracranial metastases is rare, but has been reported {148}.

Macroscopy

Due to its high connective tissue content, gliosarcoma has the gross appearance of a firm, well-circumscribed mass, which can be mistaken for a metastasis or (when attached to the dura) a meningioma. Lesions less rich in connective tissue may have features more typical of glioblastoma.

Microscopy

A mixture of gliomatous and sarcomatous tissues confers to gliosarcoma a striking biphasic tissue pattern. The glial portion is astrocytic and anaplastic, mostly showing the typical features of a glioblastoma. Epithelial differentiation, manifesting as carcinomatous features {1871} with gland-like or adenoid formations and squamous metaplasia {1250, 1734}, occurs in the glial portions of some cases. By definition, the sarcomatous component shows signs of malignant transformation (e.g. nuclear atypia, mitotic activity, and necrosis) and often demonstrates the pattern of a spindle cell sarcoma, with densely packed long bundles of spindle cells surrounded individually by reticulin fibres. Occasionally, this component has considerably more pleomorphism {779,1774}. A subset of cases show additional lines of mesenchymal differentiation, such as the formation of cartilage {119}, bone {1608}, osteoid–chondroid tissue {520,973,2487}, smooth and striated muscle {1262}, and even lipomatous features {755}. Primitive

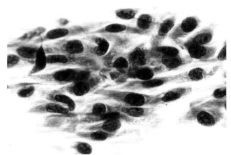

Fig. 1.44 Gliosarcoma. Spindle cells, often mitotically active, are a typical feature in smear preparations. Reprinted from Burger PC {312}.

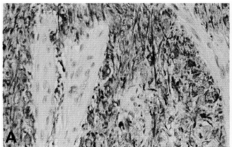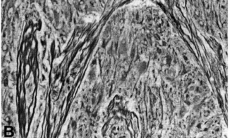

Fig. 1.45 Gliosarcoma. Biphasic pattern. Serial sections showing an alternating pattern of (**A**) GFAP-expressing glioma tissue and (**B**) sarcomatous areas that contain reticulin fibres but lack GFAP.

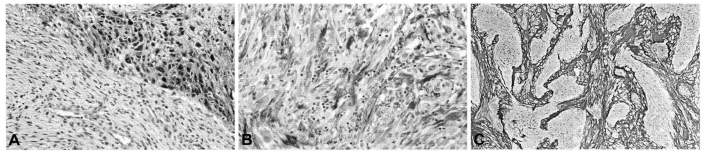

Fig. 1.46 Gliosarcoma. The gliomatous component shows strong GFAP expression and may be (**A**) geographically separated from or (**B**) intermingled with the sarcomatous tumour cells. **C** Biphasic tissue pattern denoting reticulin-rich sarcomatous and reticulin-free gliomatous elements.

neuronal components occur rarely {2349}. Distinction of the two components is facilitated by combined histochemical and immunohistochemical staining. Collagen deposition in the mesenchymal part is well demonstrated by a trichrome stain. Similarly, reticulin staining shows abundant connective tissue fibres in the mesenchymal (but not glial) component. The demonstration of a clearly malignant mesenchymal component negative for GFAP is important to distinguish true gliosarcomas from glioblastomas with florid fibroblastic proliferation (desmoplasia) elicited by meningeal invasion.

Immunophenotype
The reticulin-free glial component is positive for GFAP. The mesenchymal component is largely negative for GFAP, but isolated positive spindle cells are common. Staining for R132H-mutant IDH1 is negative in almost all cases {1183}. Immunopositivity for p53, if present, is identified in both glial and mesenchymal components {197,1038}.

Cell of origin
Originally, gliosarcoma was thought to be a collision tumour, with a separate astrocytic component and independent development of the sarcomatous portion from the proliferating vessels. Several immunohistochemical studies seemed to support this assumption, by demonstrating immunoreactivity for von Willebrand factor {2276}, UEA-I {2370}, and monohistiocytic markers {885,1312}. Another hypothesis was that the sarcomatous portion resulted from advanced glioma dedifferentiation with subsequent loss of GFAP expression and acquisition of

a sarcomatous phenotype {1179,1633}. In a study using FISH, 2 of 3 gliosarcomas showed identical numerical aberrations of chromosomes 10 and 17 in the glial and mesenchymal components, whereas in the third case, trisomy X was restricted to the chondrosarcomatous element {1913}. Similar cytogenetic patterns were observed in both glial and mesenchymal components in another study, using FISH, comparative genomic hybridization, microsatellite allelic imbalance analysis, and cytogenetic analysis {232}. These results suggested that both components were derived from neoplastic glial cells. This explanation has been further supported by the observation of p53 immunoreactivity in both tumour components {39}. Proof of a monoclonal origin has been demonstrated in 2 cases of gliosarcoma in which the gliomatous and sarcomatous components each contained an identical *TP53* mutation {197}. In addition, identical *PTEN*, *TP53*, and *TERT* mutations were detected in the gliomatous and sarcomatous tumour components of other gliosarcoma cases {2095,2679}. The monoclonality of the two components of the gliosarcomas was also confirmed by identification of *CDKN2A* deletion and *MDM2* and *CDK4* coamplification in both tumour areas {2095}. These studies strongly support the hypothesis that the sarcomatous areas are a result of a phenotypic change in the glioblastoma cells, rather than an indication of the coincidental development of two separate neoplasms.

Genetic profile
Gliosarcoma contains *PTEN* mutations, *CDKN2A* deletions, and *TP53*

mutations, but infrequent *EGFR* amplification {7,2095}, suggesting that they have a distinct profile, similar to that of IDH-wildtype glioblastoma (except for the infrequent *EGFR* amplification). Comparative genomic hybridization in 20 gliosarcomas found that several chromosomal imbalances were common: gains on chromosomes 7 (present in 75% of cases), X (20%), 9q (15%), and 20q (15%) and losses on chromosomes 10 (35%), 9p (35%), and 13q (15%) {7} [http://www.progenetix.net/progenetix/I94423]. Similar genetic alterations have been found in the gliomatous and mesenchymal components, indicating a monoclonal origin. Expression of SNAI2, TWIST, MMP2, and MMP9 is characteristic of mesenchymal tumour areas, suggesting that the mechanisms involved in epithelial–mesenchymal transition in epithelial neoplasms may also play roles in mesenchymal differentiation in gliosarcomas {1737}. Microarray-based comparative genomic hybridization analysis in glial and mesenchymal tumour areas also suggests that the mesenchymal components may be derived from glial cells with additional genetic alterations in a small proportion of gliosarcomas {1736}. See Table 1.04 on p. 47.

Prognosis and predictive factors
Large clinical trials have failed to reveal any significant differences in outcome between gliosarcoma and classic glioblastoma {779}. However, there have been multiple reports of gliosarcomas with systemic metastases and even invasion of the skull {148,1902,2302}.

Epithelioid glioblastoma

Ellison D.W.
Kleinschmidt-DeMasters B.K.
Park S.-H.

Definition

A high-grade diffuse astrocytic tumour variant with a dominant population of closely packed epithelioid cells, some rhabdoid cells, mitotic activity, microvascular proliferation, and necrosis.

Epithelioid glioblastomas occur predominantly in young adults and children, are preferentially located in the cerebrum or diencephalon, and are aggressive tumours with short survival, particularly in children. Compared with other glioblastomas, more epithelioid glioblastomas (~50%) contain a *BRAF* V600E mutation.

Epithelioid glioblastoma is distinct from gliomas or glioneuronal tumours with a poorly differentiated SMARCB1-deficient component (which may contain rhabdoid cells and exhibit a polyimmunophenotype). It is also distinct from glioblastoma with epithelial metaplasia, which exhibits glandular formations and squamous metaplasia. The term "rhabdoid glioblastoma" should be avoided. Tumours previously reported as such are either epithelioid glioblastomas without evidence of *SMARCB1* or *SMARCA4* alteration or rare glioblastomas with a population of SMARCB1-deficient cells, from which the epithelioid glioblastoma, with its different genetic profile, should be distinguished. Epithelioid glioblastoma may coexist with pleomorphic xanthoastrocytoma, but the relationship between epithelioid glioblastoma and malignant progression in pleomorphic xanthoastrocytoma requires further clarification.

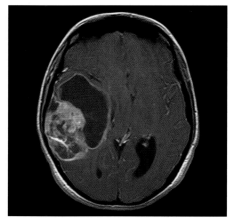

Fig. 1.47 Epithelioid glioblastoma. Complex abnormalities (including solid and cystic areas and focal enhancement) usually characterize the MRI.

ICD-O code   9440/3

Grading

Epithelioid glioblastoma corresponds histologically to WHO grade IV.

Epidemiology

Incidence data are not yet available for this uncommon variant, which has been inconsistently defined in various studies.

Etiology

The etiology and cell of origin of epithelioid glioblastoma are unknown, but most cases arise de novo. In several cases of epithelioid glioblastomas with confirmed SMARCB1 expression, a low-grade astrocytoma has been identified by biopsy as pre-existent or coexistent with the epithelioid tumour {285,1297,1735, 1795,1977}. The fact that anaplastic progression of a pleomorphic xanthoastrocytoma can manifest as an epithelioid glioblastoma raises the possibility that the two entities may be related, an association reinforced by their sharing a high frequency of *BRAF* V600E mutation {48, 2508}.

Approximately 50% of epithelioid glioblastomas harbour a *BRAF* V600E mutation, but it is unknown what genetic mechanism(s) might be responsible for the emergence of epithelioid morphology in the remainder. One microarray-based comparative genomic hybridization study of a coexistent diffuse astrocytoma and epithelioid glioblastoma identified three copy number alterations observed only in epithelioid tumour cells: a homozygous deletion in *LSAMP* and heterozygous deletions in *TENM3* and *LRP1B*. This result awaits independent validation, but suggests that *BRAF* V600E mutation alone may be permissive but not sufficient for development of epithelioid phenotype.

Localization

Epithelioid glioblastomas have been described mainly in the cerebral cortex and diencephalon. Temporal and frontal lobes are common sites, but any lobe can be affected {285,331,1297,1699}. Rare examples occur in the cerebellum, but none have been reported in the spinal cord {1302}.

Clinical features

The clinical manifestation of epithelioid glioblastoma parallels that of other glioblastomas; most patients present with symptoms and signs of raised intracranial

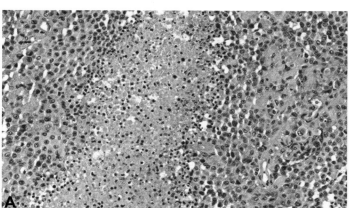
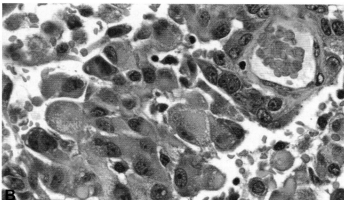

Fig. 1.48 Epithelioid glioblastoma. **A** Foci of necrosis are found in most cases. **B** Tumours may contain cells with an epithelioid, rhabdoid, or gemistocytic morphology.

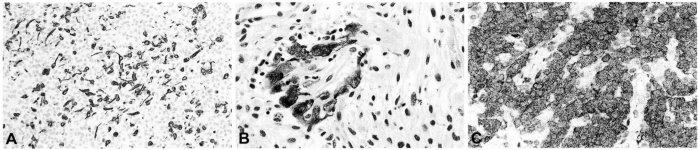

Fig. 1.49 Epithelioid glioblastoma. **A** Most tumours contain plentiful GFAP-immunopositive cells, though these may be sparse in others. **B** Focal cytokeratin expression. EMA may also be seen. **C** BRAF V600E mutations are present in about half of cases, and expression of the mutant gene product can be detected by immunohistochemistry.

pressure, although a minority of patients manifest neurological deficit or epilepsy {331,1297,1699}. Studies rarely suggest a precursor lesion, but there have been several reports of transformation from pleomorphic xanthoastrocytoma or WHO grade II astrocytoma {1297,2508}.

Imaging
On MRI, epithelioid glioblastoma characteristically presents as a gadolinium-enhancing solid mass, occasionally with cysts {285,1297,2508}. Epithelioid glioblastomas are prone to haemorrhage and often spread through the leptomeninges.

Spread
Epithelioid glioblastomas demonstrate a tendency to spread throughout the neuraxis, showing leptomeningeal dissemination in as many as one third of all patients {976,1299,1699,2755}. One reported paediatric tumour spread to the scalp via a shunt device {285}.

Macroscopy
Epithelioid glioblastomas are typically unifocal lesions, although at least one case with multifocal distribution has been reported, and metastatic disease may occur {788}. Although no feature is pathognomonic on gross examination, haemorrhage and necrosis may be prominent. A superficial location, even with dural attachment, has occasionally been noted. Leptomeningeal spread is relatively common. Cyst formation occurs, but is not a common feature.

Microscopy
Epithelioid glioblastomas are dominated by a relatively uniform population of epithelioid cells showing focal discohesion, scant intervening neuropil, a distinct cell membrane, eosinophilic cytoplasm, a paucity of cytoplasmic processes, and a laterally positioned nucleus. There is variation in how often cytoplasmic filamentous-like balls are described or sought by electron microscopy, but some rhabdoid cells are found in epithelioid glioblastoma. Less xanthomatous change is seen in epithelioid glioblastoma than in pleomorphic xanthoastrocytoma, although exceptional cases have been noted to contain giant cells {1298}, lipidization {2151}, a desmoplastic response {2151}, or cytoplasmic vacuoles {1795}. Rosenthal fibres and eosinophilic granular bodies are not features of epithelioid glioblastoma. By definition, squamous nests, glandular formation, and adenoid features are absent {2151}. Necrosis is present, but is usually of the zonal rather than palisading type. Some reports have noted a relative paucity of microvascular proliferation, but others have found no substantial difference in the vasculature patterns of epithelioid glioblastoma and classic glioblastoma {285}.

Immunophenotype
Epithelioid glioblastomas show immunoreactivity for vimentin and S100. They also show immunoreactivity for GFAP, although it is often patchy and in a few cases entirely absent from most areas of the tumour. Some epithelioid glioblastomas express epithelial markers, cytokeratins, and EMA {285,2151}. Because classic glioblastomas sometimes express cytokeratin AE1/AE3 or EMA {965,1818}, an epithelial immunophenotype should not be considered diagnostic of the epithelioid variant in isolation, without additional morphological evidence. Most authors have noted focal immunoreactivity for synaptophysin or NFP. Epithelioid glioblastomas do not express melan-A, desmin, myoglobin, or smooth muscle antigen. SMARCB1 is retained throughout the tumour cell population. In cases where it has been sought, expression of SMARCA4 has been demonstrated {285}. Immunohistochemistry using the VE1 antibody that recognizes V600E-mutant BRAF shows reactivity in about 50% of epithelioid glioblastomas, a result concordant with sequencing results {1298}.

Genetic profile
A BRAF V600E mutation is detected in about half of all epithelioid glioblastomas {285,1297}. An H3F3A K27M mutation has been reported in a single epithelioid glioblastoma, but other H3F3A and HIST1H3B mutations have not been reported {285}. Epithelioid glioblastomas also lack IDH1 and IDH2 mutations. Copy number alterations in genes involved in high-grade gliomas are occasionally present; EGFR amplification, homozygous deletion of CDKN2A, and loss of PTEN have been reported, but copy number alterations at the PDGFRA, PTEN, and MET loci are rare {285,1297}.

Genetic susceptibility
Epithelioid glioblastomas have not been reported in association with dysgenetic or hereditary tumour syndromes.

Prognosis and predictive factors
In both adult and paediatric patients, epithelioid glioblastoma has a particularly poor prognosis, even for a glioblastoma {285, 426,1299}. It demonstrates early progression and a median survival of 6.3 months (range: 0.6–82 months) in adults and 5.6 months (range: 1.5–9.7 months) in children, despite various adjuvant therapies.

Glioblastoma, IDH-mutant

Ohgaki H.
Kleihues P.
von Deimling A.
Louis D.N.

Reifenberger G.
Yan H.
Weller M.

Definition

A high-grade glioma with predominantly astrocytic differentiation; featuring nuclear atypia, cellular pleomorphism (in most cases), mitotic activity, and typically a diffuse growth pattern, as well as microvascular proliferation and/or necrosis; with a mutation in either the IDH1 or IDH2 gene.
IDH-mutant glioblastomas account for approximately 10% of all glioblastomas. Glioblastomas that develop through malignant progression from diffuse astrocytoma (WHO grade II) or anaplastic astrocytoma (WHO grade III) are almost always associated with IDH mutation and therefore carry the synonym "secondary glioblastoma, IDH-mutant". IDH-mutant glioblastoma is morphologically indistinguishable from IDH-wildtype glioblastoma, except for a lesser extent of necrosis. IDH-mutant glioblastomas manifest in younger patients (with a mean patient age at diagnosis of 45 years), are preferentially located in the frontal lobe, and carry a significantly better prognosis than IDH-wildtype glioblastomas {1797,2810}.

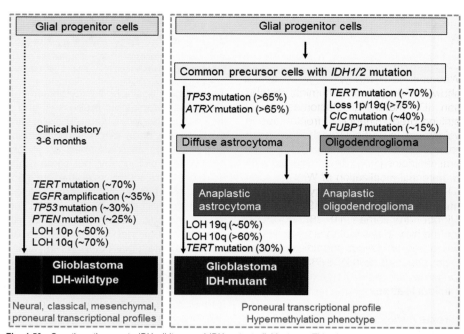

Fig. 1.50 Genetic pathways to IDH-wildtype and IDH-mutant glioblastoma. This chart is based on the hypothesis that IDH-mutant glioblastomas share common glial progenitor cells not only with diffuse and anaplastic astrocytomas, but also with oligodendrogliomas and anaplastic oligodendrogliomas. Adapted from Ohgaki H and Kleihues P {1830}.

Genetic hallmarks

The defining genetic hallmark is the presence of IDH mutations {1895}, which are associated with a hypermethylation phenotype {1810}. These mutations are the earliest detectable genetic alteration in precursor low-grade diffuse astrocytoma, indicating that these tumours are derived from common neural precursor cells that differ from those of IDH-wildtype glioblastoma. Additional typical genetic alterations are *TP53* and *ATRX* mutations and loss of chromosome arm 10q {1822,1830}.

ICD-O code   9445/3

Grading

IDH-mutant glioblastoma corresponds histologically to WHO grade IV.
The prognosis of IDH-mutant glioblastoma is considerably better than that of IDH-wildtype glioblastoma; however, WHO grading reflects the natural course of the disease rather than response to therapy. Therefore, because most patients eventually succumb to high-grade disease, IDH-mutant glioblastomas are designated as WHO grade IV.

Synonym

Secondary glioblastoma, IDH-mutant

Epidemiology

Incidence

Until the discovery of *IDH1* mutation as a molecular marker, the diagnosis of secondary glioblastomas was based on clinical observations (i.e. neuroimaging and/or histological evidence of a preceding low-grade or anaplastic astrocytoma) {1823,1827}. In a population-based study in Switzerland, using clinical criteria and histopathological evidence, only 5% of all glioblastomas diagnosed were secondary {1823,1826}. Similarly, another study showed that 19 of 392 cases (5%) of glioblastoma had a histologically proven prior low-grade glioma {605}. When *IDH1* mutations were used as a genetic marker, secondary glioblastomas accounted for 9% of all glioblastomas at the population level {1797} and for 6–13% of cases in hospital-based studies {118,1078,1417, 2810}.

Age distribution

At the population level, secondary glioblastomas develop in patients significantly younger (mean: 45 years) than do primary glioblastomas (mean: 62 years) {1823,1826}. Correspondingly, the mean age of patients with *IDH1*-mutant glioblastoma is 48 years, significantly younger than that of patients with glioblastomas that lack *IDH1* mutations (61 years) {1797}. Several hospital-based studies have also shown that patients with IDH-mutant glioblastoma were significantly younger than those with IDH-wildtype glioblastoma {214,1078,2810}.

Sex distribution

One population-based study of IDH-mutant glioblastoma found a male-to-female ratio {1830} that is significantly lower than seen in patients with IDH-wildtype glioblastoma {1823}. In a multicentre study, 49 of 618 glioblastomas (7.9%) carried an *IDH1* mutation, and the male-to-female ratio was 0.96:1, versus a ratio of 1.63:1 for IDH-wildtype glioblastomas {1417}.

Localization

Whereas IDH-wildtype glioblastomas show a widespread anatomical distribution, IDH-mutant glioblastomas have a striking predominance of frontal lobe involvement, in particular in the region surrounding the rostral extension of the lateral ventricles {1417}. This is similar to the preferential localization of WHO grade II IDH-mutant diffuse astrocytoma {2428} and IDH-mutant and 1p/19q-codeleted oligodendroglioma {1418,2871}, supporting the hypothesis that these gliomas develop from a distinct population of common precursor cells {158,1830}.

Clinical features

Clinical history

The mean length of the clinical history of patients with clinically diagnosed secondary glioblastoma was 16.8 months, significantly longer than that of patients with primary glioblastoma (6.3 months) {1823, 1826,1827}. Correspondingly, patients with secondary glioblastoma harbouring an *IDH1* mutation had a much longer mean clinical history (15.2 months) than did patients with primary IDH-wildtype glioblastomas (3.9 months) {1797}.

Symptoms

Because IDH-mutant glioblastomas are preferentially located in the frontal lobe, behavioural and neurocognitive changes are likely to predominate, although focal neurological deficits (e.g. hemiparesis and aphasia) also frequently occur. Due to the slow evolution from diffuse astrocytoma or anaplastic astrocytoma, tumour-associated oedema is less extensive and symptoms of intracranial pressure may develop less rapidly than in patients with primary IDH-wildtype glioblastoma.

Imaging

Unlike in IDH-wildtype glioblastoma, large areas of central necrosis are usually absent. Compared with IDH-wildtype glioblastoma, IDH-mutant glioblastoma presents more frequently with non-enhancing tumour components on MRI, with larger size at diagnosis, with lesser extent of oedema, and with increased prevalence of cystic and diffuse components {644,1417}.

Macroscopy

Like all glioblastomas, IDH-mutant glioblastomas diffusely infiltrate the brain parenchyma, without clear macroscopic delineation. However, large yellowish areas of central necrosis or haemorrhage, which are hallmarks of IDH-wildtype glioblastoma, are usually absent.

Microscopy

The histological features of IDH-mutant glioblastomas are similar to those of IDH-wildtype glioblastomas. However, morphological studies have revealed two significant differences. Areas of ischaemic and/or palisading necrosis have been observed in 50% of IDH-mutant glioblastomas, significantly less frequently than in IDH-wildtype glioblastomas (90%) {1797}, whereas focal

Table 1.05 Key characteristics of IDH-wildtype and IDH-mutant glioblastoma in adults

	IDH-wildtype glioblastoma	IDH-mutant glioblastoma	References
Synonym	Primary glioblastoma, IDH-wildtype	Secondary glioblastoma, IDH-mutant	{1830}
Precursor lesion	Not identifiable; develops de novo	Diffuse astrocytoma Anaplastic astrocytoma	{1827}
Proportion of glioblastomas	~90%	~10%	{1797}
Median age at diagnosis	~62 years	~44 years	{214,1078,1797, 2103}
Male-to-female ratio	1.42:1	1.05:1	{214,1417,1797}
Mean length of clinical history	4 months	15 months	{1797}
Median overall survival			
Surgery + radiotherapy	9.9 months	24 months	{1797}
Surgery + radiotherapy + chemotherapy	15 months	31 months	{2810}
Location	Supratentorial	Preferentially frontal	{1417}
Necrosis	Extensive	Limited	{1417}
TERT promoter mutations	72%	26%	{1801,1830}
TP53 mutations	27%	81%	{1797}
ATRX mutations	Exceptional	71%	{1519}
EGFR amplification	35%	Exceptional	{1797}
PTEN mutations	24%	Exceptional	{1797}

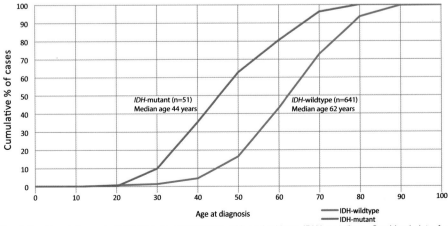

Fig. 1.51 Cumulative age distribution of glioblastomas with and without *IDH1* mutations. Combined data from Nobusawa S et al. {1797} and Cancer Genome Atlas Research Network {350}.

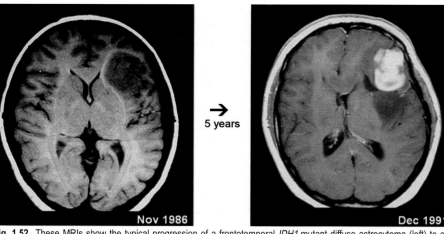

Fig. 1.52 These MRIs show the typical progression of a frontotemporal *IDH1*-mutant diffuse astrocytoma (left) to an *IDH1*-mutant secondary glioblastoma (right) over a period of 5 years {1533}. Note the absence of central necrosis.

oligodendroglioma-like components are more common in IDH-mutant glioblastomas than in IDH-wildtype glioblastomas (54% vs 20%) {1797}. A larger proportion of tumour cells with oligodendroglial morphology has also been reported in *IDH1*-mutant glioblastomas, in a large study of 618 cases {1417}.

Immunophenotype

The presence of *IDH1* R132H (the most frequent *IDH1* mutation in oligodendrogliomas, astrocytomas, and IDH-mutant glioblastomas) can be detected immunohistochemically using an antibody to the gene product, R132H-mutant IDH1 {357}. Positivity in a glioblastoma is indicative of an IDH-mutant glioblastoma, but negativity could be due to the presence of one of the less common types of *IDH1* mutation or an *IDH2* mutation {953}. Lack of immunoreactivity could also indicate the presence of a primary IDH-wildtype glioblastoma.

Mutations in the *ATRX* gene are typically present with *IDH1/2* mutations and *TP53* mutations in WHO grade II or III diffuse astrocytomas and IDH-mutant glioblastomas {1160}. Mutations in *ATRX* result in lack of expression, which can be demonstrated immunohistochemically {2750}. Immunohistochemical overexpression of p53 is frequent, reflecting the high frequency of *TP53* mutations (present in the vast majority of cases). Overexpression of EGFR is unusual; *EGFR* amplification is a hallmark of IDH-wildtype glioblastoma. GFAP expression is consistently present, although the level of expression is variable.

Cell of origin

Despite their similar histological features, IDH-mutant glioblastomas and IDH-wildtype glioblastomas seem to be derived from different precursor cells. Secondary glioblastomas, astrocytomas, and oligodendrogliomas contain IDH mutations, share a preferential frontal location, and have been hypothesized to originate from precursor cells located in (or migrating to) the frontal lobe. In contrast, IDH-wildtype glioblastomas have more widespread locations. Additional evidence supporting this hypothesis includes the observation that glioblastomas that are IDH-mutant and those that are IDH-wildtype develop in patients of different ages, have a different sex distribution, and have a significantly different clinical outcome {1830}. Their stem cells may also be different; in one study, the relative content of CD133-positive cells was significantly higher in primary glioblastomas than in secondary glioblastomas, and CD133 expression was associated with neurosphere formation only in primary glioblastomas {158}.

Genetic profile

IDH mutations

IDH mutations were first reported in 2008 {1895}, and the authors noted that "mutations in *IDH1* occurred in a large proportion of young patients and in most patients with secondary glioblastomas and were associated with an increase in overall survival". In one study, the presence of *IDH1* mutations as a genetic marker of secondary but not primary glioblastoma corresponded to the respective clinical

diagnosis in 385 of 407 cases (95%) {1797}. In this regard, IDH mutations are considered to be a defining diagnostic molecular marker of glioblastomas derived from IDH-mutant diffuse astrocytoma or IDH-mutant anaplastic astrocytoma that is more objective than clinical and/or histopathological criteria.

Timing of IDH mutation

IDH mutations are an early event in gliomagenesis and persist during progression to IDH-mutant glioblastoma. Analysis of multiple biopsies from the same patients revealed no cases in which the *IDH1* mutation occurred after the acquisition of a *TP53* mutation {2709}. An exception is *IDH1* mutations in patients with Li–Fraumeni syndrome, caused by a germline *TP53* mutation. In this inherited tumour syndrome, the *TP53* mutation is by definition the initial genetic alteration and significantly affects the subsequent acquisition of the *IDH1* mutation. The R132C (CGT→TGT) mutation, which is uncommon in sporadic cases, was the only *IDH1* mutation found in diffuse astrocytomas, anaplastic astrocytomas, and secondary glioblastomas carrying a *TP53* germline mutation {2710}.

Types of IDH mutation

All reported *IDH1* mutations are located at the first or second base of codon 132 {118,1895,2709}. The most frequent is the R132H (CGT→CAT) mutation, found in 83–91% of astrocytic and oligodendroglial gliomas {118,2709,2810}. Other mutations are rare, including R132C (CGT→TGT; found in 3.6–4.6% of cases), R132G (in 0.6–3.8%), R132S (in 0.8–2.5%), and R132L (in 0.5–4.4%) {118, 2709,2810}.

The *IDH2* gene encodes the only human protein homologous to IDH1 that uses

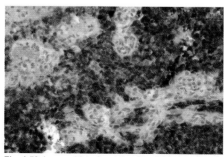

Fig. 1.53 Immunohistochemistry of a glioblastoma using an antibody to R132H-mutant IDH1. Note the strong cytoplasmic expression by tumour cells and the lack of expression in the vasculature.

NADP+ as an electron acceptor. *IDH2* mutations are all located at residue R172, which is the analogue of the R132 residue in *IDH1* {2805}. It is located in the active site of the enzyme and forms hydrogen bonds with the isocitrate substrate. *IDH2* mutations are rare in IDH-mutant glioblastoma and located at codon 172 {2810}, with the R172K mutation being the most frequent.

Secondary glioblastomas without IDH mutation
The few clinically diagnosed secondary glioblastomas that lack an IDH mutation have infrequent *TP53* mutations, and patients have a shorter clinical history and a poor prognosis {1797}. Most secondary glioblastomas lacking *IDH1* mutations develop through progression from a WHO grade III anaplastic astrocytoma, whereas the majority of secondary *IDH1*-mutant glioblastomas progress from a WHO grade II diffuse astrocytoma {1797}. Therefore, some tumours diagnosed as anaplastic astrocytoma may actually have been primary glioblastomas misdiagnosed due to a sampling error.

Primary glioblastomas with IDH mutation
In a population-based study, only 14 of 407 glioblastomas (3.4%) clinically diagnosed as primary carried an *IDH1* mutation. The patients were approximately 10 years younger than patients with secondary glioblastomas, but the genetic profiles of the two tumour groups were similar, including frequent *TP53* mutations and absence of *EGFR* amplification {1797}. Similarly, several hospital-based studies found that 3–6% of patients with *IDH1*-mutant glioblastomas clinically diagnosed as primary were 13–27 years younger than those with glioblastomas without *IDH1* mutations {118,1829, 2561,2810}. The possibility exists that these glioblastomas have rapidly progressed from precursor astrocytomas that escaped clinical diagnosis and were therefore misclassified as primary glioblastomas.

ATRX mutations
Mutations in the *ATRX* gene cause loss of expression. They are typically present with IDH and *TP53* mutations in WHO grade II IDH-mutant diffuse astrocytoma, WHO grade III IDH-mutant anaplastic astrocytoma, and IDH-mutant glioblastomas {1160,1519}.

Other genetic alterations
Genetic profiling of primary and secondary glioblastomas has shown that the frequency of *TP53* mutations is significantly higher in secondary glioblastomas (67%) than in primary glioblastomas (11%) {2705}. *EGFR* overexpression prevails in glioblastomas that are IDH-wildtype but is rare in secondary glioblastomas {2705}. In one study, only 1 of 49 glioblastomas showed both *TP53* mutation and *EGFR* overexpression, suggesting that these alterations are mutually exclusive events that could define two different genetic pathways in the evolution of glioblastoma {2705}. Subsequent studies provided evidence that primary and secondary glioblastomas develop through distinct genetic pathways.

Genetic alterations typical of IDH-wildtype glioblastoma include *EGFR* amplification, *PTEN* mutation, *TERT* promoter mutation, and complete loss of chromosome 10 {89,752,1801,1823, 1827}. Alterations more common in secondary IDH-mutant glioblastomas include *TP53* mutations and 19q loss {1754,1823,1827}. However, until the identification of IDH mutation as a molecular marker of secondary glioblastoma {118, 1797,2709,2810}, the patterns of genetic alterations, although different, did not enable unequivocal diagnosis of these two glioblastoma subtypes.

Expression profile
More than 90% of IDH-mutant glioblastomas have a proneural expression signature, and approximately 30% of glioblastomas with a proneural signature are IDH-mutant {2645}. These findings suggest that IDH-mutant glioblastomas are a relatively homogeneous group of gliomas, characterized by a proneural expression pattern. IDH-mutant diffuse astrocytoma and IDH-mutant and 1p/19q-codeleted oligodendroglioma also have the typical proneural signature {496}, further supporting the assumption that these neoplasms share common neural progenitor cells. In contrast, IDH-wildtype glioblastomas are heterogeneous, with several distinct expression profiles.

Hypermethylation phenotype
IDH-mutant glioblastomas show concerted CpG island methylation at many loci {1810}. A similar hypermethylation phenotype has been observed in IDH-mutant diffuse astrocytomas {454}

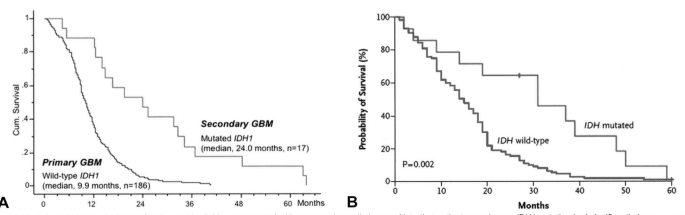

Fig. 1.54 A Cumulative survival rate of patients with glioblastoma treated with surgery plus radiotherapy. Note that patients carrying an *IDH1* mutation had significantly longer overall survival survival. Reprinted from Nobusawa S et al. {1797}. **B** In a more recent study, the median survival was 31 months for 14 patients with mutated *IDH1* or *IDH2*, versus 15 months for 115 patients with wildtype *IDH1* or *IDH2*. For patients with IDH-mutant glioblastomas, survival was calculated from the date of the secondary diagnosis. Reprinted from Yan H et al. {2810}.

and oligodendrogliomas {454}, as well as in IDH-mutant acute myeloid leukaemia {706}. The introduction of mutant IDH1 into primary human astrocytes alters specific histone markers and induces extensive DNA hypermethylation, suggesting that the presence of an *IDH1* mutation is sufficient to establish a hypermethylation phenotype {2589}. Moreover, IDH mutations disrupt chromosomal topology and thus allow aberrant chromosomal regulatory interactions that induce oncogene expression, including glioma oncogenes such as *PDGFRA* {713A}.

Genetic susceptibility
Astrocytic gliomas, including diffuse astrocytomas, anaplastic astrocytomas, and secondary glioblastomas, are the most frequent brain tumours associated with *TP53* germline mutations in families with Li–Fraumeni syndrome {1294, 1841}. In patients from three families with Li–Fraumeni syndrome, *IDH1* mutations were observed in 5 astrocytic gliomas that developed in carriers of a *TP53* germline mutation. All 5 contained the R132C (CGT→TGT) mutation {2710}, which in sporadic astrocytic tumours accounts for < 5% of all *IDH1* mutations overall {118,2709,2810}. This remarkably selective occurrence suggests a preference for R132C mutations in neural precursor cells that already carry a germline *TP53* mutation.

Prognosis and predictive factors
In his pioneering work on glioblastomas, H-J Scherer {2265} wrote, in 1940: "From a biological and clinical point of view, the secondary glioblastomas developing in astrocytomas must be distinguished from 'primary' glioblastomas. They are probably responsible for most of the 'glioblastomas of long clinical duration' mentioned in the literature." This early observation has been repeatedly confirmed. In a 1980–1994 population-based study, the median overall survival of patients with clinically diagnosed secondary glioblastoma was 7.8 months, significantly longer than that of patients with primary glioblastoma (4.7 months) {1823}. Similarly, the analysis of patients who were treated with surgery and radiotherapy showed that the mean overall survival of patients with IDH-mutant glioblastomas was 27.1 months, 2.4 times as long as that of patients with IDH-wildtype glioblastoma (11.3 months) {1797}. In another study, patients with IDH-mutant glioblastomas treated with radiotherapy/chemotherapy had an overall survival time of 31 months, twice as long as that of patients with IDH-wildtype glioblastoma {2810}.

....

Glioblastoma, NOS

Definition
A high-grade glioma with predominantly astrocytic differentiation; featuring nuclear atypia, cellular pleomorphism (in most cases), mitotic activity, and typically a diffuse growth pattern, as well as microvascular proliferation and/or necrosis; in which IDH mutation status has not been fully assessed.

Determination of IDH mutation status is important for all glioblastomas; however, if full testing is not possible (see *Genetic parameters* in *Glioblastoma, IDH-wildtype*, p. 28), the diagnosis of glioblastoma, NOS, can be made, provided that the histological variants giant cell glioblastoma, gliosarcoma, and epithelioid glioblastoma can be ruled out.

ICD-O code   9440/3

Grading
Glioblastoma, NOS, and its variants (e.g. giant cell glioblastoma that cannot be tested for IDH mutation status) correspond histologically to WHO grade IV.

Diffuse midline glioma, H3 K27M–mutant

Hawkins C.
Ellison D.W.
Sturm D.

Definition

An infiltrative midline high-grade glioma with predominantly astrocytic differentiation and a K27M mutation in either H3F3A or HIST1H3B/C.

H3 K27M–mutant diffuse midline glioma predominates in children but can also be seen in adults, with the most common locations being brain stem, thalamus, and spinal cord. Brain stem and pontine examples were previously known as brain stem glioma and diffuse intrinsic pontine glioma (DIPG), respectively. Mitotic activity is present in most cases, but is not necessary for diagnosis; microvascular proliferation and necrosis may be seen. Tumour cells diffusely infiltrate adjacent and distant brain structures. The prognosis is poor, despite current therapies, with a 2-year survival rate of < 10%.

ICD-O code   9385/3

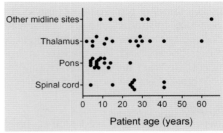

Fig. 1.56 Location of diffuse midline gliomas, H3 K27M–mutant. Pontine gliomas manifest primarily in children, whereas spinal cord lesions predominantly affect adults. Reprinted from Solomon DA et al. {2392A}.

Grading

H3 K27M–mutant diffuse midline glioma corresponds to WHO grade IV.

Epidemiology

Incidence data on diffuse gliomas specifically arising in midline structures are not available, because large brain tumour registries have not yet included these as a distinct category. The median patient age at diagnosis of diffuse midline glioma is 5–11 years, with pontine tumours arising earlier on average (at ~7 years) than their thalamic counterparts (at ~11 years). There is no clear sex predilection {1229, 1358,1863,2700,2776}.

Localization

Diffuse midline gliomas typically arise in the pons, thalamus, or spinal cord, with occasional examples involving the cerebellum.

Clinical features

Most patients with DIPG present with brain stem dysfunction or cerebrospinal fluid obstruction, typically developing over a short period of time (1–2 months). Classic clinical symptoms include the triad of multiple cranial neuropathies, long tract signs, and ataxia {2700}. With thalamic gliomas, common initial symptoms include signs of increased intracranial pressure, motor weakness/hemiparesis, and gait disturbance {1358}.

Imaging

On MRI, diffuse midline gliomas are

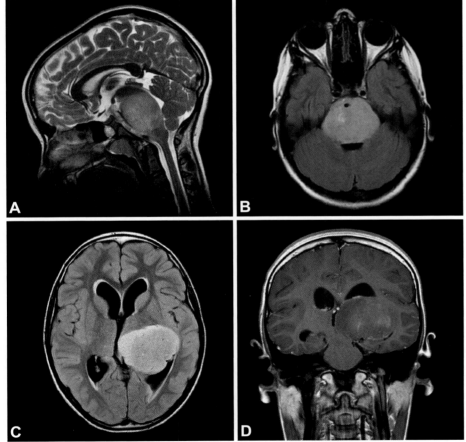

Fig. 1.55 H3 K27M–mutant diffuse midline glioma. **A** Sagittal T2-weighted MRI showing a diffusely infiltrating pontine glioma expanding the pons with crowding of the neural structures at the craniocervical junction and tonsillar herniation to the level of the C1 posterior arch. **B** Axial FLAIR MRI demonstrates a diffusely infiltrating pontine glioma expanding the pons and encasing the basilar artery. **C** Axial FLAIR MRI shows an expansile left thalamic glioma and associated obstructive hydrocephalus, with mild to moderate dilatation of the lateral ventricles, periventricular oedema, and distortion of the third ventricle. **D** Expansile thalamic glioma showing heterogeneous enhancement on the post-gadolinium coronal T1 sequence.

usually T1-hypointense and T2-hyperintense. Contrast enhancement, necrosis, and/or haemorrhage may be present. DIPG typically presents as a large, expansile, and often asymmetrical brain stem mass occupying more than two thirds of the pons {2700}. There may be an exophytic component encasing the basilar artery or protruding into the fourth ventricle. Infiltration into the cerebellar peduncles, the cerebellar hemispheres, the midbrain, and the medulla is frequent. Contrast enhancement rarely involves > 25% of the tumour volume {135}.

Spread

Two large autopsy-based studies have found that leptomeningeal dissemination of DIPG occurs in about 40% of cases {304,2831}. Diffuse tumour invasion of the brain stem is common among DIPGs, with 25% spreading to involve the upper cervical cord and thalamus as well {304, 362,2831}. Some patients exhibit distal spread as far as the frontal or (rarely) the occipital lobes, creating some phenotypic overlap with gliomatosis cerebri. No large series of diffuse midline gliomas centred in the thalamus has been reported, but some cases of gliomatosis cerebri have been reported to show an *H3F3A* K27M mutation, suggesting that the thalamic version has a similar tendency for diffuse invasion.

Macroscopy

Diffuse infiltration of CNS parenchyma by tumour cells produces distortion and enlargement of anatomical structures. Symmetrical or asymmetrical fusiform enlargement of the pons is typical in cases of diffuse pontine glioma. Tumours with

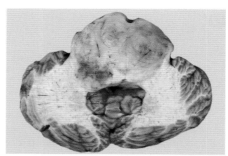

Fig. 1.57 Axial section of H3 K27M–mutant diffuse midline glioma showing expansion of the pons with areas of haemorrhage and yellowish discolouration suggesting necrosis.

areas of necrosis or haemorrhage show focal discolouration and softening.

Microscopy

Diffuse midline gliomas infiltrate grey and white matter structures. The tumour cells are generally small and monomorphic, but can be large and pleomorphic. They typically have an astrocytic morphology, although oligodendroglial morphology is also a recognized pattern. About 10% of DIPGs lack mitotic figures, microvascular proliferation, and necrosis, and thus are histologically consistent with WHO grade II. The remaining cases are high-grade, with 25% containing mitotic figures and the remainder containing mitotic figures as well as foci of necrosis and microvascular proliferation. However, for DIPG, grade does not predict the outcome in genetically classic cases (see *Prognosis and predictive factors*).

Immunophenotype

Virtually all tumour cells express NCAM1, S100, and OLIG2, but immunoreactivity for GFAP is variable in these neoplasms. MAP2 expression is common, and

synaptophysin immunoreactivity can be focal, but chromogranin-A and NeuN are not typically expressed. An *H3F3A* K27M mutation can be detected by immunohistochemistry using a mutation-specific antibody. Nuclear p53 immunopositivity may be present, suggesting an underlying *TP53* mutation, which is present in about 50% of cases. In about 10–15% of cases, an *ATRX* mutation leads to loss of nuclear ATRX expression.

Cell of origin

The common (epi)genetic features of diffuse gliomas arising in midline locations, especially the pons and the thalamus, suggest a distinct developmental origin {1175,2443}. Examination of the spatiotemporal distribution of neural precursor cells in the human brain stem indicated a nestin- and OLIG2-expressing neural precursor–like cell population in the ventral pons, which has been proposed as the possible cell of origin of diffuse pontine gliomas {1701}. However, the exact cell or cells of origin of diffuse midline gliomas remain unknown.

Genetic profile

Mutation spectrum

Sequencing studies have identified recurrent heterozygous mutations at position K27 in the histone coding genes *H3F3A*, *HIST1H3B*, and *HIST1H3C* in high-grade gliomas from the pons (in ~80% of cases), thalamus (in ~50%), and spinal cord (in ~60%) {305,721, 2304,2521,2791,2792}. Within the brain, these mutations occur exclusively in diffuse midline gliomas. K27M mutations affecting H3.3 (encoded by *H3F3A*) are about three times as prevalent as the

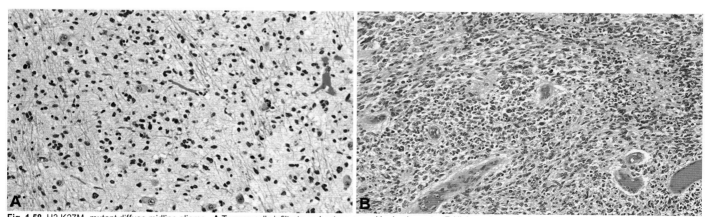

Fig. 1.58 H3 K27M–mutant diffuse midline glioma. **A** Tumour cells infiltrate and entrap normal brain elements. **B** High-grade morphological features with focal necrosis.

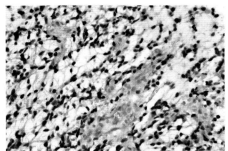

Fig. 1.59 Strong nuclear staining for K27M-mutant H3 is present in tumour cells but not in the vasculature.

same mutation in histone variant H3.1 (occurring in *HIST1H3B* or *HIST1H3C*). The K27M substitution (lysine replaced by methionine at amino acid 27) results in a decrease in H3K27me3, thought to be due to inhibition of PRC2 activity {1480}.

In addition to the specific mutations in histone variants H3.3 and H3.1, chromatin regulation is further targeted by additional non-recurrent mutations in a diverse range of chromatin readers and writers, such as members of the mixed-lineage leukaemia (MLL), lysine-specific demethylase, and chromodomain helicase DNA-binding protein families {2792}.

Other mutations in canonical cancer pathways frequently target the receptor tyrosine kinase / RAS / PI3K pathway (e.g. mutations in *PDGFRA*, *PIK3CA*, *PIK3R1*, or *PTEN*; occurring in ~50% of cases), the p53 pathway (e.g. mutations in *TP53*, *PPM1D*, *CHEK2*, or *ATM*; occurring in ~70% of cases), and to a lesser extent the retinoblastoma protein pathway {305,2521,2792}. Activating mutations or fusions targeting *FGFR1* were specifically identified in a small proportion of thalamic high-grade gliomas (10%) {721}. In contrast, recurrent mutations in *ACVR1*, the gene encoding the BMP receptor ACVR1, were detected in a subset (~20%) of DIPGs, and seem to correlate with H3.1 mutations {305,2521, 2792}.

Structural variations

High-level focal amplifications detected in diffuse midline gliomas include amplification of *PDGFRA* (in as many as 50% of DIPGs), *MYC/MYCN* (in as many as 35%), *CDK4/6* or *CCND1–3* (in 20%), *ID2* (in 10%), and *MET* (in 7%), whereas homozygous deletion of *CDKN2A/B* or loss of *RB1* or *NF1* is detected only very rarely (in < 5% of cases). Fusion events involving the tyrosine kinase receptor gene *FGFR1* occur in thalamic diffuse gliomas, and a small proportion (4%) of pontine gliomas have been found to carry neurotrophin receptor (NTRK) fusion genes. Common broad chromosomal alterations include single copy gains of chromosome 1q and chromosome 2. In addition, there may be a subset of pontine gliomas (as many as 20%) that harbour few copy number changes {251,305,2792}.

Table 1.06 Additional mutations in H3 K27M–mutant diffuse midline glioma

TP53 mutation	50%
PDGFRA amplification	30%
CDK4/6 or *CCND1–3* amplification	20%
ACVR1 mutation	20%
PPM1D mutation	15%
MYC/PVT1 amplification	15%
ATRX mutation	15%
CDKN2A/B homozygous deletion	< 5%

Genetic susceptibility

Rarely, patients with Li–Fraumeni syndrome or neurofibromatosis type 1 present with midline infiltrating gliomas, but there is no known specific genetic susceptibility for these tumours.

Prognosis and predictive factors

For diffuse midline gliomas in general, the finding of an H3 K27M mutation confers a worse prognosis than that of wildtype cases {304,1263}. In diffuse midline gliomas arising in the thalamus, high-grade histology is associated with short overall survival regardless of histone gene status. This does not seem to be the case for tumours with classic clinical and radiological features arising in the pons, but < 10% of these patients survive beyond 2 years.

Oligodendroglioma, IDH-mutant and 1p/19q-codeleted

Reifenberger G.
Collins V.P.
Hartmann C.
Hawkins C.
Kros J.M.

Cairncross J.G.
Yokoo H.
Yip S.
Louis D.N.

Definition

A diffusely infiltrating, slow-growing glioma with IDH1 *or* IDH2 *mutation and codeletion of chromosomal arms 1p and 19q.*

Histologically, IDH-mutant and 1p/19q-codeleted oligodendroglioma is composed of tumour cells morphologically resembling oligodendrocytes, with isomorphic rounded nuclei and an artefactually swollen clear cytoplasm on routinely processed paraffin sections. Microcalcifications and a delicate branching capillary network are typical. The presence of an astrocytic tumour component is compatible with the diagnosis when molecular testing reveals the entity-defining combination of IDH mutation and 1p/19q codeletion. The vast majority of IDH-mutant and 1p/19q-codeleted oligodendrogliomas occur in adult patients, with preferential location in the cerebral hemispheres (most frequently in the frontal lobe).

ICD-O code   9450/3

Grading

IDH-mutant and 1p/19q-codeleted oligodendroglioma corresponds histologically to WHO grade II.

Oligodendroglial tumours constitute a continuous spectrum ranging from well-differentiated, slow-growing neoplasms to frankly malignant tumours with rapid growth. The WHO grading system traditionally distinguished two malignancy grades for oligodendroglioma: grade II for well-differentiated tumours and grade III for anaplastic tumours. Several studies have reported WHO grading as an independent predictor of survival for patients with oligodendroglial tumours {686, 830,1446,1826}. However, these studies did not consider IDH mutation status, which is prognostically relevant. A more recent study confirmed WHO grade II as a favourable prognostic factor independent of 1p/19q codeletion in 95 patients with oligodendroglial tumours {2256}. Other authors have reported significantly

Genetic classification of oligodendroglial tumours

In contrast to the 2007 WHO classification, the current WHO classification of oligodendrogliomas requires demonstration of *IDH1* or *IDH2* mutation, typically by immunohistochemistry using the mutation-specific antibody against R132H-mutant IDH1 (followed by DNA genotyping when R132H-mutant IDH1 immunostaining is negative), as well as demonstration of 1p/19q codeletion by FISH, chromogenic in situ hybridization, or molecular genetic testing. The WHO classification does not mandate the use of a particular method for molecular testing of these markers, but recommends that 1p/19q assays be able to detect whole-arm chromosomal losses. Pathologists should have experience with their method of choice and be aware of potential methodological and interpretational pitfalls.

On the rare occasion that the entity-defining molecular markers (i.e. IDH mutation and 1p/19q codeletion) cannot be fully determined and classic histological oligodendroglioma features are present, classification of the tumour as oligodendroglioma, NOS, is recommended (see *Oligodendroglioma, NOS*, p. 69). This diagnosis indicates that the tumour is a histologically classic oligodendroglioma, which will likely exhibit a clinical behaviour similar to that of an IDH-mutant and 1p/19q-codeleted oligodendroglioma, but that could not be

analysed with comprehensive molecular testing or in which the test results were inconclusive or uninformative.

Rare tumours demonstrate classic oligodendroglial histology but lack IDH mutation and 1p/19q codeletion on molecular testing, a situation most frequently encountered in paediatric oligodendrogliomas. Such tumours should not be classified as oligodendroglioma, NOS, and must be further evaluated to exclude histological mimics, such as dysembryoplastic neuroepithelial tumour, clear cell ependymoma, neurocytoma, and pilocytic astrocytoma. Once histological mimics are excluded, such tumours can be tentatively classified as oligodendroglioma lacking IDH mutation and 1p/19q codeletion (paediatric-type oligodendroglioma). In children, most of these tumours seem to belong to a group of paediatric low-grade diffuse gliomas that are genetically characterized by *FGFR1, MYB,* or *MYBL1* alterations (see *Oligodendroglioma lacking IDH mutation and 1p/19q codeletion*, p. 68).

Tumours demonstrating evidence of 1p/19q codeletion but lacking detectable *IDH1* or *IDH2* mutations should be further evaluated to exclude the possibility of incomplete deletions on 1p and/or 19q. Such alterations may be present in subsets of IDH-wildtype (mostly high-grade) gliomas, including glioblastomas, and have been associated with poor outcome.

longer survival of patients with WHO grade II versus grade III oligodendroglial tumours with concurrent IDH mutation and *TERT* promoter mutation (with a median survival of 205.5 months with grade II tumours versus 127.3 months with grade III) {1268}. In contrast, a retrospective analysis of 212 patients with IDH-mutant and 1p/19q-codeleted oligodendroglial tumours did not find WHO grade to be a significant predictor of overall survival {1836}. Similarly, recent

data from a large combined Japanese and The Cancer Genome Atlas (TCGA) cohort suggest a limited prognostic role of histological grading in patients with WHO grade II and III oligodendroglial tumours {2464}. However, interpretation of these retrospective data requires caution, because of the potential bias due to lack of inclusion of prognostically relevant clinical information (e.g. extent of resection) and variable postoperative treatment of the patients. The current

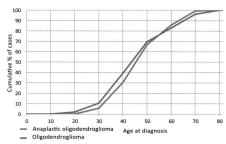

Fig. 1.60 Cumulative age distribution (both sexes) of 105 cases of IDH-mutant and 1p/19q-codeleted oligodendroglioma (mean patient age at diagnosis: 44.3 years) and 126 cases of IDH-mutant and 1p/19q-codeleted anaplastic oligodendroglioma (mean age: 45.7 years). Combined data from the German Glioma Network and the University of Heidelberg.

WHO classification adheres to the prior two-tiered histological grading of oligodendroglial tumours, with well-differentiated tumours assigned a WHO grade of II and anaplastic tumours a WHO grade of III. Future studies should investigate whether the traditional histological grading criteria should be modified and/ or complemented by molecular marker assessments, such as *CDKN2A* deletion or *TCF12* mutation, which has been linked to clinically aggressive behaviour in IDH-mutant and 1p/19q-codeleted oligodendroglioma {1407}.

Historical annotation
The first description of an oligodendroglioma was published by Bailey and Cushing {108} in 1926. This publication was followed in 1929 by the classic paper by Bailey and Bucy {107}, "Oligodendrogliomas of the brain". The association between 1p/19q codeletion and oligodendroglial histology was reported in 1994 {2091} and 1995 {161,1359}, followed in 2008 {118} and 2009 {2810} by the first reports on IDH mutation.

Epidemiology
Note that these and the following paragraphs mostly refer to epidemiological and clinical data based on histological tumour classification according to the previous WHO classification. For the most part, this information can be considered to be similar for the newly defined entity of IDH-mutant and 1p/19q-codeleted oligodendroglioma, as well as for oligodendroglioma, NOS.

Incidence
According to the Central Brain Tumor Registry of the United States (CBTRUS), the adjusted annual incidence rate of oligodendroglioma is estimated at 0.26 cases per 100 000 population {1863}. The incidence rates for anaplastic oligodendroglioma and oligoastrocytic tumours are estimated at 0.11 and 0.21 cases per 100 000 population, respectively. Oligodendroglial tumours account for 1.7% of all primary brain tumours (oligodendrogliomas for 1.2% and anaplastic oligodendrogliomas for 0.5%) and for 5.9% of all gliomas. Oligoastrocytic gliomas account for 0.9% of all primary brain tumours and for 3.3% of all gliomas.

Age and sex distribution
Epidemiological data based on histological classification indicate that most of these tumours arise in adults, with peak incidence in patients aged 35–44 years {1826,1863}. Oligodendrogliomas are rare in children, accounting for only 0.8% of all brain tumours in patients aged < 15 years and 1.8% in adolescents aged 15–19 years {1863}, with paediatric oligodendrogliomas frequently lacking IDH mutation and 1p/19q codeletion (see *Oligodendroglioma lacking IDH mutation and 1p/19q codeletion*, p. 68). With rare exceptions, children with 1p/19q-codeleted oligodendroglioma are usually older than 15 years at diagnosis {2157}. Overall, men are affected more frequently than women, with a male-to-female ratio of 1.3:1 {1863}. In the USA, oligodendroglioma is more common in Whites than in Blacks, with an incidence rate ratio of 2.5:1 {1863}.

Etiology
Rare cases of oligodendroglial tumours diagnosed after brain irradiation for other reasons have been documented {49, 600}. Although oligodendrogliomas and oligoastrocytomas are among the most frequent types of CNS tumours induced experimentally in rats by chemical carcinogens such as ethylnitrosourea and methylnitrosourea, there is no convincing evidence of an etiological role for these substances in human gliomas. Similarly, the existence of a viral etiology of oligodendroglioma is uncertain. Polyomavirus (SV40, BK virus, and JC virus) genome sequences and proteins have been detected in oligodendrogliomas {570} and a case of oligoastrocytoma {2099}. However, other authors found no frequent polyomavirus sequences in a large series of 225 gliomas {2164}. Concurrent HHV6A infection and diffuse leptomeningeal oligodendrogliomatosis has been reported in a 2-year-old boy {2445}, and there have been reports of isolated cases of oligodendroglioma arising in patients with immunodeficiency (including patients with HIV infection) {499} and after organ transplantation {2271}. Rare cases of oligodendroglioma in association with a demyelinating disease have also been reported {373}. However, epidemiological data do not indicate an increased incidence of gliomas in patients with autoimmune disease {990}.

Localization
IDH-mutant and 1p/19q-codeleted oligodendrogliomas arise preferentially in the white matter and cortex of the cerebral hemispheres. The frontal lobe is the most common location (involved in > 50% of all patients) followed in order of decreasing frequency by the temporal, parietal, and occipital lobes. Involvement of more than one cerebral lobe or bilateral tumour spread is not uncommon. Rare locations include the posterior fossa, basal ganglia, and brain stem. Leptomeningeal spread is seen in only a minority of patients {2163}. There have been rare cases of primary leptomeningeal oligodendrogliomas {1775} or oligodendroglial gliomatosis cerebri {2489}. Primary oligodendrogliomas of the spinal cord are rare, accounting for only 1.5% of all oligodendrogliomas and 2% of all spinal cord tumours {729}. Rare cases of primary spinal intramedullary oligodendroglioma and secondary meningeal dissemination have been reported, including a 1p/19q-codeleted tumour {898}. Isolated cases of oligodendroglioma arising in ovarian teratomas have been reported, although there was no assessment of IDH mutation and 1p/19q codeletion status {2592}.

Clinical features
Approximately two thirds of patients present with seizures {1680}. Other common presenting symptoms include headache and other signs of increased intracranial pressure, focal neurological deficits, and cognitive or mental changes {1446,1845}. In older studies, durations of > 5 years between the onset of symptoms and diagnosis were common, but modern neuroimaging has markedly reduced the time to diagnosis {1845}.

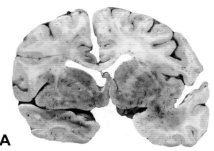 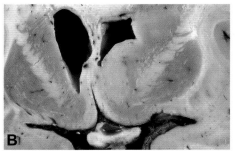 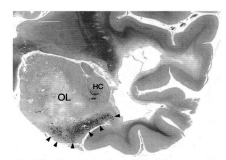

Fig. 1.61 A Recurrent oligodendroglioma with bilateral, diffuse infiltration of the frontal and temporal lobes. **B** Small oligodendroglioma of the medial basal ganglia, compressing the right lateral ventricle. Note the homogeneous cut surface.

Fig. 1.62 Oligodendroglioma (OL) of the temporal lobe with infiltration of the hippocampus (HC). Note the zone of calcification (arrowheads) at the periphery of the lesion.

Imaging

On CT, IDH-mutant and 1p/19q-codeleted oligodendrogliomas usually present as hypodense or isodense well-demarcated mass lesions, typically located in the cortex and subcortical white matter. Calcification is common but not diagnostic. MRI shows a lesion that is T1-hypointense and T2-hyperintense. The lesion is usually well demarcated and shows little perifocal oedema {2678}. Some tumours show heterogeneous features due to intratumoural haemorrhages and/or areas of cystic degeneration. Gadolinium enhancement has been detected in < 20% of WHO grade II oligodendrogliomas but in > 70% of WHO grade III anaplastic oligodendrogliomas {1260}. Contrast enhancement in low-grade oligodendrogliomas has been associated with less favourable prognosis {2621}. Demonstration of elevated 2-hydroxyglutarate levels by MR spectroscopy is a promising new means of non-invasive detection of IDH-mutant gliomas (including oligodendrogliomas) {449}. Differences in certain features between 1p/19q-codeleted and 1p/19q-intact low-grade gliomas have been reported on MR spectroscopy {292, 685,2678}, but reliable discrimination by neuroimaging is not yet possible.

Spread

IDH-mutant and 1p/19q-codeleted oligodendrogliomas characteristically extend into adjacent brain in a diffuse manner. Like other diffuse gliomas, oligodendroglioma can also (although rarely) manifest at initial clinical presentation with a gliomatosis cerebri pattern of extensive involvement of the CNS, with the affected area ranging from most of one cerebral hemisphere (three lobes or more) to both cerebral hemispheres with additional involvement of the deep grey matter

structures, brain stem, cerebellum, and spinal cord {2489}.

Macroscopy

Oligodendroglioma usually presents as a relatively well-defined, soft, greyish-pink mass. The tumour is typically located in the cortex and white matter, leading to blurring of the grey matter–white matter boundary. Local invasion into the overlying leptomeninges may be seen. Calcification is frequent and may impart a gritty texture to the tumour. Occasionally, densely calcified areas may present as intratumoural stones. Zones of cystic degeneration, as well as intratumoural haemorrhages, are common. Rare cases with extensive mucoid degeneration look gelatinous.

Microscopy

Histopathology

Oligodendrogliomas are diffusely infiltrating gliomas of moderate cellularity that in classic cases are composed of monomorphic cells with uniform round nuclei and variable perinuclear haloes on paraffin sections (a honeycomb or fried-egg appearance). Additional features include microcalcifications, mucoid/cystic degeneration, and a dense network of delicate branching capillaries. Mitotic activity is either absent or low. Nuclear atypia and an occasional mitosis are compatible with the diagnosis of a WHO grade II tumour, but brisk mitotic activity, prominent microvascular proliferation, and spontaneous necrosis are indicators of anaplasia, corresponding to WHO grade III (see *Anaplastic oligodendroglioma, IDH-mutant and 1p/19q-codeleted*, p. 70).

Cellular composition

Oligodendrogliomas are moderately

cellular tumours. Areas of increased cellularity, often in the form of circumscribed nodules, can occur in some otherwise well-differentiated tumours, so wide sampling of resection specimens is required. However, small biopsies sometimes show only scattered oligodendroglioma cells infiltrating the brain parenchyma, which are identifiable by their characteristic nuclei and (if the most common IDH mutation is present) by immunostaining for R132H-mutant IDH1 (see *Immunophenotype*). Classic oligodendroglioma cells have uniformly round nuclei that are slightly larger than those of normal oligodendrocytes and show an increase in chromatin density or a delicate salt-and-pepper pattern similar to that of neuroendocrine tumours. A distinct nuclear membrane is often apparent. In routinely formalin-fixed and paraffin-embedded material, there is a tendency for the tumour cells to undergo degeneration by acute swelling, which results in an enlarged rounded cell with a well-defined cell membrane and clear cytoplasm around a central spherical nucleus. This creates the typical honeycomb or fried-egg appearance, which although artefactual is a helpful diagnostic feature when present. However, this artefact is not seen in smear preparations or frozen sections, and may also be absent in rapidly fixed tissue and in paraffin sections made from frozen material.

Some oligodendrogliomas contain tumour cells with the appearance of small gemistocytes with a rounded belly of eccentric cytoplasm that is positive for GFAP. These cells have been referred to as minigemistocytes or microgemistocytes. Gliofibrillary oligodendrocytes are typical-looking oligodendroglioma cells on routine stains but show a thin perinuclear rim of positivity for GFAP {994}. GFAP-negative mucocytes or even signet ring cells are occasionally seen. Rare

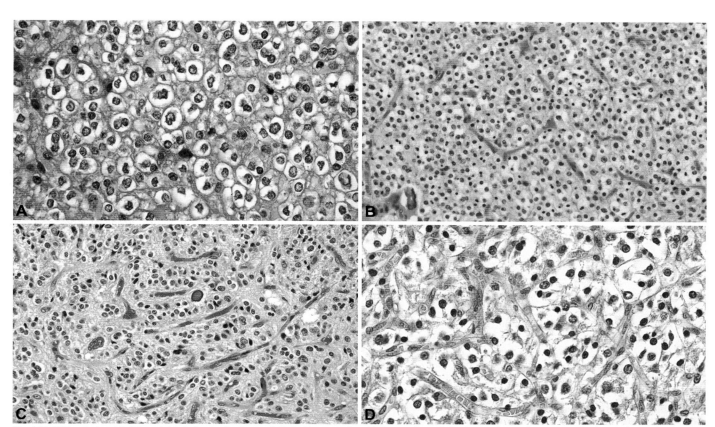

Fig. 1.63 IDH-mutant and 1p/19q-codeleted oligodendroglioma. **A** Typical honeycomb or fried-egg pattern of oligodendrogliomas: the tumour cells show a clear perinuclear halo and a sharply delineated plasma membrane; although this feature is an artefact that occurs during tissue processing, it is a hallmark of oligodendroglioma. **B** Perinuclear clearing. **C** Delicate "chicken-wire" network of branching capillaries. Note the moderate nuclear atypia and occasional microcalcification. **D** Conspicuous network of branching capillaries.

cases of oligodendroglioma consisting largely of signet ring cells (called signet ring cell oligodendroglioma) have been described {1373}, and eosinophilic granular cells are present in some oligodendrogliomas {2498}. Rare cases with neurocytic or ganglioglioma-like differentiation have also been reported {1939, 1948}. The presence of these various cellular phenotypes does not preclude an oligodendroglioma diagnosis if the tumour is positive for IDH mutation and 1p/19q codeletion. The presence of tumour cells with fibrillar or gemistocytic

astrocytic morphology is also compatible with this diagnosis when molecular testing confirms IDH mutation and 1p/19q codeletion; in other words, diffuse gliomas with oligoastrocytoma histology or with ambiguous histological features should be diagnosed as IDH-mutant and 1p/19q-codeleted oligodendroglioma when molecular testing reveals this entity-defining genotype {349,2464,2731}. Reactive astrocytes are typically scattered throughout oligodendrogliomas and may be particularly prominent at the tumour borders.

Mineralization and other degenerative features

A frequent histological feature is the presence of microcalcifications (sometimes associated with blood vessels) within the tumour tissue proper or in the invaded brain. Mineralization along blood vessels typically takes the form of small, punctate calcifications, whereas microcalcifications in the brain (called calcospherites) tend to be larger, with an irregular and sometimes laminated appearance. However, this feature is not specific for oligodendroglial tumours, and due to

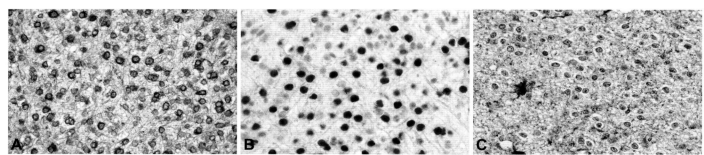

Fig. 1.64 Immunohistochemical features of IDH-mutant and 1p/19q-codeleted oligodendroglioma. **A** MAP2. **B** OLIG2. **C** GFAP.

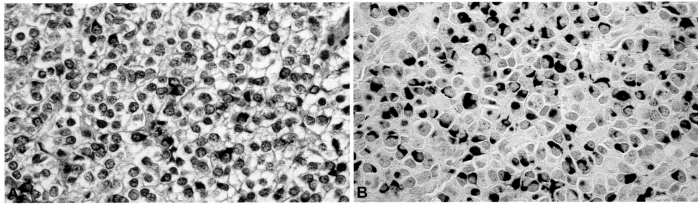

Fig. 1.65 IDH-mutant and 1p/19q-codeleted oligodendroglioma. **A** Gliofibrillary oligodendrocytes, GFAP stain. **B** This oligodendroglioma shows an unusually large number of minigemistocytes – oligodendroglioma cells with a small globular paranuclear area of strongly GFAP-positive cytoplasm.

generally incomplete tumour sampling, is sometimes not found in the available tissue sections even when clearly demonstrated on CT. Areas characterized by extracellular mucin deposition and/ or microcyst formation are frequent. Rare tumours are characterized by marked desmoplasia {1156}.

Vasculature
Oligodendrogliomas typically show a dense network of branching capillaries resembling the pattern of chicken wire. In some cases, the capillary stroma tends to subdivide the tumour into lobules. There is a tendency for intratumoural haemorrhages.

Growth pattern
Oligodendrogliomas grow diffusely in the cortex and white matter. Within the cortex, tumour cells tend to form secondary structures such as perineuronal satellitosis, perivascular aggregates, and subpial accumulations. Circumscribed leptomeningeal infiltration may induce a desmoplastic reaction. A rare spongioblastic growth pattern consists of parallel rows of tumour cells with somewhat elongated nuclei forming rhythmic palisades. Occasionally, perivascular pseudorosettes are seen, although some of these are a result of perivascular neuropil formation within foci of neurocytic differentiation {1948}. These patterns are generally present only focally.

Immunophenotype
To date, no single immunohistochemical marker has been found that is specific for oligodendroglial tumour cells. The majority of oligodendrogliomas demonstrate strong and uniform immunoreactivity with an antibody specific for R132H-mutant IDH1 {360}. Positive R132H-mutant IDH1 staining greatly facilitates the immunohistochemical differential diagnosis of oligodendroglioma versus other clear cell tumours of the CNS and non-neoplastic and reactive lesions {356,357}. However, a lack of R132H-mutant IDH1 immunopositivity does not exclude oligodendroglioma, given the possibility of less common *IDH1* and *IDH2* mutations that cannot be detected with the R132H-mutant IDH1 antibody and instead require DNA sequence analysis. Unlike most IDH-mutant diffuse astrocytomas, IDH-mutant and 1p/19q-codeleted oligodendrogliomas typically retain nuclear expression of ATRX {1519,2105}. In addition, IDH-mutant and 1p/19q-codeleted oligodendrogliomas usually lack widespread nuclear p53 staining, a finding consistent with the mutual exclusivity of *TP53* mutation and 1p/19q deletion in IDH-mutant gliomas {349,2464}.
Oligodendrogliomas are consistently immunopositive for MAP2, S100 protein, and LEU7 {221,1746,2087}. MAP2 often reveals perinuclear cytoplasmic immunostaining without significant process labelling. However, all three markers are also commonly positive in astrocytic gliomas. Similarly, the oligodendrocyte lineage–associated transcription factors OLIG1, OLIG2, and SOX10 are expressed in oligodendrogliomas but also in other gliomas {121,1500}. GFAP is detectable in intermingled reactive astrocytes but can also be found in neoplastic cells such as minigemistocytes and gliofibrillary oligodendrocytes {994, 2087}. Vimentin is infrequently expressed in well-differentiated oligodendrogliomas but more often found in anaplastic oligodendrogliomas {1336}. GFAP and vimentin immunostaining is often positive in the astrocytic-appearing tumour components of IDH-mutant and 1p/19q-codeleted oligodendrogliomas that histologically resemble oligoastrocytoma. Cytokeratins are absent, although certain antibody cocktails, such as AE1/ AE3, may give false-positive staining due to cross-reactivity {1773}.
Several antigens are specifically expressed by normal oligodendrocytes in vivo or in vitro, including myelin basic protein; proteolipid protein; myelin-associated glycoprotein; galactolipids, such as galactocerebroside and galactosulfatide; certain gangliosides; and several enzymes, such as carbonic anhydrase C, CNP, glycerol-3-phosphate dehydrogenase, and lactate dehydrogenase. However, none of these antigens has demonstrated significance as a diagnostically useful marker for oligodendrogliomas. Some are not expressed in oligodendroglioma cells (e.g. myelin basic protein {1746}), some are expressed only in a minority of cases (e.g. myelin-associated glycoprotein {1746}, galactocerebroside, proteolipid protein, and CNP {2457}), and some have expression that is not restricted to oligodendroglial tumour cells (e.g. carbonic anhydrase C {1747}).
Synaptophysin immunoreactivity of residual neuropil between the tumour cells is frequently seen in oligodendroglial tumours and should not be mistaken for evidence of neuronal or neurocytic differentiation. However, IDH-mutant and 1p/19q-codeleted oligodendroglioma may contain neoplastic cells that express synaptophysin and/or other neuronal markers, such as NeuN and neurofilaments {1939,1948}. Immunostaining for

the proneural alpha-internexin protein is frequent {607} but cannot substitute as a reliable surrogate marker for 1p/19q codeletion {625}. Similarly, NOGO-A positivity is typical of, but not exclusive to, 1p/19q-codeleted oligodendrogliomas {1600}.

Proliferation
Mitotic activity is low or absent in WHO grade II oligodendrogliomas. Accordingly, the Ki-67 proliferation index is usually < 5% (see *Prognosis and predictive factors*). On average, the Ki-67 proliferation index is significantly lower in WHO grade II oligodendrogliomas than in anaplastic oligodendrogliomas. However, a definitive diagnostic cut-off point cannot be established, due to marked variability in staining results between institutions. Nevertheless, interobserver agreement on Ki-67 proliferation index scoring as determined by MIB1 monoclonal antibody staining was good when six pathologists independently reviewed the same set of MIB1-stained slides from 30 oligodendrogliomas {2024}. Minigemistocytes are reported to be mostly MIB1-negative and thus non-proliferative, whereas gliofibrillary oligodendrocytes are more commonly positive {1371}. Other proliferation markers, such as PCNA {2096}, TOP2A {1344}, and MCM2 {2736} have been reported to correlate with WHO grade and survival in patients with oligodendroglial tumours, but do not provide clear advantages over MIB1 immunostaining in the routine setting.

Differential diagnosis
The morphological spectrum of IDH-mutant and 1p/19q-codeleted oligodendrogliomas is broad, with some similarities to a variety of reactive and neoplastic lesions. Macrophage-rich processes such as demyelinating diseases or cerebral infarcts should be readily distinguished by immunostaining for macrophage markers and lack of IDH mutation. Reactive changes such as the increased numbers of oligodendrocytes sometimes seen in partial lobectomy specimens performed for intractable seizures can also be distinguished by lack of IDH mutation.
The differential diagnosis with diffuse astrocytoma relies on histological, immunohistochemical, and molecular features. Most importantly, IDH-mutant diffuse astrocytomas lack 1p/19q codeletion. In addition, *TERT* promoter mutations

are common in IDH-mutant and 1p/19q-codeleted oligodendrogliomas but exceptional in IDH-mutant diffuse astrocytomas. The considerable overlap between *TERT* promoter mutation and 1p/19q codeletion in IDH-mutant gliomas suggests that *TERT* promoter mutation may be useful as a surrogate marker for 1p/19q codeletion. However, minor subsets of IDH-mutant and 1p/19q-codeleted oligodendrogliomas have been reported to lack *TERT* promoter mutation, and some IDH-mutant but 1p/19q-intact astrocytomas may carry *TERT* promoter mutations {89,1314,1408,2464}. Therefore, the general use of *TERT* promoter sequencing instead of 1p/19q codeletion testing is not recommended. Immunohistochemical features that may further support the differential diagnosis include frequent nuclear p53 immunostaining and loss of nuclear ATRX expression in diffuse astrocytomas.
Other neoplastic lesions that can histologically mimic oligodendroglioma are clear cell ependymoma, neurocytoma, and dysembryoplastic neuroepithelial tumour. These entities and oligodendrogliomas share the feature of neoplastic cells with uniform, round nuclei and clear cytoplasm, collectively referred to as oligodendroglial-like cells. In the routine diagnostic setting, evidence of an IDH mutation, typically demonstrated by positive R132H-mutant IDH1 immunostaining, rules out all these differential diagnoses. In the absence of IDH mutation, immunostaining for neuronal markers, in particular diffuse synaptophysin and at least focal NeuN, provides further evidence for neurocytoma. Similarly, rare cases of liponeurocytoma are distinguished from oligodendroglioma by extensive positive staining for neuronal markers, the absence of IDH mutation, and the presence of lipidized cells resembling adipocytes. Clear cell ependymomas often show at least focal perivascular pseudorosettes and dot-like or ring-shaped EMA immunoreactivity. Formation of specific glioneuronal elements, absence of IDH mutation and 1p/19q codeletion, and (in a subset) eosinophilic granular bodies, a CD34-positive cell population, and/or *BRAF* V600E mutation, distinguish dysembryoplastic neuroepithelial tumour from IDH-mutant and 1p/19q-codeleted oligodendroglioma {414}. A rare differential diagnosis is clear cell meningioma, which can be distinguished by abundant

diastase-sensitive periodic acid–Schiff positivity, immunoreactivity for EMA and desmoplakin, and lack of IDH mutation. Metastatic clear cell carcinomas differ from oligodendrogliomas in that they have sharp tumour borders, are immunoreactive for cytokeratins and EMA, and lack R132H-mutant IDH1 immunostaining or other IDH mutations.
In adult patients, the differential diagnosis with pilocytic astrocytoma rarely poses a major problem, because foci of classic pilocytic features are usually present in pilocytic astrocytomas, and IDH mutation and 1p/19q deletion are absent. Neuroradiological features, such as midline tumour location and mural nodule/cyst formation, may also provide helpful ancillary information. Molecular demonstration of *BRAF* fusion genes supports the diagnosis of pilocytic astrocytoma, although *BRAF* gain and *KIAA1549-BRAF* fusions have also been reported in some IDH-mutant and 1p/19q-codeleted oligodendroglial tumours {104,1282}. In children, the molecular distinction of oligodendroglioma from pilocytic astrocytoma is challenging because paediatric oligodendrogliomas typically lack combined IDH mutation and 1p/19q codeletion but occasionally demonstrate *BRAF* fusion genes (see *Oligodendroglioma lacking IDH mutation and 1p/19q codeletion*, p. 68). This differential diagnosis must therefore rely primarily on histological and ancillary radiological features, unless advanced molecular testing methods based on large-scale methylation and/or mutation profiling that provide entity-specific methylation or mutation profiles can be applied. The differential diagnosis of diffuse leptomeningeal glioneuronal tumour (p. 152) is facilitated by the clinical presentation and the characteristic molecular profile, with combined *KIAA1549-BRAF* gene fusion and solitary 1p deletion (or 1p/19q codeletion) but absence of IDH mutation {2156}.

Cell of origin
Although the designation of CNS neoplasms as oligodendroglial tumours could imply histogenesis from cells of the oligodendroglial lineage, the evidence supporting this assumption is circumstantial, based solely on morphological similarities of the neoplastic cells in these tumours to normal oligodendrocytes. It is also unknown whether human oligodendrogliomas arise from neoplastic

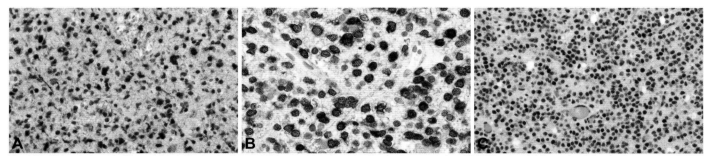

Fig. 1.66 IDH-mutant and 1p/19q-codeleted oligodendroglioma. **A,B** Immunohistochemistry showing the expression of R132H-mutant IDH1 protein. **C** Retained expression of ATRX in tumour cell nuclei.

transformation of mature oligodendrocytes, immature glial precursors, or neural stem cells. Experimental data in transgenic mice indicate that gliomas with oligodendroglial histology may originate from different cell types in the CNS, including neural stem cells, astrocytes, and oligodendrocyte precursor cells {2872}. An oligodendroglioma-like phenotype is commonly found in transgenic brain tumours, despite a variety of targeted cell types and oncogenic events {589, 2725}. Some studies have suggested a likely origin of oligodendrogliomas from NG2-positive and asymmetrical cell division–defective oligodendroglial progenitor cells {1954,2449}. However, oligodendroglial precursor cells may give rise to either oligodendroglial or astrocytic gliomas, depending on the genes driving transformation {1508}, suggesting a dominance of oncogenic signalling over cell of origin in determining the glioma phenotype.

Genetic profile

Cytogenetics

Cytogenetic studies of oligodendroglioma have revealed an unbalanced translocation between chromosomes 1 and 19 that results in loss of the der(1;19)(p10;q10) chromosome, causing whole-arm deletions of 1p and 19q, and retention of the der[t(1;19)(q10;p10)] chromosome {887,1151}.

IDH *mutation and 1p/19q codeletion*

The entity-defining alteration in oligodendrogliomas is concurrent mutation of *IDH1* or *IDH2* and whole-arm deletion of 1p and 19q. The vast majority (> 90% {953}) of IDH mutations in WHO grade II oligodendrogliomas are the *IDH1* R132H mutation, which is readily detectable by immunohistochemistry {360}. In < 10% of cases, other *IDH1* codon 132 or *IDH2*

codon 172 mutations are present, with the proportion of *IDH2* mutations being higher in oligodendroglial gliomas than in astrocytic gliomas {953}. Combined whole-arm loss of 1p and 19q is invariably associated with IDH mutation, indicating that detection of 1p/19q codeletion in the absence of IDH mutation should raise suspicion of incomplete/partial deletions, which have been detected in subsets of IDH-wildtype anaplastic astrocytomas and glioblastomas, with associated poor outcome {2658}.

Aberrant genes on 1p or 19q

Oligodendroglial tumours have frequent mutations in the human homologue of the *Drosophila* capicua gene (*CIC*) on 19q13.2 {183,2825}, with the majority of IDH-mutant and 1p/19q-codeleted oligodendrogliomas harbouring *CIC* mutations {2219,2464,2825}. A smaller subset of these tumours also carries mutations in the *FUBP1* gene on 1p31.1. One study identified IDH mutation, 1p/19q codeletion, and *TERT* promoter mutation as early genetic changes in oligodendroglioma pathogenesis, whereas *CIC* mutations may appear later in tumour progression {2464}. Other genes on 1p (e.g. *CAMTA1*, *CHD5*, *CITED4*, *DFFB*, *DIRAS3*, *PRDX1*, *ATRX*, *AJAP1*, and *TP73*) and 19q (e.g. *EMP3*, *ARHGAP35*, *PEG3*, and *ZNF296*) have been reported to show aberrant promoter methylation and/or reduced expression in IDH-mutant and 1p/19q-codeleted oligodendrogliomas {2126}. Epigenetic silencing of the pH regulator gene *SLC9A1* on 1p has been linked to lower intracellular pH and attenuation of acid load recovery in oligodendroglioma cells, which may contribute to the distinctive biology of IDH-mutant and 1p/19q-codeleted oligodendrogliomas {217}.

TERT *promoter mutations*

Unlike IDH-mutant diffuse astrocytomas,

IDH-mutant and 1p/19q-codeleted oligodendrogliomas lack *ATRX* mutation but virtually always carry activating mutations in the *TERT* promoter region, leading to increased expression of TERT {89, 1270,1314}. In fact, *TERT* promoter mutation is strongly associated with 1p/19q codeletion in IDH-mutant gliomas and is an early event in oligodendroglioma development {2464}. However, *TERT* promoter mutations are also frequent in IDH-wildtype glioblastomas {1270}. Consequently, large-scale sequencing studies have identified three major groups of cerebral gliomas, with distinct biologies and clinical outcomes. These three groups are defined, respectively, by IDH mutation associated with 1p/19q codeletion and *TERT* promoter mutation, IDH mutation associated with *TP53* and frequent *ATRX* mutation, and IDH-wildtype status associated with *TERT* promoter mutation and glioblastoma-associated genomic aberrations {349,2464}.

Other genetic alterations

Mutations in *NOTCH1*, and less commonly in other NOTCH pathway genes, have been detected in approximately 15% of oligodendrogliomas {349,2464}. Other less commonly mutated genes include epigenetic regulator genes such as *SETD2* and other histone methyltransferase genes, as well as genes encoding components of the SWI/SNF chromatin-remodelling complex {349,2464}. Unlike in IDH-mutant astrocytic tumours, *TP53* mutation is usually absent and mutually exclusive with 1p/19q deletion {349, 2464}.

Epigenetic and transcriptional changes

IDH-mutant and 1p/19q-codeleted oligodendrogliomas are characterized by widespread changes in DNA methylation, leading to concurrent hypermethylation of multiple CpG islands, a phenomenon that is referred to as G-CIMP {1810}. Mechanistically, this phenomenon has been linked with mutant IDH proteins producing 2-hydroxyglutarate, which functions as a competitive inhibitor of alpha-ketoglutarate–dependent dioxygenases including histone demethylases and the TET family of 5-methylcytosine hydroxylases {1540,2804}. This in turn leads to increased histone methylation and G-CIMP {1810,2589}. One study suggested that *CIC* mutations cooperate with IDH mutations to further increase 2-hydroxyglutarate levels {443}. In fact, DNA methylation profiles in IDH-mutant and 1p/19q-codeleted oligodendrogliomas differ from those in IDH-mutant but 1p/19q-intact astrocytomas {1723,2464, 2751}, a distinction that has been referred to as G-CIMP type A versus G-CIMP type B {2464}, and can be exploited for classification purposes (e.g. by 450k methylation bead array analysis {2751}). As a consequence of G-CIMP, many different genes may be epigenetically inactivated in oligodendrogliomas, including genes on 1p and 19q as well as genes on other chromosomes, such as the tumour suppressors *CDKN2A*, *CDKN2B*, *RB1*, and many others {2126}. *MGMT* promoter hypermethylation and reduced expression is also common {1733}. At the mRNA level, IDH-mutant and 1p/19q-codeleted oligodendrogliomas often show a proneural glioblastoma-like gene expression signature {608,2731}.

Growth factors and receptors

About half of all WHO grade II oligodendrogliomas and anaplastic oligodendrogliomas show strong expression of EGFR mRNA and protein in the absence of *EGFR* gene amplification {2090}. The simultaneous expression of the mRNAs for the pre-pro forms of EGFR and/or transforming growth factor alpha indicates the possibility of auto-, juxta-, or paracrine growth stimulation via the EGFR system {626}. One study reported that high EGFR expression was linked to shorter survival in patients with 1p/19q-codeleted oligodendrogliomas of WHO grade II but longer survival in patients with WHO grade III anaplastic oligodendrogliomas {1036}. Several other growth factors (including basic fibroblast growth factor, platelet-derived growth factors, transforming growth factor beta, IGF1, and nerve growth factor) have been reported to be involved in the regulation of proliferation

and/or maturation of oligodendroglial cells {2085}. PDGFA and PDGFB, as well as the corresponding receptors (PDGFRA and PDGFRB) are commonly co-expressed in oligodendrogliomas {582}. However, *PDGFRA* mutations are rare, and elevated expression seems to be independent of 1p/19q codeletion {955}. The functional role of PDGFB has been demonstrated by the induction of oligodendrogliomas in transgenic mice with targeted overexpression of this growth factor in neural stem or progenitor cells {521,1508}. VEGF and its receptors serve as angiogenic factors in oligodendroglial tumours, particularly in anaplastic oligodendrogliomas {402,456}.

Genetic susceptibility

Most oligodendrogliomas develop sporadically, in the absence of an obvious familial clustering or a hereditary predisposition syndrome. Large-scale genotyping data indicate a strong association between a low-frequency SNP at 8q24.21 and increased risk of IDH-mutant oligodendroglioma and astrocytoma {1152}. Other genetic polymorphisms that have been associated with increased oligodendroglioma risk include the *GSTT1* null genotype {1245} and SNPs in the *GLTSCR1* and *ERCC2* genes {2814}.

Germline mutations in shelterin complex genes, including the *POT1* gene, have been linked to familial oligodendroglioma {110}. The largest series of non-syndromic familial glioma cases published to date comprised 841 patients from 376 families with ≥ 2 affected family members each {2212}. Within this cohort, 59 patients (8%) were diagnosed with WHO grade II oligodendroglioma, 29 patients (3.9%) with WHO grade II oligoastrocytoma, 31 patients (4.2%) with WHO grade III anaplastic oligodendroglioma, and 12 patients (1.6%) with WHO grade III anaplastic oligoastrocytoma. Isolated cases of familial oligodendroglioma with 1p/19q codeletion have also been reported {713,1858}.

Only a few patients with oligodendroglial tumours have been reported in families with hereditary cancer predisposition syndromes. These include one patient manifesting *BRCA1* mutation with oligodendroglioma {1165}; one patient with Turcot syndrome, germline *PMS2* mutation, and two metachronous glioblastomas showing histological features of oligodendroglial differentiation {2525}; a

child with hereditary non-polyposis colorectal cancer and oligodendroglioma {1642}; and an adolescent with Lynch syndrome and anaplastic oligodendroglioma {978}. One child with retinoblastoma syndrome and anaplastic oligodendroglioma {16} and identical twins with Ollier-type multiple enchondromatosis and oligodendroglioma have also been documented {411}.

Prognosis and predictive factors

Prognosis

WHO grade II IDH-mutant and 1p/19q-codeleted oligodendrogliomas are typically slow-growing tumours and are associated with relatively long overall survival. A population-based study from Switzerland demonstrated a median survival time of 11.6 years for oligodendroglioma and 6.6 years for oligoastrocytoma (both defined according to histological criteria only), as well as 10-year survival rates of 51% and 49%, respectively {1826}. The CBTRUS has documented 5-year survival rates of 79.5% and 61.1%, as well as 10-year survival rates of 62.8% and 46.9%, for oligodendroglioma and oligoastrocytic glioma, respectively {1863}. However, survival estimates have varied markedly. Some single-institution studies have documented even longer median overall survival times (e.g. > 15 years {1845}) for patients with low-grade oligodendroglioma, and others have documented shorter median survivals (e.g. 3.5 years {567}). Most of the variability in these studies is likely due to differing diagnostic criteria, the absence of molecular information on IDH mutation and 1p/19q codeletion, and differing treatment approaches.

Oligodendrogliomas generally recur locally. Malignant progression of recurrence is common, although it takes longer on average than in diffuse astrocytomas {1121}. Rare cases of gliosarcoma (so-called oligosarcoma) arising from IDH-mutant and 1p/19q-codeleted oligodendroglioma have been reported {1004,2152}. Unusual cases of oligodendroglioma, including 1p/19q-codeleted tumours, have been noted in which the patients developed systemic metastases, usually at late stages of the disease {1148,1651}. It has been suggested that oligodendroglial tumours with 1p/19q codeletion may be more prone to extraneural metastasis despite their generally favourable prognosis {1651}, but this hypothesis remains unproven.

Clinical factors

Features that have been associated with more favourable outcome include younger patient age at operation, location in the frontal lobe, presentation with seizures, high postoperative Karnofsky score, lack of contrast enhancement on neuroimaging, and macroscopically complete surgical removal {2621}. One study found that a greater extent of resection was associated with longer overall and progression-free survival, but did not prolong the time to malignant progression {2386}.

Histopathology

The histological features that have been linked to worse prognosis include necrosis, high mitotic activity, increased cellularity, nuclear atypia, cellular pleomorphism, and microvascular proliferation (see Anaplastic oligodendroglioma, IDH-mutant and 1p/19q-codeleted, p. 70). However, the prognostic significance of each of these histological features requires re-evaluation in patients with molecularly characterized IDH-mutant and 1p/19q-codeleted tumours. The presence of minigemistocytes and/or gliofibrillary oligodendrocytes does not seem to influence survival {1374}. Similarly, marked desmoplasia does not relate to distinct outcome {1156}. It is assumed that an astrocytic-looking tumour component within an IDH-mutant and 1p/19q-codeleted oligodendroglioma does not indicate shorter survival, but this remains to be confirmed.

Proliferation

Several single-institution studies have found that a higher Ki-67 proliferation index, typically > 3–5%, correlates with worse prognosis in patients with oligodendroglial tumours. One study, of 32 patients with WHO grade II oligodendrogliomas, found that a Ki-67 proliferation index of > 3% was indicative of a worse prognosis {980}. Another study, of 89 patients with oligodendroglioma, reported a 5-year survival rate of 83% for patients whose oligodendrogliomas had a Ki-67 proliferation index of < 5%, versus a rate of only 24% with a Ki-67 proliferation index of > 5% {567}. This finding is similar to those of other studies {493}. In general, older studies reported

Oligodendroglioma lacking IDH mutation and 1p/19q codeletion (paediatric-type oligodendroglioma)

A small subset of histologically classic oligodendrogliomas are found to lack IDH mutation and 1p/19q codeletion on appropriate molecular testing. This group includes the majority of oligodendrogliomas in children and adolescents {1361,2057,2157}. In these cases, it is important to check carefully for and exclude histological mimics that may contain oligodendrocyte-like tumours cells, in particular dysembryoplastic neuroectodermal tumour, extraventricular neurocytoma, clear cell ependymoma, and pilocytic astrocytoma (see Differential diagnosis). However, differential diagnosis can be difficult, because individual tumours can show overlapping histological features of related tumours, such as oligodendroglioma, angiocentric glioma, and dysembryoplastic neuroepithelial tumour {1257}. Moreover, molecular studies indicate that a subset of paediatric oligodendrogliomas carry the oncogenic BRAF fusion genes {1391} that are typically detected in pilocytic astrocytoma {1176}. Thus, paediatric low-grade gliomas seem to constitute an overlapping spectrum of entities that can be difficult to distinguish by histological means alone. A careful review of 100 tumours originally classified as oligodendrogliomas in children and adolescents confirmed the diagnosis for only 50 tumours, whereas the other 50 cases showed histological features of other entities, such as pilocytic astrocytoma, dysembryoplastic neuroepithelial tumour, and oligoastrocytoma {2157}. Of the 50 confirmed cases of oligodendroglioma with classic histology, 38 tumours were low-grade and 12 tumours were anaplastic. All 50 cases were diffusely infiltrating gliomas composed of uniform round cells with perinuclear haloes and formation of secondary structures (predominantly perineuronal satellitosis). Calcifications and microcysts were also frequent. However, most tumours lacked IDH1 R132H and 1p/19q codeletion, and histological progression was rare {2157}. High-throughput molecular profiling of paediatric low-grade diffuse gliomas revealed duplications of portions of the FGFR1 gene or rearrangements of MYB in > 50% of cases, including tumours with oligodendroglial or oligoastrocytic histology {2855}. Rearrangements in the MYB-related MYBL1 transcription factor gene have also been reported {2068}. These findings indicate that the majority of diffuse gliomas in children, including tumours with oligodendroglial or oligoastrocytic histology, are genetically and biologically distinct from their adult counterparts. However, additional studies are needed to comprehensively characterize the molecular profile of these rare tumours and to clarify whether they constitute a distinct entity.

an independent prognostic value of the Ki-67 proliferation index {604}, whereas more recent data from patients with anaplastic oligodendroglioma have shown a prognostic impact of the index on univariate but not multivariate analysis {2034}. Among paediatric oligodendrogliomas, the Ki-67 proliferation index is higher in WHO grade III tumours than in WHO grade II tumours {2157}, but a study of 20 paediatric low-grade oligodendroglioma cases did not show a prognostic value for the Ki-67 proliferation index {259}.

Genetic alterations

The prognostic versus predictive role of 1p and 19q loss in WHO grade II gliomas is a matter of debate. Some studies suggested that WHO grade II gliomas with deletion of 1p or with 1p/19q codeletion are associated with longer survival independent from adjuvant therapy {686, 1216}, but others did not find longer progression-free survival when patients were not treated with upfront radiotherapy or chemotherapy {951}. Similarly, neither IDH mutation nor MGMT promoter methylation were linked to longer progression-free survival in patients with WHO grade II glioma treated by neurosurgical resection only {27,951}. In contrast, IDH mutation, 1p/19q codeletion, and MGMT promoter methylation were found to be associated with better therapeutic response and longer survival in patients with low-grade glioma treated with adjuvant radiotherapy or chemotherapy {951,1256}. A study of 360 patients with WHO grade II diffuse glioma demonstrated no prognostic role for IDH mutation, whereas 1p/19q codeletion was associated with longer overall survival and TP53 mutation with shorter overall survival {1281}. Thus, it is likely that a prognostically favourable role of IDH mutation, 1p/19q losses, and *MGMT* promoter methylation in WHO grade II glioma is linked to higher sensitivity to cytotoxic treatment rather than to generally more indolent behaviour independent of therapy. It remains to be investigated whether genetic or epigenetic alterations in other genes can improve prognostic assessment within the group of patients with IDH-mutant and 1p/19q-codeleted WHO grade II oligodendrogliomas.

Predictive factors

The optimal postoperative treatment of patients with IDH-mutant and 1p/19q-codeleted WHO grade II oligodendrogliomas is a matter of ongoing discussion. After tumour resection, radiotherapy and chemotherapy are often deferred until tumour progression because therapy-associated neurotoxicity is a major concern in patients with expected long-term survival. Patients with symptomatic residual and progressive tumours after surgery usually receive upfront treatment with radiotherapy and/or chemotherapy. The European Organisation for Research and Treatment of Cancer (EORTC) 22845 trial showed that adjuvant radiotherapy prolonged progression-free but not overall survival in patients with progressive WHO grade II gliomas {2613}. The Radiation Therapy Oncology Group (RTOG) 9802 trial initially also showed only increased progression-free survival for patients treated with radiotherapy plus PCV chemotherapy versus radiotherapy alone {2338}. However, recent long-term follow-up data also showed a major increase in overall survival after radiotherapy plus PCV chemotherapy, in particular for patients with 1p/19q-codeleted low-grade oligodendrogliomas {2481,2612}. Adjuvant chemotherapy with temozolomide may also be a feasible therapeutic strategy for patients with progressive low-grade oligodendroglioma, with 1p/19q codeletion suggested as a predictive marker for better response to temozolomide {1022, 1256,1476}. Another study reported that IDH mutation predicts better response to radiochemotherapy in patients with WHO grade II glioma {1835}. Collectively, these findings agree with data from phase III trials in patients with anaplastic gliomas (WHO grade III) that indicated IDH mutation {346} and 1p/19q codeletion as predictive markers for long-term survival after combined treatment with radiotherapy and PCV chemotherapy {344,2615}. The presence of *MSH6* mismatch repair gene mutations has been linked to temozolomide resistance independent of *MGMT* promoter methylation status {1779}. One study reported that 1p/19q codeletion predicted a lower risk of pseudoprogression in patients with oligodendroglial tumours despite being associated with longer survival {1504}.

Oligodendroglioma, NOS

Definition

A diffusely infiltrating glioma with classic oligodendroglial histology, in which molecular testing for combined IDH mutation and 1p/19q codeletion could not be completed or was inconclusive.

The diagnosis of oligodendroglioma, NOS, is reserved for diffusely infiltrating WHO grade II gliomas with classic oligodendroglial histology but without confirmation of IDH mutation and 1p/19q codeletion, due to limited tissue availability, low tumour-cell content, inconclusive test results, or other circumstances impeding molecular testing. In general, molecular testing for IDH mutation and 1p/19q codeletion is important for WHO classification of oligodendroglial tumours, implying that the diagnosis of oligodendroglioma, NOS, should be limited to a small minority of cases. Immunohistochemical demonstration of IDH mutation (in particular *IDH1* R132H) and nuclear positivity for ATRX support the diagnosis. However, unless successfully tested for 1p/19q codeletion, gliomas with oligodendroglial histology, IDH mutation, and nuclear ATRX positivity still correspond to the diagnosis of oligodendroglioma, NOS. Immunohistochemical positivity for oligodendroglioma-associated markers such as alpha-internexin {607,625} and NOGO-A {1600}, as well as immunohistochemical demonstration of loss of nuclear CIC or FUBP1 expression {146,401}, are not sufficient to substitute for 1p/19q codeletion testing.

Unlike with IDH-mutant and 1p/19q-codeleted oligodendroglioma, the presence of a conspicuous astrocytic component is not compatible with the diagnosis of oligodendroglioma, NOS (see *Oligoastrocytoma, NOS*, p. 75).

ICD-O code   9450/3

Grading

Oligodendroglioma, NOS, corresponds histologically to WHO grade II.

Anaplastic oligodendroglioma, IDH-mutant and 1p/19q-codeleted

Reifenberger G.   Cairncross J.G.
Collins V.P.   Yokoo H.
Hartmann C.   Yip S.
Hawkins C.   Louis D.N.
Kros J.M.

Definition

An IDH-mutant and 1p/19q-codeleted oligodendroglioma with focal or diffuse histological features of anaplasia (in particular, pathological microvascular proliferation and/or brisk mitotic activity).

In IDH-mutant and 1p/19q-codeleted anaplastic oligodendroglioma, necrosis (with or without palisading) may be present, but does not indicate progression to glioblastoma. The presence of an astrocytic tumour component is compatible with the diagnosis when molecular testing reveals combined IDH mutation and 1p/19q codeletion. The vast majority of IDH-mutant and 1p/19q-codeleted anaplastic oligodendrogliomas manifest in adult patients. The tumours are preferentially located in the cerebral hemispheres, with the frontal lobe being the most common location.

ICD-O code   9451/3

Grading

IDH-mutant and 1p/19q-codeleted anaplastic oligodendroglioma corresponds histologically to WHO grade III.

There is clear evidence from prospective clinical trials {344,2615,2740} and large cohort studies {2464,2731} that patients with IDH-mutant and 1p/19q-codeleted anaplastic oligodendroglial tumours have a significantly better prognosis than do patients with IDH-mutant but 1p/19q-intact or IDH-wildtype anaplastic astrocytic gliomas. In contrast, the prognostic value of WHO grading within the group of patients with IDH-mutant and 1p/19q-codeleted oligodendroglial tumours is less clear (see *Oligodendroglioma, IDH-mutant and 1p/19q-codeleted*, p. 60). Two recent uncontrolled retrospective studies suggested a limited role of WHO grading in predicting patient outcome {1836,2464}, a finding in line with retrospective data obtained from a large cohort of patients with IDH-mutant astrocytic gliomas {2103}. However, treatment regimens often differ for patients with low-grade versus high-grade oligodendroglioma, so potential bias cannot be excluded in retrospective

analyses that do not carefully control for different treatments and other prognostically relevant parameters. Histological features that have been linked to high-grade malignancy of oligodendroglioma in previous studies are high cellularity, marked cytological atypia, high mitotic activity, pathological microvascular proliferation, and necrosis with or without palisading. Anaplastic oligodendroglioma usually shows several of these features. However, the individual impact of each parameter is unclear, in particular because most of the older studies were not restricted to patients with IDH-mutant and 1p/19q-codeleted oligodendroglial tumours. Endothelial (microvascular) proliferation and brisk mitotic activity (defined as ≥ 6 mitoses per 10 high-power fields) have been suggested to be of particular importance as indicators of anaplasia in oligodendroglial tumours {830}. Thus, the diagnosis of IDH-mutant and 1p/19q-codeleted anaplastic oligodendroglioma should require at least the presence of conspicuous microvascular proliferation and/or brisk mitotic activity. Detection of a single mitosis in a resection specimen is not sufficient for classifying an oligodendroglial tumour as WHO grade III anaplastic oligodendroglioma. In borderline cases, immunostaining for MIB1 and attention to clinical and neuroradiological features, such as rapid symptomatic growth and contrast enhancement, may provide additional information for assessing the prognosis.

Epidemiology

Note that these and the following paragraphs mostly refer to epidemiological and clinical data based on histological tumour classification according to the previous WHO classification. For the most part, this information can be considered to be similar for the newly defined entity IDH-mutant and 1p/19q-codeleted anaplastic oligodendroglioma, as well as for anaplastic oligodendroglioma, NOS.

Incidence

According to a statistical report from the Central Brain Tumor Registry of the United States (CBTRUS), anaplastic oligodendroglioma (as defined by histology only) has an estimated annual incidence rate of 0.11 cases per 100 000 population and accounts for 0.5% of all primary brain tumours {1863}. Approximately one third of all oligodendroglial tumours are anaplastic oligodendrogliomas {1863}.

Age and sex distribution

Anaplastic oligodendrogliomas manifest preferentially in adults, with a median patient age at diagnosis of 49 years {1863}. Patients with anaplastic oligodendrogliomas are approximately 6 years older on average than patients with WHO grade II oligodendrogliomas, but this difference appears to be much smaller when only patients with IDH-mutant and 1p/19q-codeleted tumours are considered. Anaplastic oligodendroglioma is very rare in children. In the CBTRUS, there were no

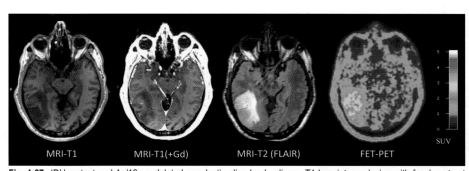

Fig. 1.67 IDH-mutant and 1p/19q-codeleted anaplastic oligodendroglioma. T1-hypointense lesion with focal contrast enhancement following gadolinium administration (+Gd). T2 (FLAIR) shows the extent of the lesion and FET-PET demonstrates increased metabolic activity.

MRI-T1   MRI-T1(+Gd)   MRI-T2 (FLAIR)   FET-PET

patients with anaplastic oligodendroglioma among the 12 103 children aged 0–14 years registered with neuroepithelial tumours, and only 32 patients with anaplastic oligodendroglioma were documented among the 3051 children registered with neuroepithelial tumours in the 15–19 years age group {1863}. In an institutional cohort of 50 paediatric patients with oligodendroglioma, 12 patients were diagnosed with anaplastic oligodendrogliomas, including 4 patients with 1p/19q codeletion {2157}.

Overall, anaplastic oligodendroglioma shows a slight male predominance, with a male-to-female ratio of 1.2:1 reported among 1650 patients {1863}. In the USA, anaplastic oligodendroglioma is more common in Whites than in Blacks, with an incidence ratio of 2.4:1 {1863}.

Etiology
See *Etiology* (p. 61) in *Oligodendroglioma, IDH-mutant and 1p/19q-codeleted.*

Localization
Anaplastic oligodendrogliomas and WHO grade II oligodendrogliomas share

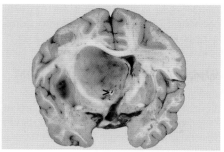

Fig. 1.68 Large, macroscopically well-delineated anaplastic oligodendroglioma of the left basal ganglia, compressing the adjacent lateral ventricle, with shift of midline structures towards the right hemisphere. The arrowhead points to a ventricular shunt.

a preference for the frontal lobe, followed by the temporal lobe. However, the tumours can also originate at other sites within the CNS, and there have been rare cases of spinal intramedullary anaplastic oligodendroglioma.

Clinical features
Patients with anaplastic oligodendroglioma commonly present with focal neurological deficits, signs of increased intracranial pressure, or cognitive deficits

{2616}. Seizures are also common but are less frequent than in patients with low-grade oligodendroglioma {933}. Anaplastic oligodendroglioma develops either de novo (typically with a short preoperative history) or by progression from a pre-existing WHO grade II oligodendroglioma. The mean time to progression from WHO grade II oligodendroglioma to WHO grade III anaplastic oligodendroglioma has been estimated at approximately 6–7 years {1446,1826}.

Imaging
Anaplastic oligodendrogliomas can show heterogeneous patterns, due to the variable presence of necrosis, cystic degeneration, intratumoural haemorrhages, and calcification. On CT and MRI, contrast enhancement is seen in most patients and can be either patchy or homogeneous {2616}. However, lack of contrast enhancement does not exclude anaplastic oligodendroglioma. Ring enhancement is less common in IDH-mutant and 1p/19q-codeleted anaplastic oligodendrogliomas than in malignant

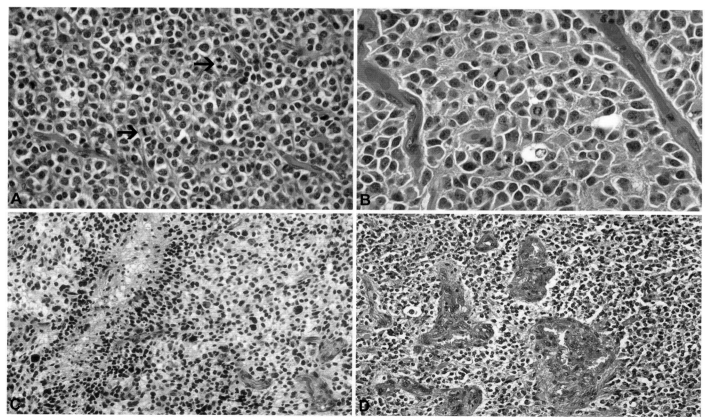

Fig. 1.69 Anaplastic oligodendroglioma. **A** Typical image of a cellular glioma with honeycomb cells and mitotic activity (arrows). **B** Marked nuclear atypia and brisk mitotic activity. **C** Focal necrosis with palisading tumour cells. **D** Marked microvascular proliferation.

gliomas, in particular glioblastomas without these molecular markers {345,2616}.

Macroscopy

The macroscopic features are similar to those of WHO grade II oligodendrogliomas, except that anaplastic oligodendrogliomas may show areas of tumour necrosis.

Microscopy

Anaplastic oligodendrogliomas are cellular, diffusely infiltrating gliomas that may show considerable morphological variation. The majority of the tumour cells typically demonstrate features that are reminiscent of oligodendroglial cells, i.e. rounded hyperchromatic nuclei, perinuclear haloes, and few cellular processes. Focal microcalcifications are often present. Mitotic activity is usually prominent, with one study suggesting a cut-off point of 6 mitoses per 10 high-power fields {830}. Occasional anaplastic oligodendrogliomas with 1p/19q codeletion are characterized by marked cellular pleomorphism, with multinucleated giant cells (called the polymorphic variant of Zülch) {1000}. Rare cases with sarcoma-like areas (called oligosarcoma) have also been observed {1004,2152}. Gliofibrillary oligodendrocytes and minigemistocytes are frequent in some anaplastic oligodendrogliomas {1374}. The characteristic vascular pattern of branching capillaries is often still recognizable, although pathological microvascular proliferation is usually prominent. Formation of secondary structures, in particular perineuronal satellitosis, is frequent in areas of cortical tumour infiltration. Anaplastic oligodendrogliomas may contain necrosis, including palisading necrosis resembling that of glioblastoma. However, as long as the tumour shows the IDH-mutant and 1p/19q-codeleted genotype, classification as

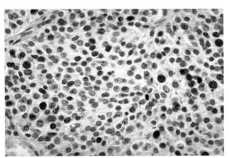

Fig. 1.70 Anaplastic oligodendroglioma. MIB1 immunohistochemistry shows high proliferative activity.

WHO grade III IDH-mutant and 1p/19q-codeleted anaplastic oligodendroglioma is appropriate. The presence of a conspicuous astrocytic component is also compatible with this diagnosis providing the tumour demonstrates IDH mutation and 1p/19q codeletion. However, in cases that cannot be conclusively tested for combined IDH mutation and 1p/19q codeletion, the presence of a conspicuous astrocytic component is not compatible with anaplastic oligodendroglioma, NOS (see *Anaplastic oligodendroglioma, NOS*, p. 74). Instead, classification as anaplastic oligoastrocytoma, NOS, or glioblastoma is more appropriate, depending on the absence or presence of necrosis.

Immunophenotype

Anaplastic oligodendrogliomas have the same immunoprofile as WHO grade II oligodendroglioma, except that proliferative activity, as most commonly determined by MIB1 immunostaining, is generally higher (i.e. MIB1-positive cells usually account for > 5% of the tumour cells). However, a definitive MIB1 cut-off point for distinction between WHO grade II and III oligodendrogliomas has not been established (see *Immunophenotype*, p. 64, in *Oligodendroglioma, IDH-mutant and 1p/19q-codeleted*).

Differential diagnosis

The differential diagnosis includes a variety of other clear cell tumour entities that can be distinguished by distinct immunohistochemical profiles and absence of combined IDH mutation and 1p/19q codeletion (see *Differential diagnosis*, p. 65, in *Oligodendroglioma, IDH-mutant and 1p/19q-codeleted*). Distinction of anaplastic oligodendroglioma from malignant small cell astrocytic tumours (including small cell glioblastoma) is of major importance, because malignant small cell astrocytic tumours behave much more aggressively, often with a clinical course typical of IDH-wildtype glioblastomas {1937}. Unlike IDH-mutant and 1p/19q-codeleted anaplastic oligodendrogliomas, small cell astrocytomas and glioblastomas lack combined IDH mutation and 1p/19q codeletion but often demonstrate *EGFR* amplification and chromosome 10 losses {1183,1937}.

Cell of origin

See *Cell of origin* (p. 65) in *Oligodendroglioma, IDH-mutant and 1p/19q-codeleted*.

Genetic profile

Cytogenetics

The hallmark cytogenetic alteration is combined whole-arm deletion of 1p and 19q, typically as a consequence of an unbalanced translocation between chromosomes 1 and 19 {887,1151}. Concurrent polysomy of 1p and 19q seems to be more common in anaplastic oligodendrogliomas than in low-grade oligodendrogliomas and has been associated with a higher Ki-67 proliferation index and less favourable clinical outcome {216,2748}. Molecular cytogenetic studies have identified various chromosomal abnormalities other than 1p/19q codeletion in anaplastic oligodendrogliomas; however, each was limited to only a small proportion of tumours. These include gains on chromosomes 7, 8q, 11q, 15q, and 20, as well as losses on chromosomes 4q, 6, 9p, 10q, 11, 13q, 18, and 22q {1084,1353, 2577}. Double-minute chromosomes, a cytogenetic hallmark of gene amplification, are rare {2537}, corresponding to

Table 1.07 Genetic profile of IDH-mutant and 1p/19q-codeleted anaplastic oligodendroglioma

Gene	Change	% of cases	References
IDH1/ IDH2	Mutation	100%	{349,2464}
1p/19q	Codeletion	100%	{349,2464}
TERT	Promoter mutation	> 95%	{349,2464}
MGMT	Promoter methylation	> 90%	{1733,2731}
CIC	Mutation	~60%	{349,2464}
CDKN2A/ p14ARF	LOH	~40%	{45A}
CDKN2A/ p14ARF	Promoter methylation	15–30%	{2702A,2779}
FUBP1	Mutation	~30%	{349,2464}
NOTCH1	Mutation	20–30%	{349,2464}
PIK3CA	Mutation	10–20%	{349,2464}
PIK3R1	Mutation	~9%	{349,2464}
TCF12	Mutation	7.5%	{1407}
ARID1A	Mutation	~7%	{349,2464}
CDKN2C	Homozygous deletion or mutation	< 5%	{1069,1993, 2464}

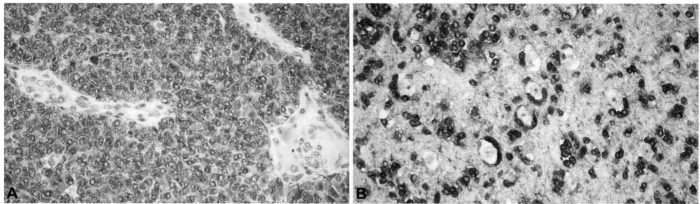

Fig. 1.71 Anaplastic oligodendroglioma. **A** R132H-mutant IDH1 stains tumour cells but is negative in blood vessels. **B** Cortical infiltration zone with tumour cells expressing R132H-mutant IDH1, including perineuronal satellitosis.

the low frequency of gene amplification detected in molecular profiling studies {2464,2731}.

Molecular genetics
As the entity name suggests, IDH mutation and 1p/19q codeletion are the defining genetic aberrations of IDH-mutant and 1p/19q-codeleted anaplastic oligodendroglioma. Promoter mutations in *TERT* are also present in the vast majority of these tumours, as is the case for IDH-mutant and 1p/19q-codeleted low-grade oligodendroglioma {89,1314, 1408,2464}. Investigation of regionally or spatially distinct tissue samples from individual patients has indicated that IDH mutation, 1p/19q codeletion, and *TERT* promoter mutation are early events in oligodendroglioma development that are shared by neoplastic cells from different tumour areas as well as between primary and recurrent tumours {2464}. As in low-grade oligodendroglioma, *CIC* mutation is frequent in anaplastic oligodendroglioma, whereas *FUBP1* mutation occurs in fewer cases. Other (less commonly) mutated genes include NOTCH pathway genes (in particular, *NOTCH1*), various epigenetic regulator genes (e.g. *SETD2*), and PI3K pathway genes (e.g. *PIK3CA*) {2464}. Mutations in the oligodendroglial lineage–associated transcription factor gene *TCF12* have been detected in a small subset (7.5%) of anaplastic oligodendrogliomas and are associated with an aggressive tumour type {1407}. Overall, the average number of chromosomes involved in copy number abnormalities is higher in anaplastic oligodendrogliomas than in low-grade oligodendrogliomas {1353,2160}. The *CDKN2A* and *CDKN2B* loci on 9p21 are altered in a subset of

anaplastic oligodendrogliomas due to homozygous deletion, mutation, or aberrant promoter methylation {666,1084,2779}. In isolated cases, homozygous deletion or mutation of the *CDKN2C* gene at 1p32 has been observed in tumours without *CDKN2A* deletions {1069,1993}. Losses of 10q, mutations of the *PTEN* tumour suppressor gene, and amplifications of proto-oncogenes are infrequent in IDH-mutant and 1p/19q-codeleted anaplastic oligodendrogliomas {666,1083,2246}. Epigenetically, these tumours are characterized by G-CIMP type A {2464} and often demonstrate a proneural glioblastoma-like expression profile. The *MGMT* promoter is typically hypermethylated {1733}.

Genetic susceptibility
See *Genetic susceptibility* (p. 67) in *Oligodendroglioma, IDH-mutant and 1p/19q-codeleted*.

Prognosis and predictive factors

Prognosis
Recent therapeutic advances have markedly improved survival times of patients with anaplastic oligodendrogliomas. Before the introduction of adjuvant treatment with combined radiochemotherapy, reported median survival times ranged from < 1 year {567} to 3.9 years {2337}. A population-based analysis from Switzerland reported a median survival time of 3.5 years for patients with anaplastic oligodendroglioma, which was markedly shorter than the median of 11.6 years for patients with WHO grade II oligodendroglioma {1826}. The CBTRUS calculated 5- and 10-year survival rates of 52.2% and 39.3%, respectively, for patients with

anaplastic oligodendroglioma {1863}. However, none of these data considered IDH mutation or 1p/19q codeletion status, which have been strongly associated with improved response to adjuvant radiotherapy/chemotherapy and longer survival {344,2615}. A retrospective analysis of 1013 adult patients with anaplastic oligodendroglial tumours found a median overall survival of 8.5 years in patients with 1p/19q-codeleted tumours, versus 3.7 years in patients with 1p/19q-intact tumours {1436}. Long-term follow-up data from the Radiation Therapy Oncology Group (RTOG) 9402 and European Organisation for Research and Treatment of Cancer (EORTC) 26951 trials indicate even higher median overall survival times (> 10 years) for patients with IDH-mutant and 1p/19q-codeleted anaplastic oligodendrogliomas who were treated with combined radiotherapy and PCV chemotherapy {344,2615}. Patients rarely develop cerebrospinal fluid spread or systemic metastases. Local tumour progression is the most common cause of death.

Predictive factors
Clinical factors that have been associated with longer survival are younger age at diagnosis, higher Karnofsky performance score, and greater extent of resection {1095,2617,2740}. Previous resection for lower-grade tumour has also been linked to more favourable prognosis {2621}. Recursive partitioning analysis of various clinical and histological parameters together with the 1p/19q codeletion status identified five distinct prognostic classes, defined mainly by patient age, tumour location, and 1p/19q status {1884}. A study based on the EORTC 26951 trial found a strong prognostic

impact of the Ki-67 proliferation index on univariate analysis but no independent influence on multivariate analysis {2034}. In addition to 1p/19q codeletion and IDH mutation, G-CIMP status and *MGMT* promoter methylation have been reported to provide prognostically relevant information for patients with anaplastic gliomas {2618,2619,2620,2740}. Long-term follow-up data from the RTOG 9402 and EORTC 26951 trials suggest not only a prognostic but also a predictive role of 1p/19q codeletion for long-term survival after aggressive multimodal treatment consisting of surgical resection followed by upfront combined radiotherapy and PCV chemotherapy {344,2615}. In the RTOG 9402 trial, patients with 1p/19q-codeleted anaplastic gliomas had median overall survival times of 14.7 years with radiotherapy plus PCV chemotherapy versus 7.3 years with radiotherapy alone. In the EORTC 26951 trial, median overall survival was not reached after > 10 years of follow-up in patients with 1p/19q-codeleted anaplastic gliomas treated by radiotherapy plus PCV chemotherapy versus 9.3 years in patients treated with radiotherapy alone. In both trials, patients with 1p/19q-intact tumours had significantly shorter overall survival in both treatment arms. These data indicate that molecular testing of anaplastic gliomas is important and can guide therapy {2730}.

Anaplastic oligodendroglioma, NOS

Definition

A diffusely infiltrating anaplastic glioma with classic oligodendroglial histology, in which molecular testing for combined IDH mutation and 1p/19q codeletion could not be completed or was inconclusive.

As with oligodendroglioma, NOS, immunohistochemical demonstration of IDH mutation (in particular *IDH1* R132H) and nuclear positivity for ATRX supports the diagnosis of an oligodendroglial tumour but cannot substitute for 1p/19q codeletion testing, because nuclear ATRX expression is retained in a subset of IDH-mutant but 1p/19q-intact anaplastic astrocytomas. Similarly, immunopositivity for alpha-internexin and loss of nuclear CIC or FUBP1 expression supports the diagnosis of anaplastic oligodendroglioma, NOS, but does not suffice for diagnosis of IDH-mutant and 1p/19q-codeleted anaplastic oligodendroglioma (see the box *Anaplastic oligodendroglioma lacking IDH mutation and 1p/19q codeletion*). The histological features of anaplastic oligodendroglioma, NOS, largely correspond to those described for IDH-mutant and 1p/19q-codeleted anaplastic oligodendroglioma. However, the presence of a conspicuous astrocytic component is not compatible with the diagnosis of anaplastic oligodendroglioma, NOS. Areas of necrosis, including palisading necrosis, are compatible with the diagnosis of anaplastic oligodendroglioma, NOS, provided the tumour shows the typical cytological characteristics and other histological hallmarks of oligodendroglioma, such as the branching capillary network and microcalcifications. However, the differential diagnosis of glioblastoma (WHO grade IV), in particular the small-cell variant, must be thoroughly considered in such cases, and is in fact more appropriate when IDH mutations are absent and genetic features of glioblastoma (such as gain of chromosome 7, loss of chromosome 10, and *EGFR* amplification) are detectable.

ICD-O code 9451/3

Grading

Anaplastic oligodendroglioma, NOS, corresponds histologically to WHO grade III.

Oligoastrocytoma, NOS

Reifenberger G.   Cairncross J.G.
Collins V.P.   Yokoo H.
Hartmann C.   Yip S.
Hawkins C.   Louis D.N.
Kros J.M.

Definition

A diffusely infiltrating, slow-growing glioma composed of a conspicuous mixture of two distinct neoplastic cell types morphologically resembling tumour cells with either oligodendroglial or astrocytic features, and in which molecular testing could not be completed or was inconclusive.

In oligoastrocytoma, NOS, tumour cells with oligodendroglial or astroglial features can be either diffusely intermingled or separated into distinct, biphasic areas. The mixed or ambiguous cellular differentiation precludes histological classification as either diffuse astrocytoma, NOS, or oligodendroglioma, NOS. Oligoastrocytoma, NOS, is an exceptional diagnosis, because most diffuse gliomas with mixed or ambiguous histology can be classified as either IDH-mutant diffuse astrocytoma or IDH-mutant and 1p/19q-codeleted oligodendroglioma, based on molecular testing. Oligoastrocytomas, NOS, usually manifest in adult patients, with preferential localization in the cerebral hemispheres.

Genetic classification of oligoastrocytomas

The WHO classification discourages the diagnosis of tumours as oligoastrocytoma or mixed glioma. Molecular genetic analyses have clearly shown that the vast majority of tumours previously classified as oligoastrocytomas have a genetic profile typical of either diffuse astrocytoma (i.e. IDH mutation combined with *TP53* mutation and *ATRX* mutation / loss of nuclear ATRX expression) or oligodendroglioma (i.e. IDH mutation combined with 1p/19q codeletion and *TERT* promoter mutation) {349,2220,2464}. The histological criteria provided in previous WHO classifications for oligoastrocytic gliomas left room for considerable interobserver variability {494,2611}. Thus, diffuse gliomas, including those with mixed or ambiguous histological features, should be

subjected to molecular testing for IDH mutation and 1p/19q codeletion. Tumours with combined IDH mutation and 1p/19q codeletion are classified as IDH-mutant and 1p/19q-codeleted oligodendroglioma, irrespective of a mixed or ambiguous histology. Tumours with IDH mutation but without 1p/19q codeletion are classified as IDH-mutant diffuse astrocytoma, also irrespective of mixed or ambiguous histology. Immunohistochemical testing for loss of nuclear ATRX expression may also provide diagnostically helpful information. Loss of ATRX positivity in the tumour cell nuclei but retained nuclear expression in non-neoplastic cells (e.g. vascular endothelia, reactive astrocytes, and activated microglial cells) supports the diagnosis of IDH-mutant diffuse astrocytoma {2105,2220}. Similarly, strong nuclear immunopositivity for p53, typically as a consequence of *TP53* mutation leading to nuclear accumulation of mutant p53 protein, is often associated with loss of nuclear ATRX expression and is virtually mutually exclusive with 1p/19q codeletion {2220}. Recent data support a diagnostic algorithm for diffuse and anaplastic gliomas based on stepwise analyses starting with immunohistochemistry for ATRX and R132H-mutant IDH1, followed by testing for 1p/19q codeletion, and then followed by IDH sequencing of the tumours that were negative for R132H-mutant IDH1 {2105}. With this approach, the vast majority of diffuse and anaplastic gliomas can be assigned to one of three major glioma classes: IDH-mutant diffuse astrocytomas, IDH-mutant and 1p/19q-codeleted oligodendrogliomas, or IDH-wildtype gliomas (including IDH-wildtype glioblastomas). Overall, the diagnosis of oligoastrocytoma, NOS, should therefore remain exceptional (i.e. restricted to diffuse gliomas in which histology does not allow for unequivocal stratification into either astrocytic or oligodendroglial lineage tumours and that cannot be subjected to appropriate molecular testing or in which molecular findings are inconclusive).

ICD-O code   9382/3

Grading

Oligoastrocytoma, NOS, corresponds histologically to WHO grade II.

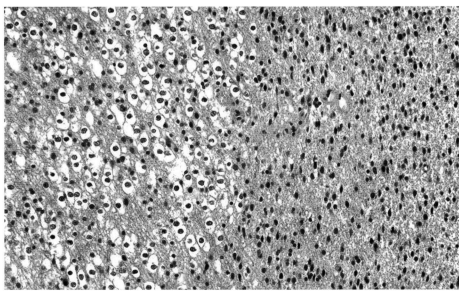

Fig. 1.72 Oligoastrocytoma. Clearly separated tumour areas displaying oligodendroglial (left) and astrocytic (right) differentiation.

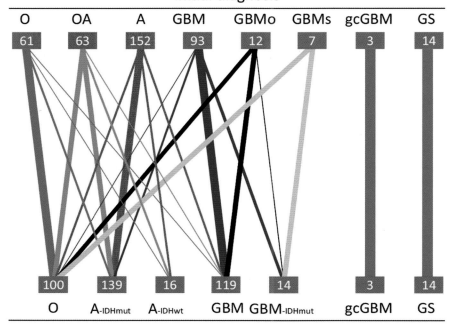

initial diagnosis

O 61 · OA 63 · A 152 · GBM 93 · GBMo 12 · GBMs 7 · gcGBM 3 · GS 14

O 100 · A-IDHmut 139 · A-IDHwt 16 · GBM 119 · GBM-IDHmut 14 · gcGBM 3 · GS 14

integrated diagnosis

Fig. 1.73 Changes from initial (purely histology-based) to integrated diagnosis in 405 adult patients with supratentorial glioma. Width of bars indicates relative proportions of the initial tumour groups. A, astrocytoma; OA, oligoastrocytoma; O, oligodendroglioma; GBM, glioblastoma; GBMo, glioblastoma with oligodendroglial component; GBMs, secondary glioblastoma; gcGBM, giant cell glioblastoma; GS, gliosarcoma. Note that all oligoastrocytomas were redistributed to other diagnoses (IDH-mutant and 1p/19q-codeleted oligodendroglioma, IDH-mutant astrocytoma, IDH-wildtype astrocytoma, or IDH-wildtype glioblastoma) after molecular marker analysis, including IDH mutation / G-CIMP, ATRX loss of nuclear expression, 1p/19q codeletion, and 7p gain / 10q loss. Reprinted from Reuss DE et al. {2105}.

Anaplastic oligoastrocytoma, NOS

Definition

An oligoastrocytoma, NOS, with focal or diffuse histological features of anaplasia, including increased cellularity, nuclear atypia, pleomorphism, and brisk mitotic activity.

Anaplastic oligoastrocytoma, NOS, is an exceptional diagnosis, because most high-grade gliomas with mixed or ambiguous histology can be classified as either IDH-mutant anaplastic astrocytoma or IDH-mutant and 1p/19q-codeleted anaplastic oligodendroglioma, based on molecular testing. Moreover, if molecular testing of an anaplastic glioma with mixed or ambiguous histology shows an IDH-wildtype status, IDH-wildtype glioblastoma must be considered as a likely differential diagnosis, because most IDH-wildtype anaplastic gliomas have genetic profiles of glioblastoma and are associated with correspondingly poor prognosis. Anaplastic oligoastrocytomas, NOS, usually manifest in adult patients, with preferential localization in the cerebral hemispheres.

ICD-O code   9382/3

Grading

Anaplastic oligoastrocytoma, NOS, corresponds histologically to WHO grade III.

Oligoastrocytoma, dual-genotype

Dual-genotype oligoastrocytoma is not considered to be a distinct entity or variant in the WHO classification. The designation refers to an IDH-mutant oligoastrocytoma of WHO grade II that is composed of a conspicuous mixture of astrocytic and oligodendroglial tumour cell populations demonstrating molecular evidence of an astrocytic genotype (i.e. IDH mutation combined with *TP53* mutation / nuclear p53 accumulation, loss of nuclear ATRX expression, and lack of 1p/19q codeletion) and an oligodendroglial genotype (i.e. IDH mutation combined with 1p/19q codeletion, lack of *TP53* mutation / nuclear p53 accumulation, and retained nuclear ATRX expression). Studies have revealed shared genetic alterations, including 1p/19q codeletion, in the oligodendroglial and astrocytic tumour components of the vast majority of oligoastrocytomas {1359, 2050}. However, a few instances of oligoastrocytoma showing evidence of genetically distinct oligodendroglial and astrocytic cell populations have been reported {1067,2050,2754}. It can be assumed that dual-genotype oligoastrocytomas are monoclonal tumours that arise from an IDH-mutant cell of origin but later during tumorigenesis develop cytologically distinct subpopulations of tumour cells with an astrocytic genotype (i.e. *TP53* and *ATRX* alteration but no 1p/19q codeletion) or an oligodendroglial genotype (i.e. 1p/19q codeletion but no *TP53* or *ATRX* alteration). Classification of dual-genotype oligoastrocytoma therefore requires detailed molecular and immunohistochemical analyses to unequivocally demonstrate the two genetically distinct tumour cell subpopulations. Care must be taken to avoid misinterpretations (e.g. due to artefactually negative nuclear immunostaining for ATRX) and false-positive detection of 1p/19q-codeleted nuclei by FISH (e.g. due to incomplete chromosomal representation in transected nuclei, aneuploidy/polyploidy, or partial hybridization failure) {763}. Overall, dual-genotype oligoastrocytoma seems to be very rare, but its true incidence is difficult to ascertain because tissue sampling is rarely comprehensive in diffuse gliomas and molecular analysis of DNA extracted from a bulk sample may not detect such molecular heterogeneity.

Genetic classification of anaplastic oligoastrocytomas

The WHO classification discourages the diagnosis of tumours as anaplastic oligoastrocytoma or anaplastic mixed glioma. Molecular genetic analyses have not demonstrated entity-specific genetic or epigenetic profiles for these tumours. Instead, large-scale molecular profiling studies have shown that the vast majority of anaplastic oligoastrocytomas have genetic alterations and DNA methylation profiles typical of either IDH-mutant anaplastic astrocytoma (with commonly associated TP53 mutation and ATRX mutation / loss of nuclear ATRX expression) or IDH-mutant and 1p/19q-codeleted anaplastic oligodendrogliomas (with commonly associated TERT promoter mutations). A third, smaller subset of cases correspond to IDH-wildtype anaplastic gliomas, which commonly demonstrate hallmark genetic aberrations of glioblastoma – in particular, gain of chromosome 7 and loss of chromosome 10 combined with TERT promoter mutation and gene amplifications (such as EGFR amplification) {349,2464,2731,2751}. The criteria provided in previous WHO classifications for anaplastic oligoastrocytoma left room for considerable interobserver variability {1370,2611}. Thus, anaplastic gliomas,

Anaplastic oligoastrocytoma, dual-genotype

Dual-genotype anaplastic oligoastrocytoma is not considered to be a distinct entity or variant in the WHO classification. The designation refers to an IDH-mutant anaplastic oligoastrocytoma of WHO grade III that demonstrates molecular evidence of genetically distinct astrocytic and oligodendroglial tumour cell populations characterized by an astrocytic genotype (i.e. IDH mutation combined with TP53 mutation / nuclear p53 accumulation, loss of nuclear ATRX expression, and lack of 1p/19q codeletion) and an oligodendroglial genotype (i.e. IDH mutation combined with 1p/19q codeletion, lack of TP53 mutation / nuclear p53 accumulation, and retained nuclear ATRX expression). To date, only isolated cases of tumours considered to be dual-genotype anaplastic oligoastrocytoma have been reported {1067, 2754}. These tumours occurred in the cerebral hemispheres of adult patients. Utmost care must be taken to exclude technical shortcomings that may lead to artefactual regional variation in immunohistochemical staining for ATRX or in FISH analysis for 1p/19q codeletion.

including those with a mixed or ambiguous histological phenotype, should be subjected to thorough molecular testing, most notably for IDH mutation and 1p/19q codeletion. As with oligoastrocytoma, NOS, immunohistochemical testing for loss of nuclear ATRX expression and nuclear accumulation of p53 may provide additional, diagnostically helpful information {2105,2220}. This integrated approach enables a clear diagnostic stratification of the vast majority of anaplastic gliomas into one of the three major classes: IDH-mutant anaplastic astrocytomas, IDH-mutant and 1p/19q-codeleted anaplastic oligodendrogliomas, or IDH-wildtype anaplastic gliomas (most of which are characterized by glioblastoma-associated genetic profiles and the associated poor prognosis). Overall, the diagnosis of anaplastic oligoastrocytoma, NOS, should therefore remain exceptional, i.e. restricted to anaplastic gliomas with astrocytic and oligodendroglial components that cannot be subjected to appropriate molecular testing or in which molecular findings are inconclusive.

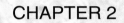

CHAPTER 2

Other astrocytic tumours
Pilocytic astrocytoma
Pilomyxoid astrocytoma
Subependymal giant cell astrocytoma
Pleomorphic xanthoastrocytoma
Anaplastic pleomorphic xanthoastrocytoma

Pilocytic astrocytoma

Collins V.P.
Tihan T.
VandenBerg S.R.
Burger P.C.
Hawkins C.

Jones D.
Giannini C.
Rodriguez F.
Figarella-Branger D.

Definition

An astrocytoma classically characterized by a biphasic pattern with variable proportions of compacted bipolar cells with Rosenthal fibres and loose, textured multipolar cells with microcysts and occasional granular bodies.

Genetically, pilocytic astrocytomas are characterized by the presence of mutations in genes coding for proteins involved in the MAPK pathway {1176,2855}. The most frequent genetic change is tandem duplication of 7q34 involving the *BRAF* gene resulting in oncogenic BRAF fusion proteins. Pilocytic astrocytomas are the most common glioma in children and adolescents, and affect males slightly more often than females. They are preferentially located in the cerebellum and cerebral midline structures (i.e. the optic pathways, hypothalamus, and brain stem) but can be encountered anywhere along the neuraxis {1533}. They are generally circumscribed and slow-growing, and may be cystic. Pilocytic astrocytoma largely behaves as is typical of a WHO grade I tumour {1533}, and patients can be cured by surgical resection. However, complete resection may not be possible in some locations, such as the optic pathways and the hypothalamus. Pilocytic astrocytomas, particularly those involving the optic pathways, are a hallmark of neurofibromatosis type 1 (NF1).

Pilomyxoid astrocytoma is considered to be a variant of pilocytic astrocytoma.

ICD-O code   9421/1

Grading

Pilocytic astrocytoma corresponds histologically to WHO grade I.

Epidemiology

Pilocytic astrocytoma accounts for 5.4% of all gliomas {1826}. According to a 2007–2011 statistical report from the Central Brain Tumor Registry of the United States (CBTRUS), pilocytic astrocytoma is most common during the first two decades of life, with an average annual age-adjusted incidence rate of 0.84 cases per 100 000 population, which declines substantially from ≤ 14 years to 15–19 years {1863}. Pilocytic astrocytoma is the most common glioma in children, without a significant sex predilection. It accounts for 33.2% of all gliomas in the 0–14 years age group {1862} and 17.6% of all childhood primary brain tumours {1863}. Similarly, in a study of 1195 paediatric tumours from a single institution, pilocytic astrocytoma was the single most common tumour (accounting for 18% of cases overall) in the cerebral compartment {2174}. In adults, pilocytic astrocytoma tends to appear about a decade earlier (mean patient age: 22 years) than does WHO grade II diffuse astrocytoma {784}, but relatively few arise in patients aged > 50 years.

Localization

Pilocytic astrocytomas arise throughout the neuraxis; however, in the paediatric population, more tumours arise in the infratentorial region. Preferred sites include the optic nerve (optic nerve glioma) {1054}, optic chiasm/hypothalamus {2159}, thalamus and basal ganglia {1622}, cerebral hemispheres {725,1994}, cerebellum (cerebellar astrocytoma) {974}, and brain stem (dorsal exophytic brain stem glioma) {311,709,1995}. Pilocytic astrocytomas of the spinal cord are less frequent but not uncommon {1677, 2186}. Large hypothalamic, thalamic, and brain stem lesions may be predominantly

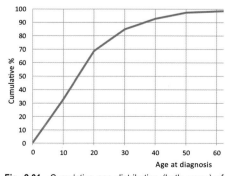

Fig. 2.01 Cumulative age distribution (both sexes) of pilocytic astrocytomas, based on biopsies from 205 patients treated at the University Hospital Zurich {1533}.

intraventricular and their site of origin difficult to define.

Clinical features

Pilocytic astrocytomas produce focal neurological deficits or non-localizing signs, such as macrocephaly, headache, endocrinopathy, and increased intracranial pressure due to mass effect or ventricular obstruction. Seizures are uncommon because the lesions involve the cerebral cortex infrequently {466, 725}. Given their slow rate of growth, pilocytic tumours' clinical presentation is generally that of a slowly evolving lesion. Pilocytic astrocytomas of the optic pathways often produce visual loss. Proptosis may be seen with intraorbital examples. Early, radiologically detected lesions may not be associated with visual symptoms or ophthalmological deficits {1054,1515}. Hypothalamic/pituitary dysfunction, including obesity and diabetes insipidus, is often apparent in patients with large hypothalamic tumours {2159}. Some hypothalamic/chiasmatic lesions in young children have been associated with leptomeningeal seeding and a poor outcome {1934}; see *Pilomyxoid astrocytoma* (p. 88), a variant of pilocytic astrocytoma. Pilocytic astrocytomas of the thalamus generally present with signs of cerebrospinal fluid obstruction or neurological deficits (such as hemiparesis) due to internal capsule compression. Cerebellar pilocytic astrocytomas usually present during the first two decades of life, with clumsiness, worsening headache, nausea, and vomiting. Brain stem examples most often cause hydrocephalus or signs of brain stem dysfunction. Unlike diffuse astrocytoma of the pons, which produces symmetrical so-called pontine hypertrophy, pilocytic tumours of the brain stem are usually dorsal and exophytic into the cerebellopontine angle. Spinal cord examples produce non-specific signs of an expanding mass {1678, 2074,2186}.

Imaging

Most cerebellar and cerebral pilocytic

astrocytomas are well demarcated, with a round or oval shape and smooth margins. Calcifications are occasionally present. Heterogeneity as a result of cyst-like areas intermixed with generally intensely enhancing soft tissue components is typical. Consistent with the tumour's low biological activity, surrounding vasogenic oedema (if present) is much less extensive than in higher-grade glial neoplasms. About two thirds of cases manifest as a cyst-like mass with an enhancing mural nodule; the other third present either as a cyst-like mass with a central non-enhancing zone or as a predominantly solid mass with a minimal or no cyst-like portion {474,1927}. In those with a cyst-like morphology, the cyst wall may or may not enhance {165}, and cyst wall enhancement may or may not indicate tumour involvement {165}. Occasional atypical imaging features of these tumours include multiple cyst-like masses and haemorrhage.

Most optic nerve gliomas are pilocytic astrocytomas, and characteristically manifest as a kinked or buckled enlargement of the optic nerve. Tumours in this location often have different imaging appearances depending on whether the patient has NF1. NF1-associated tumours more commonly affect the optic nerve, rarely extend beyond the optic pathway, and are usually not cyst-like, whereas those not associated with NF1 usually involve the optic chiasm, extend extraoptically, and are frequently cyst-like {1342}.

Spread

Otherwise typical pilocytic astrocytomas very occasionally seed the neuraxis, on rare occasions even before the primary tumour is detected {775,1934,1996}. The proliferation rate in such cases varies, but is usually low {1681}. Therefore, this atypical behaviour of pilocytic astrocytoma cannot be predicted. The hypothalamus is usually the primary site. Neuraxis seeding does not necessarily indicate future aggressive growth; both the primary lesion and the implants may grow only slowly {775,1681,1996}. The implants may be asymptomatic, and long-term survival is possible, even without adjuvant treatment {1996}. The pilomyxoid astrocytoma variant (see *Pilomyxoid astrocytoma*, p. 88), typically occurring in the hypothalamic region, more often undergoes craniospinal spread {2555}.

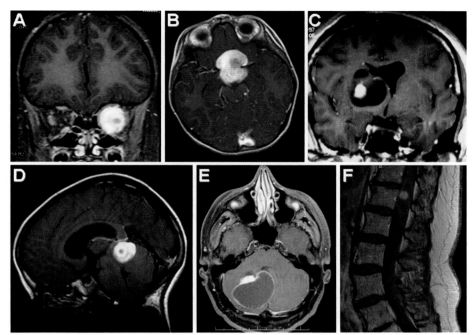

Fig. 2.02 Most pilocytic astrocytomas are strongly and diffusely enhancing. **A** Left optic nerve. **B** Hypothalamic. **C** Basal ganglia. **D** Tectal. **E** Cerebellar. **F** Spinal. Some tumours are solid (A, B, D) and others are cystic with an enhancing mural nodule (C, E, F).

Macroscopy

Most pilocytic astrocytomas are soft, grey, and relatively discrete. Intratumoural or paratumoural cyst formation is common, including with a mural tumour nodule. In spinal cord examples, syrinx formation may extend over many segments {1678}. Chronic lesions may be calcified or may stain with haemosiderin. Optic nerve tumours often circumferentially involve the subarachnoid space {2427}.

Microscopy

This astrocytic tumour of low to moderate cellularity often has a biphasic pattern, with varying proportions of compacted bipolar cells with Rosenthal fibres and loose-textured multipolar cells with microcysts. The biphasic pattern is best seen in cerebellar tumours. However, pilocytic astrocytoma can exhibit a wide range of tissue patterns, sometimes several within the same lesion. A variant of the compact, piloid pattern occurs when

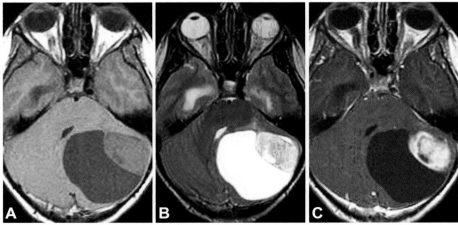

Fig. 2.03 Cerebellar pilocytic astrocytoma. **A** Axial T1-weighted MRI shows a left cerebellar cyst-like mass with slightly hyperintense mural nodule along its lateral margin. **B** Axial T2-weighted MRI shows hyperintensity of the cyst-like portion of the mass with lower signal intensity of the mural nodule. **C** Postcontrast axial T1-weighted MRI shows heterogeneous intense enhancement of the mural nodule.

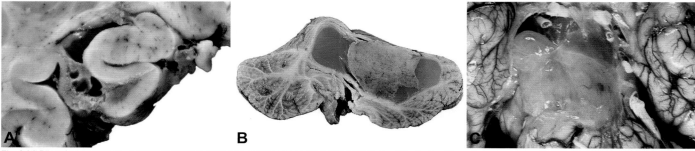

Fig. 2.04 Pilocytic astrocytoma. **A** Diffuse infiltration of the hippocampus and neighbouring structures. Note the focal formation of cysts. **B** Large, partially cystic pilocytic astrocytoma of the cerebellum with a typical mural nodule {882}. **C** Large pilocytic astrocytoma extending into the basal cisterns.

the elongated cells are less compact but separated by mucin. In such cases, individual cell processes can be seen, and cell shape varies to include more full-bodied and pleomorphic, less obviously piloid cells. A distinctive lobular pattern results when leptomeningeal involvement induces a desmoplastic reaction. At this site, tissue texture varies but Rosenthal fibres are usually abundant. Rare mitoses, hyperchromatic and pleomorphic nuclei, glomeruloid vascular proliferation, infarct-like necrosis, and infiltration of leptomeninges are compatible with the diagnosis of pilocytic astrocytoma and are not signs of malignancy.

Due to the heterogeneity of histological features, smear preparations of pilocytic astrocytomas show considerable cytological variation, and basic cytological patterns are often present in combination. Compact portions of the tumour yield bipolar piloid cells; long, hair-like processes that often extend across a full microscopic field; and Rosenthal fibres. Nuclei are typically elongated and cytologically bland. Due to their high content of refractile eosinophilic fibrils, these cells are strongly immunopositive for GFAP. Cells derived from microcystic areas have round to oval, cytologically bland nuclei; a small cell body; and relatively short, cobweb-like processes that are fibril-poor and only weakly positive for GFAP. This growth pattern may be associated with eosinophilic granular bodies. Cells indistinguishable from those of diffuse astrocytoma may populate peripheral, more infiltrative areas. Cells closely resembling oligodendrocytes are typically less frequent {480}, but can constitute a dominant component in some cases, particularly in the cerebellum. These cells strongly express OLIG2 {481}, although other tissue patterns may express OLIG2 as well. With the cells arranged in sheets or dispersed within parenchyma, the overall appearance may resemble that of an oligodendroglioma, particularly in a limited sample. The finding of foci of classic pilocytic astrocytoma usually enables the correct classification of such lesions. Regimented palisades (a so-called spongioblastoma pattern) are a striking feature in some pilocytic astrocytomas.

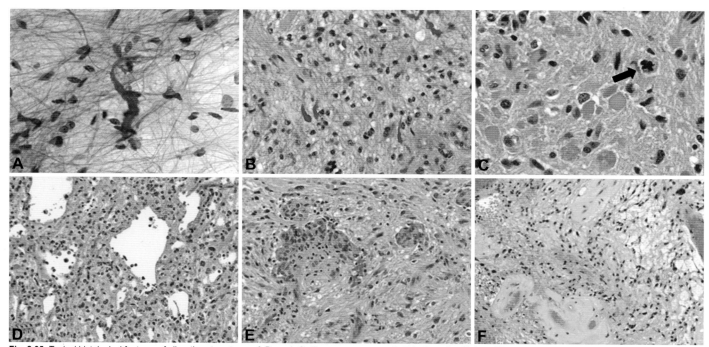

Fig. 2.05 Typical histological features of pilocytic astrocytoma. **A** Densely fibrillary areas composed of bipolar cells with long thin processes and rich in Rosenthal fibres as seen on intraoperative cytological smears and (**B**) on histological sections. **C** Eosinophilic granular bodies. Neoplastic cell nuclei are hyperchromatic. A rare mitotic figure is present (arrow). **D** Loosely arranged microcystic areas. **E** Pilocytic astrocytoma is typically a highly vascular tumour and shows both glomeruloid vessels and (**F**) thick-walled hyalinized vessels. The vascular changes correlate with the frequent presence of contrast enhancement on imaging.

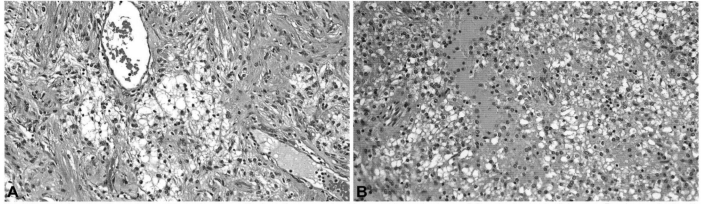

Fig. 2.06 Pilocytic astrocytoma. **A** Typical biphasic pattern with alternating compact and loose architectural patterns. **B** Pseudo-oligodendroglial pattern. Regular round cells with rounded nuclei and occasional microcystic changes.

Although many pilocytic astrocytomas are benign, some show considerable hyperchromasia and pleomorphism. Rare mitoses are present, but brisk mitotic activity, in particular diffuse brisk mitotic activity, characterizes anaplastic change, which has prognostic implications {2150} (see p. 88). In occasional (often cerebellar) tumours, a diffuse growth pattern overshadows more typical compact and microcystic features. In such cases, the presence of hyperchromatic nuclei or mitotic figures can cause confusion with high-grade diffuse astrocytoma. Less worrisome are obvious degenerative atypia with pleomorphism and nuclear–cytoplasmic pseudoinclusions, frequently seen in long-standing lesions. Multiple nuclei within large or giant cells are localized circumferentially (called a pennies-on-a-plate arrangement) {974}. Hyalinized and glomeruloid vessels are prominent features of some cases. Any necrosis is often infarct-like and non-palisading. Perivascular lymphocytes may also occur. Because pilocytic astrocytomas overrun normal tissue to some

extent, pre-existing neurons are sometimes trapped, and some lesions even demonstrate limited cytological atypia. Such lesions should be distinguished from ganglion cell tumours. The pilomyxoid variant (see *Pilomyxoid astrocytoma*, p. 88) is characterized by uniform bipolar cells in a myxoid background and frequent perivascular arrangements. Sometimes this pattern is associated with more conventional pilocytic regions or so-called intermediate tumours {1168}. Although astrocytomas in children are usually classified as either the pilocytic or the diffuse type, many cases do not in fact fit clearly into either category on the basis of histology alone. Increasingly, molecular profiling plays an ancillary role in this distinction. In some cases, small biopsy size contributes to difficulties in classification, especially in cases with a brain stem or spinal location.

Rosenthal fibres

These tapered, rounded, or corkscrew-shaped, brightly eosinophilic, hyaline masses are intracytoplasmic in location,

a property best seen in smear preparations. Rosenthal fibres are most common in compact, piloid tissue. They appear bright blue on Luxol fast blue staining. Although helpful in diagnosis, their presence is not obligatory, and they are neither specific to pilocytic astrocytoma nor indicative of neoplasia. They are often seen in ganglioglioma and are a common finding in chronic reactive gliosis. Densely fibrillar, paucicellular lesions containing Rosenthal fibres are as likely to be reactive gliosis as pilocytic astrocytoma. Ultrastructurally, Rosenthal fibres lie within astrocytic processes and consist of amorphous, electron-dense elements surrounded by intermediate (glial) filaments {588}. Being composed of alpha-B-crystallin {862}, they lack GFAP immunoreactivity except in their fibril-rich periphery.

Eosinophilic granular bodies

Eosinophilic granular bodies form globular aggregates within astrocytic processes. They are brightly eosinophilic in H&E sections, periodic acid–Schiff–positive,

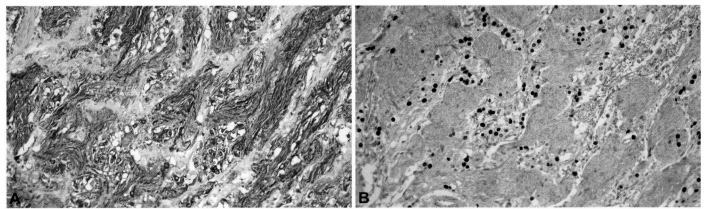

Fig. 2.07 Biphasic pilocytic astrocytoma. **A** Cells in fibrillary areas strongly express GFAP. **B** OLIG2 expression is restricted to pseudo-oligodendroglial cells.

and immunoreactive for alpha-1-antichymotrypsin and alpha-1-antitrypsin {1236}. Although eosinophilic granular bodies may be present in pilocytic astrocytoma, they are more frequent in other glial or glioneuronal neoplasms, in particular ganglion cell tumours and pleomorphic xanthoastrocytomas.

Vasculature
Pilocytic astrocytomas are highly vascular, as evidenced by their contrast enhancement {761}. Although generally obvious in H&E sections, this vascularity is accentuated on immunostains for markers of basement membrane (e.g. collagen IV and laminin) and endothelial cells (e.g. CD31 and CD34). This glomeruloid vasculature may also line tumoural cyst walls and is occasionally seen at some distance from the lesion, but this should not prompt tumour misclassification or overgrading. There may be structural and biological differences from similar vessels occurring in glioblastomas, with the microvasculature of glioblastomas exhibiting a looser, more disorganized architecture and differences in expression of angiogenesis-related genes {1727}.

Regressive changes
Given the indolent nature and often slow clinical evolution of pilocytic astrocytomas, it is not surprising that regressive features are common. Markedly hyalinized, sometimes ectatic vessels are one such feature. When neoplastic cells are scant, it can be difficult to distinguish these tumours from cavernous angiomas with accompanying piloid gliosis. Evidence of previous haemorrhage (haemosiderin) increases the resemblance. Presentation with acute haemorrhage is infrequent. Calcification, infarct-like necrosis, and lymphocytic infiltrates are additional regressive changes. Overall, calcification is an infrequent finding, and is only rarely present in optic nerve or hypothalamic/thalamic tumours or in superficially situated cerebral examples. Cysts are a common feature of pilocytic astrocytoma, especially in the locations specified above. Neovascularity often lines cyst walls, resulting in a narrow band of intense contrast enhancement at the circumference of some cysts. Dense piloid tissue with accompanying Rosenthal fibres external to this vascular layer is sometimes seen. When this layer is narrow and well demarcated from the surrounding normal tissue, it can be assumed to be reactive in nature. In other instances, the glial zone is more prominent, less demarcated, and neoplastic.

Growth pattern
Typically, pilocytic astrocytomas are macroscopically somewhat discrete. Thus, when the anatomical site permits (e.g. in the cerebellum or cerebral hemispheres), many can be removed in toto {725,974,1994}. Microscopically, however, many lesions are not well defined with respect to surrounding brain. Lesions typically permeate parenchyma for distances of millimetres to several centimetres, often entrapping normal neurons in the process. However, pilocytic tumours are relatively solid compared with diffuse gliomas, and do not aggressively overrun surrounding tissue. This property, evidenced by at least partial lack of axons on Bodian or Bielschowsky silver impregnations, and NFP immunostains, is of diagnostic value. Pilocytic astrocytomas of the optic nerve and chiasm differ somewhat in their macroscopic and microscopic patterns of growth; they are often less circumscribed and therefore difficult to delineate either macroscopically or microscopically. They share the same propensity for leptomeningeal involvement as seen in pilocytic tumours at other sites, but are somewhat more diffuse, especially within the optic nerve. This is particularly evident when pathologists attempt to determine the extent of a lesion by analysis of sequential nerve

Table 2.01 Genetic alterations affecting the MAPK pathway in pilocytic astrocytomas and their diagnostic utility; adapted from Collins VP et al. {482}

Gene	Change	% of tumours	Diagnostic utility	References
BRAF and *KIAA1549*	Tandem duplications resulting in KIAA1549-BRAF fusion proteins, all having the BRAF kinase domain and with the BRAF N-terminal regulatory domain replaced by the N-terminal end of KIAA1549	> 70%	Common in pilocytic astrocytomas, particularly cerebellar; rare in other tumour forms	{1176,1178,2855}
BRAF and various other genes	Deletions or translocations resulting in BRAF fusion proteins, all having the BRAF kinase domain and with the BRAF regulatory domain replaced by the N-terminal part of another gene	~5%	Occur in pilocytic astrocytomas; extremely rare in other entities	{1176,2855}
BRAF	V600E mutation	~5%	Occurs mainly in supratentorial pilocytic astrocytomas; also in gangliogliomas, pleomorphic xanthoastrocytomas, and dysembryoplastic neuroepithelial tumours	{1176,2855}
NF1	Loss of wild type and retained inherited mutation	~8%	Typically germline; closely associated with optic pathway pilocytic astrocytoma	{1176,2855}
FGFR1	Mutation	< 5%	Found mainly in midline pilocytic astrocytomas; frequency not established in other entities	{1176,2855}
FGFR1	Fusions / internal tandem duplication	< 5%	Rare in pilocytic astrocytoma; also observed in other low-grade gliomas	{1176,2855}
NTRK family	Fusions	~2%	Rare in pilocytic astrocytoma; frequency not established in other entities	{1176,2855}
KRAS	Mutation	Single cases	Rare in pilocytic astrocytoma; frequency not established in other entities	{1176,2855}
RAF1	Fusions with consequences similar to those of BRAF fusions, i.e. the loss of the regulatory domain and its replacement by the N-terminal end of SGRAP3	Single cases	Rare in pilocytic astrocytoma; frequency not established in other entities	{1176,2855}

margins. Microscopically, the lesion can be followed to a point beyond which it becomes less cellular, but there is no clearly defined termination.

There has been considerable discussion regarding the existence of a diffuse variant of pilocytic astrocytoma, particularly in the cerebellum {847,974,1882}. Although some such cases are simply classic pilocytic tumours in which the infiltrative edge is somewhat broader than expected or an artefact of plane of section, there are also occasional distinctly infiltrative lesions that mimic diffuse fibrillary astrocytoma, even in large specimens. In two large studies, the outcomes for children with so-called diffuse pilocytic astrocytoma of the cerebellum were favourable, supporting the idea that such tumours belong to the spectrum of pilocytic astrocytoma {974,1882}. True infiltrating diffuse astrocytomas account for as many as 15% of all astrocytic tumours of the cerebellum, but most are high-grade (i.e. WHO grade III or IV) {974}.

Infiltration of the meninges

Involvement of the subarachnoid space is common in pilocytic astrocytoma. It is not indicative of aggressive or malignant behaviour and does not portend subarachnoid dissemination; rather, it is a characteristic and even diagnostically helpful feature. Leptomeningeal invasion can occur at any tumour site, but is particularly common in the cerebellum and optic nerve. The leptomeningeal component may be reticulin-rich, more commonly in the optic nerve than in the cerebellum. Another typical pattern of extraparenchymal spread is extension into perivascular spaces.

Anaplastic transformation (pilocytic astrocytoma with anaplasia)

As a group, pilocytic astrocytomas are remarkable in that they maintain their WHO grade I {325} status over years and even decades. The alterations that occur over time are typically in the direction of regressive change rather than anaplasia. One large study found the acquisition of atypia (in particular increased cellularity, nuclear abnormalities, and occasional mitoses) to be of no prognostic significance {2565}. In a subsequent series, anaplasia in pilocytic astrocytoma was found to occur primarily in the form of diffuse, brisk mitotic activity (usually > 4 mitoses per 10 high-power fields), with or

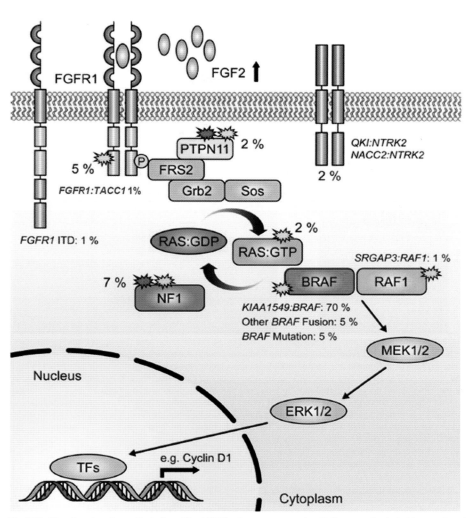

Fig. 2.08 Pilocytic astrocytoma. Illustration of the MAPK pathway components with the approximate incidence rates of the various mutations found in a series of pilocytic astrocytomas. Adapted by permission from Jones DTW et al. {1176}.

without necrosis {2150}. Tumours with these features should not be designated glioblastoma, because their prognosis is not uniformly grim. In general, the presence of necrosis in pilocytic astrocytomas with anaplasia is associated with a better prognosis than in classic cohorts of glioblastoma. The diagnosis of pilocytic astrocytoma with anaplasia may be preferable. Many such tumours had previously been irradiated {591,2565}, and therefore radiation therapy may be a factor promoting anaplastic change in some cases. However, pilocytic astrocytomas with anaplasia (including cases that develop in the setting of NF1) also occur in patients without prior irradiation {2150}. Grading criteria and nomenclature for these tumours are yet to be defined. Molecular studies, although limited, have demonstrated *BRAF* duplications

in a subset of these tumours, particularly those developing in the cerebellum {2145}, as well as absence of the R132H-mutant IDH1 protein. In the future, comprehensive molecular characterization will facilitate a more objective distinction from morphologically similar high-grade gliomas. In a recent study of 886 cases of paediatric low-grade glioma, with long clinical follow-up, there were no patients with the *KIAA1549-BRAF* fusion who underwent anaplastic transformation and died of their disease {1683}.

Immunophenotype

Pilocytic astrocytomas are well-differentiated gliomas of the astrocytic lineage, and strongly express GFAP, S100, and OLIG2 {1865}. Synaptophysin may demonstrate partial or weak reactivity, which should not be interpreted as evidence for

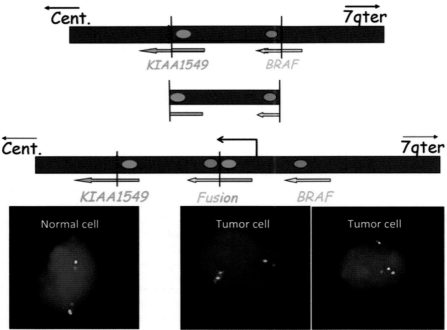

Fig. 2.09 Pilocytic astrocytoma: the development of the *KIAA1549-BRAF* fusion gene. The upper black box represents 7q34. Both *KIAA1549* and *BRAF* read towards the centromere (cent.). A fragment of approximately 2 Mb is duplicated (involving parts of both genes) and inserted at the break point, producing tandem duplication and fusion between the 5' end of *KIAA1549* and the 3' end of the *BRAF* gene (which codes for the kinase domain). The fusion gene thus codes for the BRAF kinase domain together with the N-terminal part of KIAA1549, replacing the BRAF regulatory domain. The red and green dots show the location of FISH probes that can be used to identify the occurrence of the tandem duplication, as demonstrated in the lower part of the figure, showing interphase normal and tumour nuclei with the tandem duplication hybridized with such probes. The two interphase copies of chromosome 7 in the normal nucleus each show a single red and a single green signal adjacent to each other. In contrast, the tumour cell nuclei show one pair of normal chromosomal signals, but the other copy of chromosome 7 shows an additional (yellow) signal, due to the fusion of the extra, now adjacent, red and green signals. Reprinted from Collins VP et al. {482}.

a glioneuronal tumour. NFP typically outlines a mainly solid tumour, highlighting normal surrounding axons in compressed adjacent CNS parenchyma. Optic nerve tumours generally produce a fusiform expansion of the nerve and have axons present among tumour cells, as do occasional cerebellar examples. Rosenthal fibres are positive for alpha-B-crystallin, with GFAP staining limited to their periphery. Unlike in diffuse astrocytomas, p53 protein staining is weak to absent, which is consistent with the rarity of *TP53* mutations in pilocytic astrocytoma. Immunohistochemistry for the R132H-mutant IDH1 protein has been suggested to be useful for the distinction of pilocytic astrocytomas from diffuse gliomas, given that reactivity is absent in essentially all pilocytic astrocytomas {359}. However, paediatric diffuse astrocytic tumours may also lack *IDH1* or *IDH2* mutations. In addition, reliable antibodies are currently available for only the most common IDH1 amino acid substitutions at position 132, so a negative result does

not exclude other substitutions at position 132 or mutations of the IDH2 protein. Because essentially all pilocytic astrocytomas have activating genetic alterations in components of the MAPK pathway {1176}, phosphorylated MAPK immunostaining is a consistent feature. Labelling with immunohistochemical markers of mTOR pathway activation (e.g. phosphorylated S6) is more variable {1076}. Immunohistochemistry for V600E-mutant BRAF is positive in a small subset lacking *KIAA1549-BRAF* fusion and other MAPK pathway alterations. The Ki-67 proliferation index is low in most cases of pilocytic astrocytoma, consistent with low proliferation rates {826}. Increases in the Ki-67 proliferation index have been associated with more aggressive behaviour in some studies but not others {258,2552}.

Genetic profile
The most frequent abnormality in pilocytic astrocytomas overall (found in > 70% of all cases) is an approximately 2 Mb duplication of 7q34, encompassing the *BRAF*

gene {123,575,1961}. This is a tandem duplication resulting in a transforming fusion gene between *KIAA1549* and *BRAF* {1178}. The N-terminus of the KIAA1549 protein replaces the N-terminal regulatory region of *BRAF*, retaining the *BRAF* kinase domain, which is consequently uncontrolled and constitutively activates the MAPK pathway {724,1178,2360}. This abnormality is found at all anatomical locations, but is most frequent in cerebellar tumours and somewhat less common at other sites. The gene fusions involve nine different combinations of *KIAA1549* and *BRAF* exons, making identification by RT-PCR or immunochemistry difficult, resulting in many centres accepting the demonstration of a duplication at 7q34 (usually using FISH probes) as evidence of the *KIAA1549-BRAF* fusion. In small numbers of cases, eight additional gene partners for *BRAF* fusions have also been identified (*FAM131B*, *RNF130*, *CLCN6*, *MKRN1*, *GNA11*, *QKI*, *FXR1*, and *MACF1*), with fusions occurring by various genetic rearrangements (including deletions and translocations) and all resulting in loss of the N-terminal regulatory region of the BRAF protein, with retention of the kinase domain {1176,2855}.

In addition to harbouring *BRAF* fusion genes, essentially all pilocytic astrocytomas studied in sufficient detail have been shown to have an alteration affecting some component of the MAPK pathway {1176, 2855}. These alterations include the well-documented *NF1* mutations, the hotspot *BRAF* mutation commonly known as the V600E mutation, *KRAS* mutations, recurrent aberrations affecting the *FGFR1* and the NTRK-family receptor kinase genes, and very occasional *RAF1* gene fusions with *SRGAP3*, which occur in a similar manner to the *BRAF* fusions: a tandem duplication at 3p25, with the fusion protein lacking the RAF regulatory domain but retaining the kinase domain with loss of kinase control. In cases with alterations of the NTRK genes, the alterations are also in the form of gene fusions, with several different 5' partners that contain a dimerization domain. This is presumed to lead to constitutive dimerization of the NTRK fusion proteins and activation of the kinase {1176,2855}. The changes are more varied in the case of *FGFR1*. They include hotspot point mutations (N546K and K656E), *FGFR1-TACC1* fusions similar to those seen in adult glioblastoma {2364}, a novel internal duplication of the

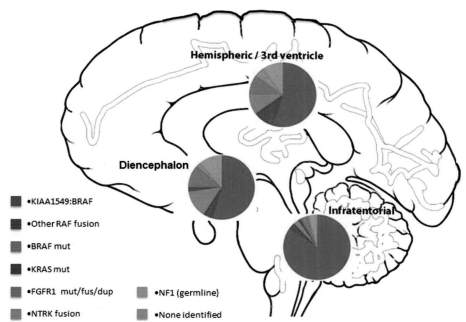

Fig. 2.10 Pilocytic astrocytoma. Pie charts summarizing the known frequencies of the various MAPK pathway alterations in different anatomical locations of the brain (i.e. posterior fossa, diencephalon, and cerebral hemispheres), calculated from a total of 188 pilocytic astrocytoma cases {482,1176,2855}. Reprinted from Collins VP et al. {482}.

Legend for pie charts:
- ■ •KIAA1549:BRAF
- ■ •Other RAF fusion
- ■ •BRAF mut
- ■ •KRAS mut
- ■ •FGFR1 mut/fus/dup
- ■ •NTRK fusion
- ■ •NF1 (germline)
- ■ •None identified

Labels: Hemispheric / 3rd ventricle, Diencephalon, Infratentorial

kinase domain of *FGFR1*, and an internal tandem duplication of *FGFR1* {1176, 2855}. A summary of the incidence of all MAPK pathway alterations identified to date in pilocytic astrocytomas of all anatomical sites is shown in Table 2.01 (p. 84). Chromosomal polysomies (in particular of chromosomes 5, 6, 7, 11, and 15) have been reported in tumours of teenagers and adults {1177,2237}.

The incidence of the various MAPK pathway alterations is not consistent across all anatomical locations {123,1113,1176, 2855}. The *KIAA1549-BRAF* fusion is extremely common in the cerebellum (found in ~90% of cases) but less common supratentorially (found in ~50%). *FGFR1* alterations are restricted mainly to midline structures, whereas the *BRAF* V600E mutation and NTRK-family fusions are more common in supratentorial tumours. Variation is also observed in the transcriptome and methylome of pilocytic astrocytomas, with infratentorial and supratentorial tumours distinguishable on the basis of their gene expression or DNA methylation signatures {1424,2335, 2527}. The reason for this relationship between site / cell of origin and certain molecular alterations is unclear. Unlike in diffuse astrocytomas, the average mutation rate is low in pilocytic astrocytomas. *TP53* mutations seem to play no role in the development of these tumours {1098,

1176,1824,2855}. Pilocytic astrocytomas with anaplastic change have yet to be studied in any detail. However, in a recent study of 26 cases that had progressed to high-grade glioma, none had a *BRAF* fusion {1683}.

The presence of the *KIAA1549-BRAF* fusion in an appropriate morphological context and together with other findings supports the diagnosis of pilocytic astrocytoma. However, the absence of such a fusion provides no diagnostic information, because there are so many other ways in which the MAPK pathway has been found to be activated in pilocytic astrocytomas. The *KIAA1549-BRAF* fusion has also been reported in several adult gliomas but rarely in other histologies, with the exception of the rare diffuse leptomeningeal glioneuronal tumour (see p. 152; formerly referred to as disseminated oligodendroglial-like leptomeningeal neoplasm), in which the fusion is frequently found together with a solitary 1p deletion {2156}. Unfortunately, many of the non–*KIAA1549-BRAF* alterations are also found to be similarly aberrant in the tumour types that are most frequently among the differential diagnosis of pilocytic astrocytoma. For example, the *BRAF* V600E mutation occurs in a small subset of pilocytic astrocytomas, but is a common alteration in gangliogliomas and pleomorphic xanthoastrocytomas

and has also been reported in dysembryoplastic neuroepithelial tumours {414, 2280}. This mutation can now be identified using a monoclonal antibody that specifically recognizes the V600E-mutant BRAF protein {355}.

A summary of genetic aberrations reported to date in pilocytic astrocytoma, as well as their diagnostic utility, is provided in Table 2.01 (p. 84).

Genetic susceptibility

Pilocytic astrocytomas are the principal CNS neoplasm associated with NF1, which occurs in approximately 1 in 3000 births. Although NF1 is inherited in an autosomal dominant manner, about half of all cases are associated with a de novo mutation (see p. 294). The *NF1* gene, located on the long arm of chromosome 17, encodes the neurofibromin protein, which acts in the MAPK pathway as a GAP for RAS, thereby facilitating the deactivation of RAS. Patients with NF1 have only one wildtype *NF1* gene copy. Subsequent functional loss of this single wildtype copy results in the absence of the *NF1*-encoded GTPase and consequent overactivity of RAS and the MAPK pathway. This so-called second hit in pilocytic astrocytomas can occur as a result of point mutation, focal or broader LOH, or DNA hypermethylation {909}. Reports have suggested that germline mutations affecting the 5′-most third of the *NF1* gene may be associated with a greater chance of developing pilocytic astrocytomas of the optic pathway {235, 2332}, although further study is needed. Approximately 15% of individuals with NF1 develop pilocytic astrocytomas {1481}, particularly of the optic nerve/ pathways (optic pathway glioma), but other anatomical sites (sometimes multiple) can also be affected. Conversely, as many as one third of all patients with a pilocytic astrocytoma of the optic nerve have NF1 {1304}. These tumours typically arise during the first decade of life; few patients with NF1 develop an optic pathway glioma after the age of 10 years.

Pilocytic astrocytomas are also associated with Noonan syndrome (a neuro-cardio-facial-cutaneous syndrome), which is caused by germline mutations of MAPK pathway genes (i.e. *PTPN11*, *SOS1*, *KRAS*, *NRAS*, *RAF1*, *BRAF*, *SHOC2*, and *CBL*) {83,2135}. The *PTPN11* gene is mutated in about 50% of patients with Noonan syndrome and is occasionally mutated (together with *FGFR1*) in sporadic pilocytic astrocytomas {1176}. However, the number of pilocytic astrocytomas reported in patients with Noonan syndrome is small {744,1743,2233,2300}.

Prognosis and predictive factors
Pilocytic astrocytoma is typically a slow-growing, low-grade tumour with a favourable prognosis. Overall survival rates at 5 and 10 years are > 95% after surgical intervention alone {291,325,688,725,1606, 1826}. Stability of WHO grade is typically maintained for decades {149,325,1878}. The tumours may even spontaneously regress, although this is rare {897,1894, 2421}. Very occasional cases progress with more anaplastic features after a variable interval, most often after irradiation or chemotherapy treatment {1957,2145}. There are few long-term studies documenting the ultimate outcome of patients with pilocytic astrocytoma.

Patient age and extent of resection are key prognostic factors {2431}. Depending on the location and size of the tumour, pilocytic astrocytoma may not be amenable to gross total resection and may either recur or progress, eventually leading to death. However, this is usually after a prolonged clinical course with multiple recurrences {725,974,1678,1996,2159}. Pilocytic astrocytomas of the optic nerve in patients with NF1 {2148} seem to have a more indolent behaviour than that of their sporadic counterparts {1516}.

Histological malignancy in pilocytic astrocytoma is rare; in one study of classic pilocytic astrocytoma, the incidence of malignancy occurring spontaneously was 0.9%, and the incidence of occurrence after radiation was 1.8% {2565}. Descriptions of anaplastic features in pilocytic astrocytomas come mainly from isolated case reports and small series {374,591,1251,2417,2682}, in which malignant histological features correlate less reliably with prognosis than those seen in patients with diffusely infiltrative astrocytomas. Malignant transformation is frequently reported in association with prior treatment {61,176,307,1296,1364,2303, 2312,2420,2565,2603}. A retrospective study of 34 pilocytic astrocytomas with spontaneous anaplastic histological features found that these tumours exhibited a wide spectrum of morphologies and behaved in a more aggressive manner, with decreased survival, than typical pilocytic astrocytomas. However, despite exhibiting morphological features of anaplasia similar to those of diffuse astrocytic tumours, they did not behave as aggressively. Even so-called high-grade pilocytic astrocytoma with anaplastic features and necrosis did not behave like a glioblastoma. Pilocytic astrocytomas with anaplastic features such as increased mitotic count (i.e. > 4 mitoses per 10 high-power fields) and necrosis behaved, in respective studies, more similarly to diffuse low-grade or anaplastic astrocytomas than to anaplastic astrocytomas or glioblastomas {2150}.

Pilomyxoid astrocytoma (see below), a recognized pilocytic astrocytoma variant typically occurring in young children, almost exclusively in the hypothalamic / third ventricular region, reportedly has a higher frequency of local recurrence and may undergo cerebrospinal fluid seeding {1534,2555}.

Pilomyxoid astrocytoma

Burger P.C. Jones D.
Tihan T. Giannini C.
Hawkins C. Rodriguez F.
VandenBerg S.R. Figarella-Branger D.

Definition
A variant of pilocytic astrocytoma histologically characterized by an angiocentric arrangement of monomorphous, bipolar tumour cells in a prominent myxoid background {2555}.

Pilomyxoid astrocytoma is preferentially located in the hypothalamic/chiasmatic region but shares other locations with pilocytic astrocytoma (e.g. the thalamus, temporal lobe, brain stem, and cerebellum) {1533}. Pilomyxoid astrocytoma predominantly affects infants and young children (with a median patient age of 10 months). It may grow more rapidly and have a less favourable prognosis than pilocytic astrocytoma, due to local recurrence and cerebrospinal spread {270}.

ICD-O code   9425/3

Grading
Although some reports have suggested an increased likelihood of recurrence, it is uncertain whether pilomyxoid astrocytoma truly corresponds histologically to WHO grade II. Therefore, a definite grade assignment is not recommended at this time.

Epidemiology
The incidence of pilomyxoid astrocytoma is unknown because this entity is typically grouped with pilocytic astrocytoma. Pilomyxoid astrocytoma accounts for a small proportion of tumours historically classified as pilocytic astrocytoma.

Localization
The hypothalamic/chiasmatic region is the most common location, although the tumour can also occur in the thalamus, cerebellum, brain stem, temporal lobe, and spinal cord {187,480,688}.

Clinical features
Pilomyxoid astrocytomas present with non-specific signs and symptoms that depend on the anatomical site. Radiological examination shows a well-circumscribed mass with relatively distinct borders. The tumour is typically T1-hypointense and T2-hyperintense. Compared with pilocytic astrocytomas, pilomyxoid astrocytomas are more likely to have necrosis and more likely to have signal intensity extending into adjacent structures. Cysts and calcifications are less common {1322}. Cerebrospinal fluid dissemination can occur before presentation.

Spread
These tumours are usually confined to the site of origin, but they may spread within cerebrospinal pathways.

Macroscopy
Intraoperative reports often describe a solid gelatinous mass. The tumours may infiltrate the parenchyma, and a clear surgical plane may not be identifiable.

Microscopy
Pilomyxoid astrocytoma is dominated by

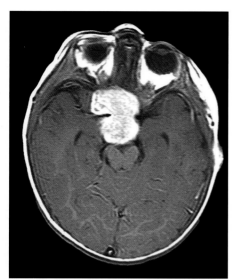

Fig. 2.11 Pilomyxoid astrocytomas are usually large, contrast-enhancing masses that are most frequent in the hypothalamic and suprasellar areas.

a markedly myxoid background, monomorphous bipolar cells, and a predominantly angiocentric arrangement. The tumour typically has a compact, non-infiltrative architecture, but some cases are infiltrative, trapping normal brain elements such as ganglion cells. The lesion is composed of small, monomorphous bipolar cells whose processes often radiate from vessels, producing a form of pseudorosette. As strictly defined, the lesion does not contain Rosenthal fibres or eosinophilic granular bodies, but mitotic figures may be present. Vascular proliferation is present in some cases, often in the form of linear glomeruloid tufts associated with cystic degeneration. Rare examples are focally necrotic. Focal pilomyxoid changes in an otherwise typical

pilocytic astrocytoma do not warrant a diagnosis of pilomyxoid astrocytoma.

Immunophenotype
Immunohistochemical staining demonstrates strong and diffuse reactivity for GFAP, S100 protein, and vimentin. Some cases are positive for synaptophysin, but staining for NFP or chromogranin-A is typically negative. CD34 expression has been reported in some cases in the hypothalamic/chiasmatic region. Staining for V600E-mutant BRAF is negative {480}. In limited studies, the Ki-67 proliferation index was found to vary substantially among pilomyxoid astrocytomas, ranging from 2% to 20% {688,1326}. There is considerable overlap of Ki-67 proliferation index values between pilomyxoid and pilocytic astrocytomas.

Cell of origin
The cell of origin for pilomyxoid astrocytoma is unclear. Some reports of pilomyxoid astrocytoma underscore its close association with pilocytic astrocytoma, suggesting a common astrocytic origin. A suggested origin is from radial glia in proximity to the optic nerve {437,2527}.

Genetic profile
Although very few pilomyxoid astrocytomas have been included in large-scale genomic studies, the data obtained to date suggest that these tumours are genetically similar to WHO grade I pilocytic astrocytomas {1034,2855}, with some showing *KIAA1549-BRAF* fusion {480}.

Genetic susceptibility
To date, no genetic susceptibility has been established for most pilomyxoid

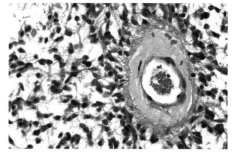

Fig. 2.12 Perivascular orientation of tumour cells is a distinctive feature of pilomyxoid astrocytoma.

astrocytomas, although cases in patients with neurofibromatosis type 1 and pilomyxoid astrocytoma have been reported {1261}. A case occurring in the context of Noonan syndrome has been reported as well {1743}.

Prognosis and predictive factors
In general, pilomyxoid astrocytomas are more aggressive and more prone to local recurrence and cerebrospinal spread than are pilocytic astrocytomas {480, 688}, but there is considerable variation in behaviour, and not all are more aggressive than WHO grade I pilocytic astrocytoma. Given the complexity of clinical, anatomical, and pathological interrelationships, it is unclear whether the more aggressive behaviour of some pilomyxoid astrocytomas is related to their intrinsic pathological features or to their unfavourable hypothalamic/chiasmatic location. Complete surgical excision, which is the most reliable prognostic factor for pilocytic astrocytoma, cannot usually be achieved in this anatomical region.

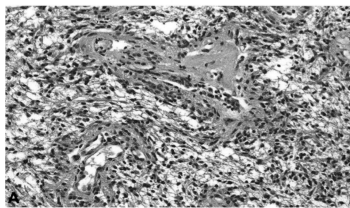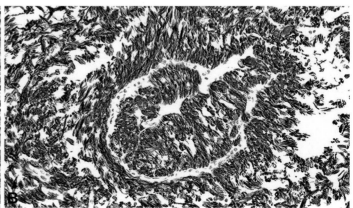

Fig. 2.13 Pilomyxoid astrocytoma. **A** Monomorphous population of small, often bipolar, cells sitting in a myxoid background. **B** Diffuse, strong immunoreactivity for GFAP.

Subependymal giant cell astrocytoma

Lopes M.B.S.
Wiestler O.D.
Stemmer-Rachamimov A.O.
Sharma M.C.
Vinters H.V.
Santosh V.

Definition

A benign, slow-growing tumour composed of large ganglionic astrocytes, typically arising in the wall of the lateral ventricles.

Subependymal giant cell astrocytoma (SEGA) has a strong association with the tuberous sclerosis syndrome (p. 306).

ICD-O code 9384/1

Grading

SEGA corresponds histologically to WHO grade I.

Epidemiology

Incidence

SEGA is the most common CNS neoplasm in patients with tuberous sclerosis, but it is uncertain whether the tumour also occurs outside this setting {26, 1809,2188}. The incidence rate of SEGA among patients with confirmed tuberous sclerosis is 5–15% {26,1809,2188}, and the tumour is one of the major diagnostic criteria of tuberous sclerosis {1809}.

Age and sex distribution

This tumour typically occurs during the first two decades of life and only infrequently arises de novo after the age of 20–25 years {1809}. However, cases can occur in infants, and several congenital cases diagnosed either at birth or by antenatal MRI have been reported {1070, 1630,1964,2067}.

Localization

SEGAs arise from the lateral walls of the lateral ventricles adjacent to the foramen of Monro.

Clinical features

Most patients present either with epilepsy or with symptoms of increased intracranial pressure. Massive spontaneous haemorrhage has been reported as an acute manifestation {2188}. With the current practice of early screening of patients with tuberous sclerosis, many SEGAs are diagnosed at an initial stage while still clinically asymptomatic {1378,2188}.

Imaging

On CT, SEGAs present as solid, partially calcified masses located in the walls of the lateral ventricles, mostly near the foramen of Monro. Ipsilateral or bilateral ventricular enlargement may be apparent. On MRI, the tumours are usually heterogeneous, isointense, or slightly hypointense on T1-weighted images, and hyperintense on T2-weighted images, with marked contrast enhancement {1094}. Prominent signal voids that represent dilated vessels are occasionally seen within the tumours. Like other brain neoplasms, SEGAs may show a high ratio of choline to creatinine and a low ratio of N-acetylaspartate to creatinine on proton MR spectroscopy, which seems to be a valuable tool for the early detection of neoplastic transformation of subependymal nodules {1979}. Leptomeningeal dissemination with drop metastases has been described {2532}.

Macroscopy

SEGAs are typically located in the walls of the lateral ventricles over the basal ganglia. The tumours are sharply demarcated multinodular lesions. Cysts of various sizes are commonly seen. Areas of remote haemorrhage may be seen due to the high vascularity of the tumour. Necrosis is rare, but focal calcifications are common.

Microscopy

SEGAs are circumscribed, often calcified tumours. They are composed mainly of large, plump cells that resemble gemistocytic astrocytes and are arranged in sweeping fascicles, sheets, and nests. Clustering of tumour cells and perivascular palisading are common features. The tumour cells show a wide spectrum of phenotypes. Typical appearances range

![Subependymal giant cell astrocytoma extending into the left ventricle and causing hydrocephalus]

Fig. 2.14 Subependymal giant cell astrocytom extending into the left ventricle and causing hydrocephalus.

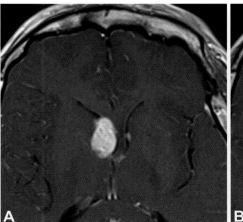
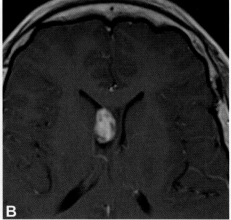

Fig. 2.15 Subependymal giant cell astrocytoma (postcontrast axial T1-weighted MRI). **A** A right subependymal giant cell astrocytoma near the foramen of Monro, with avid enhancement. **B** After 3 months of mTOR inhibitor treatment, the tumour shows decreased size and enhancement.

from polygonal cells with abundant, glassy cytoplasm (resembling gemistocytic astrocytes) to smaller, spindle cells within a variably fibrillated matrix. Giant pyramidal-like cells with a ganglionic appearance are common; these large cells often have an eccentric, vesicular nucleus with distinct nucleoli. Nuclear pseudoinclusions can be seen in some cases. Considerable nuclear pleomorphism and multinucleated cells are frequent. A rich vascular stroma with frequent hyalinized vessels and infiltration of mast cells and lymphocytes (predominantly T lymphocytes) is a consistent feature {2334}. Parenchymal or vascular calcifications are frequent {883,1964,2334}, and SEGAs may demonstrate increased mitotic activity; however, these features do not seem to denote an adverse clinical course. Similarly, the occasional presence of endothelial proliferation and necrosis are not indicative of anaplastic progression. The rare examples of SEGA outside the setting of tuberous sclerosis that recur have not been reported to show malignant transformation {2808}.

The Ki-67 proliferation index as determined by MIB1 monoclonal antibody staining is generally low (mean: 3.0%), further supporting the benign nature of these neoplasms {913,2333}. The TOP2A labelling index is also low (mean: 2.9%) {2333}. Although extremely uncommon, craniospinal dissemination has been reported in SEGA with an increased Ki-67 proliferation index but without malignant features {2532}.

Ultrastructural features of neuronal differentiation, including microtubules, occasional dense-core granules, and (rarely) synapses may be detectable, and bundles of intermediate filaments are seen in the cytoplasmic processes of the spindle astrocytic cells {302,1009,1188}.

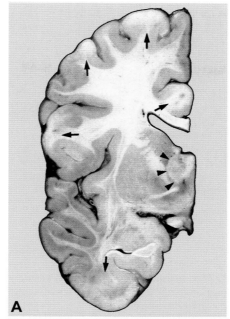

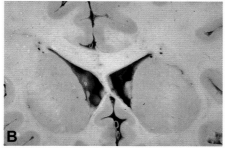

Fig. 2.16 Subependymal giant cell astrocytoma. **A** Coronal section of the left hemisphere of a patient with tuberous sclerosis, showing a subependymal giant cell astrocytoma (arrowheads) and multiple cortical tubers (arrows). **B** Multiple subependymal nodules on the walls of the lateral ventricles.

Immunophenotype
SEGA has been designated as an astrocytoma, but due to its usually mixed glioneuronal phenotype, it has also been called subependymal giant cell tumour {302,1526}. The tumour cells demonstrate variable immunoreactivity for GFAP and uniform, intense immunoreactivity for S100 protein {1526,2334,2832}. Variable immunoreactivity for neuronal markers and neuropeptides has been detected in SEGAs. The neuron-associated class III beta-tubulin is more widespread in its distribution than any other neuronal epitope, whereas neurofilament is more restricted and mainly highlights cellular processes and a few ganglionic cells {1526}. Similarly, SEGA shows variable immunoexpression for synaptophysin within the ganglionic component {2334}. Focal immunoreactivity for NeuN {2832} and neuropeptides has also been detected {1526}. Neural stem cell markers, including nestin and SOX2 are also expressed in SEGAs {1964}; however, unlike in cortical dysplasias, CD34 immunoreactivity is not seen. These findings suggest cellular lineages with a variable capacity for divergent phenotypes, including glial, neuronal, and neuroendocrine differentiation. Loss of either hamartin or tuberin immunoexpression is commonly seen in SEGAs, and combined loss occurs in rare cases {1693}.

Cell of origin
The histogenesis of SEGA is unclear. The histological and radiological features of SEGAs and subependymal nodules are similar, and there is radiological evidence supporting the development of some subependymal nodules into SEGAs over time, suggesting that these entities may constitute a continuum {241,468}. Evidence of biallelic inactivation of the *TSC1* or *TSC2* genes and activation of the mTOR pathway in SEGAs supports the hypothesis that SEGAs arise as a consequence of a two-hit mechanism {406}. SEGAs demonstrate glial, neuronal, and mixed neuroglial features (morphological, immunohistochemical, and ultrastructural), which suggests a neuroglial

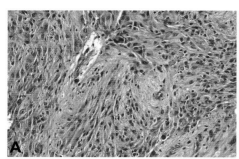

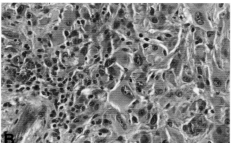

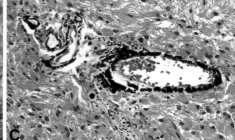

Fig. 2.17 Subependymal giant cell astrocytoma. **A** Cellular heterogeneity is typical for these tumours; elongated cells arranged within sweeping fascicles are admixed with large cells. **B** Infiltration of inflammatory cells, including mature lymphocytes and mast cells, is a consistent feature. **C** Multifocal calcification within the tumour and/or blood vessels is commonly seen.

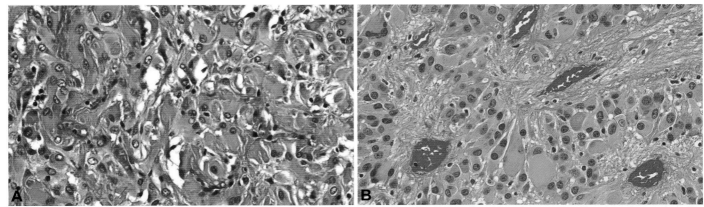

Fig. 2.18 Subependymal giant cell astrocytoma. **A** Mixed population of polygonal to ganglionic-like cells. **B** Collection of large tumour cells, with perivascular pseudorosettes reminiscent of ependymoma.

progenitor cell of origin with the capacity to undergo differentiation along glial, neuronal, and neuroendocrine lines {1526, 2334}. This hypothesis is supported by data from mouse models in which loss of *Tsc1* or activation of the mTOR pathway in subventricular zone neural progenitor cells resulted in the formation of SEGA and subependymal nodule–like lesions in the lateral ventricles {1566,2862A}.

Genetic profile
SEGA has a strong association with tuberous sclerosis, a genetic disease caused by inactivating mutations in the *TSC1* gene at 9q or the *TSC2* gene at 16p. The proteins encoded by the TSC genes, tuberin and hamartin, interact

within the cell and form a complex {486, 1212,1987}. A mutation of either gene results in disrupted function of the tuberin–hamartin complex, with similar resulting disease phenotypes.

Approximately 60% of patients with tuberous sclerosis have sporadic disease (i.e. with no family history), indicating a high rate of de novo mutations {2229A}. In affected kindreds, the disease follows an autosomal dominant pattern of inheritance, with high penetrance but considerable phenotypic variability {2354}.

In sporadic tuberous sclerosis cases, mutations in *TSC2* are 5 times more common than mutations in *TSC1* {51,516, 1174}, whereas in families with multiple members affected, the mutation ratio of

these two genes is 1:1 {2231}. *TSC1* or *TSC2* mutations are identified in about 85% of patients with tuberous sclerosis. The remaining 15% of cases may be mosaics or have a mutation in an unanalysed non-coding gene area. Mosaicism has been reported for *TSC1* and *TSC2* mutations in some parents of patients with sporadic cases and in patients with tuberous sclerosis {2229,2646}. Alternatively, there may be a third, unknown locus, although to date there is no evidence to support this possibility {2231}. Patients with tuberous sclerosis with no identified mutations have a milder phenotype than do patients with *TSC1* or *TSC2* mutations {2231}.

Like in other circumscribed astrocytomas,

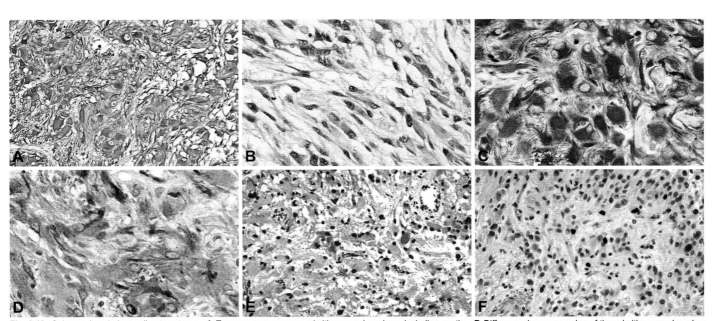

Fig. 2.19 Subependymal giant cell astrocytoma. **A** Tumours may express primitive neural markers, including nestin. **B** Diffuse nuclear expression of the primitive neural marker SOX2. **C** The majority of tumour cells are immunoreactive for GFAP. **D** Class III beta-tubulin (also called TUJ1) is the most ubiquitous neuronal-associated marker in these tumours. **E** Focal expression of NFP. **F** MIB1/Ki-67 immunohistochemistry showing a low proliferation rate.

including pilocytic astrocytoma and pleomorphic xanthoastrocytomas, *BRAF* V600E mutations have been found in SEGAs: in 6 of 14 cases in one series {1448} and in 1 of 3 cases in another {2280}, regardless of whether the tumour occurred in the setting of tuberous sclerosis. Investigations of SEGAs have also demonstrated LOH in the *TSC2* gene {992,1694}. Lost or reduced tuberin and hamartin expression has been described in SEGAs from patients with both *TSC1* and *TSC2* germline mutations, suggesting a two-hit tumour suppressor model for the pathogenesis of SEGAs {992, 1163,1255,1694}. LOH at 16p and 21q has been observed in two separate cases {2782}, and partial loss of chromosome 22q was observed in two additional paediatric patients with tuberous sclerosis {560}.

Genetic susceptibility
SEGA has a strong association with the inherited tuberous sclerosis syndrome (see *Tuberous sclerosis*, p. 306).

Prognosis and predictive factors
SEGA has a good prognosis when gross total resection is achieved. Larger or symptomatic lesions tend to have greater morbidity {551}. Careful follow-up of residual tumour is recommended because of the potential for late recurrences. Optimal outcome is associated with early detection and treatment. In individuals with tuberous sclerosis, surveillance by MRI every 1–3 years until the age of 25 years is recommended {551,1378}. Inhibition of mTOR1 with everolimus has been reported as a promising therapeutic approach in patients with inoperable tuberous sclerosis–associated SEGAs {732A,733}.

Pleomorphic xanthoastrocytoma

Giannini C.
Paulus W.
Louis D.N.
Liberski P.P.
Figarella-Branger D.
Capper D.

Definition

An astrocytic glioma with large pleomorphic and frequently multinucleated cells, spindle and lipidized cells, a dense pericellular reticulin network, and numerous eosinophilic granular bodies.

Pleomorphic xanthoastrocytoma tumour cells are neoplastic astrocytes, but there is often neuronal differentiation {828, 1007,1254}. Mitotic activity is low (< 5 mitoses per 10 high-power fields). *BRAF* V600E mutation is common in pleomorphic xanthoastrocytoma, and its presence in the absence of an IDH mutation strongly supports the diagnosis. Pleomorphic xanthoastrocytoma is rare (constituting < 1% of all astrocytic neoplasms) and most commonly affects children and young adults, with a median patient age at diagnosis of 22 years {825}. The tumour has a typical superficial location in the cerebral hemispheres, most frequently in the temporal lobe, with involvement of the adjacent leptomeninges and with cyst formation. Despite its alarming histological appearance, pleomorphic xanthoastrocytoma has a relatively favourable prognosis compared with diffusely infiltrative astrocytoma, with 70.9% recurrence-free and 90.4% overall survival rates at 5 years {1081}.

ICD-O code　　　　　　　9424/3

Grading

Pleomorphic xanthoastrocytoma corresponds histologically to WHO grade II.

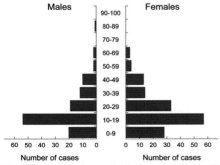

Fig. 2.20 Age and sex distribution of patients with pleomorphic xanthoastrocytoma.

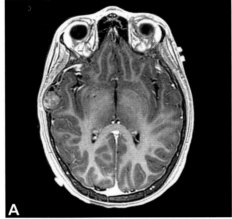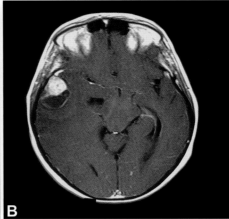

Fig. 2.21 Pleomorphic xanthoastrocytoma. T1-weighted MRI with contrast enhancement. **A,B** The neoplasms in the temporal lobe present as superficial nodular enhancing cystic tumours. Note the scalloping of overlying bone (**A**).

Epidemiology

Pleomorphic xanthoastrocytoma is a rare brain tumour, accounting for < 1% of all primary brain tumours. The 2014 statistical report published by the Central Brain Tumor Registry of the United States (CB-TRUS) lists pleomorphic xanthoastrocytoma among the "unique astrocytoma variants" and reports an annual incidence of 0.3 cases per 100 000 population {1863}.

Pleomorphic xanthoastrocytoma typically develops in children and young adults {825}, with mean and median patient ages of 25.9 and 22 years, respectively {1935}, but occurrence in older patients, including patients in their seventh and eighth decades of life, has also been reported {1935}. There is no sex bias. One study in the USA found these tumours to be more common in the Black population {1935}.

Etiology

No specific etiologies have been implicated in the genesis of pleomorphic xanthoastrocytoma. The occasional association with cortical dysplasia or with ganglion cell lesions suggests that their formation may be facilitated in malformative states {1409}. Given reports in patients with neurofibromatosis type 1 {2023}, a relation to defective *NF1*

function is also possible. The rare *TP53* mutations encountered do not suggest particular carcinogenic insults {824,1238, 1917}.

Localization

A superficial location, involving the leptomeninges and cerebrum (meningocerebral) is characteristic of this neoplasm. Approximately 98% of cases occur supratentorially, most commonly in the temporal lobe {825,1254}. Cases involving the cerebellum and spinal cord have also be reported {836,1749}, and two cases of primary pleomorphic xanthoastrocytoma of the retina in children have been reported {2847}.

Clinical features

Due to the superficial cerebral location of the lesion, many patients present with a fairly long history of seizures. Cerebellar and spinal cord cases have symptoms that reflect these sites of involvement.

Imaging

Pleomorphic xanthoastrocytoma is usually a supratentorial mass, peripherally located and frequently cystic, involving cortex and overlying leptomeninges. CT and MRI scans outline the tumour mass and/or its cyst. On CT, tumour appearance is variable (hypodense, hyperdense, or

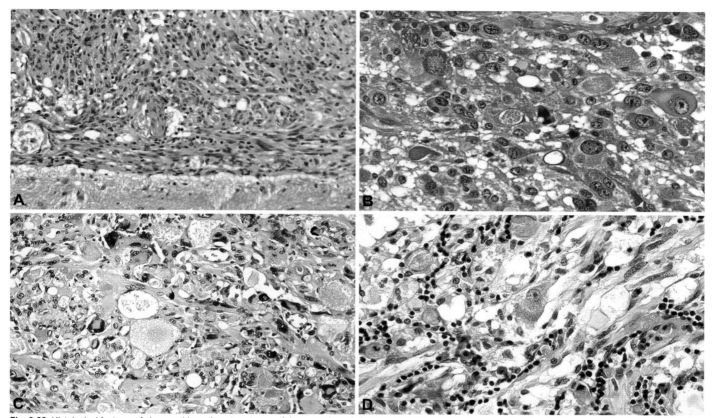

Fig. 2.22 Histological features of pleomorphicxanthoastrocytoma. **A** Leptomeningeal pleomorphic xanthoastrocytoma, sharply delineated from the underlying cerebral cortex. **B** Granular bodies, intensely eosinophilic or pale, are an almost invariable finding. **C** Tumour cells showing nuclear and cytoplasmic pleomorphism and xanthomatous change. **D** Mature ganglion cell and lymphocytic infiltrates; reprinted from Kros JM et al. {1375}.

mixed), with strong, sometimes heterogeneous contrast enhancement {1857}. Tumour cysts are hypodense. On MRI, the solid portion of the tumour is either hypointense or isointense to grey matter on T1-weighted images and shows a hyperintense or mixed signal on T2-weighted and FLAIR images, whereas the cystic component is isointense to cerebrospinal fluid. Postcontrast enhancement is moderate or strong {1857}. Perifocal oedema is usually not pronounced, due to the slow growth of the tumour.

Macroscopy

Pleomorphic xanthoastrocytomas are usually superficial tumours extending to the leptomeninges. They are frequently accompanied by a cyst, sometimes forming a mural nodule within the cyst wall. Features such as invasion of the dura {543}, predominantly exophytic growth {1688}, multifocality {1629}, and leptomeningeal dissemination {1905} are exceptional.

Microscopy

The adjective "pleomorphic" refers to the variable histological appearance of the tumour, in which spindled cells are intermingled with mononucleated or multinucleated giant astrocytes, the nuclei of which show great variation in size and staining. Intranuclear inclusions are frequent {825}, as are prominent nucleoli. In some cases, the neoplastic astrocytes are closely packed, creating a so-called epithelioid pattern {1106}. In other cases, sheets of fusiform cells are encountered. The term "xanthoastrocytoma" refers to the presence of large, often multinucleated xanthomatous cells that have intracellular accumulation of lipids. This is usually in the form of droplets, which often occupy much of the cell body, pushing cytoplasmic organelles and glial filaments to the periphery. This feature generally makes the astrocytic character easy to recognize by H&E or GFAP stains. Granular bodies (either intensely eosinophilic or pale) are a nearly invariable finding {825}. Focal collections of small lymphocytes, occasionally with plasma cells, are

also frequent {825}. The third histological hallmark of pleomorphic xanthoastrocytoma is the presence of reticulin fibres, which are best seen using silver impregnation. Reactive changes in the meninges are not the only source of reticulin fibres; individual tumour cells may be surrounded by basement membranes that also stain positively for reticulin, and these can be recognized ultrastructurally as pericellular basal laminae. By definition, the mitotic count is < 5 mitoses per 10 high-power fields. Necrosis is rarely present in WHO grade II pleomorphic xanthoastrocytoma in the absence of brisk mitotic activity, but necrosis in itself is insufficient for a WHO grade III designation (see *Anaplastic pleomorphic xanthoastrocytoma*, p. 98).

Differential diagnosis

Because pleomorphic xanthoastrocytoma often includes a diffusely infiltrating, non-pleomorphic component, diffuse astrocytoma is a common differential diagnosis. In addition to the presence of histologically more typical pleomorphic

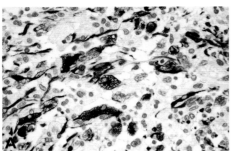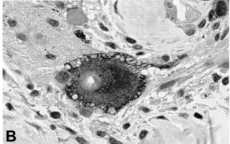

Fig. 2.23 Pleomorphic xanthoastrocytoma. **A** GFAP expression in large pleomorphic and xanthomatous cells. **B** Synaptophysin immunostaining in tumour cells {828}.

xanthoastrocytoma components, the combination of *BRAF* V600E mutation and absence of an IDH mutation supports the diagnosis of pleomorphic xanthoastrocytoma. Uncommonly, ganglioglioma can present with a glial component resembling pleomorphic xanthoastrocytoma; rare cases of composite tumours with features of pleomorphic xanthoastrocytoma and ganglioglioma in which the two neoplastic components coexist side by side with minimal intermingling have been reported {1339, 1943}. Pleomorphic xanthoastrocytoma areas showing eosinophilic granular bodies and spindle-shaped cells may be reminiscent of pilocytic astrocytoma, but areas with more typical histology, in the absence of *BRAF* translocations or other genetic aberrations leading to MAPK activation, support the diagnosis of pleomorphic xanthoastrocytoma. Mesenchymal tumours may also enter the differential diagnosis, but this consideration is usually refuted by positivity for GFAP in unequivocal tumour (non-reactive) cells, although GFAP positivity may be focal or even absent in small specimens.

Immunophenotype
Although the essential nature of pleomorphic xanthoastrocytoma is clearly and uniformly glial, with nearly invariable immunoreactivity for GFAP and S100 protein {825,828}, the tumours have a significant tendency to exhibit neuronal differentiation. Expression of neuronal markers (including synaptophysin, neurofilament, class III beta-tubulin, and MAP2) has been reported with variable frequency in tumours that have otherwise typical histological features of pleomorphic xanthoastrocytoma {828,2013}. In some cases, this biphenotypic glioneuronal appearance has been confirmed ultrastructurally {1007}. CD34 is frequently

expressed in pleomorphic xanthoastrocytoma cells {2083}. *BRAF* V600E mutation, a common alteration in pleomorphic xanthoastrocytoma, can be detected by immunohistochemistry using a specific antibody {1082,2280}. The immunophenotype with V600E-mutant BRAF expression and loss of CDKN2A expression (secondary to homozygous deletion of *CDKN2A*) is frequently observed in pleomorphic xanthoastrocytoma {1316}.

Proliferation
In most pleomorphic xanthoastrocytomas, mitotic figures are rare or absent, and the Ki-67 proliferation index is generally < 1% {825}.

Cell of origin
As originally proposed by Kepes, Rubinstein, and Eng in 1979 {1254}, it has been postulated that pleomorphic xanthoastrocytoma originates from subpial astrocytes. This hypothesis would explain the superficial location of most cases, and is supported by ultrastructural features shared between subpial astrocytes and the neoplastic cells in pleomorphic xanthoastrocytoma, in particular the presence of a basal lamina surrounding individual cells. However, the expression of neuronal markers {828} and CD34 {1316, 2083} in many pleomorphic xanthoastrocytomas, as well as the occasional association with cortical dysplasia {1271}, suggests a more complex histogenesis and a possible origin from multipotent neuroectodermal precursor cells or from a pre-existing hamartomatous lesion.

Genetic profile
Complex karyotypes have been documented, with gains of chromosomes 3 and 7 and alterations of the long arm of chromosome 1 {1495,2253,2254}, but these are not specific to pleomorphic

xanthoastrocytoma. The tumours are predominantly diploid {1047,2701}, occasionally with polyploid populations {1047}, possibly due to subgroups of particularly bizarre, multinucleated tumour cells. Comparative genomic hybridization of 50 cases identified loss of chromosome 9 as the hallmark alteration (present in 50% of cases) {2713}. Homozygous 9p21.3 deletions involving the *CDKN2A/CDKN2B* loci were identified in 6 of 10 cases (60%) {2713}. Accordingly, loss of CDKN2A protein expression was documented by immunohistochemistry in 61% of pleomorphic xanthoastrocytomas {1316}.

BRAF point mutations occur in approximately 50–78% of cases {584,601,1082, 1316,2277,2280}. Most are of the V600E type, with only a single documented exception {2280}. However, *BRAF* V600E mutations are not specific to pleomorphic xanthoastrocytoma, and are also observed in other primary CNS tumours, in particular ganglioglioma and pilocytic astrocytoma {414,599,1297,2277,2280}. The occurrence of *BRAF* mutations seems to be unrelated to the presence of histological features of anaplasia.

Two studies investigating a total of 7 non–*BRAF*-mutant pleomorphic xanthoastrocytomas identified 1 tumour harbouring a *TSC2* mutation, 1 with an *NF1* mutation, and 1 with an *ETV6-NTRK3* fusion {184, 2855}. In four series (one published only in abstract form) with a total of 123 tumours, mutations in the *TP53* gene were found in only 7 cases (6%) {824,1238, 1917}, and were unrelated to the presence of histological features of anaplasia. Amplifications of the *EGFR*, *CDK4*, and *MDM2* genes were absent in a series of 62 tumours {1238}. No *IDH1* mutations were detected in a series of 7 tumours (by sequencing) {118} or in a series of 60 cases (by immunohistochemistry for R132H-mutant IDH1) {1081}. These findings molecularly distinguish pleomorphic xanthoastrocytoma from diffusely infiltrating cerebral astrocytoma.

Although there are few data on the occurrence of *BRAF* fusions in pleomorphic xanthoastrocytoma, there was no evidence of 7q34 duplication, which is often associated with *BRAF* fusion, in a series of 10 cases analysed by microarray-based comparative genomic hybridization {1961}.

Genetic susceptibility
There are no distinct associations with

hereditary tumour syndromes, with the exception of several reports of pleomorphic xanthoastrocytoma in patients with neurofibromatosis type 1 {14,1380, 1761,1870}. Given the high frequency of MAPK pathway alterations observed in sporadic pleomorphic xanthoastrocytoma, an association with NF1 is not unexpected. Familial clustering of pleomorphic xanthoastrocytoma has not been documented. One case of a pleomorphic xanthoastrocytoma with classic histological and molecular features developing in DiGeorge syndrome has been reported {860}.

Prognosis and predictive factors

Pleomorphic xanthoastrocytoma behaves in a less malignant fashion than might be suggested by its highly pleomorphic histology {1254}, but it has an only relatively favourable prognosis. In a retrospective series of 74 cases, 54 patients with WHO grade II pleomorphic xanthoastrocytoma had an average 5-year recurrence-free survival rate of 70.9% and 5-year overall survival rate of 90.4% {1081}. Extent of resection was confirmed to be the most significant predictive factor of recurrence {825,1081}. Among patients whose tumours had low mitotic activity (i.e. < 5 mitoses per 10 high-power fields), the estimated recurrence-free survival rate was 73.7%, and was similar between paediatric patients (73.5%) and adult patients

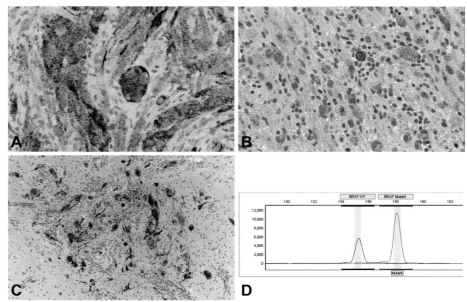

Fig. 2.24 Pleomorphic xanthoastrocytoma. Molecularly confirmed *BRAF* V600E–mutant tumours showing: (**A**) strong granular cytoplasmic immunostaining of a characteristic pleomorphic multinucleated giant tumour cell, (**B**) weak granular cytoplasmic immunostaining of pleomorphic and spindle tumour cells, and (**C**) strong granular cytoplasmic immunostaining of a cluster of isolated tumour cells (A–C: V600E-mutant BRAF immunohistochemistry). **D** The V600E-mutant BRAF peak in addition to the wildtype BRAF peak is consistent with the presence of a *BRAF* V600E mutation {1082}.

(74.4%) {1081}. The estimated 5-year overall survival rate for these patients was 89.4%, and was similar between children (92.9%) and adults (86.8%) {1081}.

BRAF V600E mutation is more common in WHO grade II pleomorphic xanthoastrocytoma than in anaplastic (WHO grade III) pleomorphic xanthoastrocytoma. *BRAF* V600E mutation status is not significantly different between paediatric and adult tumours {1081}. It is unclear whether the presence of *BRAF* V600E mutation has prognostic significance.

Anaplastic pleomorphic xanthoastrocytoma

Giannini C.
Paulus W.
Louis D.N.
Liberski P.P.
Figarella-Branger D.
Capper D.

Definition

A pleomorphic xanthoastrocytoma with ≥ 5 mitoses per 10 high-power fields.

Patients with anaplastic pleomorphic xanthoastrocytoma have significantly worse survival than those whose tumours show < 5 mitoses per 10 high-power fields {825,1081}. Necrosis may be present, but its significance in the absence of increased mitotic activity is unknown {1081}.

The frequency of *BRAF* V600E mutation is lower among anaplastic pleomorphic xanthoastrocytomas than among WHO grade II pleomorphic xanthoastrocytomas, and the prognostic significance of the mutation is unknown {1081,2290}.

ICD-O code   9424/3

Grading

Anaplastic pleomorphic xanthoastrocytoma corresponds histologically to WHO grade III.

Epidemiology

No specific epidemiological data are available regarding anaplastic pleomorphic xanthoastrocytoma compared with

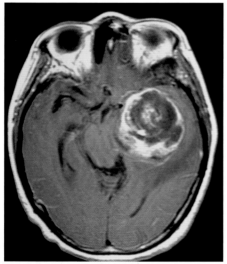

Fig. 2.25 Anaplastic pleomorphic xanthoastrocytoma. T1-weighted MRI with contrast sequences demonstrates a large non-homogeneously enhancing tumour with mass effect and moderate surrounding oedema.

pleomorphic xanthoastrocytoma. In one series of 74 cases, anaplasia was present in 23 cases (31%) at first diagnosis, in 23% of paediatric cases, and in 37% of adult cases {1081}.

Localization

Like WHO grade II pleomorphic xanthoastrocytoma, anaplastic pleomorphic xanthoastrocytoma is typically a supratentorial tumour, with the temporal lobe being the most commonly involved lobe.

Clinical features

The signs and symptoms of anaplastic pleomorphic xanthoastrocytoma are similar to those of WHO grade II pleomorphic xanthoastrocytoma. Seizures are the most common presenting symptom.

Imaging

Like WHO grade II pleomorphic xanthoastrocytoma, anaplastic pleomorphic xanthoastrocytoma is often a circumscribed supratentorial mass, peripherally located and frequently cystic, involving the cortex and overlying leptomeninges.

Microscopy

Anaplasia in pleomorphic xanthoastrocytoma typically manifests as brisk mitotic activity in a tumour that otherwise retains all the diagnostic histological features of pleomorphic xanthoastrocytoma. High levels of mitotic activity may be focal or diffuse. Necrosis is frequently present, almost always in association with brisk mitotic activity. Microvascular proliferation is uncommon and usually associated with brisk mitotic activity and necrosis. Anaplasia may be present at the time of first diagnosis or at the time of recurrence, suggesting progression from a lower-grade to an anaplastic pleomorphic xanthoastrocytoma. However, some tumours that display features of anaplasia at first resection occasionally demonstrate features at the upper limits of a WHO grade II tumour at the time of recurrence, likely reflecting tumour heterogeneity. Anaplastic pleomorphic

xanthoastrocytoma, manifesting both at initial diagnosis and at recurrence, may demonstrate less pleomorphism and a more diffusely infiltrative pattern than typical classic WHO grade II pleomorphic xanthoastrocytoma. Although histological patterns of anaplasia have not been formally studied in pleomorphic xanthoastrocytoma, small-cell, fibrillary, and epithelioid/rhabdoid transformation have been reported {1248}.

Anaplastic pleomorphic xanthoastrocytoma may be difficult to distinguish from epithelioid glioblastoma (see p. 50) both histologically and molecularly, because both tumour types commonly exhibit *BRAF* V600E mutations {1297}; in fact, pleomorphic xanthoastrocytoma recurring as epithelioid glioblastoma has also been described {2508}. Anaplastic pleomorphic xanthoastrocytomas lack the cytological uniformity typical of epithelioid glioblastomas and have eosinophilic granular bodies, which are not seen in epithelioid glioblastoma {1297,1299}. In many anaplastic pleomorphic xanthoastrocytomas, a lower-grade component with features typical of pleomorphic xanthoastrocytoma is present at least focally {825}. There have been rare reports of a SMARCB1-deficient, atypical teratoid/rhabdoid tumour–like lesion arising in pleomorphic xanthoastrocytoma, associated with loss of SMARCB1 expression in the morphologically distinct high-grade rhabdoid component {396,1157}. Such clonal evolution may be associated with a highly aggressive biology even when the original tumour is low-grade; the term "SMARCB1-deficient anaplastic pleomorphic xanthoastrocytoma" has been suggested for such a lesion.

Immunophenotype

The phenotypic profile of anaplastic pleomorphic xanthoastrocytoma is similar to that of WHO grade II pleomorphic xanthoastrocytoma.

Genetic profile

The genetic alterations specific to anaplastic pleomorphic xanthoastrocytoma

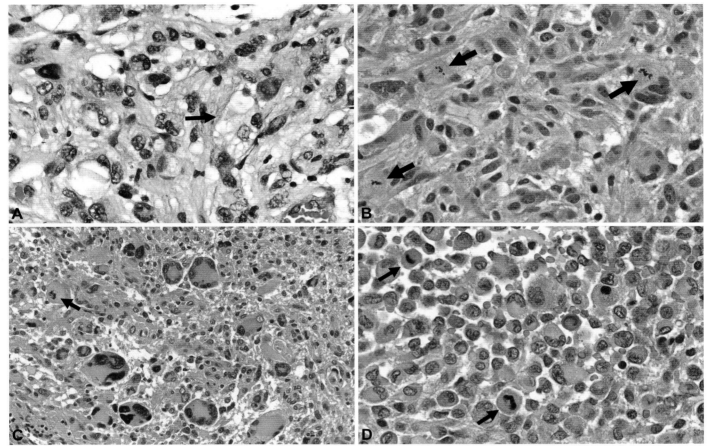

Fig. 2.26 Anaplastic pleomorphic xanthoastrocytoma. **A** The tumour shows classic features with pleomorphic and xanthomatous (arrow) cells and (**B**) brisk mitotic activity (arrows), including atypical mitoses. **C** The tumour recurred 1 year later and showed remaining areas with pleomorphic morphology and (**D**) monomorphous areas with epithelioid and rhabdoid cells with mitotic activity (arrows).

are unknown. Although some anaplastic xanthoastrocytomas may develop through malignant progression from WHO grade II pleomorphic xanthoastrocytoma, the sequence of underlying genetic events has not yet been determined. The frequency of *BRAF* V600E mutation is lower in anaplastic pleomorphic xanthoastrocytoma (9 of 19 cases [47.4%] in one study) than in pleomorphic xanthoastrocytoma (30 of 40 cases [75.0%] in a separate study), and its prognostic significance is unknown {1081,2290}. *BRAF* V600E mutation status is not significantly different between paediatric and adult cases {1081}.

Genetic susceptibility

No distinct associations between anaplastic pleomorphic xanthoastrocytoma and hereditary tumour syndromes have been reported.

Prognosis and predictive factors

A consistent relationship between mitotic activity and outcome in pleomorphic xanthoastrocytoma has emerged, whereas the relationship between necrosis and outcome remains unclear {825,1081}. One study found that a mitotic count of ≥ 5 mitoses per 10 high-power fields (with one high-power field covering 0.23 mm²) can be used to establish the diagnosis. In that study, significant mitotic activity (defined as ≥ 5 mitoses per 10 high-power fields) and/or necrosis was encountered in 31% of tumours at initial presentation {1081}. These features were found to be associated with shorter survival {1081}. The 5-year overall survival rate for patients whose tumours showed ≥ 5 mitoses per 10 high-power fields was significantly worse than that for patients whose tumours showed < 5 mitoses per 10 high-power fields (89.4% vs 55.6%, *P* = 0.0005). And the 5-year overall

survival rate for patients with tumour necrosis was worse than that for those without (42.2% vs 90.2%, *P* = 0.0002). The dataset was insufficient to detect a difference in survival between patients whose tumours had ≥ 5 mitoses per 10 high-power fields and necrosis (n = 14; 7 patients died and 6 cases recurred) and those whose tumours had ≥ 5 mitoses per 10 high-power fields but no necrosis (n = 5; 2 patients died and 3 cases recurred). Of the 2 patients whose tumours had necrosis but not increased mitotic activity, one had no evidence of disease after 10 years of follow-up; the other had only limited follow-up (1 month), but was still alive at that time. Between children and adults, there were no significant differences in 5-year recurrence-free survival (67.9% vs 62.4%, *P* = 0.39) or 5-year overall survival (87.4% vs 76.3%, *P* = 0.83). The prognostic significance of *BRAF* V600E mutation remains unknown.

CHAPTER 3

Ependymal tumours

Subependymoma

Myxopapillary ependymoma

Ependymoma

Ependymoma, *RELA* fusion–positive

Anaplastic ependymoma

Subependymoma

McLendon R.
Schiffer D.
Rosenblum M.K.
Wiestler O.D.

Rushing E.J.
Hirose T.
Santi M.

Definition

A slow-growing, exophytic, intraventricular glial neoplasm characterized by clusters of bland to mildly pleomorphic, mitotically inactive cells embedded in an abundant fibrillary matrix with frequent microcystic change.

Subependymomas are often detected incidentally, by neuroimaging or at autopsy, and have a very favourable prognosis {1126,1211,1533,2794}. Some tumours have the admixed histological features of both subependymoma and ependymoma.

ICD-O code   9383/1

Grading

Subependymoma corresponds histologically to WHO grade I.

Epidemiology

The true incidence of subependymoma is difficult to determine, because these tumours frequently remain asymptomatic and are often found incidentally at autopsy. In two studies, subependymomas accounted for approximately 8% of ependymal tumours {1398,2274}, and in one of the studies, they accounted for 0.51% of all CNS tumours resected at a single institution {1398}.

Subependymomas develop in both sexes and in all age groups, but occur most frequently in middle-aged and elderly patients. The male-to-female ratio is approximately 2.3:1 {2056,2201}.

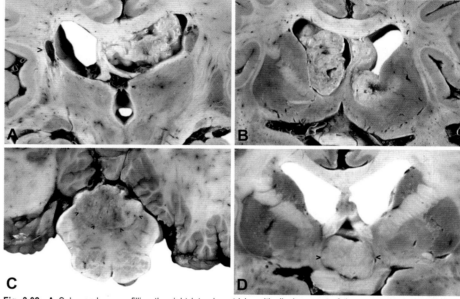

Fig. 3.02 A Subependymoma filling the right lateral ventricle, with displacement of the septum pellucidum to the contralateral hemisphere. The tumour is sharply delineated and only focally attached to the ventricular wall; the cut surface is greyish-white with some small haemorrhages; note the old cystic infarct in the left corpus caudatum (arrowhead). **B** Large subependymoma filling the left ventricle and a smaller one in the right ventricle. **C** Posterior fossa subependymoma in the caudal region of the fourth ventricle. Note the compression of the dorsal medulla (arrowheads). **D** Third ventricle subependymoma (arrowheads).

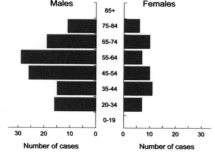

Fig. 3.01 Age and sex distribution of subependymoma, based on 167 cases; data from the Central Brain Tumor Registry of the United States (CBTRUS), 1995–2002.

Localization

Subependymomas are distinguished by their intraventricular location, sharp demarcation, slow growth, and usually non-invasive behaviour. The most frequent site is the fourth ventricle (accounting for 50–60% of cases), followed by the lateral ventricles (accounting for 30–40%). Less common sites include the third ventricle and septum pellucidum. In rare cases, tumours occur intraparenchymally in the cerebrum {1279}. In the spinal cord, subependymomas manifest as cervical and cervicothoracic intramedullary or (rarely) extramedullary masses {1130,2201}.

Clinical features

Subependymomas may become clinically apparent through ventricular obstruction and increased intracranial pressure. Spontaneous intratumoural haemorrhage has been observed {31,369}. Rare intraparenchymal tumours exhibit marked oedema and are associated with seizures {2056}. Spinal tumours manifest with motor and sensory deficits according to the affected anatomical segment. Incidental detection of asymptomatic subependymomas at autopsy is common {2201}.

Imaging

Subependymomas present as sharply demarcated nodular masses that are usually non-enhancing. Calcification and foci of haemorrhage may be apparent. Intramedullary cases are typically eccentric in location, rather than centrally positioned as is typical of intraspinal ependymomas. The lesions are hypointense to hyperintense on both T1- and T2-weighted MRI, with minimal to moderate enhancement {2056,2201}.

Macroscopy

These tumours present as firm nodules of various sizes, bulging into the ventricular lumen. In most cases, the diameter does not exceed 1–2 cm. Intraventricular and spinal subependymomas are generally

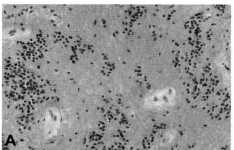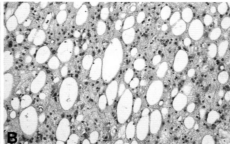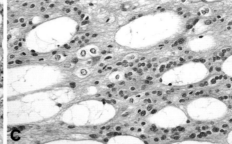

Fig. 3.03 Subependymoma. **A** Subependymomas have a coarse fibrillar matrix and contain clusters of uniform nuclei. **B** Microcysts are common. **C** Cells are uniform, often appearing as bare nuclei against the fibrillary matrix.

well demarcated. Large subependymomas of the fourth ventricle may cause brain stem compression. Rare cases arising in the cerebellopontine angle have been described in both adults and children {1048}.

Microscopy

Subependymomas are characterized by clusters of small uniform nuclei embedded in a dense fibrillary matrix of glial cell processes with frequent occurrence of small cysts, particularly in lesions originating in the lateral ventricles. Tumour cell nuclei appear isomorphic and resemble those of subependymal glia. In solid tumours, occasional pleomorphic nuclei may be encountered; however, nuclear variation is typical in multicystic tumours. Some subependymomas exhibit low-level mitotic activity, but this is exceptional. Calcifications and haemorrhage can occur. Prominent tumour vasculature may rarely be accompanied by microvascular proliferation. Occasionally, cell processes are oriented around vessels, forming ependymal pseudorosettes. In some cases, a subependymoma constitutes the most superficial aspect of a classic ependymoma or (more rarely) a tanycytic ependymoma {1279}; such combined tumours are classified as mixed ependymoma–subependymoma and are graded on the basis of the ependymoma component {2201}. In one rare example, the subependymomatous element predominated and seemed to signify a good overall prognosis {2201}. Examples of subependymoma with melanin formation {2179}, rhabdomyosarcomatous differentiation {2566}, and sarcomatous transformation of vascular stromal elements {1532} have been reported.
At the ultrastructural level, subependymomas show cells with typical ependymal characteristics, including cilium formation and microvilli, and sometimes with abundant intermediate filaments {101,1716,2274}.

Immunophenotype
Immunoreactivity for GFAP is usually present, although to various extents, and immunoreactivity can also be found for neural markers of low specificity, such as NCAM1 and neuron-specific enolase {2832}. Unlike in classic ependymomas, EMA is rarely expressed in subependymomas. One study of potential therapeutic targets reported that TOP2B, MDM2, nucleolin, HIF1-alpha, and phosphorylated STAT3 are frequently expressed in subependymomas {1329}.

Cell of origin

Proposed cells of origin include subependymal glia {101,1716}, astrocytes of the subependymal plate, ependymal cells {2205}, and a mixture of astrocytes and ependymal cells {746,2257}.

Genetic profile

A recent study using DNA methylation profiles of ependymomas from all age groups and subependymomas from adult patients to characterize the full range of disease identified nine molecular groups of ependymoma across three anatomical sites: the supratentorial compartment, posterior fossa, and spinal compartment {1880}. Groups dominated by subependymomas were found to occur in all three of these anatomical locations. Posterior fossa and spinal subependymomas harboured chromosome 6 copy number alterations, whereas supratentorial tumours showed virtually none. The supratentorial and posterior fossa subependymoma groups showed excellent overall survival.

Genetic susceptibility

Familial occurrence of subependymomas is rare, but well documented. All published cases have been located in the fourth ventricle. Reports have described the simultaneous manifestation of fourth ventricular subependymomas in

a set of 41-year-old identical twins {1799}, in a set of 22-year-old identical twins {464}, and in a brother and sister aged 28 and 31 years, respectively {430}. In a family with several brain tumours, three siblings developed subependymomas of the fourth ventricle: two brothers (aged 27 and 57 years) and a sister (aged 49 years). In addition, a younger sibling (aged 13 years) had a pontine tumour of undetermined pathology and an elder brother (aged 57 years) developed a fourth ventricular ependymoma {1032}. A prenatal, maldevelopmental origin of familial subependymomas has been suggested {464}, but the occurrence in a family with several brain tumours and in a father (aged 47 years) and son (aged 22 years) is more suggestive of a genetic susceptibility {1032,2209}.

Prognosis and predictive factors

Subependymomas have a good prognosis {1126}. To date, no recurrences after gross total resection have been reported {2257}. Complete excision may not be feasible for all tumours arising from the floor of the fourth ventricle; however, debulking alone usually yields an excellent prognosis, given that these tumours grow slowly and residual tumour may take decades to manifest as a symptomatic mass {321}. Although recurrences are generally not expected with subtotally resected tumours {2028}, rare cases have been reported, and cerebrospinal fluid spread has been documented as well {2321,2677}. Mitotic activity is usually low or absent. Scattered mitoses and cellular pleomorphism are of no clinical significance {2020,2201}. Ki-67/MIB1 immunohistochemical studies have found proliferation index values of < 1%, compatible with the slow growth of this entity, although one study of 2 cases indicated that recurrence rate may correlate with proliferation index {1354}.

Myxopapillary ependymoma

McLendon R.
Schiffer D.
Rosenblum M.K.
Wiestler O.D.

Definition
A glial tumour arising almost exclusively in the region of the conus medullaris, cauda equina, and filum terminale, and histologically characterized by elongated, fibrillary processes arranged in radial patterns around vascularized, mucoid, fibrovascular cores.

Myxopapillary ependymoma is a slow-growing variant of ependymoma. It typically occurs in young adults. The tumour generally has a favourable prognosis, but can be difficult to resect completely. When this is the case, residual tumour may recur repeatedly, as the tumour becomes entangled with spinal nerves.

ICD-O code   9394/1

Grading
Histologically, myxopapillary ependymoma corresponds to WHO grade I. However, this variant may have a more aggressive biological behaviour in children and a poor outcome after incomplete resection.

Epidemiology
Myxopapillary variants account for 9–13% of all ependymomas {1398,2274}. In the conus medullaris / cauda equina region, myxopapillary ependymomas are the most common intramedullary neoplasm, with annual incidence rates of about 0.08 cases per 100 000 males and 0.05 cases per 100 000 females {1863}.

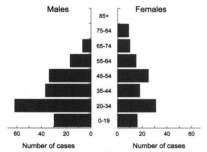

Fig. 3.04 Age and sex distribution of myxopapillary ependymoma, based on 311 cases; data from the Central Brain Tumor Registry of the United States (CBTRUS), 1995–2002.

The average patient age at presentation is 36 years, with a range of 6–82 years. In one study of 320 ependymomas of the filum terminale, 83% were of the myxopapillary type, with a male-to-female ratio of 2.2:1 {395}. The youngest patient was an infant aged 3 weeks {459}.

Localization
Myxopapillary ependymomas occur almost exclusively in the region of the conus medullaris, cauda equina, and filum terminale. They may originate from ependymal glia of the filum terminale to involve the cauda equina, and only rarely invade nerve roots or erode sacral bone. Multifocal tumours have been described {1748}. Myxopapillary ependymomas can occasionally be observed at other locations, such as the cervicothoracic spinal cord {2396}, the fourth ventricle {1502}, the lateral ventricles {2247}, and the brain parenchyma {2698}. Subcutaneous sacrococcygeal or presacral myxopapillary ependymomas constitute a distinct subgroup. They are thought to originate from ectopic ependymal remnants {1089}. Intrasacral variants can clinically mimic chordoma.

Clinical features
Myxopapillary ependymomas are typically associated with back pain, often of long duration.

Imaging
Myxopapillary ependymomas are typically sharply circumscribed and contrast-enhancing. Extensive cystic change and haemorrhage may be seen.

Spread
In a recent review of 183 patients with myxopapillary ependymomas, distant spinal metastases were found in 17 patients (9.3%) and brain metastases in 11 (6.0%). Factors associated with distant treatment failure included young age, lack of initial adjuvant radiotherapy, and incomplete excision {2711}. Paediatric patients are particularly prone to

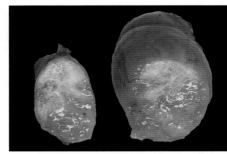

Fig. 3.05 This macroscopic photograph of a transected myxopapillary ependymoma shows its typical sausage appearance externally, with the mucinous, pinkish-white variegated appearance on cut surface.

exhibiting spinal metastatic dissemination at presentation {674,2108}.

Macroscopy
Myxopapillary ependymomas are lobulated, soft, and grey or tan. They are often encapsulated. Gelatinous alterations, cyst formation, and haemorrhage may be apparent.

Microscopy
In classic cases, cuboidal to elongated tumour cells are radially arranged in papillary fashion around hyalinized fibrovascular cores. Some examples show little or no papillary structuring and consist largely of confluent, polygonal tumour cell sheets or fascicles of spindled cells. Alcian blue–positive myxoid material accumulates between tumour cells and blood vessels, also collecting in microcysts (which help to identify largely solid, non-papillary examples). Rounded eosinophilic structures (so-called balloons) that are periodic acid–Schiff–positive and exhibit spiculated reticulin staining are seen in some cases. Mitotic activity and the Ki-67 proliferation index are low {2019}. Histological features of anaplasia are most exceptional {98}.

Ultrastructurally, the cells do not show polarity, but do show adherens junctions with cytoplasmic thickening and wide spaces containing amorphous material or loose filaments {2076,2402}. Extracellular spaces, delineated by cells with basal membranes, contain projected

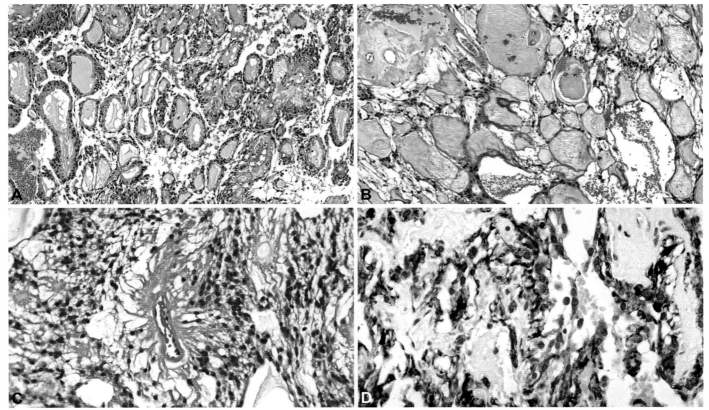

Fig. 3.06 Myxopapillary ependymoma. **A** Tumour cells accumulate around vessels with mucoid degeneration. **B** Tumour cells interspersed between large vessels with mucoid degeneration. **C** Elongated fibrillary processes extend through myxoid regions to reach a blood vessel. **D** Myxopapillary ependymoma of the cauda equina. Perivascular tumour cells consistently express GFAP.

villi {2076}. Few cilia, complex interdigitations, and abundant basement membrane structures have been described {2019}, with the distinctive feature of some examples being aggregations of microtubules within endoplasmic reticulum complexes {1018,1019}. The presence of adherens junctions and intracytoplasmic lumina with microvilli was recently confirmed {2686}.

Immunophenotype
Diffuse immunoreactivity for GFAP distinguishes myxopapillary ependymomas from metastatic carcinomas, chordomas, myxoid chondrosarcomas, paragangliomas, and schwannomas {1427,2641}. Labelling for S100 or vimentin is also typical, and reactivity for CD99 and NCAM1 is frequently seen {1427}. Immunoreactivity for the AE1/AE3 cytokeratin cocktail is a common feature of

myxopapillary ependymomas, whereas labelling for CAM5.2, CK5/6, CK7, CK20, or 34betaE12 has been reported as absent or exceptional in this setting {1427, 2641}.

Genetic profile
A recent study using DNA methylation profiles to characterize the full range of disease identified nine molecular groups of ependymoma across three anatomical sites: the supratentorial compartment, posterior fossa, and spinal compartment {1880}. Myxopapillary ependymomas were found in one molecular group from the spinal compartment. They were characterized by polyploidy (in particular gains across multiple chromosomes) and an excellent outcome.

Prognosis and predictive factors
Prognosis is favourable, with a 5-year

survival rate of 98.4% after total or partial resection {2770}. Late recurrence and distant metastases can occur after incomplete resections in both adults and children {35,674}. Children have had a less predictable outcome in some studies, even with apparent gross total resection {2216,2426}. In a series of 183 cases, treatment failure occurred in approximately one third of the patients. Recurrence was mainly local and was more frequent in younger patients and those not treated initially with adjuvant radiotherapy {1388,2711}. Gross total resection plays an important role in improving outcome, and adjuvant radiotherapy improves progression-free survival {1389,2578}.
Although age seems to be the strongest predictor of recurrence, expression of EGFR has also been cited as a potential biomarker of recurrence {2647}.

Ependymoma

Ellison D.W. Korshunov A.
McLendon R. Ng H.-K.
Wiestler O.D. Witt H.
Kros J.M. Hirose T.

Definition

A circumscribed glioma composed of uniform small cells with round nuclei in a fibrillary matrix and characterized by perivascular anucleate zones (pseudorosettes) with ependymal rosettes also found in about one quarter of cases.

Classic ependymoma generally has a low cell density and a low mitotic count. It very rarely invades adjacent CNS parenchyma to any significant extent. Cilia and microvilli are seen on ultrastructural examination.

Classic ependymomas are mainly intracranial tumours; they do occur in the spinal cord, but the myxopapillary variant is more common at this site. Classic ependymomas occur in both adults and children, although most posterior fossa tumours present in childhood. Ependymomas have a variable clinical outcome, which is primarily dependent on extent of surgical resection, the use of irradiation as an adjuvant therapy, and molecular group {857,1880}.

Three distinct histopathological phenotypes, which are classified as ependymoma variants (although without particular clinicopathological significance) can be a prominent component of both classic and anaplastic ependymoma: papillary ependymoma, clear cell ependymoma, and tanycytic ependymoma.

ICD-O code   9391/3

Grading

Traditionally, classic ependymoma and anaplastic ependymoma are considered to correspond histologically to WHO grades II and III, respectively. However, no association between grade and biological behaviour or survival has been definitively established {248,633,703}. Of the various studies of prognostic variables and outcome in ependymoma, those that have not found an association between grade (II vs III) and progression-free or overall survival outnumber those that have. The published ratios of grade II to grade III tumours in series of ependymomas vary widely, from 17:1 to 1:7, and the explanation for such inconsistent data is multifactorial {633,856,2557}. The interpretation of most histopathological variables used in this classification for grading purposes is subjective, and ependymomas are morphologically heterogeneous. For example, the significance of grading on the basis of focal microvascular proliferation or focally increased mitotic counts within large areas of bland architectural and cytological features is difficult to determine. There have been few studies of the prognostic significance of WHO grade or individual pathological features across large trial cohorts in which proper multivariate analyses of prognostic variables can be performed, and there have been only three studies in which evaluation of histological variables was defined stringently and undertaken by several observers {633,856,2557}. Due to these limiting factors, grading is almost never used for therapeutic stratification of patients with ependymoma. Given that specific genetic alterations and molecular groups have recently been proposed as prognostic or predictive factors for these tumours {1560,1880,2767}, the practice of histologically grading ependymoma may soon become obsolete altogether.

Epidemiology

Incidence

In the USA, ependymomas account for 6.8% of all neuroepithelial neoplasms. The incidence rate decreases with increasing patient age at diagnosis, from 5.6% (at 0–14 years) to 4.5% (at 15–19 years) to 4.0% (at 20–34 years) {1863}. In children aged < 3 years, as many as 30% of all CNS tumours are ependymomas. In Canada, a mean annual incidence of 4.6 cases per 100 000 population was estimated for ependymomas in infants {2046}. In the USA, ependymoma is more common in Whites than in African-Americans, with an incidence rate ratio of 1.67:1. No such difference is found between Hispanic and non-Hispanic populations {1863}. In the spinal cord, ependymomas are the most common neuroepithelial neoplasms, accounting for 50–60% of all spinal gliomas in adults {2653}, but they are rare in children {164}.

Age and sex distribution

Ependymomas can develop in patients of any age, with reported patient ages ranging from birth to 81 years [http://www.cbtrus.org]. However, incidence is greatly dependent on histological variant, molecular group, and location. Posterior fossa ependymomas are most common among children, with a mean patient age at presentation of 6.4 years {2295}, and spinal tumours dominate a second age peak at 30–40 years. Supratentorial ependymomas affect paediatric as well as adult patients. The overall male-to-female ratio is 1.77:1, but this ratio varies significantly across different anatomical sites and molecular groups {1171,1880, 2046}. In the USA, classic and anaplastic ependymoma have an approximate combined annual incidence of 0.29 cases in males and 0.22 in females.

Localization

Ependymomas may occur along the ventricular system or spinal canal, in the cerebral hemispheres, or at extra-CNS sites. Overall, 60% of the tumours develop in the posterior fossa, 30% in the supratentorial compartment, and 10% in the spinal canal [http://seer.cancer.gov/archive/csr/1975_2004]. In adult patients, infratentorial and spinal ependymomas occur with almost equal frequency, whereas infratentorial

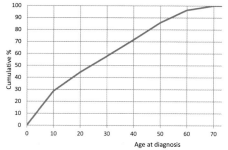

Fig. 3.07 Cumulative age distribution (both sexes) of ependymoma, based on 298 cases {2274}.

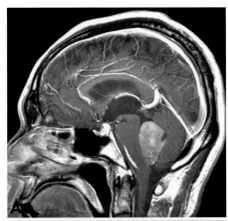

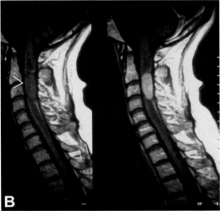

Fig. 3.08 A Fourth ventricle ependymoma. Note the enlargement of the aqueduct and hydrocephalus of the third ventricle. **B** Cervical ependymoma. Sagittal MRI shows an ependymoma in the upper cervical spinal cord (left, arrowhead) with marked gadolinium enhancement (right), delineated on both sides by a typical cyst.

ependymomas predominate in children {1385}. In children aged < 3 years at presentation, 80% of ependymomas are in the posterior fossa {2046}. Posterior fossa ependymomas are located in the fourth ventricle and sometimes involve the cerebellopontine angle; in the fourth ventricle, 60%, 30%, and 10% of the tumours originate in the floor, lateral aspect, and roof, respectively {1087,2234}. Supratentorial ependymomas arise from the lateral or third ventricles (in 60% of cases) or from the cerebral hemispheres, without obvious connection to a ventricle (in 40% of cases). In the spinal cord, cervical or cervicothoracic localization is common among classic ependymomas. In contrast, the myxopapillary variant predominantly affects the conus and cauda equina. Rare extra-CNS ependymomas have been observed in the ovaries {1327}, broad ligaments {159}, pelvic and abdominal cavities, mediastinum,

and lung. Myxopapillary ependymomas occur in the subcutaneous tissue of the sacrococcygeal area.

Clinical features

The clinical manifestations depend on tumour localization. Ependymomas of the posterior fossa can present with signs and symptoms of hydrocephalus and raised intracranial pressure, such as headache, nausea, vomiting, and dizziness. Involvement of cerebellar and brain stem structures may cause ataxia, visual disturbance, paresis, or cranial nerve deficits. Patients with supratentorial ependymomas may show focal neurological deficits or epilepsy, as well as features of raised intracranial pressure. Enlargement of the head or separation of the cranial sutures can be evident in young babies. Spinal ependymomas can present with back pain and focal motor and sensory deficits or paraparesis.

Imaging

Gadolinium-enhanced MRI shows well-circumscribed masses with various degrees of contrast enhancement. Ventricular obstruction or brain stem displacement and hydrocephalus are common accompanying features. Supratentorial tumours often exhibit cystic components. Intratumoural haemorrhage and calcification are occasionally observed. Gross infiltration of adjacent brain structures and oedema are very rare. MRI is particularly useful for determining the relationship with surrounding structures, invasion along the cerebrospinal fluid pathway, and syrinx formation. Cerebrospinal fluid spread is a key factor for staging, prognostication, and treatment.

Macroscopy

Ependymomas are well-circumscribed tumours usually arising in or near the ventricular system. They are tan-coloured and are soft and spongy, occasionally with gritty calcium deposits. Tumours arising in the caudal fourth ventricle often flow through the foramina of Luschka and Magendie to wrap around the brain stem's cranial nerves and vessels, and have been termed "plastic ependymomas" {503}. Rarely, ependymomas can occur within the cerebral hemisphere, where they are well circumscribed {2356}. Other rare examples, often recurrent tumours, infiltrate the cerebral parenchyma and

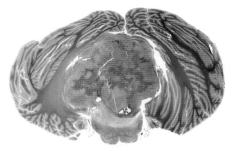

Fig. 3.09 Ependymoma in a child, filling the entire lumen of the fourth ventricle. Note the compression and displacement of the medulla.

demonstrate histopathological overlap with small cell glioblastoma {1463}.

Microscopy

Classic ependymoma is a well-delineated glioma with monomorphic cells characterized by a variable density and round to oval nuclei with speckled nuclear chromatin. The key histological features are perivascular anucleate zones (pseudorosettes) and (true) ependymal rosettes. The pseudorosettes are composed of tumour cells radially arranged around blood vessels, creating perivascular anucleate zones of fine fibrillary processes. The ependymal rosettes and tubular canals are composed of bland cuboidal or columnar tumour cells arranged around a central lumen. Pseudorosettes can be found in practically all ependymomas, whereas ependymal rosettes are present in only a minority.

Cell density can vary considerably in ependymoma, and a high nuclear-to-cytoplasmic ratio may not necessarily be associated with brisk mitotic activity or other anaplastic features, particularly in supratentorial vascular ependymoma, which demonstrates a distinctive branching network of delicate capillary blood vessels and focal clear-cell change. Some posterior fossa ependymomas contain nodules of high tumour cell density, often with an increased mitotic count. This biphasic pattern can accompany a distinctive cerebriform folding of the tumour surface.

Other histological features include regions of myxoid degeneration, intratumoural haemorrhage, dystrophic calcification, and (occasionally) metaplastic cartilage or bone. Prominent hyalinization of tumour vessels is sometimes found, especially in posterior fossa and spinal ependymomas. Regions of geographical necrosis may be observed in classic

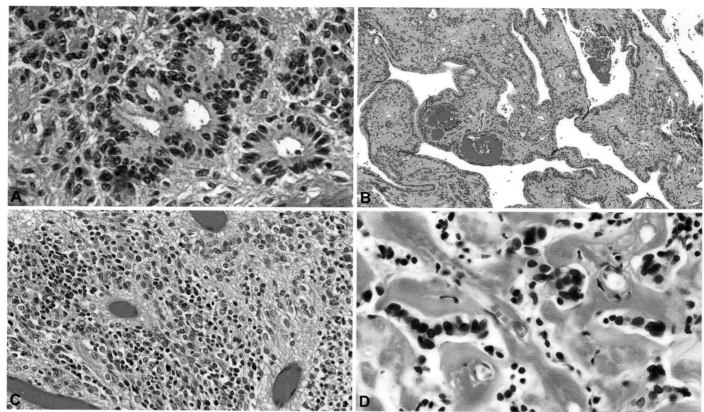

Fig. 3.10 Ependymoma. **A** Ependymal rosettes are characterized by columnar tumour cells arranged around a central lumen; they are infrequent, but a diagnostic hallmark of ependymoma {1291}. **B** Ependymal canals. **C** High tumour-cell density and perivascular pseudorosettes. **D** This ependymoma shows extensive hyalinization, which may precede calcification {1291}.

ependymoma, but palisading necrosis and microvascular proliferation are only focal features in this tumour, with its bland cytology and low mitotic count. The interface between tumour and CNS parenchyma is typically well demarcated, although evidence of brain tissue infiltration may occasionally be encountered.

Three distinct histopathological phenotypes, which are classified as ependymoma variants (although without particular clinicopathological significance) can be a prominent component of both classic and anaplastic ependymoma: papillary ependymoma, clear cell ependymoma, and tanycytic ependymoma.

Rare ependymomas have been reported with lipomatous metaplasia, widespread pleomorphic giant cells, extensive tumour cell vacuolation, melanotic differentiation, signet ring cells, and neuropil-like islands.

Ultrastructure

Ependymomas retain the characteristic ultrastructural properties of ependymal cells, such as cilia with a 9 + 2 microtubular pattern, blepharoblasts and microvilli

located at the luminal surface, junctional complexes at the lateral surface, and lack of a basement membrane at the internal surface. The cells may form microrosettes into which microvilli and cilia project. Junctional complexes (zonulae adherentes) irregularly linked by zonulae occludentes or gap junctions, as well as cell processes filled with intermediate filaments, may also be encountered {858}. A basal lamina may be present at the interface between tumour cells and vascularized stroma.

Immunophenotype

Immunoreactivity for GFAP is usually observed in pseudorosettes, but is more variable in other elements of the tumour, such as rosettes and papillae. Ependymomas typically express S100 protein and vimentin {1285}. EMA immunoreactivity can be found in most ependymomas, with expression along the luminal surface of some ependymal rosettes or manifesting as dot-like perinuclear or ring-like cytoplasmic structures {1241}. OLIG2 expression is characteristically sparse in ependymomas compared with

other gliomas {1101,1865,2031}. Focal cytokeratin immunoreactivity can be seen in some cases {2641}. Rarely, ependymomas can express neuronal antigens {72, 2036,2154}. L1CAM expression is evident in supratentorial ependymomas with a *C11orf95* rearrangement {1891}.

Cell of origin

Stem cells isolated from ependymomas have a radial glia phenotype, suggesting that radial glia cells are the histogenetic source of these tumours {2526}. Further research has implicated distinct groups of stem cells that are specific to anatomical site; cerebral neural stem cells and adult spinal neural stem cells are potential cells of origin for cerebral and spinal ependymomas, respectively, and these origins would explain the predominant locations of these tumours in the different age groups {1171,1891}. The importance of anatomical site in ependymoma biology is demonstrated by the molecular groups of the disease as defined by methylome profiling, which is considered to reflect histogenesis {1880}.

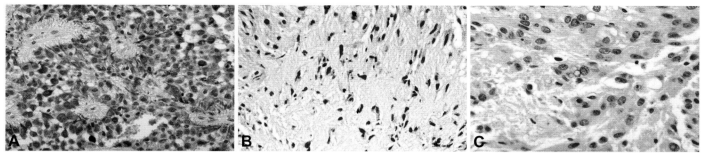

Fig. 3.11 Ependymoma. **A** GFAP immunoreactivity is largely restricted to perivascular tumour cells {1291}. **B** EMA staining with dot-like cytoplasmic reactivity; immunohistochemical detection of EMA has been used to identify intracytoplasmic microrosettes, a feature found in both typical and tanycytic ependymomas, but infrequently (if at all) in myxopapillary ependymomas. **C** EMA immunoreactivity in ependymoma demonstrates round intracytoplasmic microrosettes.

Genetic profile

Molecular alterations are very common in ependymoma and comprise cytogenetic, genetic, epigenetic, and transcriptomic changes. Ependymomas display a broad range of cytogenetic aberrations, most commonly gains of chromosomes 1q, 5, 7, 9, 11, 18, and 20 and losses of chromosomes 1p, 3, 6q, 6, 9p, 13q, 17, and 22 {1267,1351}. Supratentorial tumours preferentially show loss of chromosome 9 {372,888,1159,1171,2767,2860}; in particular, homozygous deletion of *CDKN2A* has been recurrently demonstrated in supratentorial ependymomas {1639,2008, 2526}. Gain of chromosome 1q has been reported as a reproducible prognostic marker in several trial cohorts, being associated with poor outcome in posterior fossa tumours {1266,1351,2767}. Monosomy 22 and deletions or translocations of chromosome 22q are particularly common in spinal cord tumours and tumours associated with neurofibromatosis type 2 {936}. The *NF2* gene is involved in ependymoma tumorigenesis, and *NF2* mutations occur frequently in spinal ependymomas {207,621}.

Using DNA methylation profiling, several studies have provided support for the existence of distinct molecular groups among ependymomas {1049,1424,1560, 1880}. These groups show strong relationships to certain anatomical sites (see Table 3.01, p. 110). In a large cohort (containing > 500 tumours), three groups were identified in each of the three CNS compartments (i.e. supratentorial, posterior fossa, and spinal) {1880}. Tumours with a subependymomatous morphology were classified into separate spinal, posterior fossa, and supratentorial groups, called SP-SE, PF-SE, and ST-SE, respectively. Fusion genes involving either *RELA* or *YAP1*, as previously described for a large proportion of supratentorial

ependymomas {1891}, characterize the other two supratentorial groups: ST-EPN-*RELA* and ST-EPN-*YAP1*. The other two posterior fossa groups (PF-EPN-A and PF-EPN-B) match those previously called group A and group B in some molecular studies {1026,1560,2696,2767}. The final two molecular groups for the spinal cord (including the cauda equina) contain myxopapillary ependymomas and classic ependymomas, respectively, and are termed SP-MPE and SP-EPN. In infants and young children, posterior fossa ependymomas mainly fall into the PF-EPN-A group, whereas PF-EPN-B tumours occur mainly in adolescents and adults. Copy number alterations, particularly gains and losses of whole chromosomes and chromosome arms, characterize PF-EPN-B ependymomas, whereas PF-EPN-A ependymomas show few copy number alterations. Two molecular groups, ST-EPN-*RELA* and PF-EPN-A, are associated with a particularly poor prognosis {1880,2696,2767}.

Posterior fossa ependymomas have a very low mutation rate and lack recurrent somatic mutations on analysis by whole-genome sequencing methods {1560, 1891}. Supratentorial ependymomas are characterized by a recurrent structural variant, the *C11orf95-RELA* fusion gene, which is a by-product of chromothripsis and occurs in 70% of paediatric supratentorial ependymomas.

Genetic susceptibility

Spinal ependymomas occur in neurofibromatosis type 2, indicating a role of the *NF2* gene in these neoplasms. Other hereditary forms of ependymoma are rarely observed {309}. Two patients with Turcot syndrome and ependymomas have been reported, and parental colon cancer is associated with an increased risk of ependymomas among offspring, with

a standardized incidence ratio of 3.70 {1722,2570}. However, ependymomas do not demonstrate mutations in *APC* {1849}. In a Japanese family, two of four siblings developed a cervical spinal cord ependymoma and one had a schwannoma. Neurofibromatosis type 2 was excluded, and genetic analysis revealed a common allelic loss at 22q11.2–qter in two of the affected siblings. The authors who studied this family suggested the existence of a tumour suppressor gene on chromosome 22 related to the genesis of familial ependymomas {2827}.

Prognosis and predictive factors

The identification of clinicopathological variables of prognostic value in ependymomas is an important but challenging issue {2275}. In particular, the clinical utility of individual histopathological features or tumour grade remains highly controversial {633,776}. Gain of chromosome 1q has been reported to be a potential outcome indicator among tested molecular markers {372,857,1266,1351,1639}, and outcome correlates of molecular groups may prove significant in the future {1560,1880,2696,2767}.

Patient age and extent of resection

Children with ependymoma fare worse than adults. This difference may reflect the more frequent occurrence of paediatric tumours in the posterior fossa versus the predominantly spinal location for adult tumours. Children aged < 1 year have a 5-year overall survival rate of 42.4% {791}. With increasing age, the 5-year overall survival rate improves, to 55.3% among 1–4-year-olds, 74.7% among 5–9-year-olds, and 76.2% among 10–14-year-olds. Extent of surgical resection is consistently reported to be a reliable indicator of outcome; gross total resection is associated with significantly improved survival

Table 3.01 Key characteristics of the nine molecular groups of ependymoma; based on data from a single study {1880}

Anatomical location	Group	Genetic characteristic	Dominant pathology	Age at presentation	Outcome
Supratentorial	ST-EPN-*RELA*	*RELA* fusion gene	Classic/anaplastic	Infancy to adulthood	Poor
	ST-EPN-*YAP1*	*YAP1* fusion gene	Classic/anaplastic	Infancy to childhood	Good
	ST-SE	Balanced genome	Subependymoma	Adulthood	Good
Posterior fossa	PF-EPN-A	Balanced genome	Classic/anaplastic	Infancy	Poor
	PF-EPN-B	Genome-wide polyploidy	Classic/anaplastic	Childhood to adulthood	Good
	PF-SE	Balanced genome	Subependymoma	Adulthood	Good
Spinal	SP-EPN	*NF2* mutation	Classic/anaplastic	Childhood to adulthood	Good
	SP-MPE	Genome-wide polyploidy	Myxopapillary	Adulthood	Good
	SP-SE	6q deletion	Subependymoma	Adulthood	Good

Molecular groups of ependymoma

Transcriptome and methylome profiling have established the relevance of anatomical site to ependymoma biology. In a recent study that will likely serve as the basis for the future molecular classification of the disease {1880}, nine groups of ependymoma were described; three for each of the three major CNS anatomical compartments (i.e. the supratentorial compartment, posterior fossa, and spinal compartment). The modal patient age at presentation, clinical outcome, and frequencies of histopathological variants and genetic alterations vary across these groups.

{238,1604,1644}. In the Children's Oncology Group (COG) ACNS0121 trial, resection was an independent risk factor, irrespective of pathological grade {776}. In another study, which included children aged < 3 years at presentation, a better 5-year survival rate was achieved after complete resection (43%) than after incomplete resection (36%) {2046}.

Tumour location

Tumour site has been identified as an important prognostic factor. Supratentorial ependymomas are associated with better survival rates than are posterior fossa neoplasms, especially in children {649,2060}. Spinal ependymomas have a significantly better outcome than do intracranial tumours, although late recurrences (> 5 years after surgery) can occur. Metastatic disease is associated with a poor prognosis.

Histopathology

One major and unresolved issue concerns the accurate definition of anaplasia, because an inconsistent relationship between pathological variables and outcome has emerged over several decades of study {650,704,857,1643,2178, 2778}. Of the features usually associated with anaplastic change in gliomas, only mitotic index, several other indices of proliferation, and foci of poorly differentiated tumour cells seem to be consistently associated with survival in ependymoma, and not in all studies {857,1345,1398, 2275,2557}. As a result, very few clinical trials use grade to stratify therapy, because the distinction between grade II and grade III ependymomas is so unreliable {633}.

Molecular groups

A molecular classification of the disease will likely supersede attempts to use histopathological variables in the stratification of patients for adjuvant therapy. Nine molecular groups of ependymoma have recently been identified, three from each principal anatomical compartment across the neuraxis {1880}. There is a strong association between two of these groups, ST-EPN-*RELA* and PF-EPN-A, and a poor outcome (Table 3.01).

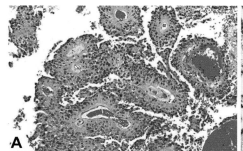
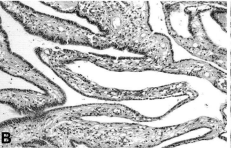
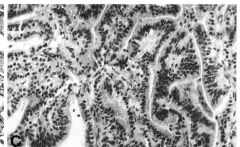

Fig. 3.12 Papillary ependymoma. **A** Discohesive growth, pseudopapillae, and perivascular pseudorosettes. **B** Finger-like projections lined by single or multiple layers of cuboidal tumour cells with smooth contiguous surfaces. **C** This ependymoma variant is characterized by well-formed papillae in which a central vessel is covered by layers of tumour cells. The differential diagnosis includes choroid plexus papilloma, the rare papillary meningioma, and metastatic carcinoma.

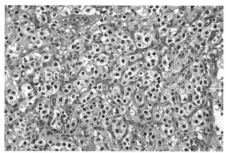

Fig. 3.13 Clear cell ependymoma, characterized by a relatively high cell density without significant increase in proliferation. Note the clear perinuclear cytoplasm resembling tumour cells in an oligodendroglioma.

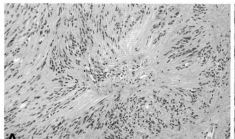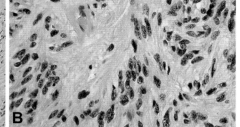

Fig. 3.14 Tanycytic ependymoma. **A** Bipolar spindle cells with elongated processes arranged around a central vessel. **B** Nuclei exhibit the typical salt-and-pepper speckling of ependymomas.

Papillary ependymoma

Definition
A rare histological variant of ependymoma characterized by well-formed papillae.

ICD-O code   9393/3

Microscopy
Ependymomas form linear, epithelial-like surfaces along their cerebrospinal fluid exposures. Some ependymomas have a papillary architecture that results when exuberant growths occasionally arise in which finger-like projections are lined by a single layer of cuboidal tumour cells with smooth contiguous surfaces and GFAP-immunopositive tumour cell processes; in contrast, choroid plexus papillomas and metastatic carcinomas form bumpy, hobnail cellular surfaces that do not feature extensive GFAP reactivity. Unlike the papillae in choroid plexus tumours, the papillae in ependymomas lack a basement membrane beneath the (neuro-)epithelial cells, which in ependymomas send fibrillary processes down to a vascular core in the same architectural arrangement as a pseudorosette.

Clear cell ependymoma

Definition
A histological variant of ependymoma characterized by an oligodendrocyte-like appearance, with perinuclear haloes due to cytoplasmic clearing.
The clear cell ependymoma variant is most frequently located in the supratentorial compartment of young patients.

ICD-O code   9391/3

Microscopy
Clear cell ependymomas display an oligodendroglial phenotype, with cytoplasmic clearing that creates clear perinuclear haloes. Most ependymomas with this phenotype are supratentorial vascular tumours in young patients {727,1673}, but the clear-cell phenotype can occasionally be found in posterior fossa or spinal tumours.
Clear cell ependymoma must be distinguished from oligodendroglioma, central neurocytoma, clear cell (renal cell) carcinoma, and haemangioblastoma. Ependymal and perivascular rosettes, immunoreactivity for GFAP and EMA, and ultrastructural studies can be helpful in this differential diagnosis. Some data suggest that clear cell ependymoma may follow a more aggressive course than other variants {727}. The clear cell tumour of the lateral ventricles once classified as ependymoma of the foramen of Monro {2876} is now recognized as central neurocytoma in most instances (see *Central neurocytoma*, p. 156).

Tanycytic ependymoma

Definition
A histological variant of ependymoma characterized by arrangement of tumour cells in fascicles of variable width and cell density and by elongated cells with spindle-shaped nuclei.

ICD-O code   9391/3

Microscopy
The tanycytic phenotype is most commonly found in spinal cord ependymomas and manifests as irregular fascicles of elongated cells. The fascicles are of variable width and cell density. Rosettes are rarely seen in these ependymomas, and pseudorosettes can be subtle. Like in other ependymomas, the nuclei display speckled (salt-and-pepper) chromatin, and anaplastic features are uncommon.
The term "tanycytic ependymoma" is used for this variant because its spindly, bipolar elements resemble tanycytes – the paraventricular cells with elongated cytoplasmic processes that extend to ependymal surfaces {711}. Because ependymal rosettes are typically absent and pseudorosettes only vaguely delineated, these lesions may be mistaken for astrocytomas, in particular pilocytic astrocytomas. However, their ultrastructural characteristics are ependymal.

Ependymoma, *RELA* fusion–positive

Ellison D.W.
Korshunov A.
Witt H.

Definition
A supratentorial ependymoma character-
ized by a RELA *fusion gene.*

The genetically defined *RELA* fusion–
positive ependymoma accounts for
approximately 70% of all childhood supratentorial tumours {1891} and a lower
proportion of such ependymomas in
adult patients {1880}. Ependymomas in
the posterior fossa and spinal compartments do not harbour this fusion gene.
RELA fusion–positive ependymomas
exhibit a range of histopathological features, with or without anaplasia.

ICD-O code   9396/3

Grading
RELA fusion-positive ependymomas are
classified according to their histopathological features into WHO grade II or
grade III. No grade I ependymoma has
been recorded as containing this genetic
alteration.

Microscopy
RELA fusion–positive ependymomas do

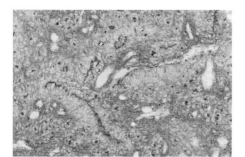

Fig. 3.15 *RELA* fusion–positive ependymoma. L1CAM
protein expression correlates well with the presence of a
RELA fusion gene.

not have a specified morphology {1891}.
They exhibit the standard range of architectural and cytological features found in
supratentorial ependymomas, but they
often have a distinctive vascular pattern of branching capillaries or clear-cell
change. Uncommon variants of ependymoma (e.g. tanycytic ependymoma) do
not tend to be *RELA* fusion–positive.

Immunophenotype
RELA fusion–positive ependymomas
demonstrate the immunoreactivities
for GFAP and EMA described in other
ependymomas. Expression of L1CAM
correlates well with the presence of a
RELA fusion in supratentorial ependymomas {1891}, but L1CAM can also be expressed by other types of brain tumours.

Genetic profile
The *C11orf95-RELA* fusion is the most
common structural variant found in
ependymomas {1880,1891,1974}. It forms
in the context of chromothripsis, a shattering and reassembly of the genome
that rearranges genes and produces
oncogenic gene products {2852}.. *RELA*
fusion–positive ependymomas show
constitutive activation of the NF-kappaB
pathway, the *RELA*-encoded transcription factor p65 being a key effector in this
pathway. Rarely, *C11orf95* or *RELA* can
be fused with other genes as a result of
chromothripsis {1891}.
The presence of a *C11orf95-RELA* fusion gene can be detected by various
methods, but a simple approach using

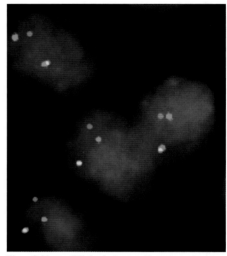

Fig. 3.16 *RELA* fusion–positive ependymoma.
Interphase FISH with break-apart probes around the
RELA gene. Overlapping probes (yellow) indicate an
intact *RELA* gene, but probe separation (red/green)
occurs with rearrangement of the *RELA* gene.

formalin-fixed, paraffin-embedded tissue is interphase FISH with break-apart
probes around both genes. Rearrangement in the context of chromothripsis
splits the dual-colour signals in probe
sets for *C11orf95* and *RELA* {1891}.

Prognosis and predictive factors
The data available to date (which come
from only a single study) suggest that
RELA fusion–positive ependymomas
have the worst outcome of the three supratentorial molecular groups {1880}.

Anaplastic ependymoma

Ellison D.W.
McLendon R.
Wiestler O.D.
Kros J.M.
Korshunov A.
Ng H.-K.
Witt H.
Hirose T.

Definition

A circumscribed glioma composed of uniform small cells with round nuclei in a fibrillary matrix and characterized by perivascular anucleate zones (pseudorosettes), ependymal rosettes in about one quarter of cases, a high nuclear-to-cytoplasmic ratio, and a high mitotic count.

A diagnosis of anaplastic ependymoma can be confidently made when an ependymal tumour shows a high cell density and elevated mitotic count alongside widespread microvascular proliferation and necrosis. Like the classic tumour, anaplastic ependymoma rarely invades adjacent CNS parenchyma to any significant extent. Cilia and microvilli are seen on ultrastructural examination.

Anaplastic ependymomas are mainly intracranial tumours; they are rare in the spinal cord. Anaplastic ependymomas occur in both adults and children, although most posterior fossa tumours present in childhood. Clear cell, papillary, or tanycytic morphology can be a feature of both classic and anaplastic ependymomas. Anaplastic ependymomas have a variable clinical outcome, which is primarily dependent on extent of surgical resection and molecular group {857,1880}.

In defining molecular groups of ependymoma, transcriptome or methylome profiling has established the relevance of anatomical site to ependymoma biology.

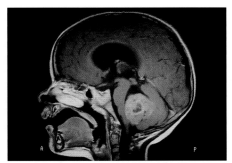

Fig. 3.17 Sagittal, gadolinium-enhanced, T1-weighted MRI of an anaplastic ependymoma of the fourth ventricle.

In a recent study that will likely serve as the basis for the future molecular classification of the disease {1880}, nine groups of ependymoma were described (three for each of the three major CNS anatomical compartments: the supratentorial compartment, posterior fossa, and spinal compartment). The modal patient age at presentation, clinical outcome, and frequencies of histopathological variants and genetic alterations vary across these groups (see Table 3.01, p. 110).

ICD-O code   9392/3

Grading

Traditionally, classic ependymoma and anaplastic ependymoma are considered to correspond histologically to WHO grades II and III, respectively. However, no association between grade

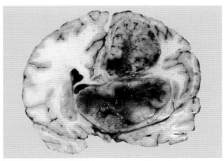

Fig. 3.18 Anaplastic ependymoma of the lateral ventricle in a 4-year-old boy, with extensive involvement of the right frontal lobe.

and biological behaviour or survival has been definitively established {248,633, 703}. Of the various studies of prognostic variables and outcome in ependymoma, those that did not find an association between grade (II vs III) and progression-free or overall survival outnumber those that did. The published ratios of grade II to grade III tumours in series of ependymomas vary widely, from 17:1 to 1:7, and the explanation for such inconsistent data is multifactorial {633,856,2557}. The interpretation of most histopathological variables used in this classification for grading purposes is subjective, and ependymomas are morphologically heterogeneous. There have been few studies of the prognostic significance of WHO grade or individual pathological features in large trial cohorts in which proper multivariate analyses of prognostic variables

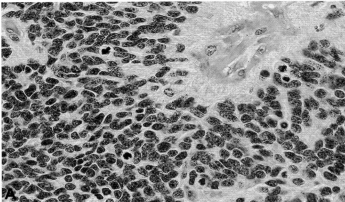
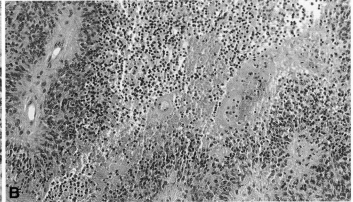

Fig. 3.19 Anaplastic ependymoma. **A** Poorly differentiated tumour cells with brisk mitotic activity. **B** Large foci of necrosis.

can be performed, and there have been only three studies in which evaluation of histological variables was defined stringently and undertaken by several observers {633,856,2557}. Due to these limiting factors, grading is hardly ever used for therapeutic stratification of patients with ependymoma. Given that specific genetic alterations and molecular groups have recently been proposed as prognostic or predictive factors for these tumours {1560,1880,2767}, the practice of histologically grading ependymoma may soon become obsolete altogether.

Microscopy

Anaplastic ependymomas almost always remain circumscribed masses, but can rarely invade adjacent brain tissue in the manner of diffuse glioma. Anaplastic ependymomas generally have a high nuclear-to-cytoplasmic ratio. Occasionally, the cell density is so high that anaplastic ependymomas can be mistaken for embryonal tumours. All anaplastic ependymomas demonstrate brisk mitotic activity, and high mitotic counts have been associated with a poor outcome in posterior fossa tumours. Microvascular proliferation and palisading necrosis often accompany the mitotic activity, although these features can also be focal in classic ependymomas with lower cell density and few mitotic figures. Pseudorosettes are a defining feature, but in some poorly differentiated supratentorial anaplastic ependymomas, they can be difficult to find.

Immunophenotype

Anaplastic ependymoma has the same immunoprofile as classic ependymoma, except that indices of tumour growth fraction, such as the Ki-67 proliferation index, are higher.

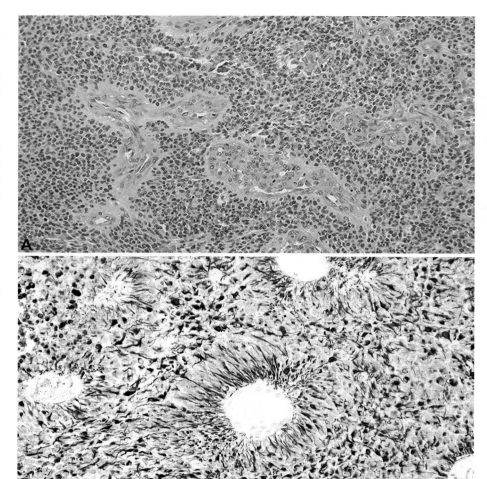

Fig. 3.20 Anaplastic ependymoma. **A** Densely packed tumour cells and microvascular proliferation. **B** GFAP highlighting radial perivascular processes.

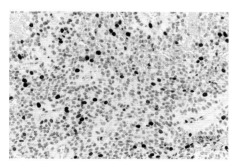

Fig. 3.19C Anaplastic ependymoma. High Ki-67 labelling index.

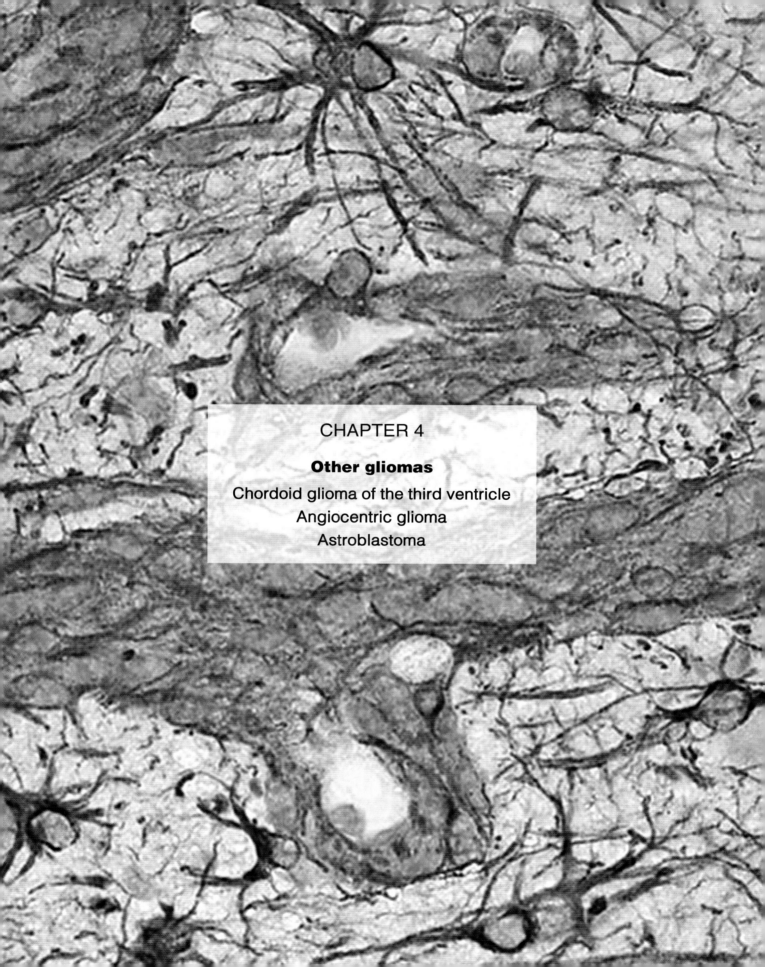

CHAPTER 4

Other gliomas

Chordoid glioma of the third ventricle
Angiocentric glioma
Astroblastoma

Chordoid glioma of the third ventricle

Brat D.J.
Fuller G.N.

Definition

A slow-growing, non-invasive glial tumour located in the third ventricle, histologically characterized by clusters and cords of epithelioid tumour cells expressing GFAP, within a variably mucinous stroma typically containing a lymphoplasmacytic infiltrate.

Chordoid gliomas of the third ventricle occur in adults and have a favourable prognosis, particularly in the setting of gross total resection.

ICD-O code   9444/1

Grading

Chordoid glioma of the third ventricle corresponds histologically to WHO grade II.

Epidemiology

These tumours are rare, with slightly more than 80 cases ever reported. Chordoid gliomas occur most frequently in adults, although patient age at presentation varies widely (5–71 years). Most patients present between the ages of 35 and 60 years (mean: 46 years), and there is a 2:1 female predominance {272,576}. Paediatric examples are rare {379}.

Localization

Chordoid gliomas occupy the anterior portion of the third ventricle, with larger tumours also filling the middle and posterior aspects {2001}. They generally arise in the midline and displace normal structures in all directions as they enlarge. Neuroimaging findings, including reports of small, localized tumours, suggest that

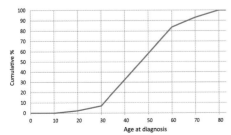

Fig. 4.01 Cumulative age distribution (both sexes) of chordoid glioma of the third ventricle, based on 43 cases.

chordoid gliomas arise in the region of the lamina terminalis in the ventral wall of the third ventricle {1461,1904}. In at least some cases, radiological studies have demonstrated an intraparenchymal hypothalamic component {2001}.

Clinical features

Chordoid gliomas occur in adults and to date have arisen only in the third ventricular region. Most cases present with signs and symptoms of obstructive hydrocephalus, including headache, nausea, vomiting, and ataxia {272,576}. Other clinical features include endocrine abnormalities reflecting hypothalamic compression (e.g. hypothyroidism, amenorrhoea, and diabetes insipidus), visual field disturbances due to compression/displacement of the optic chiasm, and personality changes including psychiatric symptoms and memory abnormalities.

Imaging

On neuroimaging, chordoid gliomas present as well-circumscribed ovoid masses within the anterior third ventricle. On MRI, they are T1-isointense to brain and show strong, homogeneous contrast enhancement {2001}. Mass effect is generally distributed symmetrically and causes vasogenic oedema in compressed adjacent CNS structures, including the optic tracts, basal ganglia, and internal capsules. Most tumours are continuous with the hypothalamus and some appear to have an intrinsic anterior hypothalamic component, suggesting a potential site of origin {1461}.

Microscopy

Chordoid gliomas are solid neoplasms, most often composed of clusters and cords of epithelioid tumour cells within a variably mucinous stroma that typically contains a lymphoplasmacytic infiltrate. Three less common histological patterns have also been reported: a solid pattern with sheets of polygonal epithelioid tumour cells without mucinous stroma, a fusiform pattern with groups of spindle-shaped cells among loose collagen, and

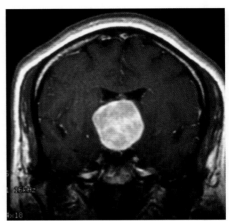

Fig. 4.02 MRI of a chordoid glioma of the third ventricle demonstrating a large, contrast-enhancing, sharply delineated mass that fills the anterior third ventricle and compresses adjacent structures.

a fibrosing pattern with abundant fibrosis. The fibrosing pattern tends to be more common in older patients {196}. Other (rare) tissue patterns include papillary, alveolar, and pseudoglandular patterns. Individual tumour cells have abundant eosinophilic cytoplasm. In some cases, limited glial differentiation in the form of coarsely fibrillar processes can also be seen {272}. Neoplastic nuclei are moderate in size, ovoid, and relatively uniform. Mitoses are absent in most tumours; when present, they are rare (< 1 mitosis per 10 high-power fields). A stromal lymphoplasmacytic infiltrate, often containing numerous Russell bodies, is a consistent finding. Consistent with their radiographical appearance, the tumours are architecturally solid and show little tendency to infiltrate surrounding brain structures. Reactive astrocytes, Rosenthal fibres, and often chronic inflammatory cells including lymphocytes, plasma cells, and Russell bodies are seen in adjacent non-neoplastic tissue.

Electron microscopy

Parallels have been drawn with the ultrastructural morphology of ependymoma {1904} and specialized ependymoma of the subcommissural organ {389}. The features of chordoid glioma include intermediate filaments, intercellular lumina, apical

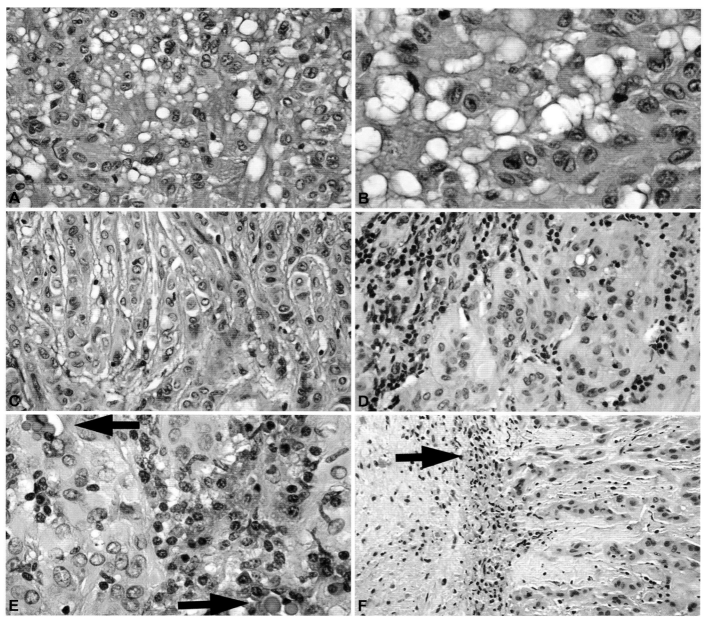

Fig. 4.03 Chordoid glioma of the third ventricle. **A** Histologically, tumours are characterized by cohesive clusters of epithelioid cells with abundant pink cytoplasm and a bubbly, bluish, mucin-rich stroma. **B** At higher magnification, nuclei are oval, moderate in size, and bland, and have dispersed chromatin. Mitotic activity and nuclear atypia are absent. **C** In almost every instance, tumour cells also form solid arrangements of either nests or linear arrays. **D,E** Lymphoplasmacytic infiltrate is present in nearly all chordoid gliomas, and Russell bodies can be identified (E, arrows). **F** The border between chordoid glioma and adjacent brain is well defined, with little evidence of tumour infiltration, often with chronic inflammation (arrow) and Rosenthal fibres in the neighbouring brain.

microvilli, hemidesmosomes, and basal lamina. Some have also been suggested to contain secretory granules {389}.

Immunophenotype

The most distinctive immunohistochemical feature of chordoid gliomas is their strong, diffuse reactivity for GFAP {272, 2235}. These tumours consistently express TTF1 in most nuclei, although the percentage of immunoreactive nuclei and the intensity of immunostaining vary depending on the antibody clone used {196}. Staining for vimentin and CD34 is also strong, whereas immunoreactivity for S100 protein, EMA, and cytokeratin is variable. Epidermal growth factor receptors and merlin are expressed, whereas nuclear accumulation of p53 is weak or absent. Neuronal and neuroendocrine markers (e.g. synaptophysin, neurofilaments, and chromogranin-A) are consistently negative {2089}. The proliferative potential of chordoid gliomas corresponds to that of other low-grade gliomas. The Ki-67 proliferation index is low, with values of 0–1.5% in one study {272} and < 5% in other reports {2089}. R132H-mutant IDH1 immunostaining is negative {196}.

Immunohistochemistry can be useful in the differential diagnosis of chordoid glioma versus other chordoid neoplasms.

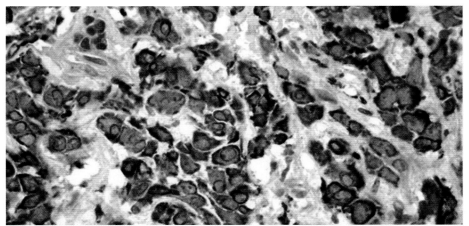
Fig. 4.04 Chordoid glioma of the third ventricle. Tumour cells with diffuse immunoreactivity for GFAP.

Chordoid meningiomas usually contain small foci of classic meningioma with whorl formation and psammoma bodies; they are also immunopositive for EMA, but negative for GFAP and CD34 {2235}. Chordomas strongly express cytokeratins and brachyury, but lack immunoreactivity for GFAP and CD34.

Cell of origin

The ultrastructural demonstration of microvilli and hemidesmosome-like structures in chordoid glioma supports an ependymal histogenesis {389}. Further evidence of ependymal or specialized ependymal differentiation has been supplied by a report of abnormal cilia in a juxtanuclear location {1904}. The presence of a cytological zonation pattern and secretory vesicles indicated a specialized ependymal differentiation, as might be expected of cells derived from a circumventricular organ such as the lamina terminalis. A recent study reported strong expression of TTF1 in both chordoid gliomas and the organum vasculosum of the lamina terminalis, suggesting an organum vasculosum origin {196}.

Genetic profile

A study using microarray-based comparative genomic hybridization and FISH demonstrated losses at 11q13 and 9p21 {1035}. No *EGFR* amplifications, chromosome 7 gain, or *TP53* mutations were noted. Another study (which used PCR-based techniques, DNA sequencing, and comparative genomic hybridization) detected no consistent chromosomal imbalances or consistent alterations of *TP53*, *CDKN2A*, *EGFR*, *CDK4*, or *MDM2* {2089}. Neither IDH mutations (i.e. *IDH1* or *IDH2* mutations) nor *BRAF* V600E mutations were found in a series of 16 chordoid gliomas {196}.

Prognosis and predictive factors

Chordoid gliomas are slow-growing and histologically low-grade. Gross total resection is the treatment of choice and can result in long-term recurrence-free survival {576}. However, the tumours' location within the third ventricle and their attachment to hypothalamic and suprasellar structures often make complete resection impossible. Postoperative tumour enlargement has been noted in half of all patients who undergo subtotal resection. Among the reported cases of chordoid gliomas, approximately 20% of the patients died in the perioperative period or from tumour regrowth {1394}. Specific postoperative complications include diabetes insipidus, amnesia, and pulmonary embolism {576}.

Angiocentric glioma

Burger P.C.
Jouvet A.
Preusser M.
Rosenblum M.K.
Ellison D.W.

Definition

An epilepsy-associated, stable or slow-growing cerebral tumour primarily affecting children and young adults; histologically characterized by an angiocentric pattern of growth, monomorphous bipolar cells, and features of ependymal differentiation.

Angiocentric glioma (also called monomorphous angiocentric glioma {2691} and angiocentric neuroepithelial tumour {1467}) has an uncertain relationship to other neoplasms exhibiting ependymal differentiation. Examples with this pattern have been reported as cortical ependymoma {1465}. Tumours harbouring both angiocentric glioma and ependymoma patterns have also been reported {2623}. The relationship between angiocentric glioma and classic ependymoma thus remains to be defined.

ICD-O code   9431/1

Grading

Angiocentric glioma corresponds histologically to WHO grade I.

Synonym

Angiocentric neuroepithelial tumour (not recommended)

Epidemiology

Incidence figures are not yet available for this uncommon lesion. Most cases

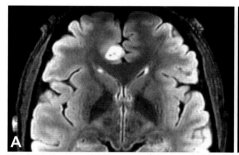
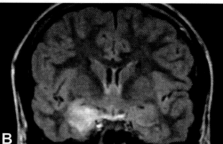

Fig. 4.05 Angiocentric glioma. **A** T2-weighted, fluid-suppressed MRI demonstrates the neoplasm as a well-defined hyperintense mass in close proximity to the cingulate gyrus of the right frontal lobe. Note the lesion's primarily cortical localization. **B** The bright lesion with little mass effect is based largely in the amygdala.

involve children. Males and females are affected equally frequently.

Localization

A superficial, cerebrocortical location is typical.

Clinical features

Angiocentric gliomas are epileptogenic lesions, with chronic and intractable partial epilepsy being particularly characteristic.

Imaging

On MRI, the superficial, if not cortically based, lesion is well circumscribed, bright on FLAIR images, and non–contrast-enhancing. A cortical band of T1-hyperintensity is present in some cases. A stalk-like extension to the subjacent lateral ventricle is another variable feature {1337}.

Spread

Angiocentric glioma has an infiltrative appearance, locally trapping neurons and other pre-existing parenchymal elements. Extensions along parenchymal vessels and the subpial zone are common {2691}.

Macroscopy

Gross features have not been detailed. One temporal lobe example was described at surgery as producing hippocampal enlargement with darkening and induration of the amygdala. The grey matter–white matter boundary may be blurred.

Microscopy

A unifying feature is the structure of remarkably monomorphic, bipolar spindled cells oriented around cortical blood

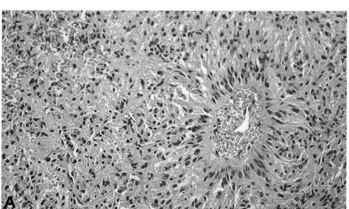
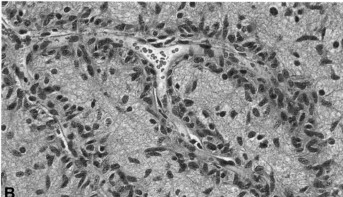

Fig. 4.06 Angiocentric glioma. **A** Elongated tumour cells forming occasionally perivascular pseudorosettes. **B** Perivascular rosettes.

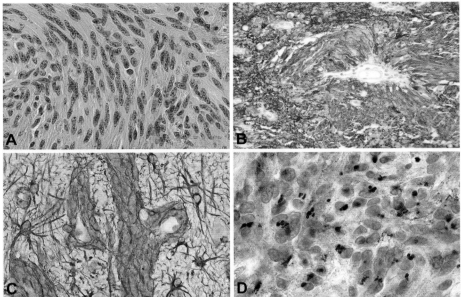

Fig. 4.07 Angiocentric glioma. **A** Compact areas that resemble schwannoma. **B** Tumour cells in perivascular pseudorosettes express GFAP. **C** Longitudinally oriented GFAP-positive cells. **D** EMA-positive dot-like structures corresponding to microlumina.

vessels (of all calibres) in single- or multilayered sleeves that extend lengthwise along vascular axes or as radial pseudorosettes of ependymomatous appearance. Cells with prominent cytoplasm and distinct cell borders give an epithelioid appearance to some cases. In such cases, perivascular formations may be similar to pseudorosettes in astroblastoma. Tumour cells often aggregate beneath the pia–arachnoid complex in horizontal streams or in perpendicular, strikingly palisading arrays, and can diffusely colonize the neuroparenchyma proper at variable density. The nuclei are slender, with granular chromatin stippling. Some examples have regions of solid growth containing more conspicuously fibrillary elements in compact, miniature schwannoma–like nodules as well as rounded epithelioid cells in nests and sheets interrupted by irregular clefts or cavities. The epithelioid cells may contain paranuclear, round, or oval eosinophilic densities with an internal granular stippling. These cytoplasmic structures correspond to EMA-immunoreactive microlumina (as seen in conventional ependymomas). Included neurons, which are interpreted either as entrapped {2691} or as possibly intrinsic to the lesion {1467}, do not exhibit significant dysmorphism. Mitoses are inapparent or rare in most cases, and neither

complex microvascular proliferation nor necrosis is seen. Examples with multiple mitoses occur, and one such case occurred as a mitotically active, anaplastic astrocytoma–like lesion {2691}.

Electron microscopy
Evidence of ependymal differentiation includes tumoural microlumina filled with microvilli and delimited by elongated intermediate junctions {2691}.

Immunophenotype
Spindled and epithelioid tumour cells are GFAP-reactive, do not label for neuronal antigens (e.g. synaptophysin, chromogranin-A, and NeuN), and frequently exhibit ependymomatous features in their dot-like, microlumen-type cytoplasmic labelling for EMA. Surface EMA expression may also be seen in epithelioid perivascular and subpial formations. Neither aberrant p53 expression by tumour cells nor anomalous labelling patterns of included neurons for synaptophysin, chromogranin-A, and NeuN have been found. R132H-mutant IDH1 staining is negative. The reported Ki-67 proliferation index in primary neurosurgical material ranges from ≤ 1% (in most reported cases) to 5%. One anaplastic recurrence exhibited elevation of the Ki-67 proliferation index to 10% (up from 1% in the primary) {2691}.

Cell of origin
It has been suggested that these tumours derive, via a maldevelopmental or neoplastic process, from the bipolar radial glia that span the neuroepithelium during embryogenesis, and that they may share similar ependymoglial traits or be capable of generating ependymocytes {1467}.

Genetic profile
Limited numbers of angiocentric gliomas have been studied for genetic alterations. However, all 4 cases analysed in two genomic studies showed copy number alterations or rearrangements at the *MYB* locus on 6q23 {2068,2855}. In the rearrangements, *MYB* was fused with *QKI* or *ESR1*. Recently, *MYB* rearrangements have been documented in all of 19 studied angiocentric gliomas, with *MYB-QKI* fusions found in 6 of 7 cases in which the fusion partner could be identified {118A}. In another study, an analysis of genomic imbalances by chromosomal comparative genomic hybridization revealed loss of chromosomal bands 6q24 to q25 as the only alteration in 1 of 8 cases. In 1 of 3 cases, a high-resolution screen by microarray-based comparative genomic hybridization identified a copy number gain of two adjacent clones from chromosomal band 11p11.2, containing the *PTPRJ* gene {2035}. Angiocentric gliomas lack *IDH1*, *IDH2*, and *BRAF* V600 mutations {300,1780,2855}.

Genetic susceptibility
Angiocentric gliomas have not been reported in association with dysgenetic syndromes or in familial forms.

Prognosis and predictive factors
These are typically indolent and radiologically stable tumours for which excision alone is generally curative, but specific prognosis and predictive factors have not been determined. One subtotally excised example recurred as an anaplastic and ultimately fatal lesion; the case exhibited typical histological features at presentation but (unusually) affected an adult {2691}. High-grade gliomas with angiocentric features have been reported, but the relationship of these to the classic lesion remains unclear {1541,1691}. Longer follow-up is needed to determine the relationship between level of mitotic activity and outcome {1490,1780}.

Astroblastoma

Aldape K.D.
Rosenblum M.K.
Brat D.J.

Definition

A rare glial neoplasm composed of cells that are positive for GFAP and have broad, non- or slightly tapering processes radiating towards central blood vessels (astroblastic pseudorosettes) that often demonstrate sclerosis.

Astroblastoma mainly affects children, adolescents, and young adults, and occurs nearly exclusively in the cerebral hemispheres. Neoplasms exhibiting foci of astroblastoma-type perivascular structuring but having components of otherwise conventional astrocytoma or ependymoma should not be given this designation.

ICD-O code   9430/3

Grading

The biological behaviour of astroblastoma varies. In the absence of sufficient clinicopathological data, it would be premature to establish WHO grade(s) at this time. However, the literature has categorized these tumours as either well differentiated or malignant (anaplastic). In one series, well-differentiated tumours had low mitotic activity (1 mitosis per 10 high-power fields) and an average Ki-67 proliferation index of 3% {267}. Regional (infarct-like) necrosis has been noted in 30% of these tumours. Neither vascular proliferation nor spontaneous necrosis with palisading has been seen.

Malignant astroblastomas are charac-terized by the presence of focal or multi-focal regions of high cellularity, anaplastic nuclear features, increased mitotic activity (> 5 mitoses per 10 high-power fields), microvascular proliferation, and necrosis with palisading. In most cases, these high-grade features are found focally in the setting of a classic, better-differentiated astroblastoma. The Ki-67 proliferation index in these malignant astroblastomas is typically > 10%.

Epidemiology

These are unusual tumours, and uniform diagnostic criteria have not been applied; therefore, definitive epidemiological data are not available. However, astroblastomas seem to be most frequent in children, adolescents, and young adults. The tumours may show a predominance in females {2204}. One report on 116 cases from the published literature suggested a substantial (70%) female predominance {2447}, which is consistent with prior conclusions {236,2539}; however, another study, which compiled 239 cases from SEER data, found an approximately equal distribution among males and females {28}.

Localization

Astroblastomas typically involve the cerebral hemispheres {28,1066,2204, 2447}. Among 177 intracranial cases in the SEER data for which the site was known, the supratentorial compartment was involved in 144 cases (81%) and the infratentorial in 33 cases (19%). The spinal cord is only rarely involved.

Imaging

On CT and MRI, astroblastomas present as well-demarcated, non-calcified, nodular or lobulated masses with frequent cystic change and conspicuous contrast enhancement {2318}.

Macroscopy

Astroblastoma is greyish pink or tan, and its consistency depends on the extent of associated collagen deposition. Foci of necrosis or haemorrhage do not necessarily indicate anaplasia.

Microscopy

Intermediate filament–laden cell processes that form parallel or radial arrays terminating on vascular basement membranes, forming astroblastic pseudorosettes, are commonly observed {1066}. These structures are composed of elongated tumour cells containing abundant eosinophilic cytoplasm, with a single, prominent process extending to a central blood vessel. Cross-sections of pseudorosettes have a radiating appearance, whereas longitudinal sections appear ribbon-like. The presence of so-called stout processes, which extend to central vessels, is critical to the definition of astroblastoma. These distinctive broad or columnar cellular processes are

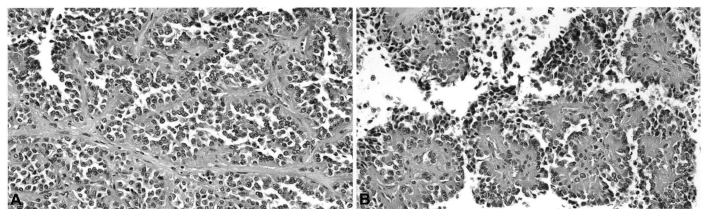

Fig. 4.08 Astroblastoma. **A** Cells oriented to central vessels. **B** Pseudorosettes with sclerosis may take a papillary form.

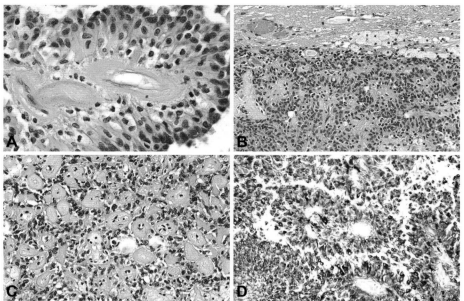

Fig. 4.09 Astroblastoma. **A** Central vessel of pseudorosette shows variable sclerosis. **B** Borders of astroblastoma with brain are generally well defined. **C** Hyaline sclerosis of central vessels is typical in astroblastomas. **D** Tumour cells strongly express GFAP.

generally positive for GFAP, whereas fibrillarity is generally lacking in the tumour stroma. Vascular hyalinization is a conspicuous feature of astroblastoma and ranges from focal and mild to extensive and severe. The combination of mild vascular hyalinization and radiating tumour cells produces a papillary architecture in a subset of tumours. In mildly hyalinized pseudorosettes, perivascular tumour cells become separated from the central vessel by a greater distance and often appear cuboidal. At low magnification, more extensive vascular hyalinization gives the impression of numerous pink hyaline rings, with a paucity of intervening tumour cells. The interface with adjacent brain is well delineated and is characterized by a pushing or non-infiltrative border. Focal infiltration of adjacent tissues by tongues of neoplastic cells is seen occasionally, but diffuse infiltration of surrounding parenchyma is not. The reported Ki-67 proliferation index varies from 1% to 18% {265,1140}. A relationship between proliferation index and outcome has not been established in the literature, although an elevated index tends to be associated with high-grade histology. Compelling evidence of neuronal differentiation has not been reported, and no ependymal features have been encountered in most studied cases. Two studies

examining ultrastructural features {1381, 1387} found cell body polarization with investing basement membranes, apical cytoplasmic blebs capped by microvilli with purse-string pedicular constrictions, and lamellar cytoplasmic interdigitations (called pleatings). Zonula adherens–type junctions framing occasional microrosettes and rare cilia were also identified in these cases.

Immunophenotype
Cytoplasmic immunoreactivity for vimentin, S100, and GFAP is characteristic, although the extent of labelling (particularly for GFAP) varies considerably {338,1984, 2204}. Cell membranes may label for EMA {338,1140}, typically as a focal phenomenon. Less-consistent immunolabelling is reported with CAM5.2 {1140,1381, 1984} and cytokeratin {1381}. Reactivity for neuron-specific enolase is variable {338,1066,1984}, and studied cases have been negative for synaptophysin {1140}. In isolated examples, neuronal cadherin {1381} and cell adhesion molecules (including CD44, NCAM1, GJB1, and GJB2) are positive {1381,1984}. Staining for OLIG2 can be present {745}.

Cell of origin
The histogenesis of astroblastoma is controversial, and the entity is not universally

accepted. Bailey and Cushing thought these tumours arose from embryonic cells programmed to become astrocytes {109}. The presence of intermediate filaments on ultrastructural examination and a lack of evidence of neuronal or (in most cases) ependymal differentiation, together with positive staining for GFAP and S100 protein, suggest that the tumour may be derived from a cell most similar to an astrocyte. The tanycyte, a cell with features intermediate between those of astrocytes and ependymal cells, has been suggested as a cell of origin for astroblastoma on the basis of ultrastructural observations {1381,1387}.

Genetic profile
DNA copy number aberrations identified by comparative genomic hybridization have been described for 7 cases {267}, and the most common alterations identified in this small series included gains of chromosomes 19 and 20q, which frequently occurred together. Less common were losses on chromosomes 10 and X, and a gain of 9q. Conventional cytogenetic studies performed on 2 cases led to the same overall conclusion {265,1140}. Although the number of cases studied to date is small, the findings are consistent with the hypothesis that astroblastoma is distinct from conventional glial neoplasms. A recent case report on a single tumour noted that neither *IDH1* nor *IDH2* mutation was detected in the tumour {745}, and a report on a series of 9 cases of astroblastoma noted a lack of positive immunostaining for R132H-mutant IDH1 in all cases {95}.

Prognosis and predictive factors
In general, high-grade histology has been found to be associated with recurrence, progression, and worse prognosis {236,2539}, although this association has recently been questioned {1135}. In one study, only a single recurrence was noted in 14 informative cases treated by gross total resection, at a mean follow-up of 24 months {265}. An analysis of the literature suggested that gross total resection resulted in a 5-year survival rate of 95% {2447}, and gross total resection of even high-grade astroblastoma may result in a favourable outcome {236}. Data from the SEER registry indicate that infratentorial location may portend improved outcome.

CHAPTER 5

Choroid plexus tumours

Choroid plexus papilloma

Atypical choroid plexus papilloma

Choroid plexus carcinoma

Choroid plexus papilloma

Paulus W.
Brandner S.
Hawkins C.
Tihan T.

Definition

A benign ventricular papillary neoplasm derived from choroid plexus epithelium, with very low or absent mitotic activity.

Histologically, choroid plexus papilloma closely resembles the non-neoplastic choroid plexus, and most tumour cells are positive for the potassium channel KIR7.1. Patients are usually cured by complete surgical resection.

ICD-O code   9390/0

Grading

Choroid plexus papilloma corresponds histologically to WHO grade I.

Epidemiology

Although choroid plexus tumours constitute 0.3–0.8% of all brain tumours overall, they account for 2–4% of those that occur in children aged < 15 years, and for 10–20% of those occurring in the first year of life. In the SEER database, choroid plexus tumours account for 0.77% of all brain tumours and for 14% of those occurring in the first year of life {351}. The average annual incidence is 0.3 cases per 1 million population {1196,2117,2777}. Choroid plexus papillomas (grade I) account for 58.2% of the choroid plexus tumours in the SEER database. Congenital tumours and fetal tumours have been observed in utero using ultrasound techniques. The overall male-to-female ratio is 1.2:1; for lateral ventricle tumours, the ratio is 1:1, and for fourth ventricle tumours, 3:2. About 80% of lateral ventricular tumours present in patients aged < 20 years, whereas fourth ventricle tumours are evenly distributed across all age groups.

Etiology

Genomic analysis of choroid plexus papilloma suggests a role of genes involved in the development and biology of plexus epithelium (i.e. *OTX2* and *TRPM3*). It is thought that their alteration may contribute to the initial steps of choroid plexus oncogenesis {1136}. Earlier reports of a possible role of SV40 {1058} have not been confirmed in more recent studies.

Localization

Choroid plexus papillomas are located within the ventricular system where the normal choroid plexus can be found. They are seen most often in the lateral ventricles, followed by the fourth and third ventricles. They are rarely found within the spinal cord or in ectopic locations {1916}. Multifocal occurrence is exceptional {1959}. A meta-analysis found that the median patient age was 1.5 years for tumours in the lateral and third ventricles, 22.5 years for those in the fourth ventricle, and 35.5 years for those in the cerebellopontine angle {2777}.

Clinical features

Choroid plexus tumours tend to block cerebrospinal fluid pathways. Accordingly, patients present with signs of hydrocephalus (in infants, increased circumference of the head), papilloedema, and raised intracranial pressure. It has

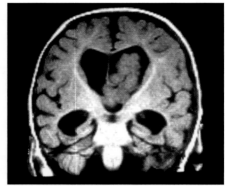

Fig. 5.02 Choroid plexus papilloma. T1-weighted MRI demonstrates a large multilobulated tumour within the left lateral ventricle.

been debated whether overproduction of cerebrospinal fluid is a major contributing factor to hydrocephalus {182}.

Imaging

On CT and MRI, choroid plexus papillomas usually present as isodense or hyperdense, T1-isointense, T2-hyperintense, irregularly contrast-enhancing, well-delineated masses within the ventricles, but irregular tumour margins and disseminated disease may occur {895}.

Spread

Even benign choroid plexus papilloma may seed cells into the cerebrospinal fluid; in rare cases, this can result in drop metastases in the surroundings of the cauda equina {2440}.

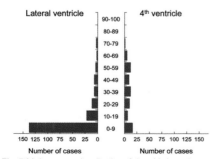

Fig. 5.01 Age versus localization of choroid plexus tumours, based on a compilation of 264 published cases {2777}.

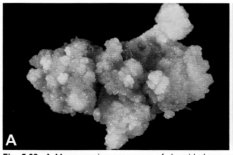

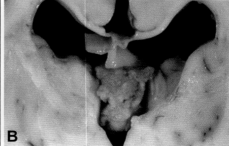

Fig. 5.03 A Macroscopic appearance of choroid plexus papilloma showing cauliflower-like appearance. **B** Choroid plexus papilloma arising in the posterior third ventricle producing partial obstruction with ventricle dilatation.

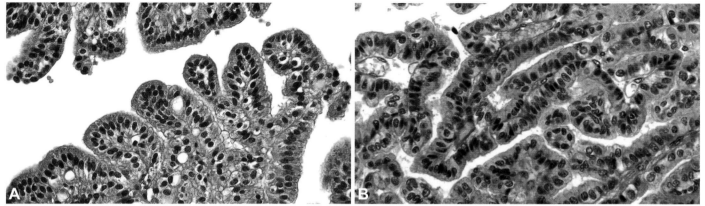

Fig. 5.04 Choroid plexus papilloma. **A** Well-differentiated papillary pattern composed of a single layer of monomorphic tumour cells. **B** Regular cuboidal cells organized in a monolayer along vessels.

Macroscopy

Choroid plexus papillomas are circumscribed cauliflower-like masses that may adhere to the ventricular wall, but are usually well delineated from brain parenchyma. Cysts and haemorrhages may occur. Intraoperative observations in rare atypical choroid plexus papillomas demonstrate a highly vascular tumour with a propensity to bleed {2494}, and this feature is also observed in some typical choroid plexus papillomas.

Microscopy

Delicate fibrovascular connective tissue fronds are covered by a single layer of uniform cuboidal to columnar epithelial cells with round or oval, basally situated monomorphic nuclei. Mitotic activity is absent or very low (< 2 mitoses per 10 high-power fields). Brain invasion with cell clusters or single cells, high cellularity, necrosis, nuclear pleomorphism, and focal blurring of the papillary pattern are unusual, but can occur. Choroid plexus papilloma closely resembles nonneoplastic choroid plexus, but the cells tend to be more crowded, elongated, or stratified in comparison with the normal

cobblestone-like surface. Rarely, choroid plexus papillomas can acquire unusual histological features, including oncocytic change, mucinous degeneration, melanization and tubular glandular architecture of tumour cells, neuropil-like islands, and degeneration of connective tissue (e.g. xanthomatous change; angioma-like increase of blood vessels; and bone, cartilage, or adipose tissue formation) {87, 299,960}.

Immunophenotype

Nearly all choroid plexus tumours express cytokeratins and vimentin {594, 912}. Most demonstrate positive staining for CK7, and positivity for CK20 is less common. In one study, none of the tumours were found to be CK20-positive when CK7-negative {1088}. EMA is often negative or only weakly and focally positive {594,1610}; strong positive staining for EMA favours other neoplasms. Transthyretin is positive in normal choroid plexus and in most choroid plexus tumours {1916}, but staining may be negative or variable among choroid plexus papillomas and choroid plexus carcinomas, and is also seen in some metastatic

carcinomas, limiting its usefulness {41}. Most choroid plexus tumours demonstrate variably positive staining for S100, possibly related to older patient age and better prognosis {1916}. Membranous expression of the inward rectifier potassium channel KIR7.1 has been found in normal choroid plexus (in 34 of 35 samples) and in choroid plexus papilloma (in 12 of 18 cases) but not in 100 cases of other primary brain tumours and cerebral metastases {958}. Another study found KIR7.1 in 30 of 30 choroid plexus tumours and the glutamate transporter EAAT1 in 32 of 35 cases, whereas these markers were absent in 4 endolymphatic sac tumours {2284}. EAAT1 has also been described to differentiate between neoplastic and non-neoplastic choroid plexus, because expression in the non-neoplastic choroid plexus was seen in only 4% of cases {180}.

Genetic profile

No large-scale sequencing studies of choroid plexus papilloma have been published to date. *TP53* mutations are rare in choroid plexus papillomas (present in < 10% of cases) {2483}. Both classic cytogenetic and genome-wide array-based approaches demonstrated hyperdiploidy in choroid plexus papilloma {598,1648, 2123}. In a series of 36 choroid plexus tumours, *MGMT* promoter methylation was found in all cases {961}.

Genetic susceptibility

Choroid plexus papilloma is a major diagnostic feature of Aicardi syndrome, a genetic but sporadic condition presumably linked to the X chromosome and defined by the triad of total or partial agenesis of the corpus callosum, chorioretinal

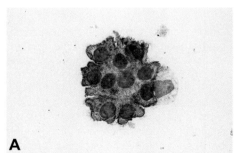
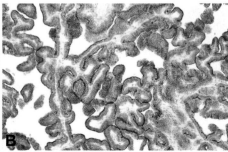

Fig. 5.05 Choroid plexus papilloma. Immunohistochemistry for the potassium channel KIR7.1. **A** Choroid plexus tumour cells in cerebrospinal fluid. **B** Typical membranous labelling of the apical cell surface of tumour cells.

lacunae, and infantile spasms {30}. In the setting of an X;17(q12;p13) translocation, hypomelanosis of Ito has been associated with the development of choroid plexus papilloma in several cases {2842}. Duplication of the short arm of chromosome 9, a rare constitutional abnormality, was associated with pathologically confirmed hyperplasia of the choroid plexus in 1 of 2 cases, and with a choroid plexus papilloma in another {1803}.

Prognosis and predictive factors

Choroid plexus papilloma can be cured by surgery alone, with a 5-year survival rate as high as 100%. In a series of 41 patients with choroid plexus papilloma, the 5-year rates of local control, control of relapse in the brain at a site distant from the initial disease, and overall survival were 84%, 92%, and 97%, respectively; the 5-year local control rate was better after gross total resection than after subtotal resection (100% vs 68%). Tumours that relapsed at sites distant from the initial disease also had local recurrence {1365}. A meta-analysis of 566 choroid plexus tumours found that 1-year, 5-year, and 10-year projected survival rates, respectively, were 90%, 81%, and 77% in choroid plexus papilloma compared with only 71%, 41%, and 35% in choroid plexus carcinoma {2777}. Choroid plexus papilloma in children aged < 36 months also had excellent prognosis after surgery alone {1415}. Malignant progression of choroid plexus papilloma is rare, but has been described {452,1147}.

Atypical choroid plexus papilloma

Paulus W.
Brandner S.
Hawkins C.
Tihan T.

Definition

A choroid plexus papilloma that has increased mitotic activity but does not fulfill the criteria for choroid plexus carcinoma. Atypical choroid plexus papillomas in children aged > 3 years and in adults are more likely to recur than their classic counterparts.

ICD-O code   9390/1

Grading

Atypical choroid plexus papilloma corresponds histologically to WHO grade II.

Epidemiology

In the SEER database, choroid plexus tumours account for 0.77% of all brain tumours and for 14% of those occurring in the first year of life, with atypical choroid plexus papilloma (grade II) accounting for 7.4% of choroid plexus tumours {351}. In the CPT-SIOP-2000 study, patients with atypical choroid plexus papilloma were younger (with a median patient age of 0.7 years) than were patients with choroid plexus papilloma or choroid plexus carcinoma (both with median patient ages of 2.3 years) {2790}.

Etiology

No differences have been established between the etiology of atypical choroid plexus papilloma and choroid plexus papilloma.

Localization

Atypical choroid plexus papillomas arise in locations where normal choroid plexus can be found. Whereas typical choroid plexus papillomas occur in the supratentorial and infratentorial regions with nearly equal frequency, atypical choroid plexus papillomas are more common within the lateral ventricles {1146}. In a large series of patients with atypical choroid plexus papillomas, 83% of the tumours were located in the lateral ventricles, 13% in the third ventricle, and 3% in the fourth ventricle {2790}.

Clinical features

Like choroid plexus papilloma, atypical choroid plexus papilloma blocks cerebrospinal fluid pathways, and patients present with hydrocephalus, papilloedema, and raised intracranial pressure.

Imaging

No differences in MRI characteristics have been reported between choroid plexus papilloma and atypical choroid plexus papilloma {2790}.

Spread

Atypical choroid plexus papilloma has been reported to present with metastasis at diagnosis in 17% of cases {2790}.

Macroscopy

Intraoperative observations in rare atypical choroid plexus papillomas demonstrate a highly vascular tumour with a propensity to bleed {2494}, but this feature is also observed in choroid plexus papillomas.

Microscopy

Atypical choroid plexus papilloma is defined as a choroid plexus papilloma with increased mitotic activity. One study found that a mitotic count of ≥ 2 mitoses per 10 randomly selected high-power fields (with 1 high-power field corresponding to 0.23 mm^2) can be used to establish this diagnosis {1146}. The same study showed that one or two of the following four features may also be present: increased cellularity, nuclear pleomorphism, blurring of the papillary pattern (solid growth), and areas of necrosis; however, these features are not required for a diagnosis of atypical choroid plexus papilloma.

Immunophenotype

Atypical choroid plexus papillomas carry a higher risk of recurrence compared with typical choroid plexus papilloma, and immunohistochemical results also correlate with recurrence. For example, negative S100 protein staining in > 50% of the tumour cells has been associated with a more aggressive clinical course {1916}. An inverse correlation has been found between transthyretin staining intensity and rate of local recurrence {1146}. In one study, positive CD44 staining was associated with atypical choroid plexus papilloma and choroid plexus carcinoma, correlating with the infiltrative nature of these tumours {2632}, but this association has not been validated. Otherwise, the immunohistochemical profile of atypical choroid plexus papilloma, including positivity for KIR7.1, is similar to that of choroid plexus papilloma {2215}.

Genetic profile

Atypical choroid plexus papillomas seem to be more similar genetically to choroid plexus papilloma than to choroid plexus carcinoma {1648}. Consistent with the entity's defining histological feature (i.e. increased mitotic activity), RNA expression profiling and gene set enrichment analysis have revealed higher expression of cell cycle–related genes in atypical choroid plexus papilloma than in choroid plexus papilloma {1136}.

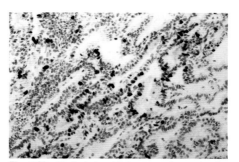

Fig. 5.06 Atypical choroid plexus papilloma showing focal increase of proliferation (Ki-67 proliferation index).

Prognosis and predictive factors

In a series of 124 choroid plexus papillomas, multivariate analysis showed that increased mitotic activity was the only histological feature independently associated with recurrence; tumours with ≥ 2 mitoses per 10 high-power fields, which constituted the definition of atypical choroid plexus papilloma, were 4.9 times as likely as those with < 2 mitoses per 10 high-power fields to recur after 5 years of follow-up {1146}. The overall and event-free survival rates for atypical choroid plexus papillomas are intermediate between those for choroid plexus papilloma and choroid plexus carcinoma; the 5-year overall survival and event-free survival rates for atypical choroid plexus papilloma are 89% and 83%, respectively {2790}. There is evidence that the diagnosis of atypical choroid plexus papilloma is prognostically relevant in children aged > 3 years and in adults, but not in children aged < 3 years, who may have good prognosis even with choroid plexus papillomas with high proliferation {2544}.

Choroid plexus carcinoma

Paulus W.
Brandner S.
Hawkins C.
Tihan T.

Definition

A frankly malignant epithelial neoplasm most commonly occurring in the lateral ventricles of children, showing at least four of the following five histological features: frequent mitoses, increased cellular density, nuclear pleomorphism, blurring of the papillary pattern with poorly structured sheets of tumour cells, and necrotic areas.

Choroid plexus carcinoma frequently invades neighbouring brain structures and metastasizes via cerebrospinal fluid. Preserved nuclear expression of SMARCB1 and SMARCA4 (i.e. no inactivation of the *SMARCB1* or *SMARCA4* gene) in virtually all tumours helps in the differential diagnosis with atypical teratoid/rhabdoid tumour.

ICD-O code   9390/3

Grading

Choroid plexus carcinoma corresponds histologically to WHO grade III.

Epidemiology

In the SEER database, choroid plexus tumours account for 0.77% of all brain tumours and for 14% of those occurring in the first year of life, with choroid plexus carcinoma (grade III) accounting for 34.4% of choroid plexus tumours {351}. About 80% of all choroid plexus carcinomas occur in children.

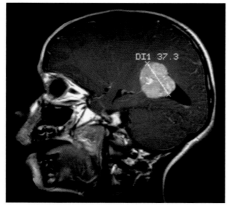

Fig. 5.07 MRI of a choroid plexus carcinoma in the lateral ventricle of a 5-year-old child with a *TP53* germline mutation.

Etiology

Most choroid plexus carcinomas occur sporadically, but they can also occur in association with hereditary syndromes such as Aicardi syndrome {2488} or (more frequently) Li–Fraumeni syndrome (LFS) {1379} (see p. 310).

Localization

The great majority of choroid plexus carcinomas are located within and around the lateral ventricles {1415}.

Clinical features

Like choroid plexus papilloma, choroid plexus carcinoma blocks cerebrospinal fluid pathways and causes symptoms related to hydrocephalus, such as increased intracranial pressure, enlarged head size, nausea, and vomiting {182}.

Imaging

On MRI, choroid plexus carcinomas typically present as large intraventricular lesions with irregular enhancing margins, a heterogeneous signal on T2-weighted and T1-weighted images, oedema in adjacent brain, hydrocephalus, and disseminated tumour {1660}.

Spread

Choroid plexus carcinoma presents with metastases at diagnosis in 21% of cases {2790}. A 20-year longitudinal cohort study of 31 patients with choroid plexus papillomas and 8 patients with choroid plexus carcinomas showed that the risk of local recurrence or metastasis associated with choroid plexus carcinoma was 20 times the risk associated with choroid plexus papilloma {182}.

Macroscopy

Choroid plexus carcinomas are highly vascular tumours with a propensity to bleed, but this feature can be seen with all types of choroid plexus tumours. Choroid plexus carcinomas are invasive tumours that may appear solid, haemorrhagic, and necrotic.

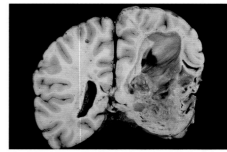

Fig. 5.08 A large choroid plexus carcinoma in the lateral ventricle with extensive invasion of brain tissue.

Microscopy

This tumour shows frank signs of malignancy. One study defined tumours as frankly malignant if they showed at least four of the following five histological features: frequent mitoses (usually > 5 mitoses per 10 high-power fields), increased cellular density, nuclear pleomorphism, blurring of the papillary pattern with poorly structured sheets of tumour cells, and necrotic areas {1146}. Diffuse brain invasion is common.

Immunophenotype

Like choroid plexus papillomas, choroid plexus carcinomas express cytokeratins, but they are less frequently positive for S100 protein and transthyretin. There is usually no membranous positivity for EMA. Positivity for p53 protein has been reported in choroid plexus carcinomas that also harboured *TP53* mutation {2483}. Choroid plexus carcinomas have a higher proliferation index than do choroid plexus papillomas and atypical choroid plexus papillomas. One study reported a mean Ki-67 proliferation index of 1.9% (range: 0.2–6%) for choroid plexus papilloma, 13.8% (range: 7.3–60%) for choroid plexus carcinoma, and < 0.1% for normal choroid plexus {2607}. Another study found a mean Ki-67 proliferation index of 4.5% (range: 0.2–17.4%) for choroid plexus papilloma, 18.5% (range: 4.1–29.7%) for choroid plexus carcinoma, and 0% for normal choroid plexus {363}. Distinct membranous staining for the potassium channel KIR7.1 is seen in about half of all choroid plexus carcinomas.

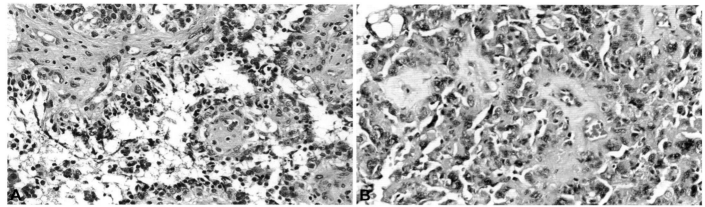

Fig. 5.09 Choroid plexus carcinoma. **A,B** Frequent mitoses, increased cellular density, nuclear polymorphism, and blurring of the papillary pattern.

Almost all choroid plexus carcinomas retain nuclear positivity for SMARCB1 and SMARCA4.

Genetic profile

Choroid plexus carcinomas are characterized by complex chromosomal alterations that are related to patient age {2198}. No large-scale sequencing studies of choroid plexus carcinoma have been published to date. About 50% of all choroid plexus carcinomas harbour *TP53* mutations. The combination of the *TP53*-R72 variant and the *MDM2* SNP309 polymorphism, which is associated with reduced *TP53* activity, was observed in the majority (> 90%) of patients with *TP53*-wildtype choroid plexus carcinomas {2483}, implicating p53 dysfunction

in virtually all choroid plexus carcinomas. Both classic cytogenetic and genome-wide array-based approaches demonstrate either hyper- or hypodiploidy in choroid plexus carcinomas {1648,2123, 2843}. *TP53* mutations in choroid plexus carcinoma are associated with increased genomic instability {2483}, in particular hypodiploidy {1648}.

Genetic susceptibility

About 40% of choroid plexus carcinomas occur in the setting of germline *TP53* mutations / LFS {2483}. Within the spectrum of tumours occurring in the setting of LFS, choroid plexus carcinomas are among the less frequent manifestations. However, the link to this inherited tumour syndrome is so strong that it has been

recommended that any patient with a choroid plexus carcinoma be tested for a *TP53* germline mutation, even in the absence of a family history of LFS {864}. Choroid plexus carcinoma has also been described in rhabdoid tumour predisposition syndrome, a familial cancer syndrome caused by germline mutation in the *SMARCB1* gene {2327}; however, these cases most likely constitute intraventricular atypical teratoid/rhabdoid tumours rather than choroid plexus carcinomas.

Prognosis and predictive factors

The 3-year and 5-year progression-free survival rates of choroid plexus carcinoma have been reported as 58% and 38%, respectively, and the overall survival rates as 83% and 62%. Deaths from disease beyond 5 years were also noted {2844}. Only extent of surgery had a significant impact on survival for choroid plexus carcinoma. The use of adjuvant radiation therapy in patients with choroid plexus carcinoma undergoing surgery was not found to be associated with improved overall survival {351}. Some children with choroid plexus carcinomas have been found to have *TP53* gene mutations in association with LFS, and several recent studies have suggested that the absence of *TP53* mutations as identified by immunohistochemical staining is associated with a more favourable outcome compared with p53-positive tumours {878,2483,2844}. One of these studies also suggested that the prognosis of *TP53*-mutant tumours may be improved with intensive chemotherapy {2844}. A more recent study demonstrated on multivariate analysis that choroid plexus carcinomas with loss of chromosome arm 12q were associated with a significantly shorter survival than were tumours without this alteration {2198}.

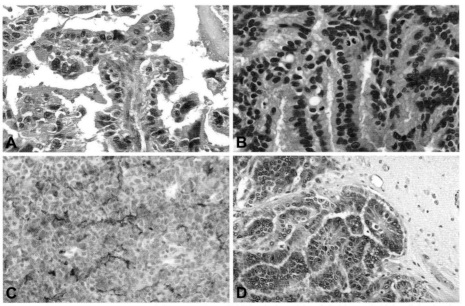

Fig. 5.10 Choroid plexus carcinoma. **A** Pleomorphism. **B** High mitotic activity. **C** Solid growth, high cellular density, and focal membranous staining for KIR7.1. **D** Infiltration of neighbouring brain tissue. Immunochemistry for transthyretin (TTR).

CHAPTER 6

Neuronal and mixed neuronal–glial tumours

Dysembryoplastic neuroepithelial tumour

Pietsch T.
Hawkins C.
Varlet P.
Blümcke I.
Hirose T.

Definition

A benign glioneuronal neoplasm typically located in the temporal lobe of children or young adults with early-onset epilepsy; predominantly with a cortical location and a multinodular architecture; and with a histological hallmark of a specific glioneuronal element characterized by columns made up of bundles of axons oriented perpendicularly to the cortical surface.

These columns are lined by oligodendrocyte-like cells embedded in a mucoid matrix and interspersed with floating neurons. If only the specific glioneuronal element is observed, the simple form of dysembryoplastic neuroepithelial tumour (DNT) is diagnosed. Complex variants of DNT additionally contain glial tumour components, often with a nodular appearance. The presence of IDH mutation or 1p/19q codeletion excludes the diagnosis of DNT. Long-term follow-up after epilepsy surgery shows an excellent outcome; recurrence or progression is exceptional.

ICD-O code   9413/0

Grading

DNT corresponds histologically to WHO grade I.

Epidemiology

Incidence

The reported incidence rates of DNTs vary widely (from 7% to 80%) in tumour series

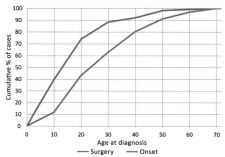

Fig. 6.01 Cumulative age distribution of dysembryoplastic neuroepithelial tumours, based on 224 cases from the German Neuropathological Reference Center for Epilepsy Surgery, University of Erlangen, Germany.

obtained from epilepsy surgery centres, depending on the histopathological diagnostic criteria used {2541}. In a series of 1511 long-term epilepsy-associated tumours reviewed at the German Neuropathological Reference Center for Epilepsy Surgery, DNTs accounted for 17.8% of the tumours in adults and 23.4% in children {219}. In another series, consisting of all neuroepithelial tumours diagnosed in a single institution since 1975, DNTs accounted for 1.2% of the tumours diagnosed in patients aged ≤ 20 years and 0.2% in patients aged > 20 years {2175}.

Age and sex distribution

Patient age at the onset of symptoms is an important diagnostic criterion. In about 90% of cases, the first seizure occurs before the age of 20 years (mean patient age at seizure onset: 15 years), with seizure onset reported in patients aged from 3 weeks {1854} to 38 years {2078}. The mean patient age at surgery and histopathological diagnosis is considerably older, with a mean age at epilepsy surgery of 25.8 years. However, earlier detection of DNTs by MRI in children and young adults with focal epilepsy, and access to paediatric and adult epilepsy surgery programmes are important factors for achieving long-term seizure control {219,251, 382,689,845,1144,1551,1745,1800}. There is a slight predominance of DNT in male patients (accounting for 56.7% of cases).

Localization

DNTs can be located in any part of the supratentorial cortex, but show a predilection for the temporal lobe {348}, preferentially involving the mesial structures {404, 530,531,532,534,537,566,1033,1903, 2026}. The second most frequent location is the frontal lobe {348}. In a meta-analysis of 624 reported DNTs, 67.3% were located in the temporal lobe, 16.3% in the frontal lobe, and 16.4% in other locations {2543}, such as the caudate nucleus {394,896} or lateral ventricles {1848}, the septum pellucidum {111,949}, the trigonoseptal region {896}, the midbrain and tectum {1399}, and the cerebellum {534,1382,2819} or

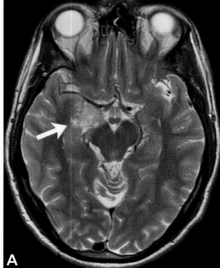

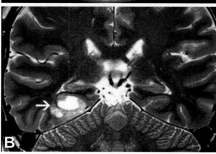

Fig. 6.02 Dysembryoplastic neuroepithelial tumour (DNT). **A** T2-weighted MRI of a tumour in the right temporal lobe with a pseudocystic appearance (arrow). **B** On MRI, a right mesiotemporal DNT is T2-hyperintense with a multicystic appearance (arrow).

brain stem {749}. Multifocal DNTs have also been reported, indicating that these tumours can also be found in the region of the third ventricle, the basal ganglia, and the pons {1376,1468,2282,2739}.

Clinical features

Patients with supratentorial DNTs typically present with drug-resistant focal epilepsy, with or without secondary seizure generalization, and with no neurological deficit. However, a congenital neurological deficit may be present in a minority of cases {404,534,537,566,689,1800,1903, 2026,2078,2177,2515}. The duration of the seizures prior to surgical intervention varies from weeks to decades (with

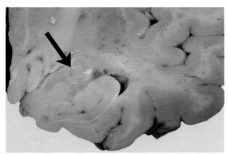

Fig. 6.03 A postmortem specimen of a dysembryoplastic neuroepithelial tumour with multinodular architecture in the mesial temporal lobe (arrow).

a mean duration of 10.8 years), resulting in variability in patient age at pathological diagnosis (with a mean age at surgery of 25.8 years).

Imaging

Cortical topography and the absence of mass effect and of significant tumoural oedema are important criteria for differentiating between DNTs and diffuse gliomas. DNTs usually encompass the thickness of the normal cortex. In a minority of cases, the area of signal abnormality also extends into the subcortical white matter {348,530,531,537,689,1395,1860, 2412}. On MRI, most DNTs present as T2-hyperintense multiple or single pseudocysts. Non-cystic tissue is hypointense or nearly isointense to grey matter on T1-weighted images and hyperintense on T2-weighted and FLAIR images {348}. In tumours that are located at the convexity, deformation of the overlying calvaria is often seen on imaging, and this finding further supports the diagnosis of DNT { 530,531,537,1395,2078,2412,2515}. Calcifications are often seen on CT. When present, they occur within more deeply located tumour portions, usually in the vicinity of contrast-enhancing regions and haemorrhages {348}. On CT and MRI, about 20% to one third of DNTs show contrast enhancement, often in multiple rings rather than homogeneously {348,1800, 2412}. Nodular or ring-shaped contrast enhancement may occur in a previously non-enhancing tumour {348,2412}, and increased lesion size, with or without peritumoural oedema, may also be observed on imaging follow-up. However, in DNTs, these changes are not signs of malignant transformation but are usually due to ischaemic and/or haemorrhagic changes {536,1155,1860}.

Macroscopy

DNTs vary in size from a few millimetres to several centimetres {1903}. In their typical location, they are often easily identifiable at the cortical surface and may show an exophytic portion. However, leptomeningeal dissemination is not a typical feature of DNTs. The appearance of the tumour on cut sections may reflect the complex histoarchitecture of the lesion. The most typical feature is the viscous consistency of the glioneuronal component, which may be associated with multiple or single firmer nodules. The affected cortex is often expanded.

Microscopy

The histopathological hallmarks are a multinodular growth pattern and the so-called specific glioneuronal element, which is characterized by columns oriented perpendicularly to the cortical surface, formed by bundles of axons lined by small oligodendrocyte-like cells. Between these columns, neurons with normal cytology (which may represent entrapped cortical neurons) appear to float in a

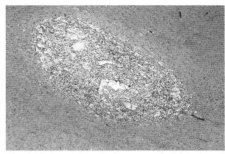

Fig. 6.04 Dysembryoplastic neuroepithelial tumour. A low-power micrograph showing a nodular growth pattern.

mucoid, alcianophilic matrix {1323}. Scattered, interspersed stellate astrocytes positive for GFAP are associated with this glioneuronal element. Constituent oligodendrocyte-like, neuronal, and astrocytic cell populations can be relatively heterogeneous from case to case and from area to area within the same tumour. DNTs do not contain dysplastic ganglion cells such as those described in gangliogliomas (i.e. binucleated neurons, large neurons that are either pyramidal or similar to resident cortical neurons, and unequivocal clustering not otherwise explicable by anatomical region). Depending on the extent of fluid extravasation, subtle variation from a columnar to an alveolar or a more compact structure may be observed {531}. Several histological forms of DNT have been described, but this subclassification has no clinical or therapeutic implications {2543}. Two histological forms of DNT (the simple form and the complex form) have been defined, but the criteria for further unspecific and diffuse forms are still under debate.

Simple form
In this morphological variant, the tumour consists of the unique glioneuronal

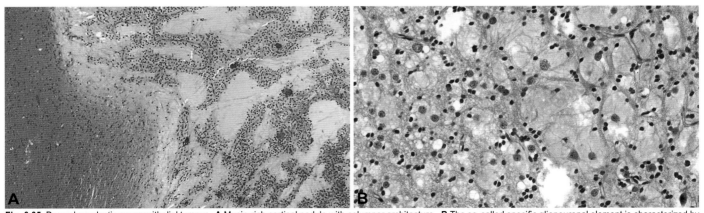

Fig. 6.05 Dysembryoplastic neuroepithelial tumour. **A** Mucin-rich cortical nodule with columnar architecture. **B** The so-called specific glioneuronal element is characterized by oligodendrocyte-like cells embedded in a mucoid matrix with interspersed floating neurons.

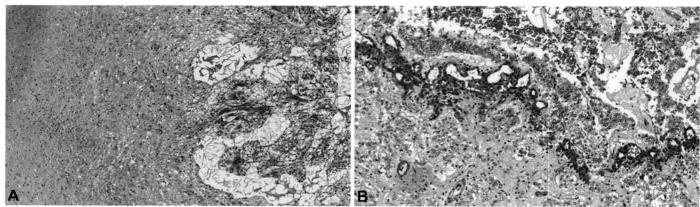

Fig. 6.06 Dysembryoplastic neuroepithelial tumour. **A** Glial nodule with piloid features can be seen in a tumour of the complex variant. **B** This glial nodule in a complex tumour shows marked endothelial proliferation.

element. It may show a patchy pattern {531}, owing to the juxtaposition of foci of tumour and of easily recognizable cortex. Other tumour components are absent.

Complex form
In this variant, glial nodules, which give the tumour its characteristic multinodular architecture, are seen in association with the specific glioneuronal element. The heterogeneous appearance of these tumours is due to the presence of additional histological components resembling astrocytic or oligodendrocytic differentiation. These constituent cell populations can vary from case to case, as well as from area to area within the same tumour. The glial components seen in the complex form of DNTs have a highly variable appearance. They may form typical nodules or may show a relatively diffuse pattern. They may closely resemble conventional categories of gliomas or may show unusual features. They often mimic pilocytic astrocytomas and may show nuclear atypia, rare mitoses, or microvascular-like proliferation and ischaemic necrosis. Their microvascular network can vary from meagre to extensive and may include glomerulus-like formations. In these vessels, the endothelial cells may be hyperplastic and mitotically active. Within the glial components, frankly hamartomatous (usually calcified) vessels are common {531,537, 2078}. Malformative vessels can cause haemorrhage {536,689,1860,2412,2542}.

Non-specific and diffuse forms
On the basis of their similar clinical presentation, cortical topography, neuroradiological features, and stability on long-term preoperative imaging follow-up, non-specific and diffuse histological variants of DNT have been described. These non-specific histological forms accounted for 20–50% of the DNTs included in three studies {537,1903,2610}. Because they lack the specific glioneuronal element, these variants of DNT are often indistinguishable from gangliogliomas or other gliomas by conventional histology, particularly when the cortical topography of the tumour is not apparent on non-representative samples. Immunohistochemistry and molecular features can help to exclude typical diffuse astrocytomas and oligodendrogliomas of adulthood (see *Genetic profile*). Criteria for the differentiation of such diffuse and non-specific variants of DNT from other long-term epilepsy-associated tumours such as gangliogliomas are not well established, and the concept of additional histological variants of DNT remains controversial. A novel classification scheme for long-term epilepsy-associated tumours has been proposed that includes these variants as well as mixed tumours {219}. It awaits further molecular–diagnostic and clinicopathological confirmation.

Cortical dysplasia
Focal cortical dysplasia is found in DNTs {2543}. It should be diagnosed only in areas of cortical abnormalities without tumour cell infiltration and classified as focal cortical dysplasia Type IIIb according to the classification proposed by the International League Against Epilepsy (ILAE) {225}.

Immunophenotype
The so-called specific glioneuronal element shows a consistent pattern in immunohistochemistry. The small oligodendrocyte-like cells express glial markers including S100 protein and the glial transcription factor OLIG2. They can also express myelin–oligodendrocyte glycoprotein, indicating oligodendroglial differentiation {2781}, as well as NOGO-A {1600}. GFAP is absent in oligodendrocyte-like cells, whereas the scattered stellate astrocytes within the specific glioneuronal element are positive for GFAP. Floating neurons can be visualized by the nuclear NeuN epitope {2772, 2773}. Variable expression of MAP2 can be found in oligodendrocyte-like cells, but staining is typically faint, and the strong perinuclear expression found in diffuse oligodendrogliomas is not detectable {224}. The oncofetal antigen CD34 has been described with variable incidences in DNTs {222,414,2543}. DNT cells should not label with antibodies against mutant IDH1 {356} or K27M-mutant H3.3 {150}. Varying proportions of DNTs have been described to stain with antibodies against V600E-mutant BRAF protein {414,2543}. The Ki-67 proliferation index of DNTs has been reported to vary from 0% to 8% focally {530,531,537,1903,2026,2515}.

Differential diagnosis
The histological diagnosis of DNT may be difficult, in particular with limited material. En bloc resection during epilepsy surgery is therefore recommended {219}. The typical columnar architecture of the specific glioneuronal element can be obscured when the samples are not adequately oriented, and due to its semiliquid consistency, this element can be lost as a result of inadvertent surgical aspiration and/or fragmentation during fixation. It is therefore important that the diagnosis of DNT be considered in any case in which all of the following features are

present: history of focal seizures (usually beginning before the age of 20 years), no progressive neurological deficit, predominantly cortical topography of a supratentorial lesion, no mass effect (except if related to a cyst), and no peritumoural oedema {530,532,537}.

Dysembryoplastic neuroepithelial tumour versus low-grade diffuse glioma

DNTs lack mutations in *IDH1* or *IDH2*, which are found in a large proportion of diffuse astrocytomas and oligodendrogliomas of adults {2810}. However, in the paediatric setting, such mutations are rare in diffuse oligodendrogliomas {2157}.

Clinical and radiological criteria help in distinguishing these benign tumours from diffuse gliomas. Diffusely infiltrating low-grade gliomas with a microcystic matrix may mimic a so-called specific glioneuronal element. Residual neurons may appear as floating neurons overrun by glioma cells. Oligodendroglioma may exhibit a nodular pattern and can induce secondary architectural changes of the cortex, which can make this tumour difficult to distinguish from a focal cortical dysplasia. Immunohistochemistry for GFAP and MAP2 is very helpful, because the oligodendrocyte-like cells of the specific glioneuronal element lack GFAP (which is typically seen in diffuse astrocytomas) and they also lack the strong ring-shaped cytoplasmic staining for MAP2 observed in diffuse oligodendrogliomas {224}.

Dysembryoplastic neuroepithelial tumour versus ganglioglioma

Gangliogliomas can also pose a challenge for the differential diagnosis of DNTs, because (1) the dysplastic ganglion cells of gangliogliomas may not be present in small or non-representative samples, (2) these tumours may show a multinodular architecture, (3) small gangliogliomas may show predominant cortical topography, and (4) the clinical presentation of gangliogliomas is often similar to that of DNTs. However, ganglioglioma should be suspected when the tumour shows perivascular lymphocytic infiltration, a network of reticulin fibres, and/or a large cystic component, or when the tumour has prominent immunoreactivity for the class II epitope of CD34. Because gangliogliomas can undergo malignant transformation, their distinction

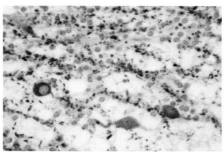

Fig. 6.07 Dysembryoplastic neuroepithelial tumour. Floating neurons show immunoreactivity for synaptophysin, whereas small oligodendrocyte-like cells are immunonegative.

from DNTs is prognostically important. However, examples of composite/mixed ganglioglioma and DNT have been reported and were considered to constitute a transitional form between the two tumours {229,404,1008,2021,2346,2543}. Such cases should be diagnosed as mixed forms. In a recent proposal for a neuropathology-based classification of long-term epilepsy-associated tumours, the term "composite neuroepithelial tumours" was proposed for such lesions {219}.

Cell of origin

Several factors suggest that DNTs have a dysontogenetic/malformative origin, such as the young age at onset of symptoms and bone deformity adjacent to the tumours {530,531,534,537}. However, the exact histogenesis of DNT remains unknown {219,2543}.

Genetic profile

Paediatric DNTs have been shown to have stable genomes {1874}, whereas recurrent gains of whole chromosomes 5 and 7 were found in approximately 20% and 30% of cases, respectively, in a series of adult DNTs {2016}. As in other glioneuronal tumours, recurrent *BRAF* V600E mutations were identified in 30% of DNTs {414,2015}. These mutations were associated with activation of mTOR signalling {2015}. Neither *TP53* mutations {751} nor *IDH1*/*IDH2* mutations have been detected in DNTs {2810}. Similarly, codeletion of whole chromosome arms 1p/19q has not been demonstrated in DNT {1874,2016}. These markers of diffuse gliomas were also found to be absent in 2 cases of DNT of the septum pellucidum {2800}. *H3F3A* K27M mutations were not present in DNT {833}.

Genetic susceptibility

DNTs occasionally occur in patients with neurofibromatosis type 1 or XYY syndrome {1218,1376,1468}.

Prognosis and predictive factors

DNTs are benign lesions, and their stability has been demonstrated in a study that included 53 patients for whom successive preoperative CT or MRI was available, with a mean duration of follow-up of 4.5 years {2412}. However, variable histomorphological features and diagnoses of multiple variants of DNT overlapping with other glioneuronal tumour entities make reliable analysis of prognostic and predictive factors difficult {219}. Long-term clinical follow-up usually demonstrates no evidence of recurrence, even in patients with only partial surgical removal {530,531, 534,537,689,1287,1451,1551,2078,2232, 2412}. Ischaemic or haemorrhagic changes may occur, with or without an increase in size of the lesion or peritumoural oedema {536,689,1155,1860,2412}. Reported risk factors for the development of recurrent seizures during long-term follow-up after operation include a longer preoperative history of seizures {94,991}, the presence of residual tumour {1800}, and the presence of cortical dysplasia adjacent to DNT {2224}.

Among the > 1000 DNTs that have been reported, malignant transformation is a rare event. MRI may reveal tumour recurrence, but histopathology often remains benign. Only 20 histologically proven cases have exhibited clear in situ tumour recurrence, and only 6 showed malignant transformation {413}. Ray et al. {2077} reported that the prognosis can be favourable after gross resection of the recurrent DNT. Anaplastic transformation has occurred after radiation and/or chemotherapy {2077,2203}. Atypical clinical presentation and ambiguous histopathological diagnosis must also be taken into account, and have interfered with reliable prediction of the biological behaviour of DNT from published case series {219, 2541}. Patients with DNT recurrence may require closer follow-up. These biological events further support the neoplastic (rather than dysplastic or hamartomatous) nature of DNT.

Gangliocytoma

Capper D.
Becker A.J.
Giannini C.
Figarella-Branger D.
Huse J.T.
Rosenblum M.K.
Blümcke I.
Wiestler O.D.

Definition
A rare, well-differentiated, slow-growing neuroepithelial neoplasm composed of irregular clusters of mostly mature neoplastic ganglion cells, often with dysplastic features.

The stroma consists of non-neoplastic glial elements. Transitional forms between gangliocytoma and ganglioglioma exist, and the distinction of these two entities is not always possible.

ICD-O code   9492/0

Grading
Gangliocytoma corresponds histologically to WHO grade I.

Epidemiology
Gangliocytomas are rare tumours predominantly affecting children. The relative incidence reported in epilepsy surgical series ranges from 0% to 3.2% {2541}.

Localization
Like gangliogliomas, these tumours can occur throughout the CNS. Dysplastic cerebellar gangliocytoma (Lhermitte–Duclos disease) is discussed in separate sections of this volume (see pp. 142, 314). Gangliocytoma of the pituitary is reviewed in the volume *WHO classification of tumours of the endocrine organs*.

Clinical features
Gangliocytomas share the clinical features of gangliogliomas.

Imaging
Radiological data specifically addressing gangliocytoma have not been reported.

Microscopy
Gangliocytomas are composed of irregular groups of large, multipolar neurons (often with dysplastic features). Binucleated neurons are commonly observed. The density of dysplastic ganglion cells is typically low; it may be close to the density of neurons in grey matter, but is higher in some cases. Some ganglionic cells

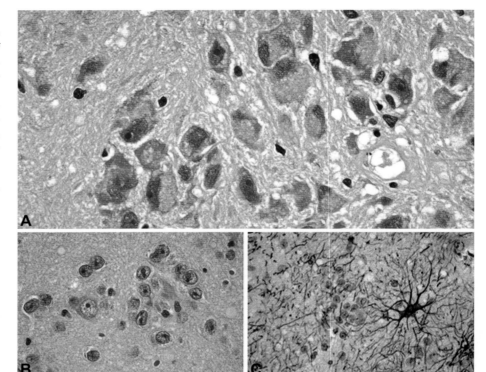

Fig. 6.08 Gangliocytoma. **A** Focal accumulation of multipolar, dysplastic neurons. **B** Clusters of mature neurons are embedded in an otherwise normal brain matrix. **C** Stellate ramification of GFAP-positive astrocytes is compatible with non-neoplastic nature in a gangliocytoma.

may show a lower degree of differentiation, but the presence of mitotically active neuroblasts is not compatible with the diagnosis of gangliocytoma and should prompt the differential diagnosis of CNS ganglioneuroblastoma (see p. 207). The stroma consists of non-neoplastic glial elements but may be difficult to distinguish from a low-cellularity glial component of a ganglioglioma. A network of reticulin fibres may be present, particularly in a perivascular location.

Immunophenotype
The neoplastic ganglion cells are typically positive (to various degrees) for synaptophysin, neurofilament, chromogranin-A, and MAP2. The neuronal nuclear antigen NeuN is often only weakly expressed, or may be negative.

Genetic profile
Genetic data specifically addressing gangliocytomas have not been reported. A close genetic relationship to ganglioglioma seems possible.

Genetic susceptibility
Dysplastic cerebellar gangliocytoma (Lhermitte–Duclos disease), which is associated with Cowden syndrome, is covered in separate sections of this volume (see pp. 142, 314). No distinct genetic susceptibility factors have been reported for classic gangliocytoma.

Prognosis and predictive factors
Gangliocytomas are benign tumours with favourable outcome. Specific prognostic or predictive factors have not been reported.

Multinodular and vacuolating neuronal tumour of the cerebrum

Multinodular and vacuolating neuronal tumour of the cerebrum is a recently reported clinicopathological lesion with uncertain class assignment {1068}. A total of 14 cases have been reported; they typically occurred in adults, predominantly in the temporal lobe, and were most frequently associated with seizures or seizure equivalents {228,759,1068, 1738}. Multinodular and vacuolating neuronal tumours can also present incidentally, without seizures {228}. On T2-weighted and FLAIR MRI, this tumour is characterized by hyperintensity and absence of enhancement, often showing a subtle or conspicuous internal nodularity. Histologically, it is composed of small to medium-sized neuroepithelial cells with globose amphophilic cytoplasm and large nuclei with vesicular chromatin and distinctive nucleoli resembling small neurons. The cells do not display the multinucleation or conspicuous dysmorphism associated with neoplastic ganglion cells {1068}. The cells are arranged in nodules involving the deep half of the cortex and/or subcortical white matter, showing prominent intracellular and stromal vacuolation. The cells express neuronal markers, including synaptophysin and the neuronal protein ELAV3/4, but not the neuronal nuclear protein NeuN, chromogranin, or the glial marker GFAP. They frequently express OLIG2. The lesions are frequently associated with the presence of ramified, CD34-positive neural elements in neighbouring cerebral cortex.

It is not clear whether multinodular and vacuolating neuronal tumour is a neoplastic process or a hamartomatous/malformative process. Mutation testing has shown no *BRAF* V600 hotspot mutations (7 cases tested) {228,759,1068} or *IDH1/IDH2* mutations (3 cases tested) {228,759}. The single point mutation *MAP2K1* Q56P (c.167A→C) has been reported in 1 case, and there was no obvious evidence of copy number variation by microarray-based comparative genomic hybridization analysis in 2 other cases {1068}. The behaviour of multinodular and vacuolating neuronal tumour is benign, and gross total removal or substantial resection provides disease control.

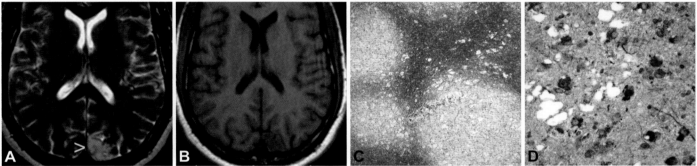

Fig. 6.09 Multinodular and vacuolating neuronal tumour of the cerebrum. **A** On MRI, the tumour presents as a superficial lesion with a high T2 signal (arrowhead) and (**B**) with a somewhat nodular appearance on T1-weighted images. **C** Nodular pattern. Nissl stain. **D** Small neurons are neurofilament-positive.

Ganglioglioma

Becker A.J.
Wiestler O.D.
Figarella-Branger D.
Blümcke I.
Capper D.

Definition

A well-differentiated, slow-growing glio-neuronal neoplasm composed of dysplastic ganglion cells (i.e. large cells with dysmorphic neuronal features, without the architectural arrangement or cytological characteristics of cortical neurons) in combination with neoplastic glial cells.

Gangliogliomas preferentially present in the temporal lobe of children or young adults with early-onset focal epilepsy. Intracortical cystic structures and a circumscribed area of cortical (and subcortical) signal enhancement are characteristic on FLAIR and T2-weighted MRI. *BRAF* V600E mutation occurs in approximately 25% of gangliogliomas, whereas IDH mutation or combined loss of chromosomal arms 1p and 19q exclude a diagnosis of a ganglioglioma. The prognosis is favourable, with a recurrence-free survival rate as high as 97% at 7.5 years.

ICD-O code   9505/1

Grading

Most gangliogliomas correspond histologically to WHO grade I. Some gangliogliomas with anaplastic features in their glial component (i.e. anaplastic gangliogliomas) are considered to correspond histologically to WHO grade III {1552,1570} (see p. 141). Criteria for WHO grade II have been discussed but not established {1552,1570}.

Epidemiology

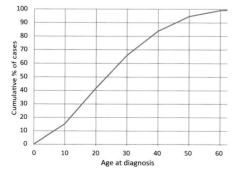

Fig. 6.10 Cumulative age distribution of ganglioglioma at diagnosis, based on 602 cases from the German Neuropathological Reference Center for Epilepsy Surgery.

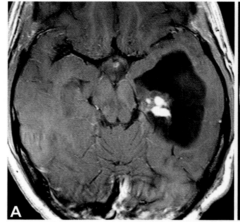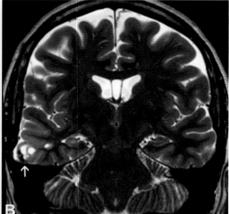

Fig. 6.11 Ganglioglioma. **A** Relatively small enhancing nodule and a large, associated septated cyst in a 15-year-old male. The cyst wall is not enhancing. **B** Coronal T2-weighted imaging shows a cortical/subcortical lesion with intracortical cysts, bony remodelling, and a hypointense portion suggesting calcification (arrow).

The available data indicate that gangliogliomas and gangliocytomas together account for 0.4% of all CNS tumours and 1.3% of all brain tumours {1207,1552}. There are no population-based epidemiological data on gangliogliomas.

Patient age at presentation ranges from 2 months to 70 years. Data from several large series with a total of 626 patients indicate a mean/median patient age at diagnosis of 8.5–25 years. The male-to-female ratio is 1.1–1.9:1 {1428,2027, 2541,2774}. In a survey conducted by the German Neuropathological Reference Center for Epilepsy Surgery of 212 children with gangliogliomas, the mean patient age at surgery was 9.9 years and 48% of the patients were girls.

Localization

These tumours can occur throughout the CNS, including in the cerebrum, brain stem, cerebellum, spinal cord, optic nerves, pituitary, and pineal gland. The majority (> 70%) of gangliogliomas occur in the temporal lobe {226,1010,1428, 2027,2774}.

Clinical features

The symptoms vary according to tumour size and site. Tumours in the cerebrum are frequently associated with a history of focal seizures ranging in

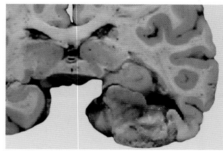

Fig. 6.12 Ganglioglioma of the right temporal lobe also involving the hippocampal formation.

duration from 1 month to 50 years before diagnosis, with a mean/median duration of 6–25 years {1428,2027,2774}. For tumours involving the brain stem and spinal cord, the mean durations of symptoms

Table 6.01 Localization of gangliogliomas

Localization	Tumours	
Temporal	509	84%
Frontal	28	5%
Parietal	17	3%
Occipital	12	2%
Multiple lobes	30	5%
Other	6	1%
Based on 602 surgical specimens submitted to the German Neuropathological Reference Center for Epilepsy Surgery.		

before diagnosis are 1.25 and 1.4 years, respectively {1428}. Gangliogliomas have been reported in 15–25% of patients undergoing surgery for control of seizures {2541}. They are the tumours most commonly associated with chronic temporal lobe epilepsy {219}.

Imaging

Classic imaging features include intracortical cyst(s) and a circumscribed area of cortical (and subcortical) signal increase on FLAIR and T2-weighted images {2602}. Contrast enhancement varies in intensity from none to marked, and may be solid, rim, or nodular. Tumour calcification can be detected in 30% of tumours. Scalloping of the calvaria may be seen adjacent to superficially located cerebral tumours.

Macroscopy

Gangliogliomas are macroscopically well-delineated solid or cystic lesions, usually with little mass effect. Calcification may be observed. Haemorrhage and necrosis are rare.

Microscopy

The histopathological hallmark of gangliogliomas is a combination of neuronal and glial cell elements, which may exhibit marked heterogeneity. The spectrum of ganglioglioma varies from tumours with a predominantly neuronal phenotype to variants with a dominant glial population. Some cases also contain cells of intermediate differentiation. Dysplastic neurons in gangliogliomas may be characterized by clustering, a lack of cytoarchitectural organization, cytomegaly, perimembranous aggregation of Nissl substance, or the presence of binucleated forms (seen in < 50% of cases). The glial component of gangliogliomas shows substantial variability, but constitutes the proliferative cell population of the tumour. It may include cell types resembling fibrillary astrocytoma, oligodendroglioma, or pilocytic astrocytoma. Eosinophilic granular bodies are encountered more often than Rosenthal fibres. A fibrillary matrix is usually prominent and may contain microcystic cavities and/ or myxoid degeneration. Rarefaction of white matter is another common feature. Gangliogliomas may develop a reticulin fibre network apart from the vasculature. Occasional mitoses and small foci of necrosis are compatible with the diagnosis

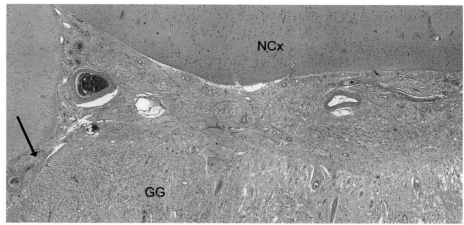

Fig. 6.13 Ganglioglioma (GG) with sharp demarcation from the adjacent brain parenchyma (NCx) and infiltration into subarachnoid space (arrow).

of ganglioglioma. Some additional histopathological features frequently identified in gangliogliomas are dystrophic calcification, either within the matrix or as neuronal/capillary incrustation; extensive lymphoid infiltrates along perivascular spaces or within the tumour/brain parenchyma; and a prominent capillary network. In a few cases, the prominent capillary network manifests as a malformative angiomatous component.

Some tumours also display a clear-cell morphology, which raises the differential diagnoses of oligodendroglioma and dysembryoplastic neuroepithelial tumour. Ganglion cells may also be a component of extraventricular neurocytic tumours and papillary glioneuronal tumours. Focal cortical dysplasia is an uncommon finding in gangliogliomas {225}. It should be diagnosed only in areas of cortical abnormalities without tumour cell infiltration and classified as focal cortical dysplasia Type IIIb according to the classification proposed by the International League Against Epilepsy (ILAE) {127,225}.

Immunophenotype

Antibodies to neuronal proteins such as MAP2, neurofilaments, chromogranin-A, and synaptophysin demonstrate the neuronal component in gangliogliomas and highlight its dysplastic nature. To date, there is no specific marker to differentiate dysplastic neurons from their normal counterparts; however, chromogranin-A expression is usually very weak or absent in normal neurons, whereas diffuse and strong expression suggests a dysplastic neuron. For cases with *BRAF* V600E mutation, a mutation-specific antibody

has been used for the identification of lesional ganglion cells in gangliogliomas {1318}. Immunostains for the oncofetal marker CD34 can also be helpful. CD34 is not present in neurons in adult brain, but is consistently expressed in 70–80% of gangliogliomas, especially variants emerging from the temporal lobe. CD34-immunopositive neural cells are prominent not only in confluent areas of the tumour, but also in peritumoural satellite lesions {222}. Immunoreactivity for GFAP characterizes the cells that form the neoplastic glial component of gangliogliomas. Unlike in diffuse gliomas, MAP2 immunoreactivity is faint or absent in the astrocytic component of gangliogliomas {224}. Ki-67/MIB1 labelling involves only the glial component, with the mean Ki-67 proliferation index ranging from 1.1% to 2.7% {1010,1552,2027,2774}.

Genetic profile

Cytogenetic alterations

About 100 gangliogliomas have been studied cytogenetically {188,1029,2408, 2674,2824}. Of these, chromosomal abnormalities were found in about one third. Gain of chromosome 7 is the most common alteration, although the structural and numerical abnormalities differ from case to case. Associations between cytogenetic data and outcome have not been fully addressed, but the karyotype was abnormal in 3 cases with adverse outcome {1141,1142,2674}. In one study, chromosomal imbalances were detected in 5 of 5 gangliogliomas by comparative genomic hybridization {2824}.

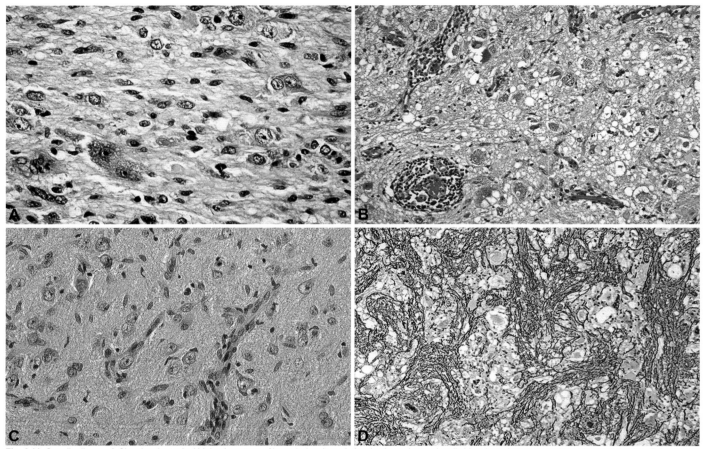

Fig. 6.14 Ganglioglioma. **A** Showing the typical biphasic pattern of irregularly oriented, dysplastic, and occasionally binucleated neurons and neoplastic glial cells. **B** Prominent dysplastic neuronal component and perivascular inflammatory exudates. **C** Biphasic composition of dysplastic neurons and neoplastic glial cells. **D** Occasionally, gangliogliomas develop a reticulin fibre network apart from the vasculature.

Molecular genetics

A *BRAF* V600E mutation is the most common genetic alteration in gangliogliomas, occurring in 20–60% of investigated cases {414,601,2280}. This broad range of reported mutation frequency is probably related to the sensitivity of the detection methods used, as well as the patient age range in the investigated series, given that *BRAF* point mutations are particularly frequent in younger patients {1318}. *BRAF* V600E is not specific for gangliogliomas; it is also observed in other brain tumours, in particular pleomorphic xanthoastrocytomas, pilocytic astrocytomas, and dysembryoplastic neuroepithelial tumours {414,2280}. V600E-mutant BRAF protein is localized mainly to ganglion cells, but can also be found in cells of intermediate differentiation, as well as in the glial compartment, suggesting that ganglion and glial cells in ganglioglioma may derive from a common precursor cell {1318}. One study identified fusions of *BRAF* to *KIAA1549*, *FXR1*, and *MACF1* in 3 gangliogliomas not harbouring a *BRAF* V600E mutation, indicating alternative mechanisms for MAPK pathway activation in some cases {2855}. The presence of a *BRAF* V600E mutation was associated with shorter recurrence-free survival in one series of paediatric gangliogliomas. The tumours in this series were mainly extratemporal and not related to long-term epilepsy {518}. Transcriptomic profiles indicate

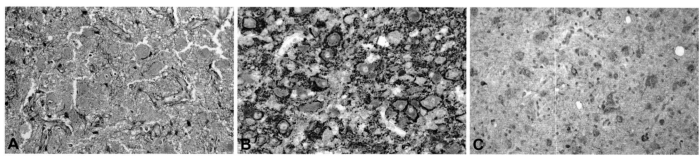

Fig. 6.15 Ganglioglioma. **A** GFAP expression. **B** Synaptophysin expression. **C** Strong expression of V600E-mutant BRAF protein.

reduced expression of some neurodevelopmental genes, including *LDB2* in neuronal components {93,675}. Detection of an *IDH1/2* mutation excludes the diagnosis of ganglioglioma or gangliocytoma and strongly supports the diagnosis of diffuse glioma {601,1037}. Detection of *TP53* or *PTEN* mutations or *CDK4* or *EGFR* amplification does not support a diagnosis of ganglioglioma.

Genetic susceptibility
One case of ganglioglioma of the optic nerve was reported in a patient with neurofibromatosis type 1 {1657}, and one case of spinal cord ganglioglioma was reported in a child with neurofibromatosis type 2 {2252}. Ganglioglioma has also been reported in two patients with Peutz–Jeghers syndrome {553,2101}.

Prognosis and predictive factors
Gangliogliomas are benign tumours, with a 7.5-year recurrence-free survival rate of 97% {1552}. Good prognosis is associated with tumours in the temporal lobe, complete surgical resection, and chronic epilepsy. Anaplastic changes in the glial component and a high Ki-67 proliferation index and p53 labelling index may indicate aggressive behaviour and less favourable prognosis {1010,1207,2027}.

However, any correlation between histological anaplasia and clinical outcome is inconsistent {1207,1428,1552}, and most studies lack molecular analysis to exclude high-grade gliomas. In a series of paediatric gangliogliomas, shorter recurrence-free survival was associated with absence of oligodendroglial morphology, higher glial cell density, microvascular proliferation, and a prominent lymphoplasmacytic inflammatory infiltrate {518}, as well as absence of chronic epilepsy, extratemporal localization, a gemistocytic cell component, and intratumoural expression of CD34 {1570}.

Anaplastic ganglioglioma

Becker A.J.
Wiestler O.D.
Figarella-Branger D.
Blümcke I.
Capper D.

Definition
A glioneuronal tumour composed of dysplastic ganglion cells and an anaplastic glial component with elevated mitotic activity.

ICD-O code   9505/3

Grading
Anaplastic gangliogliomas correspond histologically to WHO grade III {1552,1570}.

Microscopy
In anaplastic gangliogliomas, malignant changes almost invariably involve the glial component and include increased cellularity, pleomorphism, and increased numbers of mitotic figures. Other potential anaplastic features include vascular proliferation and necrosis {1010,1552, 2027,2774}. Few cases have been observed in which a malignant glioma arose from the site of a previously resected ganglioglioma {226}. Exclusion of diffuse glioma with entrapped pre-existing neuronal cells is obligatory for the diagnosis of anaplastic ganglioglioma and may be facilitated by additional genetic analysis {1037}.

Genetic profile

Cytogenetics
Analyses of 2 gangliogliomas and their anaplastic recurrences (WHO grade III) have been reported. The losses of *CDKN2A/B* and *DMBT1* or gain/amplification of *CDK4* found in the anaplastic tumours were already present in the respective low-grade gangliogliomas, as detected by microarray-based comparative genomic hybridization and interphase FISH {1029}.

Molecular genetics
In one study, *CDKN2A* deletion was observed in 2 of 3 anaplastic gangliogliomas {2660}. In another study, *BRAF* V600E mutation was found in 3 of 6 cases {2280}.

Prognosis and predictive factors
Two studies suggested that patients with anaplastic gangliogliomas had substantially reduced 5-year overall and progression-free survival rates and increased recurrence rates {1552,1570}. Another study did not find histological grade to be predictive of outcome {1428}. However, the low numbers of anaplastic gangliogliomas included in these studies may limit the generalizability of these cliniconeuropathological correlations. Intriguingly, a paediatric series of gangliogliomas reported favourable 5-year overall and event-free survival rates despite anaplastic neuropathological features {1227}.

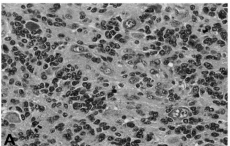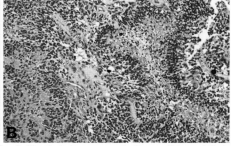

Fig. 6.16 Anaplastic ganglioglioma. **A** Dysplastic, occasionally binucleated neurons and mitoses within a relatively cellular and pleomorphic astroglial matrix. **B** The same tumour contains palisading tumour cells around necrotic foci.

Dysplastic cerebellar gangliocytoma (Lhermitte–Duclos disease)

Eberhart C.G.
Wiestler O.D.
Eng C.

Definition

A rare, benign cerebellar mass composed of dysplastic ganglion cells that conform to the existing cortical architecture.

In dysplastic cerebellar gangliocytoma (Lhermitte–Duclos disease), the enlarged ganglion cells are predominantly located within the internal granule layer and thicken the cerebellar folia. The mass is a major CNS manifestation of Cowden syndrome (see p. 314), an autosomal dominant condition that causes a variety of hamartomas and neoplasms.

Historical annotation

Dysplastic cerebellar gangliocytoma was first described in 1920 by Lhermitte and Duclos {1482} and by Spiegel {2406}. The disease has also been called "cerebellar granule cell hypertrophy", "diffuse hypertrophy of the cerebellar cortex", and "gangliomatosis of the cerebellum". Eventually, the association between Cowden syndrome and dysplastic cerebellar gangliocytoma was recognized {641,1873,2654,2656}.

ICD-O code   9493/0

Grading

It is not yet clear whether dysplastic cerebellar gangliocytoma (Lhermitte–Duclos disease) is neoplastic or hamartomatous. If neoplastic, it corresponds histologically to WHO grade I.

Epidemiology

Due to the rarity of Lhermitte–Duclos disease, there has not been a systematic study to determine the distribution of patient age at onset, but most cases have been identified in adults. A review of the literature indicates that Lhermitte–Duclos disease can be diagnosed in patients as young as 3 years old and as old as in the eighth decade of life {641,1525,2864}. *PTEN* mutations have been identified in virtually all cases of adult-onset Lhermitte–Duclos disease but not in childhood-onset cases {2864}, suggesting that the biologies of the two are different.

The single most comprehensive clinical epidemiological study estimated the prevalence of Cowden syndrome to be 1 case per 1 million population {2414}. However, after identification of the gene for Cowden syndrome {1499}, a molecular-based estimate of prevalence in the same population was 1 case per 200 000 population {1764}. Due to difficulties in recognizing this syndrome, prevalence figures are likely to be underestimates. In one study of 211 patients with Cowden syndrome, 32% developed Lhermitte–Duclos disease {2125}.

Localization

Dysplastic cerebellar gangliocytoma (Lhermitte–Duclos disease) lesions are found in the cerebellar hemispheres.

Clinical features

The most common clinical presentations of Lhermitte–Duclos disease include dysmetria; other cerebellar signs; and signs and symptoms of mass effect, obstructive hydrocephalus, and increased intracranial pressure. Cranial nerve deficits, macrocephaly, and seizures are also often

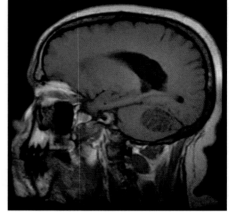

Fig. 6.18 MRI of dysplastic cerebellar gangliocytoma (Lhermitte–Duclos disease).

present. Variable periods of preoperative symptoms have been reported, with a mean length of approximately 40 months {2654}. Because cerebellar lesions may develop before the appearance of other features of Cowden syndrome, patients with Lhermitte–Duclos disease should be monitored for the development of additional tumours, including breast cancer in females.

Imaging

Neuroradiological studies demonstrate distorted architecture in the affected cerebellar hemisphere, with enlarged cerebellar folia and cystic changes in some cases. MRI is particularly sensitive in depicting the enlarged folia, with alternating T1-hypointense and T2-hyperintense tiger-striped striations {843,1664,2718}. The lesions typically do not enhance.

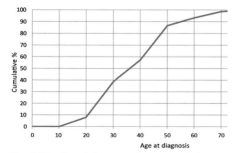

Fig. 6.17 Cumulative age distribution of Cowden syndrome (both sexes) in 75 cases.

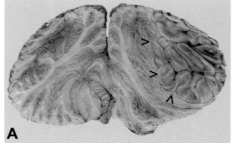
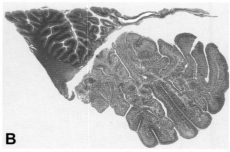

Fig. 6.19 Dysplastic cerebellar gangliocytoma (Lhermitte–Duclos disease). **A** Macroscopy with delineated enlargement of cerebellar folia (arrowheads). **B** Low-power microscopy showing enlargement and distortion of cerebellar cortex.

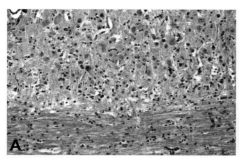
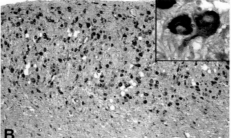
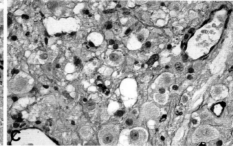

Fig. 6.20 Dysplastic cerebellar gangliocytoma. **A** The internal granule layer of the cerebellum at the top of the image is filled with dysplastic ganglion cells. **B** The dysplastic ganglion cells are strongly immunopositive for phosphorylated S6. **C** Immunohistochemical stains for PTEN show loss of expression in the enlarged neurons, with preserved staining in vessels.

Advanced techniques (including FDG-PET {972}, MR spectroscopy {679}, and diffusion-weighted imaging {1686}) have also been used to characterize Lhermitte–Duclos disease. Infiltrating medulloblastomas have been reported to mimic dysplastic cerebellar gangliocytoma on imaging {602,1686}.

Spread

Dysplastic cerebellar gangliocytoma can recur locally, but it does not spread to other structures in the brain or outside of the CNS.

Macroscopy

The affected cerebellum displays a discrete region of hypertrophy and a coarse gyral pattern that extends into deeper layers. Dysplastic cerebellar gangliocytomas are usually confined to one hemisphere, but they can occasionally be multifocal.

Microscopy

The dysplastic gangliocytoma of Lhermitte–Duclos disease causes diffuse enlargement of the molecular and internal granular layers of the cerebellum, which are filled by ganglionic cells of various size {3}. An important diagnostic feature is the relative preservation of the cerebellar architecture; the folia are enlarged and distorted but not obliterated. A layer of abnormally myelinated axon bundles in parallel arrays is often observed in the outer molecular layer. Scattered cells morphologically consistent with granule neurons are also sometimes found under the pia or in the molecular layer. The resulting structure of these dysmorphic cerebellar folia has been referred to as inverted cerebellar cortex. Purkinje cells are reduced in number or absent. Calcification and ectatic vessels are commonly present within the lesion. Vacuoles are sometimes observed in the molecular layer and white matter {3}.

Immunophenotype

The dysplastic neuronal cells are immunopositive for synaptophysin. Antibodies specific to the Purkinje cell antigens LEU4, PCP2, PCP4, and calbindin have been found to label a minor subpopulation of large atypical ganglion cells, but not to react with the majority of the neuronal elements, suggesting that only a small proportion of neurons are derived from a Purkinje cell source {926,2351}. Immunohistochemistry also demonstrates loss of PTEN protein expression in most dysplastic cells and increased expression of phosphorylated AKT and S6, reflecting aberrant signalling that is predicted to result in increased cell size and lack of apoptosis {3, 2864}. Undetectable or very low proliferative activity has been reported in the few cases analysed with proliferation markers {3,926}.

Cell of origin

It remains unclear whether Lhermitte–Duclos disease is hamartomatous or neoplastic in nature. Malformative histopathological features, very low or absent proliferative activity, and the absence of progression support classification as hamartoma. However, recurrent growth has occasionally been noted, and dysplastic gangliocytomas can develop in adult patients with previously normal MRI scans {3,926,1580}. It has been suggested that the primary cell of origin is the cerebellar granule neuron {926}, and that a combination of aberrant migration and hypertrophy of granule cells is responsible for formation of the lesions {3}. Murine transgenic models based on localized PTEN loss support this hypothesis {1401}.

Genetic profile

Approximately 85% of Cowden syndrome cases, as strictly defined by the International Cowden Consortium (ICC) criteria,

have a germline mutation in *PTEN*, including intragenic mutations, promoter mutations, and large deletions/rearrangements {1499,1589,2865}. Pilot data suggest that a subset of individuals with Cowden syndrome and Cowden syndrome–like symptoms but without *PTEN* mutations instead have germline variants of *SDHB* (on 1p35-36) or *SDHD* (on 11q23), both of which have been shown to affect the same downstream signalling pathways as *PTEN* (AKT and MAPK) {1782}.

Genetic susceptibility

Dysplastic cerebellar gangliocytoma (Lhermitte–Duclos disease) is a component of Cowden syndrome (also called *PTEN* hamartoma syndrome). Cowden syndrome is an autosomal dominant disorder characterized by multiple hamartomas involving tissues derived from all three germ cell layers. The classic hamartoma associated with Cowden syndrome is trichilemmoma. People with Cowden syndrome also have a high risk of breast and thyroid carcinomas, mucocutaneous lesions, non-malignant thyroid abnormalities, fibrocystic disease of the breast, gastrointestinal hamartomas, early-onset uterine leiomyomas, macrocephaly, and mental retardation. The syndrome is caused by germline mutations of the *PTEN* gene. A subset of individuals with Cowden syndrome and Cowden syndrome–like symptoms but without germline *PTEN* mutations have been found to harbour germline variants of *SDHB* or *SDHD* {245}.

Prognosis and predictive factors

Although several recurrent Lhermitte–Duclos disease lesions have been reported, no clear prognostic or predictive factors have emerged. However, patients should be followed for other potential manifestations of Cowden syndrome, particularly breast cancer in female patients.

Desmoplastic infantile astrocytoma and ganglioglioma

Brat D.J.
VandenBerg S.R.
Figarella-Branger D.
Reuss D.E.

Definition

A benign glioneuronal tumour composed of a prominent desmoplastic stroma with a neuroepithelial population restricted either to neoplastic astrocytes – desmoplastic infantile astrocytoma (DIA) – or to astrocytes together with a variable mature neuronal component – desmoplastic infantile ganglioglioma (DIG) – sometimes with aggregates of poorly differentiated cells {1533}.

DIA and DIG typically occur in infants, most often as a large and cystic lesion involving the superficial cerebral cortex and leptomeninges, often attached to dura.

ICD-O code   9412/1

Grading

DIA and DIG correspond histologically to WHO grade I.

Synonyms and historical annotation

DIA was first described in the literature by Taratuto et al. {2514}, as superficial cerebral astrocytoma attached to dura with desmoplastic stromal reaction. It was included in the first edition of the WHO classification in 1993 under the term "desmoplastic cerebral astrocytoma of infancy" {1290}. In 1987, VandenBerg et al. {2629} described desmoplastic supratentorial neuroepithelial tumours of infancy with divergent differentiation (DIG), occurring in the same clinical setting. Unlike DIA, DIG was described as having a neuronal component with variable differentiation, and this description

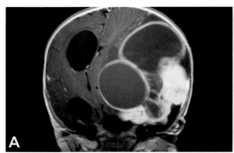
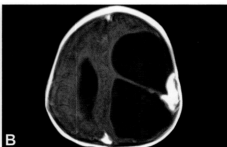

Fig. 6.22 A Desmoplastic infantile astrocytoma. Coronal contrast-enhanced T1-weighted MRI in a 10-month-old child with a large head, showing a mixed cystic and solid mass in the left cerebral hemisphere. The solid portion enhances strongly, abutting and thickening the adjacent meninges. **B** Desmoplastic infantile ganglioglioma. Postcontrast axial MRI demonstrating a superficial enhancing component of a desmoplastic infantile ganglioglioma together with a large septated cystic component that enlarges the skull and displaces the midline.

also stressed the presence of immature neuroepithelial cell aggregates. Because both lesions have similar clinical, neuroimaging, and pathological features (including a favourable prognosis), they are now categorized together as DIA and DIG in the WHO classification.

Epidemiology

DIAs and DIGs are rare neoplasms of early childhood. Their incidence can only be estimated from their frequency in institutional series. One series of 6500 CNS tumours from patients of all ages reported 22 cases of DIG (0.3%) {2628}. In a series of CNS intracranial tumours limited to children, 6 DIAs were found, accounting for 1.25% of all paediatric brain tumours {2514}. In studies limited to brain tumours of infancy, DIA and DIG accounted for 15.8% of the tumours {2875}.

The age range for 84 reported cases of DIA/DIG was 1–24 months, with a median age of 6 months and a male-to-female ratio of 1.5:1 {1533}. The large majority of infantile cases present within the first year of life. Several non-infantile cases, with patient ages ranging from 5 to 25 years, have more recently been reported. There is a strong male predominance in the non-infantile cases reported to date {1928}.

Localization

DIAs and DIGs invariably arise in the supratentorial region and commonly involve

more than one lobe; preferentially the frontal and parietal, followed by the temporal, and (least frequently) the occipital.

Clinical features

The signs and symptoms are of short duration and include increasing head circumference, tense and bulging fontanelles, lethargy, and the setting-sun sign. Occasionally, patients present with seizures, focal motor signs, or skull bossing over the tumour.

Imaging

On CT, DIAs and DIGs present as large, hypodense cystic masses with a solid isodense or slightly hyperdense superficial portion that extends to the overlying meninges and displays contrast enhancement. The cystic portion is usually located deep in the cerebrum, whereas the solid portion is peripheral. On MRI, T1-weighted images show a hypointense cystic component with an isointense peripheral solid component that enhances with gadolinium. On T2-weighted images, the cystic component is hyperintense and the solid portion is heterogeneous. Oedema is usually absent or modest {2571}.

Macroscopy

These tumours are large (measuring as much as 13 cm in diameter) and have deep uniloculated or multiloculated cysts filled with clear or xanthochromic fluid.

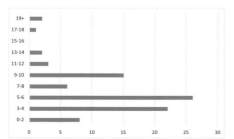

Fig. 6.21 Age distribution (months, both sexes) of desmoplastic infantile astrocytoma and ganglioglioma, based on 84 published cases.

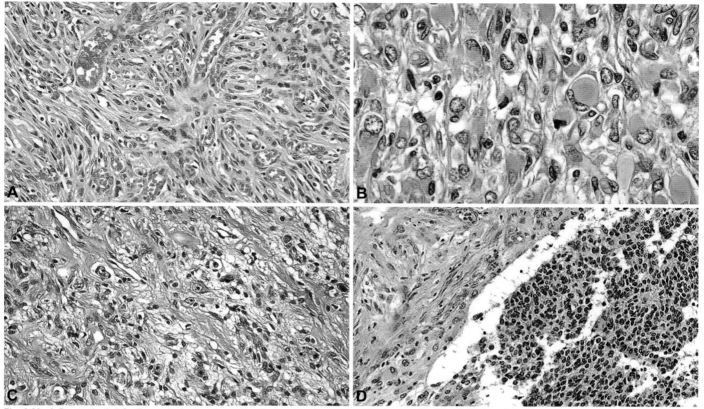

Fig. 6.23 A Desmoplastic infantile cerebral astrocytoma. Neoplastic astrocytes arranged in streams with (**B**) a field of gemistocytic neoplastic astrocytes. **C** Desmoplastic infantile ganglioglioma with scattered ganglion cells and (**D**) low-grade spindle cells in a collagen-rich matrix and a component of primitive small blue round cells.

The solid superficial portion is primarily extracerebral, involving leptomeninges and superficial cortex. It is commonly attached to the dura, firm or rubbery in consistency, and grey or white in colour. There is no gross evidence of haemorrhage or necrosis.

Microscopy

The diagnostic features are those of a slow-growing superficial neuroepithelial tumour composed of a dominant desmoplastic leptomeningeal component and most often containing a variable poorly differentiated neuroepithelial component. The desmoplastic leptomeningeal component consists of a mixture of fibroblast-like spindle-shaped cells, often with a wavy pattern with abundant connective tissue, intermixed with slightly pleomorphic neoplastic neuroepithelial cells with eosinophilic cytoplasm arranged in fascicles or demonstrating storiform or whorled patterns {2514,2629}. Reticulin impregnations show a prominent reticulin-positive network surrounding almost every cell and mimicking a mesenchymal tumour. Astrocytes are the sole tumour

cell population in DIA. In DIG, neoplastic astrocytes are predominant, but a neoplastic neuronal component with variable differentiation is also present, most often taking the form of ganglion cells {2628}. In addition to this desmoplastic leptomeningeal component, both DIA and DIG contain a population of poorly differentiated neuroepithelial cells with small, round, deeply basophilic nuclei and minimal surrounding cytoplasm. This immature component, lacking desmoplasia, may predominate in some areas. A cortical component devoid of desmoplasia may also be observed; this component is often multinodular, with some nodules being microcystic.

There is a sharp demarcation between the cortical surface and the desmoplastic tumour, although Virchow–Robin spaces in the underlying cortex are often filled with tumour cells. Calcifications are common, but mononuclear inflammatory infiltrates are usually lacking. Mitotic activity and necrosis are uncommon and are mostly restricted to the population of poorly differentiated neuroepithelial cells {2628}. Some tumours contain

angiomatoid vessels, but microvascular proliferation is not evident {539,1538}.

Electron microscopy

Astrocytic tumour cells are characterized by intermediate filaments that are typically arranged in bundles and by scattered cisternae of rough endoplasmic reticulum and mitochondria. An extensive basal lamina surrounds individual tumour cells. Fibroblasts containing granular endoplasmic reticulum and well-developed Golgi complexes are also apparent, particularly in collagen-rich areas {539, 1538}. The neuronal cells of DIG contain dense-core secretory granules and may develop small processes containing neurofilaments. In neuronal cells, immuno-electron microscopy has shown filamentous reactivity to neurofilament heavy polypeptide in cell bodies and processes lacking a basal lamina.

Immunophenotype

In the desmoplastic leptomeningeal component, fibroblast-like cells express vimentin, most express GFAP, and a few express SMA. Most neuroepithelial cells

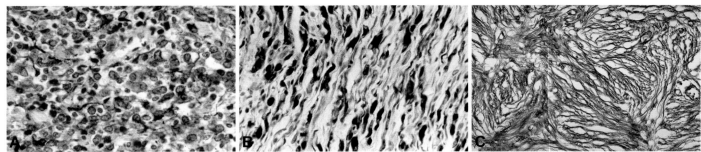

Fig. 6.24 **A** Desmoplastic infantile ganglioglioma. The poorly differentiated component is immunoreactive for the neuronal marker MAP2. **B** Desmoplastic infantile cerebral astrocytoma. GFAP-expressing neoplastic astrocytes arranged in streams; the desmoplastic component remains unstained with (**C**) a marked desmoplastic component demonstrated by reticulin staining.

also react with GFAP. Astrocytes largely predominate in this component. Antibodies to collagen IV react in a reticulin-like pattern around the tumour cells {99, 1538}. Expression of neuronal markers (e.g. synaptophysin, neurofilament heavy polypeptide, and class III beta-tubulin) is observed in neoplastic neuronal cells; mostly in ganglion cells, but also in cells lacking overt neuronal differentiation on routine stains {1918}. In the poorly differentiated neuroepithelial component, cells react with GFAP {1776} and vimentin, but also with neuronal markers and MAP2 {1918,2628}. Desmin expression may be encountered, but epithelial markers (e.g. cytokeratins and EMA) are not expressed.

The Ki-67 proliferation index ranges from < 0.5% to 5%, with the majority of reported values being < 2% {1369}. In the unusual DIAs and DIGs that show histological anaplasia, mitotic activity is readily identified and a Ki-67 proliferation index as high as 45% has been reported {547,1963}.

Cell of origin

The exact cellular origins of DIAs and DIGs have not been established. The presence of primitive small-cell populations that express both glial and neuronal proteins might suggest that these are progenitor cells to the better-differentiated neuroepithelial components and supports the hypothesis that DIAs and DIGs are embryonal neoplasms programmed to progressive maturation. The specialized subpial astrocytes of the developing brain have been suggested as a potential cell of origin, given that they are superficially localized and form a continuous, limiting basal lamina, similar to the abundant basal lamina production of DIA

and DIG {99,1538}. The absence of the genetic alterations typical of most diffuse astrocytomas suggests that diffuse astrocytomas are not related to these neoplasms.

Genetic profile

Classic cytogenetic analysis has been carried out on only a limited number of cases, in which either a normal karyotype or non-clonal abnormalities were described {393}. A comparative genomic hybridization study of 3 cases of DIA and DIG did not reveal any consistent chromosomal gains or losses {1369}. One case of DIG showed a loss on 8p22-pter, and one DIA showed a gain on 13q21. A more recent genome-wide DNA copy number analysis of 4 DIAs and 10 DIGs found that large chromosomal alterations were rare, but demonstrated focal recurrent losses at 5q13.3, 21q22.11, and 10q21.3 {832}. Frequent gains were seen at 7q31, which includes the gene for hepatocyte growth factor receptor (*MET*), and less-frequent gains were noted at 4q12 (*KDR*, *KIT*, and *PDGFRA*) and 12q14.3 (*MDM2*). No evidence of *KIAA1549-BRAF* fusions was noted in these cases. Unsupervised clustering and principal component analysis of the copy number alterations in this group of DIAs and DIGs did not separate the tumours based on histological class, suggesting that they constitute a single molecular genetic entity with a spectrum of histological features {832}.

Early molecular studies of DIA did not uncover any LOH on chromosomes 10 and 17 or any *TP53* mutations {1538}. More recently, the mutational status of *BRAF* has been investigated in two relatively large series of DIAs and DIGs. In one study, *BRAF* V600E mutations were found in 1 of 14 tumours. In the other, pyrosequencing

identified the *BRAF* V600E mutation in 2 of 18 DIAs/DIGs {808,1315}. The authors of both studies concluded that this activating mutation was an uncommon finding in DIA/DIG.

Prognosis and predictive factors

Most studies indicate that gross total resection results in long-term survival in cases of DIA and DIG. In one study of 8 patients with DIA (median follow-up: 15.1 years), 6 patients survived to the end of follow-up (the other 2 died perioperatively) {2514}. In another study, no deaths or evidence of tumour recurrence were observed among 14 patients with DIG (median follow-up: 8.7 years) {2628}. Thus, surgery alone, with total removal, seems to provide local tumour control. In cases of subtotal resection or biopsy, most tumours are stable or regrow only slowly. There have been reports of radiological regression of some tumours after subtotal resection {2500}. Dissemination of these tumours through the cerebrospinal fluid has been reported, but should be considered a rare event {527,547}.

Long-term tumour control can be achieved by total surgical resection of DIA and DIG despite the presence of primitive-appearing cellular aggregates with mitotic activity or foci of necrosis. Among the DIGs that show foci of frank anaplasia (i.e. with high mitotic rate, microvascular proliferation, and perinecrotic palisading tumour cells), there have been reports of long-term survival after gross total resection {2451,2500}. Tumour progression has been reported in DIGs that could not be completely resected, especially in those with a high proliferation index and anaplastic features. Histological features of glioblastoma have been described in the recurrence {547,1523,1963}.

Papillary glioneuronal tumour

Nakazato Y.
Figarella-Branger D.
Becker A.J.
Rosenblum M.K.
Komori T.
Park S.-H.

Definition

A low-grade biphasic neoplasm with astrocytic and neuronal differentiation and histopathological features including a pseudopapillary structure composed of flat to cuboidal astrocytes that are positive for GFAP lining hyalinized vessels, interpapillary collections of synaptophysin-positive neurocytes, and occasional ganglion cells; with low mitotic activity and infrequent necrosis or microvascular proliferation.

Papillary glioneuronal tumour (PGNT) is a rare glioneuronal tumour that preferentially occurs in the supratentorial compartment in young adults, with no sex preference. A circumscribed cystic or solid mass with contrast enhancement is characteristic on MRI. A novel translocation, t(9;17)(q31;q24), which results in an *SLC44A1-PRKCA* fusion oncogene, is present in a high proportion of cases. The prognosis is good.

ICD-O code   9509/1

Grading

Most PGNTs correspond histologically to WHO grade I and behave in a manner consistent with this grade {2285}, but a minority of cases show atypical histological features or late biological progression {1102,1139,1731}.

Synonyms and historical annotation

PGNT was established as a clinicopathological entity by Komori et al. {1324} in 1998, but was previously described under other designations, including "pseudopapillary ganglioglioneurocytoma" and "pseudopapillary neurocytoma with glial differentiation" {1274}.

Epidemiology

Incidence

PGNTs are rare neoplasms, accounting for < 0.02% of intracranial tumours {22}.

Age and sex distribution

The median patient age at diagnosis is 23 years (range: 4–75 years). A recent review of the literature showed that 35% of patients were aged < 18 years and 60% were aged < 26 years. No sex predilection has been found {2285}.

Localization

PGNTs are typically located in the cerebral hemispheres, often in proximity to the ventricles, and with a predilection for the temporal lobe {283,1324,2022}. Occasionally, they grow intraventricularly {572,2011}. On MRI and CT, the tumours present as demarcated, solid to cystic, contrast-enhancing masses with little mass effect. A cystic or mural nodule architecture may be seen.

Clinical features

The principal manifestations include headaches and seizures. Rarely, neurological deficits, such as disturbances of vision, gait, sensation, cognition, and emotional affect have also been encountered. Haemorrhage as the initial presentation has been reported {303,1888}. Some cases are asymptomatic and discovered incidentally, even when the tumour is large (as large as 6 cm in one case) {572,586,1324}.

Imaging

Radiologically, a cystic component is typical, but the tumours can be broadly classified into four groups: cysts with mural nodules, masses that are cystic only, mixed cystic and solid masses, and masses that are solid only {2285}. The tumours are usually located in the white matter, frequently near the ventricle {65, 2285}. On MRI, the solid portion is isointense or hypointense on T1-weighted images and diffusion-weighted images, and hyperintense on T2-weighted images and FLAIR images {65,1439}. Most of the tumours (85%) have no (or only minimal) peritumoural oedema, even when they are large in volume {2285,2606}. About 10% of the reported cases showed overt or occult signs of intratumoural haemorrhage {169}. Calcification has also been reported in some cases {2505,2757}.

Spread

To date, leptomeningeal or cerebrospinal fluid seeding has not been reported. Only one case has shown primary extraneural metastases, which involved bilateral pleura, pericardium, and the left

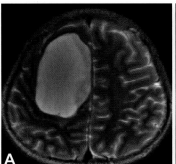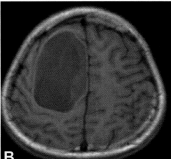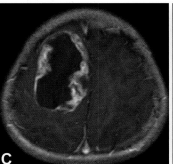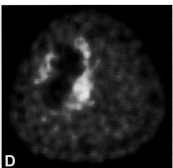

Fig. 6.25 Papillary glioneuronal tumour. **A** T2-weighted MRI shows a solid and cystic mass in the right frontal lobe. **B** This mass is hypointense on T1-weighted MRI. **C** Peripheral enhancement is noted in the solid portion on postcontrast T1-weighted MRI. **D** ¹¹C-methionine PET reveals that this mass has high uptake in the peripheral portion.

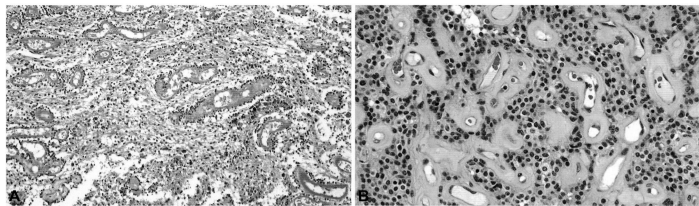

Fig. 6.26 Papillary glioneuronal tumour. **A** At low magnification, the tumour shows typical papillary structures; vessels are hyalinized and haemosiderin deposits are obvious. **B** Characteristic pseudopapillary structure with hyalinized blood vessels.

breast and occurred 4.5 years after initial resection {250}.

Macroscopy

PGNTs are usually composed of solid and cystic elements {2285}. Almost all cases are supratentorial. Most occur within the cerebral hemisphere (especially the frontal or temporal lobe), but some are intraventricular {1731}. They are usually grey and friable and may be calcified. Rare cases have presented with extensive haemorrhage, mimicking a cavernoma {169}.

Microscopy

Histopathology

PGNT is characterized by a prominent pseudopapillary architecture, a single or pseudostratified layer of flattened or cuboidal glial cells with round nuclei and scant cytoplasm around hyalinized blood vessels, and intervening collections of neurocytes and medium-sized ganglion cells with accompanying neuropil.

The background can be fibrillary or microcystic. Neurocytes often resemble oligodendrocyte-like cells {1324,1484, 1731}. Interpapillary neuronal cells show considerable variation in size and shape {1324,2633}. Vascular structures can be prominent and occasionally manifest as a mass of hyalinized material without much intervening tumour {2583}.

In addition to neuronal cells, minigemistocytes with eccentrically located nuclei and eosinophilic cytoplasm are occasionally observed in interpapillary spaces {1102,2509}. At the periphery of the lesion, scattered tumour cells are intermingled with gliotic brain tissue, which contains Rosenthal fibres, eosinophilic granular bodies, haemosiderin pigment, and microcalcifications {1324,2583}. These glial elements lack both nuclear atypia and mitotic activity. Microvascular proliferation or necrosis is exceptional, even in cases with relatively increased proliferative activity {1484}, although there have been a few reports of examples with frank anaplasia {9,1102}.

Electron microscopy

The limited ultrastructural studies on these tumours have identified three cell types: astrocytic, neuronal, and poorly differentiated {257,1324,1731}. Astrocytes contain cytoplasmic bundles of intermediate filaments and are separated from vascular adventitia by a basal lamina. Neurons are characterized by neuronal processes filled with parallel microtubules, their terminations with clear vesicles, and occasional synapses. Poorly differentiated cells are polygonal and contain dense bodies and free ribosomes but no intermediate filaments in the cytoplasm. Minigemistocytes with numerous bundles of glial filaments have also been reported {1102}.

Immunophenotype

The cytoplasm and processes of flattened to cuboidal cells covering hyalinized vessels are immunostained by antibodies to GFAP, S100 protein, and nestin {1324,1484,2509}. In some cases, oligodendrocyte-like cells that are positive for OLIG2 and negative for GFAP surround

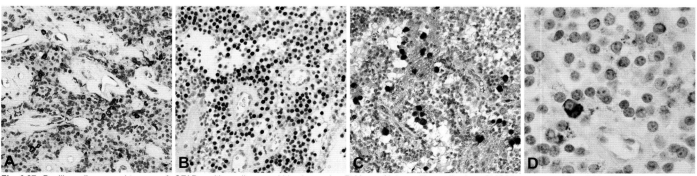

Fig. 6.27 Papillary glioneuronal tumour. **A** GFAP-positive cells around blood vessels. **B** Many of interpapillary cells show OLIG2 immunoreactivity. **C** NeuN positivity is found in some interpapillary cells. **D** Ganglioid cells and neurocytes show NFP immunoreactivity.

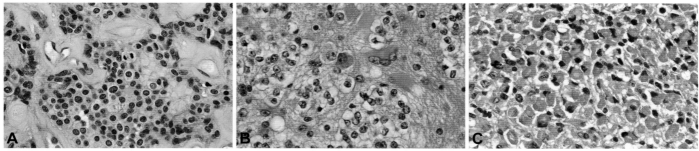

Fig. 6.28 Papillary glioneuronal tumour. **A** Mitotic figures are rarely seen. **B** Ganglioid cells and neurocytes with fibrillary neuropil. **C** Minigemistocytes are occasionally observed in some cases.

this layer {2509}. The minigemistocytes demonstrate intense immunoreactivity for GFAP. The neuronal cells and neuropil stain with antibodies to synaptophysin, neuron-specific enolase, and class III beta-tubulin {1324,2509}. The majority of the neuronal cells are positive for NeuN; however, NFP expression is mostly confined to large ganglion cells, and chromogranin-A expression is absent {1324}.

Proliferation
The Ki-67 proliferation index generally does not exceed 1–2%, but cases displaying elevated activity (ranging from 10% to > 50%) have been reported {250}.

Cell of origin
An origin from multipotent precursors capable of divergent glioneuronal differentiation is presumed, with paraventricular examples possibly deriving from the subependymal matrix {1324}.

Genetic profile / genetic susceptibility
The translocation t(9;17)(q31;q24), resulting in an *SLC44A1-PRKCA* fusion oncogene, is present in a high proportion of cases. The prognosis is good.
To date, no familial or syndrome-associated cases of PGNTs have been reported. An initial series of 6 patients reported no 1p abnormalities in PGNTs {2509}. Recently, an *FGFR1* N546K mutation was observed in a single PGNT {800}. Another study described recurrent *SLC44A1-PRKCA* fusions {278}. To date, comparative genomic hybridization has not revealed an aberration profile characteristic of this tumour {670,1731}.

Prognosis and predictive factors
In most cases, gross total resection without adjuvant therapy results in long-term recurrence-free survival. Therefore, surgical removal is the main prognostic factor. Anaplastic features (e.g. mitoses, microvascular proliferation, necrosis, and a high proliferation rate) have been reported in rare cases and were variably associated with aggressive behaviour {1139, 1772}. There have been no reported cases that progressed or recurred after surgery when the Ki-67 proliferation index was < 5.0% {1888}. However, > 20 cases have been reported to have atypical features, with an elevated Ki-67 proliferation index (of > 5.0%). Of these tumours, 50% eventually progressed or recurred {9,22, 250,1102,1139,1439,1888,1976}.

Rosette-forming glioneuronal tumour

Hainfellner J.A.
Giangaspero F.
Rosenblum M.K.
Gessi M.
Preusser M.

Definition

A neoplasm composed of two distinct histological components: one containing uniform neurocytes forming rosettes and/ or perivascular pseudorosettes and the other being astrocytic in nature and resembling pilocytic astrocytoma.

Rosette-forming glioneuronal tumour is slow-growing, preferentially affects young adults, and occurs predominantly in the fourth ventricle, but can also affect other sites such as the pineal region, optic chiasm, spinal cord, and septum pellucidum.

ICD-O code   9509/1

Grading

Rosette-forming glioneuronal tumour corresponds histologically to WHO grade I, and its generally favourable postoperative course is consistent with this grade.

Epidemiology

Rosette-forming glioneuronal tumour is known to be rare, but specific population-based incidence rates are not yet available.

Localization

Rosette-forming glioneuronal tumours arise in the midline, usually occupy the fourth ventricle and/or aqueduct, and can extend to involve adjacent brain stem, cerebellar vermis, pineal gland, or thalamus. Secondary hydrocephalus may be seen. Localization outside the fourth ventricle (e.g. in the pineal region, optic chiasm, spinal cord, and septum pellucidum) has been described, and in rare cases, dissemination throughout the ventricular system can occur {58,68, 2285,2803}.

Clinical features

Patients most commonly present with headache (a manifestation of obstructive hydrocephalus) and/or ataxia. Cervical pain is occasionally experienced. Rare cases are asymptomatic and discovered as incidental imaging findings.

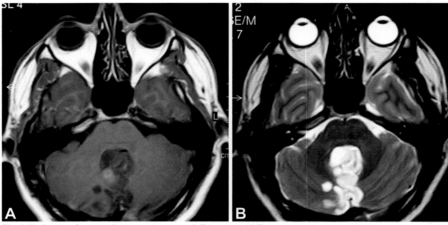

Fig. 6.29 Rosette-forming glioneuronal tumour. **A** T1-weighted MRI shows low intensity of the tumour mass and focal gadolinium enhancement. **B** T2-weighted MRI demonstrates a relatively hyperintense midline tumour occupying the fourth ventricle and involving cerebellar vermis.

Imaging

On MRI, rosette-forming glioneuronal tumour presents as a relatively circumscribed, solid tumour showing T2-hyperintensity, T1-hypointensity, and focal/multifocal gadolinium enhancement.

Spread

Localization outside of the fourth ventricle (e.g. in the pineal region, optic chiasm, spinal cord, and septum pellucidum) has been described. In rare cases, dissemination throughout the ventricular system can occur {58,68,2285,2803}.

Macroscopy

Rosette-forming glioneuronal tumour most commonly involves the cerebellum and wall or floor of the fourth ventricle. An intraventricular component is typical, occasionally with aqueductal extension.

Microscopy

Rosette-forming glioneuronal tumours are generally demarcated, but limited infiltration may be seen. They are characterized by a biphasic neurocytic and glial architecture {1119,1325,2033}. The neurocytic component consists of a uniform population of neurocytes forming neurocytic rosettes and/or perivascular pseudorosettes. Neurocytic rosettes feature ring-shaped arrays of neurocytic nuclei around delicate eosinophilic neuropil cores. Perivascular pseudorosettes feature delicate cell processes radiating

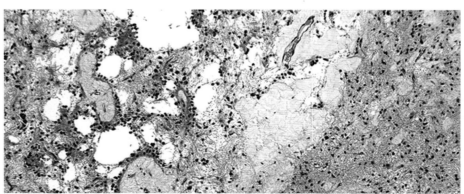

Fig. 6.30 Rosette-forming glioneuronal tumour consists of two components: neurocytic (left) and astrocytic (right).

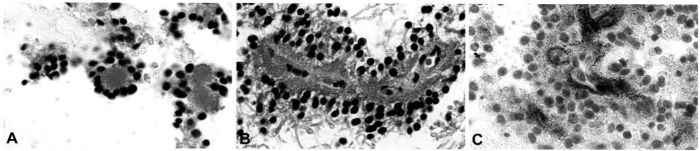

Fig. 6.31 Rosette-forming glioneuronal tumour. **A** Neurocytic rosette: a ring-like array of neurocytic tumour cell nuclei around an eosinophilic neuropil core. **B** Perivascular pseudorosette with delicate cell processes radiating towards a capillary. **C** Synaptophysin immunoreactivity in the pericapillary area of a perivascular pseudorosette.

towards vessels. Both patterns, when viewed longitudinally, may show a columnar arrangement. Neurocytic tumour cells have spherical nuclei with finely granular chromatin and inconspicuous nucleoli, scant cytoplasm, and delicate cytoplasmic processes. These neurocytic structures may lie in a partly microcystic, mucinous matrix. The glial component of rosette-forming glioneuronal tumour typically dominates and in most areas resembles pilocytic astrocytoma. Astrocytic tumour cells are spindle to stellate in shape, with elongated or oval nuclei and moderately dense chromatin. Cytoplasmic processes often form a compact to loosely textured fibrillary background. In some areas, the glial component may be microcystic, containing round to oval, oligodendrocyte-like cells with occasional perinuclear haloes. Rosenthal fibres, eosinophilic granular bodies, microcalcifications, and haemosiderin deposits may be encountered. Overall, cellularity is low. Mitoses and necroses are absent. Vessels may be thin-walled and dilated or hyalinized. Thrombosed vessels and glomeruloid vasculature may also be seen. Ganglion cells are occasionally present, but adjacent, perilesional cerebellar cortex does not show dysplastic changes.

Electron microscopy
Astrocytic cells of the glial component contain dense bundles of glial filaments. Rosette-forming neurocytic cells are intimately apposed and feature spherical nuclei with delicate chromatin, cytoplasm containing free ribosomes, scattered profiles of rough endoplasmic reticulum, prominent Golgi complexes, and occasional mitochondria. Loosely arranged cytoplasmic processes form the centres of rosettes and contain aligned microtubules as well as occasional dense-core granules. Presynaptic specializations may be seen, and mature synaptic terminals may

form surface contacts with perikarya and other cytoplasmic processes.

Immunophenotype
Immunoreactivity for synaptophysin is present at the centres of neurocytic rosettes and in the neuropil of perivascular pseudorosettes {1119,1325,2033}. Both the cytoplasm and processes of neurocytic tumour cells may express MAP2 and neuron-specific enolase. In some cases, NeuN positivity can be observed in neurocytic tumour cells. GFAP and S100 immunoreactivity is present in the glial component, but absent in rosettes and pseudorosettes. The Ki-67 proliferation index is low: < 3% in reported cases.

Cell of origin
Neuroimaging, histological findings, and molecular evidence indicate that rosette-forming glioneuronal tumour may arise from brain tissue surrounding the ventricular system. For cases affecting the fourth ventricle, an origin from the subependymal plate or the internal granule cell layer of cerebellum has been suggested {1325,2547}.

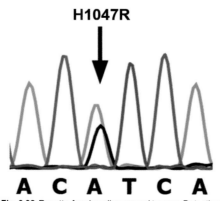

H1047R

A C A T C A

Fig. 6.32 Rosette-forming glioneuronal tumour. Detection of a missense mutation in exon 20 of *PIK3CA* by Sanger sequencing.

Genetic profile
PIK3CA and *FGFR1* mutations (in hotspot codons Asn546 and Lys656) have been found in rosette-forming glioneuronal tumours {340,629,804,2547}. Despite the histological similarity between rosette-forming glioneuronal tumours and pilocytic astrocytomas, *KIAA1549-BRAF* fusions and *BRAF* V600E mutations have not been described in rosette-forming glioneuronal tumour {629,803,807,1220}, and the tumour has not shown evidence of *IDH1/2* mutations {629,2392,2547,2801} or 1p/19q codeletion {2694,2801}. Mass spectrometry array mutation profiling with a panel covering multiple hotspots for single-nucleotide variants did not reveal mutations in *AKT1*, *AKT2*, *AKT3*, *EGFR*, *GNAQ*, *GNAS*, *KRAS*, *MET*, *NRAS*, or *RET* {629}.

Genetic susceptibility
One reported patient with rosette-forming glioneuronal tumour had a type I Chiari malformation {1325}. Rosette-forming glioneuronal tumours have also been described in patients with neurofibromatosis type 1 {2263}, as well as Noonan syndrome {1220}.

Prognosis and predictive factors
The clinical outcome of these generally benign lesions is favourable in terms of survival, but disabling postoperative deficits have been reported in approximately half of cases. In rare cases, tumour dissemination and progression is possible {58,2285}.

Diffuse leptomeningeal glioneuronal tumour

Reifenberger G.
Rodriguez F.
Burger P.C.
Perry A.
Capper D.

Definition

A rare glioneuronal neoplasm characterized by predominant and widespread leptomeningeal growth, an oligodendroglial-like cytology, evidence of neuronal differentiation in a subset of cases, and a high rate of concurrent KIAA1549-BRAF gene fusions and either solitary 1p deletion or 1p/19q codeletion in the absence of IDH mutation.

Diffuse leptomeningeal glioneuronal tumours preferentially occur in children but have also been reported in young adults. The characteristic widespread leptomeningeal tumour growth is readily detectable as diffuse leptomeningeal enhancement on MRI. An associated parenchymal, typically intraspinal mass is sometimes present. The oligodendroglial-like tumour cells show frequent immunopositivity for OLIG2 and S100, whereas GFAP and synaptophysin expression is more variable. Most tumours are histologically low-grade lesions, but a few demonstrate features of anaplasia. Most tumours show slow clinical progression, with a more aggressive course occasionally encountered.

Grading

The vast majority of diffuse leptomeningeal glioneuronal tumours present histologically as low-grade lesions. However, a subset of tumours show features of anaplasia with increased mitotic and proliferative activity as well as glomeruloid microvascular proliferation, which

have been associated with more aggressive clinical behaviour {2149}. Due to the limited patient numbers and inadequate clinical follow-up reported to date, the WHO classification does not yet assign a distinct WHO grade to this entity.

Synonyms

Disseminated oligodendroglioma-like leptomeningeal neoplasm; primary leptomeningeal oligodendro-gliomatosis

Historical annotation

In 1942, Beck and Russell reported 4 cases of oligodendrogliomatosis of the cerebrospinal pathway that would correspond to diffuse leptomeningeal glioneuronal tumours {151}.

Epidemiology

Diffuse leptomeningeal glioneuronal tumours are rare, and data on incidence are not available. In the largest published series, of 36 patients {2149}, the median age at diagnosis was 5 years, with the patient ages ranging from 5 months to 46 years. Only 3 of the 36 patients were aged > 18 years, supporting the preferential manifestation in children also found in other, smaller studies. Males are more commonly affected than females. Among the 60 patients reported in seven independent studies, 38 patients were male (a male-to-female ratio of 1.7:1) {446, 786,1258,2030,2109,2149,2294}.

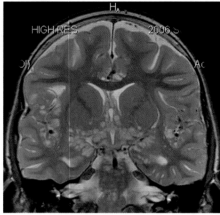

Fig. 6.33 Diffuse leptomeningeal glioneuronal tumour. Numerous superficial hyperintense cystic-like lesions are best appreciated on T2-weighted MRI.

Etiology

The etiology of diffuse leptomeningeal glioneuronal tumours is unknown. The vast majority of tumours develop spontaneously, without evidence of genetic predisposition or exposure to specific carcinogens. One patient with a 5p deletion syndrome has been reported {2149}.

Localization

These tumours preferentially involve the spinal and intracranial leptomeninges. In the intracranial compartment, leptomeningeal growth is most commonly seen in the posterior fossa, around the brain stem, and along the base of the brain. One or more circumscribed, intraparenchymal, cystic or solid tumour nodules may be seen, with

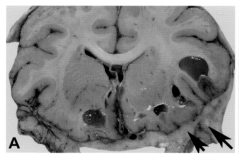
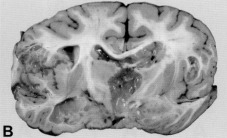
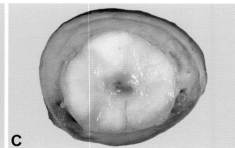

Fig. 6.34 Diffuse leptomeningeal glioneuronal tumour. **A** Diffuse leptomeningeal thickening (arrows) is a consistent feature on postmortem studies; parenchymal cysts may also be encountered in some cases, usually in a superficial location. **B** Note the extensive intraventricular involvement, as well as the parenchymal cysts. **C** Extensive spinal leptomeningeal involvement.

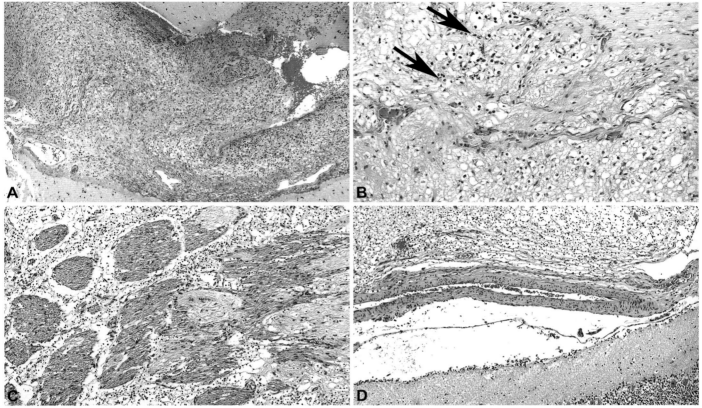

Fig. 6.35 Diffuse leptomeningeal glioneuronal tumour. **A** Marked expansion and hypercellularity of the leptomeninges. **B** A small intraparenchymal component may be present, usually in the spinal cord. Infiltration of overlying leptomeninges by neoplastic cells (arrows) is typical. **C** Extensive leptomeningeal dissemination in spinal cord may result in intimate coating of nerve roots. **D** Cerebellar leptomeninges. Infiltration by bland oligodendroglial-like cells throughout the CNS is a key histological feature.

spinal intramedullary lesions being more common than intracerebral masses.

Clinical features
Patients often present with acute onset of signs and symptoms of increased intracranial pressure due to obstructive hydrocephalus, including headache, nausea, and vomiting. Opisthotonos and signs of meningeal or cranial nerve damage may be present. Some patients show ataxia and signs of spinal cord compression. Rare patients present with seizures.

Imaging
MRI shows widespread diffuse leptomeningeal enhancement and thickening along the spinal cord, often extending intracranially to the posterior fossa, brain stem, and basal brain. Small cystic or nodular T2-hyperintense lesions along the subpial surface of the spinal cord or brain are frequent. Discrete intraparenchymal lesions, most commonly in the spinal cord, were found in 25 of 31 patients (81%) in the largest reported cohort {2149}. Patients also commonly

demonstrate obstructive hydrocephalus with associated periventricular T2-hyperintensity.

Macroscopy
Postmortem investigations have confirmed radiological findings and demonstrated widespread diffuse leptomeningeal tumour spread in the spinal and intracranial compartments {2149}. Multifocal extension of tumour tissue along Virchow–Robin spaces and areas of limited brain invasion are common. Tumour growth along peripheral

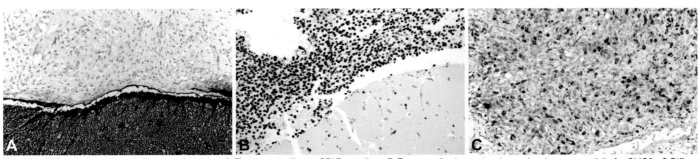

Fig. 6.36 Diffuse leptomeningeal glioneuronal tumour. **A** The tumour cells are GFAP-negative. **B** Tumour cells show extensive nuclear immunoreactivity for OLIG2. **C** Diffuse leptomeningeal glioneuronal tumour with anaplastic features. The Ki-67 proliferation index is elevated, suggestive of a more aggressive clinical behaviour.

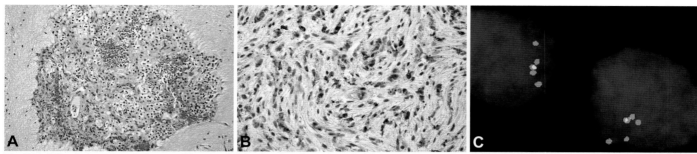

Fig. 6.37 Diffuse leptomeningeal glioneuronal tumour. **A** Extension along the perivascular Virchow–Robin space is evident within the adjacent brain parenchyma of this tumour. **B** Synaptophysin positivity is seen in this tumour. **C** FISH studies using *BRAF* (red) and *KIAA1549* (green) probes show increased copy numbers and yellow fusion signals.

nerve roots and infiltration of basal cranial nerves and ganglia may also be seen.

Microscopy

Cerebrospinal fluid examination demonstrates elevated protein levels, although cytology is often negative {2149,2294}. Therefore, the diagnosis usually requires a meningeal tumour biopsy. Histologically, diffuse leptomeningeal glioneuronal tumours are low- to moderate-cellularity neoplasms composed of relatively monomorphic oligodendroglial-like tumour cells with uniform, medium-sized round nuclei and inconspicuous nucleoli. Like in oligodendroglioma, artificial perinuclear haloes and cytoplasmic swelling are commonly seen in formalin-fixed, paraffin-embedded tissue sections. The tumour cells grow diffusely or in small nests in the leptomeninges, with desmoplastic and myxoid changes commonly present. A storiform pattern may be observed in desmoplastic areas. Mitotic activity is usually low, and other histological features of anaplasia are absent in most cases. However, rare examples show histological evidence of anaplasia either at primary presentation or after tumour progression {2149}. Anaplastic features include brisk mitotic activity (defined as ≥ 4 mitoses per 10 high-power fields) {2149}. Areas of necrosis are usually absent on biopsies but have been detected in individual cases at autopsy {2149}. A small subset of tumours contain ganglion or ganglioid cells. Neuropil associated with ganglion cells and neuropil-like islands have also been observed. Rarely, eosinophilic granular bodies are observed. Rosenthal fibres are usually absent. The intraparenchymal component resembles a diffusely infiltrative glioma, mostly oligodendroglioma-like, although astrocytic features occasionally predominate.

Immunophenotype

The oligodendroglial-like tumour cells typically express OLIG2, MAP2, and S100 protein {2030,2149}. GFAP immunopositivity in tumour cells is seen in < 50% of the cases and is often restricted to a minor proportion of neoplastic cells. Expression of synaptophysin is detectable in as many as two thirds of the tumours, and is particularly common in those containing neuropil aggregates and ganglion cells. Immunostaining for NeuN, neurofilaments, EMA, and R132H-mutant IDH1 is

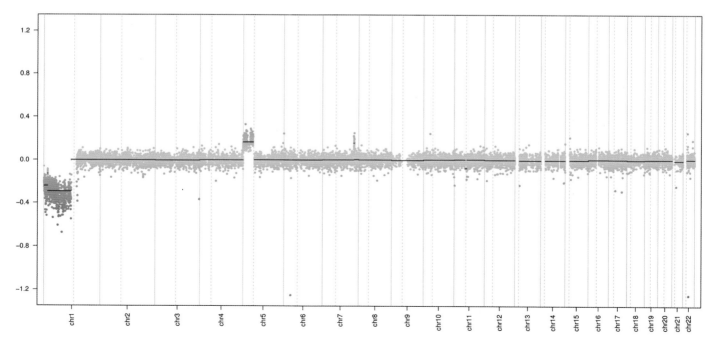

Fig. 6.38 Diffuse leptomeningeal glioneuronal tumour. DNA copy number profile determined by 450k methylation bead array analysis; note the deletion of 1p and the circumscribed gains on 5p and 7q in a case with *KIAA1549-BRAF* fusion.

negative. The Ki-67 proliferation index is usually low, with a median value of 1.5% reported in one series {2149}. However, a subset of cases have an elevated Ki-67 proliferation index {2030,2149,2294}, with one study reporting less favourable outcome associated with a proliferation index of > 4% {2149}.

Differential diagnosis

The differential diagnosis includes leptomeningeal dissemination of primarily intraparenchymal diffuse astrocytic or oligodendroglial gliomas. Pilocytic astrocytoma may also show leptomeningeal dissemination. The absence of morphological features of pilocytic differentiation, the lack of (or only focal) GFAP immunoreactivity, the presence of synaptophysin-positive cells, and the characteristic molecular profile of *KIAA1549-BRAF* fusion combined with isolated 1p deletion or 1p/19q codeletion {2156} suggest that diffuse leptomeningeal glioneuronal tumour is a distinct entity. Pleomorphic xanthoastrocytomas are readily distinguished by their pleomorphic histology. Diffuse leptomeningeal glioneuronal tumours also lack *BRAF* V600E mutations {2156}, a molecular marker found in most pleomorphic xanthoastrocytomas and a subset of gangliogliomas {2280}.

Cell of origin

The cellular origin of diffuse leptomeningeal glioneuronal tumours is unknown. The absence of obvious parenchymal lesions in some patient suggests an origin from displaced neuroepithelial cells within the meninges. However, an intraparenchymal origin is also possible, given that small intraparenchymal foci are frequently present in addition to the diffuse leptomeningeal tumour spread.

Genetic profile

The most frequent genetic alteration in diffuse leptomeningeal glioneuronal tumours reported to date is *KIAA1549-BRAF* fusion, with 12 of 16 investigated cases (75%) showing this alteration {2156}. Deletions of chromosomal arm 1p are also frequently observed in FISH analysis and were reported in 10 of 17 tumours (59%) in one series {19, 253,786,2149,2156}. In single cases with SNP array data, complete 1p arm loss was demonstrated {2149,2156}. Codeletions of 1p and 19q have been observed at a lower frequency, present in 3 of 17 tumours (18%) in one series {2156}. In one case with 1p/19q codeletion, a t(1p;19q)(q10;p10) translocation was demonstrated by FISH {2185}. *BRAF* V600E point mutations were not observed in a series of 9 cases {2156}, and immunohistochemistry for R132H-mutant IDH1 was negative in 14 cases {2030,2149}. DNA sequencing revealed neither *IDH1* nor *IDH2* mutations in 6 cases investigated (D. Capper, University of Heidelberg, personal communication, September 2015).

Genetic susceptibility

In a series of 36 cases, no evidence of recognized genetic predisposing features or other tumour syndromes was observed, although one patient had a constitutional 5p deletion, one a coexisting type I Chiari malformation, and one a factor V Leiden mutation {2149}.

Prognosis and predictive factors

Diffuse leptomeningeal glioneuronal tumours may go through periods of stability or slow progression over many years, although often with considerable morbidity {2149}. In a retrospective series of 24 cases, with a median available follow-up of 5 years, 9 patients (38%) died between 3 months and 21 years after diagnosis (median: 3 years) {2149}, and 8 of the 24 patients lived for > 10 years after diagnosis {2149}. Mitotic activity of any degree ($P = 0.045$), a Ki-67 proliferation index of $\geq 4\%$ ($P = 0.01$), and glomeruloid microvascular proliferation ($P = 0.009$) at the initial biopsy were each associated with decreased overall survival {2149}.

Central neurocytoma

Figarella-Branger D.
Söylemezoglu F.
Burger P.C.
Park S.-H.
Honavar M.

Definition

An uncommon intraventricular neoplasm composed of uniform round cells with a neuronal immunophenotype and low proliferation index.

Central neurocytoma is usually located in the region of the foramen of Monro, predominantly affects young adults, and has a favourable prognosis.

ICD-O code   9506/1

Grading

Central neurocytoma corresponds histologically to WHO grade II. The tumours are usually benign, but some recur, even after total surgical removal. Because the prognostic values of anaplastic features and the Ki-67 proliferation index are still uncertain, it is not yet possible to attribute two distinct histological grades (I and II) to central neurocytoma variants.

Synonyms and historical annotation

The term "central neurocytoma" was coined by Hassoun et al. {967} to describe a neuronal tumour with pathological features distinct from cerebral neuroblastomas, occurring in young adults, located in the third ventricle, and histologically mimicking oligodendroglioma. These tumours had been previously reported as ependymomas of the foramen of Monro or intraventricular oligodendrogliomas. Central neurocytomas were then reported in other intraventricular locations, mainly in the lateral and third ventricles, but also the fourth ventricle.

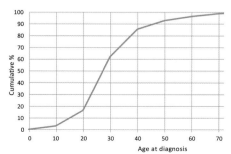

Fig. 6.39 Cumulative age distribution (both sexes) of central neurocytoma (excluding extraventricular neurocytoma), based on 201 cases.

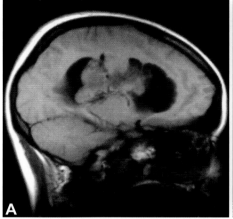 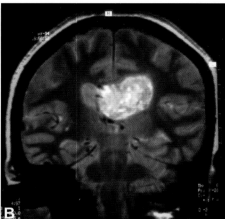

Fig. 6.40 Central neurocytoma. **A** Large intraventricular tumour of the lateral ventricle with hypointensity on T1-weighted MRI. **B** Strong contrast enhancement on T1-weighted MRI after gadolinium injection.

The diagnosis of central neurocytoma should be restricted to neoplasms located within the intracerebral ventricles. Tumours mimicking central neurocytomas but occurring within the cerebral hemispheres (so called cerebral neurocytomas) {1792} or the spinal cord {476,2519} were later documented. Neoplasms that arise within the CNS parenchyma and share histological features with the more common central neurocytomas but exhibit a wider morphological spectrum are now called extraventricular neurocytomas {816} (see p. 159). Some tumours have neurocytic tumour cells but are not classified as central or extraventricular neurocytomas; for example, neurocytic differentiation has been reported in an increasing number of tumours with distinctive morphological features, some of these tumours emerging as new entities, such as cerebellar liponeurocytoma and papillary glioneuronal tumour {1324} and variants {387}.

Epidemiology

In an analysis of > 1000 cases, the mean patient age at clinical manifestation was 28.5 years; 46% of patients were diagnosed in the third decade of life and 70% between the ages of 20 and 40 years. Patient ages reported in the literature range from 8 days to 82 years, although paediatric cases are rare. Both sexes are equally affected, with a male-to-female ratio of 1.02:1. Population-based incidence rates for central neurocytoma are not available. In large surgical series, central neurocytomas account for 0.25–0.5% of all intracranial tumours {969}.

Localization

Central neurocytomas are typically located supratentorially in the lateral ventricle(s) and/or the third ventricle. The most common site is the anterior portion of one of the lateral ventricles, followed by combined extension into the lateral and third ventricles, and by a bilateral intraventricular location. Attachment to the septum pellucidum seems to be a feature of the tumour {1462,2047,2690}. Isolated third and fourth ventricular occurrence is rare {491,2638}.

Clinical features

Most patients present with symptoms of increased intracranial pressure, rather than with a distinct neurological deficit. The clinical history is short (median: 1.7–3 months) {1462}.

Imaging

On CT, the masses are usually isodense or slightly hyperdense. Calcifications and cystic changes may be seen {597}. On MRI, central neurocytomas are T1-isointense to brain and have a so-called

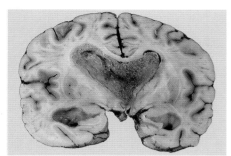

Fig. 6.41 A large central neurocytoma filling both lateral ventricles and extending into the third ventricle and the temporal horn of the left ventricle {1291}.

soap-bubble multicystic appearance on T2-weighted images. They often exhibit FLAIR hyperintensity, with a well-defined margin. In all cases, heterogeneous enhancement after gadolinium injection is observed, and the tumour may show vascular flow voids. Haemorrhage may be seen {597,1788,2690}. An inverted alanine peak and a notable glycine peak on proton MR spectroscopy are useful in the differential diagnosis of intraventricular neoplasms {597,1571}.

Spread
Craniospinal dissemination is exceptional {643,2567}.

Macroscopy
Central neurocytoma is greyish and friable. Calcifications and haemorrhages can occur.

Microscopy
Neurocytoma is a neuroepithelial tumour composed of uniform round cells that show immunohistochemical and ultrastructural features of neuronal differentiation. Additional features include fibrillary areas mimicking neuropil and a low proliferation rate. Various architectural patterns

may be observed, even in the same specimen. These include an oligodendroglioma-like honeycomb architecture, large fibrillary areas mimicking the irregular rosettes in pineocytomas, cells arranged in straight lines, and perivascular pseudorosettes as observed in ependymomas. The cells are isomorphous, with a round or oval nucleus with finely speckled chromatin and variably present nucleoli. Capillary blood vessels, usually arranged in an arborizing pattern, give the tumours a neuroendocrine appearance. Calcifications are seen in half of all cases, usually distributed throughout the tumour. Rarer findings include Homer Wright rosettes and ganglioid cells {2134,2661}. Mitoses are exceptional, and necrosis or haemorrhage is rare.

In rare instances, anaplastic histological features (i.e. brisk mitotic activity, microvascular proliferation, and necrosis) can occur in combination, and tumours with these features are called atypical central neurocytomas {969,2661,2818}. This term is also used for central neurocytomas with a Ki-67 proliferation index of ≥ 2% or 3% {2053,2478}, even when there are no associated anaplastic histological features.

Electron microscopy
Although it was electron microscopy that allowed Hassoun et al. {969} to discover the neuronal differentiation of cells forming central neurocytomas, electron microscopy is no longer required for the diagnosis of central neurocytoma, due to the tumour's characteristic clinicopathological features and immunohistochemical profile. When performed, electron microscopy shows regular round nuclei with finely dispersed chromatin and a small distinct nucleolus in a few cells. The cytoplasm contains mitochondria, a

prominent Golgi complex, and some cisternae of rough endoplasmic reticulum, often arranged in concentric lamellae. Numerous thin and intermingled cell processes containing microtubules, dense-core vesicles, and clear vesicles are always observed {388,969}. Well-formed or abnormal synapses may be present, but are not required for the diagnosis.

Immunophenotype
Synaptophysin is the most suitable and reliable diagnostic marker, with immunoreactivity diffusely present in the tumour matrix, especially in fibrillary zones and perivascular nucleus-free cuffs {705,969}. Most cases are also immunoreactive for NeuN, although the intensity and extent of the labelling vary {2399,2638}. Other neuronal epitopes (e.g. class III beta-tubulin and MAP2) are also usually expressed, whereas expression of chromogranin-A, NFP, and alpha-internexin is lacking, except in very rare cases showing gangliocytic differentiation. Although most studies have found GFAP to be expressed only in entrapped reactive astrocytes, this antigen has been reported in tumour cells by some authors {2478,2582,2661, 2662}. OLIG2 has also been reported in tumour cells in some cases {1500}. This immunoprofile helps to distinguish central neurocytoma from ependymoma and pineocytoma; ependymoma is synaptophysin-negative and more diffusely positive for GFAP than is central neurocytoma, and pineocytoma expresses NFPs and synaptophysin {1187,2638}. Central neurocytomas are not immunoreactive for the R132-mutant IDH1 gene product {356}, and p53 expression is usually lacking {2638}.

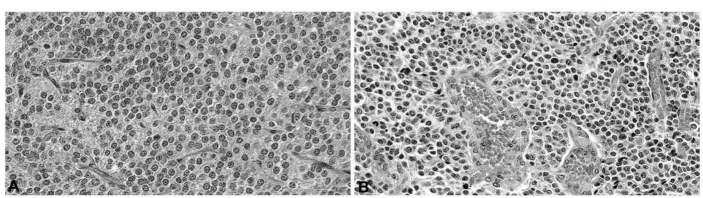

Fig. 6.42 Central neurocytoma. **A** Round monomorphic cells and vascularized thin-walled capillaries. **B** Central neurocytoma with anaplastic histological features. Microvascular proliferation associated with mitotic activity.

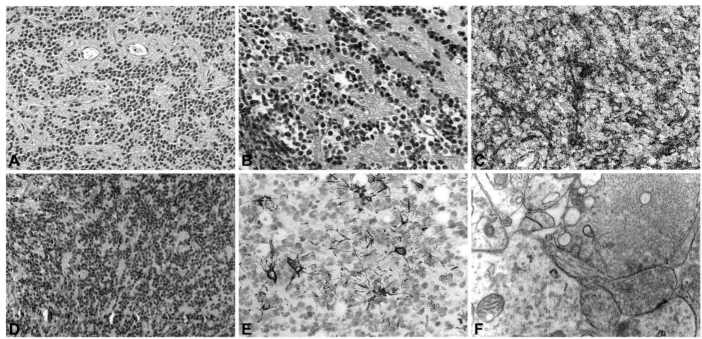

Fig. 6.43 Central neurocytoma. **A,B** Round cells with nucleus-free areas of neuropil. **C** Synaptophysin is consistently expressed by the tumour cells, including in their processes {1291}. **D** NeuN is diffusely expressed in all tumour nuclei. **E** GFAP is seen in only a few reactive astrocytes. **F** Ultrastructure showing numerous cell processes filled with neurotubules and synaptic structures containing dense-core granules and clear vesicles.

Proliferation

The Ki-67 proliferation index is usually low (< 2%), but higher values can occur in atypical central neurocytomas {2053,2478}.

Cell of origin

The cell of origin is still unknown. Because of the frequent involvement of the septum pellucidum and the predominant neuronal differentiation of the tumour, central neurocytoma was first thought to derive from the nuclei of the septum pellucidum {967}. However, given the evidence for both glial and neuronal differentiation in some tumours, central neurocytoma may in fact derive from neuroglial precursor cells with the potentiality of dual differentiation. These tumours could originate from the subependymal plate of the lateral ventricles {2662}. An origin from circumventricular organs has also been proposed {1186}.

Genetic profile

Central neurocytomas contain numerous DNA copy number alterations {1350}, including *MYCN* gain. A transcriptomic study showed overexpression of genes involved in the WNT signalling pathway, calcium function, and maintenance of neural progenitors {2637}. These genes may contribute to central neurocytoma tumorigenesis.

Central neurocytomas have not been reported to exhibit 1p/19q codeletion, with the exception of a single case of atypical neurocytoma located in the insular cortex {1718}.

Prognosis and predictive factors

The clinical course of central neurocytoma is usually benign, with the extent of resection being the most important prognostic factor. Craniospinal dissemination is exceptional {643,2567}. In a meta-analysis of 310 cases of central neurocytoma, the local control rates at 3 and 5 years after gross total resection were 95% and 85%, respectively, versus 55% and 45% after subtotal resection {2052}. Although most clinical studies support the assumption that radiotherapy is not necessary after gross total resection, many authors have recommended postoperative radiotherapy after incomplete resection to prevent recurrence {1907}. The prognostic relevance of atypical histological features in central neurocytomas and any consequent treatment strategy is more controversial; there have been reports of central neurocytoma devoid of anaplastic histological features but associated with adverse outcome {2638}.

Shorter recurrence-free intervals have been reported by some authors for central neurocytomas with a Ki-67 proliferation index of > 2% or 3% {1561,2478}, but this was not found by others {2638}. Anaplastic histological features are not generally associated with poor prognosis. However, a mitotic count of ≥ 3 mitoses per 10 high-power fields has been found to be a predictor of higher risk of recurrence {1462,2638}. In one multicentre study of 71 patients, incomplete resection was predictive of poor outcome {2638}.

Extraventricular neurocytoma

Figarella-Branger D.
Söylemezoglu F.
Burger P.C.
Park S.-H.
Honavar M.

Definition

A tumour composed of small uniform cells that demonstrate neuronal differentiation but are not IDH-mutant, and that presents throughout the CNS, without apparent association with the ventricular system.

Extraventricular neurocytoma is usually well circumscribed and slow-growing, and shares most histological features with central neurocytoma. Because some tumours (including pilocytic astrocytomas, dysembryoplastic neuroepithelial tumours, gangliogliomas, papillary glioneuronal tumours [PGNTs], oligodendrogliomas with neurocytic features, and diffuse leptomeningeal glioneuronal tumours) show synaptophysin expression, synaptophysin expression is not sufficient to establish a diagnosis of extraventricular neurocytoma. Strong and diffuse OLIG2 expression is not compatible with a diagnosis of extraventricular neurocytoma. Some entities that are genetically well defined (e.g. IDH-mutant and 1p/19q-codeleted oligodendroglioma and PGNTs) should be excluded by appropriate genetic testing. However, the genetic characteristics of extraventricular neurocytoma are not yet well defined.

ICD-O code   9506/1

Grading

Extraventricular neurocytomas correspond histologically to WHO grade II. There have been suggestions for further grading on the basis of mitotic rate, Ki-67 proliferation index, and the presence or absence of vascular proliferation and/or necrosis {769}. The term "atypical" has been used for lesions with an elevated mitotic rate and Ki-67 proliferation index {1213}. There is some evidence that each of these factors is associated with risk of recurrence, but definitive grading criteria have not yet been established.

Epidemiology

Extraventricular neurocytoma can present in patients of any age. The patient age at diagnosis of cases reported in the

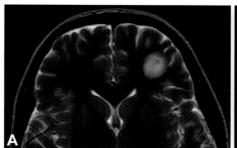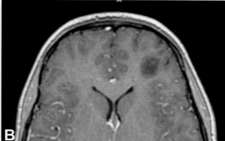

Fig. 6.44 Extraventricular neurocytoma. **A** Hyperintense frontal mass on T2-weighted MRI. **B** Hypointense mass with no contrast enhancement is seen on T1-weighted MRI after gadolinium administration.

literature ranges from 1 to 79 years, with the median age in the fourth decade of life {938,2470}.

There does not seem to be a significant relationship between sex and the incidence of extraventricular neurocytoma. The male-to-female ratio is about 1:1, with a slight female predominance seen in some series and a slight male predominance seen in others {269,769, 938}. However, because most cases reported before 2012 were not screened for IDH mutations, it is difficult to be certain of the diagnosis of extraventricular neurocytoma.

Etiology

No specific etiology has been implicated in the genesis of extraventricular neurocytoma.

Localization

The cerebral hemispheres are the most common site for extraventricular neurocytoma (affected in 71% of cases). The tumours most often affect the frontal lobes (in 30% of cases), followed by the spinal cord (in 14%). These tumours can occur in the thalamus, hypothalamic region, cerebellum, and pons, with isolated cases reported in cranial nerves, the cauda equina, the sellar region, and even outside the craniospinal compartment {769,2470}.

Clinical features

The clinical presentation varies according to the location of the tumour and whether it exerts a mass effect. Cerebral

extraventricular neurocytomas have been associated with seizures, headaches, visual disturbances, hemiparesis, and cognitive disturbances; thalamic and hypothalamic lesions with increased intracranial tension; and spinal lesions with motor, sensory, and sphincter dysfunction {769,2470}.

Imaging

On MRI, extraventricular neurocytoma presents as a solitary, well-demarcated mass of non-specific signal intensity and variable contrast enhancement, with a cystic component in 58% of cases, mild perilesional oedema in 51.5%, and calcification in 34% {269,1518,2822}. The solid component is predominantly isointense on T1-weighted images, but may be hypointense. On T2-weighted and FLAIR images, the signal is predominantly hyperintense.

Spread

Extraventricular neurocytoma spread is particularly rare, although craniospinal dissemination can occur as remote metastasis or along the surgical route {938}. Cases of diffuse leptomeningeal neuroepithelial tumour have been reported mainly in children. These cases share with extraventricular neurocytoma some histological and immunohistochemical features, including proliferation of a uniform population of oligodendrocyte-like cells expressing synaptophysin but not R132H-mutant IDH1 {2294}. These tumours represent a new entity (see *Diffuse leptomeningeal glioneuronal tumour*, p. 152).

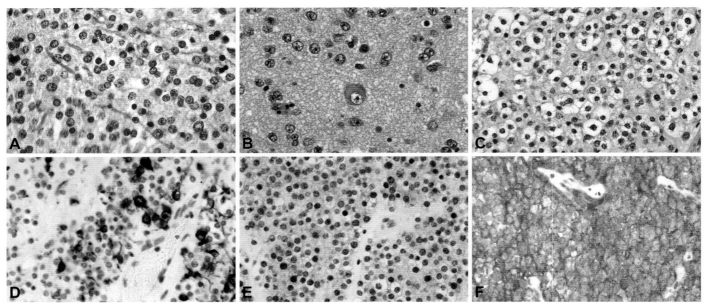

Fig. 6.45 Extraventricular neurocytoma. **A** Spinal extraventricular neurocytoma composed of monomorphic cells that have round nuclei with fine nuclear chromatin. **B** Focal ganglionic differentiation. **C** The cells, often with perinuclear haloes, have round nuclei with finely stippled chromatin and small nucleoli. **D** Occasional neoplastic cells express GFAP. **E** Nuclear expression of NeuN. **F** Diffuse cytoplasmic immunoreactivity for synaptophysin is characteristic of extraventricular neurocytoma. The sparse neuropil between tumour cells is also stained.

Macroscopy

Some examples are well circumscribed (sometimes with a cyst–mural nodule configuration), whereas others are more infiltrative and therefore less discrete.

Microscopy

A wide variety of histopathological appearances have been reported in this histologically heterogeneous lesion, which is usually more complex than the highly cellular, cytologically monomorphous central neurocytoma {269,816}. Tumours with the dense cellularity and neuropil islands common in central neurocytoma are diagnostically straightforward, but uncommon. More often, the tumours are less cellular and have an oligodendroglioma-like appearance due to small, uniform round cells with artefactually cleared cytoplasm embedded in a fibrillar matrix. Unlike in central neurocytoma, ganglion cell differentiation is common. Ganglioid cells – neurons intermediate in size between ganglion cells and neurocytes – are also frequent. Hyalinized vessels and calcifications may be present. A glial astrocytic component is uncommon, and can be difficult to distinguish from reactive gliosis. Cases with a convincing ganglion cell component can be labelled ganglioneurocytoma.

Immunophenotype
Immunoreactivity for synaptophysin is essential for the diagnosis of extraventricular neurocytoma and is present in oligodendroglioma-like cells and larger neurons. Clusters of neurosecretory granules are visualized by chromogranin-A staining in some cases with ganglion cells. In lesions with a glial component, these cells may be positive for GFAP. R132-mutant IDH1 protein is absent {21, 2822}. Expression of OLIG2 has been reported in some cases, but a more convincing example was immunonegative for this marker. IDH and 1p/19q status were not reported for these cases {1714,1832}.

Cell of origin

There is no consensus on the putative cell of origin. Extraventricular neurocytoma may arise from mislocated neural progenitor cells in the brain parenchyma {269}. These neural progenitor cells differentiate into distinct cell lineages (neurocytic and astrocytic) in this particular microenvironment {1876}.

Genetic profile

Although deletion of chromosome arms 1p and 19q (either in isolation or in combination) has been found in extraventricular neurocytoma, neither *IDH1/2* mutation nor *MGMT* methylation has been reported {21,356,1206,1718,1732}. Therefore, if extraventricular neurocytoma is suspected on pathological examination, investigation for IDH mutation is mandatory, to rule out diffuse glioma with neurocytic differentiation {356,2822}. Because 1p/19q codeletion is a hallmark of oligodendroglioma, it is likely that presumed extraventricular neurocytomas exhibiting 1p/19q codeletion are in fact oligodendrogliomas {2147}. The differential diagnosis also includes ganglioglioma, dysembryoplastic neuroepithelial tumour, and even PGNT, so it is recommended to test for *BRAF* V600E mutation and for *SLC44A1-PRKCA* fusion, a recurrent genetic alteration reported in PGNT {278}.

To date, neither high-throughput genotyping nor sequencing studies have been carried out. Microarray-based comparative genomic hybridization has been performed in 2 cases, revealing distinct profiles, with loss and gain of multiple chromosomal loci {1732}.

Prognosis and predictive factors

Although extraventricular neurocytoma is generally benign and has a low rate of recurrence, outcomes are known to vary considerably. In one study, the presence of 1p/19q codeletion was a poor prognostic factor {2147}. Gross total resection has been associated with a low rate of recurrence {269,769,1213}. Subtotally resected lesions are often stable, but recurrence is possible {269,769,1213}.

Cerebellar liponeurocytoma

Kleihues P.
Giangaspero F.
Chimelli L.
Ohgaki H.

Definition

A rare cerebellar neoplasm with advanced neuronal/neurocytic differentiation and focal lipoma-like changes.

Cerebellar liponeurocytoma affects adults, has low proliferative activity, and usually has a favourable prognosis. However, recurrence can occur and malignant progression has been reported.

ICD-O code   9506/1

Grading

Cerebellar liponeurocytoma corresponds histologically to WHO grade II. Recurrences have been reported in almost 50% of cases. Recurrent tumours may display increased mitotic activity, an increased Ki-67 proliferation index, vascular proliferation, and necrosis {817,1900, 2054}. The time to clinical progression is often long (mean: 6.5 years), but in some cases relapse occurs within a few months {1153}.

Synonyms

The terms "neurolipocytoma" {635}, "medullocytoma" {817}, "lipomatous glioneurocytoma" {57}, and "lipidized mature neuroectodermal tumour of the cerebellum" {866} have been proposed. The term "cerebellar liponeurocytoma" is now widely accepted and is supported by genetic analyses that indicate that this lesion is a rare but distinct clinicopathological entity {1044,1790,2400}.

Epidemiology

More than 40 cases of cerebellar

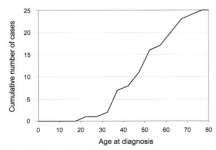

Fig. 6.46 Age distribution of cerebellar liponeurocytoma, based on 25 published cases.

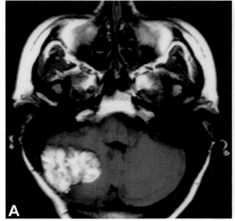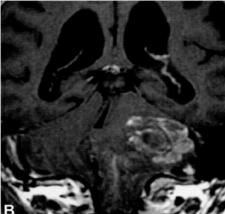

Fig. 6.47 Cerebellar liponeurocytoma. **A** T1-weighted MRI (with gadolinium) of a recurrent liponeurocytoma, presenting as an irregular, strongly enhancing lesion in the right cerebellar hemisphere. Reprinted from Jenkinson MD et al. {1153}. **B** Axial T1-weighted MRI after gadolinium administration shows areas of prominent hypointense signal within a well-demarcated isodense tumour {53}.

liponeurocytoma have been reported in the English-language literature {1790}. The mean patient age is 50 years (range: 24–77 years), with peak incidence in the third to sixth decades of life. There is no significant sex predilection {1044,1908}.

Localization

Cerebellar liponeurocytoma most commonly involves the cerebellar hemispheres, but can also be located in the paramedian region or vermis and extend to the cerebellopontine angle or fourth ventricle {1790}.

Clinical features

Headache and other symptoms and signs of raised intracranial pressure (either from the lesion itself or due to obstructive hydrocephalus) are common presentations. Cerebellar signs, including ataxia and disturbed gait, are also common {1867}.

Imaging

On CT, the tumour is variably isodense or hypodense, with focal areas of marked hypoattenuation corresponding to fat density {53,1790}. On T1-weighted MRI, the tumour is isointense to hypointense, with patchy areas of hyperintensity corresponding to regions of high lipid content.

Enhancement with gadolinium is usually heterogeneous, with areas of tumour showing variable degrees of enhancement. On T2-weighted MRI, the tumour is slightly hyperintense to the adjacent brain, with focal areas of marked hyperintensity. Associated oedema is minimal or absent {34}. Fat-suppressed images may be helpful in supporting a preoperative diagnosis {53}.

Microscopy

Cerebellar liponeurocytoma is a very rare adult cerebellar neoplasm composed of a uniform population of small neurocytic cells arranged in sheets and lobules and with regular round to oval nuclei, clear cytoplasm, and poorly defined cell membranes. The histological hallmark of this entity is focal accumulation of lipid-laden cells that resemble adipocytes but constitute lipid accumulation in neuroepithelial tumour cells.

Electron microscopy shows dense-core and clear vesicles, microtubule-containing neurites, and (occasionally) synapse-like structures {766,817}.

The growth fraction of the small-cell component, as determined by the Ki-67 proliferation index, is usually in the range of 1–3%, but can be as high as 6%, with a mean value of 2.5% {635,1200,2400}. In

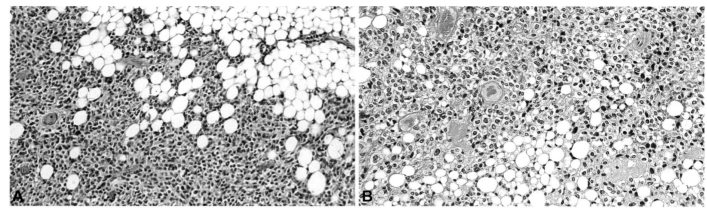

Fig. 6.48 Cerebellar liponeurocytoma. **A** Typical histology of cerebellar liponeurocytoma with focal accumulation of adipocytic tumour cells on a background of densely packed small round neoplastic cells, which often show a perinuclear halo. **B** Note the typical focal lipomatous differentiation of tumour cells, with displacement of nuclei to the cell periphery.

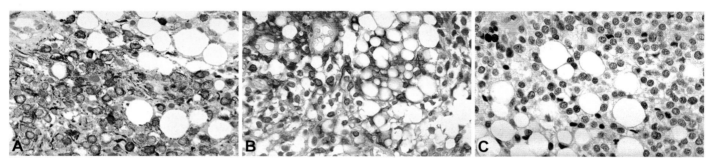

Fig. 6.49 Cerebellar liponeurocytoma. **A** Small tumour cells and neoplastic cells with lipomatous differentiation express MAP2; similarly, liponeurocytomas also express synaptophysin. **B** Expression of the astrocytic marker GFAP is observed in most cases, but only focally. **C** The Ki-67 proliferation index (as determined by nuclear MIB1 monoclonal antibody staining) is usually low.

the adipose component, the Ki-67 proliferation index is even lower. Features of anaplasia such as nuclear atypia, necrosis, and microvascular proliferation are typically absent in primary lesions, but may be found in recurrent tumours {817, 2054}. Similarly, the lipidized component may be markedly reduced or even absent {2054} in recurrent lesions.

Immunophenotype
Immunohistochemically, there is consistent expression of neuronal markers, including neuron-specific enolase, synaptophysin, and MAP2. Focal GFAP expression by tumour cells, which indicates astrocytic differentiation, is observed in most cases {2400}. One report

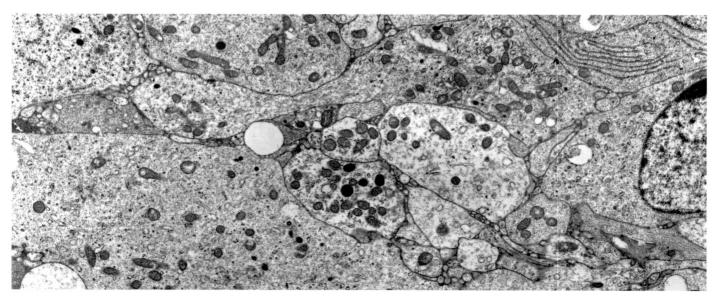

Fig. 6.50 Cerebellar liponeurocytoma. Electron microscopy shows dense-core and clear vesicles, microtubule-containing neurites, and occasionally synapse-like structures.

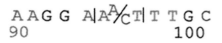

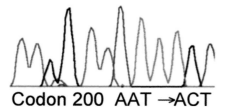

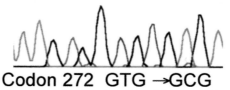

Codon 200 AAT →ACT   Codon 272 GTG →GCG

Fig. 6.51 Cerebellar liponeurocytoma. Examples of *TP53* missense mutations in codons 200 and 272 detected in cerebellar liponeurocytoma {1044}.

mentioned immunoreactivity to desmin and morphological features of incipient myogenic differentiation {866}.

The growth fraction as determined by the Ki-67 proliferation index is usually in the range of 1–3%, but can be as high as 10% in recurrent lesions {2054}. In the adipose component, the Ki-67 proliferation index is lower.

Cell of origin

A recent study demonstrated that the transcription factor NGN1, but not ATOH1, is expressed in cerebellar liponeurocytoma (unlike in normal adult cerebellum) and that adipocyte fatty acid–binding protein, typically found in adipocytes, is significantly overexpressed in cerebellar liponeurocytoma compared with both normal adult cerebellum and human medulloblastoma. These findings suggest an origin of cerebellar liponeurocytoma from cerebellar progenitors, which are distinct from cerebellar granule progenitors and aberrantly differentiate into adipocyte-like tumour cells {73}.

Genetic profile

Genetic analysis of 20 cases showed the presence of *TP53* missense mutations in 20%. The absence of isochromosome 17q and the lack of *PTCH*, *CTNNB1*, and *APC* mutations suggest that liponeurocytomas are not likely a variant of medulloblastoma. This assumption was further supported by gene expression profiles suggesting that this neoplasm is closer to neurocytoma than to the medulloblastoma subgroups {1044}. However, the presence of *TP53* mutations, which are absent in central neurocytomas, indicates development through different genetic pathways {1044}. *BRAF* and IDH mutations were absent in a recently reported case in which the recurrent lesion showed anaplastic changes {2054}.

Prognosis and predictive factors

The low proliferative activity is accompanied by a favourable clinical outcome. Most patients with sufficient follow-up survived > 5 years, largely irrespective of whether adjuvant radiotherapy was administered. The longest known survival is 18 years, in a patient whose treatment was limited to surgical excision. However, recurrence and radioresistance have been reported {1153}. Of 21 patients with follow-up data, 6 (29%) died between 6 months and 2 years after surgical intervention, 5 (24%) died 2–4 years after surgical intervention, and 10 (48%) survived for 5–16 years after surgical intervention. The 5-year survival rate was 48%, and the mean overall survival was 5.8 years {32,1044}. However, 62% of the patients developed a recurrence, after 1–12 years (mean: 6.5 years). In 3 patients, there was a second relapse 1–5 years later (mean: 3 years). Recurrent tumours may show increased mitotic activity, increased proliferative activity, vascular proliferation, and necrosis {817,2054}, although some tumour recurrences lack these atypical histopathological features {1153}. Histopathological properties predicting recurrence have not been identified.

Paraganglioma

Brandner S.
Soffer D.
Stratakis C.A.
Yousry T.

Definition

A unique neuroendocrine neoplasm, usually encapsulated and benign, arising in specialized neural crest cells associated with segmental or collateral autonomic ganglia (paraganglia); consisting of uniform chief cells exhibiting neuronal differentiation forming compact nests (Zellballen) surrounded by sustentacular cells and a delicate capillary network.

In the CNS, paragangliomas primarily affect the cauda equina / filum terminale and jugulotympanic regions.

ICD-O code   8693/1

Grading

Paragangliomas of the filum terminale correspond histologically to WHO grade I.

Epidemiology

Paragangliomas of the CNS are uncommon. Most present as spinal intradural tumours in the region of the cauda equina / filum terminale. Almost 300 cases have been reported since 1970, when cauda equina region paraganglioma was first described {1666}. Many other cases have undoubtedly gone unreported. Cauda equina paragangliomas generally affect adults, with peak incidence in the fourth to sixth decades of life. Patient age ranges from 9 to 75 years (mean age: 46 years) {2811}, with a slight male predominance (male-to-female ratio: 1.4–1.7:1) {2790}. Jugulotympanic paragangliomas are more common in Caucasians, have a strong female predilection, and occur mainly in the fifth and sixth decades of life {1111}. In a series of 200 cases of paragangliomas, 9% were located intraspinally {2790}. Phaeochromocytomas and paragangliomas are rare tumours with a combined estimated annual clinical incidence of 3 cases per 1 million population {147}.

Localization

Overall, paragangliomas of the cauda equina region constitute 3.4–3.8% of all tumours affecting this location {2765, 2815}. Other spinal levels are involved far less often; 19 paragangliomas have been reported in the thoracic region, most of which were extradural with an intravertebral and paraspinal component {397,489, 795,2363,2531} and 5 of which involved the cervical region {211,422,1542,1831, 2456}. Intracranial paragangliomas are usually extensions of jugulotympanic paragangliomas {1111}. However, rare examples of purely intracranial tumours have been situated in the sellar region {417,592,1742}, cerebellopontine angle {559,844}, cerebellar parenchyma {1496, 2025,2226}, and various locations in the forebrain {638,1646,2097,2828}.

Clinical features

Like other spinal tumours, cauda equina paragangliomas exhibit no distinctive clinical features. Common presenting symptoms include a history of low-back pain and sciatica. Less common manifestations are numbness, paraparesis, and sphincter symptoms. Fully developed cauda equina syndrome is uncommon. Signs of increased intracranial pressure and papilloedema are an unusual presentation {15,120,328,794,2236}. Endocrinologically, functional paragangliomas of the cauda equina region are extremely rare {794}. They present with signs of catecholamine hypersecretion, such as episodic or sustained hypertension, palpitations, diaphoresis, and headache. Another unusual presentation of cauda equina paraganglioma is with subarachnoid haemorrhage {1492}. Cerebrospinal fluid protein levels are usually markedly increased {2389,2395}.

The reported paragangliomas of the thoracic spine presented with signs of spinal cord compression or signs of catecholamine hypersecretion {1143,2363}. About 36% of all jugulotympanic paragangliomas extend into the cranial cavity {1111}. These most often present with pulsatile tinnitus and lower cranial nerve dysfunction {1111}.

Imaging

MRI is the investigative procedure of choice, although the findings are non-specific {15}; the appearance of paraganglioma is indistinguishable from that of schwannoma or ependymoma {1682}.

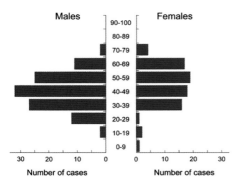

Fig. 6.52 Age and sex distribution of spinal paraganglioma, based on 71 published cases.

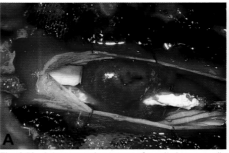 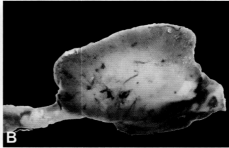

Fig. 6.53 **A** Intraoperative aspect of a spinal paraganglioma attached to the filum terminale. **B** Macroscopic aspect of a spinal paraganglioma attached to a nerve root. A well-circumscribed, solid tumour, partly attached to a spinal root; formalin fixed.

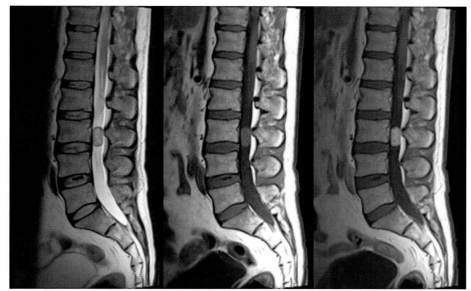

Fig. 6.54 MRI of spinal paraganglioma: a T2-weighted image (left), a T1-weighted image (centre), and a T1-weighted image with gadolinium contrast enhancement (right) show the encapsulated, well-demarcated tumour.

The tumour can be hypointense, isointense, or hyperintense on T1- and T2-weighted images, and gadolinium enhancement may be present or absent. Typically, paraganglioma presents as a sharply circumscribed, occasionally partly cystic mass that is hypointense or isointense to spinal cord on T1-weighted images, markedly contrast-enhancing, and hyperintense on T2-weighted images. The presence of a T2-hypointense rim (the so-called cap sign, related to haemosiderin content) is considered diagnostically helpful {1478,2811,2815}.

A salt-and-pepper appearance, caused by the hypervascular structure, can be seen on T2-weighted images. Cystic changes can be caused by intratumoural haemorrhage. Plain X-rays are usually non-informative, but rarely show erosion (scalloping) of vertebral laminae due to chronic bone compression.

Spread
The vast majority of cauda equina paragangliomas are slow-growing and curable by total excision; with long-term follow-up, it is estimated that 4% recur after

gross total removal {2438}. Cerebrospinal fluid seeding of spinal paragangliomas has occasionally been documented {487,2144,2438,2540}. Although paragangliomas in general are considered benign, about 10–20% of them have metastatic potential {1437}. In contrast, metastasis outside the CNS (to the bone) from cauda equina paragangliomas has been reported only once {1712}. As is the case in paragangliomas in general, there is no single histological parameter that can predict malignant behaviour in cauda equina paragangliomas {1655}. Numerous factors have been associated with malignancy in paragangliomas in general, including *SDHB* mutations, high proliferation index, and large tumour size. Tumour size cut-off points of 5–6 cm of diameter and 80–150 g of weight have been suggested to predict malignant behaviour {1655}. However, the only accepted criterion for malignancy is the presence of distant metastasis {378,1655}.

Macroscopy
Generally, paragangliomas are oval to sausage-shaped, delicately encapsulated, soft, reddish-brown masses that bleed freely. The 59 spinal tumours included in one group of five series measured 10–112 mm in greatest dimension {1609,1682,2811}. Capsular calcification and cystic components may be found. The tumours occasionally penetrate dura and invade bone. Most paragangliomas of the cauda equina are entirely intradural and are attached either to the filum terminale or (less often) to a caudal nerve root {2395}.

Microscopy
Paragangliomas are well-differentiated tumours resembling normal paraganglia. They are composed of chief (type I) cells arranged in nests or lobules (called Zellballen) surrounded by an inconspicuous single layer of sustentacular (type II) cells. The Zellballen are also surrounded by a delicate capillary network and a delicate supporting reticulin fibre network that may undergo sclerosis. The uniform round or polygonal chief cells have central, round to oval nuclei with finely stippled chromatin and inconspicuous nucleoli. Degenerative nuclear pleomorphism is typically mild. The cytoplasm is usually eosinophilic and finely granular. In some cases, it is amphophilic or clear. Sustentacular cells are spindle-shaped;

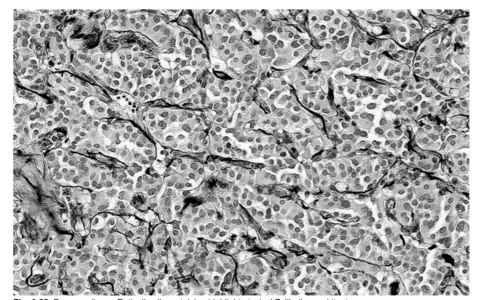

Fig. 6.55 Paraganglioma. Reticulin silver staining highlights typical Zellballen architecture.

encompassing the lobules, their long processes are often so attenuated that they are not visible on routine light microscopy and can be detected only on immunostains for S100 protein. Approximately 25% of all cauda equina paragangliomas are so-called gangliocytic paragangliomas, containing mature ganglion cells and a Schwann cell component {313}. Ependymoma-like perivascular formations are also common. Some tumours show architectural features reminiscent of carcinoid tumours, including angiomatous, adenomatous, and pseudorosette patterns {2395}. Tumours composed predominantly of spindle {1712} and melanin-containing cells (called melanotic paragangliomas) {773,1712} have also been described at this site, as has oncocytic paraganglioma {1889}. Foci of haemorrhagic necrosis may occur, and scattered mitotic figures can be seen. Neither these features nor nuclear pleomorphism is of prognostic significance {2395}.

Ultrastructure

The distinctive ultrastructural feature of chief cells is the presence of dense-core (neurosecretory) granules measuring 100–400 nm (mean: 140 nm). Sustentacular cells are characterized by an elongated nucleus with marginal chromatin, increased cytoplasmic electron density, relative abundance of intermediate filaments, and lack of dense-core granules {647,2395}.

Immunophenotype

Consistent with their neuroendocrine differentiation, the chief cells of paragangliomas are immunoreactive for the commonly used neuroendocrine markers chromogranin-A and synaptophysin {1303,1655,2395}. The diagnosis of paraganglioma in other sites is confirmed by positivity for tyrosine 3-monooxygenase, the rate-limiting enzyme in catecholamine synthesis {1655}. However, this test is usually not required for cauda equina paragangliomas, because it distinguishes paragangliomas from other neuroendocrine carcinomas, which are not considered in the differential diagnosis in this location. Whereas paragangliomas in other sites are cytokeratin-immunonegative, those arising from the cauda equina can show positivity for cytokeratins, typically in the form of perinuclear immunoreactivity {432,894,1655,2438}.

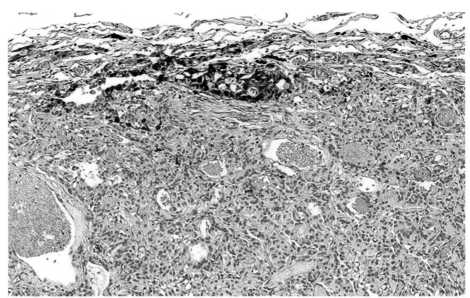

Fig. 6.56 This paraganglioma shows subcapsular haemosiderin, visualized with Perls Prussian blue stain.

Gangliocytic paragangliomas containing a variable mixture of epithelioid neuroendocrine cells, Schwann cell–like cells, and scattered ganglion cells can show cytokeratin positivity in the epithelioid cells {894,2328}. Expression of 5-HT and various neuropeptides (e.g. somatostatin and met-enkephalin) has been demonstrated in paragangliomas of the cauda equina region {1712,2395}. Loss of SDHB expression is considered a surrogate marker for familial paraganglioma syndromes caused by any SDH mutation. Although SDHB immunohistochemistry has become part of the routine assessment of paragangliomas in many centres {1655}, it is probably of limited value in cauda equina paragangliomas given the very low rate of SDH mutations {1420,1955}.

Sustentacular cells show inconsistent (sometimes only focal) S100 protein reactivity {313} and usually show staining for GFAP as well. Chief cells may also

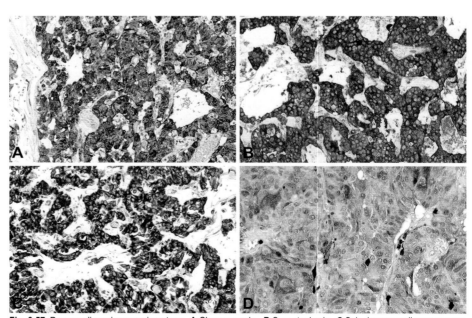

Fig. 6.57 Paraganglioma immunophenotype. **A** Chromogranin. **B** Synaptophysin. **C** Spinal paragangliomas express cytokeratins. **D** S100 is expressed by sustentacular cells and occasional chief cells.

show variable S100 immunoreactivity. Recent guidelines suggest that proliferation rate (mitotic activity and Ki-67 proliferation index) should be recorded for paragangliomas as well as for other neuroendocrine tumours {1655}; however, the value of proliferation markers in cauda equina paragangliomas has not been established.

Cell of origin

The histogenesis of cauda equina paraganglioma is a matter of debate. Some authors favour an origin from paraganglion cells associated with regional autonomic nerves and blood vessels, despite the fact that such cells have not been identified at this site {1513}. Others have suggested that peripheral neuroblasts normally present in the adult filum terminale undergo paraganglionic differentiation {339,2204}. Jugulotympanic paragangliomas presumably arise from microscopic paraganglia within the temporal bone {1412}. Of interest, although perhaps not relevant to histogenesis, are reports of the coexistence of paraganglioma and myxopapillary ependymoma in the cauda equina region {1243} and of a biphasic tumour consisting primarily of paraganglioma and to a lesser extent ependymoma {339}.

Genetic profile

The mutations found in paragangliomas are described in *Genetic susceptibility*. The genetic and epigenetic profiles (i.e. methylation, expression {930,1475}, microRNA {540}, and metabolomics {381,1090}) of phaeochromocytomas/paragangliomas with succinate dehydrogenase defects differ dramatically from those with other genetic causes.

Genetic susceptibility

It is estimated that as many as half of all phaeochromocytomas/paragangliomas in adults and > 80% of these tumours in children are inherited {2139}.

To date, autosomal dominant germline mutations of > 10 genes have been described in association with these tumours: *VHL* (associated with von Hippel–Lindau disease); *RET* (associated with multiple endocrine neoplasia type 2); *NF1* (associated with neurofibromatosis type 1); genes coding for the subunits of the succinate dehydrogenase enzyme – *SDHD* (associated with inherited paraganglioma-1), *SDHA* and *SDHAF2* (associated with paraganglioma-2), *SDHC* (associated with paraganglioma-3), and *SDHB* (associated with paraganglioma-4) – which forms part of mitochondrial complex II {778,840}; and the tumour suppressors *TMEM127* {2049} and *MAX* {484}. Multiple paragangliomas and/or phaeochromocytomas are often caused by *SDHD*, *SDHAF2*, *SDHB*, *SDHC*, and *SDHA* mutations, whereas isolated phaeochromocytomas are also associated with *TMEM127* and *MAX* mutations {778}. An association between paragangliomas/phaeochromocytomas and fumarase defects was recently reported {380}. *NF1* mutations seem to be more frequent than previously thought {2726}. Genes with roles in multiple neoplasia syndromes, such as the *VHL* gene, may also be epigenetically modified {71}; the *VHL* gene is epigenetically inactivated in phaeochromocytomas and abdominal paragangliomas {71}.

Spinal paragangliomas may be non-familial in most cases, but a study of 22 spinal paragangliomas showed an *SDHD* germline mutation in one patient with recurrent spinal paraganglioma and a cerebellar metastasis {1605}. Systemic paragangliomas may be multifocal, but no association has been reported between cauda equina paragangliomas and other spinal paragangliomas. Concurrent cases of spinal paraganglioma with brain tumours {339,487}, spinal epidural haemangioma {2735}, syringomyelia {2419}, and intramedullary cysts {672} have been reported, but these associations may be coincidental.

Paraganglioma and gastrointestinal stromal tumour are associated as characteristics of Carney–Stratakis syndrome, a familial syndrome inherited in an autosomal dominant manner {2436}. The disease is caused by mutations and/or deletions of *SDHA*, *SDHB*, *SDHC*, and *SDHD*, in > 90% of the described cases {1898}. Paragangliomas or phaeochromocytomas can also be found as part of an allelic condition called Carney triad. This sporadic syndrome is seen almost exclusively in females and may be due to epigenetic alterations of *SDHC* {930} or other defects of the *SDHC* chromosomal locus on 1q {1614}. Paragangliomas and/or phaeochromocytomas can also be seen in association with renal cancer {841}, pituitary tumours {2798}, and possibly thyroid tumours {1777}.

In general, a single benign paraganglioma may not be indicative of any genetic predisposition, whereas multiple paragangliomas or an association of a paraganglioma with another neoplasia (e.g. phaeochromocytoma, gastrointestinal stromal tumour, renal cancer, pituitary adenoma, or thyroid cancer) should prompt investigation of a possible genetic syndrome underlying the presentation.

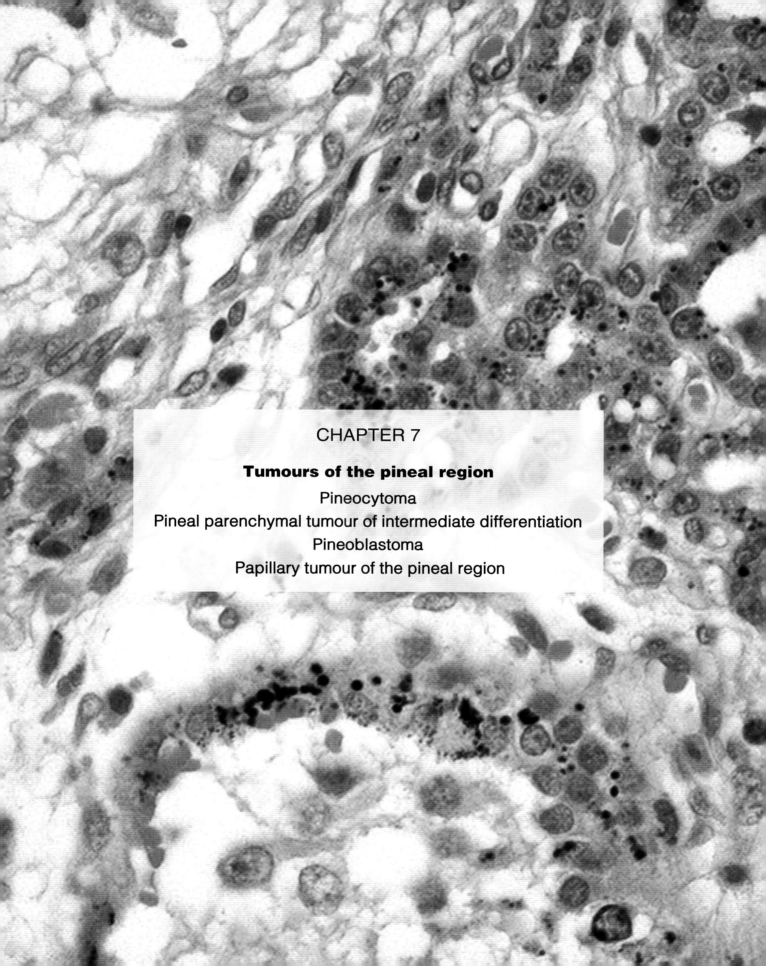

CHAPTER 7

Tumours of the pineal region

Pineocytoma

Pineal parenchymal tumour of intermediate differentiation

Pineoblastoma

Papillary tumour of the pineal region

Pineocytoma

Nakazato Y.
Jouvet A.
Vasiljevic A.

Definition

A well-differentiated pineal parenchymal neoplasm composed of uniform cells forming large pineocytomatous rosettes and/or of pleomorphic cells showing gangliocytic differentiation.

Pineocytoma is a rare neoplasm. It accounts for about 20% of all pineal parenchymal tumours and typically affects adults, with a mean patient age at diagnosis of 43 years. There is a female predominance, with a male-to-female ratio of 0.6:1. Other characteristics are exclusive localization in the pineal region and a well-demarcated solid mass without infiltrative or disseminating growth. Specific genetic alterations have not yet been identified. The prognosis is good after total surgical removal.

ICD-O code   9361/1

Grading

Pineocytoma corresponds histologically to WHO grade I.

Epidemiology

Pineal region tumours account for < 1% of all intracranial neoplasms, and approximately 27% of pineal region tumours are of pineal parenchymal origin {1332, 2458}. Of these, pineocytomas account for 17–30% (mean: 20%) {91,1187,2279, 2809}. Before the classification of pineal parenchymal tumour of intermediate differentiation as a distinct entity, as many as 60% of pineal parenchymal tumours were classified as pineocytomas {997, 1638}. Pineocytomas can occur in patients of any age, but most frequently

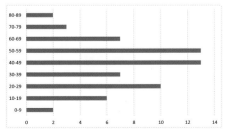

Fig. 7.01 Age distribution of patients with pineocytoma, based on 63 cases, both sexes.

affect adults, with a mean patient age of 42.8 years {91,1187,1674,2279,2809}. There is a female predominance, with a male-to-female ratio of 0.6:1.

Localization

Pineocytomas typically remain localized in the pineal area, where they compress adjacent structures, including the cerebral aqueduct, brain stem, and cerebellum. Protrusion into the posterior third ventricle is common.

Clinical features

Because of expansile growth in the pineal region, pineocytomas present with signs and symptoms related to increased intracranial pressure due to aqueductal obstruction, neuro-ophthalmological dysfunction (i.e. Parinaud syndrome), and brain stem or cerebellar dysfunction {240,445,465,927,2279}. Common presentations include headache, papilloedema, ataxia, impaired vision, nausea and vomiting, impaired ambulation, loss of upward gaze, dizziness, and tremor.

Imaging

On CT, pineocytomas usually present as globular, well-delineated masses < 3 cm in diameter. They appear hypodense and homogeneous, some harbouring either peripheral or central calcification {435}. Occasional cystic changes may be seen and are usually not easily confused with typical pineal cysts {665}. Most tumours exhibit heterogeneous contrast enhancement. Isodense to slightly hyperdense appearance and homogeneous contrast enhancement on CT have also been reported {1751}. Accompanying hydrocephalus is a common feature {2279}. On MRI, the tumours tend to be hypointense or isointense on T1-weighted images and hyperintense on T2-weighted images, with strong, homogeneous contrast enhancement {1751}. The margins with surrounding structures are usually well defined, and are best analysed by MRI.

Spread

Strictly defined pineocytomas grow

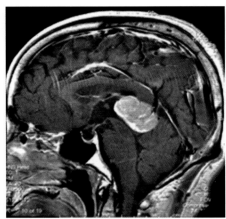

Fig. 7.02 Sagittal gadolinium-enhanced T1-weighted MRI of a pineocytoma in the pineal region.

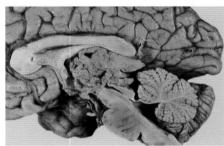

Fig. 7.03 Sagittal section of a large pineocytoma extending into the third ventricle. Note the granular cut surface with occasional cysts.

locally but are not associated with cerebrospinal fluid seeding {677}.

Macroscopy

Pineocytomas are well-circumscribed lesions with a greyish-tan, homogeneous or granular cut surface {240,997,2258}. Degenerative changes, including cyst formation and foci of haemorrhage, may be present {1638}.

Microscopy

Histopathology

Pineocytoma is a well-differentiated, moderately cellular neoplasm composed of relatively small, uniform, mature cells resembling pinealocytes. It grows primarily in sheets, and often features large pineocytomatous rosettes composed of

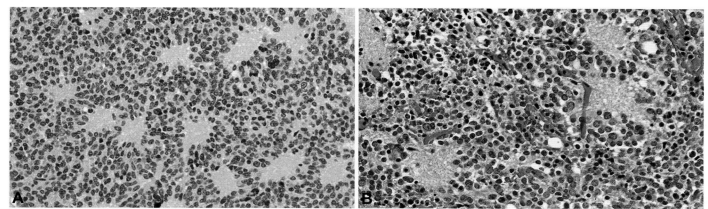

Fig. 7.04 A Typical pineocytoma. A sheet of tumour cells with scattered pineocytomatous rosettes. **B** Pineocytoma. Uniform tumour cells resembling pinealocytes.

abundant delicate tumour cell processes. Pineocytomatous rosettes are not seen in normal pineal gland. In pineocytoma, poorly defined lobules may be seen, but a conspicuous lobular architecture is instead a feature of normal pineal gland. Most nuclei are round to oval, with inconspicuous nucleoli and finely dispersed chromatin. Cytoplasm is moderate in quantity and homogeneously eosinophilic. Processes are conspicuous and short, often ending in club-shaped expansions that are optimally demonstrated by neurofilament immunostaining or silver impregnation. Mitotic figures are lacking (with < 1 mitosis per 10 high-power fields) in all but occasional large specimens {1187}. Pineocytomatous rosettes vary in number and size. Their anucleate centres are composed of delicate, enmeshed cytoplasmic processes resembling neuropil {240,1187,1811,2279}. The nuclei surrounding the periphery of the rosette are not regimented. A pleomorphic cytological variant is encountered in some pineocytomas {701}. This variant

is characterized by large ganglion cells and/or multinucleated giant cells with bizarre nuclei {240,997,1384,1638,2279}. The mitotic activity of this pattern is still low, despite the tumours' ominous nuclear appearance. The stroma of pineocytoma consists of a delicate network of vascular channels lined by a single layer of endothelial cells and supported by scant reticulin fibres. Microcalcifications are occasionally seen but usually correspond to calcifications of the remaining pineal gland.

Electron microscopy

Ultrastructurally, pineocytomas are composed of clear and various numbers of dark cells joined with zonulae adherentes {968,997,1185,1674}. The cells extend tapering processes that occasionally terminate in bulbous ends. Their cytoplasm is relatively abundant and contains well-developed organelles. Pineocytoma cells share numerous ultrastructural features with normal mammalian pinealocytes, such as paired twisted filaments,

annulate lamellae, cilia with a 9 + 0 microtubular pattern, microtubular sheaves, fibrous bodies, vesicle-crowned rodlets, heterogeneous cytoplasmic inclusion, and membrane whorls, as well as mitochondrial and centriolar clusters. Membrane-bound dense-core granules and clear vesicles are present in the cytoplasm and cellular processes. The cellular processes show occasional synapse-like junctions.

Immunophenotype

Pineocytoma cells usually show strong immunoreactivity for synaptophysin, neuron-specific enolase, and NFP. Variable staining has also been reported for other neuronal markers, including class III beta-tubulin, microtubule-associated protein tau, UCHL1, chromogranin-A, and the neurotransmitter 5-HT {477,1185,1187, 1384,1811,2809}. Photosensory differentiation is associated with immunoreactivity for S-arrestin and rhodopsin {1638, 1811,1933}. In pleomorphic variants, the

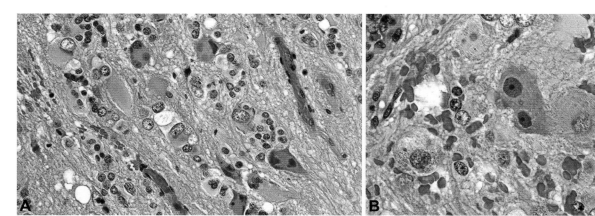

Fig. 7.05 Pleomorphic pineocytoma. **A** Pleomorphism and gangliocytic differentiation. **B** Mono- and multinucleated ganglion cells.

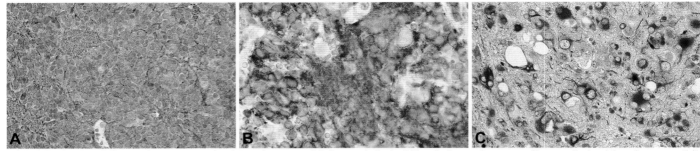

Fig. 7.06 Pineocytoma. **A** Pineocytomatous rosettes show intense immunoreactivity for synaptophysin. **B** The cytoplasm and processes of tumour cells show intense immunoreactivity for NFP. **C** Pleomorphic cells often show immunoreactivity for NFP.

ganglioid cells usually express several neuronal markers, especially NFP.

Proliferation

In most cases, mitotic figures are very rare or absent {702,1187,1217}. The mean Ki-67 proliferation index is < 1% {91,702, 1217}.

Cell of origin

The histogenesis of pineal parenchymal tumours is linked to the pinealocyte, a cell with photosensory and neuroendocrine functions. The ontogeny of the human pineal gland recapitulates the phylogeny of the retina and the pineal organ {1675}. During the late stages of intrauterine life and the early postnatal period, the human pineal gland consists primarily of cells arranged in rosettes similar to those of the developing retina. These feature abundant melanin pigment as well as cilia with a 9 + 0 microtubular pattern. By the age of 3 months, the number of pigmented cells gradually decreases so that pigment becomes undetectable by histochemical methods {1675}. As differentiation progresses, cells that are strongly immunoreactive for neuron-specific enolase accumulate. By the age of 1 year,

pinealocytes predominate. To a variable extent, pineal parenchymal tumours mimic the developmental stages of the human pineal gland. In tissue culture, pineocytoma cells are also capable of synthesizing 5-HT and melatonin {700}.
The immunoexpression of CRX and ASMT in pineocytoma is an additional indication that these tumours are biologically linked to pinealocytes {754,2241}. CRX is a transcription factor involved in the development and differentiation of pineal cell lineage, and ASMT is a critical enzyme for the synthesis of melatonin (a hormone produced by the pineal gland).

Genetic profile

Conventional cytogenetic studies based on karyotypes are rare. Karyotype analysis of 3 pineocytomas demonstrated a pseudodiploid or hypotriploid profile with various numerical and structural abnormalities, including loss of all or part of chromosome 22, loss or partial deletion of chromosome 11, loss of chromosome 14, and gain of chromosomes 5 and 19 {162,525,2061}. However, no chromosomal gains or losses were found by comparative genomic hybridization analysis {2122}. A relationship between

the *RB1* gene and pineocytoma has not been established. A microarray analysis of pineocytoma has shown high-level expression of genes coding for enzymes related to melatonin synthesis (i.e. *TPH1* and *ASMT*) and genes involved in retinal phototransduction (i.e. *OPN4*, *RGS16*, and *CRB3*). These reactivities indicate bidirectional neurosecretory and photosensory differentiation {698}.

Genetic susceptibility

No syndromic associations or genetic susceptibilities have been demonstrated. The occurrence of pineocytoma in siblings was reported in one family {796}.

Prognosis and predictive factors

The clinical course of pineocytomas is characterized by a long interval (4 years in one series) between the onset of symptoms and surgery {240}. No strictly classified pineocytomas have been shown to metastasize {677,2278}. The reported 5-year survival rate of patients with pineocytoma ranges from 86% to 91% {677, 2278}. In one series, the 5-year event-free survival rate was 100% {677}. Extent of surgery is considered to be the major prognostic factor for pineocytoma {465}.

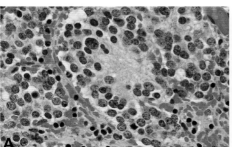
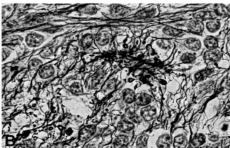
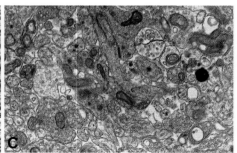

Fig. 7.07 Pineocytoma. **A** In a pineocytomatous rosette, tumour cells surround an eosinophilic fibrillated core. **B** Argyrophilic tumour cell processes end with club-shaped expansions in the pineocytomatous rosettes (Bodian silver impregnation). **C** Ultrastructure of a pineocytomatous rosette, showing numerous cell processes filled with clear vesicles, dense-core granules, and mitochondria.

Pineal parenchymal tumour of intermediate differentiation

Jouvet A.
Nakazato Y.
Vasiljevic A.

Definition

A tumour of the pineal gland that is intermediate in malignancy between pineocytoma and pineoblastoma and is composed of diffuse sheets or large lobules of monomorphic round cells that appear more differentiated than those observed in pineoblastomas.

Pleomorphic cytology may be present. Pineal parenchymal tumours of intermediate differentiation (PPTIDs) occur mainly in adults (mean patient age: 41 years), and show variable biological and clinical behaviour, from low-grade tumours with frequent local and delayed recurrences to high-grade tumours with risk of craniospinal dissemination. Accordingly, mitotic activity, Ki-67 proliferation index, and neuronal and neuroendocrine differentiation are also variable, and reported 5-year overall survival rates range from 39% to 74% {677,1187}.

ICD-O code   9362/3

Grading

The biological behaviour of pineal parenchymal tumour of intermediate differentiation is variable and may correspond to WHO grades II or III, but definite histological grading criteria remain to be defined.

Synonyms and historical annotation

The category of PPTID was first clearly introduced in 1993 by Schild et al. {1185, 1674,2279}. PPTIDs have been reported under various names, such as "malignant pineocytoma" {997}, "pineocytoma with anaplasia" {2586}, and "pineoblastoma with lobules" {240}. These terms have obscured the value of the designation, and they are not recommended.

In earlier studies, no true PPTID group was identified. However, mixed pineocytoma–pineoblastoma was sometimes described as an intermediate tumour between pineocytoma and pineoblastoma {1638,2279}. By definition, this tumour is composed of clearly delineated areas of pineoblastoma admixed with well-demarcated areas of pineocytoma. Neoplastic cells lack the so-called intermediate morphology that is required for a diagnosis of PPTID. Mixed pineocytoma–pineoblastoma should not be included in the PPTID group, but rather belongs in the pineoblastoma group (see *Pineoblastoma*, p. 176).

Epidemiology

PPTIDs account for approximately 45% of all pineal parenchymal tumours, with a range of 21–54% in most recent series {91,1105,2809,2868}. Earlier reported incidence rates of PPTID were even more variable, from 0% to 59%, reflecting the general ignorance of this pineal parenchymal tumour, the frequent misdiagnosis of the entity, and/or the inclusion of mixed pineocytoma–pineoblastomas and other unusual pineal parenchymal tumours in this group {240,1187,1638,1811}. PPTIDs can occur in patients of any age, but most frequently affect adults, with a mean patient age of 41 years (range: 1–83 years) {754,1105,1187,2809}. There is a slight female preponderance, with a male-to-female ratio of 0.8:1.

Localization

PPTIDs are localized in the pineal region.

Clinical features

The clinical presentation is similar to that of other pineal parenchymal tumours. The main symptoms are headaches and vomiting, related to increased intracranial pressure caused by obstructive hydrocephalus. Hydrocephalus is the consequence of tumoural extension of the pineal gland into the posterior third ventricle, with compression of the corpora quadrigemina and compromise of cerebrospinal fluid flow through the aqueduct. Compression of the superior colliculus by the expanding mass may cause ocular movement abnormalities (i.e. Parinaud syndrome), including paralysis of upward gaze, pupillary abnormalities (i.e. slightly dilated pupils that react to accommodation but not to light), and nystagmus retractorius {69,195,757,2319}. A rare case of apoplectic haemorrhage of a PPTID with sudden-onset symptoms has been reported {2684}.

Imaging

On imaging, PPTIDs usually present as bulky masses with local invasion. They are more rarely circumscribed. On CT, the tumours may show occasional peripheral so-called exploded calcifications {1321}. On MRI, PPTIDs are heterogeneous and mostly hypointense on T1-weighted images and hyperintense on T2-weighted images. On both CT and MRI, postcontrast enhancement is usually marked and heterogeneous {1105,1321}.

Spread

PPTIDs have a potential for local recurrence and craniospinal dissemination {677,1105,2708,2835}. Local recurrence occurs in approximately 22% of cases {677}. Craniospinal dissemination may be observed at the time of diagnosis (in 10% of cases) or may occur during the course of the disease (in 15% of cases) {677}.

Macroscopy

The gross appearance of PPTIDs is similar to that of pineocytomas. They are circumscribed, soft in texture, and lacking gross evidence of necrosis. An irregular tumour surface was observed by endoscopy in a case with spinal metastasis {1105}.

Microscopy

PPTID may exhibit two architectural patterns: diffuse (neurocytoma- or oligodendroglioma-like) and/or lobulated

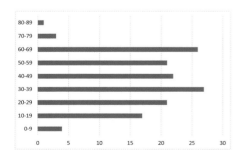

Fig. 7.08 Age distribution of pineal parenchymal tumours of intermediate differentiation, based on 142 published cases, both sexes.

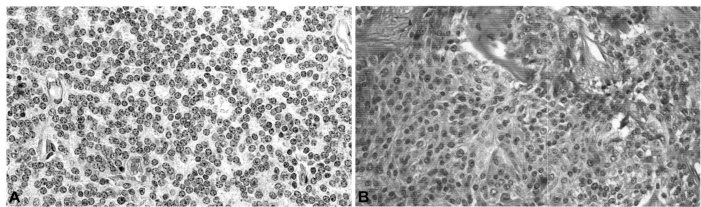

Fig. 7.09 Pineal parenchymal tumour of intermediate differentiation. **A** Neurocytoma-like appearance in a pineal parenchymal tumour of intermediate differentiation. Tumour with moderate cellularity and round nuclei harbouring salt-and-pepper chromatin; the fibrillary background is characterized by small pseudorosettes; larger pseudorosettes, as seen in pineocytomas, are not observed. **B** Pseudolobulated pineal parenchymal tumour of intermediate differentiation. In this tumour, large fibrous vessels delineate poorly defined lobules of neoplastic cells.

(with vessels delineating vague lobules) {1187}. Transitional cases also exist, defined as tumours in which typical pineocytomatous areas are associated with a diffuse or lobulated pattern more consistent with PPTID. PPTIDs are characterized by moderate to high cellularity. The neoplastic cells usually harbour round nuclei showing mild to moderate atypia and a so-called salt-and-pepper chromatin. The cytoplasm of cells is more easily distinguishable than in pineoblastoma. A pleomorphic cytological variant may be encountered in PPTIDs as well as in pineocytomas {701,1384}. This variant is characterized by bizarre ganglioid cells with single or multiple atypical nuclei and abundant cytoplasm. Mitotic activity is low to moderate.

Proliferation

PPTID is a potentially aggressive neoplasm. In a large published series, the wide range of reported mitotic counts reflects the difficulty in making the diagnosis (often in a small biopsy); there were 0 mitoses per 10 high-power fields in 54% of cases, 1–2 in 28%, 3–6 in 15%, and rarely > 6 {1187}.

In the PPTID group, the mean Ki-67 proliferation index is usually significantly different from those of pineocytomas and pineoblastomas, ranging from 3.5% to 16.1% {91,1105,2122,2835,2868}.

Immunophenotype

Immunohistochemistry shows synaptophysin positivity {91,754,1105,1187}. Variable labelling is also seen with antibodies to NFP and chromogranin-A {1185, 1187,2586,2809}. GFAP and S100 protein are usually expressed in astrocytic interstitial cells {91,1187}. Ganglion cells in pleomorphic variants may also express S100 protein {1187}. Like in other pineal parenchymal tumours, there is no nuclear NeuN staining in PPTID {1217, 1487,2684}. ASMT-positive cells are significantly more numerous in PPTIDs than in pineoblastomas {754}. In pleomorphic variants, the ganglioid cells usually express several neuronal markers, especially NFP {701,1384}.

Cell of origin

Pineal parenchymal tumours arise from pinealocytes or their precursor cells, and the close kinship among pineocytoma, PPTID, and pineoblastoma is evidenced by several shared clinical, morphological, and genetic features {698,1187,1674, 2279}. The immunoexpression of cone-rod homeobox (CRX) and acetylserotonin methyltransferase (ASMT) proteins in PPTID is an additional indication that PPTIDs are biologically linked to pinealocytes {754,2241}. CRX is a transcription factor involved in the development and differentiation of pineal cell lineage, and

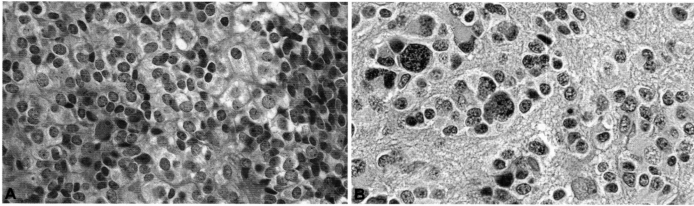

Fig. 7.10 Pineal parenchymal tumour of intermediate differentiation. **A** Diffuse pineal parenchymal tumour of intermediate differentiation. This tumour is composed of round cells with a conspicuous cytoplasm and round to oval nuclei with delicate chromatin. **B** Pleomorphic cells in a low-grade pineal parenchymal tumour of intermediate differentiation.

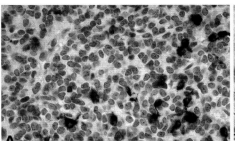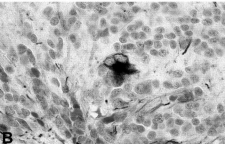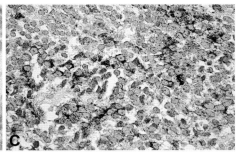

Fig. 7.11 Pineal parenchymal tumour of intermediate differentiation. **A** Focal NFP expression in a low-grade tumour. **B** Strong expression of NFP in a ganglion cell. **C** Focal expression of chromogranin-A.

ASMT is a critical enzyme for the synthesis of melatonin (a hormone produced by the pineal gland).

Genetic profile

By comparative genomic hybridization, frequent chromosomal changes have been identified in PPTIDs. An average of 3.3 gains and 2 losses has been reported {2122}. The most common chromosomal imbalances in PPTID are 4q gain, 12q gain, and 22 loss. In one RT-PCR analysis, the expression of four genes (*PRAME*, *CD24*, *POU4F2*, and *HOXD13*) in high-grade PPTID was high, almost to the levels seen in pineoblastoma, and in contrast to the low expression of these genes in pineocytoma and low-grade PPTID {698}. One analysis showed expression of EGFRvIII in a PPTID without concomitant *EGFR* gene amplification {1487}.

Genetic susceptibility

No syndromic associations or genetic susceptibilities have been reported for PPTID.

Prognosis and predictive factors

Compared with pineoblastomas, PPTIDs are more likely to present with localized disease, and they have a better prognosis, with a median overall survival of 165 months (vs 77 months for pineoblastoma) and a median progression-free survival of 93 months (vs 46 months for pineoblastoma) {1549}. In one study, prognosis was related to mitotic count and to neuronal differentiation as assessed by anti-NFP immunohistochemistry {677,1187}. Low-grade PPTIDs were defined as tumours showing < 6 mitoses per 10 high-power fields and expression of NFP in numerous cells {1187}. In this group, the 5-year overall survival rate was 74%. Recurrences occurred in 26% of patients and most were mainly local and delayed {677}. High-grade PPTIDs were defined as tumours showing < 6 mitoses per 10 high-power fields but no or only rare expression of NFP, or showing ≥ 6 mitoses per 10 high-power fields and NFP expression in numerous cells {1187}. In this group, the 5-year overall survival rate was 39%. Risk of recurrence was higher (56%), as was risk of

spinal dissemination (28%) {677}. The low-grade and high-grade prognostic groups also showed a significantly different mean Ki-67 proliferation index (5.2% vs 11.2%) {702}. Although an association has been found in some studies between NFP immunopositivity and a better prognosis, the use of this criterion to assess prognosis in pineal parenchymal tumours remains controversial {91,1187, 2835}. In another study, PPTIDs in the low-risk group (defined by < 3 mitoses per 10 high-power fields and a Ki-67 proliferation index of < 5%) had better overall survival and progression-free survival than did PPTIDs in the high-risk group (defined by ≥ 3 mitoses per 10 high-power fields or a Ki-67 proliferation index of ≥ 5%) {2835}. The relevance of these criteria (mitotic count, NFP immunoexpression, and Ki-67 proliferation index) requires confirmation by further studies; consequently, there are currently no recommended criteria for grading PPTID (see *Grading*, p. 173). Transformation of PPTID into pineoblastoma has been rarely reported {1050,1272}.

Pineoblastoma

Jouvet A.
Vasiljevic A.
Nakazato Y.
Tanaka S.

Definition

A poorly differentiated, highly cellular, malignant embryonal neoplasm arising in the pineal gland.

Pineoblastoma usually occurs within the first two decades of life (mean patient age: 17.8 years), with a predilection for children. It is histologically characterized by the presence of patternless sheets of small immature neuroepithelial cells with a high nuclear-to-cytoplasmic ratio, hyperchromatic nuclei, and scant cytoplasm. Proliferation activity is high, with frequent mitoses and a Ki-67 proliferation index of > 20%. SMARCB1 nuclear expression is retained, enabling distinction from atypical teratoid/rhabdoid tumour. Isochromosome 17q or amplification of 19q13.42 are usually not seen. Pineoblastomas tend to spread via cerebrospinal fluid pathways and often follow aggressive clinical courses.

ICD-O code   9362/3

Grading

Pineoblastoma corresponds histologically to WHO grade IV.

Epidemiology

Pineoblastomas are rare, accounting for approximately 35% of all pineal parenchymal tumours (from 24% to 61% depending on the series) {91,1187,2279, 2651,2809}. They can occur at any age, but most present in the first two decades of life, with a distinct predilection for children (mean patient age: 17.8 years) {91, 1187,2279,2809}. There is a slight female

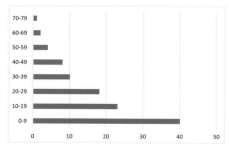

Fig. 7.12 Age distribution of pineoblastoma, based on 113 published cases, both sexes.

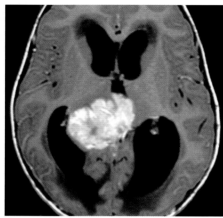

Fig. 7.13 Pineoblastoma. Axial contrast-enhanced T1-weighted MRI in a 3-year-old child with large head shows severe obstructive hydrocephalus and a heterogeneously enhancing pineal mass.

predominance, with a male-to-female ratio of 0.7:1.

Localization

Pineoblastomas are localized in the pineal region.

Clinical features

The clinical presentation of pineoblastoma is similar to that of other tumours of the pineal region. The main symptoms are related to elevated intracranial pressure (primarily from obstructive hydrocephalus) and include headaches and vomiting {508,671,1457}. Ocular symptoms and signs may also be observed, such as decreased visual acuity and Parinaud syndrome. The interval between initial symptoms and surgery may be < 1 month {508}.

Imaging

On neuroimaging, pineoblastomas present as large, multilobulated masses in the pineal region and show frequent invasion of surrounding structures, including the tectum, thalamus, and splenium of the corpus callosum {435,1751,2093, 2553}. Small cystic/necrotic areas and oedema may be observed {1343,2093, 2553}. On CT, pineoblastomas are usually slightly hyperdense, with postcontrast enhancement {435,1751}. Calcifications

are infrequent {435,1751}. Nearly all patients show obstructive hydrocephalus {435,1751,2373}. On T1-weighted MRI, the tumours are often hypointense to isointense, with heterogeneous contrast enhancement. They are isointense to mildly hyperintense on T2-weighted images {435,1751,2093,2553}.

Spread

Pineoblastomas directly invade neighbouring brain structures (including the leptomeninges, third ventricle, and tectal plate) and tend to disseminate along cerebrospinal fluid pathways {240}. Craniospinal dissemination is observed in 25–33% of patients at initial diagnosis {677,1457,2517,2651}.

Macroscopy

Pineoblastomas are poorly demarcated, invasive masses of the pineal region. They are soft, friable, and pinkish grey {240,2258}. Haemorrhage and/or necrosis may be present, but calcification is rarely seen. Invasion of surrounding structures is a common finding.

Microscopy

Pineoblastomas resemble other so-called small blue round cell or primitive neuroectodermal tumours of the CNS and are composed of highly cellular, patternless sheets of densely packed small cells. The cells feature somewhat irregular nuclear shapes, a high nuclear-to-cytoplasmic ratio, hyperchromatic nuclei with

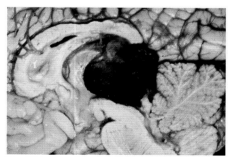

Fig. 7.14 Pineoblastoma. A large and haemorrhagic tumour localized in the pineal region and invading the third ventricle.

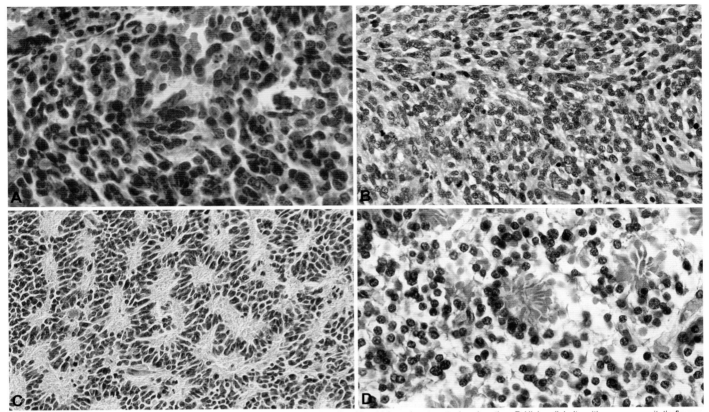

Fig. 7.15 Pineoblastoma. **A** Marked proliferation of undifferentiated neoplastic cells with a high nuclear-to-cytoplasmic ratio. **B** High cellularity with numerous mitotic figures. **C** Homer Wright rosettes. **D** Fleurettes.

an occasional small nucleolus, scant cytoplasm, and indistinct cell borders. The diffuse growth pattern is interrupted only by occasional rosettes. Pineocytomatous rosettes are lacking, but Homer Wright and Flexner–Wintersteiner rosettes may be seen. Flexner–Wintersteiner rosettes indicate retinoblastic differentiation, as do highly distinctive but infrequently occurring fleurettes. Mitotic activity varies, but is generally high, and necrosis is common {997,1187,1674,2279}.

Mixed pineocytoma–pineoblastoma
Mixed tumours are somewhat controversial neoplasms showing a biphasic pattern with distinct alternating areas resembling pineocytoma and pineoblastoma. Most importantly, areas resembling pineocytoma must be distinguished from overrun normal parenchyma {997,1638, 1811,2279}.

Pineal anlage tumours
Pineal anlage tumours are extremely rare neoplasms of the pineal region. They are often considered a peculiar variant of

pineoblastoma because of their pineal localization, primitive neuroectodermal tumour–like component, and highly aggressive clinical course. Historically, pineal anlage tumours were named after their shared histological features with melanotic neuroectodermal tumour of infancy (or retinal anlage tumour, a benign tumour typically located in the maxilla with local aggressiveness). Despite shared features with pineoblastomas, pineal anlage tumours have a distinct morphology. They are characterized by a combination of neuroectodermal and

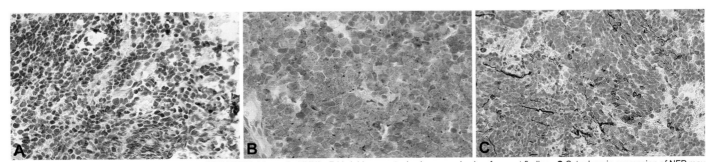

Fig. 7.16 Pineoblastoma. **A** Nuclear expression of SMARCB1 (also called INI1). **B** Variable synaptophysin expression is a frequent finding. **C** Cytoplasmic expression of NFP may be focally observed, but is rare.

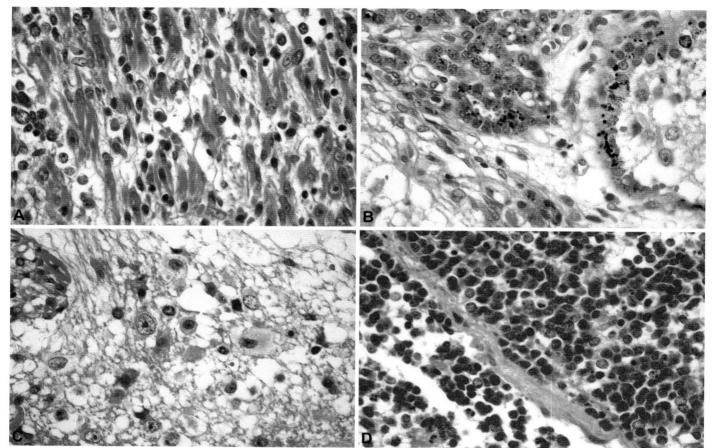

Fig. 7.17 Pineal anlage tumour. **A** Striated muscle cells. **B** Tubular structures composed of epithelioid cells containing melanin pigment. **C** Ganglion cells may be seen. **D** Area resembling pineoblastoma with sheets of small blue round cells.

heterologous ectomesenchymal components. The neuroepithelial component is characterized by pineoblastoma-like sheets or nests of small blue round cells, neuronal ganglionic/glial differentiation, and/or melanin-containing epithelioid cells. The ectomesenchymal component contains rhabdomyoblasts, striated muscle, and/or cartilaginous islands {29,177, 2288}. Given these distinctive characteristics, it is likely that pineal anlage tumour constitutes a separate entity.

Proliferation
The mean Ki-67 proliferation index in pineoblastoma ranges from 23.5% to 50.1% {91,702,754,2122}.

Electron microscopy
Characterized by a relative lack of significant differentiation, the fine structure of pineoblastoma is similar to that of any poorly differentiated neuroectodermal neoplasm. The cells are round to oval, with slightly irregular nuclei and abundant euchromatin as well as heterochromatin. The cytoplasm is scant and contains polyribosomes, few profiles of rough endoplasmic reticulum, and small mitochondria, as well as occasional microtubules, intermediate filaments, and lysosomes {1587,1674,1811}. Dense-core granules are rarely seen in the cell body {1587,1674}. Cell processes, which are poorly formed and short, may contain microtubules as well as scant dense-core granules {1587}. Bulbous endings are not seen {1674}. Junctional complexes of zonula adherens and zonula occludens type may be present between cells and processes {1185,1587,1674,1811}. Synapses are absent {1811}. Cilia with a 9 + 0 microtubular pattern are occasionally seen {1587}. Rarely, cells radially arranged around a small central lumen are encountered {1811}.

Immunophenotype
The immunophenotype of pineoblastomas is similar to that of pineocytomas and includes reactivity for neuronal, glial, and photoreceptor markers. Positivity for synaptophysin, neuron-specific enolase, NFP, class III beta-tubulin, and chromogranin-A may also be seen, as may S-arrestin staining {1187,1638,1811, 1933,2809}. Reactivity for GFAP should prompt the exclusion of entrapped reactive astrocytes. SMARCB1 is consistently expressed in pineoblastomas {1669, 2497}.

Cell of origin
Pineoblastomas share morphological and immunohistochemical features with cells of the developing human pineal gland and retina. Evidence of this ontogenetic concept includes the expression of ASMT, CRX, S-arrestin, and rhodopsin in pineal parenchymal tumours {754,1638, 2241} and the occasional association between bilateral retinoblastoma and pineoblastoma (a condition called trilateral retinoblastoma syndrome) {544}. The occasional progression from lower-grade

pineal parenchymal tumours to pineoblastomas also supports this concept {1050,1272}.

Genetic profile

Conventional cytogenetic studies in pineoblastomas have shown various numerical and structural abnormalities, but non-random aberration has not been consistently described {286}. Isochromosome 17q, a common chromosomal abnormality in medulloblastoma, has been observed in a few karyotypes of pineoblastomas, but was absent in microarray-based comparative genomic hybridization studies {1668,2122,2206}. On comparative genomic hybridization analysis, the genomic imbalance in pineoblastomas is less than has been observed in CNS primitive neuroectodermal tumours, with an average of 5.6 chromosomal changes in one study and with the changes observed being unrelated to lower-grade tumours of the pineal region {1668,2122}. No amplicon of the 19q13.42 region has been detected to date in pineal neoplasms diagnosed as pineoblastomas. Conventional cytogenetic studies and comparative genomic hybridization analyses have shown frequent structural alterations of chromosome 1 and losses involving all or part of chromosomes 9, 13, and 16 {286,1668, 2122,2206}. No aberrations of the $TP53$ or $CDKN1A$ genes have been detected {2584,2585}. Pineoblastomas are known to occur in patients with $RB1$ gene abnormalities, and the prognosis of such cases is significantly worse than that of sporadic cases {1991}; however, the status of $RB1$ in sporadic pineoblastomas is not clearly defined. In one microarray analysis of pineal parenchymal tumours, four genes ($PRAME$, $CD24$, $POU4F2$, and $HOXD13$) were significantly upregulated in pineoblastomas and high-grade pineal parenchymal tumours of intermediate differentiation {698}.

Genetic susceptibility

Pineoblastomas can occur in patients with familial (bilateral) retinoblastoma, a condition called trilateral retinoblastoma syndrome {544}, and these tumours have also been reported in patients with familial adenomatous polyposis {772,1086}. Pineoblastomas can also occur in patients with $DICER1$ germline mutations {545,2210}; in these cases, the biallelic inactivation of $DICER1$, mainly by allelic loss of the wild-type allele, may play a role in pineoblastoma pathogenesis {545,2210}.

Prognosis and predictive factors

Pineoblastoma is the most aggressive of the pineal parenchymal tumours, as evidenced by the occurrence of craniospinal seeding and (rarely) extracranial metastasis {677,997,1114,2279}. Overall survival has been short; older studies reported median values ranging from 1.3 to 2.5 years {412,677,1638}, but recent studies have reported improved median overall survival times reaching 4.1–8.7 years {671,1128}. Similarly, reported 5-year overall survival rates vary from 10% to 81%. Disseminated disease at the time of diagnosis (as determined by cerebrospinal fluid examination and MRI of the spine) {412,671,2517}, young patient age {610,1005,2517}, and partial surgical resection {1128,1457,2517} are negative prognostic predictors. Radiotherapy treatment seems to positively affect prognosis {671,1457,2279}. The 5-year survival of patients with trilateral retinoblastoma syndrome has significantly increased in the past decade (from 6% to 44%), probably due to better chemotherapy regimens and earlier detection of pineal disease {544}.

Papillary tumour of the pineal region

Jouvet A.
Vasiljevic A.
Nakazato Y.
Paulus W.
Hasselblatt M.

Definition
A neuroepithelial tumour localized in the pineal region and characterized by a combination of papillary and solid areas, with epithelial-like cells and immunoreactivity for cytokeratins (especially CK18).
Papillary tumour of the pineal region affects children and adults (mean patient age: 35 years) and presents as a large, well-circumscribed mass, often with T1-hyperintensity. The tumours are associated with frequent recurrence (occurring in 58% of cases by 5 years), but spinal dissemination is rare. Overall survival is 73% at 5 years and 71.6% at 10 years.

ICD-O code   9395/3

Grading
The biological behaviour of papillary tumour of the pineal region is variable and may correspond to WHO grades II or III, but definite histological grading criteria remain to be defined.

Epidemiology
Because these tumours are so rare, incidence data are not available. The 181 papillary tumours of the pineal region reported in the literature include examples in both children and adults {697,699,872,957,984}. Reported patient ages range from 1 to 71 years, with a median of 35 years. No sex predilection has been shown, with a male-to-female ratio of 1.06:1.

Localization
By definition, papillary tumours of the pineal region arise in the pineal region.

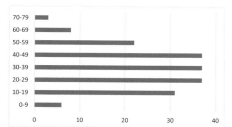

Fig. 7.18 Age distribution of papillary tumours of the pineal region, based on 181 published cases, both sexes.

Clinical features
Symptoms are non-specific, may be of short duration, and include headache due to obstructive hydrocephalus and Parinaud syndrome {676}.

Imaging
On neuroimaging, papillary tumours of the pineal region present as well-circumscribed heterogeneous masses composed of cystic and solid portions and centred by the posterior commissure or the pineal region. Aqueductal obstruction with hydrocephalus is a frequent associated finding {65,2012,2114,2248}. The tumours may demonstrate intrinsic T1-hyperintensity {392,408,2248}. In the absence of calcification, haemorrhage, melanin, or fat on imaging, this T1-hyperintensity may be related to secretory material with high protein and glycoprotein content {408}. However, others have found this feature to be absent {65,1280}. Postcontrast enhancement is usually heterogeneous.

Spread
Papillary tumour of the pineal region is characterized by frequent local recurrence (with at least one relapse in 57% of patients in one series). Spinal dissemination is reported rarely (in 7% of cases in one series) {676,1280}.

Macroscopy
Papillary tumours of the pineal region present as relatively large (20–54 mm) {696}, well-circumscribed tumours indistinguishable grossly from pineocytoma.

Microscopy
Papillary tumour of the pineal region is an epithelial-looking tumour with papillary features and more densely cellular areas, often exhibiting ependymal-like differentiation (true rosettes and tubes). Papillary tumour of the pineal region may exhibit a prominent papillary architecture or, conversely, a more solid morphology in which papillae are barely recognizable {696,984}. In papillary areas, the vessels are covered by layers of large, pale to

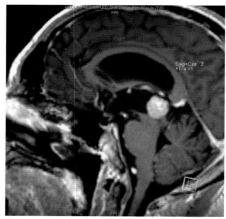

Fig. 7.19 MRI of papillary tumour of the pineal region, located in the posterior part of the third ventricle, showing contrast enhancement.

eosinophilic columnar cells. In cellular areas, cells with a somewhat clear or vacuolated cytoplasm (and occasionally with an eosinophilic periodic acid–Schiff–positive cytoplasmic mass) may also be seen. The nuclei are round to oval, with stippled chromatin; pleomorphic nuclei may be present. The mitotic count ranges from 0 to 13 mitoses per 10 high-power fields {984}. Necrotic foci may be seen. Vessels are hyalinized and often have a pseudoangiomatous morphology, with multiple lumina {696}. Microvascular proliferation is usually absent. When the pineal gland is present, there is a clear demarcation between the tumour and the adjacent gland.

Proliferation
Mitotic activity is moderate in most cases {872,1184}, with a median of 2 mitoses per 10 high-power fields reported in the largest published series {696}. Increased mitotic activity (≥ 3 mitoses per 10 high-power fields) was observed in 48% of tumours in one series {984} and in 33% of tumours in another study {696}. Marked mitotic activity (≥ 10 mitoses per 10 high-power fields) was reported in only 9% of papillary tumours of the pineal region {696,985}. In one series of 33 papillary tumours of the pineal region, the Ki-67 proliferation index ranged from 1.0% to 29.7% (median: 7.5%) {696}. In two

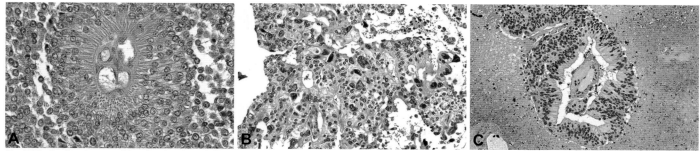

Fig. 7.20 Papillary tumour of the pineal region. **A** The vascular axes of neoplastic papillae often harbour multiple capillaries, resulting in a pseudoangiomatous appearance. **B** In some tumours, bizarre pleomorphic cells are observed; this nuclear atypia is more dystrophic in nature than related to anaplasia. **C** Neoplastic cells detached from the papillary vascularized core, leading to an apparent clear perivascular space. Note the extensive necrosis.

other series, increased proliferative activity (defined as a Ki-67 proliferation index of ≥ 10%) was observed in 39% and 40% of cases, respectively {696,984}. High proliferative activity has been linked to younger patient age {699}.

Electron microscopy
On electron microscopy, papillary tumours of the pineal region show combined ependymal, secretory, and neuroendocrine features. Papillary tumours of the pineal region are usually composed of alternating clear and dark epithelioid cells adjoined at the apical region by well-formed intercellular junctional complexes. Apical poles of cells show numerous microvilli with occasional cilia. The nuclei are oval, indented, or irregular and are frequently found at one pole of the cell. Interdigitated ependymal-like processes are seen at the basal pole of some cells and are bordered by a basement membrane. Zonation of organelles may be observed. The cytoplasm is usually rich in organelles, which include numerous clear and coated vesicles, mitochondria, and rare dense-core vesicles. Rough endoplasmic reticulum is abundant, and dilated cisternae filled with a granular secretory product may be seen. Perinuclear intermediate filaments are present in some cells {512,696,1184}.

Immunophenotype
The most distinctive immunohistochemical feature of papillary tumours of the pineal region is their reactivity for keratins (KL1, AE1/AE3, CAM5.2, and CK18), particularly in papillary structures. GFAP expression is less common than in ependymomas. Papillary tumours of the pineal region also stain for vimentin, S100 protein, neuron-specific enolase, MAP2, NCAM1, and transthyretin {957,2344}. Focal membrane or dot-like EMA staining as encountered in ependymomas is rare {957,1184,1383}. NFP immunolabelling is never seen, whereas the neuroendocrine markers synaptophysin and chromogranin-A are sometimes weakly and focally expressed {1184}. Most papillary tumours of the pineal region are characterized by the absence of staining for membranous KIR7.1, cytoplasmic stanniocalcin-1, cadherin-1, and claudin-2, markers that are frequently present in choroid plexus tumours {696,699,957}.

Cell of origin
Immunohistochemical findings (i.e. cytokeratin positivity) and ultrastructural demonstration of ependymal, secretory, and neuroendocrine organelles suggest that papillary tumours of the pineal region may originate from remnants of the specialized ependymal cells of the subcommissural organ {1184}. Further evidence for a putative origin from specialized ependymocytes of the subcommissural organ comes from the high levels of expression in papillary tumour of the pineal region of genes expressed in the subcommissural organ, including *ZFHX4*, *SPDEF*, *RFX3*, *TTR*, and *CALCA* {698, 986}. Papillary tumours of the pineal region have a claudin expression profile similar to that of the subcommissural organ in human fetuses (i.e. claudin-1 and -3 positivity and claudin-2 negativity) and rats (i.e. claudin-3 positivity) {696,2474}.

Genetic profile
In two comparative genomic hybridization studies, recurrent chromosomal imbalances included losses of chromosome 10 (in 7 of 8 cases) as well as gains on chromosomes 4 (in 6 of 8 cases) and 9 (in 7 of 8 cases) {902,957}. On high-resolution copy number analysis, losses affecting chromosome 10 were observed in all 5 cases examined; losses of chromosomes 3, 14, and 22 and gains of whole chromosomes 8, 9, and 12 were observed in > 1 case. These findings were confirmed in a recent study that

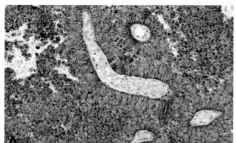
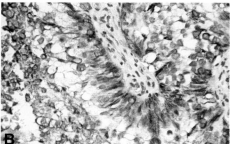
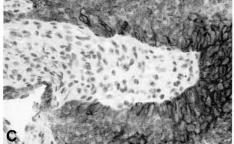

Fig. 7.21 Papillary tumour of the pineal region. **A** CK18 is expressed in the epithelial-like neoplastic cells. Immunoexpression may be diffuse (as in this example) or may predominate in perivascular areas. **B** Expression of CK18 predominates in perivascular areas. **C** NCAM1 (also called CD56) is usually strongly expressed, whereas only faint and focal immunopositivity is reported in choroid plexus tumours.

also showed distinct DNA methylation profiles differentiating papillary tumours of the pineal region from ependymomas {986}. Genetic alterations of *PTEN* (one homozygous deletion and two exon 7 point mutations) have been encountered {872}. No expression of the V600E-mutant BRAF protein has been detected by immunohistochemistry in these tumours {460}.

Genetic susceptibility

No syndromic association or evidence of genetic susceptibility has been documented.

Prognosis and predictive factors

The clinical course of papillary tumours of the pineal region is often complicated by local recurrences. In a retrospective multicentre study of 31 patients, tumour progression occurred in 72% of cases, and the 5-year estimates of overall and progression-free survival were 73% and 27%, respectively. Incomplete resection tended to be associated with decreased survival and with recurrence {699}. In an updated retrospective series of 44 patients, only gross total resection and younger patient age were associated with overall survival; radiotherapy and chemotherapy had no significant impact {676}. Another study, of 19 patients, also found no significant effect of clinical factors on overall survival or progression-free survival {984}. In that series, increased mitotic activity was significantly associated with shorter progression-free survival; patients whose tumours showed ≥ 3 mitoses per 10 high-power fields had a median progression-free survival time of 52 months (range: 8–96 months) versus 68 months (range: 66–70 months) for those whose tumours showed < 3 mitoses. Similarly, increased proliferative activity was associated with shorter progression-free survival; patients whose tumours had a Ki-67 proliferation index of ≥ 10% had a median progression-free survival time of 29 months (range: 0–64 months) versus 67 months (range: 44–90 months) for those whose tumours had a Ki-67 proliferation index of < 10%. The tumours of the 3 patients who succumbed to disease all showed increased mitotic and proliferative activity {984}. The usefulness of mitotic count or proliferation index in defining a more aggressive subset of papillary tumours of the pineal region requires confirmation in further studies. Recurrences might show higher proliferative activity {902,1447}.

CHAPTER 8

Embryonal tumours

Medulloblastomas, genetically defined

Medulloblastoma, WNT-activated

Medulloblastoma, SHH-activated

Medulloblastoma, non-WNT/non-SHH

Medulloblastomas, histologically defined

Medulloblastoma, classic

Desmoplastic/nodular medulloblastoma

Medulloblastoma with extensive nodularity

Large cell / anaplastic medulloblastoma

Embryonal tumour with multilayered rosettes, C19MC-altered

Medulloepithelioma

CNS neuroblastoma

CNS ganglioneuroblastoma

CNS embryonal tumour, NOS

Atypical teratoid/rhabdoid tumour

Medulloblastoma

Ellison D.W.
Eberhart C.G.
Pietsch T.
Pfister S.

Introduction

In this update of the WHO classification, medulloblastomas are classified according to molecular characteristics in addition to histopathological features. The molecular classification relates to the clustering of medulloblastomas into groups on the basis of transcriptome or methylome profiling and has been introduced because of its increasing clinical utility {1804}. A histopathological classification has also been retained, due to its clinical utility when molecular analysis is limited or not feasible.

Transcriptome profiling studies of medulloblastomas indicate that these tumours can be separated into several distinct molecular clusters {2524}, which by consensus have been distilled into four principal groups: WNT-activated medulloblastomas, SHH-activated medulloblastomas, group 3 medulloblastomas, and group 4 medulloblastomas.

Tumours in the WNT-activated and SHH-activated groups show activation of their respective cell signalling pathways. The four principal groups emerged from clustering analyses following transcriptome, microRNA, and methylome profiling, and there is excellent concordance across these platforms for the assignment of individual tumours {142,1804}. There are also significant associations between the four groups and specific genetic alterations and clinicopathological variables.

In the updated WHO classification, WNT-activated medulloblastomas (accounting for ~10% of cases) and SHH-activated medulloblastomas (~30% of cases) are listed separately from non-WNT/non-SHH tumours, which comprise group 3 tumours (~20% of cases) and group 4 tumours (~40% of cases). Group 3 and group 4 medulloblastomas are listed as provisional variants, because they are not as well separated as WNT-activated and SHH-activated medulloblastomas in molecular clustering analyses and by current clinical laboratory assays {448, 1335}.

2016 WHO classification of medulloblastomas
Medulloblastomas, genetically defined
Medulloblastoma, WNT-activated
Medulloblastoma, SHH-activated and *TP53*-mutant
Medulloblastoma, SHH-activated and *TP53*-wildtype
Medulloblastoma, non-WNT/non-SHH
Medulloblastoma, group 3
Medulloblastoma, group 4
Medulloblastomas, histologically defined
Medulloblastoma, classic
Desmoplastic/nodular medulloblastoma
Medulloblastoma with extensive nodularity
Large cell / anaplastic medulloblastoma
Medulloblastoma, NOS

Medulloblastoma has always been considered to be an embryonal tumour of the cerebellum. However, WNT-activated medulloblastomas are thought to arise from cells in the dorsal brain stem {831}, although not all brain stem embryonal tumours are WNT-activated medulloblastomas.

The established morphological variants of medulloblastoma (i.e. desmoplastic/nodular medulloblastoma, medulloblastoma with extensive nodularity, and large cell or anaplastic medulloblastomas) have their own particular clinical associations {619, 1603,1626,1627}. Large cell and anaplastic medulloblastomas were listed as separate variants in the previous version of the classification, but because nearly all large cell tumours also demonstrate an anaplastic component and both variants are associated with a poor outcome, they are commonly considered for clinical purposes as being in a single combined category of large cell / anaplastic medulloblastoma {2208,2664}. This association and its designation have been recognized in the update of the classification.

The molecular and morphological variants of medulloblastoma listed in the new classification demonstrate particular relationships {631}. All true desmoplastic/nodular medulloblastomas and medulloblastomas

Table 8.01 Medulloblastoma subtypes characterized by combined genetic and histological parameters

Genetic profile	Histology	Prognosis
Medulloblastoma, WNT-activated	Classic	Low-risk tumour; classic morphology found in almost all WNT-activated tumours
	Large cell / anaplastic (very rare)	Tumour of uncertain clinicopathological significance
Medulloblastoma, SHH-activated, *TP53*-mutant	Classic	Uncommon high-risk tumour
	Large cell / anaplastic	High-risk tumour; prevalent in children aged 7–17 years
	Desmoplastic/nodular (very rare)	Tumour of uncertain clinicopathological significance
Medulloblastoma, SHH-activated, *TP53*-wildtype	Classic	Standard-risk tumour
	Large cell / anaplastic	Tumour of uncertain clinicopathological significance
	Desmoplastic/nodular	Low-risk tumour in infants; prevalent in infants and adults
	Extensive nodularity	Low-risk tumour of infancy
Medulloblastoma, non-WNT/non-SHH, group 3	Classic	Standard-risk tumour
	Large cell / anaplastic	High-risk tumour
Medulloblastoma, non-WNT/non-SHH, group 4	Classic	Standard-risk tumour; classic morphology found in almost all group 4 tumours
	Large cell / anaplastic (rare)	Tumour of uncertain clinicopathological significance

Table 8.02 Characteristics of genetically defined medulloblastomas

	WNT-activated	SHH-activated		Non-WNT/non-SHH	
		TP53-wildtype	TP53-mutant	Group 3	Group 4
Predominant age(s) at presentation	Childhood	Infancy Adulthood	Childhood	Infancy Childhood	All age groups
Male-to-female ratio	1:2	1:1	1:1	2:1	3:1
Predominant pathological variant(s)	Classic	Desmoplastic/nodular	Large cell / anaplastic	Classic Large cell / anaplastic	Classic
Frequent copy number alterations	Monosomy 6	PTCH1 deletion 10q loss	MYCN amplification GLI2 amplification 17p loss	MYC amplification Isodicentric 17q	MYCN amplification Isodicentric 17q
Frequent genetic alterations	CTNNB1 mutation DDX3X mutation TP53 mutation	PTCH1 mutation SMO mutation (adults) SUFU mutation (infants) TERT promoter mutation	TP53 mutation	PVT1-MYC GFI1/GFI1B structural variants	KDM6A GFI1/GFI1B structural variants
Genes with germline mutation	APC	PTCH1 SUFU	TP53		
Proposed cell of origin	Lower rhombic lip progenitor cells	Cerebellar granule neuron cell precursors of the external granule cell layer and cochlear nucleus (Neural stem cells of the subventricular zone)*		CD133+/lineage− neural stem cells (Cerebellar granule neuron cell precursors of the external granule cell layer)*	Unknown

*Parentheses indicate a less likely origin.

with extensive nodularity align with the SHH-activated molecular group. Virtually all WNT-activated tumours have classic morphology. Most large cell / anaplastic tumours belong either to the SHH-activated group or to group 3.

Integrated diagnosis

This updated classification is intended to encourage an integrated approach to diagnosis {1535}. When molecular analysis is feasible, combined data on both molecular group and morphological variant provide optimal prognostic and predictive information. This approach is further enhanced when specific genetic data are integrated into the diagnosis, e.g. by the inclusion of TP53 gene status in the classification.

SHH-activated medulloblastomas are a heterogeneous group; a tumour with TP53 mutation and large cell / anaplastic morphology has an abysmal prognosis, in contrast to SHH-activated and TP53-wildtype medulloblastomas with extensive nodularity, which have a good clinical outcome if treated appropriately {2870}.

Some molecular genetic alterations currently used in the risk stratification of medulloblastomas, such as MYC amplification, are not included in the classification, but could nevertheless be incorporated

into an integrated diagnosis that brings together molecular group, histopathological variant, and specific genetic alteration to enhance the level of diagnostic precision.

Immunohistochemical assays that work on formalin-fixed paraffin-embedded tissue and are readily available worldwide can be used to discern some genetically defined variants of medulloblastoma and genetic alterations with clinical utility {1240}. However, the updated classification does not make specific recommendations regarding the merits of the various methods for determining molecular groups or genetic alterations.

Definition

An embryonal neuroepithelial tumour arising in the cerebellum or dorsal brain stem, presenting mainly in childhood and consisting of densely packed small round undifferentiated cells with mild to moderate nuclear pleomorphism and a high mitotic count.

Medulloblastoma is the most common CNS embryonal tumour and the most common malignant tumour of childhood. It is now classified into molecular (i.e. genetic) variants as well as morphological variants, all with clinical utility. Most medulloblastomas arise in the cerebellum, but the WNT-activated variant has

its origins in cells of the dorsal brain stem that are derived from the lower rhombic lip. Medulloblastoma variants show a broad range of morphological features, including neurocytic and ganglionic differentiation, and distinct biological behaviours. In making a diagnosis medulloblastoma, it is important to exclude histopathologically similar entities that arise in the posterior fossa, such as high-grade small cell gliomas, embryonal tumour with multilayered rosettes, and atypical teratoid/rhabdoid tumours.

Grading

Irrespective of their histological or genetic characterization, medulloblastomas correspond histologically to WHO grade IV.

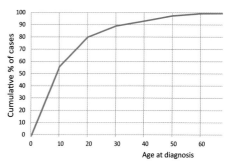

Fig. 8.01 Cumulative age distribution of medulloblastoma (both sexes), based on 831 cases (2008–2015). Data from the Brain Tumor Reference Center, Bonn.

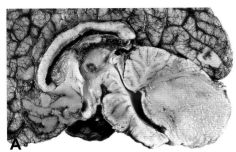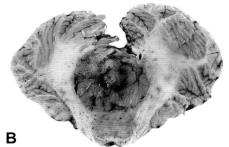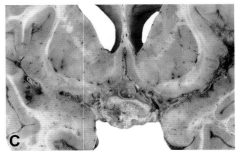

Fig. 8.02 Medulloblastoma. **A** Sagittal section. The tumour occupies mostly the lower part of the cerebellum. **B** Typical gross postmortem appearance of a medulloblastoma in the cerebellar midline, occupying the cerebellar vermis. **C** Diffuse CSF seeding by a medulloblastoma into the basal cisterns and meninges.

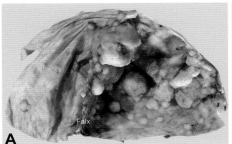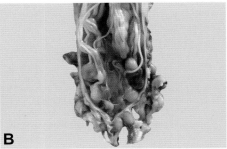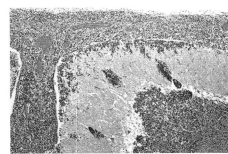

Fig. 8.03 **A** Numerous medulloblastoma metastases of various sizes on the falx cerebri and the inner surface of the dura mater covering the left cerebral hemisphere. Some smaller dural metastases are present on the contralateral side. **B** Multiple nodules in the cauda equina of the spinal cord representing CSF drop metastases of a medulloblastoma.

Fig. 8.04 Infiltration by a cerebellar medulloblastoma of the subarachnoid space. Note the clusters of tumour cells in the molecular layer, particularly in the subpial region.

Medulloblastoma, NOS

The diagnosis of medulloblastoma, NOS, is appropriate when an embryonal neural tumour is located in the fourth ventricle or cerebellum and the nature of biopsied tissue prevents classification of the tumour into one of the genetically or histologically defined categories of medulloblastoma. This situation usually arises when there is uncertainty about a tumour's architectural and cytological features as a result of insufficient tissue sampling or the presence of tissue artefacts. For the diagnosis of medulloblastoma, NOS, it is important to exclude histopathologically similar entities, such as high-grade small cell gliomas, embryonal tumour with multilayered rosettes, and atypical teratoid/rhabdoid tumours.

ICD-O code 9470/3

Epidemiology

Incidence

Medulloblastoma is the most common CNS embryonal tumour of childhood. Of all paediatric brain tumours, medulloblastoma is second in frequency only to pilocytic astrocytoma, and accounts for 25% of all intracranial neoplasms {673}. The annual overall incidence of medulloblastoma is 1.8 cases per 1 million population, whereas the annual childhood incidence is 6 cases per 1 million children; these incidence rates have not changed over time {1896}. As is the case with other high-grade brain tumours, the incidence of medulloblastoma differs across ethnicities. In the USA, overall annual incidence is highest among White non-Hispanics (2.2 cases per 1 million population), followed by Hispanics (2.1 per 1 million) and African Americans (1.5 per 1 million) [http://www.cbtrus.org/2011-NPCR-SEER/WEB-0407-Report-3-3-2011.pdf]. As many as a quarter of all medulloblastomas occur in adults, but < 1% of adult intracranial tumours are medulloblastomas {1645}.

Age and sex distribution

The median patient age at diagnosis of medulloblastoma is 9 years, with peaks in incidence at 3 and 7 years of age {2138}. Of all patients with medulloblastoma, 77% are aged < 19 years {673}. The tumour has an overall male-to-female ratio of 1.7:1. Among patients aged > 3 years, the male-to-female ratio is 2:1, but the incidence rates among boys and girls aged ≤ 3 years are equal {511,899}. The various molecular groups and histopathological variants of medulloblastoma have different age distributions {631, 1334,2524}.

Localization

Medulloblastomas grow into the fourth ventricle or are located in the cerebellar parenchyma {213}. Some cerebellar tumours can be laterally located in a hemisphere.

Clinical features

Medulloblastomas growing in the fourth ventricle cause increased intracranial pressure by exerting mass effect and blocking cerebrospinal fluid pathways. Therefore, most patients present with a short history of raised intracranial pressure: headaches that have increased in frequency and severity, frequent nausea upon waking, and bouts of vomiting. Cerebellar ataxia is common. Symptoms and signs relating to compression of cranial nerves or long tracts passing through the brain stem are uncommon.

Spread

Like other embryonal tumours, medulloblastoma has a propensity to spread through cerebrospinal fluid pathways to seed the neuraxis with metastatic tumour deposits. Rarely, it spreads to organ systems outside the CNS, particularly to bones and the lymphatic system. Reports of metastasis to the peritoneum implicate ventriculoperitoneal shunts.

Macroscopy

Most medulloblastomas arise in the region of the cerebellar vermis, as pink or grey often friable masses that fill the fourth ventricle. Medulloblastomas located in the cerebellar hemispheres tend to be firm and more circumscribed, and generally correspond to the desmoplastic/nodular variant with SHH pathway activation. Small foci of necrosis can be grossly evident, but extensive necrosis is rare. In disseminated medulloblastoma, discrete tumour nodules are often found in the craniospinal leptomeninges or cerebrospinal fluid pathways.

Microscopy

Several morphological variants of medulloblastoma are recognized, alongside the classic tumour: desmoplastic/nodular medulloblastoma, medulloblastoma with extensive nodularity, and large cell / anaplastic medulloblastoma. Their specific microscopic architectural and cytological features are described in the corresponding sections of this volume. A dominant population of undifferentiated cells with a high nuclear-to-cytoplasmic ratio and mitotic figures is a common feature, justifying the designation "embryonal", but it is important to consider other entities in the differential diagnosis. High-grade small cell gliomas and some ependymomas have an embryonal-like cytology, and elements of the embryonal tumour with multilayered rosettes or atypical teratoid/rhabdoid tumour can be identical to medulloblastoma. Any of these entities can be confused with medulloblastoma, especially in small biopsies, so determining a tumour's immunophenotype or genetic profile is an important part of working through the differential diagnosis.

Two distinctive morphological variants of medulloblastoma are described in this section, because they may occur in the

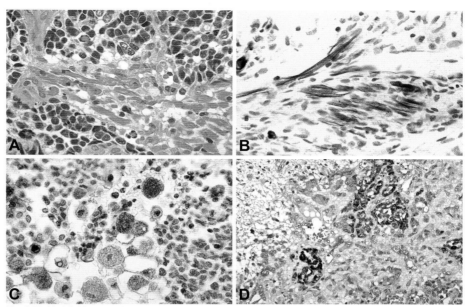

Fig. 8.05 Medulloblastoma with myogenic or melanotic differentiation. **A** Striated muscle fibres. **B** Anti–fast myosin immunostaining of highly differentiated, striated myogenic cells. **C** Biphasic pattern of small undifferentiated embryonal cells and large rhabdomyoblasts immunostaining for myoglobin. **D** Melanotic cells commonly appear as tubular epithelial structures, which are immunopositive for HMB45 and cytokeratins.

setting of a classic or large cell / anaplastic tumour and are no longer considered distinct histopathological variants. These are the rare (accounting for < 1% of cases) medulloblastoma with myogenic differentiation (previously called medullomyoblastoma) and medulloblastoma with melanotic differentiation (previously called melanocytic medulloblastoma). Although these tumours are very rare, it is not uncommon for their phenotypes to occur together.

In addition to a conventional embryonal element, medulloblastoma with myogenic differentiation contains a variable number and distribution of spindle-shaped rhabdomyoblastic cells and sometimes large cells with abundant eosinophilic cytoplasm {2211,2383}. Occasionally, elongated differentiated strap cells, with the cross-striations of skeletal muscle, are evident.

Medulloblastoma with melanotic differentiation contains a small number of melanin-producing cells, which sometimes form clumps {730,1965}. These may appear entirely undifferentiated (like other embryonal cells) or have an epithelioid phenotype. Epithelioid melanin-producing cells may form tubules, papillae, or cell clusters.

Immunophenotype

Although a few medulloblastomas express no neural antigens, the expression of markers of neuronal differentiation is common. Immunoreactivity for synaptophysin, class III beta-tubulin, or NeuN is demonstrated at least focally in most medulloblastomas. Homer Wright rosettes and nodules of neurocytic differentiation are immunopositive for these markers. In contrast, expression of NFPs is rare. GFAP-immunopositive cells are often found among the undifferentiated embryonal cells of a medulloblastoma; however, they generally show the typical spider-like appearance of reactive astrocytes and tend to be more abundant near blood vessels. These cells are usually considered to be entrapped astrocytes, although the observation of similar cells in extracerebral metastatic deposits raises the possibility that at least some are well-differentiated neoplastic astrocytes. Cells showing GFAP immunoreactivity and the cytological features of bona fide neoplasia can be observed in approximately 10% of medulloblastomas. In medulloblastoma with myogenic differentiation, cells demonstrating myogenic differentiation are immunopositive for desmin or myogenin, but not alpha-SMA. In medulloblastomas with melanotic differentiation, melanin-producing cells express HMB45 or melan-A, and the clumps of epithelioid cells associated with focal melanin production generally show immunoreactivity for cytokeratins. Nuclear SMARCB1 and SMARCA4 expression is retained in all medulloblastoma variants; the loss of expression of one of these SWI/SNF complex proteins in the context of an embryonal tumour is characteristic of atypical teratoid/rhabdoid tumour.

Genetic susceptibility

Medulloblastomas occur in the setting of several inherited cancer syndromes: naevoid basal cell carcinoma syndrome (also called Gorlin syndrome; see p. 319), Li–Fraumeni syndrome; see p. 310), mismatch repair cancer syndrome (Turcot syndrome, p. 317), Rubinstein–Taybi syndrome {249A}, and Nijmegen breakage syndrome {1058A}.

Genetic susceptibility to medulloblastoma has been documented in monozygotic twins {434}, siblings, and relatives {1065,2666}. Association with other brain tumours {673} and Wilms tumour {1846, 2062} has also been reported.

Medulloblastomas, genetically defined

Medulloblastoma, WNT-activated

Ellison D.W.
Giangaspero F.
Eberhart C.G.
Haapasalo H.
Pietsch T.
Wiestler O.D.
Pfister S.

Definition

An embryonal tumour of the cerebellum / fourth ventricle composed of small uniform cells with round or oval nuclei that demonstrate activation of the WNT signalling pathway.

Nearly all WNT-activated medulloblastomas are classic tumours. WNT-activated tumours with an anaplastic morphology have been reported, but are very rare. The WNT pathway activation that is characteristic of this medulloblastoma can be demonstrated by the accumulation of beta-catenin immunoreactivity in tumour cell nuclei, but an optimal evaluation combines this method with detection of monosomy 6 or *CTNNB1* mutation; approximately 85% of WNT-activated medulloblastomas defined by immunohistochemistry or gene expression profiling demonstrate monosomy 6 and/or harbour a *CTNNB1* mutation.

WNT-activated medulloblastoma is thought to originate from the dorsal brain stem to fill the fourth ventricle. WNT-activated tumours account for approximately 10% of all medulloblastomas. Most cases present in children aged between 7 and 14 years, but they can also occur in young adults. This variant has an excellent prognosis with standard therapeutic approaches. Besides *CTNNB1*, genes that are recurrently mutated in WNT-activated medulloblastomas include *TP53*, *SMARCA4,* and *DDX3X*.

ICD-O code   9475/3

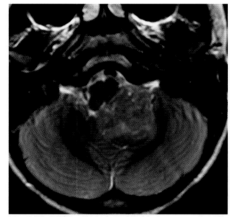

Fig. 8.06 WNT-activated medulloblastomas are usually centred on the foramen of Luschka, but tumours frequently spread along the lateral wall of the fourth ventricle and appear intraventricular.

Grading

WNT-activated medulloblastoma corresponds histologically to WHO grade IV. However, this genetically defined variant

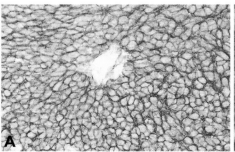
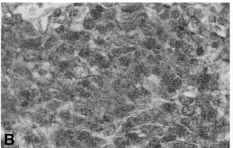
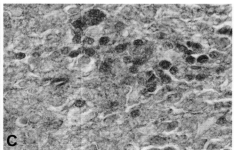

Fig. 8.07 **A** Non-WNT medulloblastoma often shows beta-catenin immunoreactivity restricted to the plasma membrane and cytoplasm. **B** WNT-activated medulloblastoma. Nuclear immunoreactivity for beta-catenin indicates activation of the WNT pathway. **C** WNT-activated medulloblastoma. Immunoreactivity for beta-catenin manifests as groups of positive nuclei in some WNT-activated medulloblastomas.

has an excellent prognosis with standard therapeutic approaches.

Epidemiology
WNT-activated tumours account for about 10% of all medulloblastomas {634, 777,1972}. They typically occur in older children and also account for a significant proportion (~15%) of adult medulloblastomas, but hardly ever occur in infants.

Localization
Some reports indicate that WNT-activated medulloblastomas are all located in the cerebellar midline, with or without close contact to the brain stem {831,2534}, and one report suggests that these tumours are more precisely localized to the cerebellar peduncle or cerebellopontine angle {1936}.

Imaging
MRI of WNT-activated medulloblastomas shows tumours located in the cerebellar midline / cerebellopontine angle, with many in close contact to the brain stem {831}.

Microscopy
Nearly all WNT-activated medulloblastomas have a classic morphology; anaplastic WNT-activated tumours have been reported, but are very rare {631}. Desmoplastic/nodular medulloblastomas do not occur in this group.

Immunophenotype
WNT-activated medulloblastomas have the same neural protein immunoprofile as other classic medulloblastomas. Their growth fraction as estimated by the Ki-67 proliferation index is also the same. Nearly all medulloblastomas show some cytoplasmic immunoreactivity for beta-catenin, but WNT-activated tumours show nuclear beta-catenin immunoreactivity in most cells, although staining can be patchy in about one quarter of cases {630,631}.

Cell of origin
WNT-activated medulloblastomas are thought to arise from cells in the dorsal brain stem that originate from the lower rhombic lip {831}. The DNA methylation fingerprint of these tumours, which might be the best evidence for cell of origin in human tissues, indicates that WNT-activated medulloblastoma has a profile distinct from those of other medulloblastoma subgroups {1049,1972,2345}.

Genetic profile
A recent meta-analysis of all large next-generation sequencing datasets showed that approximately 90% of WNT-activated medulloblastomas contained somatic mutations in exon 3 of *CTNNB1* {1804}. Other recurrently mutated genes in WNT-activated medulloblastomas include *DDX3X* (in 50% of cases), *SMARCA4* (in 26.3%), *KMT2D* (in 12.5%), and *TP53* (in 12.5%). In addition to *CTNNB1* mutation, monosomy 6 has long been established as a hallmark genetic aberration in WNT-activated medulloblastomas, occurring in approximately 85% of cases {472,1334}.

Genetic susceptibility
There is a rare association between *APC* germline mutation and WNT-activated medulloblastoma {937,1057}.

Prognosis and predictive factors
The prognosis of patients with WNT-activated medulloblastoma is excellent; with current surgical approaches and adjuvant therapy regimens, overall survival is close to 100% {634,2549}. Unlike in SHH-activated medulloblastomas, *TP53* mutations in WNT-activated medulloblastomas (which are all somatic and most commonly heterozygous) do not confer a worse prognosis {2870}. Predictive biomarkers have not yet been established within the WNT-activated molecular group.

Medulloblastoma, SHH-activated

Eberhart C.G.
Giangaspero F.
Ellison D.W.
Haapasalo H.
Pietsch T.
Wiestler O.D.
Pfister S.

Medulloblastoma, SHH-activated and TP53-mutant

Definition

An embryonal tumour of the cerebellum with evidence of SHH pathway activation and either germline or somatic TP53 mutation.

In large series of tumours, SHH-activated medulloblastomas tend to have similar transcriptome, methylome, and micro-RNA profiles. SHH pathway activation in *TP53*-mutant tumours is associated with amplification of *GLI2*, *MYCN*, or *SHH*. Mutations in *PTCH1*, *SUFU*, and *SMO* are generally absent. Large cell / anaplastic morphology and chromosome 17p loss are also common in SHH-activated and *TP53*-mutant tumours. Patterns of chromosome shattering known as chromothripsis are often present.

SHH-activated tumours account for approximately 30% of all medulloblastomas and originate from rhombic lip–derived cerebellar granule neuron precursors, the proliferation of which is dependent on SHH signalling activity. SHH-activated and *TP53*-mutant medulloblastomas are rare and generally found in children aged 4–17 years. Clinical outcomes in patients with SHH-activated and *TP53*-mutant tumours are very poor.

ICD-O code   9476/3

Medulloblastoma, SHH-activated and TP53-wildtype

Definition

An embryonal tumour of the cerebellum with molecular evidence of SHH pathway activation and an intact TP53 locus.

SHH pathway activation in *TP53*-wildtype tumours can be associated with germline or somatic mutations in the negative regulators *PTCH1* or *SUFU*, as well as activating somatic mutations in *SMO* or (rarely) amplification of *GLI2*. Desmoplastic/nodular medulloblastomas and medulloblastomas with extensive nodularity are always included in the SHH-activated group, but tumours with a hedgehog signalling pathway signature can also have

a classic or large cell / anaplastic morphology, particularly in older children. Patients with SHH-activated and *TP53*-wildtype medulloblastomas are generally children aged < 4 years, adolescents, or young adults. In addition to genetic changes activating SHH signalling, mutations in *DDX3X* or *KMT2D* and amplification of *MYCN* or *MYCL* are sometimes seen, as are deletions of chromosomal arms 9q, 10q, and 14q. Clinical outcomes in patients with SHH-activated tumours are variable.

ICD-O code   9471/3

Grading

Like all medulloblastomas, SHH-activated and *TP53*-mutant medulloblastoma and SHH-activated and *TP53*-wildtype medulloblastoma correspond histologically to WHO grade IV.

Epidemiology

SEER data from 1973–2007 suggest medulloblastoma incidence rates of 6.0 cases per 1 million children aged 1–9 years and 0.6 cases per 1 million adults aged > 19 years {2382}. SHH-activated medulloblastomas in general show a bimodal age distribution, being most common in infants and young adults, with a male-to-female ratio of approximately 1.5:1 {1804}. In contrast, SHH-activated and *TP53*-mutant tumours are generally found in children aged 4–17 years {1333}. In one study that included 133 SHH-activated medulloblastomas, 28 patients (21%) had a *TP53* mutation, and the median age of these patients was approximately 15 years {2870}.

Localization

SHH-activated medulloblastomas were proposed in one report to involve mainly the lateral cerebellum, a finding related to their origin from granule neuron precursors {831}. A subsequent study that included 17 SHH-activated medulloblastomas found that although 9 of those tumours were hemispheric, the other 8 were centred in, or significantly involved, the vermis {2534}. The localization of SHH-activated tumours may

be age-dependent. A third study found that in older children and young adults, SHH-activated medulloblastomas grow predominantly in the rostral cerebellar hemispheres, whereas in infants they more frequently involve the vermis {2716}. Specific data on the localization of SHH-activated and *TP53*-mutant or *TP53*-wildtype medulloblastoma are not yet available.

Imaging

On CT and MRI, medulloblastomas present as solid, intensely contrast-enhancing masses. SHH-activated medulloblastomas are most often identified in the lateral hemispheres, but can also involve midline structures {831,2534}. Oedema was relatively common in one imaging series that included 12 desmoplastic/nodular medulloblastomas and 9 medulloblastomas with extensive nodularity {743}. A nodular, so-called grape-like pattern on MRI often characterizes medulloblastoma with extensive nodularity because of the tumour's distinctive and diffuse nodular architecture {820,1744}. Medulloblastomas involving the peripheral cerebellar hemispheres in adults occasionally present as extra-axial lesions resembling meningiomas or acoustic nerve schwannomas {154}.

Spread

Medulloblastomas have the potential to invade locally, metastasize through the cerebrospinal fluid, or (more rarely) spread outside the CNS. Overall, SHH-activated medulloblastomas are less frequently metastatic than group 3 tumours, but spread within the neuraxis is often a presenting feature of SHH-activated and *TP53*-mutant medulloblastoma. The molecular groups of medulloblastoma, including SHH-activated tumours, have been shown to remain stable in

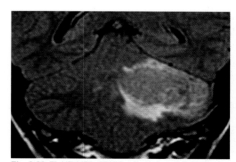

Fig. 8.08 FLAIR MRI of SHH-activated medulloblastoma. These tumours often originate from the cerebellar hemisphere.

comparisons of primary and metastatic lesions {2692}. However, *TP53* mutation can sometimes be seen in a local or distant relapse even when it is not present in the primary medulloblastoma {1003}.

Macroscopy
Some SHH-activated medulloblastomas tend to be firm and more circumscribed than other tumours, reflecting intratumoural desmoplasia. Small foci of necrosis can be grossly evident, but extensive necrosis is rare in SHH-activated tumours.

Microscopy
Desmoplastic/nodular and medulloblastoma with extensive nodularity variants of medulloblastoma are always included in the SHH-activated group, but this molecular group can also have a classic or large cell / anaplastic morphology. In one study, diffuse anaplasia was seen in 66% of all SHH-activated and *TP53*-mutant medulloblastomas, but in less than 10% of *TP53*-wildtype tumours {2870}.

Immunophenotype
Gene expression and methylation profiling remain the gold standard for defining molecular groups of medulloblastoma. However, SHH-activated medulloblastomas express a signature of activated hedgehog signalling, and several proteins have been found to be useful as surrogate markers for this activity, including GAB1 {631}, TNFRSF16 {332,1402}, and SFRP1 {1805}. One study defined a diagnostic immunohistochemical method that can distinguish between WNT-activated, SHH-activated, and non-WNT/non-SHH tumours using formalin-fixed paraffin-embedded material {631}. GAB1 and YAP1 are the immunohistochemical markers indicating SHH activation. The anti-GAB1 antibody labelled only tumours with an SHH-activated profile or *PTCH1* mutation, whereas the anti-YAP1 antibody labelled tumour cells in both WNT-activated and SHH-activated medulloblastomas, but not non-WNT/non-SHH medulloblastomas. Non-desmoplastic SHH-activated medulloblastomas generally show widespread and strong immunoreactivities for GAB1 and YAP1, whereas desmoplastic/nodular tumours display stronger staining for these proteins within internodular regions {631, 1670}.

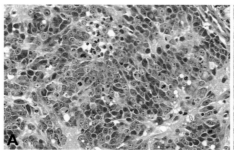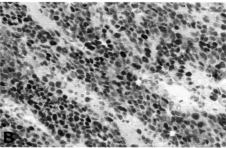

Fig. 8.09 SHH-activated and *TP53*-mutant medulloblastoma. **A** Marked anaplasia and mitotic activity, consistent with large cell / anaplastic medulloblastoma. **B** Immunoreactivity for p53, reflecting the presence of a *TP53* mutation.

Like other medulloblastomas, SHH-activated medulloblastomas can express MAP2 and synaptophysin. In SHH-activated medulloblastomas with features of medulloblastoma with extensive nodularity, strong NeuN nuclear labelling can be seen in large islands with advanced neurocytic differentiation. Pathological p53 accumulation can be detected in a small proportion of SHH-activated medulloblastomas, frequently in association with signs of cytological anaplasia. This is correlated with somatic *TP53* mutation {2482}, and can also be linked to germline *TP53* mutations (Li–Fraumeni syndrome) {2075}.

Cell of origin
SHH-activated medulloblastomas are thought to derive from ATOH1-positive cerebellar granule neuron precursors {2310,2817}. It has also been suggested that a proportion of SHH-activated medulloblastomas could arise from granule neuron precursors of the cochlear nuclei, a derivative of the auditory lower rhombic lip of the brain stem {884}. Approximately half of all patients with SHH-activated and *TP53*-mutant medulloblastoma have *TP53* mutations in the germline {2870}. This suggests that this mutation may play a key role in early transformation.

Genetic profile
Mutations and other genetic alterations activating hedgehog signalling are the main molecular drivers of SHH-activated medulloblastoma, with alterations involving known pathway genes in 116 (87%) of 133 SHH-activated tumours in a recent study {1333}. *PTCH1*, the principal gene underlying naevoid basal cell carcinoma syndrome, which predisposes patients to developing basal cell carcinoma and medulloblastoma, was mapped to 9q22 by linkage analysis. LOH in this region has also been demonstrated in many sporadic

desmoplastic/nodular medulloblastomas {2296}. PTC1 is an inhibitor of hedgehog signalling and is particularly important in cerebellar development. The pathway ligand SHH is secreted by Purkinje cells and is a major mitogen for cerebellar granule cell progenitors in the external germinal layer {2715}. Activation of the pathway occurs when the SHH ligand binds to PTC1, releasing PTC1 from SMO inhibition and activating GLI transcription factors in the primary cilia {280}. The SHH pathway can thus be aberrantly activated by loss of PTC1 function or increased activity of SHH, SMO, or GLI factors.

Early array-based expression studies identified active SHH signalling in a subset of medulloblastomas, which were often desmoplastic/nodular or medulloblastomas with extensive nodularity {2000, 2549}. Larger mRNA expression profiling experiments confirmed the existence of this group, and it was adopted as one of four principal molecular groups by an international consensus panel {2524}. Analyses of genome-wide methylation profiles have also supported the existence of a distinct SHH-activated group, and can be performed in formalin-fixed tissue {1049}. Smaller sets of SHH-associated genes measured using gene counting technology or quantitative RT-PCR can also be used to define this molecular group for the purpose of clinical classification {1808, 2355}.

Structural variations or mutations in DNA are often distinct across the various medulloblastoma molecular groups. High-level amplifications associated with the SHH-activated group include loci containing *MYCL*, *GLI2*, *PPM1D*, *YAP1*, and *MDM4* {1807}. The *MYCN* locus is often amplified in both SHH-activated and group 4 medulloblastomas. Many of these altered loci have known links to the SHH pathway. *MYCN* expression is directly regulated by GLI transcription factors in both granule cell precursors and tumours {1839}. YAP1 is also a known target and important effector of hedgehog signalling in neoplastic and non-neoplastic cerebellar progenitors {690}. Homozygous deletions at the *PTEN* and *PTCH1* loci have also been found preferentially or exclusively in SHH-activated tumours compared with other molecular groups {1807}.

Somatic mutations are relatively rare in medulloblastoma compared with other tumours, with a median of 12 non-silent and 4 silent mutations reported in one study of coding regions across 92 primary medulloblastoma/normal sample pairs {2042}. In this and a similar study {2142}, mutations in *PTCH1*, *SUFU*, and other genes associated with the hedgehog signalling pathway were found exclusively in SHH-activated tumours. However, in some SHH-activated tumours, no clear genetic explanation for SHH pathway activation can be determined.

The most common somatic point mutations are in the *TERT* promoter, resulting in increased telomerase activity. An analysis of 466 medulloblastomas revealed *TERT* mutations in 21% overall, with the highest frequency – 83% (55 of 66 cases) – identified among the adult cases of the SHH-activated group, in which they were linked to good outcomes {2098}. Point mutations in *TP53*, particularly in SHH-activated rather than WNT-activated medulloblastomas, are associated with chromothripsis, in which chromosomes shatter and acquire multiple rearrangements simultaneously in a single catastrophic event {2075}. Overall, the frequency of specific genetic changes in SHH-activated medulloblastomas seems to be somewhat different in infants, children, and adults {1333}.

Genetic susceptibility

Inherited point mutations in *TP53* in Li–Fraumeni syndrome can result in medulloblastoma, and it has been shown that these medulloblastomas belong to the SHH-activated group and are prone to chromothripsis {2075}. Patients whose SHH-activated tumours harbour *TP53*

mutation or chromothripsis should be tested for germline alterations, and this high-risk group of tumours is considered a distinct variant. Mutations in *TP53* are most commonly found in the DNA binding regions encoded by exons 4 through 8 {2870}. Approximately half of all SHH-activated and *TP53*-mutant medulloblastomas have been shown to have germline rather than somatic alterations. Although some WNT-activated medulloblastomas have mutations in *TP53*, these changes have so far been somatic {2870}.

Another inherited syndrome associated with SHH-activated medulloblastoma is naevoid basal cell carcinoma syndrome (also called Gorlin syndrome). It is characterized by multiple basal cell carcinomas of the skin, odontogenic jaw keratocysts, medulloblastoma, and developmental abnormalities. Most naevoid basal cell carcinoma syndrome cases are due to heterozygous germline mutations in *PTCH1*, with mutations identified in 97 of 171 patients (56%) in one study {2376}. However, mutations in *PTCH1* and *TP53* are thought to be mutually exclusive {1333}. The age distributions of these groups also differ; medulloblastomas with germline *PTCH1* or *SUFU* mutations present in infants and children aged < 4 years, whereas those with a germline *TP53* mutation occur in older children.

Prognosis and predictive factors

SHH-activated and *TP53*-mutant medulloblastomas are associated with a very poor outcome. In one study, the 5-year overall survival of patients with an SHH-activated medulloblastoma was 76% for those with a *TP53*-wildtype tumour and 41% for those with a *TP53*-mutant tumour {2870}. Known clinical high-risk factors, such as metastatic disease, are also associated with *TP53* mutation within the SHH-activated group. It is becoming increasingly clear that some genetic prognostic markers must be interpreted within the context of molecular group. For example, although *TP53* mutations were found in 16% of WNT-activated tumours and 21% of SHH-activated

tumours, they were significantly associated with a poor prognosis only in SHH-activated tumours {2870}.

Patient outcome with SHH-activated and *TP53*-wildtype medulloblastomas is varied and shows a significant association with pathological features. Medulloblastomas with extensive nodularity in infants are noted for a good prognosis, and most desmoplastic/nodular tumours in this young age group also have a relatively good outcome {2208}. The situation for SHH-activated and *TP53*-wildtype medulloblastomas with a classic or large cell / anaplastic morphology is less clear, though these appear to have a worse outcome than the two types of desmoplastic medulloblastoma, at least in infancy.

Molecular factors predicting response to therapies targeting SHH are beginning to emerge. Small-molecule inhibitors that act on the SMO receptor have been shown to be effective in some medulloblastomas with hedgehog activation, but not in other molecular groups {2143,2355}. However, SHH-activated medulloblastoma can also be resistant to SMO inhibitors, due to activation of the pathway downstream of pharmacological blockade. Such downstream activation can be present at diagnosis or can develop as a therapeutic resistance mechanism. It has been suggested that the genetic mechanism of pathway activation is linked to the likelihood of response to SMO inhibition {1333,2143}. Adults with SHH-activated medulloblastoma are more likely to harbour activating alterations in *PTCH1* or *SMO* resulting in tumours sensitive to SMO inhibitors, whereas SHH-activated medulloblastomas from infants and children (including SHH-activated and *TP53*-mutant tumours) often contain downstream alterations in *SUFU*, *GLI2*, and *MYCN* that are refractory to these pharmacological agents. It has been suggested that DNA-damaging alkylating agents and radiation should be avoided whenever possible when treating patients with a germline *TP53* mutation {2075}.

Medulloblastoma, non-WNT/non-SHH

Ellison D.W.
Eberhart C.G.
Pfister S.

Definition

An embryonal tumour of the cerebellum consisting of poorly differentiated cells and excluded from the WNT-activated and SHH-activated groups by molecular testing.
Non-WNT/non-SHH medulloblastomas are either group 3 or group 4 medulloblastomas. These are classic or large cell / anaplastic tumours that cluster into two groups in terms of transcriptome, methylome, and microRNA profiles as analysed across large series of medulloblastomas. Distinct methylome profiles probably reflect a different histogenesis of the four medulloblastoma groups, although tumours from groups 3 and 4 are more similar to each other than to WNT-activated or SHH-activated medulloblastomas (see Table 8.01, p. 184).

The group 3 transcriptome profile is characterized by relatively high expression of *MYC*, and *MYC* amplification is overrepresented in this molecular group. Group 4 tumours are characterized by recurrent alterations in *KDM6A* and *SNCAIP*, as well as in other genes. Non-WNT/non-SHH tumours account for approximately 60% of all medulloblastomas and typically have classic histopathological features. Most non-WNT/non-SHH tumours present in childhood; they are relatively uncommon in infants and adults.

ICD-O code   9477/3

Epidemiology

Group 3 medulloblastomas account for approximately 20% of all cases, and for a higher proportion of cases (~45%) in infants. Group 3 medulloblastoma is exceedingly rare in adults {1334}. Group 4 medulloblastomas are the largest molecular group, accounting for about 40% of all tumours. Peak incidence occurs in patients aged 5–15 years, with lower incidence in infants and adults {1807}.

Spread

Metastatic disease is present in about 40% of group 3 tumours at the time of diagnosis, a presentation that is a particular feature of group 3 medulloblastomas in infancy {1334,1804}.

Microscopy

Most non-WNT/non-SHH medulloblastomas have a classic morphology. These tumours occasionally exhibit areas of rosette formation or a palisading pattern of tumour cell nuclei. Nodule formation can occur in the absence of desmoplasia in non-WNT/non-SHH medulloblastomas. A reticulin preparation demonstrates no strands of collagen around or between the nodules, which otherwise show neurocytic differentiation and a reduced growth fraction, in a similar manner to nodules associated with desmoplasia in desmoplastic/nodular medulloblastoma or medulloblastoma with extensive nodularity. Large cell / anaplastic tumours in the non-WNT/non-SHH molecular group generally belong to group 3.

Immunophenotype

The neural marker immunohistochemical profile of non-WNT/non-SHH medulloblastoma is the same as those of classic or large cell / anaplastic tumours in the WNT-activated or SHH-activated groups. The tumours express synaptophysin to

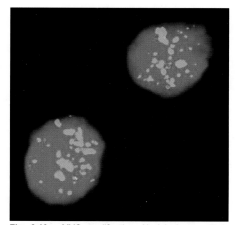

Fig. 8.10 *MYC* amplification. Nuclei show multiple clumped *MYC* signals indicative of double minutes (green). The red signals from centromeric probes indicate chromosome 8 copy number.

a variable extent, and tumour cells are rarely immunopositive for GFAP. With a panel of three antibodies (to beta-catenin, GAB1, and YAP1), non-WNT/non-SHH tumours show cytoplasmic (but not nuclear) beta-catenin immunoreactivity, and the tumour cells are immunonegative for GAB1 and YAP1 {631}.

Genetic profile

Overexpression of *MYC* is a cardinal feature of group 3 medulloblastomas, and *MYC* amplification (often accompanied by *MYC-PVT1* fusion {1807}) is relatively common among group 3 medulloblastomas. However, *MYC* amplification is found mainly in infant disease, and occurs in < 25% of group 3 tumours overall {632, 1426}. Other recurrently mutated or focally amplified genes include *SMARCA4* (altered in 10.5% of cases), *OTX2* (in 7.7%), *CTDNEP1* (in 4.6%), *LRP1B* (in 4.6%), and *KMT2D* (in 4%) {1804}. Two recurrent oncogenes in group 3 medulloblastomas are the homologues *GFI1* and *GFI1B*, which are activated through a mechanism called enhancer hijacking {1806}. By far the most common cytogenetic aberrations in medulloblastoma (occurring in ~80% of group 4 tumours) involve copy number alterations on chromosome 17: 17p deletion, 17q gain, or a combination of these in the form of an isodicentric 17q {631,1334, 1804}. The most frequently mutated or focally amplified genes in group 4 tumours are *KDM6A* (altered in 13% of cases), the locus around *SNCAIP* (in 10.4%), *MYCN* (in 6.3%), *KMT2C* (in 5.3%), *CDK6* (in 4.7%), and *ZMYM3* (in 3.7%) {1804}. Activated GFI oncogenes have also been observed in a subset of group 3/4 tumours that do not cluster reliably into one or other group {1806}.

Prognosis and predictive factors

MYC amplification has long been established as a genetic alteration associated with poor outcome in patients with medulloblastoma {620,632,2268}. This observation is reflected in the relatively poor outcome of group 3 medulloblastomas, but *MYC* amplification has prognostic significance even among group 3 tumours {2345}. Metastatic disease at the time of presentation, which is associated with poor outcome, seems to be the most robust prognostic marker among group 4 tumours {2345}.

Medulloblastomas, histologically defined

Medulloblastoma, classic

Ellison D.W.
Eberhart C.G.
Giangaspero F.
Haapasalo H.

Pietsch T.
Wiestler O.D.
Pfister S.

Definition
An embryonal neuroepithelial tumour arising in the cerebellum or dorsal brain stem, consisting of densely packed small round undifferentiated cells with mild to moderate nuclear pleomorphism and a high mitotic count.

Classic medulloblastomas lack significant intratumoural desmoplasia, the marked nuclear pleomorphism of the anaplastic variant, and the cytological features of the large cell variant. Classic medulloblastomas account for 72% of all medulloblastomas. They occur throughout the patient age range of medulloblastoma, from infancy to adulthood, but predominantly in childhood, and are found in all four molecular medulloblastoma groups.

ICD-O code
9470/3

Epidemiology
The classic medulloblastoma is more frequent than its variants in childhood, but is less common than desmoplastic/nodular medulloblastoma in infants and adults.

Microscopy
Classic medulloblastomas are the archetypal CNS small blue round cell tumour. They consist of a syncytial arrangement of densely packed undifferentiated embryonal cells. Mitotic figures and apoptotic bodies are found among the tumour cells. Intratumoural desmoplasia is lacking, but pericellular desmoplasia is induced where tumour cells invade the leptomeninges. Homer Wright rosettes are found in some classic (and large cell / anaplastic) medulloblastomas.

Occasionally, nodules of neurocytic differentiation and reduced cell proliferation are evident in some areas of classic tumours, but these are never associated with internodular desmoplasia or perinodular collagen when examined in a reticulin preparation. Additionally, these non-desmoplastic nodular medulloblastomas are non-WNT/non-SHH tumours, unlike desmoplastic/nodular tumours, which belong to the SHH-activated group.

Immunophenotype
Classic medulloblastomas express various non-specific neural markers, such as NCAM1, MAP2, and neuron-specific enolase. Most cases are immunopositive for synaptophysin and NeuN, but these neuronal markers may also be absent. Immunoreactivity for NFPs is very rare. Cells showing GFAP expression and an embryonal morphology can be observed in as many as 10% of medulloblastomas {314}. When present, these cells are infrequent and tend to be scattered throughout the tumour, which is unlike the pattern of GFAP immunoreactivity in small-cell astrocytic tumours.

Nuclear SMARCB1 and SMARCA4 expression is retained in all medulloblastoma types; the loss of expression of one of these SWI/SNF complex proteins is diagnostic of atypical teratoid/rhabdoid tumour.

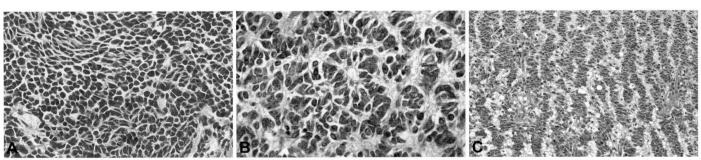

Fig. 8.11 Histopathological features of the classic medulloblastoma. **A** Typical syncytial arrangement of undifferentiated tumour cells. **B** Area with Homer Wright (neuroblastic) rosettes. **C** Arrangement of tumour cells in parallel rows (spongioblastic pattern).

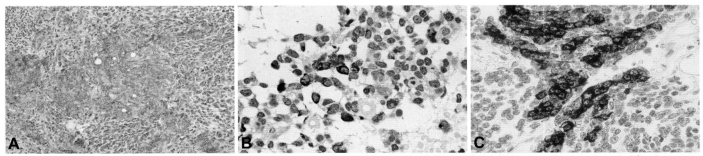

Fig. 8.12 Medulloblastoma. **A** Focal expression of synaptophysin. **B** Focal GFAP staining of tumour cells. **C** Clusters of medulloblastoma cells expressing retinal S-antigen.

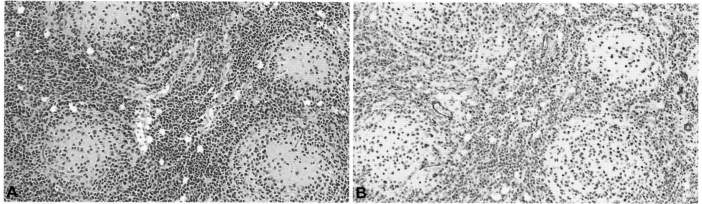

Fig. 8.13 A Classic medulloblastoma with nodules but (B) no desmoplasia. Reticulin stain. These medulloblastomas belong to the non-WNT/non-SHH molecular group and should not be confused for desmoplastic/nodular medulloblastomas.

Desmoplastic/nodular medulloblastoma

Pietsch T.
Ellison D.W.
Haapasalo H.
Giangaspero F.
Wiestler O.D.
Pfister S.
Eberhart C.G.

Definition

An embryonal neural tumour arising in the cerebellum and characterized by nodular, reticulin-free zones and intervening densely packed, poorly differentiated cells that produce an intercellular network of reticulin-positive collagen fibres.

Desmoplastic/nodular medulloblastoma is characterized by specific clinical, genetic, and biological features. It occurs in the cerebellar hemispheres and the midline and has a bimodal patient age distribution, with a relatively high incidence in young children and adolescents, as well as among adults. In early childhood, it is associated with naevoid basal cell carcinoma syndrome (also called

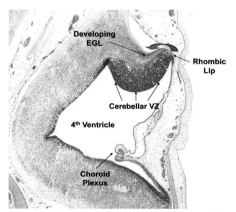

Fig. 8.14 The developing human posterior fossa. EGL, external granule layer; VZ, ventricular zone.

Gorlin syndrome). Desmoplastic/nodular medulloblastoma displays pathological activation of the SHH pathway, which is caused by mutations in genes that encode components of the pathway, such as *PTCH1*, *SMO*, and *SUFU*. Genetic and histological features of classic medulloblastoma, such as isochromosome 17q and neuroblastic rosettes, are absent. Desmoplastic/nodular medulloblastoma overlaps histologically with MBEN, which contains large irregular reticulin-free regions of neurocytic differentiation between narrow desmoplastic strands of proliferating embryonal cells. Desmoplastic/nodular medulloblastoma is associated with a more favourable outcome in young children than are non-desmoplastic variants of medulloblastoma.

ICD-O code   9471/3

Grading

Like all medulloblastomas, desmoplastic/nodular medulloblastoma corresponds histologically to WHO grade IV.

Epidemiology

Desmoplastic/nodular medulloblastomas are estimated to account for 20% of all medulloblastomas {1972}. In children aged < 3 years, desmoplastic/nodular medulloblastoma accounts for 47–57% of

all cases {1627,2207}. In one retrospective cohort of adult patients, desmoplastic/nodular medulloblastoma constituted 21% of all medulloblastomas {1347}.

Localization

Unlike most classic (non-WNT) medulloblastomas, which are restricted to the midline, desmoplastic/nodular medulloblastoma may arise in the cerebellar hemispheres and in the vermis. Most medulloblastomas occurring in the cerebellar hemispheres are of the desmoplastic/nodular type {332}.

Imaging

On MRI, desmoplastic/nodular medulloblastomas present as solid, frequently contrast-enhancing masses. Tumours involving the peripheral cerebellar hemispheres in adults occasionally present as extra-axial lesions.

Spread

Tumours can relapse locally, metastasize via cerebrospinal fluid pathways, and in rare cases spread to extra-CNS sites

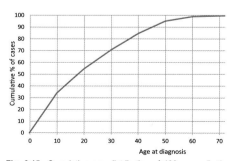

Fig. 8.15 Cumulative age distribution of 180 cases (both sexes). Data from the Brain Tumor Reference Center, Bonn.

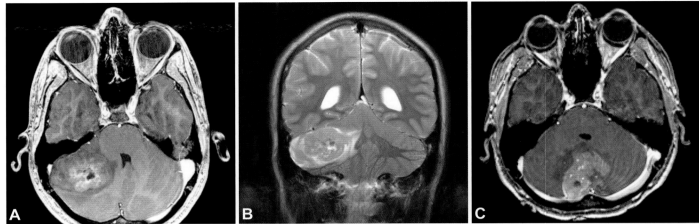

Fig. 8.16 Desmoplastic/nodular medulloblastoma. **A** T1-weighted, (**B**) T2-weighted contrast-enhanced MRI of tumours in the cerebellar hemisphere. **C** T1-weighted, contrast-enhanced MRI of a tumour in the vermis.

such as the skeletal system. At diagnosis, metastatic disease is found less frequently with desmoplastic/nodular medulloblastomas than with other variants.

Microscopy

Desmoplastic/nodular medulloblastoma is characterized by nodular, reticulin-free zones (so-called pale islands) surrounded by densely packed, undifferentiated, highly proliferative cells with hyperchromatic and moderately pleomorphic nuclei, which produce a dense intercellular reticulin fibre network {818, 1234}. In rare cases, this defining pattern is not present throughout the entire tumour and there is instead a more

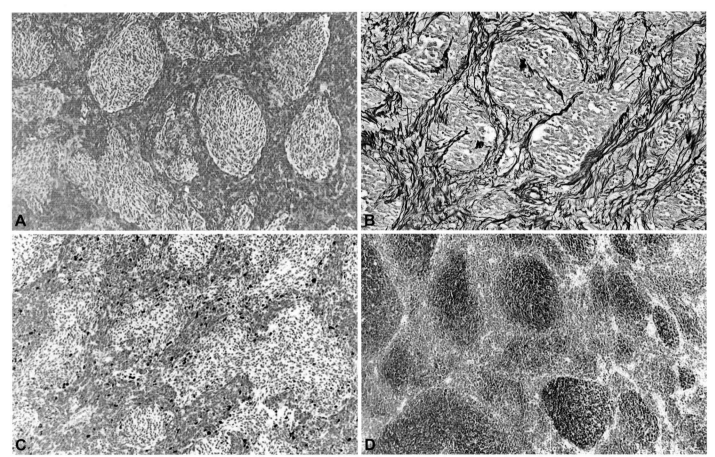

Fig. 8.17 Desmoplastic/nodular medulloblastoma. **A** Pale nodular areas surrounded by densely packed hyperchromatic cells. **B** Reticulin silver impregnation showing the reticulin-free pale islands. **C** MIB1 monoclonal antibody staining shows that the proliferative activity predominates in the highly cellular, intermodal areas. **D** Neuronal differentiation, shown by immunoreactivity for neuron-specific enolase, occurs mainly in the pale islands.

syncytial arrangement of non-desmoplastic embryonal cells present in a few areas. The nodules contain tumour cells with features of variable neurocytic maturation embedded in a neuropil-like fibrillary matrix. The level of mitotic activity in the nodules is lower than in the internodular areas. Neuroblastic rosettes are not found in desmoplastic/nodular medulloblastoma. Tumours with small nodules can easily be overlooked if no reticulin staining is performed. Medulloblastomas that show only an increased amount of reticulin fibres (without a nodular pattern) or that show a focal nodular pattern without desmoplasia are not classified as desmoplastic/nodular medulloblastoma {1627}; the two characteristic features must occur together for a diagnosis of desmoplastic/nodular medulloblastoma.

Immunophenotype
The nodules in desmoplastic/nodular medulloblastoma show variable expression of neuronal markers, including synaptophysin and NeuN. Nodules with very strong NeuN expression, which is an indicator of advanced neurocytic differentiation, are typical of medulloblastoma with extensive nodularity, but can also occur in the desmoplastic/nodular variant. The Ki-67 proliferation index is much higher in internodular areas than in nodules {1627}. Activation of the SHH pathway can be inferred by immunohistochemistry for specific targets, such as GAB1 and TNFRSF16 {631,1402}. These markers are expressed predominantly in internodular areas. GFAP expression can be found specifically in tumour cells in a subset of cases {332}. Widespread and strong nuclear accumulation of p53, suggesting a *TP53* mutation, can be detected in rare desmoplastic/nodular medulloblastomas, frequently in association with signs of cytological anaplasia. This finding can accompany either somatic or germline *TP53* alteration (Li–Fraumeni syndrome) {2075,2482}.

Cell of origin
Desmoplastic/nodular medulloblastomas are derived from granule cell progenitor cells forming the external granule cell layer during cerebellar development {332}. These progenitors are dependent

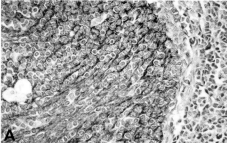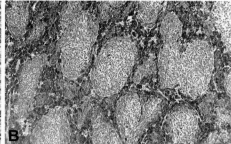

Fig. 8.18 Desmoplastic/nodular medulloblastoma. **A** The nodules represent zones of neuronal maturation and show intense immunoreactivity for synaptophysin. **B** SHH activation can be visualized by immunohistochemistry with antibodies against SHH targets, in this case, with antibodies against TNFRSF16 (also called p75-NGFR) {332,1401}, which is strongly expressed in the synaptophysin-negative internodular areas.

on SHH (produced by Purkinje cells) as a mitogen {2715}.

Genetic profile
Desmoplastic/nodular medulloblastoma displays pathological activation of the SHH pathway, which is often caused by mutations in genes encoding members of the pathway, including *PTCH1*, *SMO*, and *SUFU* {1422,1973,2523}. In a recent analysis using next-generation sequencing, 85% of desmoplastic/nodular medulloblastomas carried genetic alterations in *PTCH1*, *SUFU*, *SMO*, *SHH*, *GLI2*, or *MYCN*. This study showed a predominance of *SUFU* and *PTCH1* mutations in young children, whereas *PTCH1* and *SMO* mutations were more common in adults {1333}. Rare mutations in other genes (e.g. *LDB1*) have also been described. Recurrent *DDX3X* mutations, as well as *TERT* promoter mutations, have been identified. Allelic losses of regions on chromosomes 9q and 10q are found in some desmoplastic/nodular medulloblastomas {2296}, whereas isochromosome 17q, which is a marker of midline classic (non-WNT) and large cell / anaplastic medulloblastomas, is absent from desmoplastic/nodular medulloblastoma {1334}.

Genetic susceptibility
Naevoid basal cell carcinoma syndrome (also called Gorlin syndrome) is caused mainly by heterozygous germline mutations in *PTCH1* and rarely by germline mutations in *SUFU* or *PTCH2* {2376}. Medulloblastomas occurring in the context of naevoid basal cell carcinoma

syndrome are mainly desmoplastic variants (i.e. desmoplastic/nodular medulloblastoma or medulloblastoma with extensive nodularity) {67}. It has been shown that the risk of medulloblastoma in *PTCH1*-related naevoid basal cell carcinoma syndrome is approximately 2%, and that the risk is 20 times the value in *SUFU*-related naevoid basal cell carcinoma syndrome {2376}. In children with *SUFU*-related naevoid basal cell carcinoma syndrome, brain MRI surveillance is highly recommended {2376}. Germline mutations of *SUFU* have also been described in patients with desmoplastic medulloblastomas that do not fulfil the diagnostic criteria for naevoid basal cell carcinoma syndrome {294}. The families of infants with desmoplastic medulloblastomas should be offered genetic counselling because of the high frequency of germline alterations and naevoid basal cell carcinoma syndrome {787}.

Prognosis and predictive factors
In most cases, desmoplastic/nodular medulloblastoma in early childhood has an excellent outcome with surgery and chemotherapy alone {2207}. In a meta-analysis of prognostic factors in infant medulloblastoma, progression-free or overall survival at 8 years was significantly better for desmoplastic variants than for other medulloblastomas {2208}. No survival difference between desmoplastic/nodular medulloblastoma and classic medulloblastoma was found in a European multicentre trial involving older children with standard-risk medulloblastoma {1431}.

Medulloblastoma with extensive nodularity

Giangaspero F.
Ellison D.W.
Eberhart C.G.
Haapasalo H.

Pietsch T.
Wiestler O.D.
Pfister S.

Definition

An embryonal tumour of the cerebellum characterized by many large reticulin-free nodules of neurocytic cells against a neuropil-like matrix and by narrow internodular strands of poorly differentiated tumour cells in a desmoplastic matrix.

In the medulloblastoma with extensive nodularity (MBEN), the internodular reticulin-rich component with embryonal cells is a minor element. This variant occurs predominantly in infants and is associated with a favourable outcome with current treatment regimens.

MBEN is closely related to desmoplastic/nodular medulloblastoma, with which it overlaps histopathologically and genetically; both variants are SHH-activated tumours. MBEN is associated with naevoid basal cell carcinoma syndrome (also called Gorlin syndrome).

ICD-O code   9471/3

Grading

Like all medulloblastomas, MBEN corresponds histologically to WHO grade IV.

Epidemiology

In large series, medulloblastomas with extensive nodularity account for 3.2–4.2% of all medulloblastoma variants overall {619,1972}, but in children aged

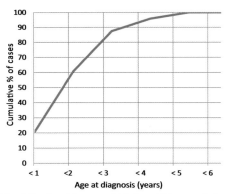

Fig. 8.19 Cumulative age distribution of 24 cases (both sexes). Data from the Brain Tumor Reference Center, Bonn.

< 3 years (in whom desmoplastic/nodular medulloblastomas account for as many as 50% of cases {1627,2207}), medulloblastoma with extensive nodularity has been reported to account for 20% of all cases {787}.

Localization

More than 80% of medulloblastomas with extensive nodularity are located in the vermis {787}. This localization contrasts with that of desmoplastic/nodular medulloblastoma, which more frequently involves the cerebellar hemispheres.

Imaging

On MRI, medulloblastoma with extensive nodularity presents as a very large multinodular lesion with enhancing grape-like structures involving the vermis and sometimes the cerebellar hemispheres {2821}. Rare cases have a peculiar gyriform presentation, in which the cerebellar folia are well-delineated and enlarged, with contrast enhancement {25,787}. Downward herniation of the cerebellar tonsils and effacement of the cisternal spaces of the posterior fossa can be observed.

Spread

Medulloblastoma with extensive nodularity can relapse locally or (rarely) can metastasize via cerebrospinal fluid pathways. However, such cases seem to respond well to subsequent treatment and have a favourable prognosis {820,2208}.

Microscopy

Medulloblastoma with extensive nodularity differs from the related desmoplastic/nodular variant in that is has an expanded lobular architecture due to the fact that the reticulin-free zones become unusually enlarged and rich in neuropil-like tissue. These zones contain a population of small cells with round nuclei, which show neurocytic differentiation and exhibit a streaming pattern. Mitotic activity is low or absent in these neurocytic areas. The internodular component is markedly reduced in some areas {820,1627,2459}. After radiotherapy and/or chemotherapy, medulloblastomas with extensive nodularity occasionally undergo further

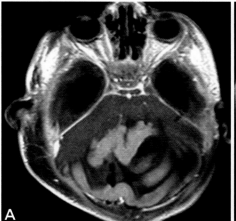
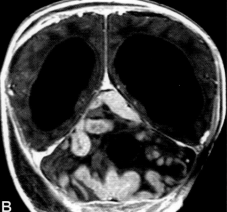
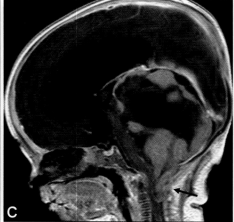

Fig. 8.20 Medulloblastoma with extensive nodularity. **A** Multinodular and gyriform pattern. **B** In a 1-month-old girl, the gadolinium-enhanced sagittal T1-weighted MRI shows a huge lesion involving both cerebellar hemispheres and the vermis. The lesion has a multinodular and gyriform pattern of enhancement. **C** Note the downward herniation of the tumour through the foramen magnum (arrow) and the marked effacement of the cisternal spaces of the posterior fossa. There is also supratentorial hydrocephalus and macrocrania.

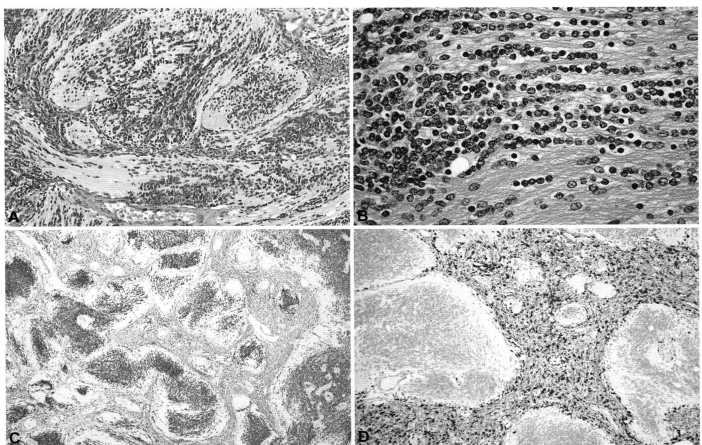

Fig. 8.21 Medulloblastoma with extensive nodularity. **A** Lobular architecture with large, elongated, reticulin-free zones. **B** Elongated, reticulin-free zones containing streams of small round neurocytic cells on a fibrillary background. **C** Strong immunoreactivity for NeuN in neurocytic cells of pale islands. **D** High MIB1 immunolabelling in internodular regions, contrasting with minimal proliferation in pale islands.

maturation into tumours dominated by ganglion cells {419,538}.

Immunophenotype

Like in desmoplastic/nodular medulloblastomas, the neuropil-like tissue and the differentiated neurocytic cells within nodules are strongly immunoreactive for synaptophysin and NeuN and the Ki-67 proliferation index is much higher in internodular areas {1627}. Activation of the SHH pathway can be demonstrated by immunohistochemistry for specific targets such as GAB1 {631} or TNFRSF16 {1402}.

Cell of origin

Medulloblastoma with extensive nodularity, like most SHH-activated medulloblastomas, seems to be derived from ATOH1-positive cerebellar granule neuron precursors {2310,2817}.

Genetic profile

Medulloblastoma with extensive nodularity carries mutations in genes encoding members of the SHH pathway. Most cases harbour a *SUFU* mutation {294}. However, a recent study of 4 medulloblastomas with extensive nodularity found a *PTCH1* mutation in 2 of the tumours and an *SUFU* and *SMO* mutation in one each of the other 2 tumours {1333}.

Genetic susceptibility

In the majority of cases, naevoid basal cell carcinoma syndrome is caused by germline mutations of *PTCH1*. In a few cases, germline mutations instead occur in *SUFU* {2376} or *PTCH2* {667,747}. Naevoid basal cell carcinoma syndrome is diagnosed in 5.8% of all patients with medulloblastoma, but in 22.7% of patients with a desmoplastic/nodular tumour variant and 41% of patients with medulloblastoma with extensive nodularity. The risk of medulloblastoma in *PTCH1*-related naevoid basal cell carcinoma syndrome is approximately 2%, and the risk is 20 times the value in *SUFU*-related naevoid basal cell carcinoma syndrome {294,1333}. In children with

SUFU-related naevoid basal cell carcinoma syndrome, neuroimaging surveillance is recommended {2376}. Families with children that present with MBEN should be offered genetic counselling because of the high frequency of naevoid basal cell carcinoma syndrome {787,2376}.

Prognosis and predictive factors

Medulloblastoma with extensive nodularity has an excellent outcome in the majority of cases {787,1603,2208}. In an international meta-analysis of survival and prognostic factors in infant medulloblastoma, the progression-free and overall survival rates of 21 cases of medulloblastoma with extensive nodularity at 8 years were 86% and 95%, respectively {2208}. Metastatic disease at presentation did not affect the favourable prognosis, suggesting that a diagnosis of medulloblastoma with extensive nodularity confers a better outcome regardless of adverse clinical features {2208}.

Large cell / anaplastic medulloblastoma

Ellison D.W.
Giangaspero F.
Eberhart C.G.
Haapasalo H.

Pietsch T.
Wiestler O.D.
Pfister S.

Definition
An embryonal neural tumour of the cerebellum or dorsal brain stem characterized by undifferentiated cells with marked nuclear pleomorphism, prominent nucleoli, cell wrapping, and high mitotic and apoptotic counts.

Large cell / anaplastic (LC/A) medulloblastoma demonstrates severe anaplasia or a large cell phenotype across the majority of the tumour. 'Severe anaplasia' combines marked nuclear pleomorphism with abundant mitotic activity and apoptosis {619,1626}. The large cell phenotype manifests uniform round nuclei with prominent nucleoli. Intratumoural desmoplasia is not a feature of this variant, but desmoplasia can be evident when tumour cells overrun the leptomeninges. By definition, classic morphology, with only mild to moderate nuclear pleomorphism, cannot be present across a majority of the tumour.

Anaplastic and large cell medulloblastomas were initially described as separate variants, but the pure large cell tumour is extremely rare; most large cell medulloblastomas also contain regions of anaplasia {288,619,821,1626}. Both morphological variants are associated with a poor outcome with standard therapies, as well as with amplification of *MYC* or *MYCN*, although these associations are not strong and depend on the tumour's molecular group. For clinical purposes, the two variants are regarded as equivalent, so are now combined as the large cell / anaplastic (LC/A) variant {822,1671, 2664}. This variant accounts for approximately 10% of all medulloblastomas and occurs across the patient age range of the medulloblastoma.

ICD-O code   9474/3

Grading
Like all medulloblastomas, LC/A medulloblastoma corresponds histologically to WHO grade IV.

Epidemiology
Large cell / anaplastic medulloblastomas are found across all molecular groups of the disease, accounting for about 10% of all tumours {619,1626}. They can occur in patients of any age. Considered separately, anaplastic medulloblastomas are about 10 times as prevalent as large cell medulloblastomas {630}. They are most frequent among group 3 and SHH-activated medulloblastomas; LC/A tumours hardly ever occur in the WNT-activated group.

Microscopy
Anaplasia as a feature of an embryonal tumour was first proposed for medulloblastomas with marked nuclear pleomorphism accompanied by particularly high mitotic and apoptotic counts {288, 619}. Nuclear moulding and cell wrapping are additional features. Large cell medulloblastoma lacks the variability in cell size and shape that characterizes the anaplastic variant {821,1626}; its cells are large and monomorphic with prominent nucleoli, but it shows the high rate of cell turnover seen in anaplastic tumours. Nearly all large cell medulloblastomas contain regions with an anaplastic phenotype; the pure form is rare.

Genetic profile
Large cell / anaplastic medulloblastomas are found mainly among group 3 or SHH-activated medulloblastomas. Among group 3 medulloblastomas, which overexpress *MYC*, large cell / anaplastic morphology (in particular the large cell phenotype) is associated with *MYC* amplification {620}. SHH-activated LC/A tumours are particularly associated with *GLI2* and *MYCN* amplification, *TP53* mutations (which are often germline), and specific patterns of chromosome shattering called chromothripsis {1333,2075}.

Prognosis and predictive factors
At the time the tumours were first described, large cell and anaplastic medulloblastomas were strongly suspected to behave more aggressively than classic tumours, often presenting with metastatic disease {288,821}. In retrospective studies of patients in trial cohorts, large cell / anaplastic morphology has been shown to be an independent prognostic indicator of outcome {619,632}; in current trials, LC/A tumours are regarded as high-risk tumours warranting intensified adjuvant therapy. The 5-year progression-free survival rate for LC/A medulloblastomas is 30–40% {632,2192}, although SHH-activated LC/A tumours with a *TP53* mutation and group 3 tumours with *MYC* amplification can behave even more aggressively {2192,2870}.

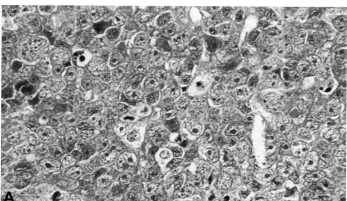
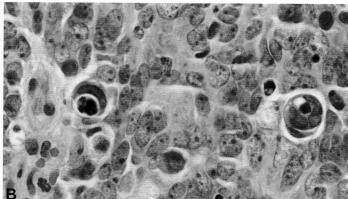

Fig. 8.22 Large cell / anaplastic medulloblastoma. **A,B** Increased nuclear size, pleomorphism, and prominent nucleoli. Tumour "cell wrapping" is also evident (B).

Embryonal tumour with multilayered rosettes, C19MC-altered

Korshunov A.
McLendon R.
Judkins A.R.
Pfister S.
Eberhart C.G.
Fuller G.N.
Sarkar C.
Ng H.-K.
Huang A.
Kool M.
Wesseling P.

Definition

An aggressive CNS embryonal tumour with multilayered rosettes and alterations (including amplification and fusions) in the C19MC locus at 19q13.42.

C19MC-altered embryonal tumours with multilayered rosettes (ETMRs) can develop in the cerebrum, brain stem, or cerebellum and span a broad histological spectrum. As well as multilayered rosettes, many tumours also contain both primitive embryonal regions and differentiated areas with broad swaths of neoplastic neuropil. Most paediatric CNS embryonal tumours previously classified as embryonal tumour with abundant neuropil and true rosettes, ependymoblastoma, and medulloepithelioma are included in this group {1349,2403}. However, any CNS embryonal tumour with C19MC amplification or fusion qualifies for this designation, including those without distinctive histopathological features.

ICD-O code   9478/3

Grading

Like other CNS embryonal tumours, C19MC-altered ETMR corresponds histologically to WHO grade IV.

Epidemiology

The true incidence of C19MC-altered ETMR is difficult to determine due to the varied terminology previously applied to these tumours, their rarity, and the fact that some lack signature microscopic features and must be distinguished genetically from other CNS embryonal lesions. Initially, most ETMRs were described as single cases, and the largest cumulative series includes approximately 100 samples. With few exceptions, ETMRs affect children aged < 4 years, the vast majority of cases occurring during the first 2 years of life. There is an almost equal distribution between males and females, with a male-to-female ratio of 1.1:1 {801,1349,2403}.

Localization

ETMRs develop in both the supratentorial and infratentorial compartments. The most common site is the cerebral hemisphere (affected in 70% of cases), with frequent involvement of the frontal and parietotemporal regions {801,1349}. Occasionally, these tumours can be very large, involving multiple lobes and even both cerebral hemispheres. An infratentorial location is less frequent, with either cerebellum or brain stem affected in 30% of cases. Tumour protrusion into the cerebellopontine cistern may be observed. Some extracranial tumours (e.g. intraocular medulloepithelioma and sacrococcygeal ependymoblastoma) share some

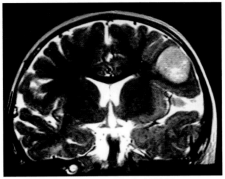

Fig. 8.23 Well-circumscribed cortical ETMR.

histopathological features with intracranial ETMR but disclose striking molecular diversity and consequently deserve a separate nosological designation {1129, 1345A}.

Clinical features

The most common clinical manifestations are symptoms and signs of increased intracranial pressure (i.e. headache, vomiting, nausea, and visual disturbances). Focal neurological signs (i.e. ataxia or weakness) are more common in older children and in cases with infratentorial location.

Imaging

CT and MRI usually show contrast-enhancing large tumour masses,

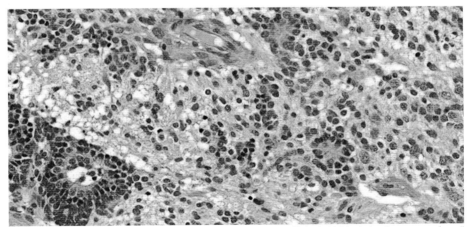

Fig. 8.24 Embryonal tumour with abundant neuropil and true rosettes. Biphasic histological pattern: areas of small embryonal cells with multilayered rosettes and neuropil-like areas with neoplastic neurocytic cells.

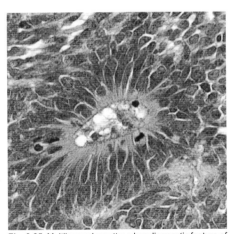

Fig. 8.25 Multilayered rosette: a key diagnostic feature of embryonal tumours with multilayered rosettes.

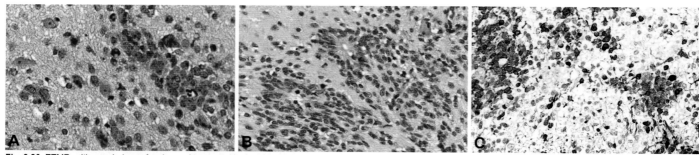

Fig. 8.26 ETMR, with morphology of embryonal tumour with abundant neuropil and true rosettes. **A** Neoplastic neurons between aggregates of small cells. **B** Rosettes in neuropil-like areas. **C** Single cells and clusters of LIN28A-positive tumour cells.

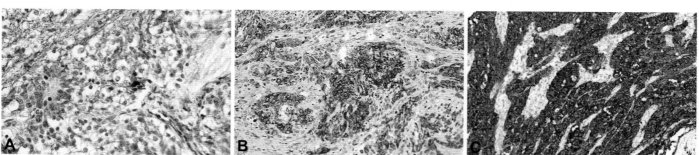

Fig. 8.27 ETMR, with morphology of embryonal tumour with abundant neuropil and true rosettes. **A** Synaptophysin expression within neuropil areas. **B** Vimentin expression. **C** Intense LIN28A immunoreactivity.

sometimes containing cysts or calcification. The radiological differential diagnosis of these lesions includes other CNS embryonal tumours, desmoplastic infantile ganglioglioma and supratentorial anaplastic ependymoma.

Spread

The tumour may be locally and widely infiltrative. Widespread leptomeningeal dissemination, extracranial invasive growth in the soft tissues, and extracranial metastases have all been reported {1300,1349,2771}.

Macroscopy

ETMR is usually greyish pink, and well circumscribed, with areas of necrosis and haemorrhage and minute calcifications. Some tumours are cystic. Widespread leptomeningeal dissemination and extraneural metastases are frequent in the terminal stage of disease.

Microscopy

Rosettes are a frequent and characteristic histopathological feature of C19MC-altered embryonal tumours. They are multilayered and mitotically active structures consisting of pseudostratified neuroepithelium with a central, round, or slit-like lumen. The lumen of the rosette is either empty or filled with eosinophilic

debris. The cells facing the lumen have a defined apical surface with a prominent internal limiting membrane in some rosettes. The nuclei of the rosette-forming cells tend to be pushed away from the lumen towards the outer cell border. In most tumours, a defined outer membrane around rosettes is lacking. There are three histological patterns found in ETMR , C91MC-altered. On the basis of their molecular commonality, these are now considered to constitute either various points along a morphological spectrum or diverse differentiation within a single tumour entity, rather than distinct nosological categories {1191,1349}.

Embryonal tumour with abundant neuropil and true rosettes
This pattern of ETMR shows a biphasic architecture featuring dense clusters of small cells with round or polygonal nuclei, scanty cytoplasm, and indistinct cell bodies, as well as large, paucicellular, fibrillar/neuropil-like areas, infrequently containing neoplastic neurocytic and ganglion cells {618,801}. In some cases, the neuropil has a fascicular quality. Hypercellular areas contain numerous mitoses and apoptotic bodies. In the aggregates of small cells, multilayered rosettes are often present. In some cases, these rosettes are observed as highly cellular

structures in the otherwise paucicellular neuropil-like areas, and rarely neoplastic ganglion cells can be found between the cells composing the layers of the rosettes.

Ependymoblastoma
This pattern of ETMR features sheets and clusters of poorly differentiated cells incorporating numerous multilayered rosettes, but typically lacks a neuropil-like matrix and ganglion cell elements. Rosettes are intermixed with small to medium-sized embryonal cells that have a high nuclear-to-cytoplasmic ratio and variably developed fibrillary processes.

Medulloepithelioma
This pattern of ETMR typically presents as a distinct cerebral mass in young children. It is characterized by papillary, tubular, and trabecular arrangements of neoplastic pseudostratified epithelium with an external (periodic acid–Schiff–positive and collagen IV–positive) limiting membrane, resembling the primitive neural tube. On the luminal surface of these tubules, cilia and blepharoblasts are absent. Mitotic figures are abundant and tend to be located near the luminal surface. In zones away from tubular and papillary structures, there are large sheets of poorly differentiated cells with

hyperchromatic nuclei and a high nuclear-to-cytoplasmic ratio. Clusters of multilayered rosettes may be seen here. Tumour cells range from embryonal cells to mature neurons and astrocytes. Rare tumours display mesenchymal differentiation or contain melanin pigment {36,301}. During tumour progression (local or distant recurrence), ETMRs with abundant neuropil tend to show loss of neuropil-like foci and may exhibit either extended clusters of embryonal cells with multilayered rosettes or prominent papillary and tubular structures {1346,1349}. In a few embryonal tumours with abundant neuropil and rosettes, post-treatment neuronal and glial/astrocytic maturation resembling a low-grade glioneuronal tumour has been reported {78,611,1413}. Other tumours show complete loss of key histopathological patterns of ETMR during progression and instead resemble other embryonal neoplasms {2771}.

Electron microscopy
The tumour cells that make up the embryonal areas and rosettes have a compact arrangement. They have large nuclei and scanty cytoplasm with only a few organelles {1429,1997,2576}. The cells forming rosettes are joined with junctional complexes and show abortive cilia and a few basal bodies at an apical site. On the luminal side, there is an amorphous surface coating but no true membrane. Tubular and papillary structures in the medulloepithelioma pattern show extensive lateral junctions (zonulae adherentes) and a basal lamina on the outer surface, consisting of a distinct continuous basement membrane. The neuropil-like tumour component shows long cellular processes containing numerous microtubules as well as neurosecretory granules in ganglion-like tumour cells.

Immunophenotype
The primitive neuroepithelial component of ETMR is intensely immunoreactive for nestin and vimentin {618,801}. Multilayered rosettes and tubular structures are also positive for these markers and frequently demonstrate an expression gradient, with basal labelling greater than luminal labelling. The small-cell areas and true rosettes may also show focal expression of cytokeratins, EMA, and CD99, but are usually negative for neuronal and glial markers. In contrast, the neuropil-like areas (including neoplastic neurons) stain

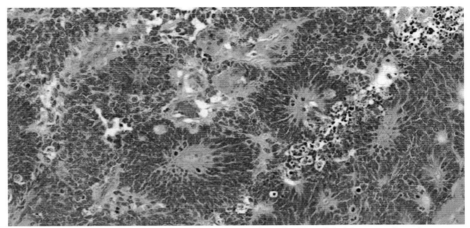

Fig. 8.28 ETMR, ependymoblastoma morphology. Nests of poorly differentiated tumour cells and numerous multilayered rosettes.

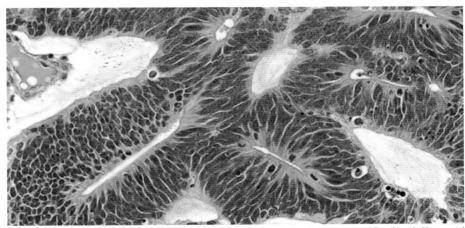

Fig. 8.29 ETMR, medulloepithelioma morphology. Papillary-like and tubular structures resembling the primitive neural tube.

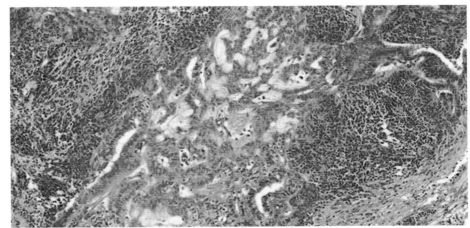

Fig. 8.30 ETMR, medulloepithelioma morphology. Coexistence of tubular structures, trabecular structures, and multilayered rosettes.

strongly for synaptophysin, NFPs, and NeuN. Immunoreactivity for GFAP highlights scattered cells resembling reactive astrocytes, but may also be present in some embryonal cells. ETMRs show strong and diffuse nuclear immunoreactivity for INI1 throughout all components. The Ki-67 proliferation index ranges from 20% to 80%, with the immunolabelling highlighting cellular areas; rosettes and tubular structures are also proliferative. Recently, the LIN28A protein has been suggested as an immunohistochemical diagnostic marker for ETMR {1348,1349, 1967,2403}. LIN28A is a protein that binds small RNAs, and it is known to be a negative regulator of the let-7 family of microRNAs, which may act as tumour suppressor microRNAs. LIN28A is a conserved cytoplasmic protein, but may be transported to the nucleus, where it seems to regulate the translation and stability of mRNA. Strong and diffuse LIN28A cytoplasmic immunostaining is found in ETMRs irrespective of their morphology {1349,2403}. LIN28A immunoreactivity is most prominent and intense in multilayered rosettes and poorly differentiated small-cell areas, as well as in the papillary and tubular structures of the medulloepithelioma pattern, whereas only single collections of positive cells are observed within the neuropil-like tumour areas. However, LIN28A expression is not specific for ETMR; it is also found in some gliomas, atypical teratoid/rhabdoid tumours, germ cell tumours, teratomas, and non-CNS neoplasms {2403,2723}. Nevertheless, this immunohistochemical marker can be very useful in support of a diagnosis of ETMR.

Cell of origin

A shared molecular signature between the histological types of ETMR suggests that they may share a common origin, such as a primitive cell population in the subventricular zone, with further evolution into a wider range of morphological appearances and mimics {1349}.

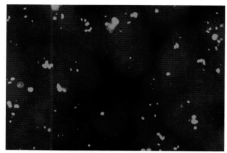

Fig. 8.31 C19MC-altered embryonal tumour with multilayered rosettes. Amplification of the C19MC locus at 19q13.42.

Genetic profile

Various high-resolution cytogenetic techniques (e.g. microarray-based comparative genomic hybridization, SNP arrays, and methylation arrays) disclose recurrent copy number aberrations in ETMRs: gains of chromosomes 2, 7q, and 11q and loss of 6q {384,1349,2115,2403}. These methods also reveal a focal high-level amplicon at 19q13.42, spanning a 0.89 Mb region {1346,1349,1491,1798, 1962,2403}. This amplicon is identified in the majority of ETMRs and seems to be a specific and sensitive diagnostic marker for these tumours. This unique amplicon covers a cluster of microRNAs (a polycistron) named C19MC, which is clearly upregulated in these tumours {1491, 1962}. This genetic aberration has not been detected in other paediatric brain tumours {1346,1491}. A recent study also demonstrated complex rearrangements at 19q13.42, as well as fusion of C19MC to the *TTYH1* gene {1295}. As a result, the promoter of *TTYH1* drives expression of C19MC microRNAs.

FISH analysis applying a target probe to the C19MC locus is a very helpful tool for the diagnosis of ETMR in routine neuropathological practice {1346,1349,1796, 1798}. In a series of 97 histologically typical ETMRs, FISH revealed the prototypic C19MC amplification in 96% of samples, irrespective of the histological type {1349}. All supratentorial ETMRs demonstrated amplification of C19MC, whereas a small subset of infratentorial tumours disclosed only gain of 19q. Another study evaluated the specificity of C19MC amplification in a series of > 400 paediatric brain tumours and found that the amplification was restricted to CNS embryonal tumours with increased expression of LIN28A {2403}. Gene expression and methylation profiling reveals a common molecular signature for ETMR, regardless of morphological pattern or tumour location {1349,2403}. Unsupervised clustering analysis showed that the methylation and gene expression profiles generated for ETMRs are clearly distinct from other paediatric brain tumours, confirming their nosological status as a single CNS tumour entity {1349}.

Prognosis and predictive factors

ETMRs demonstrate rapid growth and are associated with an aggressive clinical course, with reported survival times typically averaging 12 months after combination therapies {801,1349,2403}. Many patients experience local tumour regrowth, and a smaller number develop widespread tumour dissemination and systemic metastases. Gross total tumour resection and radiation may provide some benefit {10,50,1578,1762}. Patient survival does not differ significantly between the three histological types of ETMR {1349}. Recurrent chromosomal aberrations are also not associated with clinical outcome. In extremely rare cases with a long-term survival, post-treatment neuronal differentiation has been proposed as a favourable indicator of outcome {78,611,1413}.

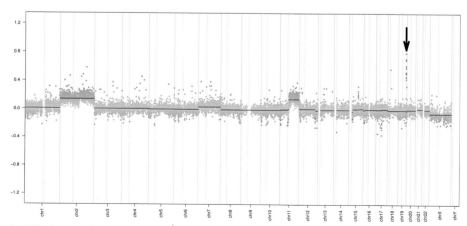

Fig. 8.32 Cytogenetic profile (methylation array) prototypic for ETMR: amplification of C19MC (arrow) and gain of chromosome 2.

Embryonal tumour with multilayered rosettes, NOS

Definition

An aggressive CNS embryonal tumour with multilayered rosettes, in which copy number at the 19q13 C19MC locus either shows no alteration or has not been tested.

Embryonal tumours with multilayered rosettes (ETMRs), NOS, can develop in the cerebrum, brain stem, and cerebellum and span a broad histological spectrum. However, many have the morphological features of tumours previously classified as ependymoblastoma or embryonal tumour with abundant neuropil and true rosettes. These tumours are now regarded as patterns of ETMR. Medulloepitheliomas in which copy number at the 19q13 C19MC locus shows no alteration or is not tested are considered separately, because they are considered genetically distinct (see p. 207).

ICD-O code   9478/3

Other CNS embryonal tumours

McLendon R.
Judkins A.R.
Eberhart C.G.
Fuller G.N.
Sarkar C.

Ng H.-K.
Huang A.
Kool M.
Pfister S.

Definition

A group of rare, poorly differentiated embryonal neoplasms of neuroectodermal origin that lack the specific histopathological features or molecular alterations that define other CNS tumours.

Currently, the medulloblastoma, the embryonal tumour with multilayered rosettes (ETMR) characterized by genetic alterations at the C19MC locus on 19q.13.42, and the atypical teratoid/rhabdoid tumour (AT/RT) characterized by loss of SMARCB1 (INI1) or SMARCA4 (BRG1) expression, represent genetically defined embryonal tumours of the CNS. There remain several CNS embryonal tumours for which no genetic data have yet facilitated a molecular classification. Histologically, one resembles ETMR and has been included alongside that tumour as ETMR, NOS. The other resembles AT/RT and is designated CNS embryonal tumour with rhabdoid features. Others are included here: medulloepithelioma, CNS neuroblastoma, CNS ganglioneuroblastoma, and CNS embryonal tumour, NOS.

The introduction of ETMR, C19MC-altered into this updated classification has complicated the presentation of epidemiological and clinical data for embryonal tumours that are not defined genetically, because it is not yet clear whether such data for C19MC-altered ETMR differ significantly from the broader category of CNS embryonal tumours.

Data based on the broad category of CNS embryonal tumours and probably applicable to medulloepithelioma, CNS neuroblastoma, CNS ganglioneuroblastoma, and CNS embryonal tumour, NOS, are presented in this overarching section of the chapter ahead of the definitions and specific information on microscopy and immunophenotype for each tumour.

Grading

All CNS embryonal tumours correspond histologically to WHO grade IV.

Epidemiology

CNS embryonal neoplasms account for approximately 1% of brain tumours overall, but constitute 13% of neoplasms arising in children aged 0–14 years {1863}. In one study, they constituted about 3–5% of all paediatric brain tumours (i.e. those in patients aged ≤ 18 years) {1967}.
Shifting diagnostic criteria and nomenclature make precise analysis of CNS embryonal tumour epidemiology difficult, but at least one study has found an increase in the incidence of medulloblastomas and other embryonal tumours over the past two decades {1896}. The Central Brain Tumor Registry of the United States (CBTRUS) reports an overall average annual age-adjusted incidence rate in childhood of 0.12 cases per 100 000 population, with a median patient age at onset of 3.5 years and no significant sex predominance {1862}. Although most CNS embryonal tumours occur in infancy and childhood, some cases do arise in adults {157,806,1273,1968}. However, the incidence of adult CNS embryonal tumours is difficult to determine because of their rarity and lack of signature biomarkers.

Localization

CNS embryonal tumours are typically located in the cerebral hemispheres, with rare examples occurring in the brain stem {741} and spinal cord {2643}.

Imaging

On CT, CNS embryonal tumours have similar appearances, regardless of site. They are isodense to hyperdense, and density increases after injection of contrast material. They can present as solid masses or may contain cystic or necrotic areas. Between 50% and 70% of all CNS embryonal tumours contain calcification. Oedema surrounding parenchymal masses is not usually extensive. MRI appearances can vary, depending on the site of origin. The tumours are T1-hypointense relative to cortical grey matter. They look similar on T2-weighted imaging, but cystic or necrotic areas are hyperintense. There is contrast enhancement with gadolinium on T1-weighted imaging. Regions of haemorrhage (if present) are T2-hypointense.

Spread

Metastatic dissemination is evident in 25–35% of CNS embryonal tumours at presentation, mostly in the subarachnoid space, including the spinal canal. Therefore, diagnostic lumbar puncture for cytology, as well as spinal MRI, is mandatory for all patients {1045}. Extraneural metastases to the bone, liver, and cervical lymph nodes have been reported {167}.

Macroscopy

CNS embryonal tumours are found most commonly in the cerebrum, but can also occur in the brain stem, spinal cord, or suprasellar region {805}. Those in the suprasellar region tend to be smaller than those in the cerebrum. The tumours are typically well-circumscribed pink masses, and demarcation between tumour and brain ranges from indistinct to clear cut. The tumours are most often solid, but can contain cystic areas as well as areas of haemorrhage and necrosis. They are soft unless they contain a prominent desmoplastic component, in which case they are firm and often have a tan colour.

Cell of origin

The histogenesis of CNS embryonal tumours other than medulloblastoma has been controversial for many years, and the only point on which consensus has been achieved is that these poorly differentiated tumours arise from primitive neuroepithelial cells {1289,2171}.

Table 8.03 Biomarkers useful in the characterization of small cell, embryonal-appearing tumours

Biomarker	Associated tumour
C19MC amplification or LIN28A expression	Embryonal tumour with multilayered rosettes
SMARCB1 loss or SMARCA4 loss	Atypical teratoid/rhabdoid tumour
H3 K27 and G34 mutations	Paediatric-type glioblastomas
C11orf95-RELA fusion gene or L1CAM expression	Supratentorial ependymoma
IDH1 or *IDH2* mutation	Adult-type diffuse gliomas

Prognosis and predictive factors

Overall, CNS embryonal tumours show aggressive clinical behaviour and have a very poor prognosis, with multiple local relapses and widespread leptomeningeal dissemination. Overall survival at 5 years in paediatric patients with CNS embryonal tumours is reported to be 29–57% {43, 440,478,590,1173,2082,2558}, which is poorer than the survival rate for children with medulloblastoma {809,2558}. Factors associated with poor prognosis in paediatric patients include young age, metastatic disease, and incomplete resection {440,478,806,810,1173,1474,2082,2558}.

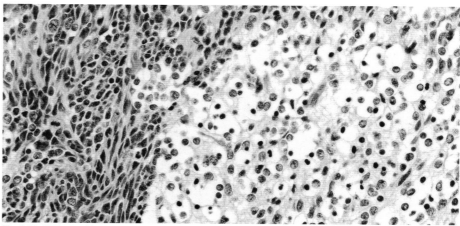

Fig. 8.33 CNS neuroblastoma. Abrupt transition from undifferentiated embryonal cells to cells with variable neurocytic differentiation and cytoplasmic clearing.

Medulloepithelioma

Definition

A CNS embryonal tumour with a prominent pseudostratified neuroepithelium that resembles the embryonic neural tube in addition to poorly differentiated neuroepithelial cells.

Even though medulloepithelioma is a very rare tumour, a significant proportion of those analysed genetically have not shown C19MC alterations {2403}. Although a diagnostic genetic signature has yet to be defined for such tumours, they are grouped as a tumour entity, distinct from ETMR.

ICD-O code   9501/3

Microscopy

Medulloepithelioma consists of sheets of embryonal cells interspersed to a variable extent by tubular and trabecular arrangements of a neoplastic pseudostratified neuroepithelium, which appears similar to embryonic neural tube. This has a periodic acid–Schiff–positive external limiting membrane, and its luminal surface lacks cilia and blepharoblasts. Neural differentiation may occasionally be found in the form of cells with a dystrophic neuronal or astrocytic morphology. Mitotic figures are readily found.

Immunophenotype

Embryonal cells in medulloepithelioma rarely show immunoreactivity for neuronal markers, such as synaptophysin and NFPs, and GFAP-positive tumour cells are exceptional. The neuroepithelium may show patchy expression of cytokeratins and, less often, EMA. Ki-67

immunolabelling is uniformly high among embryonal cells. LIN28A is expressed by medulloepitheliomas that lack C19MC amplification {2403}.

CNS neuroblastoma

Definition

A CNS embryonal tumour characterized by poorly differentiated neuroepithelial cells, groups of neurocytic cells, and a variable neuropil-rich stroma.

This exceedingly rare tumour shows a distinctive pattern of differentiation, not unlike some peripheral neuroblastomas.

ICD-O code   9500/3

Microscopy

Zones of neurocytic differentiation are found among sheets of densely packed primitive embryonal cells. Neurocytic differentiation manifests as cells with slightly larger nuclei and variably distinct cytoplasm set against a faintly fibrillar matrix at lower density than the embryonal cells. Architectural features include Homer Wright rosettes, palisading patterns of cells, and regions of necrosis with granular calcification. Exceptionally, a Schwannian stroma may be present.

Immunophenotype

The embryonal cells may be immunonegative for neural markers, such as synaptophysin or GFAP, but some might show weak expression of synaptophysin. Very rarely, GFAP expression is found in a few tumour cells, but GFAP-positive cells are

generally reactive astrocytes. Groups of neurocytic cells express synaptophysin or NeuN. Ki-67 immunolabelling is high in embryonal cells, but lower elsewhere.

CNS ganglioneuroblastoma

Definition

A CNS embryonal tumour characterized by poorly differentiated neuroepithelial cells and groups of neurocytic and ganglion cells.

This rare tumour shows varying degrees of neuronal differentiation, but dystrophic ganglion cells are a prominent element.

ICD-O code   9490/3

Microscopy

Varying degrees of neuronal differentiation characterize this tumour, which also contains sheets of primitive embryonal cells. Neurocytic and ganglion cells, the latter occasionally binucleated, are usually present as small groups, rather than dispersed diffusely among the embryonal cells. Dispersed cells with a neuronal morphology and appearing to form a pattern are more likely to be entrapped neurons. Mitotic figures and apoptotic bodies are readily found among embryonal cells. Architectural features include Homer Wright rosettes, palisading patterns of cells, and regions of necrosis with granular calcification.

Immunophenotype

Embryonal cells may be immunonegative for neural markers, such as

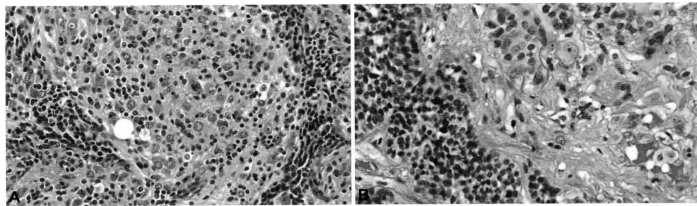

Fig. 8.34 CNS ganglioneuroblastoma. **A** Nodule of admixed neurocytic and ganglion cells among embryonal cells. **B** Embryonal cells next to large cells with variable neuronal differentiation embedded in a fibrillary stroma.

synaptophysin or GFAP, but some usually show weak expression of synaptophysin. Groups of neurocytic and ganglion cells express synaptophysin, NFPs, MAP2, and NeuN. Ki-67 immunolabelling is high in embryonal cells, but lower elsewhere.

CNS embryonal tumour, NOS

Definition
A rare, poorly differentiated embryonal neoplasm of neuroectodermal origin that lacks the specific histopathological features or molecular alterations that define other CNS tumours.

ICD-O code 9473/3

CNS embryonal tumours, NOS, are characterized by poorly differentiated neuroepithelial cells with a variable capacity for divergent differentiation along neuronal, astrocytic, myogenic, or melanocytic lines. CNS embryonal tumours can have histological features overlapping those of other brain tumours, many of which have been reclassified from this group through the identification of unique molecular biomarkers.

The current definition of CNS embryonal tumour, NOS, is more circumscribed than in prior WHO classifications, in which the umbrella designation "CNS primitive neuroectodermal tumour (PNET)" was used. Embryonal tumours such as medulloepitheliomas, ependymoblastomas, and embryonal tumours with abundant neuropil and true rosettes, which exhibit alterations at the 19q13 C19MC locus and were previously included within the broad CNS PNET designation, are now considered to be a distinct genetically defined entity, called embryonal tumour with multilayered rosettes (ETMR), C19MC-altered. Molecular genetic advances now permit the improved classification of other CNS embryonal tumours as well; for example, the diagnosis of atypical teratoid/rhabdoid tumour is made by demonstrating mutation of *SMARCB1* or *SMARCA4* or loss of expression of SMARCB1 (INI1) or SMARCA4 (BRG1). Other high-grade undifferentiated neural neoplasms that are composed of small uniform cells and enter the differential diagnosis of CNS embryonal tumour often have their own molecular signatures (see Table 8.03, p. 206).

Malignant gliomas with primitive neuronal components, though rare, constitute a separate entity and were initially described in adults {1099,1625,1946,2343}. This entity is considered a variant of glioblastoma rather than a CNS embryonal tumour (see p. 33).

Microscopy
CNS embryonal tumours are poorly differentiated neoplasms composed of cells with round to oval nuclei and a high nuclear-to-cytoplasmic ratio. Commonly encountered features include frequent mitoses and apoptotic bodies. More tightly packed regions with angular or moulded cells may also be identified, and Homer Wright rosettes can be found. Necrosis and vascular endothelial proliferation may also be seen. Calcification is relatively common within degenerative regions. A fibrous stroma is occasionally present and can vary from a delicate lobular framework to dense fibrous cords.

Some variants of CNS embryonal tumour display distinctive architectural or cytological features. The latter often manifests as neuronal differentiation.

Immunophenotype
CNS embryonal tumour can show variable expression of divergent neuroepithelial markers, including proteins associated with both glial differentiation (GFAP) and neuronal differentiation (synaptophysin, NFP, and NeuN) {875}. Expression of these markers is typically present in a thin rim of cytoplasm, although NeuN is nuclear. Antibodies that recognize GFAP may also label reactive astrocytes. However, poorly differentiated regions of the neoplasm often predominate, in which no immunohistochemical signs of neural differentiation are apparent. The Ki-67 proliferation index is typically variable, but a very high growth fraction, often with > 50% of immunopositive tumour cells, is usual.

Atypical teratoid/rhabdoid tumour

Judkins A.R.
Eberhart C.G.
Wesseling P.
Hasselblatt M.

Definition

A malignant CNS embryonal tumour composed predominantly of poorly differentiated elements and frequently including rhabdoid cells, with inactivation of SMARCB1 (INI1) or (extremely rarely) SMARCA4 (BRG1).

Atypical teratoid/rhabdoid tumours (AT/RTs) occur most frequently in young children. Neoplastic cells demonstrate histological and immunohistochemical evidence of polyphenotypic differentiation along neuroectodermal, epithelial, and mesenchymal lines. Diagnosis of AT/RT requires demonstration of inactivation of *SMARCB1* or, if intact, *SMARCA4* genes, either by routine immunohistochemical staining for their proteins or by other appropriate means. Tumours with this morphology but lacking this molecular genetic confirmation should be classified as CNS embryonal tumours with rhabdoid features (p. 212).

ICD-O code   9508/3

Grading

AT/RT corresponds histologically to WHO grade IV.

Epidemiology

In several large series, AT/RTs accounted for 1–2% of all paediatric brain tumours {2116,2783}. AT/RT is very rare in adult patients {2063}. However, due to the preponderance of cases in children aged < 3 years, AT/RTs are estimated to account for ≥ 10% of all CNS tumours in infants {192}.

Age and sex distribution

AT/RT is a paediatric tumour. It most often presents in patients aged < 3 years and rarely in children aged > 6 years. There is a male predominance, with a male-to-female ratio of 1.6–2:1 {1002,2530}. AT/RT rarely occurs in adults {2063}.

Localization

In two large series of paediatric cases, the ratio of supratentorial to infratentorial tumours was 4:3 {1002,2530}. Supratentorial tumours are often located in the cerebral hemispheres and less frequently in the ventricular system, suprasellar region, or pineal gland. Infratentorial tumours can be located in the cerebellar hemispheres, cerebellopontine angle, and brain stem, and are relatively prevalent in the first 2 years of life. Infrequently, AT/RT arises in the spinal cord. Seeding of AT/RT via the cerebrospinal fluid pathways is common and is found in as many as one quarter of all patients at presentation {1002}. Infratentorial localization is very rare in adult patients diagnosed with AT/RT {646}.

Clinical features

The clinical presentation is variable, depending on the age of the patient and the location and size of the tumour. Infants, in particular, present with non-specific signs of lethargy, vomiting, and/or failure to thrive. More specific problems include head tilt and cranial nerve palsy, most commonly sixth and seventh nerve paresis. Headache and hemiplegia are more commonly reported in children aged > 3 years.

Imaging

CT and MRI findings are similar to those in patients with other embryonal tumours. AT/RTs are isodense to hyperintense on FLAIR images and show restricted diffusion. Cystic and/or necrotic regions are apparent as zones of heterogeneous signal intensity. Almost all tumours are

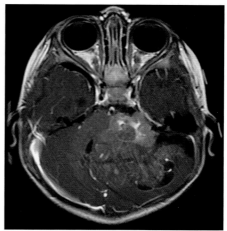

Fig. 8.36 AT/RT. Axial T1-weighted contrast-enhanced image demonstrates a heterogeneously enhancing left cerebellar mass.

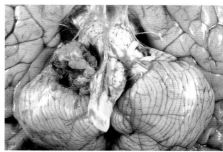

Fig. 8.37 AT/RT with multiple haemorrhages, arising in the right cerebellopontine angle.

variably contrast-enhancing, and leptomeningeal dissemination can be seen in as many as a quarter of cases at presentation {1659}.

Macroscopy

These tumours (and their deposits along the cerebrospinal fluid pathways) generally have a gross appearance similar to that of medulloblastoma and other CNS embryonal tumours. They tend to be soft, pinkish-red, and often appear to be demarcated from adjacent parenchyma. They typically contain necrotic foci and may be haemorrhagic. Those with significant amounts of mesenchymal tissue may be firm and tan-white in some regions. Tumours arising in the

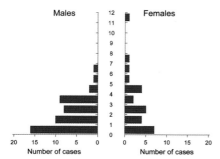

Fig. 8.35 Age and sex distribution of atypical teratoid/rhabdoid tumour, based on 73 cases {1002,2530}.

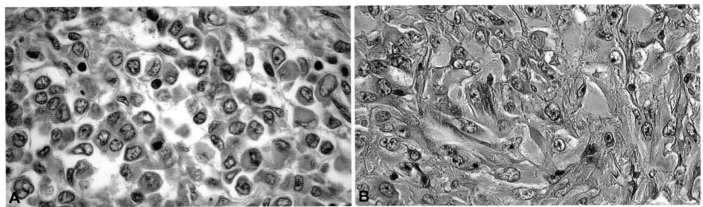

Fig. 8.38 Atypical teratoid/rhabdoid tumour. **A** Rhabdoid cells with vesicular chromatin, prominent nucleoli, and eosinophilic globular cytoplasmic inclusions. **B** Tumour cells with abundant, pale eosinophilic neoplasm.

cerebellopontine angle wrap themselves around cranial nerves and vessels and invade brain stem and cerebellum to various extents. Rarely, AT/RT can show bony involvement {2697}.

Microscopy

AT/RTs are heterogeneous lesions that can often be difficult to recognize solely on the basis of histopathological criteria {324,2172}. The most striking feature in many cases is a population of cells with classic rhabdoid features, eccentrically located nuclei containing vesicular chromatin, prominent eosinophilic nucleoli, abundant cytoplasm with an obvious eosinophilic globular cytoplasmic inclusion, and well-defined cell borders. The cells typically fall along a spectrum ranging from those with a classic rhabdoid phenotype to cells with less striking nuclear atypia and large amounts of pale eosinophilic cytoplasm. The cytoplasm of these cells has a finely granular, homogeneous character or may contain a poorly defined, dense, pink body resembling an inclusion. Ultrastructurally, rhabdoid cells typically contain whorled bundles of intermediate filaments filling much of the perikaryon {202,916}. A frequently encountered artefact in these cells is cytoplasmic vacuolation. Rhabdoid cells may be arranged in nests or sheets and often have a jumbled appearance. However, these cells are the exclusive or predominant histopathological finding in only a minority of cases.

Most tumours contain variable components with primitive neuroectodermal, mesenchymal, and epithelial features. A small-cell embryonal component is the most commonly encountered, present in two thirds of all tumours. Mesenchymal differentiation is less common and typically presents as areas with spindle cell features and a basophilic or mucopolysaccharide-rich background. Epithelial differentiation is the least common histopathological feature. It can take the form of papillary structures, adenomatous areas, or poorly differentiated ribbons and cords. A myxoid matrix occurs uncommonly; in cases where this is the predominant histopathological pattern, distinction from choroid plexus carcinoma can be challenging. Mitotic figures are usually abundant. Broad areas of geographical necrosis and haemorrhage are commonly encountered in these tumours.

Immunophenotype

AT/RTs demonstrate a broad spectrum of immunohistochemical reactivities that align with their histological diversity. However, the rhabdoid cells characteristically demonstrate expression of EMA, SMA, and vimentin. Immunoreactivities for GFAP, NFP, synaptophysin, and cytokeratins are also commonly observed. In contrast, germ cell markers and markers of skeletal muscle differentiation are not typically expressed. Immunohistochemical staining for expression of the SMARCB1 protein (INI1) has been shown to be a sensitive and specific test for the diagnosis of AT/RT. In normal tissue and most neoplasms, SMARCB1 is a constitutively expressed nuclear protein; in AT/RT, there is loss of nuclear expression of SMARCB1 {1192}. Paediatric CNS embryonal tumours without rhabdoid features, but with loss of SMARCB1 expression in tumour cells, qualify as AT/RTs as well {918}. Rare SMARCB1-deficient non-rhabdoid tumours forming cribriform strands, trabeculae, and well-defined

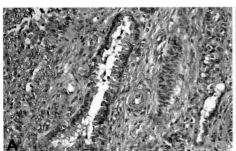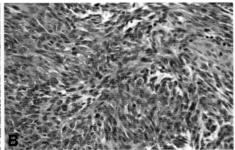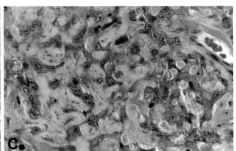

Fig. 8.39 Atypical teratoid/rhabdoid tumour. **A** Gland-like component. **B** Spindle cell morphology. **C** Mucopolysaccharide-rich background.

surfaces are called cribriform neuroepithelial tumours {964}. Cribriform neuroepithelial tumour is most likely an epithelioid variant of AT/RT but is characterized by a relatively favourable prognosis {92,612, 964}. Some authors have reported inactivation of SMARCB1 in choroid plexus carcinomas, but others believe that such tumours have histopathological features justifying a diagnosis of AT/RT, and that classic choroid plexus carcinomas do not lose SMARCB1 expression {802,1190}. Rarely, tumours with clinical and morphological features of AT/RT and retained SMARCB1 expression are encountered. Loss of nuclear expression of SMARCA4 (BRG1) is rarely seen in such cases {959}. AT/RTs in children have marked proliferative activity; often having a Ki-67 proliferation index of > 50% {1016}. Limited data are available on adult patients, but in some cases the proliferation index is significantly lower {1550}.

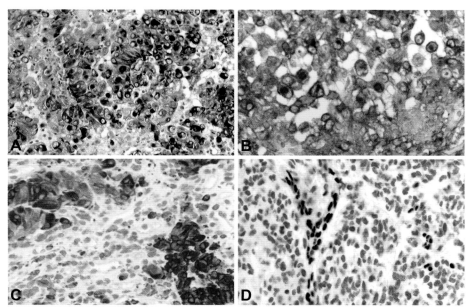

Fig. 8.40 Atypical teratoid/rhabdoid tumour. **A** Strong expression of vimentin. **B** Membranous and cytoplasmic expression of EMA. **C** Expression of GFAP (brown) and NFP (red). **D** Loss of expression of SMARCB1 (INI1) in nuclei of tumour cells, with retained expression in intratumoural blood vessels.

Cell of origin

The histogenesis of rhabdoid tumours is unknown. Neural, epithelial, and mesenchymal markers can all be expressed, and given these tumours' association with young children, it has been suggested that they derive from pluripotent fetal cells {247,1864}. Meningeal, neural crest, and germ cell origins have also been proposed {451,1887,2172}. AT/RTs arising in the setting of ganglioglioma, or other low-grade CNS lesions, suggest the possibility of progression from other tumour types {55,1157}.

Genetic profile

AT/RTs can occur sporadically or as part of a rhabdoid tumour predisposition syndrome {192}. Mutation or loss of the SMARCB1 locus at 22q11.2 is the genetic hallmark of this tumour {194,2649}. Whole-exome sequencing demonstrates that the genomes of AT/RTs are remarkably simple; they have an extremely low rate of mutations, with loss of SMARCB1 being the primary recurrent event. The SMARCB1 protein is a component of the mammalian SWI/SNF complex, which functions in an ATP-dependent manner to alter chromatin structure {2137}. Loss of SMARCB1 expression at the protein level is seen in almost all AT/RTs, and most of the tumours have detectable deletions or mutations of SMARCB1; the other cases exhibit loss of SMARCB1 function due to reduced RNA or protein

expression {192}. Homozygous deletions of the SMARCB1 locus are detected in 20–24% of cases {192,2530}. In other cases, one SMARCB1 allele is mutated and the second allele is lost by deletion or mitotic recombination. Rare tumours demonstrate two coding sequence mutations. Nonsense and frameshift mutations that are predicted to lead to truncations of the protein are identified in the majority of these cases {192}. Localization of mutations within the SMARCB1 gene seems to vary somewhat between rhabdoid tumours arising at various sites in the body, and exons 5 and 9 contain hotspots in CNS AT/RT. Because expression of SMARCB1 is sometimes decreased in AT/RT in the absence of genetic alterations, its promoter was analysed in 24 cases, using bisulfite sequencing and methylation-sensitive PCR, but no evidence of hypermethylation was detected {2853}. No relationship between the type of SMARCB1 alteration and outcome could be established.

Very infrequently, tumours are encountered that have features of AT/RT and intact SMARCB1 protein expression; these may instead have mutation and inactivation of SMARCA4, another component of the SWI/SNF complex {2293}. These tumours are associated with very young patient age and a poor prognosis {962}. In one family with a germline SMARCA4 mutation, AT/RT and ovarian cancer were

diagnosed in a newborn and his mother, respectively, providing a link between AT/RT and small cell carcinoma of the ovary of hypercalcaemic type {728}.

The specific functions of SMARCB1 and SMARCA4 and their role in malignant transformation are not entirely clear, but loss of SMARCB1 seems to result in widespread but specific deregulation of genes and pathways associated with cell cycle, differentiation, and cell survival {1458,2579}. Cell cycle regulatory genes that are overexpressed in AT/RT include CCND1 and AURKA {2858}. Loss of SMARCB1 leads to transcriptional activation of EZH2, as well as repression and increased H3K27me3 of polycomb gene targets as part of the broader SWI/SNF modulation of the polycomb complex to maintain the epigenome {52,2761}. The Hippo signalling pathway is involved in the detrimental effects of SMARCB1 deficiency, and its main effector, YAP1, is overexpressed in AT/RT {1145}.

Genetic susceptibility

In familial cases of rhabdoid tumours, i.e. in rhabdoid tumour predisposition syndrome 1 (involving the SMARCB1 gene) and rhabdoid tumour predisposition syndrome 2 (involving the SMARCA4 gene), unaffected adult carriers and gonadal mosaicism have been identified {962, 1133,2327}. Because the risk of germline mutations has been reported to be ≥ 33%

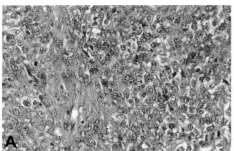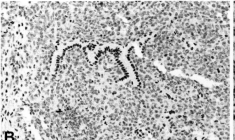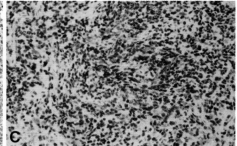

Fig. 8.41 Atypical teratoid/rhabdoid tumour. **A** Tumour cells with abundant pale eosinophilic cytoplasm and vesicular chromatin staining. **B** Loss of expression of SMARCA4 (BRG1); only non-neoplastic cells are labelled. **C** Retained expression of SMARCB1 (also called INI1), for comparison.

in SMARCB1-deficient AT/RT and may be substantially higher in SMARCA4-deficient tumours {962}, it is important to perform molecular genetic studies in all newly diagnosed cases {192,962}.

Prognosis and predictive factors
Although overall the prognosis of AT/RTs is poor, emerging data from a series of clinical trials have demonstrated that not all AT/RTs share the same uniformly dismal prognosis. Retrospective analysis of children with AT/RTs who were enrolled at the German HIT trial centre between 1988 and 2004 demonstrated a 3-year overall survival rate of 22% and an event-free survival rate of 13%, and also identified a subset of patients (14%) who were long-term event-free survivors {2665}. In a large prospective trial incorporating chemotherapy in an intensive multimodal treatment approach that included radiation, a 2-year progression-free survival rate of 53% ± 13% and an overall survival rate of 70% ± 10% were found {433}. Further demonstrating the overall efficacy of high-dose chemotherapy with radiation, a retrospective review of the Canadian Brain Tumour Consortium data found, that children who received high-dose chemotherapy, and in some cases radiation, had a 2-year overall survival rate of 60% ± 12.6% versus 21.7% ± 8.5%

among children on standard-dose therapy {1414}. In contrast, the Children's Cancer Group study CCG-9921, with standard-dose chemotherapy alone, reported a 5-year event-free survival rate of 14% ± 7% and an overall survival rate of 29% ± 9% {809}.

The results of global genomic and transcriptional analysis of AT/RT suggest that these tumours may constitute at least two different molecular classes, with distinct outcomes. One study suggested that tumours with enrichment of neurogenic or forebrain markers are associated with supratentorial location, more favourable response to therapy, and better long-term survival, whereas AT/RT with mesenchymal lineage markers are more frequently infratentorial and associated with worse long-term survival {2569}. It may ultimately be possible to risk-stratify AT/RTs on the basis of molecular group, location, extent of resection, and disease stage. However, even for the favourable subgroup this remains an aggressive disease, with 5-year progression-free and overall survival rates of 60% and recurrence occurring in about one third of patients.

CNS embryonal tumour with rhabdoid features

Definition
A highly malignant CNS embryonal tumour composed predominantly of poorly differentiated elements and including rhabdoid cells, either with expression of SMARCB1 (INI1) and SMARCA4 (BRG1) or in which SMARCB1 and SMARCA4 status cannot be confirmed.

In CNS embryonal tumour with rhabdoid features, neoplastic cells demonstrate histological and immunohistochemical evidence of polyphenotypic differentiation along neuroectodermal, epithelial, and mesenchymal lines.

Thus, the pathological features of these tumours are the same as those for AT/RTs. Because of the extreme rarity of CNS embryonal tumour with rhabdoid features, no data are available to determine whether its epidemiological or clinical characteristics are significantly different from those of AT/RTs.

ICD-O code   9508/3

Grading
CNS embryonal tumour with rhabdoid features corresponds histologically to WHO grade IV.

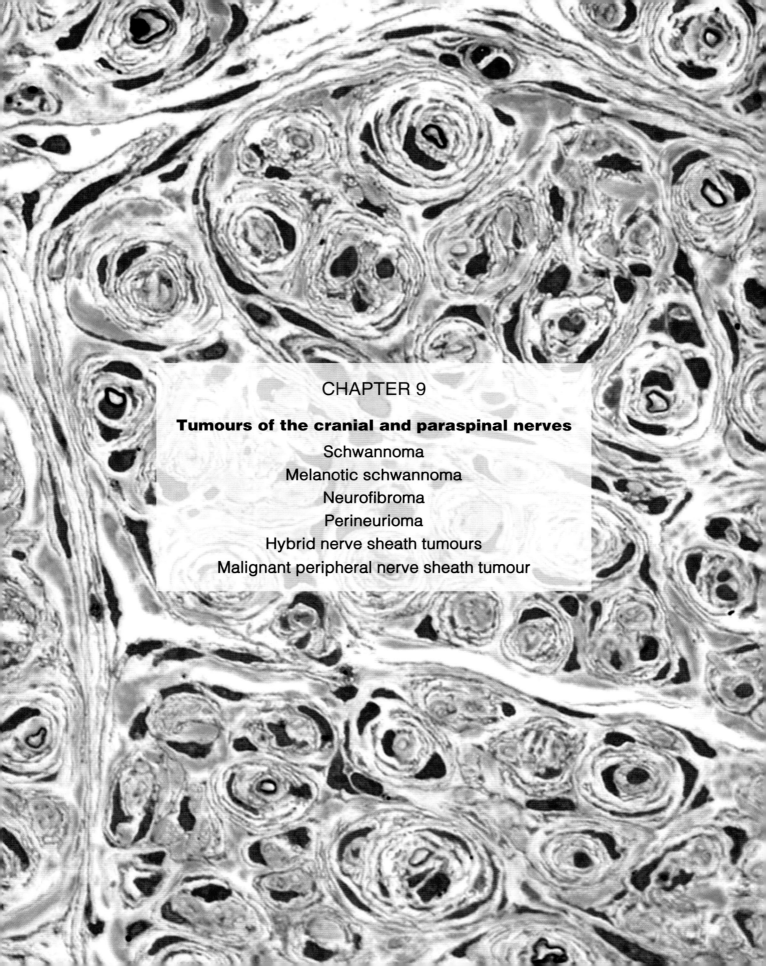

CHAPTER 9

Tumours of the cranial and paraspinal nerves

Schwannoma

Melanotic schwannoma

Neurofibroma

Perineurioma

Hybrid nerve sheath tumours

Malignant peripheral nerve sheath tumour

Schwannoma

Antonescu C.R.
Louis D.N.
Hunter S.
Perry A.
Reuss D.E.
Stemmer-Rachamimov A.O.

Definition

A benign, typically encapsulated nerve sheath tumour composed entirely of well-differentiated Schwann cells, with loss of merlin (the NF2 gene product) expression in conventional forms.

Schwannomas are solitary and sporadic in the vast majority of cases, can affect patients of any age, and follow a benign clinical course. Multiple schwannomas are associated with neurofibromatosis type 2 (NF2) and schwannomatosis.

ICD-O code   9560/0

Grading

Conventional, non-melanotic schwannomas and their variants correspond histologically to WHO grade I.

Synonyms

Neurilemoma; neurinoma

Epidemiology

Schwannomas account for 8% of all intracranial tumours, 85% of cerebellopontine angle tumours, and 29% of spinal nerve root tumours {2204}. Approximately 90% of cases are solitary and sporadic and 4% arise in the setting of NF2. Of the 5% of schwannomas that are multiple but not associated with NF2 {375}, some may be associated with schwannomatosis {1558}. Patients of any age can be affected, but paediatric cases are rare. The peak incidence is in the fourth to sixth decades of life. Most studies show no sex

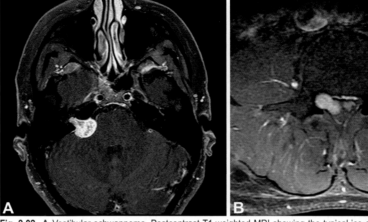

Fig. 9.02 A Vestibular schwannoma. Postcontrast T1-weighted MRI showing the typical ice-cream-cone shape of a vestibular schwannoma, with the cone representing the portion within the internal auditory canal and the scoop of ice cream the portion in the cerebellopontine angle. **B** Paraspinal schwannoma. Postcontrast T1-weighted MRI showing both intraspinal extramedullary and extraspinal components, with a point of constriction at the nerve exit.

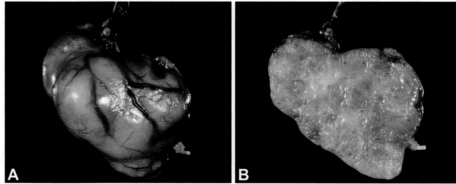

Fig. 9.03 Schwannoma. **A** External surface showing the parent nerve of origin and a variably translucent capsule. **B** On cut surface, schwannomas often show a glistening to mucoid appearance, variable cystic degeneration, and yellow spots reflecting collections of xanthomatous macrophages.

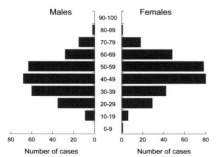

Fig. 9.01 Age and sex distribution of schwannomas, based on 582 patients treated at the University Hospital Zurich.

predilection, but some series have shown a female predominance among intracranial tumours {526,1613,2204}. Cerebral intraparenchymal schwannomas are associated with a younger patient age and a male predominance {375}. Schwannomas of spinal cord parenchyma are too rare for their epidemiology to be assessed {996}.

Localization

The vast majority of schwannomas occur outside the CNS. Peripheral nerves in the skin and subcutaneous tissue are most often affected. Intracranial schwannomas

show a strong predilection for the eighth cranial nerve in the cerebellopontine angle, particularly in NF2 {1893}. They arise at the transition zone between central and peripheral myelination and affect the vestibular division. The adjacent cochlear division is almost never the site of origin. This characteristic location, which is not shared by neurofibromas or malignant peripheral nerve sheath tumours, results in diagnostically helpful enlargement of the internal auditory meatus on neuroimaging. Intralabyrinthine schwannomas are uncommon {1763}. Intraspinal schwannomas show a strong predilection

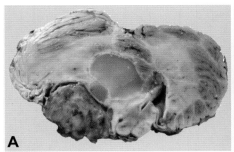
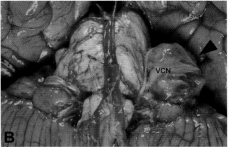

VCN

Fig. 9.04 Vestibular schwannoma. **A** Large vestibular schwannoma compressing neighbouring cerebellar structures and the brain stem. Note the pressure-induced cyst formation in the cerebellar white matter. **B** Schwannoma (arrowhead) originating from the left vestibulocochlear nerve (VCN).

for sensory nerve roots; motor and autonomic nerves are affected far less often. Occasional CNS schwannomas are not associated with a recognizable nerve; these include approximately 70 reported cases of spinal intramedullary schwannomas and 40 cases of cerebral parenchymal or intraventricular schwannomas {375,528,1278,2722}. Dural examples are rare {77}. Peripheral nerve schwannomas, unlike neurofibromas, tend to be attached to nerve trunks, most often involving the head and neck region or flexor surfaces of the extremities. Visceral schwannomas are rare, as are osseous examples {1662,2038}.

Clinical features

Peripherally situated schwannomas may present as incidental (asymptomatic) paraspinal tumours, as spinal nerve tumours with radicular pain and signs of nerve root / spinal cord compression, or as eighth cranial nerve tumours with related symptoms (including hearing loss, tinnitus, and occasional vertigo). Motor symptoms are uncommon because schwannomas favour sensory nerve roots. Bilateral vestibular tumours are the hallmark of NF2. Pain is the most common presentation for schwannomas in patients with schwannomatosis.

Imaging

MRI shows a well-circumscribed, sometimes cystic and often heterogeneously enhancing mass {375}. Vestibular schwannomas often display a classic ice-cream-cone sign, with the tapered intraosseous cone exiting the internal auditory canal and expanding out to a rounded cerebellopontine angle mass. Masses in paraspinal and head and neck sites may be associated with bone erosion, which is sometimes evident on plain X-ray. Paraspinal examples may also show a dumbbell shape, with a point of constriction at the neural exit foramen.

Macroscopy

Most schwannomas are globoid masses measuring < 10 cm. With the exception of rare examples arising at intraparenchymal CNS sites, viscera, skin, and bone, they are usually encapsulated. In peripheral tumours, a nerve of origin is identified in less than half of cases, often draped over the tumour capsule. The cut surface of the tumour typically shows light-tan glistening tissue interrupted by bright yellow patches, with or without cysts and haemorrhage. Infarct-like necrosis related to degenerative vascular changes may be evident in sizable tumours, such as the giant lumbosacral, retroperitoneal, and pelvic schwannomas that often erode adjacent vertebral bodies.

Microscopy

Conventional schwannoma is composed entirely of neoplastic Schwann cells, other than inflammatory cells, which may be focally numerous. Two basic architectural patterns, in varying proportions, are typically present: areas of compact, elongated cells with occasional nuclear palisading (Antoni A pattern) and less cellular, loosely textured cells with indistinct processes and variable lipidization (Antoni B pattern). A retiform pattern is uncommonly seen. The Schwann cells that make up the tumour have moderate quantities of eosinophilic cytoplasm without discernible cell borders. Antoni A tissue features normochromic spindle-shaped or round nuclei approximately the size of those of smooth muscle cells, but tapered instead of blunt-ended. In Antoni B tissue, the tumour cells have smaller, often round to ovoid nuclei. The Antoni A pattern consists of densely packed spindled tumour cells arranged in fascicles running in different directions. The tumour nuclei may show a tendency to align in alternating parallel rows, forming nuclear palisades. When marked, nuclear palisades are referred to as Verocay bodies. All schwannoma cells show a pericellular reticulin pattern corresponding to surface basement membranes. In Antoni B areas, the tumour cells are loosely arranged.

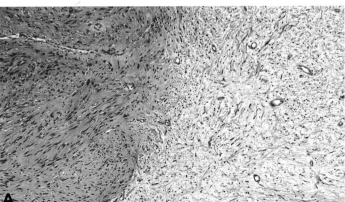
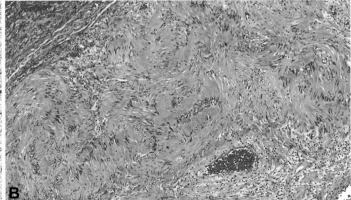

Fig. 9.05 Schwannoma. **A** Compact Antoni A (left) and loose Antoni B (right) areas. **B** A capsule (upper left) surrounds a compact Antoni A region with nuclear palisades, consistent with Verocay bodies.

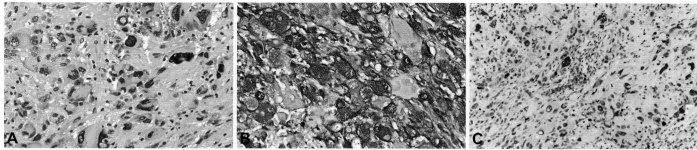

Fig. 9.06 Ancient schwannoma. **A** Marked degenerative atypia may induce concern for malignant transformation, but other features of malignancy are lacking. **B** Diffuse S100 expression. **C** The markedly atypical tumour cells are negative for Ki-67, providing further support that they are degenerative in nature.

Collections of lipid-laden cells may be present within either Antoni A or Antoni B tissue. Schwannoma vasculature is typically thick-walled and hyalinized. Dilated blood vessels surrounded by haemorrhage are common. In the setting of NF2, vestibular schwannomas may show a predominance of Antoni A tissue, whorl formation, and a lobular grape-like growth pattern on low-power examination {2387}. Molecular data suggest that these are polyclonal and likely constitute the confluence of multiple small schwannomas {578}. Malignant transformation, less often microscopic than extensive and transcapsular {1628,2789}, rarely occurs in conventional schwannomas.

Ancient schwannoma

Nuclear pleomorphism, including bizarre forms with cytoplasmic–nuclear inclusions, and the occasional mitotic figure may be seen, but should not be misinterpreted as indicating malignancy. Analogous to other schwannomas, there is typically diffuse S100 and collagen IV positivity, extensive SOX10 expression, and a low Ki-67 proliferation index in the enlarged atypical cells.

Cellular schwannoma

ICD-O code   9560/0

The cellular schwannoma variant is defined as a hypercellular schwannoma

composed exclusively or predominantly of Antoni A tissue and devoid of well-formed Verocay bodies {2786}. The most common location of cellular schwannoma is at paravertebral sites in the pelvis, retroperitoneum, and mediastinum {2786}. Cranial nerves, especially the fifth and eighth, may be affected {376}. The clinical presentation of cellular schwannoma is similar to that of conventional schwannoma, but the histological features of hypercellularity, fascicular cell growth, occasional nuclear hyperchromasia and atypia, and low to medium mitotic activity (usually < 4 mitoses per 10 high-power fields, but occasionally as many as ≥ 10 mitoses per 10 high-power fields) may lead to a misdiagnosis of malignancy (malignant peripheral

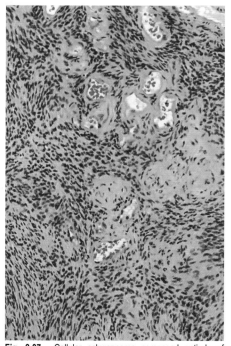

Fig. 9.07 Cellular schwannoma composed entirely of compact Antoni A tissue, but with other common features of conventional schwannoma, such as hyalinized blood vessels.

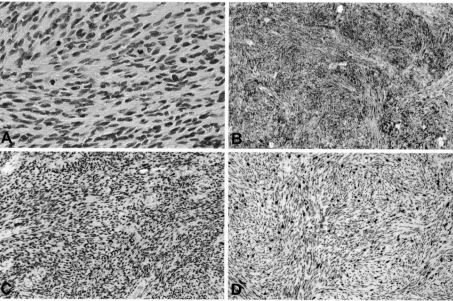

Fig. 9.08 Cellular schwannoma. **A** An increased mitotic index is often seen in cellular schwannoma and should not be taken as evidence of malignant peripheral nerve sheath tumour (MPNST) when other classic features of schwannoma are also found. **B** Diffuse expression of S100 protein helps to distinguish cellular schwannoma from MPNST. **C** Extensive nuclear positivity for SOX10 helps distinguish this cellular schwannoma from MPNST. **D** A moderate Ki-67 proliferation index is not uncommon in cellular schwannoma, but the proliferation index is usually still lower than that encountered in most MPNSTs.

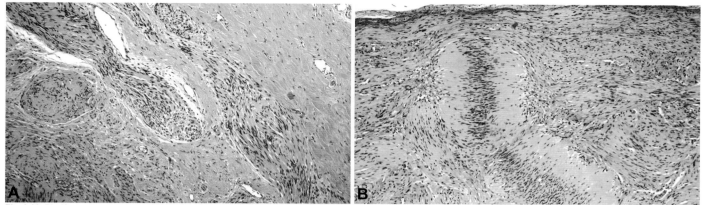

Fig. 9.09 Plexiform schwannoma. **A** Multiple fascicle involvement (plexiform pattern) in a schwannoma. **B** At higher magnification, Verocay bodies can be seen.

nerve sheath tumour) {1924}. In one series, cellular schwannomas were found to differ from malignant peripheral nerve sheath tumours in that the schwannomas had Schwannian whorls, a peritumoural capsule, subcapsular lymphocytes, macrophage-rich infiltrates, and an absence of fascicles, as well as strong, widespread expression of S100, SOX10, neurofibromin, and CDKN2A (p16), with a Ki-67 proliferation index < 20% in most examples {1924}. Cellular schwannomas are benign. Although recurrences are seen, notably in intracranial, spinal, and sacral examples {376}, no cellular schwannoma is known to have metastasized or to have followed a clinically malignant, fatal course. Only two examples of cellular schwannoma, one associated with NF2, have been reported to have undergone malignant transformation {82}.

Plexiform schwannoma

ICD-O code   9560/0

The plexiform schwannoma variant is defined as a schwannoma growing in a plexiform or multinodular manner and can be of either conventional or cellular type {20,2787}. Presumably involving multiple nerve fascicles or a nerve plexus, the vast majority arise in skin or subcutaneous tissue of an extremity, the head and neck, or the trunk, with deep-seated examples also documented {20}. These tumours have been described both in childhood and at birth {2788}. Despite an often rapid growth, hypercellularity, and increased mitotic activity, the behaviour is that of a benign tumour, prone to local recurrence but with no metastatic potential {2788}.

The tumour has a rare association with NF2 (but not with NF1) and has also been noted to occur in patients with schwannomatosis {1108}. Cranial and spinal nerves are usually spared.

Electron microscopy
Ultrastructural features are diagnostic. The cells have convoluted, thin cytoplasmic processes that are nearly devoid of pinocytotic vesicles but are lined by a continuous basal lamina. Stromal long-spaced collagen (called Luse bodies) is a common finding in conventional schwannoma but less so in the cellular variant.

Immunophenotype
The tumour cells strongly and diffusely express S100 protein {2724}; often express SOX10, LEU7, and calretinin {707, 1924}; and may focally express GFAP {1635}. All schwannoma cells have surface basal lamina, so membrane staining for collagen IV and laminin is extensive and most commonly pericellular. Low-level p53 protein immunoreactivity may be seen, particularly in cellular schwannomas {376}. NFP-positive axons are generally absent, but small numbers may be encountered in schwannomas, particularly in tumours associated with NF2 or schwannomatosis {2714}. A mosaic pattern of SMARCB1 (INI1) expression is seen in 93% of tumours from patients with familial schwannomatosis, 55% of tumours from patients with sporadic schwannomatosis, 83% of NF2-associated tumours, and only 5% of solitary, sporadic schwannomas {1909}.

Genetic profile
Extensive analyses have implicated the

NF2 gene as a tumour suppressor integral to the formation of sporadic schwannomas {1117,2314}. The NF2 gene and the merlin protein (also called schwannomin) that it encodes are discussed in detail in the chapter on neurofibromatosis type 2. Inactivating mutations of the NF2 gene have been detected in approximately 60% of all schwannomas {204,1116,1117,2190,2575}. These genetic events are predominantly small frameshift mutations that result in truncated protein products {1536}. Although not described for exons 16 or 17, mutations occur throughout the coding sequence of the gene and at intronic sites. In most cases, such mutations are accompanied by loss of the remaining wildtype allele on chromosome 22q. Other cases demonstrate loss of chromosome 22q in the absence of detectable NF2 gene mutations. Nevertheless, loss of merlin expression, shown by western blotting or immunohistochemistry, appears to be a universal finding in schwannomas, regardless of their mutation or allelic status {1014,1074,2222}. This suggests that abrogation of merlin function is an essential step in schwannoma tumorigenesis. Loss of chromosome 22 has also been noted in cellular schwannoma {1522}. Other genetic changes are rare in schwannomas, although small numbers of cases with loss of chromosome 1p, gain of 9q34, and gain of 17q have been reported {1471,2699}.

Genetic susceptibility
Although most schwannomas are sporadic in occurrence, multiple schwannomas may occur in the setting of two tumour syndromes. Bilateral vestibular schwannomas are pathognomonic of

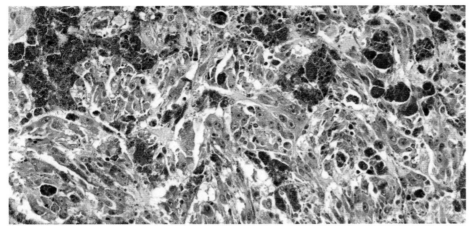

Fig. 9.10 Melanotic schwannoma with clusters of plump, spindled, and epithelioid, heavily pigmented tumour cells.

NF2, whereas multiple, mostly non-vestibular schwannomas in the absence of other NF2 features are characteristic of schwannomatosis (see *Schwannomatosis*, p. 301). Patients with schwannomatosis present with multiple, often painful schwannomas, which in some cases are segmental in distribution. Germline *SMARCB1* mutations at 22q11.23 have been found in half of all familial and < 10% of all sporadic schwannomatosis cases {1064,2325,2381}. Somatic *NF2* inactivation has been shown in tumours, but germline NF2 mutations are absent {1115,1557}. Germline loss-of-function mutations in *LZTR1* predispose individuals to an autosomal dominant inherited disorder of multiple schwannomas, and are identified in approximately 80% of 22q-related schwannomatosis cases that lack mutations in *SMARCB1* {1980}. The presence of *LZTR1* mutations also confers an increased risk of vestibular schwannoma, constituting further overlap with NF2 {2377}.

Prognosis and predictive factors

Schwannomas are benign, slow-growing tumours that infrequently recur and only very rarely undergo malignant change {2789}. Recurrences are more common (occurring in 30–40% of cases) for cellular schwannomas of the intracranial, spinal, and sacral regions {376} and for plexiform schwannoma {2788}.

....

Melanotic schwannoma

Definition

A rare, circumscribed but unencapsulated, grossly pigmented tumour composed of cells with the ultrastructure and immunophenotype of Schwann cells but that contain melanosomes and are reactive for melanocytic markers.

In melanotic schwannoma, cytological atypia (including hyperchromasia and macronucleoli) is common. Unlike in conventional schwannomas, collagen IV and laminin usually envelop cell nests rather than showing extensive pericellular

deposition. Similarly, melanotic schwannomas feature true melanosomes and less-uniform envelopment of individual cells by basal lamina on electron microscopy.

The peak age incidence of melanotic schwannoma is a decade younger than that of conventional schwannoma. Melanotic schwannomas occur in both non-psammomatous {720} and psammomatous {368,624} varieties. The vast majority of non-psammomatous tumours affect spinal nerves and paraspinal ganglia, whereas psammomatous lesions also involve autonomic nerves of viscera, such as the intestinal tract and heart. Cranial nerves may also be affected. Distinguishing between the two varieties of melanotic schwannoma is important, because about 50% of patients with psammomatous tumours have Carney complex, an autosomal dominant disorder {367} characterized by lentiginous facial pigmentation, cardiac myxoma, and endocrine hyperactivity. Endocrine hyperactivity includes Cushing syndrome associated with adrenal hyperplasia and acromegaly due to pituitary adenoma {368}. Slightly more than 10% of all melanotic schwannomas follow a malignant course {367}.

ICD-O code   9560/1

Genetic susceptibility

Allelic loss of the *PRKAR1A* region on 17q has been reported in tumours from patients with Carney complex, but has not been documented in non-psammomatous melanotic schwannomas {2435}. Psammomatous melanotic schwannoma is a component of Carney complex, in which patients have loss-of-function germline mutations of the *PRKAR1A* gene on chromosome 17q, encoding the cAMP-dependent protein kinase type I-alpha regulatory subunit {2435}.

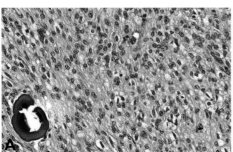
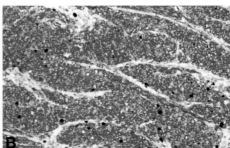
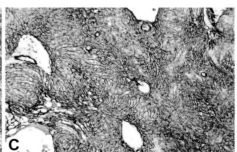

Fig. 9.11 Melanotic schwannoma. **A** Psammomatous calcification is a diagnostically useful feature of psammomatous melanotic schwannomas. **B** This dual stain reveals diffuse immunoreactivity for melan-A (in red) and a low Ki-67 proliferation index, with positive nuclei (in brown). The low proliferation index helps distinguish this lesion from melanoma. **C** Psammomatous melanotic schwannoma. The extensive pericellular collagen-IV expression in this case supports its Schwannian nature, given that melanocytic tumours are not associated with basement membrane deposition.

Neurofibroma

Perry A.
von Deimling A.
Louis D.N.
Hunter S.
Reuss D.E.
Antonescu C.R.

Definition

A benign, well-demarcated, intraneural or diffusely infiltrative extraneural nerve sheath tumour consisting of neoplastic, well-differentiated Schwann cells intermixed with non-neoplastic elements including perineurial-like cells, fibroblasts, mast cells, a variably myxoid to collagenous matrix, and residual axons or ganglion cells.

Multiple and plexiform neurofibromas are typically associated with neurofibromatosis type 1 (NF1), whereas sporadic neurofibromas are common, mostly cutaneous tumours that can affect patients of any age and any area of the body.

ICD-O code   9540/0

Grading

Neurofibroma corresponds histologically to WHO grade I.

Epidemiology

Neurofibromas are common and occur either as sporadic solitary nodules unrelated to any apparent syndrome or (far less frequently) as solitary, multiple, or numerous lesions in individuals with NF1. Patients of any race, age, or sex can be affected.

Localization

Neurofibroma presents most commonly as a cutaneous nodule (localized cutaneous neurofibroma), less often as a circumscribed mass in a peripheral nerve (localized intraneural neurofibroma), or as a plexiform mass within a major nerve trunk or plexus. Least frequent is diffuse but localized involvement of skin and subcutaneous tissue (diffuse cutaneous neurofibroma) or extensive to massive involvement of soft tissue of a body area (localized gigantism and elephantiasis neuromatosa). Neurofibromas rarely involve spinal roots sporadically, but commonly do so in patients with NF1, in which multiple bilateral tumours are often associated with scoliosis and risks of malignant transformation {1778}; in contrast, they almost never involve cranial nerves.

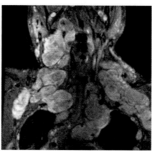
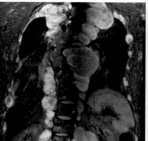
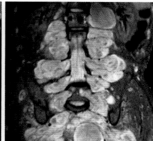

Fig. 9.12 Total spine MRI in a patient with neurofibromatosis type 1 with extensive bilateral paraspinal disease burden. Neurofibromas involve nearly every nerve root; also note the thoracic spine curvature defect.

Clinical features

Rarely painful, neurofibroma presents as a mass. Deeper tumours, including paraspinal forms, present with motor and sensory deficits attributable to the nerve of origin. The presence of multiple neurofibromas is the hallmark of NF1, in association with many other characteristic manifestations (see *Neurofibromatosis type 1*, p. 294).

Macroscopy

Cutaneous neurofibromas are nodular to polypoid and circumscribed, or are diffuse, and involve skin and subcutaneous tissue. Neurofibromas confined to nerves are fusiform and (in all but their proximal and distal margins) well circumscribed. Plexiform neurofibromas consist either of multinodular tangles (resembling a bag of worms), when involving multiple trunks of a neural plexus, or of rope-like lesions, when multiple fascicles of a large, non-branching nerve such as the sciatic

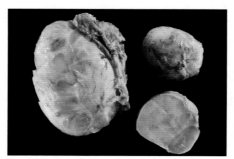

Fig. 9.13 Neurofibroma of a spinal root, with a firm consistency and homogeneous cut surface.

nerve are affected. On cut surface, they are firm, glistening, and greyish tan.

Microscopy

Neurofibromas are composed in large part of neoplastic Schwann cells with thin, curved to elongated nuclei and scant cytoplasm, as well as fibroblasts in a matrix of collagen fibres and Alcian blue–positive myxoid material. These cells have considerably smaller nuclei than those of schwannomas. The cell processes are thin and often not visible on routine light microscopy. Residual axons are often present within neurofibromas, and can be highlighted with neurofilament immunohistochemistry or Bodian silver impregnations. Large diffuse neurofibromas often contain highly characteristic tactile-like structures (specifically pseudo-Meissner corpuscles) and may also contain melanotic cells. Stromal collagen formation varies greatly in abundance and sometimes takes the form of dense, refractile bundles with a so-called shredded-carrot appearance. Intraneural neurofibromas often remain confined to the nerve, encompassed by its thickened epineurium. In contrast, tumours arising in small cutaneous nerves commonly spread diffusely into surrounding dermis and soft tissues. Unlike in schwannomas, blood vessels in neurofibromas generally lack hyalinization, and although neurofibromas sometimes resemble the Antoni B regions of a schwannoma, they generally lack Antoni A–like regions and Verocay bodies.

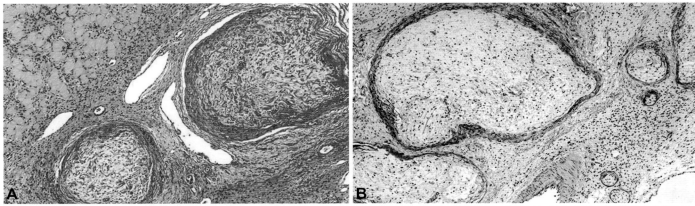

Fig. 9.14 Plexiform neurofibroma. **A** Multinodular pattern from involvement of multiple fascicles. Note the associated diffuse neurofibroma in the background, with pseudo-Meissner corpuscles (upper left). **B** EMA immunostaining highlights the perineurium surrounding multiple involved fascicles, whereas the tumour cells are mostly negative.

Ancient neurofibroma

This pattern is defined by degenerative nuclear atypia alone (analogous to ancient schwannoma) and should be distinguished from atypical neurofibroma, given the lack of any associated clinical relevance {2146}; this is similar to ancient schwannoma, which has degenerative atypia but lacks any other features of malignancy.

Atypical neurofibroma

Atypical neurofibroma is a variant defined by worrisome features such as high cellularity, scattered mitotic figures, monomorphic cytology, and/or fascicular growth in addition to cytological atypia, may show premalignant features (see Genetic profile) and is notoriously difficult to distinguish from low-grade malignant peripheral nerve sheath tumour (MPNST) {178}.

ICD-O code   9540/0

Plexiform neurofibroma

Plexiform neurofibroma is a variant defined by involvement of multiple fascicles, which are expanded by tumour cells and collagen, but commonly demonstrate residual, bundled nerve fibres at their centres. Rare neurofibromas are thought to exhibit limited perineurial differentiation {2845} or form a hybrid neurofibroma/perineurioma {2146}.

ICD-O code   9550/0

Electron microscopy

Electron microscopy shows a mixture of cell types, the two most diagnostically important being the Schwann cell and the perineurial-like cell {648}. The perineurial-like cell features long, very thin cell processes, pinocytotic vesicles, and interrupted basement membrane. Fibroblasts and mast cells are least frequent.

Immunophenotype

Staining for S100 protein is invariably positive, but the proportion of reactive cells is smaller than in schwannoma. A similar pattern is seen with nuclear SOX10 positivity {1222}. Expression of basement membrane markers is more variable than in schwannoma. Unlike perineuriomas, neurofibromas contain only limited numbers of EMA-positive cells, with reactivity most apparent in residual perineurium. Scattered cells, presumably the perineurial-like cells seen ultrastructurally also show GLUT1 {1012} or claudin positivity {2044}. Neurofilament staining reveals entrapped axons in intraneural and plexiform neurofibromas, whereas KIT staining highlights recruited mast cells and a subset of stromal cells may stain for CD34. Like in other nerve sheath tumours, GFAP expression may be seen.

Genetic profile

Given their mixed cellular composition, it has been difficult to determine whether neurofibromas are monoclonal. Notably, allelic loss of the *NF1* gene region of

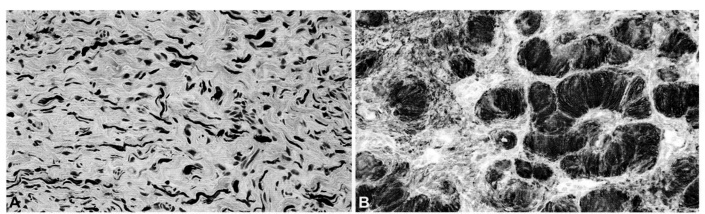

Fig. 9.15 Neurofibroma. **A** Strong, but patchy S100 positivity is seen, the stain generally labelling a smaller proportion of cells than in schwannoma. **B** In pseudo-Meissner corpuscles, S100 staining is diffuse.

17q seems to be confined to the S100-positive Schwann cells in neurofibromas {1947}, suggesting that they are the clonal neoplastic element. This is further supported by in vitro experiments showing biallelic inactivation of the *NF1* gene in cultured Schwann cells from neurofibromas {1564}, confirming the two-hit hypothesis for the genesis of these lesions, at least those arising from patients with NF1. However, some data also suggest that S100-negative perineurial-like cells are neoplastic, and that neurofibromas arise from dedifferentiated myelinating Schwann cells in a process similar to wound healing in peripheral nerve {2112}. The situation in sporadic tumours has yet to be fully elucidated, but the morphological similarity between sporadic and inherited neurofibromas, as well as the clear involvement of the *NF1* gene in sporadic MPNSTs, suggests that *NF1* alterations are also involved in the genesis of sporadic neurofibromas, and this has in fact been documented in rare cases {156,2434}. Neurofibromas do not normally develop in mouse models with inactivation of *NF1* in Schwann cells, unless the mouse itself is also *NF1* haploinsufficient, analogous to human patients with NF1; evidence suggests that haploinsufficient mast cells within the tumour microenvironment stimulate *NF1*-deficient Schwann cells to grow and form neurofibromas {2869} or that additional signalling pathways of nerve injury are required for tumour formation. The downstream

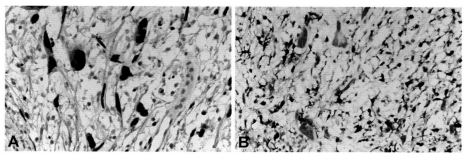

Fig. 9.16 Atypical neurofibroma. **A** Retained SOX10 expression in cytologically atypical nuclei. **B** Loss of expression of CDKN2A (p16) in cytologically atypical nuclei, possibly representing a premalignant change.

effects of *NF1* loss include activation of the RAS/MAPK and AKT/mTOR pathways. Less is known about cutaneous neurofibromas, although evidence suggests a similar mechanism but with a different cell of origin (e.g. dermal skin-derived precursors) and different hotspot mutations {1442,2545}.

Additional chromosomal losses are not common in neurofibromas, but have been noted on 19p, 19q, and 22q in NF1-associated neurofibromas and on 19q and 22q in sporadic neurofibromas {1320}. *CDKN2A/CDKN2B* losses are generally considered a sign of malignant transformation, and these losses are also commonly found in tumours diagnosed as atypical neurofibromas in patients with NF1, suggesting that such tumours may be premalignant lesions {155}.

Genetic susceptibility

The occurrence of multiple and plexiform neurofibromas is a hallmark of NF1 (see *Neurofibromatosis type 1*, p. 294). Neurofibromas are exceptionally uncommon in NF2 and schwannomatosis.

Prognosis and predictive factors

Plexiform neurofibromas and neurofibromas of major nerves are considered potential precursors of MPNST. Malignant transformation occurs in 5–10% of large plexiform tumours, but is a rare event in diffuse cutaneous and massive soft tissue neurofibromas. A patient with a sizable plexiform neurofibroma is highly likely to have NF1 and should be investigated for other evidence of the disorder. Similar to low-grade MPNST, an atypical neurofibroma that extends to a surgical margin has a low risk of subsequent recurrence, but essentially no associated mortality {179}.

Perineurioma

Antonescu C.R.
Perry A.
Reuss D.E.

Definition

A tumour composed entirely of neoplastic perineurial cells.

Intraneural perineuriomas are benign and consist of proliferating perineurial cells within the endoneurium, forming characteristic pseudo–onion bulbs. Soft tissue perineuriomas are typically not associated with nerve, are variably whorled, and are usually benign. Malignant soft tissue perineurioma is a rare variant of malignant peripheral nerve sheath tumour displaying perineurial differentiation. Intraneural perineurioma, long mistakenly considered a form of hypertrophic neuropathy, is now recognized as a neoplasm {637}.

ICD-O code   9571/0

Grading

Intraneural perineuriomas correspond histologically to WHO grade I. Soft tissue perineuriomas range from benign (corresponding histologically to WHO grade I) to variably malignant (corresponding histologically to WHO grades II–III).

Epidemiology

Intraneural perineuriomas typically present in adolescence or early adulthood and show no sex predilection. Soft tissue perineuriomas occur in adults, predominantly females (with a female-to-male ratio of 2:1), and present with non-specific mass effects. Both the intraneural and soft tissue variants of perineurioma are rare, accounting for approximately 1% of nerve sheath and soft tissue neoplasms, respectively. More than 50 cases of intraneural perineurioma have been reported to date, including cranial nerve examples. More than 100 cases of soft tissue perineurioma have been described {695, 827,879,1042,2070}, including an intraosseous example surrounding a cranial nerve {134}.

Localization

Intraneural perineuriomas primarily affect peripheral nerves of the extremities; cranial nerve lesions are rare {59,515,1483}. One example was reportedly associated with Beckwith–Wiedemann syndrome {424}. Soft tissue perineuriomas are located in the deep soft tissue and are grossly unassociated with nerve. Visceral involvement is rare {1041,2608}. One example involving the CNS arose within a lateral ventricle {829}.

Clinical features

In intraneural perineuriomas, progressive muscle weakness (with or without obvious atrophy) is more frequent than are sensory disturbances. Malignant examples of soft tissue perineuriomas prone to recurrence and occasional metastasis

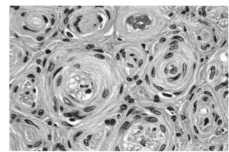

Fig. 9.18 Intraneural perineurioma. Pseudo–onion bulb formation is seen at high magnification.

have been reported {756,1011,1221,2176, 2460} and are apparently unassociated with neurofibromatosis type 1 {1011}.

Macroscopy

Intraneural perineurioma produces a segmental, tubular, several-fold enlargement of the affected nerve. Individual nerve fascicles appear coarse and pale. Most lesions are < 10 cm long, but one 40-cm-long sciatic nerve example has been reported {637}. Although multiple fascicles are often involved, a bag-of-worms plexiform growth is not seen. Involvement of two neighbouring spinal nerves has been reported {637}. Soft tissue perineuriomas are solitary, generally small (1.5–7 cm), and well circumscribed but unencapsulated. Rarely, the tumours can be multinodular {82}. On cut

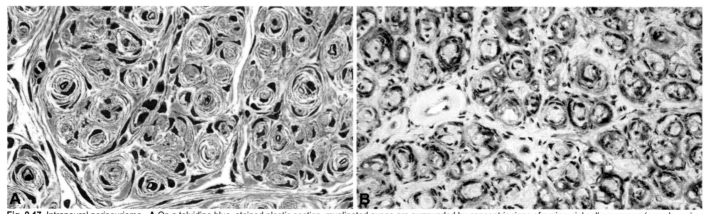

Fig. 9.17 Intraneural perineurioma. **A** On a toluidine blue–stained plastic section, myelinated axons are surrounded by concentric rings of perineurial cell processes (pseudo–onion bulbs). **B** EMA staining highlights concentric layers of perineurial cells in pseudo–onion bulbs.

surface, they are firm and greyish white to infrequently focally myxoid. Malignant soft tissue perineuriomas are usually not associated with a nerve and may feature invasive growth and variable necrosis.

Microscopy

Intraneural perineurioma consists of neoplastic perineurial cells proliferating throughout the endoneurium. These cells form concentric layers around axons, causing enlargement of fascicles and forming characteristic pseudo-onion bulbs. This distinctive architectural feature is best seen on cross-section, wherein fascicles vary in cellularity. The proliferation of cytologically normal-looking perineurial cells largely takes place within endoneurium, but perineurium is often affected as well. Particularly large whorls can envelop numerous nerve fibres. Occasionally, perineurial cells enclosing one or several axons contribute to an adjacent onion bulb as well. Thus, pseudo-onion bulbs anastomose, forming a complex endoneurial network. Even within a single fascicle, cell density and the complexity of the lesion can vary. Mitotic activity is rare. In early lesions, axonal density and myelination may be almost normal, whereas in fully developed lesions, when most fibres are surrounded by perineurial cells and therefore widely separated, myelin is often scant or absent on Luxol fast blue staining. At late stages, only Schwann cells without accompanying axons may remain at the centre of the perineurial whorls. Hyalinization may be prominent.

Soft tissue perineuriomas are composed of spindled, wavy cells with remarkably thin cytoplasmic processes arranged in lamellae and embedded in collagen fibres. Crude whorls or storiform arrangements are commonly seen. Aggregates of collagen fibres are often encircled by long, remarkably narrow tumour cell processes. Nuclei are elongate with tapered ends and are often curved or wrinkled. Nucleoli are inconspicuous. Granular cells are a very uncommon feature of perineurioma {585}. Mitoses vary in number. In the largest published series {1042}, the mitotic count ranged from 0 to 13 (mean: 1) mitoses per 30 high-power fields, with 65% of the tumours showing none. Degenerative atypia (i.e. nuclear pleomorphism, hyperchromasia, and cytoplasmic–nuclear inclusions) is seen primarily in long-standing tumours {1042}.

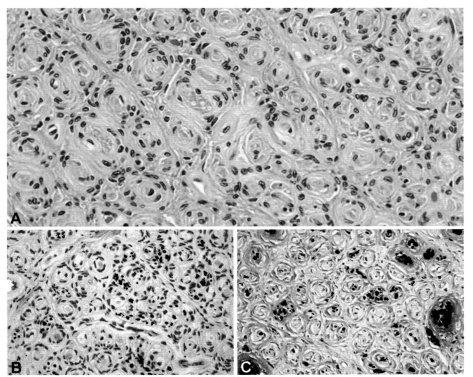

Fig. 9.19 Intraneural perineurioma. **A** Pseudo–onion bulbs and variable collagenization on cross-section. **B** NFP staining highlights entrapped centrally placed axons in pseudo–onion bulbs. **C** S100 staining shows entrapped centrally placed Schwann cells in pseudo–onion bulbs.

Necrosis is typically lacking. The sclerotic variant, characterized by an abundant collagenous stroma, has been described occurring mainly in the fingers of young male patients {695}. This variant features only crude whorl formation, occasionally centred on a minute nerve. A reticular variant that occurs at a variety of anatomical sites and primarily affects adults features a lace-like or reticular growth pattern composed of anastomosing cords of fusiform cells {879}. Malignant soft tissue perineuriomas (i.e. perineurial malignant peripheral nerve sheath tumours) are uncommon and characterized by hypercellularity, hyperchromasia, and often brisk (but variable) mitotic activity (WHO grade II), necrosis usually being a feature of WHO grade III tumours. Progressive malignant change of WHO grade II to grade III lesions may be seen, but transformation of benign soft tissue perineuriomas to malignant examples has not been documented.

Electron microscopy

Intraneural perineuriomas feature myelinated nerve fibres circumferentially surrounded by ultrastructurally normal-looking perineurial cells. The cells have long, thin cytoplasmic processes bearing numerous pinocytotic vesicles and are lined by patchy surface basement membrane. Stromal collagen may be abundant.

Soft tissue perineuriomas typically consist of spindle-shaped cells with long, exceedingly thin cytoplasmic processes embedded in an abundant collagenous stroma. Cytoplasm is scant and contains sparse profiles of rough endoplasmic reticulum, occasional mitochondria, and a few randomly distributed intermediate filaments. The processes exhibit numerous pinocytotic vesicles and a patchy lining of basement membrane. Intercellular tight junctions are relatively frequent. One example featuring ribosome–lamella complexes has been reported {580}. Malignant soft tissue perineuriomas show similar ultrastructural features {1011, 2176,2460}, only a subset being poorly differentiated {1011}.

Immunophenotype

Like normal perineurial cells, all intraneural perineuriomas are immunoreactive for vimentin. The pattern of EMA staining is membranous, as are those of collagen IV and laminin. Axons at the centre of pseudo–onion bulbs and residual Schwann cells stain for NFP and S100 protein, respectively. Staining for p53 protein has also been reported {637}. Soft tissue perineurioma features the same basic immunophenotype. Claudin-1 {719,2070} and GLUT1 {1012} are also diagnostically useful markers. Unlike various other soft tissue tumours, perineuriomas generally lack reactivity for CD34, MUC4, and in particular, S100 protein. Malignant soft tissue perineuriomas usually show at least some EMA staining and lack S100 protein reactivity.

Proliferation
Intraneural perineuriomas, despite a paucity of mitoses, may show a Ki-67 proliferation index of 5–15% {637}. In contrast to benign soft tissue perineuriomas,

which often have a low mitotic index, malignant soft tissue perineuriomas are more proliferative, with mitotic counts of 1–85 mitoses (median: 16) per 10 high-power fields in the largest reported series {1011}.

Genetic profile
Both intraneural and soft tissue perineuriomas feature the same cytogenetic abnormality: monosomy of chromosome 22 {637,827}. Loss of chromosome 13, an abnormality found in several soft tissue tumours, has also been described in soft tissue perineurioma {1717}. Loss of chromosome 10 and a small chromosome 22q deletion involving *NF2* have also been reported {281,2311}. No genetic

studies of malignant soft tissue perineuriomas have been reported.

Prognosis and predictive factors
Intraneural perineuriomas are benign. Long-term follow-up indicates that they do not have a tendency to recur or metastasize. Biopsy alone is sufficient for diagnosis. Conventional soft tissue perineuriomas are usually amenable to gross total removal. Recurrences are very infrequent, even in cases with histological atypia, and none have been reported to metastasize. Neither sclerotic nor reticular tumours are prone to recurrence {695,879}. Malignant perineuriomas are far less prone to metastasize {756,1011, 1221} than are conventional malignant peripheral nerve sheath tumours {1011}.

Hybrid nerve sheath tumours

Antonescu C.R.
Stemmer-Rachamimov A.O.
Perry A.

Definition
Benign peripheral nerve sheath tumours (PNSTs) with combined features of more than one conventional type (i.e. neurofibroma, schwannoma, and perineurioma).
Two of the more common types of hybrid nerve sheath tumours are schwannoma/perineurioma, which typically occurs sporadically, and neurofibroma/schwannoma, which is typically associated with schwannomatosis, neurofibromatosis type 1 (NF1) or neurofibromatosis type 2 (NF2). Rare cases of neurofibroma/perineurioma have also been described, usually associated with NF1.

Etiology
Hybrid schwannoma/perineurioma occurs sporadically {1040}, whereas neurofibroma/schwannoma can occur in the setting of either schwannomatosis or neurofibromatosis {945}. Similarly, hybrid neurofibroma/perineurioma tumours are more commonly reported in association with NF1 {1091,1199}.

Localization
Hybrid nerve sheath tumours show a wide anatomical distribution and often involve the dermis and subcutis {681,

1040}. They are rarely associated with cranial or spinal nerves. Most tumours showing biphasic schwannoma and reticular perineurioma have been reported on the digits {1661}.

Clinical features
The clinical features of peripheral nerve sheath hybrid tumours are similar to or indistinguishable from those of other benign PNSTs and largely depend on the site of origin. Hybrid nerve sheath tumours (including spinal examples) may cause neurological deficit or pain when they involve a large peripheral nerve.

Macroscopy
The gross appearance and radiological findings of hybrid tumours are indistinguishable from those of other PNSTs (i.e. schwannomas and neurofibromas).

Microscopy
Hybrid schwannoma/perineurioma tumours show predominantly Schwannian cytomorphology but have a perineurioma-like architecture. These tumours are usually well circumscribed but unencapsulated, and composed of spindle cells with plump, tapering nuclei and palely

eosinophilic cytoplasm with indistinct cell borders, arranged in a storiform, whorled, and/or lamellar architecture {1040}. The tumours may exhibit myxoid stromal changes (seen in half of all cases) and often display degenerative cytological atypia similar to the ancient changes seen in schwannoma.
Hybrid neurofibromas/schwannomas are tumours in which two distinct components are recognized: a schwannoma-like component with nodular Schwann cell proliferation (which may contain Verocay bodies) and a neurofibroma-like component with a mixed cellular population, myxoid change, and collagen {681, 945}. Plexiform architecture is common. The schwannoma-like component is mainly composed of cellular Antoni A areas, often containing Verocay bodies with Schwann cells demonstrating nuclear palisading. In contrast, the neurofibroma-like component may demonstrate abundant fibroblasts, collagen, and myxoid changes, with Schwannian cells having a distinctive elongated and wavy appearance.
The few examples of hybrid neurofibroma/perineurioma that have been described consisted of plexiform neurofibromas

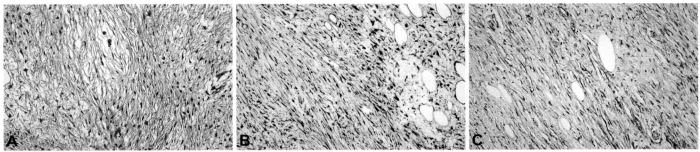

Fig. 9.20 Hybrid schwannoma/perineurioma. **A** Benign spindle cell nerve sheath tumour with loose myxoid stroma that is difficult to classify on H&E alone. **B** S100 immunostaining highlights about two thirds of the hybrid nerve sheath tumour cells, identifying the Schwann cell component. **C** EMA staining highlights about one third of the tumour cells, identifying the perineurial component.

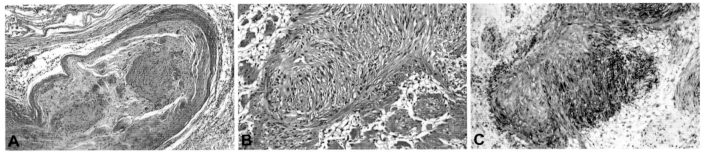

Fig. 9.21 Hybrid neurofibroma/schwannoma. **A,B** Schwann cell micronodules. **C** S100-positive Schwann cell micronodules.

with considerable areas of perineuriomatous differentiation, in patients with NF1 {1199}. In these lesions, biphasic (Schwannian and perineuriomatous) differentiation was apparent mainly on immunohistochemistry, with rare cases in which the neurofibromatous and perineuriomatous areas were recognizable on routine H&E stains {1199}.

Immunophenotype
Schwannoma/perineurioma hybrid tumours show dual differentiation by immunohistochemistry, with the Schwannian cells (plump-spindled) being positive for S100 protein whereas the perineurial cells (slender-spindled) show variable immunoreactivity for EMA, claudin-1, and GLUT1 {2816}. Using double staining for EMA and S100 protein, parallel layers of alternating S100-positive and EMA-positive cells can be seen, with no coexpression of antigens by the same cells {1040}. On the basis of these dual-labelling results, most tumours were found to be composed of about two thirds Schwann cells and one third perineurial cells.

The most helpful stains for the work-up of a neurofibroma/schwannoma are those that highlight the presence of a monomorphic Schwann cell population in the schwannoma component (i.e. S100 and SOX10) or a polymorphic cell population in the neurofibroma component, including Schwann cells (S100 and SOX10), perineurial cells (EMA and GLUT1), and fibroblasts. Entrapped axons may be seen in neurofibromatosis-associated schwannomas, but the presence of entrapped large bundles of axons is more common in neurofibromas {681}.
In neurofibroma/perineurioma, the biphasic Schwannian and perineuriomatous differentiation is apparent by immunohistochemistry, with the perineuriomatous areas staining positively for EMA, GLUT1, and claudin-1 and negatively for S100 protein {1199}. In fact, intraneural perineurial proliferations have been documented by screening neurofibromatous lesions and normal nerves in patients with NF1 using a battery of perineurial markers, supporting the existence of both pure and hybrid perineuriomatous

lesions within the spectrum of PNSTs in NF1 {17}.

Genetic susceptibility
More than half of all patients with hybrid PNSTs have multiple PNSTs, suggesting a tumour syndrome. Hybrid neurofibroma/schwannoma is a common tumour type in schwannomatosis, occurring in 71% of patients. There is also a striking association with neurofibromatosis {945} where this hybrid lesion is more common in NF2 (occurring in 26% of cases) than in NF1 (occurring in 9% of cases). Within patients with schwannomatosis, 61% of the developed tumours had the appearance of schwannoma-like nodules within a neurofibroma-like tumour, corresponding to hybrid neurofibroma/schwannoma {945}. The presence of hybrid morphology and/or mosaic SMARCB1 (INI1) expression on immunohistochemistry suggests that a schwannoma may be associated with a form of neurofibromatosis, in particular NF2 and schwannomatosis {1909,1990}. Similarly, hybrid neurofibroma/perineurioma occurs mostly in association with NF1 {1199}.

Malignant peripheral nerve sheath tumour

Reuss D.E.
Louis D.N.
Hunter S.

Perry A.
Hirose T.
Antonescu C.R.

Definition

A malignant tumour with evidence of Schwann cell or perineurial cell differentiation, commonly arising in a peripheral nerve or in extraneural soft tissue.

Malignant peripheral nerve sheath tumours (MPNSTs) primarily affect young to middle-aged adults, but also affect adolescents; about 50% of MPNSTs are associated with neurofibromatosis type 1 (NF1), in which they often arise from a pre-existing plexiform or intraneural neurofibroma and affect younger patients. In contrast, most sporadic cases arise from large peripheral nerves without an associated benign precursor. Most MPNSTs show combined inactivation of *NF1*, *CDKN2A*, and PRC2 component genes.

ICD-O code   9540/3

Grading

Clinically validated and reproducible grading systems for MPNST are generally lacking. One approach to MPNST grading is to divide the tumours into low-grade (~15% of cases) and high-grade (~85% of cases) {2146}, albeit without robust and validated criteria. Low-grade MPNSTs are well-differentiated tumours most often arising in transition from neurofibroma. An increased mitotic rate is often seen but is not required for the diagnosis {1166}. Conventional monomorphous spindle cell MPNSTs, highly pleomorphic MPNSTs, and MPNSTs with divergent differentiation (e.g. malignant triton tumour; glandular MPNST; and osteosarcomatous, chondrosarcomatous, and angiosarcomatous differentiation) are all considered high-grade.

Epidemiology

MPNSTs are uncommon, accounting for ≤ 5% of all malignant soft tissue tumours {1479}. MPNSTs primarily affect adults in the third to the sixth decades of life. The mean age of patients with MPNSTs associated with NF1 is approximately a decade younger (28–36 years) than that of patients with sporadic cases (40–44 years) {606,1055}. There is no sex pre-

dilection. Childhood and adolescent cases account for 10–20% of MPNSTs {66}.

Etiology

About 50% of all MPNSTs are associated with NF1, in which setting they typically arise from deep-seated plexiform neurofibromas or large intraneural neurofibromas. About 40% of MPNSTs arise in patients without known predisposition {606,1055}, and 10% of MPNSTs are associated with previous radiation therapy {1416}. Only rare examples develop from conventional schwannoma {1628}, ganglioneuroblastoma/ganglioneuroma {2113}, or phaeochromocytoma {2223}.

Localization

Large and medium-sized nerves are distinctly more prone to involvement than are small nerves. The most commonly involved sites include the buttock and thigh, brachial plexus and upper arm, and paraspinal region. The sciatic nerve is most frequently affected. Cranial nerve MPNSTs are rare, and more commonly arise from schwannomas than do MPNSTs located elsewhere {2260}. Primary intraparenchymal MPNST is rare {129}.

Clinical features

The most common presentation in the extremities is a progressively enlarging mass, with or without neurological symptoms. Spinal tumours often present with radicular pain {2439}.

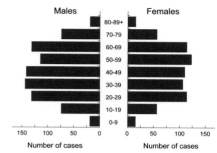

Fig. 9.22 Age and sex distribution of MPNST, based on 1711 histologically confirmed cases. Data from the Surveillance, Epidemiology, and End Results Program (SEER), National Cancer Institute, Washington DC.

Imaging

Imaging findings correspond to those of soft tissue sarcoma. Inhomogeneous contrast enhancement and irregularity of contour (a reflection of invasion) are commonly seen. FDG-PET is a sensitive tool for the detection of MPNSTs in patients with NF1 {441,574}.

Spread

MPNSTs often infiltrate adjacent soft tissues and may spread along intraneural and haematogenous routes. About 20–25% of patients develop metastases, most commonly to the lungs {2874}.

Macroscopy

The gross appearance of MPNST varies greatly. Because a significant proportion of these tumours arise in neurofibroma,

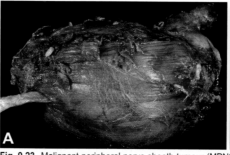
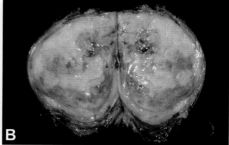

Fig. 9.23 Malignant peripheral nerve sheath tumour (MPNST). **A** Resected MPNST with its parent nerve on the left. Note the skeletal muscle that forms part of the surgical margin, indicating invasion into the surrounding soft tissues. **B** On cut surface, this tumour shows the classic variegated appearance, with fleshy soft cellular regions alternating with yellow foci of necrosis.

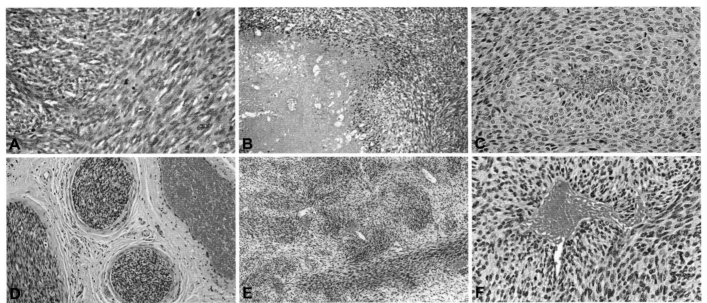

Fig. 9.24 Malignant peripheral nerve sheath tumour (MPNST). **A** Brisk mitotic activity. **B** Well-delineated geographical necrosis. **C** A pattern of perivascular hypercellularity and slight intraluminal herniation. **D** Intraneural spread of tumour into small neural fascicles. **E** Marbled, alternating light (loose) and dark (compact) appearance is typical of some MPNSTs. **F** Intraluminal vascular herniation of tumour cells is seen in this tumour.

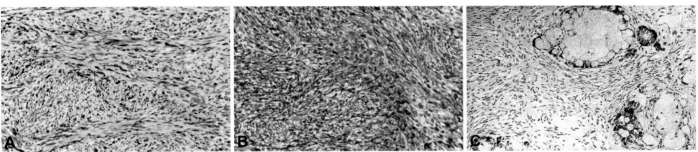

Fig. 9.25 Malignant peripheral nerve sheath tumour (MPNST). **A** Patchy S100 expression. **B** EGFR immunoreactivity. **C** Glandular MPNST, containing neuroendocrine cells immunoreactive to chromogranin.

some as focal transformations, the process may be minimally apparent on gross examination. In contrast, larger, typically high-grade tumours originating in or unassociated with a nerve produce either fusiform, expansile masses or globular, entirely unencapsulated soft tissue tumours. Both types infiltrate surrounding structures. The vast majority of tumours are > 5 cm, and examples > 10 cm are common. Their consistency ranges from soft to hard, and the cut surface is typically cream-coloured or grey. Foci of necrosis and haemorrhage are common and may be extensive.

Microscopy
MPNSTs vary greatly in appearance. Many exhibit a herringbone (fibrosarcoma-like) or interwoven fasciculated pattern of cell growth. Both patterns feature tightly packed spindle cells with variable quantities of eosinophilic cytoplasm. Nuclei are typically elongated and wavy and (unlike those of smooth muscle) have tapered ends. The tumours show either alternating loose and densely cellular areas or a diffuse growth pattern. Perivascular hypercellularity and tumour aggregates appearing to herniate into vascular lumina are also common {1924}. Unusual growth patterns may be seen, including haemangiopericytoma-like areas or rarely, nuclear palisading. MPNSTs grow within nerve fascicles but commonly invade adjacent soft tissues. A pseudocapsule of variable thickness is often present. Three quarters of these tumours have geographical necrosis and mitotic activity, often showing > 4 mitoses per high-power field (high-grade).

Malignant peripheral nerve sheath tumour with divergent differentiation

Synonyms
Malignant triton tumour; glandular malignant peripheral nerve sheath tumour

A variety of mesenchymal tissues such as cartilage, bone, skeletal muscle, smooth muscle, and angiosarcoma-like areas can be present in MPNSTs. MPNSTs showing rhabdomyosarcomatous differentiation are called malignant triton tumours. Nearly 60% of patients with malignant triton tumour have NF1. Glandular MPNST is a variant containing glandular epithelium that resembles that of intestine. Neuroendocrine differentiation is frequently seen, whereas squamous epithelium is far less often encountered. Three quarters of the patients have NF1 {2785}.

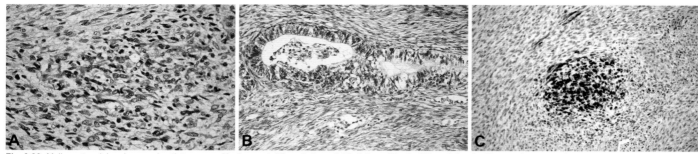

Fig. 9.26 Malignant peripheral nerve sheath tumours with divergent differentiation. **A** Rhabdomyoblastic differentiation (malignant triton tumour). **B** Formation of glands. **C** Focal myogenic differentiation visualized by desmin-positive tumour cells.

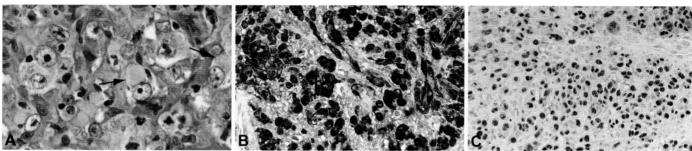

Fig. 9.27 Epithelioid malignant peripheral nerve sheath tumour. **A** Some tumours include rhabdoid cells with eosinophilic paranuclear globular to fibrillar inclusions (arrows). **B** Extensive S100 positivity. **C** Marked nuclear immunoreactivity for SOX10.

The common association with NF1 and a spindle-cell background indistinguishable from that of ordinary MPNST suggest a close relationship between high-grade MPNST with divergent differentiation and conventional high-grade MPNST.

The following two variants are likely to be different not only in their histological characteristics but also in their genetics, lack of syndromic association, and/or biological behaviour, and should therefore be strictly distinguished from conventional MPNST: epithelioid MPNST and perineurial MPNST (malignant perineurioma).

Epithelioid malignant peripheral nerve sheath tumour

ICD-O code   9540/3

Less than 5% of MPNSTs are either partially or purely epithelioid {718,1162, 1435}. This variant shows no association with NF1 and can arise from malignant transformation of a schwannoma {1628, 2789}. Both superficial (above the fascia) and deep-seated examples have been reported. The risks of recurrence, metastasis, and disease-related death seem to be lower than those associated with conventional MPNST {1162}.

MPNST with perineurial differentiation (malignant perineurioma)

ICD-O code   9540/3

Rare MPNSTs show histological and ultrastructural features of perineurial differentiation. Like benign perineuriomas, these tumours are EMA–positive and S100-negative, but show hypercellularity, nuclear atypia, and increased mitotic activity. Perineurial MPNSTs have the potential to metastasize, but appear to be less aggressive than conventional MPNSTs {1011,2176}.

Differential diagnosis of MPNSTs

The distinction of MPNSTs from other high-grade sarcomas relies mainly on demonstration of tumour origin from either a peripheral nerve or a benign precursor, or on immunohistochemical or genetic features. Until proven otherwise, malignant spindle cell tumours in patients with NF1 should be considered to be MPNSTs. One particular entity to consider in the differential diagnosis of MPNST is synovial sarcoma of nerve. Synovial sarcomas are common soft tissue sarcomas but can also occur as distinct rare primary tumours of nerve. These tumours show considerable morphological and immunohistochemical overlap with

conventional MPNSTs, but unlike MPNSTs, they carry an *SS18-SSX2* or *SS18-SSX1* fusion gene {2259}.

Immunophenotype
Only 50–70% of MPNSTs exhibit S100 protein staining. Reactivity is grade-related. In high-grade tumours reactivity is either patchy or found only in individual cells, whereas in low-grade examples it may be extensive {2724}. However, in epithelioid MPNST, diffuse S100 protein expression is common and SMARCB1 (INI1) is lost in 50% of cases {718}. Lack of immunostaining for HMB45 and melan-A, taken together with origin from a peripheral nerve or a benign nerve sheath tumour may help distinguish epithelioid MPNST from malignant melanoma. Immunostaining for p53 protein is positive in 75% of all MPNSTs, in contrast to the infrequent staining in neurofibromas {931}, although cellular schwannomas can also be positive {1924}. Most MPNSTs are also negative for CDKN2A (p16), in contrast to the consistent but often patchy expression in cellular schwannomas {1785,1924}. However, some atypical neurofibromas also show CDKN2A (p16) loss {2862}. EGFR is expressed in about one third of MPNSTs but is absent in cellular schwannomas. Diffuse loss of SOX10 occurs in 75% of MPNSTs, but

SOX10 is retained in cellular schwannomas {1924}. Full-length neurofibromin is absent in about 90% of MPNSTs associated with NF1 and 43% of sporadic MPNSTs. Diffuse loss of neurofibromin is not observed in synovial sarcoma, solitary fibrous tumour, dedifferentiated liposarcoma, myxoid liposarcoma, cellular schwannoma, or low-grade fibromyxoid sarcoma, but may occur in myxofibrosarcoma, pleomorphic liposarcoma, and undifferentiated pleomorphic sarcoma {1924,2102}. MPNSTs with divergent differentiation show expression of related differentiation markers (e.g. desmin in malignant triton tumour or keratin, carcinoembryonic antigen, and neuroendocrine markers in glandular MPNST). In most MPNSTs, the Ki-67 proliferation index is > 20% {1924}.

Loss of H3K27me3 expression was recently shown to be a highly specific marker for MPNST, although only modestly more sensitive than S100 protein and SOX10, being documented in >90% of radiation-associated MPNST and in >60% of NF1-related MPNST {2038A, 2254A}. The H3K27me3 loss of expression is more variable within the sporadic MPNST, ranging from 49-95% among the 2 recent studies, most likely related to the different criteria applied in diagnosis.

Cell of origin

Mouse models of peripheral nerve sheath tumours associated with NF1 suggest that MPNSTs do not directly derive from neural crest stem cells, but instead from more differentiated Schwann cells {1182, 2793,2859}. Embryonic Schwann cell precursors have been identified (using cell-lineage tracing) as cells of origin in a mouse model of plexiform neurofibroma {429}.

Genetic profile

MPNST associated with NF1, sporadic MPNST, and radiation-induced MPNST share highly recurrent genetic inactivation in NF1, CDKN2A, and the PRC2 components SUZ12 and EED {1460,2857}. Biallelic inactivation of NF1 is present in benign neurofibromas, but mutations in additional genes are rarely found. However, atypical neurofibromas, which are presumed to be MPNST precursors, often show additional deletions in CDKN2A {155}. These genetic data suggest that the combined inactivation of NF1, CDKN2A, and PRC2 components is critical for the

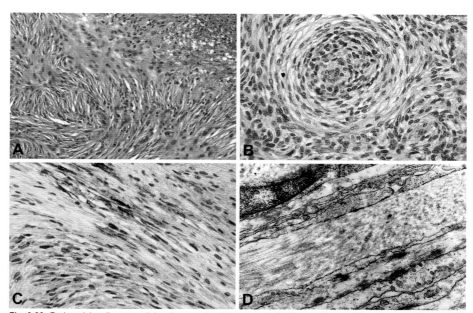

Fig. 9.28 Perineurial malignant peripheral nerve sheath tumour. **A** Storiform pattern and focal necrosis (upper right). **B** A whorling pattern. **C** Patchy immunoreactivity for EMA and (**D**) the presence of long thin processes, pinocytotic vesicles, and patchy basement membrane support perineurial differentiation.

pathogenesis of most MPNSTs, a hypothesis that is also supported by functional data. NF1 encodes for the important RasGAP neurofibromin, and its inactivation increases the levels of active RAS. Loss of function of PRC2 through deletion/mutation of SUZ12 or EED leads to decreased levels of H3K27me3 and increased levels of H3K27ac, thereby amplifying the transcription of RAS target genes {548}. CDKN2A encodes for the important cell cycle regulators p16 and p14ARF, and deletion of the CDKN2A locus enables evasion from hyperactive RAS-induced senescence, promoting sustained proliferation {2324,2336}. In addition, genetic alterations in TP53 are found in about 42% of all MPNSTs, further supporting tumour progression {1460}. MPNSTs typically have complex numerical and structural karyotypic abnormalities. Common abnormalities include gains of chromosomes 2, 7p, 8q, 14, and 17q and losses of chromosomes 9p, 11q, 13q, 17p, and 18 {1362}. Gains at 16p or losses from 10q or Xq have been reported as negative prognostic factors {274}. Gene amplifications that occur in a subset of tumours include ITGB4, PDGFRA, BIRC5, CCNE2, EGFR, HGF, MET, TERT, and CDK4, with CDK4 amplifications being an independent predictor of poor survival {1579,2834}. No cytogenetic differences have been noted between sporadic and NF1-associated

tumours. Although only a small number of cases have been analysed to date, epithelioid MPNSTs do not have the same genetic profile as conventional MPNSTs, suggesting that they may constitute a distinct entity {1460}. Molecular data on perineurial MPNST are lacking.

Genetic susceptibility

Approximately half of all MPNSTs manifest in patients with NF1 (see *Neurofibromatosis type 1*, p. 294). This association is particularly strong for malignant triton tumour and glandular MPNST. Patients with NF1 and plexiform neurofibromas have the highest risk of developing MPNST {2588}.

Prognosis and predictive factors

MPNSTs (except those with perineurial differentiation) are highly aggressive tumours with a poor prognosis. In a large retrospective study, truncal location, tumour size ≥ 5 cm, local recurrence, and high-grade designation had adverse impacts on disease-specific survival {2439}. The study also reported a trend towards decreased survival in patients with cases associated with NF1 compared with sporadic cases. Gains at 16p, losses from 10q or Xq, and CDK4 amplifications have been reported as negative prognostic factors {274,2834}.

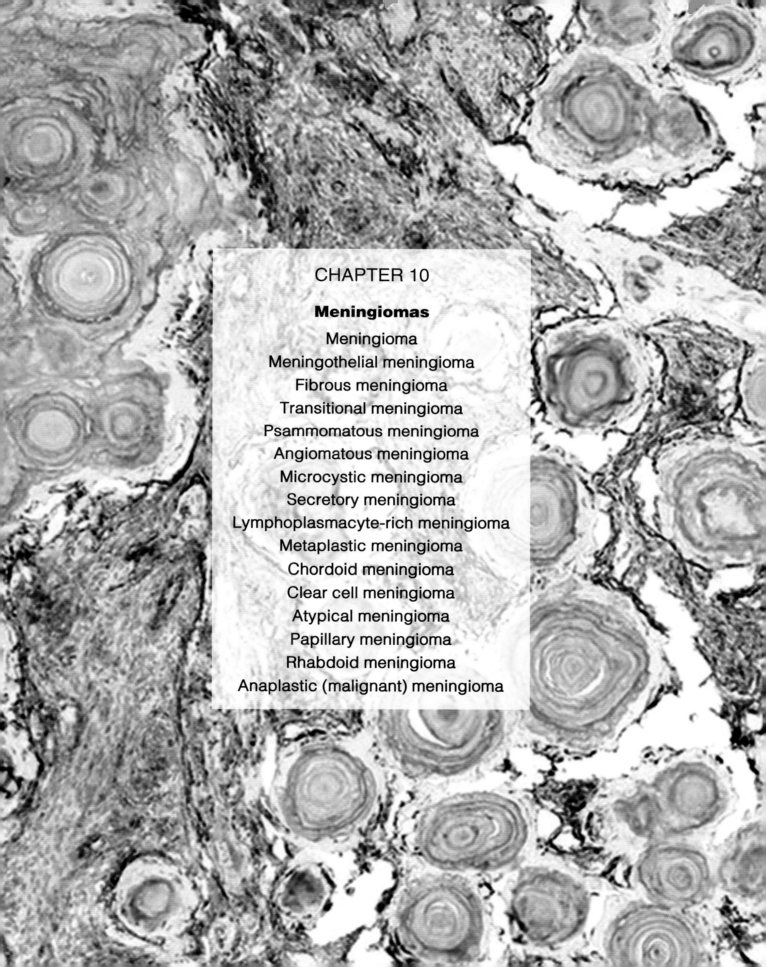

CHAPTER 10

Meningiomas

Meningioma
Meningothelial meningioma
Fibrous meningioma
Transitional meningioma
Psammomatous meningioma
Angiomatous meningioma
Microcystic meningioma
Secretory meningioma
Lymphoplasmacyte-rich meningioma
Metaplastic meningioma
Chordoid meningioma
Clear cell meningioma
Atypical meningioma
Papillary meningioma
Rhabdoid meningioma
Anaplastic (malignant) meningioma

Meningioma

Perry A.
Louis D.N.
Budka H.
von Deimling A.
Sahm F.

Rushing E.J.
Mawrin C.
Claus E.B.
Loeffler J.
Sadetzki S.

Definition

A group of mostly benign, slow-growing neoplasms that most likely derive from the meningothelial cells of the arachnoid layer.

There are three major groups of meningiomas, which differ in grade and biological behaviour (see Table 10.01).

ICD-O code   9530/0

Grading

Most meningiomas correspond histologically to WHO grade I (benign). Certain histological subtypes or meningiomas, with specific combinations of morphological parameters, are associated with less favourable clinical outcomes and correspond histologically to WHO grades II and III (Table 10.01).

Epidemiology

Incidence

The lifetime risk of developing meningioma is approximately 1%. It is the most frequently reported brain tumour in the USA, accounting for 36% of all brain tumours overall, although tumours of the meninges account for just 2.8% of all paediatric primary brain tumours {596}. More than 90% of all meningiomas are solitary. About 20–25% and 1–6% of meningiomas are WHO grades II and III, respectively {1837,1951,2448}.

Age and sex distribution

The median age of patients with meningioma is 65 years, with risk increasing with age {596}. Age-adjusted incidence rates vary significantly by sex. Females are at greater risk than males, with annual incidence rates of 10.5 cases per 100 000 females and 4.8 cases per 100 000 males {596}. This difference is greatest prior to menopause, with the highest female-to-male ratio (3.15:1) in the 35–44 years age group {2746}. Grade II and III lesions occur at higher rates in males. Incidence also varies significantly by race, with reported annual incidence rates per 100 000 population of 9.1, 7.4, and 4.8 in Blacks, Whites, and Asians / Pacific Islanders, respectively, in the USA {596}.

Etiology

Ionizing radiation is the only established environmental risk factor for meningioma, with higher risk among people who were exposed in childhood than as adults. At high dose levels, data exist for patients treated with therapeutic radiation to the head {189,1001,2213}. Evidence also exists for lower dose levels {470,1607,1920}. Two studies of imaging technologies (e.g. CT) that use diagnostic levels of radiation higher than those used for dental or plain X-rays reported links with subsequent brain tumours (glioma and meningioma) {1607,1920}. Researchers from the Tinea Capitis Cohort Study have studied genetic predisposition for radiation-associated meningioma and have found strong support for genetic susceptibility to the development of meningioma after exposure to ionizing radiation {717}.

An association between hormones and meningioma risk is suggested by several findings, including the increased incidence of the disease in women versus men; the presence of progesterone receptors in most meningiomas; and reports of modestly increased risk associated with the use of endogenous/exogenous hormones, body mass index, and current smoking, as well as decreased risk associated with breastfeeding for ≥ 6 months {471}. A recent large case–control study found that among female subjects, members of the case group were more likely than members of the control group to report hormonally related conditions, including uterine fibroids (OR: 1.2, 95% CI: 1.0–1.5), endometriosis (OR: 1.5, 95% CI: 1.5–2.1), and breast cancer (OR: 1.4, 95% CI: 0.8–2.3) {469}. Evidence of a possible interaction between smoking and sex was also reported {716}. Attempts to link specific chemicals, dietary factors, and occupations, as well as head trauma and mobile phone use, with meningiomas have provided inconclusive findings. However, allergic conditions (e.g. asthma and eczema) have been associated with reduced risk of meningioma {2747}.

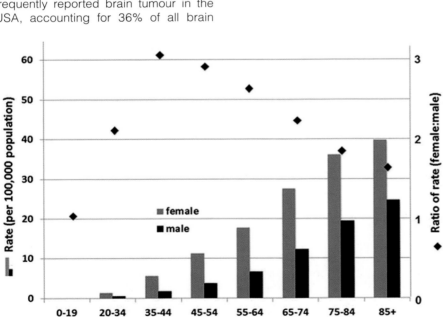

Fig. 10.01 Age- and sex-specific incidence rates (per 100 000 population) of meningioma in the USA (2002–2006). The left scale refers to the bar graph, the right scale to the female-to-male incidence ratio, which is indicated for each age group by a diamond {2746}.

Table 10.01 Meningioma variants grouped by WHO grade and biological behaviour

Meningiomas with low risk of recurrence and aggressive behaviour:		
		ICD-O code
Meningothelial meningioma	WHO grade I	9531/0
Fibrous (fibroblastic) meningioma	WHO grade I	9532/0
Transitional (mixed) meningioma	WHO grade I	9537/0
Psammomatous meningioma	WHO grade I	9533/0
Angiomatous meningioma	WHO grade I	9534/0
Microcystic meningioma	WHO grade I	9530/0
Secretory meningioma	WHO grade I	9530/0
Lymphoplasmacyte-rich meningioma	WHO grade I	9530/0
Metaplastic meningioma	WHO grade I	9530/0
Meningiomas with greater likelihood of recurrence and aggressive behaviour:		
Chordoid meningioma	WHO grade II	9538/1
Clear cell meningioma	WHO grade II	9538/1
Atypical meningioma	WHO grade II	9539/1
Papillary meningioma	WHO grade III	9538/3
Rhabdoid meningioma	WHO grade III	9538/3
Anaplastic meningioma	WHO grade III	9530/3
Meningiomas of any subtype with high proliferation index		

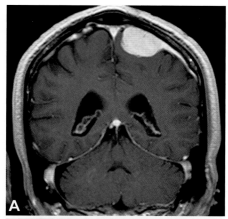
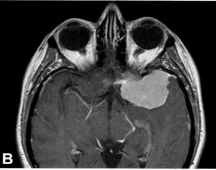

Fig. 10.02 Meningioma. **A** T1-weighted, post-constrast coronal MRI showing a meningioma of the cerebral convexity with a prominent dural 'tail'. **B** Postcontrast T1-weighted MRI of a meningioma with homogeneous contrast enhancement. The adjacent cortex appears to mould around the tumour. The trailing contrast into adjacent dura is referred to as the dural tail sign and corroborates the impression of an extra-axial mass.

Localization

The vast majority of meningiomas arise in intracranial, intraspinal, or orbital locations. Intraventricular and epidural examples are uncommon. Rare examples have been reported outside the neural axis (e.g. in the lung). Within the cranial cavity, common sites include the cerebral convexities (with tumours often located parasagittally, in association with the falx and venous sinus), olfactory grooves, sphenoid ridges, para-/suprasellar regions, optic nerve sheath, petrous ridges, tentorium, and posterior fossa. Most spinal meningiomas occur in the thoracic region. Atypical and anaplastic meningiomas most commonly affect the convexities and other non–skull base sites {1214}. Metastases of malignant meningiomas most often involve lung, pleura, bone, or liver.

Clinical features

Meningiomas are generally slow-growing and produce neurological signs and symptoms due to compression of adjacent structures; the specific deficits depend on tumour location. Headache and seizures are common (but non-specific) presentations.

Imaging

On MRI, meningiomas typically present as isodense, uniformly contrast-enhancing dural masses. Calcification is common, and is best seen on CT. A characteristic feature is the so-called dural tail surrounding the dural perimeter of the mass. This familiar imaging sign corresponds to reactive fibrovascular tissue and does not necessarily predict foci of dural involvement by tumour. Peritumoural cerebral oedema is occasionally prominent, in particular with certain histological variants and high-grade examples {1856}. Cyst formation may occur within or at the periphery of a meningioma. Neuro-imaging features are not entirely specific for identifying meningiomas, predicting tumour behaviour, or excluding other diagnoses.

Spread

Even benign meningiomas commonly invade adjacent anatomical structures (especially dura), although the rate and extent of local spread are often greater in the more aggressive subtypes. Thus, depending on location and grade, some meningiomas produce considerable patient morbidity and mortality. Extracranial metastases are extremely rare, occurring in about 1 in 1000 meningiomas and most often in association with WHO grade III tumours. The rare metastases of histologically benign meningiomas typically occur after surgery, but can arise de novo as well.

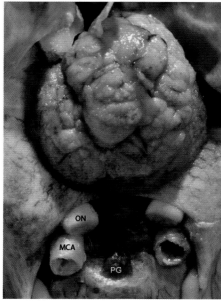

Fig. 10.03 Large meningioma originating from the olfactory groove. Note the smooth, slightly lobulated surface. MCA, middle cerebral artery; ON, optic nerve; PG, pituitary gland.

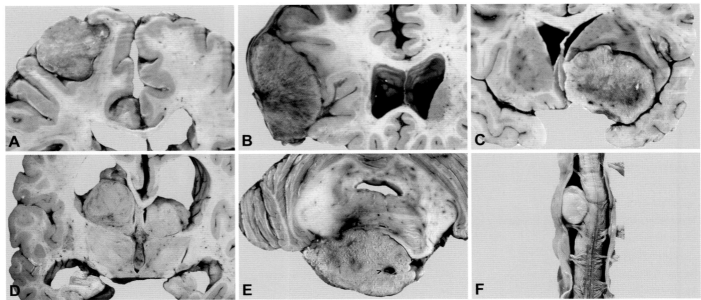

Fig. 10.04 Macroscopy of meningioma. **A** Meningioma of the left parasagittal region of the parietal lobe. The tumour compresses the cerebral cortex, but does not infiltrate. **B** Large lateral meningioma compressing the left frontal cortex. Note the attachment to the dura mater and the sharp delineation from brain structures. In this location, meningiomas are often flat rather than round. **C** Meningioma of the medial sphenoid wing encasing the carotid artery. **D** Large meningioma of the lateral ventricles and the third ventricle causing a hydrocephalus. **E** Large meningioma originating from the clivus. Note the compression of the brain stem with residual haemorrhage. The basilar artery (arrowhead) is entrapped by the tumour but not occluded. **F** Spinal meningioma compressing the spinal cord.

Macroscopy

Most meningiomas are rubbery or firm, well-demarcated, sometimes lobulated, rounded masses that feature broad dural

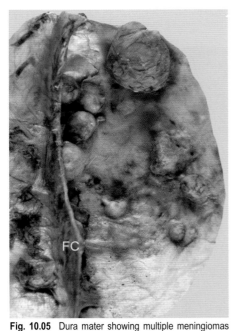

Fig. 10.05 Dura mater showing multiple meningiomas that differ greatly in size. They are located unilaterally, without extending beyond the falx cerebri (FC) to the contralateral side. Multiple dural meningiomas have been shown to be of clonal origin and probably result from spread through the dura {2413}.

attachment. Invasion of dura or dural sinuses is fairly common. Occasional meningiomas invade into the adjacent skull, where they may induce characteristic hyperostosis, which is highly indicative of bone invasion. Meningiomas may attach to or encase cerebral arteries, but only rarely infiltrate arterial walls. They may also infiltrate the skin and extracranial compartments, such as the orbit. Adjacent brain is often compressed but rarely frankly invaded. In certain sites, particularly along the sphenoid wing, meningiomas may grow as a flat, carpet-like mass, a pattern called en plaque meningioma. Some meningiomas appear gritty on gross inspection, implying the presence of numerous psammoma bodies. Bone formation is far less common. Atypical and anaplastic meningiomas tend to be larger and often feature necrosis.

Microscopy

Meningiomas exhibit a wide range of histological appearances. Of the subtypes in the WHO classification, the most common are meningothelial, fibrous, and transitional meningiomas. Most of the subtypes behave in a benign fashion, but four distinct variants, which are categorized as WHO grade II and III, are more likely to recur and to follow a more aggressive clinical course (see the following

sections and Table 10.01). The criteria used to diagnose atypical and anaplastic meningiomas are applied independent of specific meningioma subtype.

Immunophenotype

The vast majority of meningiomas stain for EMA, although this immunoreactivity is less consistent in atypical and malignant lesions. Vimentin positivity is found in all meningiomas, but is relatively nonspecific. Somatostatin receptor 2A is expressed strongly and diffusely in almost all cases (including anaplastic meningiomas), but can also be encountered in neuroendocrine neoplasms {1641}. S100 protein positivity is most common in fibrous meningiomas, but is not usually diffuse, as it is in schwannomas. Other potentially useful immunohistochemical markers in selected cases include Ki-67 and progesterone receptor (see *Prognosis and predictive factors*).

Diagnostic ultrastructural features of meningiomas include abundance of intermediate filaments (vimentin), complex interdigitating cellular processes (particularly in meningothelial variants), and desmosomal intercellular junctions. These cell surface specializations, as well as intermediate filaments, are few in fibrous meningiomas, the cells being separated by collagen. Secretory meningiomas feature single or multiple epithelial-like lumina within single cells. These cell surfaces show short apical microvilli and surround electron-dense secretions {1393}. Microcystic meningiomas feature long cytoplasmic processes enclosing intercellular electron-lucent matrix, with cells joined by desmosomes.

Proliferation

In general, cellular proliferation increases in proportion to grade. The mitotic index and Ki-67 proliferation index correlate approximately with volume growth rate. Studies have suggested that meningiomas with an index of > 4% have an increased risk of recurrence similar to that of atypical meningioma, whereas those with an index of > 20% are associated with death rates analogous to those associated with anaplastic meningioma {1953}. However, significant differences in technique and interpretation make it difficult to establish definitive cut-off points that would translate accurately from one laboratory to another.

Cell of origin

Meningiomas are thought to be derived from meningothelial (arachnoid) cells.

Genetic profile

The current model of meningioma genetics in WHO grades I–III is summarized in Fig. 10.06.

Meningiomas were among the first solid tumours recognized as having cytogenetic alterations, the most consistent change being monosomy 22 {2846}. In general, karyotypic abnormalities are more extensive in atypical and anaplastic meningiomas {1615}. Other cytogenetic changes associated with meningioma include deletion of chromosome 1p (which is associated with poor outcome) {1132} and losses of chromosomes 6q, 9p, 10, 14q, and 18q (which occur in higher-grade tumours) {2846}. Chromosomal gains reported in higher-grade meningiomas include gains of chromosomes 1q, 9q, 12q, 15q, 17q, and 20q.

The NF2 gene

Mutations in the *NF2* gene are detected in most meningiomas associated with neurofibromatosis type 2 (NF2) and as many as 60% of sporadic meningiomas {1466,2727}. In most cases, such mutations are small insertions or deletions or are nonsense mutations that affect splice

sites, create stop codons, or result in frameshifts occurring mainly in the 5'-most two thirds of the gene {1536}. The common, predictable effect of these mutations is a truncated and presumably non-functional merlin protein (also called schwannomin). The frequency of *NF2* mutations varies among meningioma variants. Fibroblastic and transitional meningiomas, which are preferentially located at the convexity, often carry *NF2* mutations {954,1367,2727}. In contrast, meningothelial, secretory, and microcystic meningiomas located at the skull base only rarely harbour *NF2* mutations, but are driven by other genetic alterations (see *Other genes*). In line with this, most non-NF2 meningioma families develop meningothelial tumours {1536}. Furthermore, reduced expression of merlin has been observed in various histopathological variants of meningiomas, but seems to be rare in meningothelial tumours {1455}. In atypical and anaplastic meningiomas, *NF2* mutations occur in approximately 70% of cases, matching the frequency of *NF2* mutations in benign fibroblastic and transitional meningiomas. This indicates that *NF2* inactivation is an early tumorigenic event, a theory supported by findings in mouse models {1204}. Mouse models have also indicated an origin from prostaglandin-D synthase–positive meningeal precursor cells with inactivated *NF2* {1205}. *NF2*-driven meningiomas with malignant progression show more genetic instability than do *NF2*-intact meningiomas {877}. In radiation-induced meningiomas, the frequencies of *NF2* mutations and loss of chromosome 22 are lower, whereas structural abnormalities of chromosome 1p are more common, suggesting a different molecular pathogenesis {1164,1501}.

Other genes

The close association of *NF2* mutations in meningiomas with allelic loss on chromosome 22 and mouse modelling of meningioma development clearly suggest that *NF2* is the major meningioma tumour suppressor gene on that chromosome {2727}. However, deletion studies of chromosome 22 have also detected losses and translocations of genetic material outside the *NF2* region, raising the possibility that other tumour-associated genes are located there. Candidate genes include *LARGE*, *MN1*, *AP1B1*, and *SMARCB1*, although these show only

rare alterations {1615,2291}. Additional altered genes have been identified using genomic and targeted sequencing strategies in a subset of *NF2*-wildtype meningiomas {262,467,2217}. These alterations preferentially affect WHO grade I meningiomas at the skull base. A hotspot mutation in the *AKT1* gene (*AKT1* E17K) is found in about 13% of meningiomas, mostly of meningothelial or transitional subtype. Another mutation affects the *TRAF7* gene (mutated in 8–24% of cases), almost always occurring in combination with *KLF4* mutations, which are also found in 93–100% of secretory meningiomas {2104}. Mutations in the *SMO* gene are found in 4–5% of WHO grade I meningiomas, mostly those located in the medial anterior skull base. Additionally, *SMARCE1* mutations have recently been identified in clear cell meningiomas {2375}.

Deletions of the 9p21 region, including the *CDKN2A* gene, are particularly common in anaplastic meningiomas and are associated with shortened survival {246, 1938}. Mouse models have also shown that adding *CDKN2A/B* loss to *NF2* loss enhances the rate of formation of meningiomas, including high-grade forms {1960}. Additionally, higher-grade meningiomas escape senescence due to overexpression of telomerase, which in a subset of cases occurs due to *TERT* promoter mutations {876}. The potential prognostic value of this marker was shown in a study of 252 meningiomas revealing hotspot C228T and C250T mutations in 1.7%, 5.7%, and 20.0% of WHO grade I, II, and III meningiomas respectively, with median progression free survival times of 10.1 versus 179 months in mutant versus wildtype tumours {2220A}. Other molecular alterations associated with high tumour grade and aggressive clinical behaviour include losses of the *NDRG2* gene on 14q11.2 and the *MEG3* gene on 14q32, gains of the *RPS6KB1* gene and other loci on the 17q23 amplicon, loss of various *NF2* homologues within the erythrocyte membrane protein band 4.1 family (e.g. the *EPB41L3* gene on chromosome 18p11.3), and loss of the protein 4.1B binding partner, CADM1 {116,333,343,1548,1615}.

Clonality of solitary, recurrent, and multiple meningiomas

Studies of X chromosome inactivation using Southern blot analysis indicate that

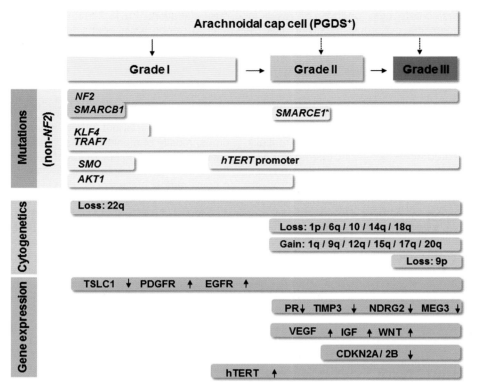

Fig. 10.06 Genetic model of meningioma tumorigenesis and progression; figure adapted from Karajannis MA and Zagzag D (eds): Molecular Pathology of Nervous System Tumors. Chapter 17. Springer 2015. Mutations are labelled in grey, with light grey indicating mutations occurring in meningiomas without *NF2* alterations. Cytogenetic aberrations are labelled in blue, and gene expression changes are labelled in green. Bar length indicates the relative frequency of an alteration within the given tumour grade. *SMARCE1* mutations have been found nearly exclusively in clear cell meningiomas. EGFR, epidermal growth factor receptor; IGF, insulin-like growth factor; PDGFR, platelet-derived growth factor receptor; PGDS+, prostaglandin D2 synthase–positive precursor cells in murine meningioma models; PR, progesterone receptor.

meningiomas are monoclonal tumours {1118}, although PCR-based assays have suggested that a small proportion could be polyclonal {2867}. Nevertheless, both the Southern blot data {1118} and the finding that the overwhelming majority of meningiomas with NF2 mutations only have a single mutation {2727} indicate that meningiomas are clonal. Similarly, all recurrent meningiomas have been found to be clonal with respect to the primary tumour {2663}. The clonality of multiple meningiomas has also been analysed using studies of X chromosome inactivation and by mutation analysis of the NF2 gene in multiple tumours from the same patient {1433,2413}. In these studies, the majority of lesions from patients with ≥ 3 meningiomas were shown either to have the same copy of the X chromosome inactivated or to carry the same NF2 mutation. These data provide strong evidence for a clonal origin of multiple meningiomas in most patients. They also suggest that multiple lesions arise

through dural spread, a hypothesis also supported by the common findings of peritumoural implants in 10% of meningiomas {244} and of small meningothelial nests in grossly unremarkable dural strips from the convexities of patients with meningiomas {244}. Nevertheless, it is possible that some cases with multiple meningiomas constitute genetic mosaics, with segmental, dural constitutional NF2 mutations. Germline mutations in the SMARCB1 gene can also give rise to multiple schwannomas and meningiomas {2622}.

Genetic susceptibility

Although the vast majority of meningiomas are sporadic, rare examples occur as part of tumour predisposition syndromes, with NF2 being by far the most common. However, family history studies have also suggested a role for inherited susceptibility beyond NF2, including one study in which patients with meningioma were 4.4 times as likely as

controls to report a first-degree family history of meningioma {469}. In the Interphone Study, the largest study of genetic polymorphisms and meningioma risk, investigators found a significant association with meningioma for 12 SNPs drawn from DNA repair genes {181}. The group reported a novel and biologically intriguing association between meningioma risk and three variants in *BRIP1* (17q22), the gene encoding the FACJ protein, which interacts with BRCA1. A genome-wide association study identified a single susceptibility locus at 10p12.31 (*MLLT10*) {593}. *MLLT10* is implicated in various leukaemias and activates the WNT pathway. A rare association with naevoid basal cell carcinoma syndrome (also called Gorlin syndrome) has also been suggested, based on germline *SUFU* or *PTCH1* mutations {1265,2202}. The relationship between meningioma and other inherited tumour syndromes, such as Werner syndrome and Cowden syndrome, is less defined.

Prognosis and predictive factors
The major prognostic questions regarding WHO grade II and III meningiomas involve estimates of recurrence and overall survival, respectively.

Clinical factors
In most cases, meningiomas can be removed entirely, as assessed by operative or neuroradiological criteria. In one series, 20% of gross totally resected benign meningiomas recurred within 20 years {1197}. The major clinical factor in recurrence is extent of resection, which is influenced by tumour site, extent of invasion, attachment to vital intracranial structures, and the skill of the surgeon. Other clinical factors, such as young patient age and male sex are less powerful predictors of recurrence; both are partially explained by the increased frequency of high-grade meningiomas in such patients.

Histopathology and grading
Some histological variants of meningioma are more likely to recur. However, overall, WHO grade is the most useful morphological predictor of recurrence (Table 10.01). Benign meningiomas have recurrence rates of about 7–25%, whereas atypical meningiomas recur in 29–52% of cases, and anaplastic meningiomas at rates of 50–94%. Even within the benign meningiomas however, the

presence of some atypical features (but not enough for WHO grade II designation) increases the risk of subsequent progression/recurrence over those with no atypical features at all {1581A}. Malignant histological features are associated with shorter survival times: 2–5 years depending largely on the extent of resection {30A,483A,1951}.

Progesterone receptor status
Progesterone receptor expression is inversely associated with meningioma grade. Its absence negatively impacts disease-free intervals in some series, but in most, it is not independent of other known prognostic factors, such as grade {1940,2181}. Almost all WHO grade III meningiomas are receptor negative, but because a significant subset of histologically and clinically benign meningiomas also lack the receptor, the significance of this finding in the absence of other prognostic features should not be overstated.

Meningioma variants

Perry A.
Louis D.N.
Budka H.
von Deimling A.

Sahm F.
Mawrin C.
Rushing E.J.

Meningothelial meningioma

Definition
A classic and common variant of meningioma, with medium-sized epithelioid tumour cells forming lobules, some of which are partly demarcated by thin collagenous septa.

Like normal arachnoid cap cells, the tumour cells of meningothelial meningioma are largely uniform, with oval nuclei with delicate chromatin and variable nuclear holes (i.e. empty-looking clear spaces) and nuclear pseudoinclusions (i.e. cytoplasmic invaginations). Eosinophilic cytoplasm is abundant, and the delicate, intricately interwoven tumour cell processes seen ultrastructurally cannot be discerned on light microscopy, explaining the outdated synonym "syncytial meningioma". Whorls and psammoma bodies are infrequent in meningothelial meningioma; when present, they tend to be less formed than in transitional, fibrous, or psammomatous subtypes. Larger lobules should not be confused with the sheeting or loss of architectural pattern seen in atypical meningioma. This subtype is encountered most often in the anterior skull base and is less likely to be driven by *NF2* mutations {942,1367}.

Because the tumour cells so closely resemble those of the normal arachnoid cap, reactive meningothelial hyperplasia occasionally resembles this meningioma variant. The most florid examples of meningothelial hyperplasia are typically found adjacent to optic nerve gliomas, other tumour types, or haemorrhage; meningothelial hyperplasia is also commonly found in the setting of chronic renal disease, advanced patient age, arachnoiditis ossificans, spontaneous intracranial haemorrhage, and occasionally in patients with diffuse dural thickening and contrast enhancement on neuroimaging {1945}.

ICD-O code   9531/0

Grading
Meningothelial meningioma corresponds histologically to WHO grade I.

Fibrous meningioma

Definition
A variant of meningioma that consists of spindled cells forming parallel, storiform, and interlacing bundles in a collagen-rich matrix.

In fibrous meningioma, whorl formation and psammoma bodies are infrequent. Nuclear features characteristic of meningothelial meningioma are often found focally. The tumour cells form fascicles with various amounts of intercellular collagen, which are striking in some cases. These fascicles may raise the differential diagnosis of solitary fibrous tumour / haemangiopericytoma (SFT/HPC), but only SFT/HPC expresses nuclear STAT6 {2308}. Rare fibrous meningiomas also include nuclear palisades resembling Verocay bodies, a diagnostic pitfall exacerbated by frequent S100 expression in this subtype, albeit not as diffusely staining as most schwannomas. Like other subtypes, most fibrous meningiomas express EMA.

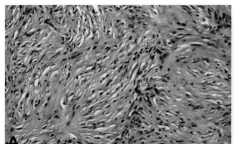

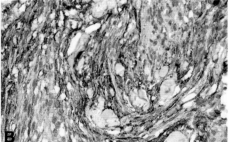

Fig. 10.07 Meningothelial meningioma with lobular growth pattern, syncytium-like appearance due to poorly defined cell borders, scattered clear nuclear holes, and occasional intranuclear pseudoinclusions (arrows).

Fig. 10.08 Fibrous meningioma. **A** A distinctive feature of this variant is the development of abundant reticulin and collagen fibres between the individual cells. **B** Most fibrous meningiomas express EMA.

NF2 mutations and convexity locations are common.

ICD-O code   9532/0

Grading

Fibrous meningioma corresponds histologically to WHO grade I.

Transitional meningioma

Definition

A common variant of meningioma that contains meningothelial and fibrous patterns as well as transitional features.

In transitional meningioma, lobular and fascicular foci appear side by side with conspicuous tight whorls and psammoma bodies. *NF2* mutations and origin from the convexity are common {942,1367}.

ICD-O code   9537/0

Grading

Transitional meningioma corresponds histologically to WHO grade I.

Psammomatous meningioma

Definition

A designation applied to meningiomas

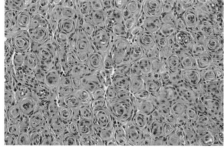

Fig. 10.09 Transitional meningioma with prominent whorl formation.

(usually of the transitional type) containing a predominance of psammoma bodies over tumour cells.

In psammomatous meningioma, the psammoma bodies often become confluent, forming irregular calcified masses and occasionally bone. In some tumours, the tumour cells are almost completely replaced by psammoma bodies, and intervening meningothelial cells are hard to find. Psammomatous meningiomas characteristically occur in the thoracic spinal region of middle-aged to elderly women, and the majority of these tumours behave in an indolent fashion.

ICD-O code   9533/0

Grading

Psammomatous meningioma corresponds histologically to WHO grade I.

Angiomatous meningioma

Definition

A variant of meningioma that features numerous blood vessels, which often constitute a greater proportion of the tumour mass than do the intermixed meningioma cells.

Angiomatous meningioma is also known as vascular meningioma. The tumour cells may be hard to recognize as meningothelial, with cytological features often overlapping with those of the microcystic meningioma. The vascular channels are small to medium-sized, thin- or thick-walled, and variably hyalinized. Moderate to marked degenerative nuclear atypia is common, but the vast majority of these tumours are histologically and clinically benign {963}. The differential diagnosis includes vascular malformations and haemangioblastoma, although the stromal cells of haemangioblastoma feature

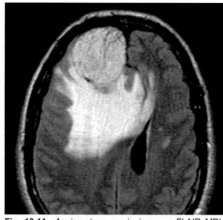

Fig. 10.11 Angiomatous meningioma on FLAIR MRI, showing marked peritumoural brain oedema.

inhibin alpha and brachyury expression {133} rather than meningothelial markers such as EMA and somatostatin receptor 2A. The designation "angiomatous" should not be equated with the obsolete term "angioblastic meningioma" (see *Solitary fibrous tumour / haemangiopericytoma*, p. 249). Angiomatous meningiomas do not exhibit aggressive behaviour, although adjacent cerebral oedema may be out of proportion to tumour size {1856}. Unlike most meningiomas, which have a normal diploid or monosomy 22 karyotype, angiomatous meningiomas are often aneuploid and commonly have polysomies, particularly for chromosomes 5, 13, and 20 {2}.

ICD-O code   9534/0

Grading

Angiomatous meningioma corresponds histologically to WHO grade I.

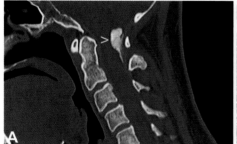
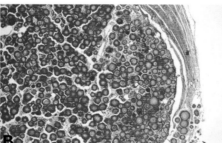
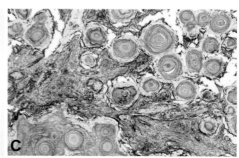

Fig. 10.10 Psammomatous meningioma. **A** CT showing bone-like density of a psammomatous meningioma (arrowhead) involving the cervicomedullary junction. **B** Almost complete replacement of the meningioma by psammomatous calcifications (postdecalcification specimen). **C** EMA immunostaining reveals meningioma cells between psammoma bodies.

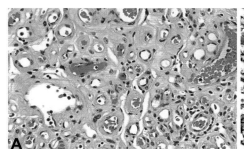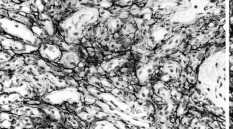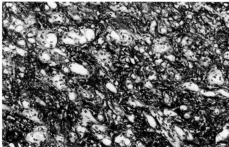

Fig. 10.12 Angiomatous meningioma. **A** Blood vessels constitute most of the mass. The intervening tumour cells are difficult to recognize as meningothelial. **B** Tumour cells showing positivity for EMA. **C** Strong immunoreactivity for somatostatin receptor type 2A.

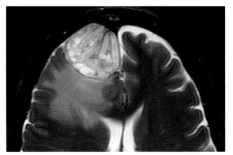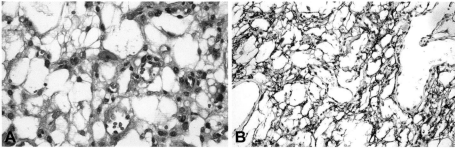

Fig. 10.13 Microcystic meningioma on T2-weighted MRI, with macrocysts and adjacent brain oedema.

Fig. 10.14 Microcystic meningioma. **A** Cobweb-like background with numerous delicate processes. **B** Thin processes are often evident on EMA immunostaining.

Microcystic meningioma

Definition
A variant of meningioma characterized by cells with thin, elongated processes encompassing microcysts and creating a cobweb-like background.

Occasionally, grossly or radiologically discernible macrocysts are also evident in microcystic meningioma. Degenerative nuclear atypia is common, but microcystic meningiomas are typically benign. Like in the angiomatous variant with which microcystic meningioma is often intermixed, accompanying cerebral oedema is common {1875}.

ICD-O code   9530/0

Grading
Microcystic meningioma corresponds histologically to WHO grade I.

Secretory meningioma

Definition
A variant of meningioma characterized by the presence of focal epithelial differentiation in the form of intracellular lumina containing periodic acid–Schiff–positive eosinophilic secretions called pseudopsammoma bodies.

These pseudopsammoma bodies show immunoreactivity for carcinoembryonic antigen and a variety of other epithelial and secretory markers, and the surrounding tumour cells are positive for both carcinoembryonic antigen and cytokeratin. Secretory meningiomas may be associated with elevated blood levels of carcinoembryonic antigen that drop with resection and rise with recurrence {1531}. Mast cells may be numerous and there is often peritumoural oedema {2560}. Genetically, secretory meningiomas are characterized by the combination of *KLF4* K409Q and *TRAF7* mutations {2104}.

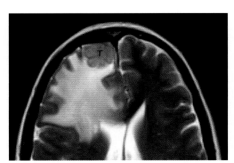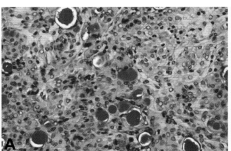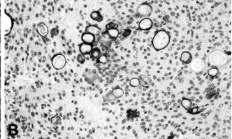

Fig. 10.15 Small secretory meningioma (T) on T2-weighted MRI, showing extensive peritumoural brain oedema.

Fig. 10.16 Secretory meningioma. **A** The pseudopsammoma bodies are periodic acid–Schiff–positive. **B** Evidence of epithelial metaplasia includes cytokeratin positivity in tumour cells forming gland-like spaces.

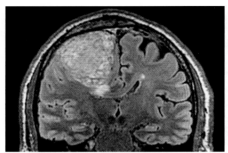

Fig. 10.17 Lymphoplasmacyte-rich meningioma. Signal heterogeneity on FLAIR MRI likely corresponds to pockets of inflammation.

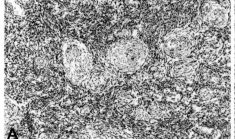

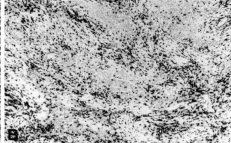

Fig. 10.18 Lymphoplasmacyte-rich meningioma. **A** Macrophages immunoreactive for CD68 are the dominant inflammatory component. Note the immunonegative meningothelial nests. **B** Immunostaining for CD3 shows abundant reactive T cells.

ICD-O code   9530/0

Grading
Secretory meningioma corresponds histologically to WHO grade I.

Lymphoplasmacyte-rich meningioma

Definition
A rare variant of meningioma that features extensive chronic inflammatory infiltrates, often overshadowing the inconspicuous meningothelial component.

Some previously reported cases of lymphoplasmacyte-rich meningioma likely constitute inflammatory processes with associated meningothelial hyperplasia, although cases behaving similarly to conventional meningioma have also been described {1421}. Neuroimaging features vary widely, with frequent peritumoural oedema and occasional multifocality or diffuse carpet-like meningeal involvement resembling pachymeningitis. Systemic haematological abnormalities, including hyperglobulinaemia and iron-refractory anaemia have also been reported {2866}. Because macrophages

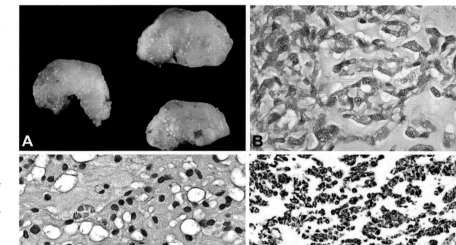

Fig. 10.20 Chordoid meningioma. **A** On cut surface, the mucoid matrix is grossly evident. **B** Eosinophilic tumour cells in a mucous-rich matrix. **C** Trabeculae of eosinophilic and vacuolated epithelioid cells associated with a basophilic mucin-rich stroma. **D** Vimentin immunohistochemistry highlights the ribbon-like architecture.

often predominate and plasma cells are not always conspicuous, the alternative term "inflammation-rich meningioma" has also been proposed {1421}.

ICD-O code   9530/0

Grading
Lymphoplasmacyte-rich meningioma corresponds histologically to WHO grade I.

Metaplastic meningioma

Definition
A variant of meningioma with striking focal or widespread mesenchymal components including osseous, cartilaginous, lipomatous, myxoid, and xanthomatous tissue, either singly or in combinations.

These alterations have no known clinical significance, and many probably do not constitute true metaplasia (e.g. lipid accumulation rather than true lipomatous metaplasia {483}). Clinical correlation is occasionally needed to distinguish ossified meningiomas from meningiomas exhibiting bone invasion.

ICD-O code   9530/0

Grading
Metaplastic meningioma corresponds histologically to WHO grade I.

Chordoid meningioma

Definition
A rare variant of meningioma that histologically resembles chordoma, featuring

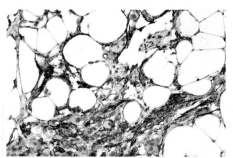

Fig. 10.19 Lipoma-like metaplastic meningioma. Positivity for EMA in lipoma-like cells suggests fat accumulation in meningioma cells rather than true adipocyte metaplasia.

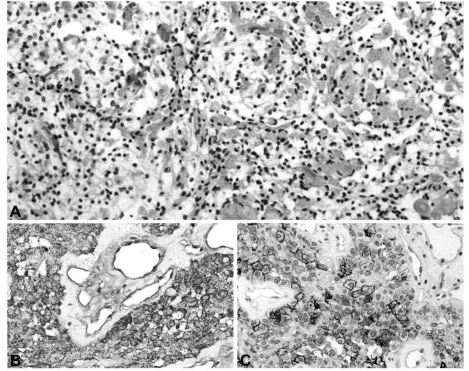

Fig. 10.21 Clear cell meningioma. **A** Sheets of rounded clear cells and perivascular interstitial collagenization. **B** Abundant periodic acid–Schiff–positive intracytoplasmic glycogen. **C** Immunoreactivity for EMA.

patternless (commonly) or sheeting architecture and round to polygonal cells with clear, glycogen-rich cytoplasm and prominent blocky perivascular and interstitial collagen.

The perivascular and interstitial collagen occasionally coalesces into large acellular zones of collagen or forms brightly eosinophilic amianthoid-like collagen. It shows prominent periodic acid–Schiff–positive and diastase-sensitive cytoplasmic glycogen. Whorl formation is vague at most and psammoma bodies are inconspicuous. Clear cell meningioma has a proclivity for the cerebellopontine angle and spine, especially the cauda equina region. It also tends to affect younger patients, including children and young adults. Clear cell meningiomas are associated with more aggressive behaviour, including frequent recurrence and occasional cerebrospinal fluid seeding {2873}. Familial examples have been reported in association with *SMARCE1* mutations {2379}. The more aggressive behaviour of these tumours, corresponding to WHO grade II, has been most clearly demonstrated when the clear-cell pattern is predominant and well developed.

ICD-O code   9538/1

Grading
Clear cell meningioma corresponds histologically to WHO grade II.

Atypical meningioma

Definition
A meningioma of intermediate grade between benign and malignant forms, with increased mitotic activity, brain invasion on histology, or at least three of the following features: increased cellularity, small

cords or trabeculae of eosinophilic, often vacuolated cells set in an abundant mucoid matrix.

In chordoid meningioma, chordoid areas are often interspersed with more typical meningioma tissue; pure examples are uncommon. Chronic inflammatory infiltrates are often patchy when present, but may be prominent. Chordoid meningiomas are typically large, supratentorial tumours. They have a very high rate of recurrence after subtotal resection {501}. Infrequently, patients have associated haematological conditions, such as anaemia or Castleman disease {1249}. The more aggressive behaviour

of these tumours, corresponding to WHO grade II, has been most clearly demonstrated when the chordoid pattern is predominant and well developed.

ICD-O code   9538/1

Grading
Chordoid meningioma corresponds histologically to WHO grade II.

Clear cell meningioma

Definition
A rare variant of meningioma with a

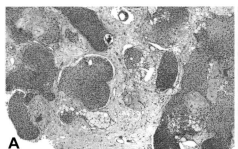
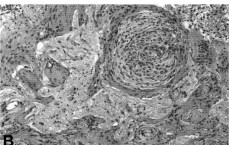
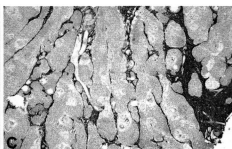

Fig. 10.22 Brain-invasive meningioma. **A** Tongue-like protrusions into adjacent brain parenchyma. **B** Leptomeningeal meningioma in a child, with extensive perivascular spread along Virchow–Robin spaces and hyalinization mimicking meningioangiomatosis. This unusual pattern of spread should not be misinterpreted as true brain invasion. **C** Entrapped GFAP-positive islands of gliotic brain parenchyma at periphery of the tumour.

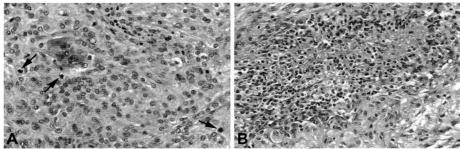

Fig. 10.23 Atypical meningioma. **A** Atypical meningioma is most reliably identified by increased mitotic activity (arrows). Note the absence of nuclear atypia in this example. **B** The micronecrosis seen in this image is considered spontaneous in that it was not iatrogenically induced (e.g. by embolization).

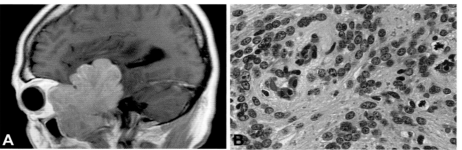

Fig. 10.24 Papillary meningioma. **A** Postcontrast T1-weighted MRI. Occasional papillary meningiomas feature a cauliflower-like imaging appearance. **B** Nucleus-free perivascular zone resembling the pseudorosette of an ependymoma; the additional presence of mitotic figures is evident on the right.

cells with a high nuclear-to-cytoplasmic ratio, prominent nucleoli, sheeting (i.e. uninterrupted patternless or sheet-like growth), and foci of spontaneous (i.e. not iatrogenically induced) necrosis.

In one series, increased mitotic activity was defined as ≥ 4 mitoses per 10 high-power (40× magnification, 0.16 mm²) fields {1952}. An alternative grading approach simply combines hypercellularity with a mitotic count of ≥ 5 mitoses per 10 high-power fields {1569}. Despite the tumour's name, nuclear atypia itself is not useful in grading atypical meningioma,

because it results more commonly from degenerative changes. Clinical risk factors for atypical meningioma include male sex, non–skull base location, and prior surgery {1214}. Atypical meningiomas have been associated with high recurrence rates, even after gross total resection {23}. Bone involvement has been associated with increased recurrence rates in the setting of atypical meningioma {771}.

Invasion of the brain by meningioma is characterized by irregular, tongue-like protrusions of tumour cells infiltrating

underlying parenchyma, without an intervening layer of leptomeninges. This causes reactive astrocytosis, with entrapped islands of GFAP-positive parenchyma at the periphery of the tumour. Extension along perivascular Virchow–Robin spaces does not constitute brain invasion because the pia is not breached in this form of spread; perivascular spread and hyalinization can mimic meningioangiomatosis, but does not constitute true brain invasion. Such examples are most commonly encountered in children {819,1944}. Brain invasion can occur in meningiomas that otherwise appear benign, atypical, or anaplastic (malignant). The presence of brain invasion is associated with a higher likelihood of recurrence. Because histologically benign and histologically atypical brain-invasive meningiomas both have recurrence and mortality rates similar to those of atypical meningiomas as defined using other criteria {1952}, brain invasion is a criterion for atypical meningioma.

ICD-O code   9539/1

Grading

Atypical meningioma corresponds histologically to WHO grade II.

Papillary meningioma

Definition

A rare variant of meningioma defined by the presence of a perivascular pseudopapillary pattern constituting most of the tumour.

This pseudopapillary architecture is characterized by loss of cohesion, with clinging of tumour cells to blood vessels and a perivascular nucleus-free

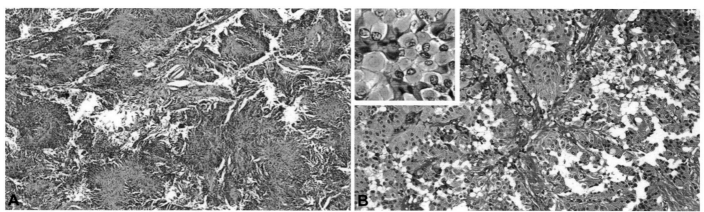

Fig. 10.25 Papillary meningioma. **A** At low magnification, the pseudopapillary pattern is evident, with loss of cellular cohesion away from central vascular cores. **B** This meningioma combines a papillary growth pattern with rhabdoid cytology, including globular paranuclear inclusions (inset).

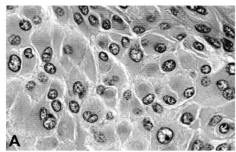
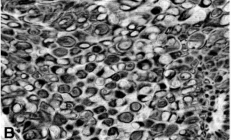
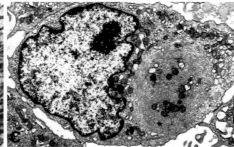

Fig. 10.26 Rhabdoid meningioma. **A** Eccentrically placed vesicular nuclei, prominent nucleoli, and eosinophilic globular/fibrillar paranuclear inclusions. **B** Vimentin-positive paranuclear inclusions. **C** Rhabdoid meningioma cell showing a paranuclear whorled bundle of intermediate filaments with entrapped organelles.

zone resembling the pseudorosettes of ependymoma. This feature frequently increases in extent with recurrences, and other high-grade histological features are almost always found. Papillary meningiomas tend to occur in young patients, including children {1545}. An invasive tendency, including brain invasion, has been noted in 75% of cases, recurrence in 55%, metastasis (mostly to lung) in 20%, and death of disease in about half {1368, 1901}. Some meningiomas combine a papillary architecture with rhabdoid cytology {2796}. The more aggressive behaviour of these tumours, corresponding to WHO grade III, has been most clearly demonstrated when the papillary pattern is predominant and well developed.

ICD-O code   9538/3

Grading

Papillary meningioma corresponds histologically to WHO grade III {1545}.

Rhabdoid meningioma

Definition

An uncommon variant of meningioma that consists primarily of rhabdoid cells: plump cells with eccentric nuclei, open chromatin, a prominent nucleolus, and prominent eosinophilic paranuclear inclusions, appearing either as discernible whorled fibrils or compact and waxy.

These rhabdoid cells resemble those described in other tumours, including atypical teratoid/rhabdoid tumour of the brain; however, unlike in atypical teratoid/rhabdoid tumour, SMARCB1 expression is retained in rhabdoid meningioma {1941}. Rhabdoid cells may become increasingly evident with tumour recurrences. Most rhabdoid meningiomas have a high proliferation index and other histological features of malignancy. Some combine a papillary architecture with rhabdoid cytology (see *Papillary meningioma*, p. 242). When the rhabdoid features are

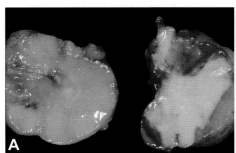
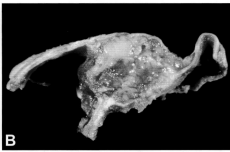
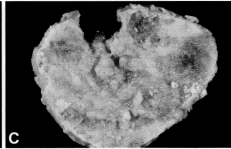

Fig. 10.27 Anaplastic (malignant) meningioma (common, albeit non-specific macroscopic features). **A** Note the soft, gelatinous consistency on cut surface, as well as the large yellow zone of necrosis on the right. **B** The superior sagittal sinus is occluded by tumour. **C** The inner surface of the skull is moth-eaten due to extensive bone invasion by an adjacent meningioma.

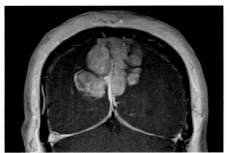
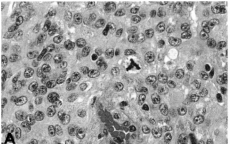
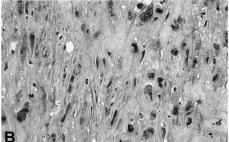

Fig. 10.28 Bilateral parasagittal anaplastic (malignant) meningioma. Irregular borders and highly invasive growth pattern on postcontrast T1-weighted MRI.

Fig. 10.29 Anaplastic (malignant) meningioma. **A** An atypical mitotic figure and prominent nucleoli. **B** Sarcoma-like anaplastic (malignant) meningioma. Spindled morphology, increased matrix deposition, and poorly differentiated cytology.

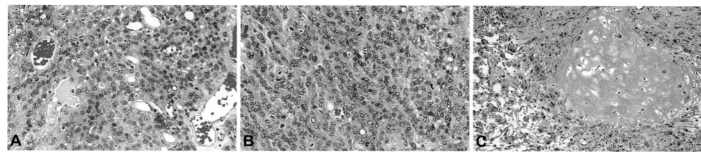

Fig. 10.30 Anaplastic (malignant) meningioma. **A** Carcinoma-like anaplastic meningioma. Sheet-like growth with large epithelioid cells, abundant cytoplasm, and prominent nucleoli. **B** More than 20 mitoses per 10 high-power fields. Eight mitotic figures can be seen in this single high-power field. **C** Chondrosarcoma-like focus.

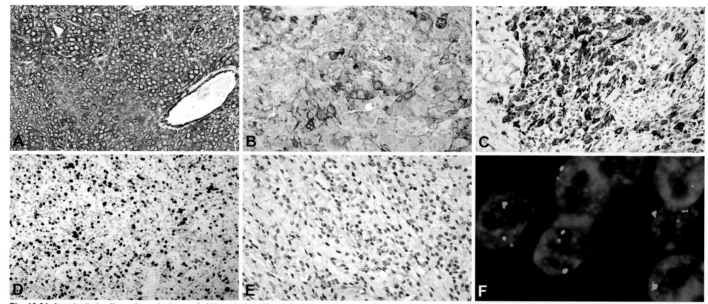

Fig. 10.31 Anaplastic (malignant) meningioma. **A** Although vimentin positivity is not very specific, even the most poorly differentiated meningiomas are typically strongly and diffusely positive. This can be helpful in the differential diagnosis with metastatic carcinomas, most of which are negative or only focally positive for vimentin. **B** Positivity for EMA is typically patchy in meningiomas of all grades. Because 10–20% are negative, a lack of EMA staining does not exclude the diagnosis of meningioma. **C** Strong positivity for CK7 (and other cytokeratins) in this example represented a diagnostic pitfall for metastatic carcinoma; however, other morphological, immunohistochemical, and genetic features were characteristic of meningothelial origin. **D** Ki-67 proliferation index > 20%. **E** Rare nuclei are positive for progesterone receptor. **F** Most tumour nuclei display two green centromere 9 signals, but only one red 9p21 (*CDKN2A*) signal, consistent with deletion.

fully developed and combined with other malignant features, these meningiomas often have an aggressive clinical course consistent with WHO grade III {1252, 1950}. However, some meningiomas show rhabdoid features only focally and/ or lack other histological features of malignancy; such cases are less aggressive as a group {2639A}. Therefore, it is suggested that they be graded as normally, but with the added descriptor of "with rhabdoid features" and a comment that closer follow-up may be warranted {2639A}. Rare forms appear rhabdoid on histology, but ultrastructurally show interdigitating processes rather than the typical paranuclear aggregates of intermediate filaments {823}.

ICD-O code 9538/3

Grading

Rhabdoid meningioma corresponds histologically to WHO grade III.

Anaplastic (malignant) meningioma

Definition

A meningioma that exhibits overtly malignant cytology (resembling that of carcinoma, melanoma, or high-grade sarcoma) and/or markedly elevated mitotic activity. In one study, markedly elevated mitotic activity was defined as ≥ 20 mitoses per 10 high-power (0.16 mm²) fields {1951}. Anaplastic (malignant) meningiomas

account for 1–3% of meningiomas overall. In addition to high mitotic counts, most also show extensive necrosis and a Ki-67 proliferation index > 20%. Rare cases show true epithelial or mesenchymal metaplasia {1910}. Confirmation of the meningothelial origin of cases with diffuse anaplasia often requires either a history of meningioma at the same site or immunohistochemical, ultrastructural, and/or genetic support.

Anaplastic meningiomas are often fatal, with average survival times ranging from < 2 years to > 5 years, depending greatly on the extent of resection {1951, 2448}. Clinical risk factors for anaplastic meningioma include a non–skull base origin, male sex, and prior surgery {1214}. Because malignant progression in meningiomas, as in gliomas, is a continuum of increasing anaplasia, determining the cut-off point between atypical and anaplastic meningioma is sometimes challenging.

ICD-O code

9530/3

Grading

Anaplastic (malignant) meningioma corresponds histologically to WHO grade III.

Other morphological variants

Due to the wide morphological spectrum that can be encountered in meningiomas, rare examples are difficult to classify as any of the well-accepted variants. These include meningiomas with oncocytic, mucinous, sclerosing, whorling–sclerosing, GFAP-expressing, and granulofilamentous inclusion–bearing features {46,173,781,917,1039,2168}. However, there is currently insufficient evidence that these tumours constitute distinct variants. Another rare pattern encountered secondarily in a variety of meningiomas is that of meningothelial rosettes, which are composed mostly of cell processes and collagen, with or without a central gland-like lumen {1520}. Most tumours once called pigmented meningiomas are now known to be melanocytomas. However, the recruitment of melanocytes from the adjacent meninges into the substance of a true meningioma accounts for dark pigmentation in rare cases {1768}.

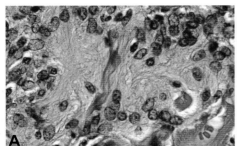
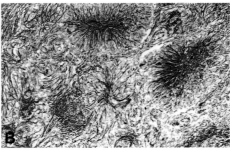
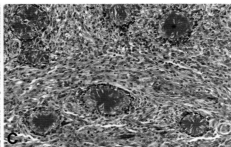

Fig. 10.32 Rosette-forming meningioma. **A** Meningioma with rosette formation composed mostly of cell processes. **B** Vimentin immunostaining emphasizes the cell processes in meningothelial rosettes. **C** Trichrome staining highlights the dense collagen in the centre of some meningothelial rosettes.

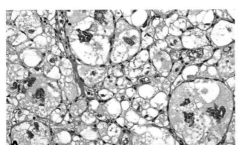
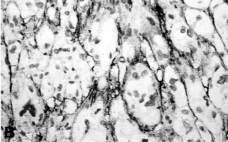
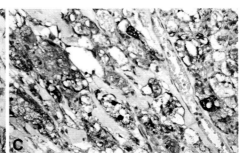

Fig. 10.33 Meningioma with oncocytic features. **A** Marked degenerative nuclear atypia. **B** EMA expression. **C** Immunostain for antimitochondrial antigen confirms the oncocytic changes.

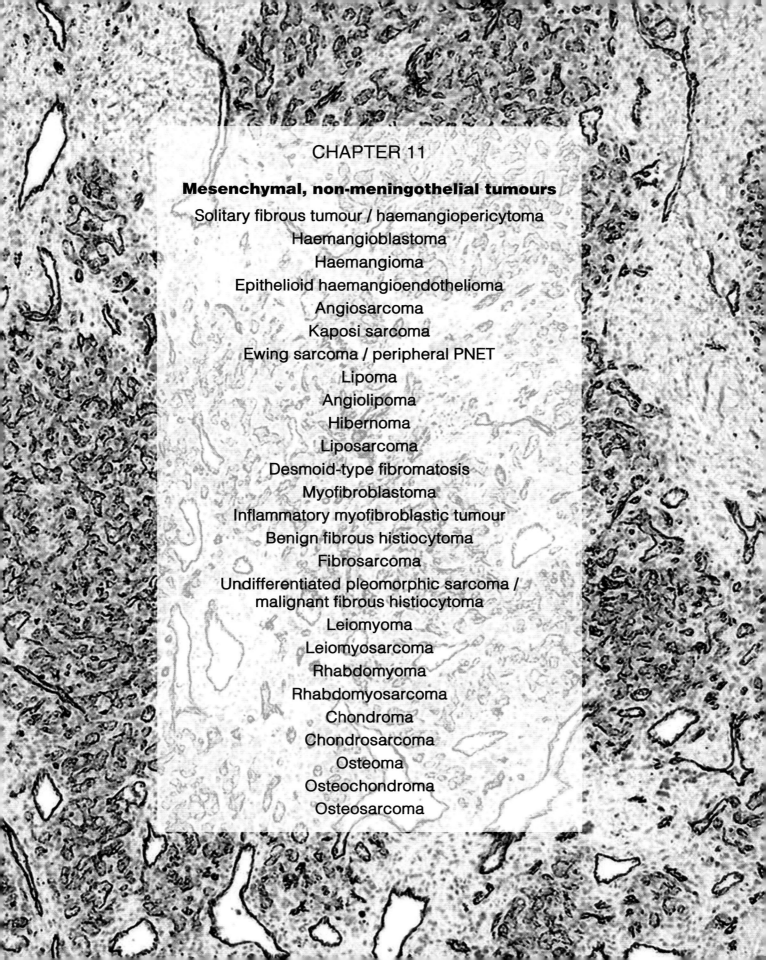

CHAPTER 11

Mesenchymal, non-meningothelial tumours

Solitary fibrous tumour / haemangiopericytoma

Haemangioblastoma

Haemangioma

Epithelioid haemangioendothelioma

Angiosarcoma

Kaposi sarcoma

Ewing sarcoma / peripheral PNET

Lipoma

Angiolipoma

Hibernoma

Liposarcoma

Desmoid-type fibromatosis

Myofibroblastoma

Inflammatory myofibroblastic tumour

Benign fibrous histiocytoma

Fibrosarcoma

Undifferentiated pleomorphic sarcoma /
malignant fibrous histiocytoma

Leiomyoma

Leiomyosarcoma

Rhabdomyoma

Rhabdomyosarcoma

Chondroma

Chondrosarcoma

Osteoma

Osteochondroma

Osteosarcoma

Mesenchymal, non-meningothelial tumours

Antonescu C.R.
Paulus W.
Perry A.
Rushing E.J.
Hainfellner J.A.

Bouvier C.
Figarella-Branger D.
von Deimling A.
Wesseling P.

Definition

Benign and malignant mesenchymal tumours originating in the CNS, with terminology and histological features corresponding to their soft tissue and bone counterparts.

Mesenchymal tumours arise more commonly in the meninges than in the CNS parenchyma or choroid plexus. In principle, any mesenchymal tumour may arise within or secondarily impact on the nervous system, but the primary mesenchymal CNS tumours are very rare. They can occur in patients of any age and arise more commonly in supratentorial than in infratentorial or spinal locations. The clinical symptoms and neuroradiological appearance of most tumours are non-specific.

The histological features of mesenchymal tumours affecting the CNS are similar to those of the corresponding extracranial soft tissue and bone tumours {714}. Solitary fibrous tumour / haemangiopericytoma (by far the most common mesenchymal, non-meningothelial neoplasm) and peripheral nerve sheath tumours (the most common neoplasms of cranial and paraspinal nerves) are described separately. Antiquated nosological terms, such as "spindle cell sarcoma", "pleomorphic sarcoma," and "myxosarcoma" have been replaced by designations indicating more specific differentiation or updated terminology {714}. The non-specific diagnostic term "meningeal sarcoma" is also to be avoided, because it has been used in the past to denote both sarcomatoid anaplastic meningiomas and various types of sarcomas.

Grading

Mesenchymal, non-meningothelial tumours range from benign neoplasms (corresponding histologically to WHO grade I) to highly malignant sarcomas (corresponding histologically to WHO grade IV).

Epidemiology

The various forms of lipoma account for only 0.4% of all intracranial tumours, and the other benign mesenchymal tumours are even rarer. In two series, of 19 and 17 cases, sarcomas accounted for < 0.1–0.2% of the intracranial tumours {1838,1919}. The higher values that have been reported in the past are a reflection of overdiagnosis related to historical classification schemes. The most common tumour types include fibrosarcoma and undifferentiated pleomorphic sarcoma / malignant fibrous histiocytoma (MFH) {1838,1919}.

Mesenchymal tumours can occur in patients of any age. Rhabdomyosarcoma occurs preferentially in children, whereas undifferentiated pleomorphic sarcoma / MFH and chondrosarcoma usually manifest in adults. As a whole, sarcomas show no obvious sex predilection.

Etiology

Intracranial fibrosarcoma, undifferentiated pleomorphic sarcoma / MFH, chondrosarcoma, and osteosarcoma can occur several years after irradiation {453, 1791}. Isolated cases of intracranial and spinal fibrosarcoma, undifferentiated pleomorphic sarcoma / MFH, and angiosarcoma have also been related to previous trauma or surgery {1020}, an etiology that may be more common to desmoid-type fibromatosis {1684}. EBV is associated with the development of intracranial smooth muscle tumours in immunocompromised patients {287}.

Localization

Tumours arising in meninges are more common than those originating within CNS parenchyma or in choroid plexus. Most mesenchymal tumours are supratentorial, but rhabdomyosarcomas are more often infratentorial. Chondrosarcomas involving the CNS arise most often in the skull base. Among benign mesenchymal lesions, intracranial lipomas have a characteristic location and typically occur at midline sites, such as the anterior corpus callosum, quadrigeminal plate, suprasellar and hypothalamic regions, and auditory canal. Spinal cord examples involve the conus medullaris–filum terminale and also occur at the thoracic level. Intraventricular and tuber cinereum lipomas are rare {233}. Occasional CNS lipomas have a fibrous connection with surrounding soft or subcutaneous tissue. Osteolipomas have predilection for the suprasellar/interpeduncular regions {233,2367}. Most spinal lipomas (in particular angiolipomas) arise in the epidural space.

Clinical features

The clinical symptoms and signs are variable and non-specific, and depend largely on tumour location. Spontaneous regression is rare {1390}. Whereas the neuroradiological appearance of most mesenchymal tumours is non-specific, the neuroimaging characteristics of lipoma are virtually diagnostic; on MRI, T1-weighted images show the high signal intensity of fat, which then disappears with fat-suppression techniques. Speckled calcifications are typical of chondroid and osseous tumours.

Spread

Primary meningeal sarcomatosis is a diffuse leptomeningeal sarcoma lacking circumscribed masses {2598}. Although this entity is strictly defined as a non-meningothelial mesenchymal tumour, most published cases have not been diagnosed according to modern nomenclature. Re-examination of published cases using immunohistochemistry has revealed that most cases actually constitute carcinoma, lymphoma, glioma, or embryonal tumour.

Macroscopy

The macroscopic appearance of mesenchymal tumours depends entirely on their differentiation and is similar to that of the corresponding extracraniospinal soft tissue tumours. Lipomas are bright yellow, lobulated lesions. Epidural lipomas are delicately encapsulated and discrete, whereas intradural examples are often intimately attached to leptomeninges and CNS parenchyma. Chondromas are demarcated, bosselated, greyish-white, and variably translucent, and typically form large, dural-based masses indenting brain parenchyma. Meningeal sarcomas are firm in texture and tend to invade adjacent brain. Intracerebral sarcomas appear well delineated, but parenchymal invasion is a feature. The cut surface of sarcomas is typically firm and fleshy; high-grade lesions often show necrosis and haemorrhage.

Cell of origin
Mesenchymal tumours affecting the CNS are thought to arise from craniospinal meninges, vasculature, and surrounding osseous structures. Given that cranial and intracranial mesenchymal structures (e.g. bone, cartilage, and muscle) are in part derived from the neuroectoderm (ectomesenchyme), development of the corresponding sarcoma types could also constitute reversion to a more primitive stage of differentiation. Lipomas arising within the CNS are often associated with developmental anomalies, and may be congenital malformations rather than true neoplasms, in particular those with partial or complete agenesis of the corpus callosum and spinal dysraphism with tethered cord {218,998,2823}. Intracranial rhabdomyosarcoma may also be associated with malformations of the CNS {999}.

Genetic profile
The molecular genetic alterations of intracranial sarcomas may be similar to those of corresponding extracranial soft tissue tumours {79}, but few data are available to date. However, examples of meningeal-based Ewing sarcoma / peripheral primitive neuroectodermal tumour have shown the typical *EWSR1*-type rearrangements found in bone and soft tissue counterparts {565,1617}.

Genetic susceptibility
Several associations with inherited disease have been noted. Intracranial cartilaginous tumours may be associated with Maffucci syndrome and Ollier disease; lipomas with encephalocraniocutaneous lipomatosis; and osteosarcoma with Paget disease.

Prognosis and predictive factors
Whereas most benign mesenchymal tumours can be completely resected and have a favourable prognosis, primary intracranial sarcomas are aggressive and associated with a poor outcome. Local recurrence and/or distant leptomeningeal seeding are typical. For example, despite aggressive radiation and chemotherapy, almost all reported cases of CNS rhabdomyosarcoma have been fatal within

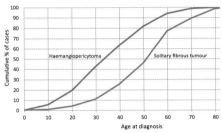

Fig. 11.01 Cumulative age distribution (both sexes) of haemangiopericytoma phenotype (186 cases) and solitary fibrous tumour phenotype (157 cases). Data derived from Fargen KM et al. {669}.

2 years. Systemic metastasis of intracranial sarcoma is relatively common. Nevertheless, primary CNS sarcomas are less aggressive than glioblastomas; in a series of 18 cases, the estimated 5-year survival rates for high-grade and low-grade primary CNS sarcomas were 28% and 83%, respectively {1838}.

Solitary fibrous tumour / haemangiopericytoma

Giannini C.
Rushing E.J.
Hainfellner J.A.
Bouvier C.
Figarella-Branger D.
von Deimling A.
Wesseling P.
Antonescu C.R.

Definition
A mesenchymal tumour of fibroblastic type, often showing a rich branching vascular pattern, encompassing a histological spectrum of tumours previously classified separately as meningeal solitary fibrous tumour and haemangiopericytoma.

Most meningeal solitary fibrous tumours / haemangiopericytomas harbour a genomic inversion at the 12q13 locus, fusing the *NAB2* and *STAT6* genes {444, 2141}, which leads to STAT6 nuclear expression that can be detected by immunohistochemistry. Detection of STAT6 nuclear expression or *NAB2-STAT6* fusion is highly recommended to confirm the diagnosis.

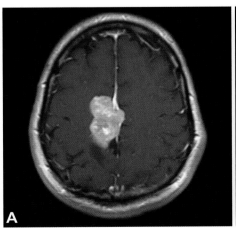
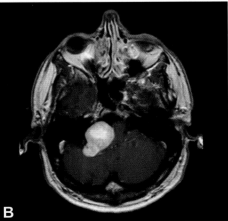
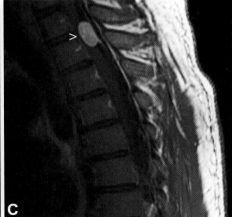

Fig. 11.02 Solitary fibrous tumour / haemangiopericytoma. **A** The falcine tumour in a 51-year-old man shows postgadolinium enhancement to a variable extent. **B** The tumour of the posterior fossa / cerebellopontine angle in a 55-year-old man shows postgadolinium enhancement. **C** Tumour of the upper thoracic spine in a 45-year-old man (a T1 mass, 1.6 cm in length) shows postgadolinium enhancement and a dural tail, mimicking meningioma.

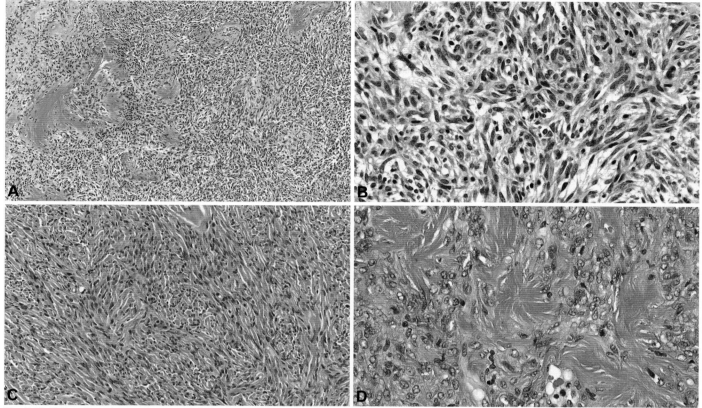

Fig. 11.03 Solitary fibrous tumour phenotype. **A** Patternless architecture characteristic of this phenotype. **B** The tumour is composed of cells with bland ovoid to spindle-shaped nuclei and scant eosinophilic cytoplasm. **C** Stromal and perivascular hyaline collagen deposition and (**D**) keloidal or amianthoid-like collagen are common.

A negative result should prompt consideration of alternative diagnoses (see *Differential diagnosis*). When STAT6 immunohistochemistry or *NAB2-STAT6* fusion testing are not or cannot be performed, this should be indicated in the report.

The histological spectrum encompasses two main morphological variants: the solitary fibrous tumour phenotype characterized by a patternless architecture or short fascicular pattern, with alternating hypocellular and hypercellular areas with thick bands of collagen, and the haemangiopericytoma phenotype characterized by high cellularity and a delicate, rich network of reticulin fibres typically investing individual cells. Thin-walled branching haemangiopericytoma-like (staghorn) vessels are a feature shared by both phenotypes.

Solitary fibrous tumour / haemangiopericytoma (SFT/HPC) is rare (accounting for < 1% of all primary CNS tumours) and most commonly affects adults (in the fourth to sixth decade of life). The tumours are typically dural-based and often supratentorial, with about 10% being spinal. The clinical behaviour of tumours with the solitary fibrous tumour phenotype is generally benign, provided gross total resection can be achieved, whereas tumours with the haemangiopericytoma phenotype have a high rate of recurrence (> 75% at 10 years) and may develop extracranial metastases, especially in bones, lungs, and liver (in ~20% of cases).

ICD-O codes

Solitary fibrous tumour / haemangiopericytoma

Grade 1	8815/0
Grade 2	8815/1
Grade 3	8815/3

Grading

Outside the CNS (e.g. in the soft tissue, pleura, and other visceral sites), the term "haemangiopericytoma" has long been subsumed into the designation "solitary fibrous tumour", with unified criteria for malignancy. These criteria include hypercellularity and necrosis in addition to elevated mitotic count (which remains the best indicator of poor outcome) {714, 861}. A mitotic count of > 4 mitoses per

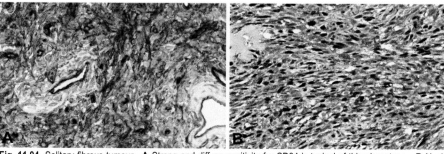

Fig. 11.04 Solitary fibrous tumour. **A** Strong and diffuse positivity for CD34 is typical of this phenotype. **B** Nuclear localization of STAT6 protein detected by immunohistochemistry.

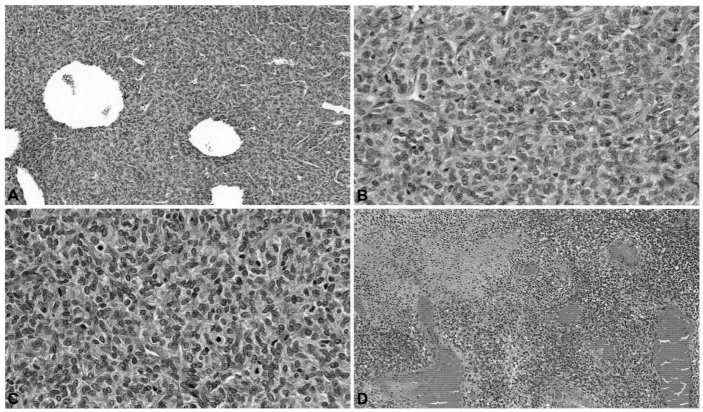

Fig. 11.05 The haemangiopericytoma phenotype. **A** Diffuse high cellularity, with thin-walled, branching vessels. **B** Closely apposed cells with round to ovoid nuclei arranged in a haphazard pattern, with limited intervening stroma. **C** Numerous mitoses. **D** Focal necrosis is typically present.

10 high-power fields is required for the designation of solitary fibrous tumour as malignant, irrespective of solitary fibrous tumour or haemangiopericytoma histopathological phenotype {714}. In the CNS, the classification and grading of these tumours has been somewhat different, resulting in a three-tiered system, with grade I tumours considered benign and typically treated by surgical resection alone, and grade II and III tumours considered malignant and treated with adjuvant therapy, typically radiotherapy. A hypocellular, collagenized tumour with a classic solitary fibrous tumour phenotype is considered to correspond histologically to grade I, whereas more densely cellular tumours mostly corresponding to the haemangiopericytoma phenotype are considered malignant. Tumours with a haemangiopericytoma phenotype are subclassified as grade II or grade III (anaplastic) depending on mitotic count (< 5 vs ≥ 5 mitoses per 10 high-power fields) {1533,1637}. Patients diagnosed with grade II or III haemangiopericytoma benefit from adjuvant radiotherapy {813, 814}.

One study proposed a three/four-tiered grading scheme (grades I, IIa, IIb, and III) after combining the solitary fibrous tumour and haemangiopericytoma designations and applying common (but slightly different) criteria based on hypercellularity, necrosis, and mitotic count (≤ 5 vs > 5 mitoses per 10 high-power fields). In that study, mitotic count was found to be the only independent prognostic factor for progression-free and overall survival in multivariate analysis {256}. Because the distinction between grade I versus grades II and III meningeal

solitary fibrous tumours / haemangiopericytomas has significant therapeutic implications, the current consensus is that it is still premature to consider replacing the current three-tiered with another grading system. Larger studies are needed to determine whether the malignancy definition (i.e. > 4 mitoses per 10 high-power fields), which is applied to non-CNS sites irrespective of solitary fibrous tumour or haemangiopericytoma histopathological phenotype, is relevant to meningeal locations.

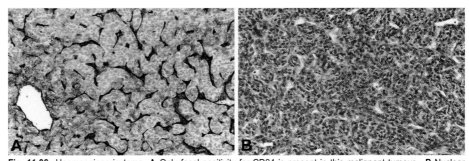

Fig. 11.06 Haemangiopericytoma. **A** Only focal positivity for CD34 is present in this malignant tumour. **B** Nuclear localization of STAT6 protein is detected by immunohistochemistry.

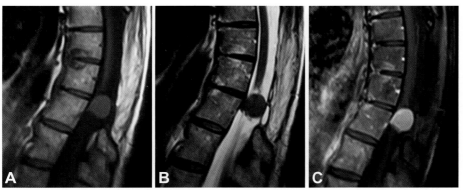

Fig. 11.07 Intradural extramedullary solitary fibrous tumour / haemangiopericytoma. **A** T1-weighted MRI. Isointense tumour (15 mm × 15 mm × 15 mm) located at T10–T11. **B** T2-weighted MRI. **C** Postcontrast T1-weighted MRI. The lesion is homogeneously and diffusely enhanced after gadolinium injection.

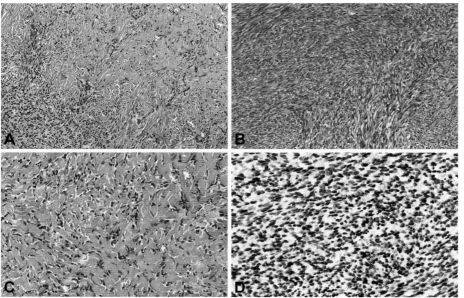

Fig. 11.08 Solitary fibrous tumour / haemangiopericytoma. **A** Patternless architecture with alternating hypocellular and hypercellular areas. **B** Highly cellular area. **C** Hypocellular areas with thick bands of collagen. **D** STAT6 is strongly expressed in all tumour nuclei.

Epidemiology

The true incidence and prevalence of this entity are difficult to ascertain, due to inconsistent nomenclature. In the 2014 statistical report published by the Central Brain Tumor Registry of the United States (CBTRUS), because of their rarity, solitary fibrous tumour / haemangiopericytomas are grouped with other mesenchymal tumours of the meninges, which as a group have an average annual age-adjusted incidence rate of 0.08 cases per 100 000 population {1863}. Data from large series suggest that solitary fibrous tumour / haemangiopericytomas constitute < 1% of all CNS tumours {522,859, 1637,2269}.

Age and sex distribution

Peak incidence occurs in the fourth to fifth decade of life, and males are affected slightly more frequently than females {522,1637,2269}. Primary CNS solitary fibrous tumours / haemangiopericytomas have been reported in the paediatric population, although they are exceedingly rare {1623,2550}.

Localization

Most solitary fibrous tumours / haemangiopericytomas are dural-based (often supratentorial), and about 10% are spinal. Skull base, parasagittal, and falcine locations are especially common {1637, 2269}. Uncommon locations include the cerebellopontine angle {2516}, pineal gland {2854}, and sellar region {1189}.

Clinical features

In most cases, the symptoms and signs are consistent with their localization, accompanied by mass effect, with increased intracranial pressure due to tumour size {859,1637}. Massive intracranial haemorrhage {1602} and hypoglycaemia from tumours that release insulin-like growth factor {2391} are rare complications.

Imaging

Plain CT images show solitary, irregularly contoured masses without calcifications or hyperostosis of the adjacent skull. On MRI, the tumours are isointense on T1-weighted images, with high or mixed intensity on T2-weighted images, along with variable contrast enhancement. Dural contrast enhancement at the periphery of the lesion (dural tail) and flow voids may be observed {2693}. Arteriography reveals a hypervascular mass with prominent draining veins.

Macroscopy

Solitary fibrous tumours / haemangiopericytomas are usually well-circumscribed, firm white to reddish-brown masses, depending on the degree of collagenous stroma and cellularity. Occasionally, they show infiltrative growth or lack dural attachment {365,377,1656}. Variable myxoid or haemorrhagic changes may be present.

Microscopy

Solitary fibrous tumour / haemangiopericytoma shows two main distinct histological phenotypes, although cases with intermediate/hybrid morphology are also seen. The classic solitary fibrous tumour phenotype shows a patternless architecture characterized by a combination of hypocellular and hypercellular areas separated by thick bands of hyalinized, sometimes keloidal or amianthoid-like collagen and thin-walled branching haemangiopericytoma-like (staghorn) vessels. The tumour cells have a monomorphic ovoid to spindle-shaped cytomorphology, with scant eosinophilic cytoplasm. The nuclei are round or oval, with moderately dense chromatin and inconspicuous nucleoli lacking the pseudoinclusions characteristic of meningiomas. Mitoses are generally scarce, rarely exceeding 3 per 10 high-power fields {365,714}. In contrast, the classic haemangiopericytoma phenotype is characterized by high cellularity, with closely apposed ovoid cells arranged in a haphazard pattern with limited intervening stroma {1637}. Mitotic activity and necrosis are often present, but are variable. A rich network of reticulin fibres typically invests individual or small groups of tumour cells. Invasion of brain parenchyma or engulfment of vessels or nerves may be noted in either pattern {1656}. Calcifications, including psammoma bodies, are not seen. Rarely, a variably prominent adipocytic component may be present.

Differential diagnosis
The differential diagnosis includes both meningothelial and soft tissue neoplasms. Fibrous meningioma is a close mimic of solitary fibrous tumour {365}, but typically expresses EMA and is negative for CD34 and nuclear STAT6 expression. Dural-based Ewing sarcoma / peripheral primitive neuroectodermal tumour shares the hypercellularity and CD99 positivity of haemangiopericytoma, but lacks nuclear STAT6 staining and is characterized by *EWSR1* gene rearrangement in the great majority of cases {565}. Both primary and metastatic monophasic synovial sarcomas can simulate solitary fibrous tumour / haemangiopericytoma. Immunoreactivity for EMA and TLE1 and/or FISH analysis for the presence of *SS18* gene rearrangement support this diagnosis {1507}. Mesenchymal chondrosarcoma, a rare malignant tumour with a bimorphic pattern, is composed of sheets and nests of poorly differentiated small round cells interrupted by islands of well-differentiated hyaline cartilage and a branching vasculature. Because the cartilage islands can be extremely focal, this entity may be mistaken for malignant solitary fibrous tumour / haemangiopericytoma if insufficiently sampled {714}. Malignant peripheral nerve sheath tumour rarely occurs in the meninges and may resemble the haemangiopericytoma phenotype. However, malignant peripheral nerve sheath tumour is usually negative for CD34 and STAT6 and may show focal expression of S100 protein and SOX10.

Electron microscopy
Solitary fibrous tumours / haemangiopericytomas are composed of closely apposed elongated cells with short processes that contain small bundles of intracytoplasmic intermediate filaments.

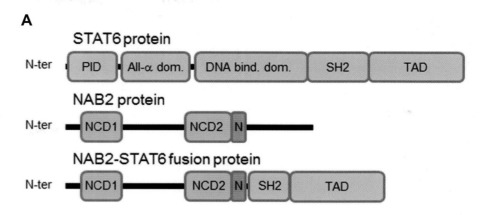

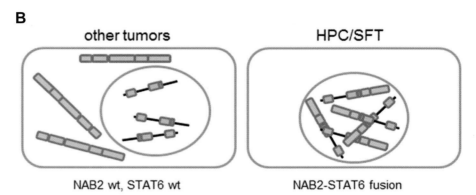

Fig. 11.09 Solitary fibrous tumour / haemangiopericytoma (HPC/SFT). **A** The break point in STAT6 varies, but is within or N-terminal to the SH2 domain. The break point in NAB2 also varies, but is usually C-terminal to the nuclear localization sequence (N). **B** Preservation of the NAB2 nuclear localization signal results in nuclear localization of the fusion protein {2308}. All-α dom., all-alpha domain; DNA bind. dom., DNA-binding domain; NCD1, NAB-conserved domain 1; NCD2, NAB-conserved domain 2; N-ter, N-terminus; PID, protein interaction domain; SH2, SRC homology domain; TAD, transcriptional activator domain; wt, wildtype.

The individual tumour cells are surrounded by electron-dense, extracellular basement membrane–like material – the ultrastructural equivalent of the reticulin network visible on light microscopy. True desmosomes and gap junctions (as seen in meningiomas) are absent {524}.

Immunophenotype
Solitary fibrous tumours / haemangiopericytomas are typically diffusely positive for vimentin and CD34 {1949}, although loss of CD34 expression is common in malignant tumours. The *NAB2-STAT6* fusion leads to nuclear relocalization of STAT6 protein and can be detected with very high specificity and sensitivity by immunohistochemistry {1317,1866,2308}. Meningiomas show faint nuclear and/or cytoplasmic positivity, but no strong isolated nuclear STAT6 immunostaining {2308}. The *NAB2-STAT6* fusion can also be detected at the protein level with high specificity and sensitivity by

proximity ligation assay {1317,2308}. Other markers, such as desmin, SMA, cytokeratin, EMA, and progesterone receptor, may be rarely encountered as a focal finding {1656,1949,2066,2764}. *ALDH1A1* gene overexpression, which was initially detected by microarray analysis, can be demonstrated by immunohistochemistry showing ALDH1 positivity in 84% of cases, compared to only 1% of meningiomas {255}.

Proliferation
The median Ki-67 proliferation index was 10% (range: 0.6–36%) in a series of 31 haemangiopericytomas {2039}. Another study reported a median Ki-67 proliferation index of 5% in a series of 29 solitary fibrous tumours and 10% in a series of 43 cellular solitary fibrous tumours / haemangiopericytomas {256}.

Cell of origin
The histogenesis of CNS solitary fibrous

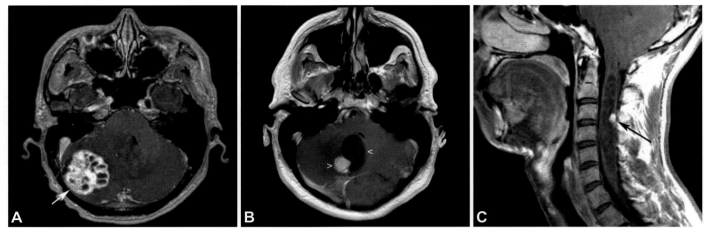

Fig. 11.10 Haemangioblastoma. **A** MRI of a cerebellar haemangioblastoma. The tumour is multicystic and enhancing. **B** MRI shows a cerebellar haemangioblastoma with an enhancing mural nodule. Note the compressed fourth ventricle in front of the tumour. **C** MRI of a cervical spinal cord haemangioblastoma. There is an associated large cyst around the enhancing mural nodule (arrow).

tumour/haemangiopericytoma remains a matter of debate. Their fibroblastic nature and the presence of a common *NAB2-STAT6* gene fusion {444,2141,2308} are strong arguments for grouping CNS solitary fibrous tumour and haemangiopericytoma together under the term "solitary fibrous tumour / haemangiopericytoma".

Genetic profile
The central (and to date specific) genetic abnormality in solitary fibrous tumour / haemangiopericytoma is a genomic inversion at the 12q13 locus, fusing the *NAB2* and *STAT6* genes in a common direction of transcription {444,2141}. This gene fusion is present in most cases, regardless of histological grade or anatomical location (meningeal, pleural, or soft tissue). The recent discovery of *NAB2-STAT6* fusion in the majority of solitary fibrous tumours / haemangiopericytomas has provided strong evidence for a morphological continuum. The presence of the NAB2-STAT6 fusion protein results in nuclear localization of STAT6 and strong nuclear positivity for STAT6 by immunohistochemistry {2308}.
In contrast, the rare sinonasal haemangiopericytoma does not exhibit the *NAB2-STAT6* fusion, but instead harbours *CTNNB1* mutations {18,929}.

Genetic susceptibility
There is no evidence of familial clustering of meningeal solitary fibrous tumour / haemangiopericytoma.

Prognosis and predictive factors
The clinical behaviour of tumours with the solitary fibrous tumour phenotype

is traditionally considered to be benign, provided that gross total resection can be achieved and atypical histological features are absent {365}. The prognostic significance of focal (rather than generalized) atypia in these tumours and of invasion in bone and dural sinuses is unclear {209,669}. In contrast, even after gross total resection, tumours with the haemangiopericytoma phenotype have a high rate of recurrence (> 75% in patients followed for > 10 years). In addition, about 20% of patients with tumours of the haemangiopericytoma phenotype develop extracranial metastases, especially to bone, lung, and liver {209,815,903,2673}. Gross total resection favourably affects recurrence and survival, and patients benefit from adjuvant radiotherapy {813,814,815,903}. As discussed previously, the historical three-tiered grading system (in which the solitary fibrous tumour phenotype is

considered to be grade I and the haemangiopericytoma phenotype grade II or III) may need to be adapted to improve the prognostic significance.

Haemangioblastoma

Plate K.H.
Aldape K.D.
Vortmeyer A.O.
Zagzag D.
Neumann H.P.H.

Definition
A tumour histologically characterized by neoplastic stromal cells and abundant small vessels.
Haemangioblastoma is a benign slow-growing tumour of adults, typically occurring in the brain stem, cerebellum, and spinal cord. Haemangioblastomas

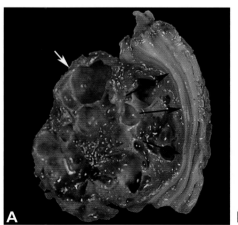
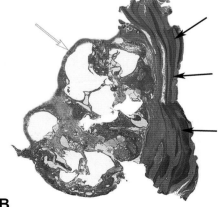

Fig. 11.11 Haemangioblastoma. **A,B** The tumour is multicystic (white arrow) and well demarcated from the surrounding cerebellum (black arrows).

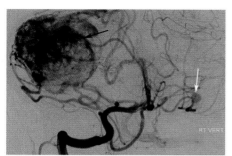

Fig. 11.12 Haemangioblastoma. Cerebral angiogram demonstrates two tumours; the larger one is in the right cerebellar hemisphere (black arrow) and the smaller one is in the left cerebellar hemisphere (white arrow); both are hypervascular.

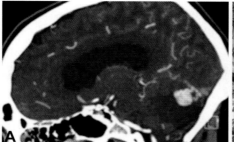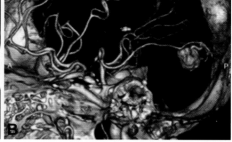

Fig. 11.13 Cerebellar haemangioblastoma. **A** CT image. **B** CT angiography shows the tumour receiving vascularization from the left superior cerebellar artery.

occur in sporadic forms (accounting for ~70% of cases) and in association with the inherited von Hippel–Lindau disease (VHL) (accounting for ~30% of cases). The *VHL* tumour suppressor gene is inactivated both in VHL-associated cases and in most sporadic cases.

ICD-O code   9161/1

Grading

Haemangioblastoma corresponds histologically to WHO grade I.

Epidemiology

Haemangioblastomas are uncommon tumours that occur as sporadic lesions and in familial forms associated with VHL. Accurate incidence rates are not available. Haemangioblastomas usually occur in adults. The average patient age at presentation of VHL-associated tumours is approximately 20 years younger than that of sporadic tumours {1567}. The male-to-female ratio is approximately 1:1.

Localization

Haemangioblastomas can occur in any part of the nervous system. Sporadic tumours occur predominantly in the cerebellum, usually in the hemispheres (in ~80% of cases). Haemangioblastomas associated with VHL are often multiple (in 65% of patients) and affect the brain stem, spinal cord, and nerve roots in addition to the cerebellum. Supratentorial and peripheral nervous system lesions are rare.

Clinical features

Symptoms of intracranial haemangioblastoma generally arise from impaired cerebrospinal fluid flow due to a cyst or solid tumour mass, resulting in an increase of intracranial pressure and hydrocephalus. Cerebellar deficits such as dysmetria and ataxia can also occur. Spinal tumours become symptomatic due to local compression resulting in symptoms such as pain, hypaesthesia, and incontinence. Haemangioblastomas produce erythropoietin, which causes secondary polycythaemia in about 5% of patients {853}. Haemorrhage is a rare complication of CNS haemangioblastoma {639,855}.

Imaging

Haemangioblastomas have a characteristic radiographical appearance on both CT and MRI, as well as a distinct prolonged vascular stain on cerebral angiography {112}. MRI is the preferred imaging modality, but in rare cases angiography better detects occult vascular nodules that may not be apparent on standard imaging. MRI studies typically show a gadolinium-enhancing mass, with an associated cyst in approximately 75% of cases. The solid component is usually peripherally located within the cerebellar hemisphere. Flow voids may be seen within the nodule due to enlarged feeding/draining vessels. Evidence of calcification is usually absent on imaging. Spinal cord haemangioblastomas are often associated with a syrinx.

Macroscopy

Most haemangioblastomas (60%) present as well-circumscribed, partly cystic, highly vascularized lesions; about 40% are completely solid. Occasionally, the tumour is yellow due to rich lipid content. The classic appearance is that of a cyst with a solid vascular nodule that abuts a pial surface {2683}.

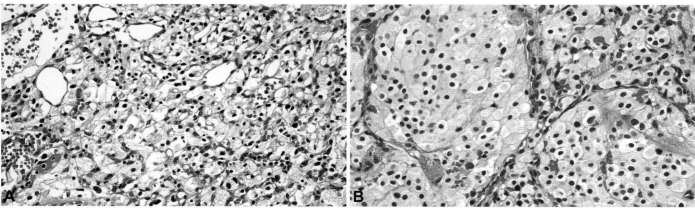

Fig. 11.14 Haemangioblastoma. **A** Stromal cells with clear, vacuolated cytoplasm due to accumulation of lipid droplets. **B** The cellular variant is a closer mimic of metastatic renal cell carcinoma and is characterized by cohesive nests of epithelioid stromal cells, with less-vacuolated cytoplasm and fewer intervening capillaries.

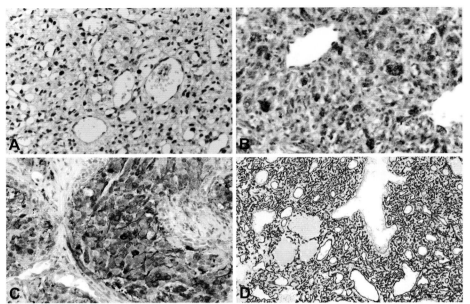

Fig. 11.15 Haemangioblastoma. **A** Nuclear expression of HIF1A in stromal cells. **B** Immunostaining for inhibin highlights the stromal cells. **C** Unlike in metastatic renal cell carcinoma, the tumour cells of this cellular haemangioblastoma are inhibin-positive. **D** CD34 immunostaining highlights the rich vascular network, whereas intervening stromal cells are negative.

Microscopy

Haemangioblastomas are characterized by two main components: (1) stromal cells that are characteristically large and vacuolated but can show considerable cytological variation and (2) abundant vascular cells. Cellular and reticular variants of haemangioblastoma are distinguished by the abundance and morphology of the stromal cell component.

Numerous thin-walled vessels are apparent and are readily outlined by a reticulin stain. In accordance with the highly vascular nature of haemangioblastoma, intratumoural haemorrhage may occur. In adjacent reactive tissues, particularly in cyst and syrinx walls, astrocytic gliosis and Rosenthal fibres are frequently observed. The tumour edge is generally well demarcated, and infiltration into

surrounding neural tissues rarely occurs. Mitotic figures are rare. Stromal cells account for only 10–20% of the cells and constitute the neoplastic component of the tumour. Their nuclei can vary in size, with occasional atypical and hyperchromatic nuclei. However, haemangioblastoma's most characteristic and distinguishing morphological feature is numerous lipid-containing vacuoles, resulting in the typical clear-cell morphology of haemangioblastoma, which may resemble metastatic renal cell carcinoma (RCC). The fact that patients with VHL are also prone to RCC adds to the complexity of this differential diagnosis. Cases of tumour-to-tumour metastasis (RCC metastatic to haemangioblastoma) have also been reported in this setting {934}.

Immunophenotype

The stromal and capillary endothelial cells differ significantly in their expression patterns. Stromal cells lack endothelial cell markers, such as von Willebrand factor and CD34, and do not express endothelium-associated adhesion molecules such as CD31 {336,2769}. Unlike endothelial cells, stromal cells variably express neuron-specific enolase, NCAM1, S100, and ezrin {336,337,1100}. Vimentin is the major intermediate filament expressed by stromal cells. Stromal cells also express a variety of other proteins, including CXCR4 {1498,2839}, aquaporin-1 {1524}, brachyury, several carbonic anhydrase isozymes {2040}, and EGFR {335}, but they do not usually express GFAP {2769}. Both HIF1A {2841} and HIF2A {712} have been detected in stromal cells, and they may drive the expression of VEGF, which is also abundant in stromal cells {1363}. The corresponding receptors VEGFR1 and VEGFR2 {2768}, are expressed on endothelial cells, suggesting a paracrine mode of angiogenesis activation {971, 2437}. The endothelial cells of haemangioblastomas also express receptors for other angiogenic growth factors, including platelet-derived growth factors {335}. Immunohistochemistry is useful for distinguishing haemangioblastoma from RCC. RCCs are positive for epithelial markers such as EMA, whereas haemangioblastomas are negative. Additional potentially useful markers include D2-40 {2193} and inhibin alpha {1021}, which are both positive in haemangioblastoma but generally negative in RCC. CD10 staining shows the opposite results {1193}.

Table 11.01 Common immunohistochemical profiles of haemangioblastoma and renal cell carcinoma

Molecule	Haemangioblastoma	Renal cell carcinoma
Aquaporin-1	+ {428,2720}	+/– {2720}
Brachyury	+ {133}	– {133}
CD10	– {1999,2720}; +/– {2132}	+ {1999,2132,2720}
AE1/AE3	– {577,2720}	+ {577,2720}
CAM5.2	– {1999}	+ {1999}
D2-40	+/– {2132}; + {2193}	+/– {2132}; – {2193}
EMA	+/– {2720}	+ {2720}
Inhibin alpha	+ {366,577,1021,1999,2132,2720}	– {366,577,1021,1999}; +/– {2132,2720}
LEU7	+/– {1061}; + {1999}	– {1061}; +/– {1999}
NCAM1 (also called CD56)	+ {1999}	– {1999}
Neuron-specific enolase	+/– {1061}	+/– {1061}
PAX2	– {366,2132}	+ {366,2132}
PAX8	– {366}	+ {366}
Renal cell carcinoma marker	– {1093,2132}	+ {1093}; +/– {2132}
S100	+/– {1061}	+/– {1061}

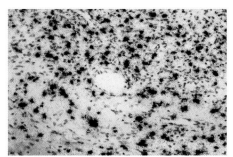
Fig. 11.16 Haemangioblastoma. VEGF mRNA expression in stromal cells.

Cell of origin

Stromal cells constitute the neoplastic cell type in haemangioblastoma {2437, 2670} and are surrounded by abundant non-neoplastic cells, including endothelial cells, pericytes, and lymphocytes. This intercellular genomic heterogeneity suggests that the majority of nucleated cells in the tumour mass do not arise from a common ancestral clone, supporting the hypothesis that the tumour mass histology is a consequence of reactive angiogenesis resulting from paracrine signalling mediated by the VHL tumour suppressor protein–deficient HIF1A-expressing stromal cells {2329,2437}. The exact origin of these stromal cells is still controversial, but on the basis of immunohistochemical expression data, various cell types have been suggested, including glial cells {56}, endothelial cells {1194}, arachnoid cells {1695}, embryonic choroid plexus cells {215}, neuroendocrine cells {153}, fibrohistiocytic cells {1767}, cells of neuroectodermal derivation {12}, and heterogeneous cell populations {2512}. More recent study reports have noted that the stromal cells of haemangioblastoma express proteins common to embryonal haemangioblast progenitor cells {854}. One such protein, SCL, has a distribution of expression in the developing nervous system that is similar to the topographical distribution of haemangioblastoma tumours in patients, suggesting that stromal cells may be haemangioblasts or haemangioblast progenitor cells {854,2352,2669}.

Genetic profile

Biallelic inactivation of the *VHL* gene is a frequent occurrence in familial haemangioblastomas, but is not common in sporadic tumours. However, studies on sporadic tumours (including somatic mutation analyses, assessments of allelic loss, deep-coverage DNA sequencing, and hypermethylation studies) have found loss or inactivation of the *VHL* gene in as many as 78% of cases {851,1456, 2329}, suggesting that loss of function of *VHL* is a central event in haemangioblastoma formation. No other gene has been found to be significantly mutated {2329}. The VHL tumour suppressor protein forms a ternary complex (called the VCB complex) with TCEB1 and TCEB2 {873}. The VHL tumour suppressor protein controls cell cycle regulation and, in a prolyl hydroxylase–dependent manner, the degradation of HIF1A and HIF2A. As a consequence, loss of function of *VHL* leads to upregulation of hypoxia-responsive genes such as those encoding VEGF and erythropoietin, despite the absence of tumour hypoxia. This condition is called pseudohypoxia {680}.

Genetic susceptibility

Haemangioblastoma is a frequent manifestation of VHL (occurring in 60% of patients) {850}. Genetic counselling and molecular genetic screening for germline mutations in the *VHL* gene are therefore essential for patients with haemangioblastoma {850}.

Prognosis and predictive factors

The prognosis of sporadic CNS haemangioblastoma is excellent if surgical resection can be performed successfully, which is typically possible. Permanent neurological deficits are rare {490} and can be avoided when CNS haemangioblastomas are diagnosed and treated early {852}. Patients with sporadic tumours have a better outcome than those with tumours associated with VHL, because patients with VHL tend to develop multiple lesions {1687}.

Other mesenchymal tumours

Antonescu C.R.
Paulus W.
Perry A.
Rushing E.J.
Hainfellner J.A.

Bouvier C.
Figarella-Branger D.
von Deimling A.
Wesseling P.

Haemangioma

Definition

A benign vascular neoplasm greatly varying in size. Most haemangiomas affecting the CNS are primary lesions of bone that impinge on the CNS secondarily. Dural {1, 1244} and parenchymal {2361} haemangiomas are less common.

Histologically, haemangiomas have predominantly capillary-type growth and occur mostly in the paediatrics age group. Infantile haemangiomas are consistently positive for GLUT1, a marker that is typically used to distinguish haemangioma from arteriovenous malformation in extracranial locations {409}. However, in a recent study, both cerebral cavernous malformations and cerebral arteriovenous malformations showed endothelial immunoexpression of GLUT1 and thus seemed to differ from most other arteriovenous malformations {1632}.

Malformative vascular lesions

Most vascular lesions of the CNS are malformative in nature, including cerebral cavernous malformation (also called cavernous angioma or cavernoma), arteriovenous malformation, venous angioma, and capillary telangiectasia. Cerebral cavernous malformations typically occur in the brain, but the spinal cord and the eye may also be involved. Histologically, cerebral cavernous malformations are composed of an admixture of capillary-type and large saccular vessels with

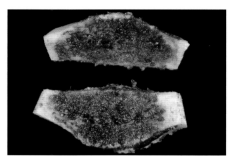

Fig. 11.17 Capillary haemangioma. Reddish-brown sponge-like appearance of an intraosseous capillary haemangioma on cut surface of a skull resection specimen.

fibrotic walls. Cerebral cavernous malformations can be inherited as an autosomal dominant disorder (accounting for 20% of cases), but most are sporadic. Biallelic somatic and germline mutations in one of the cerebral cavernous malformation genes have been implicated as a two-hit mechanism of inherited cerebral cavernous malformation pathogenesis {33}. Another tumefactive vascular lesion that can occur in the brain or meninges is intravascular papillary endothelial hyperplasia, a papillary proliferation of endothelium associated with thrombosis {1366}.

ICD-O code   9120/0

Epithelioid haemangioendothelioma

Definition

A low-grade malignant vascular neoplasm characterized by the presence of epithelioid endothelial cells, arranged in cords and single cells embedded in a distinctive chondromyxoid or hyalinized stroma.

Epithelioid haemangioendothelioma is rarely located in the skull base, dura, or brain parenchyma {106,1802}. Its cells contain relatively abundant eosinophilic cytoplasm, which may be vacuolated. In general, the nuclei are round or occasionally indented or vesicular, and show only minor atypia. Mitoses and limited necrosis may be seen. Small intracytoplasmic lumina (blister cells) are seen, but well-formed vascular channels are typically absent. Immunohistochemical studies (e.g. for CD31 and ERG) confirm these tumours' endothelial nature. Approximately 90% of epithelioid haemangioendotheliomas harbour the recurrent t(1;3)(p36;q25) translocation, which results in a *WWTR1-CAMTA1* fusion {651, 2510}. A smaller subset of epithelioid haemangioendotheliomas have a t(x;11)

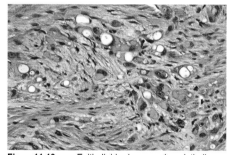

Fig. 11.18 Epithelioid haemangioendothelioma. Intracytoplasmic lumina and a basophilic stroma are prominent features of this example.

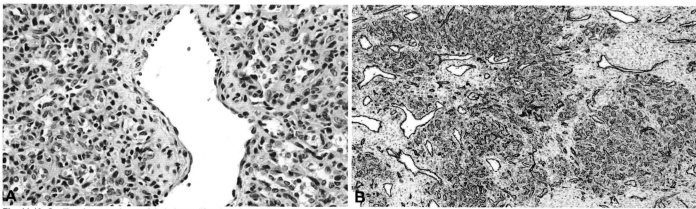

Fig. 11.19 Capillary haemangioma. **A** Lobular proliferation of small thin-walled blood vessels. **B** The lobular growth pattern is visualized on this immunostain for CD31.

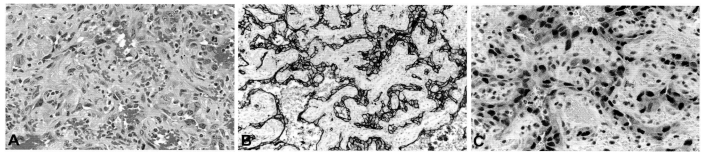

Fig. 11.20 Angiosarcoma. **A** Anastomosing vascular channels lined by large, cytologically atypical tumour cells. **B** Immunostaining for CD34 highlights the anastomosing vascular pattern. **C** Immunostaining for FLI1 marks the cytologically atypical angiosarcoma nuclei.

(p11;q22) translocation, which results in a *YAP1-TFE3* fusion {80}.

ICD-O code   9133/3

Angiosarcoma

Definition

A high-grade malignant neoplasm with evidence of endothelial differentiation.

The rare examples of angiosarcoma that originate in brain or meninges {1636} vary in differentiation from patently vascular tumours with anastomosing vascular channels lined by mitotically active, cytologically atypical endothelial cells to poorly differentiated, often epithelioid solid lesions, in which immunoreactivity for vascular markers (e.g. CD31, CD34, ERG, and FLI1) is required for definitive diagnosis. Occasional cytokeratin reactivity complicates the distinction of poorly differentiated angiosarcoma from metastatic carcinoma {2131}. No genetic abnormalities have been described for CNS angiosarcomas.

ICD-O code   9120/3

Kaposi sarcoma

Definition

A malignant neoplasm characterized by spindle-shaped cells forming slit-like blood vessels, which is only rarely encountered as a parenchymal or meningeal tumour, typically in the setting of HIV type 1 infection or AIDS {115,334}.

In this setting, it is often difficult to determine whether a Kaposi sarcoma lesion is primary or metastatic. The tumour is almost always immunopositive for HHV8 {2140}.

ICD-O code   9140/3

Ewing sarcoma / peripheral primitive neuroectodermal tumour

Definition

A small round blue cell tumour of neuroectodermal origin that involves the CNS either as a primary dural neoplasm {565, 1617,1696,2358} or by direct extension from contiguous bone or soft tissue (e.g. skull, vertebra, or paraspinal soft tissue). Radiologically, primary CNS Ewing sarcoma / peripheral primitive neuroectodermal tumour can mimic meningioma.

A wide patient age range has been reported, although peak incidence occurs in the second decade of life. The histology, immunophenotype, and biology are essentially identical to those of tumours encountered in bone or soft tissue {714}. The tumour is composed of sheets of small, round, primitive-appearing cells with scant clear cytoplasm and uniform nuclei with fine chromatin and smooth nuclear contours. Homer Wright rosettes are occasionally seen, but are usually not prominent. Most tumours stain at least focally with synaptophysin and neuron-specific enolase, whereas cytokeratin is only focally seen (in as many as 20% of cases). CD99 shows strong and diffuse membranous immunoreactivity in the vast majority. CD99 can also be expressed (although this expression is usually more patchy and cytoplasmic) in other tumour types, including solitary fibrous tumour / haemangiopericytoma and (less commonly), medulloblastoma or other embryonal CNS neoplasms. Therefore, most Ewing sarcoma / peripheral primitive neuroectodermal tumours must be confirmed at the molecular level either by RT-PCR for the presence of an *EWSR1-FLI1* or *EWSR1-ERG* fusion transcript or by FISH for *EWSR1* gene rearrangement {279}. Alternative gene fusions in the

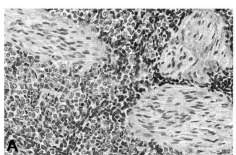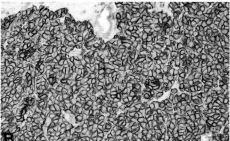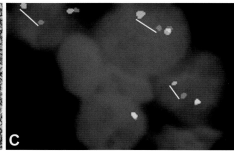

Fig. 11.21 Ewing sarcoma / peripheral primitive neuroectodermal tumour. **A** Invasion of nerve roots. **B** Diffuse membrane immunoreactivity for CD99. **C** FISH results positive for *EWSR1* (*EWS*) gene rearrangement, with split of paired red and green signals (white lines).

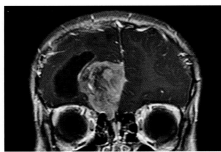
Fig. 11.22 Postcontrast T1-weighted MRI of a dural-based Ewing sarcoma / peripheral primitive neuroectodermal tumour mimicking meningioma.

Ewing sarcoma–like family of tumours have also been described, including *CIC-DUX4* {1104} and the *BCOR-CCNB3* intrachromosomal inversion {1971}.

ICD-O code   9364/3

Lipoma

Definition
A benign lesion that microscopically resembles normal adipose tissue {306}.
Intracranial lipomas are believed to be congenital malformations rather than true neoplasms, resulting from abnormal differentiation of the meninx primitiva (the undifferentiated mesenchyme) {1203}.

ICD-O code   8850/0

Microscopy

Lipoma
Most lipomas show lobulation at low magnification. Lipomas have an inconspicuous capillary network. Patchy fibrosis is a common feature, and calcification and myxoid change are occasionally seen. Osteolipomas are exceedingly rare and may show zonation, with central adipose tissue and peripheral bone {2367}.

Complex lipomatous lesions
Complex lipomatous lesions vary considerably in terms of their histological composition. For example, lumbosacral lipomas (leptomyelolipomas) that occur in the context of tethered spinal cord syndrome are likely malformative and may consist of subcutaneous and intradural components linked by a fibrolipomatous stalk that may attach to the dorsum of the cord or to the filum terminale {998}. Lipomas of the cerebellopontine angle {201}, an uncommonly affected off-midline

site, may incorporate intradural portions of cranial nerve roots and their ganglia. Many also feature striated muscle or other mesenchymal tissues. Some of these lesions have been referred to as choristomas. It has even been suggested that intracranial lipomas containing various other tissue types represent a transition between lipoma and teratoma {2572}. Whether these various lesions are neoplasms or malformative overgrowths is yet to be determined.

Epidural lipomatosis
Epidural lipomatosis is a rare lesion that consists of diffuse hypertrophy of spinal epidural adipose tissue. As such, it is not a neoplasm but a metabolic response, often to chronic administration of steroids {919}.

Angiolipoma

Definition
A lipoma variant with prominent vascularity; by definition, the vessels are of capillary type and are generally most prominent in the periphery, often containing dispersed fibrin thrombi.
The proportions of adipose cells and vasculature in angiolipoma vary {1982, 2367}. With time, interstitial fibrosis may ensue. Angiolipomas may be overdiagnosed because ordinary haemangiomas are often accompanied by fat; however, ordinary haemangiomas have a more heterogeneous spectrum of vascular channels, including thick-walled venous-type vascular channels and cavernous spaces.

ICD-O code   8861/0

Hibernoma

Definition
A very rare lipoma variant within the CNS, composed of uniform granular or multivacuolated cells with small, centrally located nuclei, resembling brown fat {442}.

ICD-O code   8880/0

Liposarcoma

Definition
A malignant tumour composed entirely or partly of neoplastic adipocytes.
Intracranial liposarcoma is extremely rare. An example associated with subdural haematoma has been described {461}, and an example of gliosarcoma with a liposarcomatous element has been reported {242}.

ICD-O code   8850/3

Desmoid-type fibromatosis

Definition
A locally infiltrative but cytologically benign lesion composed of uniform myofibroblastic-type cells in an abundant collagenous stroma, arranged in intersecting fascicles {1684}.
Desmoid-type fibromatosis must be distinguished from cranial fasciitis of childhood, a process histologically related to nodular fasciitis, featuring rapid growth within the deep scalp, lacking an intradural component, and having no malignant potential {1438}. Cranial infantile myofibromatosis also enters into the differential diagnosis but often displays a biphasic pattern, with alternating haemangiopericytoma-like areas and myoid components {2479}.

ICD-O code   8821/1

Myofibroblastoma

Definition
A benign mesenchymal neoplasm composed of spindle-shaped cells with features of myofibroblasts embedded in a stroma that contains coarse bands of hyalinized collagen and conspicuous mast cells, admixed with a variable amount of adipose tissue {714}.
Myofibroblastomas of the CNS are similar to their mammary-type counterparts, being part of a larger spectrum of CD34-positive lesions (including spindle cell lipoma and cellular angiofibroma) that show common 13q14 losses by FISH or loss of RB immunoexpression {420,742}. Myofibroblastomas are also strongly positive for desmin {2348}.

ICD-O code   8825/0

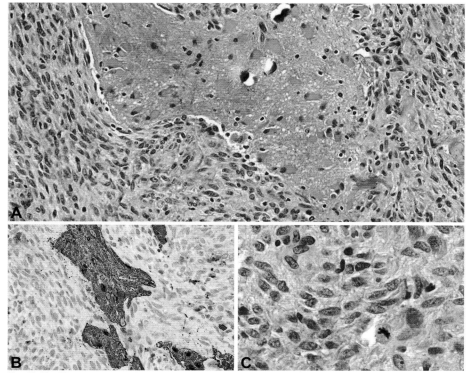

Fig. 11.23 Fibrosarcoma. **A** This hypercellular radiation-induced neoplasm shows features of fibrosarcoma with intersecting fascicles of spindled cells; note the entrapped island of gliotic brain tissue. **B** Immunostain for GFAP highlights entrapped islands of gliotic brain, whereas tumour cells are negative. **C** Increased mitotic activity.

Inflammatory myofibroblastic tumour

Definition

A distinctive neoplastic proliferation, usually composed of bland myofibroblastic-type cells intimately associated with a variable lymphoplasmacytic infiltrate and arranged in loose fascicles within an oedematous stroma.

The term "inflammatory myofibroblastic tumour" was once considered to be synonymous with inflammatory pseudotumour or plasma cell granuloma and to be a variant of inflammatory fibrosarcoma. Inflammatory myofibroblastic tumour of the CNS is rare and can occur in patients of any age. The radiological characteristics of these tumours are often similar to those of meningiomas. All three patterns reported in inflammatory myofibroblastic tumours of soft tissue (myxoid–nodular fasciitis–like, fibromatosis-like, and scar-like) have also been observed in the CNS. Approximately 50% of all inflammatory myofibroblastic tumours harbour *ALK* gene rearrangement and overexpress ALK {81}. Gene fusions involving other kinases have also been implicated in the pathogenesis of

inflammatory myofibroblastic tumour, including *ROS1*, *PDGFRB*, and *RET* {81, 1539}. Most inflammatory myofibroblastic tumours have favourable outcomes after gross total resection.

ICD-O code   8825/1

The differential diagnosis of inflammatory myofibroblastic tumour includes hypertrophic intracranial pachymeningitis, a pseudotumoural lesion that entails progressive dural thickening due to pachymeningeal fibrosis and chronic inflammation. These lesions are often associated with autoimmune disorders {2507}, and some have recently been reclassified as IgG4-related disease {1509}.

Benign fibrous histiocytoma

Definition

A lesion composed of a mixture of spindled (fibroblast-like) and plump (histiocyte-like) cells arranged in a storiform pattern.

Benign fibrous histiocytoma (also called fibrous xanthoma or fibroxanthoma) may involve dura or cranial bone {2604}.

Scattered giant cells and/or inflammatory cells are commonly seen. Many tumours that had an intraparenchymal component and were initially described as fibrous xanthoma were subsequently shown to be GFAP-positive and reclassified as pleomorphic xanthoastrocytoma {1254}.

ICD-O code   8830/0

Fibrosarcoma

Definition

A rare sarcoma type showing monomorphic spindle cells arranged in intersecting fascicles (a so-called herringbone pattern).

Fibrosarcomas are markedly cellular, exhibit brisk mitotic activity, and often feature necrosis {789}. Similar histological features are seen in adult-type fibrosarcoma; congenital/infantile fibrosarcoma; and fibrosarcomatous transformation in the setting of a solitary fibrous tumour / haemangiopericytoma or dermatofibrosarcoma protuberans. Sclerosing epithelioid fibrosarcoma affecting the CNS has also been reported {205}.

ICD-O code   8810/3

Undifferentiated pleomorphic sarcoma / malignant fibrous histiocytoma

Definition

A malignant neoplasm composed of spindled, plump, and pleomorphic giant cells that can be arranged in a storiform or fascicular pattern.

Most cases of undifferentiated pleomorphic sarcoma / malignant fibrous histiocytoma are overtly malignant, featuring

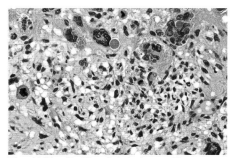

Fig. 11.24 Undifferentiated pleomorphic sarcoma. This highly pleomorphic dural-based sarcoma shows immunoreactivity for vimentin, but no expression of more specific lineage markers.

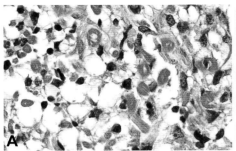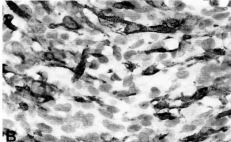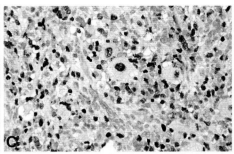

Fig. 11.25 Meningeal rhabdomyosarcoma. **A** Rhabdomyoblasts are evident in this primitive-appearing meningeal tumour from a child. **B** Desmin positivity highlights the rhabdomyoblasts. **C** Extensive myogenin immunoreactivity.

numerous mitoses as well as necrosis. Only isolated cases of the inflammatory variant of this entity have been reported to involve brain {1598}.

ICD-O code   8802/3

Leiomyoma

Definition
A benign smooth muscle tumour that can typically be readily recognized by its pattern of intersecting fascicles, being composed of eosinophilic spindle cells with blunt-ended nuclei {1506}.

As a rule, leiomyomas lack mitotic activity and cytological atypia. Occasional examples feature nuclear palisading and should not be mistaken for schwannoma. Diffuse leptomeningeal leiomyoma {1195} and an angioleiomyomatous variant {1410} have been described. EBV- and AIDS-associated cases have also been reported {1225}.

ICD-O code   8890/0

Leiomyosarcoma

Definition
A malignant neoplasm with predominantly smooth muscle differentiation.

The morphological variants of leiomyosarcoma include epithelioid leiomyosarcoma, myxoid leiomyosarcoma, granular cell leiomyosarcoma, and inflammatory leiomyosarcoma {715}.
Intracranial leiomyosarcomas {555, 1537}, like their soft tissue counterparts, retain the intersecting fascicles at 90° angles and eosinophilic cytoplasm, but show marked nuclear pleomorphism, increased mitotic activity, and necrosis. Most intracranial leiomyosarcomas arise in or adjacent to the dura (e.g. in

the paraspinal region or epidural space) {1595,2851}. Parenchymal examples are rare {623}. An association with EBV and immunosuppression has been established {2851}, but leiomyosarcomas arising in these settings are less clearly malignant and may respond to immune reconstitution. Most leiomyosarcomas diffusely express desmin and SMA.

ICD-O code   8890/3

Rhabdomyoma

Definition
A benign lesion consisting of mature striated muscle.

One reported case of rhabdomyoma associated with a cranial nerve also featured a minor adipose tissue component {2630}. However, most reported intraneural examples are in fact neuromuscular choristoma (also called benign triton tumour). This is an important diagnostic distinction given the high risk of postoperative fibromatosis associated with neuromuscular choristoma {979}. CNS rhabdomyomas must also be distinguished from skeletal muscle heterotopia, most of which occur within prepontine leptomeninges {710}.

ICD-O code   8900/0

Rhabdomyosarcoma

Definition
A malignant neoplasm with predominantly skeletal muscle differentiation.

Whether meningeal or parenchymal, nearly all primary CNS rhabdomyosarcomas are of the embryonal type {2069,2513}; alveolar rhabdomyosarcoma {1259} and a rhabdomyosarcomatous element in gliosarcoma {2465} are

exceptionally rare. Most tumours consist primarily of undifferentiated small cells, whereas strap cells with cross striations are only occasionally observed. Immunostaining for desmin and myogenin usually confirms the diagnosis. Rhabdomyosarcomas must be differentiated from other brain tumours that occasionally show skeletal muscle differentiation, such as medullomyoblastomas, gliosarcomas, MPNSTs, germ cell tumours, and even rare meningiomas {1120}. Malignant ectomesenchymoma, a mixed tumour composed of ganglion cells or neuroblasts and one or more mesenchymal elements (usually rhabdomyosarcoma) may also occur in the brain {1919}.

ICD-O code   8900/3

Chondroma

Definition
A benign, well-circumscribed neoplasm composed of low-cellularity hyaline cartilage.

Isolated cases of intracranial chondroma (usually dural-based) have been reported {500,1397}. Outside the CNS, chondromas often develop in the skull and only secondarily displace dura and brain. Malignant transformation of a large

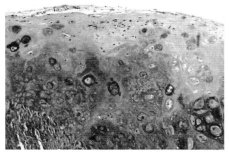

Fig. 11.26 Dural chondroma, a meningeal tumour composed of mature hyaline cartilage.

CNS chondroma to chondrosarcoma has been documented over a long clinical course {1689}.

ICD-O code 9220/0

Chondrosarcoma

Definition
A malignant mesenchymal tumour with cartilaginous differentiation.
Most chondrosarcomas arise de novo, but some develop in a pre-existing benign cartilaginous lesion.

ICD-O code 9220/3

Microscopy

Conventional chondrosarcoma
Intracranial, extraosseous chondrosarcomas of the classic type are rare {407, 1352,1855,1919}. The same is true for extraskeletal myxoid chondrosarcoma, which has been reported to arise within the brain {416} as well as in the leptomeninges of the brain. Chondrosarcomas arising in the skull base, in particular in the midline, should be distinguished from (chondroid) chordoma. Unlike chordomas, chondrosarcomas are non-reactive for keratin, EMA {1685}, and brachyury {2672}.

Mesenchymal chondrosarcoma
Mesenchymal chondrosarcoma also arises more often in bones of the skull or spine than within dura or brain parenchyma {2200,2262,2820}. Some tumours consist primarily of the small-cell component, punctuated by scant islands of atypical hyaline cartilage, whereas in others the chondroid element predominates. The histological pattern of the mesenchymal component resembles either a Ewing sarcoma–like small blue cell malignancy or a solitary fibrous tumour / haemangiopericytoma, due to its distinctive staghorn vascular network. The transition between the chondroid and mesenchymal component is typically abrupt; however, a more gradual transition can also occur, and this pattern is more challenging to distinguish from small cell osteosarcomas. When the cartilage is not obvious, SOX9 immunostaining may be useful, because it is positive in the undifferentiated mesenchymal component {668}. In difficult cases, the diagnosis can be

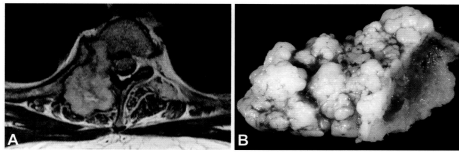

Fig. 11.27 Chondrosarcoma. **A** MRI of a low-grade chondrosarcoma arising from the vertebral column. Note the lobulated contours and invasion into adjacent soft tissues. **B** Meningeal low-grade chondrosarcoma showing glistening nodules of hyaline cartilage with focal softening and liquefaction.

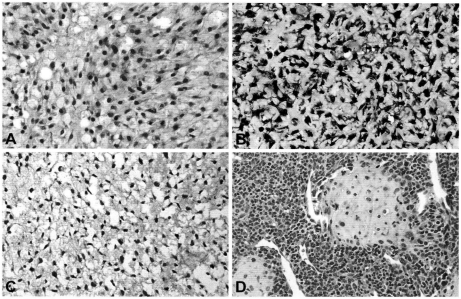

Fig. 11.28 Chondrosarcoma. **A** Low-grade chondrosarcoma may show small stellate to epithelioid cells set within a myxoid background, overlapping morphologically with chordoma. **B** S100 immunoreactivity is typically strong in low-grade chondrosarcomas, but is not very specific, because it may also be seen in other diagnostic considerations, such as chordoma. **C** Lack of nuclear brachyury expression helps distinguish chondrosarcoma from chordoma. **D** The combination of a small blue cell tumour with well-formed hyaline cartilage is characteristic of mesenchymal chondrosarcoma.

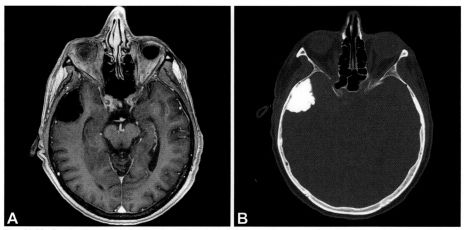

Fig. 11.29 Dural osteoma. **A** Postcontrast T1-weighted MRI reveals a non-enhancing extra-axial mass. **B** Bone-window CT reveals an osseous mass involving the dura and inner table of the skull.

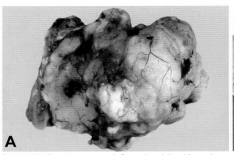 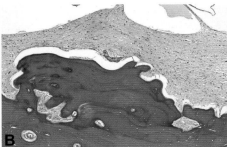

Fig. 11.30 Dural osteoma. **A** Bosselated dural-based osseous tumour. **B** On microscopy, gliotic brain parenchyma is seen adjacent to the dense bone of the dural osteoma.

confirmed by the presence of *NCOA2* gene rearrangements {2688}.

Osteoma

Definition
A benign bone-forming tumour with limited growth potential.

Isolated cases of intracranial osteoma (usually dural-based) have been reported {427}. Outside the CNS, osteomas often develop in the skull and only secondarily displace dura and brain. Histologically, they correspond to similar tumours arising in bone and must be distinguished from asymptomatic dural calcification, ossification related to metabolic disease or trauma, and rare examples of astrocytoma and gliosarcoma with osseous differentiation.

ICD-O code   9180/0

Osteochondroma

Definition
A benign cartilaginous neoplasm, which may be pedunculated or sessile, arising on the surface of the bone.

Osteochondroma is characterized by the presence of a cartilaginous cap and a fibrous perichondrium that extends to the periosteum of the bone.

ICD-O code   9210/0

Osteosarcoma

Definition
A malignant bone-forming mesenchymal tumour.

Osteosarcoma predominantly affects adolescents and young adults. The preferred sites are the skull and the spine and more rarely the meninges and the brain {144,352,2214,2227,2326}. Bone matrix or osteoid deposition by the proliferating tumour cells is required for the diagnosis. Osteosarcomatous elements may exceptionally be encountered as components of germ cell tumour and gliosarcoma {132}.

ICD-O code   9180/3

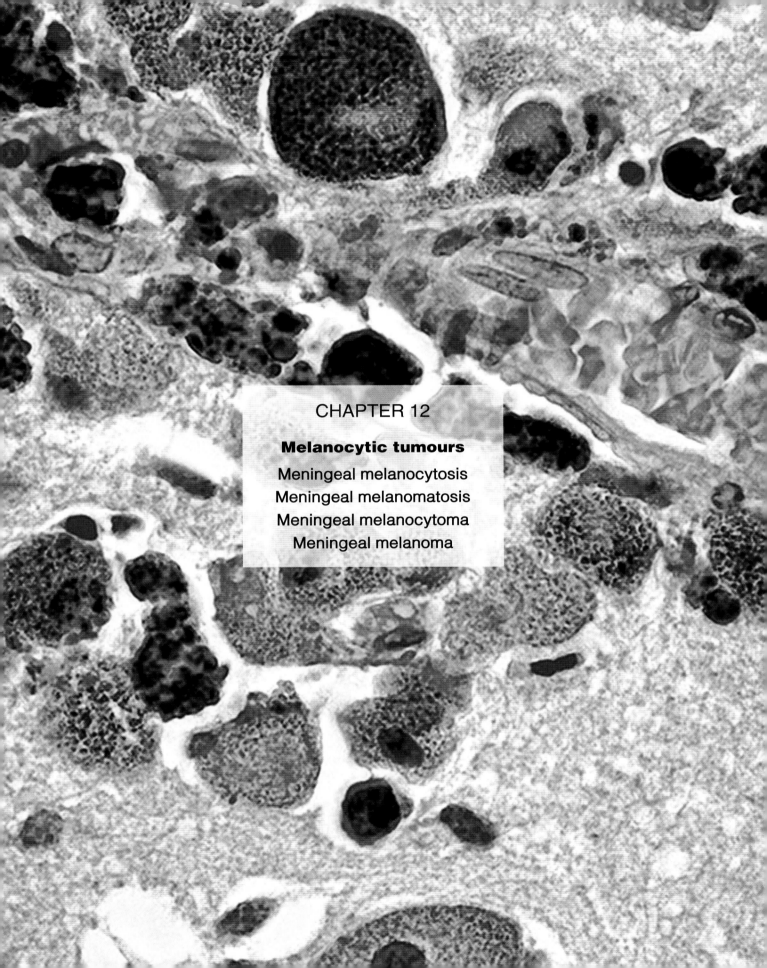

CHAPTER 12

Melanocytic tumours

Meningeal melanocytosis
Meningeal melanomatosis
Meningeal melanocytoma
Meningeal melanoma

Melanocytic tumours

Brat D.J.
Perry A.
Wesseling P.
Bastian B.C.

Definition
Primary melanocytic neoplasms of the CNS are diffuse or localized tumours that presumably arise from leptomeningeal melanocytes.

Benign lesions that are diffuse without forming macroscopic masses are termed melanocytosis, whereas malignant diffuse or multifocal lesions are termed melanomatosis. Benign or intermediate-grade tumoural lesions are termed melanocytomas. Malignant lesions that are discrete tumours are termed melanomas.

Microscopy
Diagnosis of this family of neoplasms hinges on the recognition of tumour cells that have melanocytic differentiation. Most melanocytic neoplasms display melanin pigment finely distributed within the tumour cytoplasm and coarsely distributed within the tumour stroma and the cytoplasm of tumoural macrophages (melanophages). Rare melanocytomas and occasional primary melanomas do not demonstrate melanin pigment; diagnosis then relies more heavily on immunohistochemistry and mutation profile. Identification of melanocytic lesions usually requires histopathological examination, but the diagnosis of melanocytosis and melanomatosis has occasionally been made by cerebrospinal fluid cytology {2106}.

Differential diagnosis
Primary CNS melanocytic neoplasms must be distinguished from other melanotic tumours that involve the CNS, including metastatic melanoma and other primary tumours undergoing melanization, as can occur in melanotic schwannoma, medulloblastoma, paraganglioma, and various gliomas {266,1405}. There is little evidence supporting the existence of a true melanotic meningioma, although rare melanocytic colonization of meningiomas has been documented {1768}. Melanotic neuroectodermal tumour of infancy (retinal anlage tumour) has also been reported at intracranial locations {1219}.

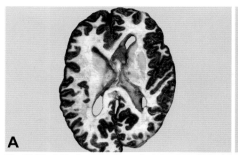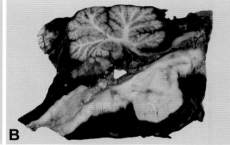

Fig. 12.01 A Meningeal melanocytosis involving the subarachnoid space of the cerebral hemispheres. **B** Meningeal melanomatosis infiltrating the meninges around the brain stem and cerebellum.

Immunophenotype
Most tumours react with the anti-melanosomal antibodies HMB45, melan-A, and microphthalmia-associated transcription factor (MITF). They also express S100 protein. Staining for vimentin and neuron-specific enolase are variable. Among the discrete melanocytic tumours (melanocytoma and melanoma), expression of collagen IV and reticulin is lacking around individual tumour cells, but is present around blood vessels and larger tumoural nests {1406}. There is only rare expression of GFAP, NFPs, cytokeratins, or EMA. The Ki-67 proliferation index is typically < 1–2% in melanocytomas and averages about 8% in primary melanomas {266}.

Cell of origin
Melanocytic neoplasms of the nervous system and its coverings are thought to arise from leptomeningeal melanocytes that are derived from the neural crest {1405}. These melanocytes may differ developmentally from melanocytes in epithelia (e.g. the epidermis and mucosal membrane) and seem to be more closely related to melanocytes in the uveal tract {139}. In the normal CNS, melanocytes are preferentially localized at the base of the brain, around the ventral medulla oblongata, and along the upper cervical spinal cord. Melanocytic neoplasms associated with neurocutaneous melanosis likely derive from melanocyte precursor cells that reach the CNS after acquiring somatic mutations, mostly of *NRAS*.

Genetic susceptibility
Little is known regarding the inherited susceptibility of these neoplasms, if any. Both the cutaneous naevi and the CNS melanocytic neoplasms that arise in the setting of neurocutaneous melanosis are strongly associated with activating somatic mutations of *NRAS*, most often involving codon 61 {1921,2225}. *BRAF* V600E mutations have also been identified in the cutaneous naevi of patients with neurocutaneous melanosis (albeit less frequently), but mutations have not yet been described in CNS melanocytic neoplasms in this setting. Although the *NRAS* mutations are not inherited, they are thought to occur early in embryogenesis, prior to the migration of melanocyte precursors to their locations in the skin and leptomeninges {1405}. In patients with neurocutaneous melanosis, the multiple congenital melanocytic naevi and associated leptomeningeal melanocytic lesions contain the same *NRAS* mutation, whereas the normal skin and blood cells are not mutated, suggesting that a single postzygotic mutation of *NRAS* is responsible for the multiple cutaneous and leptomeningeal melanocytic lesions in this phacomatosis {1286}.

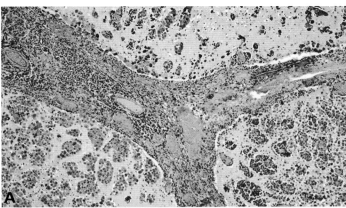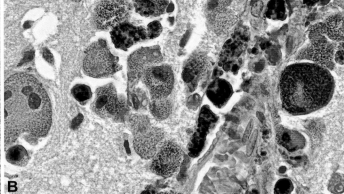

Fig. 12.02 Meningeal melanomatosis. **A** Extensive invasion of the subarachnoid space with perivascular infiltration of cerebral cortex. **B** Highly pleomorphic melanin-laden cells invading the cerebral cortex.

Meningeal melanocytosis and meningeal melanomatosis

Meningeal melanocytosis

Definition
Meningeal melanocytosis is a diffuse or multifocal proliferation of cytologically bland melanocytic cells that arises from the leptomeninges and involves the subarachnoid space.

Meningeal melanocytosis cells can spread into the perivascular spaces without frank invasion of the brain {1533}.

ICD-O code   8728/0

Meningeal melanomatosis

Definition
A primary CNS melanoma that arises from leptomeningeal melanocytes and displays a diffuse pattern of spread throughout the subarachnoid space and Virchow–Robin spaces, often with CNS invasion.

ICD-O code   8728/3

Epidemiology
Diffuse meningeal melanocytic neoplasms are rare, and population-based incidence is not available {1201}. Meningeal melanocytosis and melanomatosis are strongly linked with neurocutaneous melanosis, a rare phacomatosis that is typically associated with giant congenital naevi and presents before the age of 2 years. In one series of 39 such cases, the age at presentation for CNS manifestations ranged from stillbirth to the second

decade, with an equal sex distribution and no racial predisposition {1201}.

Localization
Melanocytosis and melanomatosis involve the supratentorial leptomeninges, the infratentorial leptomeninges, and may involve the superficial brain parenchyma by extending into perivascular Virchow-Robin spaces. They generally involve large expanses of the subarachnoid space with focal or multifocal nodularity occasionally seen. The sites of highest frequency include the cerebellum, pons, medulla, and temporal lobes.

Clinical features
Neurological symptoms associated with melanocytosis or melanomatosis arise secondarily to either hydrocephalus or local effects on the CNS parenchyma. Neuropsychiatric symptoms, bowel and bladder dysfunction, and sensory and motor disturbances are common. Once malignant transformation occurs, symptoms progress rapidly, with increasing intracranial pressure resulting in irritability, vomiting, lethargy, and seizures.

Neurocutaneous melanosis is a combination of melanocytosis or melanomatosis with giant or numerous congenital melanocytic naevi of the skin, usually involving the trunk or head and neck, and with various other malformative lesions, such as Dandy–Walker syndrome, syringomyelia, and lipomas {563,564, 1574}. Approximately 25% of patients with meningeal melanocytosis have significant concomitant cutaneous lesions. Conversely, about 10–15% of patients with large congenital melanocytic naevi of the skin develop clinical symptoms related to CNS melanocytosis {564}, and

radiological evidence of CNS involvement has been reported in as many as 23% of asymptomatic children with giant congenital naevi {726}. As part of a completely distinct clinical entity, melanocytosis may also be associated with congenital naevus of Ota {117}.

Imaging
CT and MRI of melanocytosis and melanomatosis show diffuse thickening and enhancement of the leptomeninges, often with focal or multifocal nodularity {1981}. Depending on melanin content, diffuse and circumscribed melanocytic tumours of the CNS may have a characteristic appearance on MRI due to the paramagnetic properties of melanin, resulting in an isodense or hyperintense signal on T1-weighted images and a hypointense signal on T2-weighted images {2372}.

Macroscopy
Diffuse melanocytic neoplasms present as dense black replacement of the subarachnoid space or as dusky clouding of the meninges.

Microscopy
The pathological proliferation of leptomeningeal melanocytes and their production of melanin account for the main microscopic findings in these diseases {583}. Tumour cells diffusely involving the leptomeninges assume a variety of shapes, including spindled, round, oval, and cuboidal. In melanocytosis, individual cells are cytologically bland and accumulate within the subarachnoid space and Virchow–Robin spaces without demonstrating overt CNS invasion {2372}. Unequivocal CNS parenchymal invasion

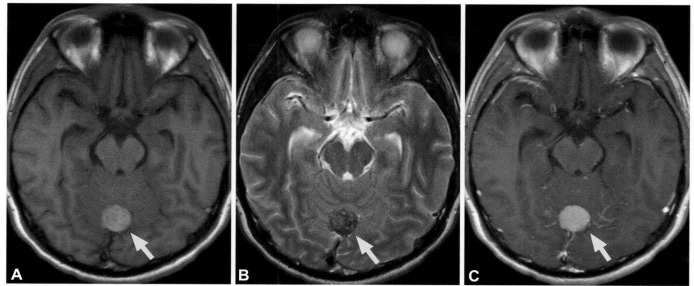

Fig. 12.03 MRI features of meningeal melanocytoma. A T1-weighted axial images (pre-contrast) reveal a hyperintense, well-circumscribed mass in the midline of the cerebellum arising from the dura. B On T2-weighted images, the mass is hypointense. C Following the administration of contrast agent, the melanocytoma shows homogeneous enhancement.

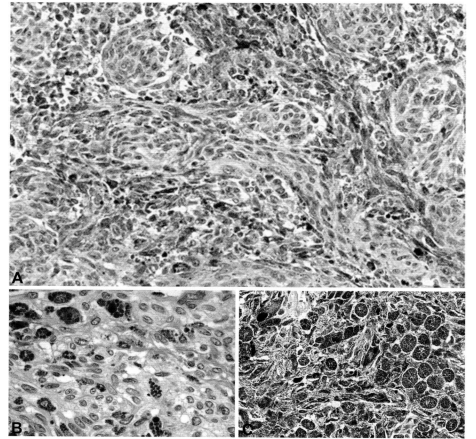

Fig. 12.04 Meningeal melanocytoma. A Loose or tight nests of low-grade, pigmented spindle cells with intervening stroma containing higher levels of melanin pigment. Note the vague, loosely formed whorls and fascicles. B Accumulation of large, melanin-containing macrophages (melanophages) is seen between tumour cells with a more spindled phenotype. The nuclei of tumour cells are bean-shaped and have micronucleoli. Melanin within the cytoplasm of melanophages is typical in larger aggregates. C Melanin-containing macrophages (melanophages).

should not be seen in melanocytosis; if it is identified, the tumour must be considered melanomatosis. Similarly, the presence of mitotic activity, severe cytological atypia, or necrosis also warrants a diagnosis of melanomatosis.

Prognosis and predictive factors

Diffuse melanocytic neoplasms of the leptomeninges generally carry a poor prognosis even in the absence of histological malignancy {2106}.

Meningeal melanocytoma

Definition

A well-differentiated, solid, and non-infiltrative melanocytic neoplasm that arises from leptomeningeal melanocytes.

Meningeal melanocytoma is characterized by the presence of epithelioid, fusiform, polyhedral, or spindled melanocytes, without evidence of anaplasia, necrosis, or elevated mitotic activity.

ICD-O code   8728/1

Epidemiology

Melanocytomas account for 0.06–0.1% of brain tumours, and the annual incidence has been estimated at 1 case per 10 million population {1149}. Melanocytomas can occur in patients of any age (range: 9–73 years), but are most frequent in the fifth decade of life (mean age: 45–50 years). There is a slight female predominance, with a female-to-male ratio of 1.5:1 {266,2687}.

Localization
Most melanocytomas arise in the extramedullary, intradural compartment at the cervical and thoracic spine. They can be dural-based or associated with nerve roots or spinal foramina {266,849}. Less frequently, they arise from the leptomeninges in the posterior fossa or supratentorial compartments. The trigeminal cave is a site with a peculiar predilection for primary melanocytic neoplasms, and tumours at this site are associated with an ipsilateral naevus of Ota {117,1970}.

Clinical features
Melanocytomas present with symptoms related to compression of the spinal cord, cerebellum, or cerebrum by an extra-axial mass, with focal neurological signs depending on location {266}.

Imaging
Melanocytomas and melanomas generally show homogeneous enhancement on postcontrast images. Tumours with abundant melanin will show a characteristic pattern of T1 hyperintensity (precontrast) and T2 hypointensity.

Macroscopy
Melanocytoma are solitary mass lesions, generally extra-axial, that may be black, reddish brown, blue, or macroscopically non-pigmented.

Microscopy
Melanocytomas are solitary low-grade tumours with no invasion of surrounding structures {266,1405,2687}. Slightly spindled or oval tumour cells containing variable melanin often form tight nests with a superficial resemblance to the whorls of meningioma. Heavily pigmented tumour cells and tumoural macrophages are especially seen at the periphery of nests. Other melanocytoma variants demonstrate storiform, vasocentric, and sheet-like arrangements. Only rare amelanotic melanocytomas have been described. The nuclei are oval or bean-shaped, occasionally showing grooves, with small eosinophilic nucleoli. Cytological atypia and mitoses are generally absent (on average, < 1 mitosis per 10 high-power fields). It has been suggested that melanocytic tumours with bland cytological features, such as those of melanocytoma, but showing CNS invasion or elevated mitotic activity, should be classified as intermediate-grade melanocytic neoplasms {266}.

Electron microscopy
The cells of melanocytoma lack junctions and contain melanosomes at various stages of development. Unlike in schwannomas, a well-formed pericellular basal lamina is lacking, but groups of melanocytoma cells may be ensheathed {38}. Unlike in meningioma, no desmosomes or interdigitating cytoplasmic processes are present.

Genetic profile
Hotspot mutations of *GNAQ* or *GNA11*, most often involving codon 209, are frequent in melanocytoma, similar to those present in uveal melanoma and blue naevus {1313,1404,1405,1724}. Cytogenetic losses involving chromosome 3 and the long arm of chromosome 6 have been reported for melanocytoma as well.

Prognosis and predictive factors
Melanocytoma lacks anaplastic features, but a few undergo local recurrences; intermediate-grade melanocytic tumours typically invade the CNS, although too few have been reported to reliably predict the biology of these tumours {266}. Rare examples of malignant transformation of a melanocytoma have been reported {2182}.

Meningeal melanoma

Definition
A primary malignant neoplasm of the CNS that arises from leptomeningeal melanocytes, presents as a solitary mass lesion, and displays aggressive growth properties.

ICD-O code   8720/3

Epidemiology
Primary meningeal melanomas have been reported in patients aged 15–71 years (mean: 43 years). An annual incidence of 0.5 cases per 10 million population has been reported{988}.

Localization
Meningeal melanomas are dural-based and occur throughout the neuraxis,

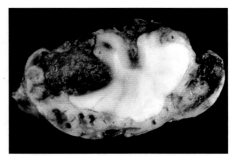

Fig. 12.05 Spinal meningeal melanoma with diffuse infiltration of the leptomeninges and focal infiltration of the medulla.

showing a slight predilection for the spinal cord and posterior fossa {760}.

Clinical features
Like melanocytomas, melanomas present with focal neurological signs depending on location {266}.

Imaging
CNS structures adjacent to a melanoma are often T2-hyperintense, indicating vasogenic oedema generated in response to rapid tumour growth.

Macroscopy
Malignant melanomas are typically solitary, with extra-axial location. Pigmentation may vary from black to reddish brown, blue, or macroscopically non-pigmented.

Microscopy
Primary meningeal melanoma is histologically similar to melanomas arising in other sites. Anaplastic spindled or epithelioid cells arranged in loose nests, fascicles, or sheets display variable cytoplasmic melanin {266,760}. Some melanomas contain large cells with bizarre nuclei, numerous typical and atypical mitotic figures, significant pleomorphism, and large nucleoli; others are densely cellular and less pleomorphic, usually consisting of tightly packed spindle cells with a high nuclear-to-cytoplasmic ratio. Melanomas are more pleomorphic, anaplastic, and mitotically active, and have a higher cell density, than melanocytoma and often demonstrate unequivocal tissue invasion or coagulative necrosis. Meningeal melanomatosis may arise from diffuse spreading of a primary malignant meningeal melanoma through the subarachnoid space.

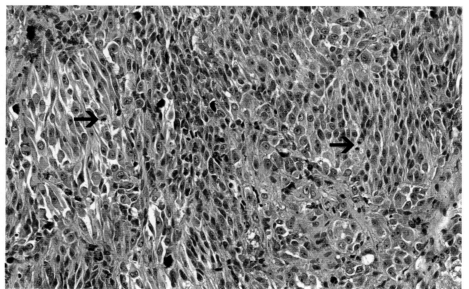

Fig. 12.06 Thoracic meningeal melanoma. The epithelioid and spindled tumour cells have ample, eosinophilic cytoplasm and a large vesicular nucleus with prominent nucleolus, and show marked mitotic activity (arrows). Dispersed melanophages are present between the tumour cells; in this tumour, a *GNA11* mutation was identified.

Genetic profile

In the case of childhood CNS melanomas and neurocutaneous melanosis, there is a strong link to mutations in *NRAS*, especially codon 61 {1921}. Less frequently, *BRAF* V600E mutations have been described in the congenital melanocytic naevi of patients with neurocutaneous melanosis {2225}.

Primary CNS melanomas also harbour *GNAQ* or *GNA11* mutations, albeit at a lower frequency than do melanocytomas. These tumours appear to progress to melanoma analogous to uveal melanoma, in which *GNAQ* or *GNA11* mutations arise early, and are followed by inactivation of *BAP1* or mutation of *SF3B1* or *EIF1AX* as they evolve into malignant tumours. Mutations in genes typically seen in cutaneous or acral melanomas, such the *TERT* promoter, *NRAS*, *BRAF*, and *KIT*, are rare in primary CNS melanocytic neoplasms of adults, and when encountered raise suspicion of a metastasis. However, the uncertainty involved in establishing the primary versus metastatic nature of a melanoma may confound interpretation of molecular studies.

Genomic alterations may be helpful in distinguishing between different types of melanotic tumours of the CNS; in particular, DNA methylation patterns have been shown to identify melanotic neoplasms in a manner concordant with mutation spectrum and histological classes {498, 1313,1406}.

Prognosis and predictive factors

Malignant melanoma is a highly aggressive and radioresistant tumour with poor prognosis, and it can metastasize to remote organs. Nevertheless, the prognosis of the primary meningeal melanoma seems to be better than that of metastatic examples, particularly if localized and complete resection is possible {739}. Considering the close relationship to uveal melanoma, BAP1 loss is likely an adverse prognostic markers in those primary CNS melanomas that are not associated with congenital naevi.

CHAPTER 13

Lymphomas

Diffuse large B-cell lymphoma of the CNS
Immunodeficiency-associated CNS lymphomas
Intravascular large B-cell lymphoma
Low-grade B-cell lymphomas
T-cell and NK/T-cell lymphomas
Anaplastic large cell lymphoma
MALT lymphoma of the dura

Lymphomas

Deckert M.
Paulus W.
Kluin P.M.
Ferry J.A.

Diffuse large B-cell lymphoma of the CNS

Definition
A diffuse large B-cell lymphoma (DLBCL) confined to the CNS at presentation.
Excluded from this entity are lymphomas arising in the dura, intravascular large B-cell lymphoma, and lymphomas of T-cell or NK-cell lineage (which may also present in the CNS), as well as lymphomas with systemic involvement or with secondary involvement of the CNS. Immuno-deficiency-associated primary CNS lymphomas are discussed separately.

ICD-O code   9680/3

Epidemiology
Primary CNS lymphomas (PCNSLs) account for 2.4–3% of all brain tumours and 4–6% of all extranodal lymphomas {2286}. The overall annual incidence rate of PCNSL is 0.47 cases per 100 000 population {2652}. In the past two decades, an increased incidence has been reported in patients aged > 60 years {2652}. PCNSL can affect patients of any age, with a peak incidence during the fifth to seventh decade of life. The median patient age is 56 years, and the male-to-female ratio is 3:2.

Etiology
In immunocompetent individuals, etiological factors are unknown. Viruses (e.g. EBV, HHV6 {1915}, HHV8 {1704}, and the

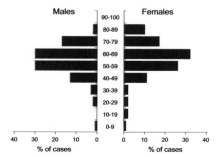

Fig. 13.01 Age and sex distribution of primary CNS lymphomas in immunocompetent patients.

polyomaviruses SV40 and BK virus {1702, 1725}) do not play a role.

Localization
About 60% of all PCNSLs involve the supratentorial space, including the frontal lobe (in 15% of cases), temporal lobe (in 8%), parietal lobe (in 7%), and occipital lobe (in 3%), basal ganglia and periventricular brain parenchyma (in 10%), and corpus callosum (in 5%). The posterior fossa and spinal cord are less frequently affected (in 13% and 1% of cases, respectively) {562}. A single tumour is encountered in 60–70% of patients, with the remainder presenting with multiple tumours {562}. The leptomeninges may be involved, but exclusive meningeal manifestation is unusual. Ocular manifestation (i.e. in the vitreous, retina, or optic nerve) occurs in 20% of patients and may antedate intracranial disease {1123}. Extraneural dissemination is very rare. In cases with systemic spread, PCNSL has a propensity to home to the testis, another immunoprivileged organ {237,1124}.

Clinical features
Patients present with cognitive dysfunction, psychomotor slowing, and focal neurological symptoms more frequently than with headache, seizures, and cranial nerve palsies. Blurred vision and eye floaters are symptoms of ocular involvement {140,1340,1926}.

Imaging
MRI is the most sensitive technique to detect PCNSL, which is hypointense on T1-weighted images, isointense to hyperintense on T2-weighted images, and densely enhancing on postcontrast images. Peritumoural oedema is relatively limited and is less severe than in malignant gliomas and metastases {1340}. Meningeal involvement may present as hyperintense enhancement {1403}. With steroid therapy, lesions may vanish within hours {562}.

Spread
The diagnostic value of cerebrospinal

fluid (CSF) analysis is limited {1340}. Meningeal dissemination is diagnosed in 15.7% of cases (12.2% by CSF cytomorphology, 10.5% by PCR, and 4.1% by MRI) {1341}. Pleocytosis is found in 35–60% of PCNSL cases and correlates with meningeal dissemination {1341}. Cell counts may even be normal. The CSF harbours neoplastic cells in a minority of patients with leptomeningeal involvement, and their detection may require repeated lumbar puncture. The combination of cytological and immunohistochemical analysis with multiparameter flow cytometry may enhance detection of CSF lymphoma cells {2299}. PCR analysis of the CDR3 region of the *IGH* gene region followed by sequencing of the PCR products may identify a clonal B-cell population in the CSF, but does not enable lymphoma classification. Elevated CSF levels of miR-21, miR-19, and miR-92a have been reported to differentiate PCNSL from inflammatory and other CNS disorders {124}; however, the diagnostic usefulness of this parameter and its potential as a marker during follow-up {125} are yet to be definitively established.

Macroscopy
As observed on postmortem examination, PCNSLs occur as single or multiple masses in the brain parenchyma, most frequently in the cerebral hemispheres. Often, they are deep-seated and adjacent to the ventricular system. The tumours can be firm, friable, granular, haemorrhagic, and greyish tan or yellow, with central necrosis. Or they can be virtually indistinguishable from the adjacent neuropil. Demarcation from surrounding parenchyma is variable. Some tumours appear well delineated, like metastases. When diffuse borders and architectural effacement are present, the lesions resemble gliomas. Like malignant gliomas, these tumours may diffusely infiltrate large areas of the hemispheres without forming any distinct mass, a manifestation which has been referred to as 'lymphomatosis cerebri'. However, this term

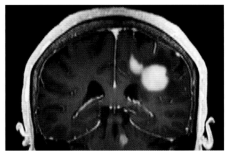

Fig. 13.02 Primary CNS lymphoma. Postcontrast T1-weighted MRI showing multifocal disease with homogeneous contrast enhancement and relatively little surrounding oedema. Periventricular disease is evident in both the frontoparietal region and the brain stem.

does not define a distinct disease entity, so it should not replace the specific diagnosis (i.e. DLBCL of the CNS). Meningeal involvement may resemble meningitis or meningioma, or can even be inconspicuous macroscopically.

Microscopy

Stereotactic biopsy

Stereotactic biopsy is the gold standard for establishing the diagnosis and classification of CNS lymphoma. It is important to withhold corticosteroids before biopsy, because they induce rapid tumour waning. Corticosteroids have been shown to prevent diagnosis in as many as 50% of cases {298}.

Histopathology

PCNSLs are highly cellular, diffusely growing, patternless tumours. Centrally, large areas of geographical necrosis are common, and may harbour viable perivascular lymphoma islands. At the periphery, an angiocentric infiltration pattern is frequent. Infiltration of cerebral blood vessels causes fragmentation of the argyrophilic fibre network. From these perivascular cuffs, tumour cells invade the neural parenchyma, either with a well-delineated invasion front with small clusters or with single tumour cells diffusely infiltrating the tissue, which shows a prominent astrocytic and microglial activation and harbours reactive inflammatory infiltrates consisting of mature T and B cells. Morphologically, PCNSLs consist of large atypical cells with large round, oval, irregular, or pleomorphic nuclei and distinct nucleoli, corresponding to centroblasts or immunoblasts. Some cases show a relatively monomorphic cell population, with intermingled macrophages mimicking the appearance of Burkitt lymphoma.

Immunophenotype

The tumour cells are mature B cells with a PAX5-positive, CD19-positive, CD20-positive, CD22-positive, CD79a-positive phenotype. IgM and IgD, but not IgG, are expressed on the surface {1707}, with either kappa or lambda light chain restriction. Most express BCL6 (60–80%) and MUM1/IRF4 (90%), whereas plasma cell markers (e.g. CD38 and CD138) are usually negative. Less than 10% of all PCNSLs express CD10 {561}. CD10 expression is more frequent in systemic DLBCL; therefore, CD10 positivity in a CNS lymphoma with DLBCL characteristics should prompt a thorough investigation for systemic DLBCL that might have metastasized to the CNS. HLA-A/B/C and HLA-DR are variably expressed, with approximately 50% of PCNSLs having lost HLA class I and/or II expression {237,

2128}. BCL2 expression is common; 82% of PCNSLs have a BCL2-high, MYC-high phenotype {296}. Mitotic activity is brisk; accordingly, the Ki-67 proliferation index usually exceeds 70% or even 90% {296}. Apoptotic cells may be frequent. With the exception of isolated cases, there is no evidence of EBV infection {1705}, and the presence of EBV should prompt evaluation for underlying immunodeficiency.

Genetic profile

PCNSLs are mature B-cell lymphomas. The tumour cells correspond to late germinal centre exit B cells with blocked terminal B-cell differentiation. Thus, they carry rearranged and somatically mutated immunoglobulin (IG) genes with evidence of ongoing somatic hypermutation {1705,1925,2548}. Consistent with the ongoing germinal centre programme, they show persistent BCL6 activity {296}. The process of somatic hypermutation is not confined to its physiological targets (IG and *BCL6* genes), but extends to other genes that have been implicated in tumorigenesis, including *BCL2*, *MYC*, *PIM1*, *PAX5*, *RHOH*, *KLHL14*, *OSBPL10*, and *SUSD2* {297,1709,2639}. These data indicate that aberrant somatic hypermutation has a major impact on the pathogenesis of PCNSL. The fixed IgM/IgD phenotype of the tumour cells is in part due to miscarried IG class switch rearrangements during which the Smu region is deleted {1707}. *PRDM1* mutations also contribute to impaired IG class switch recombination {502}.

Translocations affect the IG genes (in 38% of cases) and *BCL6* (in 17–47%) recurrently, whereas *MYC* translocations are rare and translocations of the *BCL2*

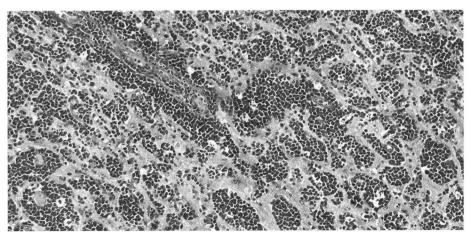

Fig. 13.03 Primary malignant CNS lymphoma with characteristic perivascular spread of tumour cells.

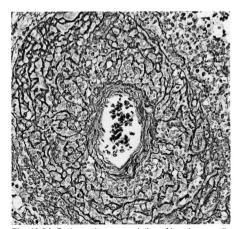

Fig. 13.04 Perivascular accumulation of lymphoma cells embedded in a concentric network of reticulin fibres.

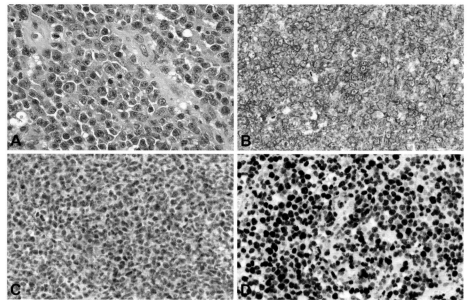

Fig. 13.05 Primary CNS lymphoma. **A** Diffuse large B-cell lymphoma. **B** Tumour cells express the pan–B-cell marker CD20. **C** Expression of the BCL6 protein by the tumour cells. **D** Strong nuclear expression of the MUM1 protein by the majority of tumour cells of a primary CNS lymphoma.

gene are absent {296,341,1710}. FISH and genome-wide SNP analyses have shown recurrent gains of genetic material, most frequently affecting 18q21.33-q23 (in 43% of cases), including the *BCL2* and *MALT1* genes; chromosome 12 (in 26%); and 10q23.21 (in 21%) {2309}. Losses of genetic material most frequently involve 6q21 (in 52% of cases), 6p21 (in 37%), 8q12.1-q12.2 (in 32%), and 10q23.21 {2309}. Heterozygous or homozygous loss or partial uniparental disomies of chromosomal region 6p21.32 affect 73% of PCNSLs; this region harbours the HLA class II–encoding genes *HLA-DRB*, *HLA-DQA*, and *HLA-DQB* {1181,2127, 2309}. Correspondingly, 55% and 46%

of PCNSLs have lost expression of HLA class I and II gene products, respectively {237}.

Several important pathways (i.e. the B-cell receptor, the toll-like receptor, and the NF-kappaB pathway) are frequently activated due to genetic alterations affecting the genes *CD79B* (in 20% of cases), *INPP5D* (in 25%), *CBL* (in 4%), *BLNK* (in 4%), *CARD11* (in 16%), *MALT1* (in 43%), *BCL2* (in 43%), and *MYD88* (in > 50%), which may foster proliferation and prevent apoptosis {865,1357,1703, 1706,1708,2309}.

Epigenetic changes may also contribute to PCNSL pathogenesis, including epigenetic silencing by DNA methylation.

DNA hypermethylation of *DAPK1* (in 84% of cases), *CDKN2A* (in 75%), *MGMT* (in 52%), and *RFC* (in 30%) may be of potential therapeutic relevance {457,475, 692,2309}.

Genetic susceptibility

In immunocompetent individuals, genetic predispositions to PCNSL have not been described. About 8% of patients with PCNSL have had a prior extracranial tumour {2100}, most of which arose in the haematopoietic system. In patients with PCNSL with preceding extraneural lymphoma, comparative molecular analyses of primary and secondary lymphomas may confirm or exclude a common clonal origin of these tumours, distinguishing CNS relapse from an unrelated secondary cerebral lymphoma. However, because these analyses are not routinely performed, information about a possible association is usually lacking. In individual patients, associations between PCNSL and other tumours (e.g. carcinoma, meningioma, and glioma) or hereditary tumour syndromes (e.g. neurofibromatosis type 1) are likely to be coincidental.

Folate and methionine metabolism has been proposed to be relevant to PCNSL susceptibility. The G allele of the methyltetrahydrofolate homocysteine S-methyltransferase c.2756A→G (D919G) missense polymorphism was found to be underrepresented among patients with PCNSL, suggesting a protective function of this allele {1512}.

Prognosis and predictive factors

PCNSL has a considerably worse outcome than does systemic DLBCL. Older

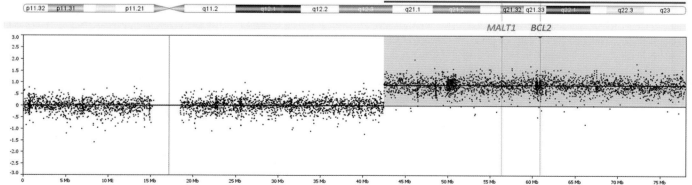

Fig. 13.06 Primary CNS lymphoma. Microarray-based comparative genomic hybridization demonstrating copy number and allelic profile of a sample with a gain in 18q. The log2 ratio is displayed from the p arm to the q arm of the chromosome, showing a gain of two copies of the same allele in 18q12.3qter (shaded region: log2 ratio = 1; four allele states).

patient age (> 65 years) is a major negative prognostic factor and is associated with reduced survival and an increased risk of neurotoxicity {4,1340}.

High-dose methotrexate-based polychemotherapy is currently the treatment of choice {1340}. The inclusion of whole-brain irradiation may improve outcome, but bears the risk of neurotoxicity resulting in severe cognitive, motor, and autonomic dysfunction, particularly in elderly patients {4}. The missense variant Tc2c.776C→G mutation of transcobalamin C is associated with shorter survival and neurotoxicity {1511}. Most protocols report a median progression-free survival of about 12 months and an overall survival of approximately 3 years. In a subgroup of elderly patients with PCNSL with methylated *MGMT*, temozolomide monotherapy appeared to be therapeutically effective {1400}.

The presence of reactive perivascular CD3 T-cell infiltrates on biopsy has been associated with improved survival {2004}. LMO2 protein expression by the tumour cells has been associated with prolonged overall survival {1528}. BCL6 expression has been suggested as a prognostic marker in several studies, although conflicting conclusions as to whether it is a favourable or unfavourable marker have been reported {1700,2037, 2071,2393}. In one study, del(6)(q22) was associated with inferior overall survival {341}.

Corticoid-mitigated lymphoma

Because the tumour cells are highly susceptible to steroid-induced apoptosis, PCNSL may vanish rapidly on MRI and within biopsies following corticosteroid administration. Microscopically, neoplastic B cells may be present in only small numbers or may even be absent. Samples may show non-specific inflammatory and reactive changes and/or necrosis; foamy macrophages are frequent {298, 561}. In some cases, PCR analysis of the CDR3 region of the *IGH* gene may reveal a monoclonal B-cell population. However, pseudoclonality due to very low numbers of B cells poses a problem.

Sentinel lesions

In rare cases, PCNSL has been reported to be preceded (by as long as 2 years) by demyelinating and inflammatory lesions similar to multiple sclerosis {45, 1071,1386}.

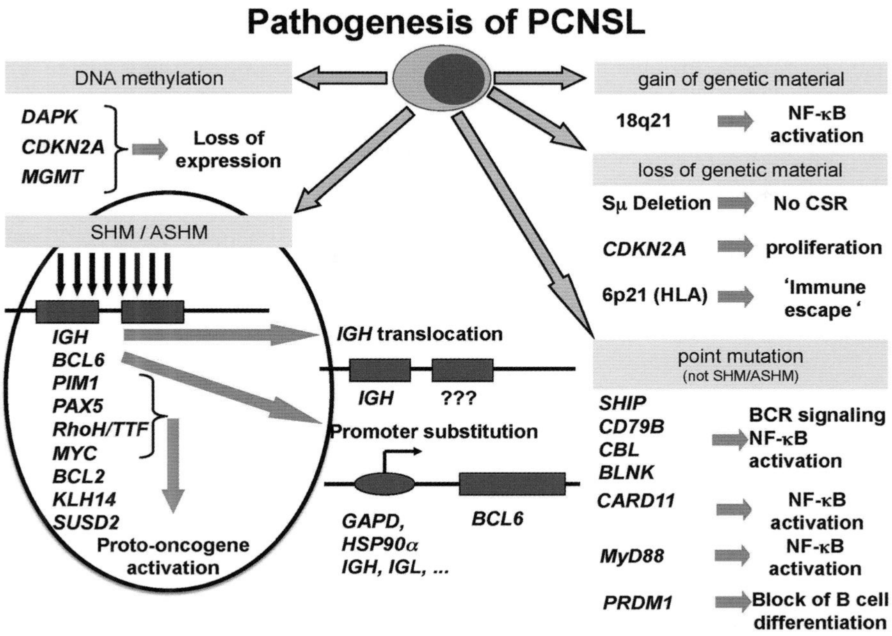

Pathogenesis of PCNSL

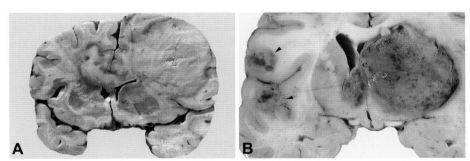

Fig. 13.07 Pathogenesis of primary CNS lymphoma (PCNSL). Alterations of specific pathways contribute to the lymphomagenesis of PCNSL. ASHM, aberrant somatic hypermutation; BCR, B-cell receptor; CSR, class-switch recombination; SHM, somatic hypermutation.

Fig. 13.08 A Large, necrotizing diffuse large B-cell lymphoma of the right hemisphere, extending via the corpus callosum into the white matter of the left hemisphere. The patient was an HIV-1-infected infant. **B** Primary malignant CNS lymphomas of the basal ganglia. Note the additional foci in the left insular region (arrowheads).

Immunodeficiency-associated CNS lymphomas

Inherited or acquired immunodeficiency predisposes patients to CNS lymphoma. Immunodeficiency syndromes include ataxia-telangiectasia, Wiskott–Aldrich syndrome, and IgA deficiency. Autoimmune disorders (e.g. systemic lupus erythematosus and Sjögren syndrome), iatrogenic immunosuppression (either for the purpose of organ transplantation or due to treatment with drugs such as methotrexate, azathioprine, or mycophenolate for a wide variety of other diseases), and immune system senescence are associated with an increased risk of CNS lymphoma. HIV infection was largely responsible for the significant increase in the incidence of CNS lymphoma in the 1980s. Generally, immunosuppression-associated CNS lymphoma is EBV-related. Thus, the lymphoma cells express EBNA1–6, LMP1, EBER1, and EBER2 {1310}.

AIDS-related diffuse large B-cell lymphoma

Within this category, AIDS-related diffuse large B-cell lymphoma (DLBCL) of the CNS, EBV-positive DLBC, NOS , lymphomatoid granulomatosis, and monomorphic or polymorphic post-transplant lymphoproliferative disorders may primarily manifest within the CNS.

AIDS-related DLBCL of the CNS shares the morphological features of primary CNS lymphoma in immunocompetent patients, with the exception of a more frequent multifocal presentation, EBV association, and a tendency to contain more and larger areas of necrosis. These areas of necrosis may simulate necrotizing cerebral toxoplasmosis, which may occur concomitantly {2425}. HIV-associated primary CNS lymphoma has become rarer with the introduction of HAART therapy {2652}.

EBV+ diffuse large B-cell lymphoma, NOS

EBV-positive DLBCL, NOS, may affect the CNS in elderly patients with no known immunodeficiency. Lymphomagenesis is attributed to the immunosenescence that can develop with advancing age {1131}.

Lymphomatoid granulomatosis

This affects the brain in 26% of cases {1911}. The lesions are characterized by angiocentric and angiodestructive lymphoid infiltrates. The proportion of EBV-expressing CD20-positive, CD30-positive or -negative, CD15-negative large neoplastic B cells contributing to these infiltrates is variable and may be small. They are admixed with CD4 and CD8 T lymphocytes. The infiltrates invade blood vessel walls and may induce infarct-like necrosis of tumour and/or brain tissue.

The CNS may be the only part of the body affected by post-transplant lymphoproliferative disorder, although CNS involvement is not frequent. For more details on morphology and grading, see the *WHO classification of tumours of haematopoietic and lymphoid tissues* {2473}.

ICD-O code   9766/1

Intravascular large B-cell lymphoma

Definition

A distinctive lymphoma characterized by exclusively intravascular growth.
Except for the solely cutaneous cases CNS involvement occurs in > 75–85% of cases {174}. The brain is nearly always involved, and spinal cord involvement is less common. The hallmark intravascular growth leads to clinical symptoms

mimicking those of cerebral infarction or subacute encephalopathy.
Macroscopy reveals infarcts (acute and/or old), necrosis, and/or haemorrhage, although abnormalities may be inconspicuous. Microscopically, large atypical B cells can be seen occluding cerebral blood vessels. Lack of CD29 and ICAM1 (CD54) expression is thought to underlie the tumour cells' inability to migrate transvascularly {2003}.

ICD-O code   9712/3

Miscellaneous rare lymphomas in the CNS

Other than diffuse large B-cell lymphoma of the CNS (i.e. primary CNS lymphoma), lymphomas manifesting primarily in the CNS are rare {1503}. They include low-grade B-cell and T-cell lymphomas, very rare Burkitt lymphoma {1503}, and high-grade T-cell and NK/T-cell lymphomas {893,1503,1529,1817,2017}. Low-grade lymphomas account for approximately 3% of all CNS lymphomas; the majority are of B-cell lineage {1125,1503}. Convincing cases of Hodgkin lymphoma primary to the CNS are vanishingly rare {799}. The differential diagnosis includes secondary CNS involvement by a systemic lymphoma and a chronic inflammatory process, and likely also EBV-positive DLBCL, NOS. Meticulous staging to exclude a systemic lymphoma is essential. For low-grade lymphomas, careful pathological evaluation to confirm a neoplastic process is critical.

Low-grade B-cell lymphomas

Low-grade B-cell lymphomas of the CNS almost exclusively affect adults. Patients present with seizures, visual defects, focal neurological findings, and/or memory impairment {100,1125,1886,2368,2593}. There is no association with immunodeficiency, but one patient with MALT lymphoma had a long history of white matter disease with some features of multiple sclerosis {2270}, and another patient with MALT lymphoma had *Chlamydophila psittaci* infection {2005}. Treatment has varied widely and has included complete or partial resection, steroids, radiation, chemotherapy, and combinations of these. The behaviour is indolent compared with that of usual primary CNS diffuse large B-cell lymphoma, and patients

usually do well {100,1503,1886,2005, 2270,2368,2593}
Microscopic examination reveals a dense, diffuse, or perivascular infiltrate, predominantly of small lymphocytes, with variable numbers of plasma cells admixed. Immunophenotyping shows a predominance of CD20-positive B cells (usually CD5-negative and CD10-negative), sometimes with a component of monotypic plasma cells, with a low proliferation index. These lymphomas, when subclassified, have been designated as small lymphocytic lymphoma (positive for CD5 and CD23) {100}, lymphoplasmacytic lymphoma {1125,1503,2368}, extranodal MALT lymphoma {1125,1503, 2368}, and follicular lymphoma {1125}.

T-cell and NK/T-cell lymphomas

Primary T-cell lymphoma of the CNS is very rare, accounting for approximately 2% of all primary lymphomas in the CNS {693,2341}. These lymphomas appear to be more common in Asia than elsewhere {450} and mainly affect young to middle-aged adults {1503}. Reported cases are often not subclassified except that they are generally reported to be peripheral T-cell lymphomas. They occur as single or multiple tumours in the cerebral hemispheres (in 64% of cases), basal ganglia (11%), corpus callosum (13%), brain stem (9%), cerebellum (7%), meninges (2%), and spinal cord (4%). Microscopically, malignant T cells express CD45 and T-cell antigens (CD2, CD3, CD4 or CD8, CD5, and CD7), although loss of T-cell antigens may occur. Some cases are positive for the cytotoxic granule proteins granzyme B and perforin. Molecular genetic demonstration of T-cell monoclonality can be helpful in distinguishing T-cell lymphoma from T-cell–rich large B-cell lymphoma and inflammation. Their histological and immunophenotypic features may vary, but low-grade appearance is relatively common {450,1503,2341}. The prognosis appears to be similar to or perhaps slightly better than that of diffuse large B-cell lymphoma. Anaplastic large cell lymphoma arising in the CNS has distinctive features and is discussed separately.
EBV-positive nasal-type extranodal NK/T-cell lymphoma primary to the CNS mainly affects young to middle-aged adult men, has pathological features similar to those seen in other sites, and

is associated with a very poor prognosis {893,1817,2017}.

Anaplastic large cell lymphoma

Primary CNS anaplastic large cell lymphoma, ALK-positive
Primary CNS anaplastic large cell lymphoma (ALCL) is rare. Of all cases of ALCL, < 1% are primary in the CNS {2756}. Patients are children and young adults, with reported patient ages ranging from 23 months to 31 years and with a male preponderance {770,797,1650, 1890,2657}. There are no known risk factors. Patients present with headache, seizures, nausea, fever, or a combination of these {174,1890}. They are often initially thought to have an infection rather than a neoplasm {693,770,1890}. Patients usually have one or more intracerebral masses, often accompanied by involvement of the leptomeninges and occasionally even the dura or skull {1890,2199,2756}. Rarely, lymphoma is confined to the leptomeninges {1650,1890}.

This is an aggressive lymphoma, but with prompt diagnosis and administration of appropriate chemotherapy, complete remission and long-term survival can often be achieved {770,797,1890,2756}.

Most cases of ALCL are of the common type {1890}, but primary CNS ALCL of the lymphohistiocytic variant {2756} and combined lymphohistiocytic and small-cell variants {693} have also been reported. Biopsy shows large atypical cells, including hallmark cells, with a variable admixture of reactive cells. The tumour cells are positive for CD30, ALK, and usually EMA, and show variable expression of T-lineage antigens {770,1890, 2657}. The underlying genetic abnormality is a translocation of the *NPM1* and *ALK* genes {1890}.

ICD-O code 9714/3

Primary CNS anaplastic large cell lymphoma, ALK-negative
Primary CNS ALK-negative anaplastic large cell lymphoma is a rare neoplasm that affects adults of both sexes. Patients present with one or more intraparenchymal lesions, which are usually supratentorial {797}. Diffuse white matter

Fig. 13.09 MALT lymphoma of the dura. Vaguely nodular and diffuse proliferation of lymphoid cells in the frontal dura.

involvement has been reported {2450}. The pathological findings are similar to those of ALK-positive anaplastic large cell lymphoma, except that ALK is not expressed. The prognosis appears to be worse than that of ALK-positive anaplastic large cell lymphoma {797}.

ICD-O code 9702/3

Extranodal marginal zone lymphoma of mucosa-associated lymphoid tissue (MALT lymphoma) of the dura

Lymphomas primary in the dura mater are much less frequent than those primary in the brain {1107}. By far the most common dural lymphoma is MALT lymphoma {1392,1464}. Exceedingly rare cases of MALT lymphoma arising in the brain have also been reported {2270, 2717}. Dural MALT lymphoma affects adults, and women are affected more often than men, with a male-to-female ratio of approximately 1:5 {1107,2587,2642}. Most MALT lymphomas arise in the cranial dura; patients present with symptoms that include headache, seizures, dizziness, focal neurological defects, and visual changes {63,1107,1208,1209, 1392,2642}. MALT lymphoma arising in the dura over the spinal cord is much less common {2642} and may be associated with spinal cord compression {1209}. Radiographical evaluation reveals a mass or plaque-like thickening of the dura,

often mimicking a meningioma {1107, 1209,1392,2587,2642}. Lymphomas are typically localized at presentation {1107, 1392,2587,2642}; in a small minority of cases, extradural disease is identified {2642}. Treatment has varied, but nearly all patients achieve complete remission and typically remain well on follow-up {1107,1208,1209,1392,1464,2587,2642}.

The histological and immunophenotypic findings are similar to those of MALT lymphomas in other sites. The lymphomas are composed of small lymphocytes, marginal zone cells with slightly irregular and pale cytoplasm, few large cells, and, frequently, many plasma cells, sometimes with remnants of reactive follicles {1107,1208,1392,2587,2642} and occasionally with amyloid {1464,2587}. Dural lymphoma may invade adjacent brain, with a tendency to involve Virchow–Robin spaces {1107,1209,2642}. The neoplastic cells are CD5-negative and CD10-negative B cells, often with a component of monotypic plasma cells, indicating plasmacytic differentiation {1209,2642}. The monotypic plasma cells are IgG4-positive in some cases (6 of 19 cases in one series), but evidence of systemic IgG4-related disease is absent {2642}. Trisomies, most often of chromosome 3, are occasionally detected {2587,2642}. MALT lymphoma–associated translocations are rare {186,2642}.

ICD-O code 9699/3

CHAPTER 14

Histiocytic tumours

Langerhans cell histiocytosis
Erdheim–Chester disease
Rosai–Dorfman disease
Juvenile xanthogranuloma
Histiocytic sarcoma

Histiocytic tumours

Paulus W.
Perry A.
Sahm F.

Langerhans cell histiocytosis

Definition
A clonal proliferation of Langerhans-type cells that express CD1a, langerin (CD207), and S100 protein.

Langerhans cell histiocytosis most frequently affects children. The CNS can be affected via direct invasion from craniofacial bone and skull base or from meninges, via extra-axial masses of the hypothalamic–pituitary region, or in a leukoencephalopathy-like pattern, and primary intraparenchymal CNS masses may also occur. This entity was previously referred to as eosinophilic granuloma and/or histiocytosis X.

ICD-O code   9751/3

Epidemiology
Most cases of Langerhans cell histiocytosis occur in childhood, with an annual incidence of 0.5 cases per 100 000 individuals aged < 15 years.

Etiology
The etiology of Langerhans cell histiocytosis is largely unknown. In most patients, there is either mild or no underlying defect in immunological integrity. Nevertheless, an abnormal immune response is thought to play a potentially important etiological role; for example, data suggest defective interactions between T cells and macrophages.

Localization
Imaging studies of Langerhans cell histiocytosis have shown that the most common presentation of CNS involvement is as lesions of the craniofacial bone and skull base (seen in 56% of cases), with or without soft-tissue extension. Intracranial, extra-axial masses are also common, particularly in the hypothalamic–pituitary region (seen in 50% of all cases), meninges (in 29%), and choroid plexus (in 6%). A leukoencephalopathy-like pattern, with or without dentate nucleus or basal ganglia neurodegeneration, is seen in 36% of all Langerhans cell histiocytosis

cases, and cerebral atrophy occurs in 8% {2018}. Rare intraparenchymal CNS masses have also been described.

Clinical features
The most common neurological sign of Langerhans cell histiocytosis is diabetes insipidus (occurring in 25% of cases overall and 50% of cases of multisystemic disease), with about 60% of patients also showing signs of hypothalamic dysfunction (e.g. obesity, hypopituitarism, and growth retardation). The clinical features of Langerhans cell histiocytosis–associated neurodegenerative lesions range from asymptomatic imaging abnormalities to tremors, gait disturbances, dysarthria, dysphagia, motor spasticity, ataxia, behavioural disturbances, learning difficulties, global cognitive deficits, and/or psychiatric disease {889}.

Imaging
Histiocytic lesions of the skull present as patchy T2-hyperintense lesions, eventually resulting in a punched-out or geographical appearance of the bone {2848}.
Within the CNS parenchyma, Langerhans cell histiocytosis presents as hyperintense lesions with non-specific enhancement on T2-weighted images. Involvement of the pituitary region may be associated with loss of the posterior pituitary bright spot in T1-weighted images and thickening of the pituitary stalk in contrast-enhanced images {513,2848}.

Macroscopy
Intracranial Langerhans cell histiocytosis lesions are often yellow or white and range from discrete dural-based nodules to granular parenchymal infiltrates. CNS lesions may be well delineated or poorly defined.

Microscopy
Langerhans cell histiocytosis infiltrates are composed of Langerhans cells, macrophages, lymphocytes, plasma cells, and variable eosinophils. The nuclei of Langerhans cells are typically slightly

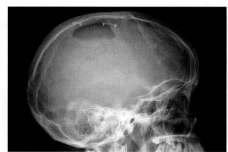

Fig. 14.01 Langerhans cell histiocytosis. X-ray showing bone lucency at site of disease.

eccentric, ovoid, and reniform or convoluted, with linear grooves and inconspicuous nucleoli. There is abundant pale to eosinophilic cytoplasm, and Touton giant cells may be seen. Copious collagen deposition is common. In the neurodegenerative lesions of the cerebellum and brain stem, there are often no Langerhans cells, but marked inflammation accompanies severe neuronal and axonal loss {889}. Eosinophils may aggregate and undergo necrosis, producing granulomas or abscesses.

Immunophenotype
Neoplastic Langerhans cells consistently express CD1a, S100 protein, vimentin, and usually langerin (CD207) {438}. CD68 and HLA-DR content is low and generally paranuclear. Expression of PTPRC and lysozyme is low. The Ki-67 proliferation index is highly variable and can reach 50%.

Genetic profile
Langerhans cell histiocytosis lesions carry *BRAF* V600E mutations in 38–58% of cases {103,2218,2249}. Of the *BRAF*-wildtype Langerhans cell histiocytosis cases, 33–50% harbour *MAP2K1* mutations {290,398}.

Genetic susceptibility
The occurrence of multifocal Langerhans cell histiocytosis in monozygotic twins, sometimes with simultaneous onset of disease, has been repeatedly reported and suggests genetic susceptibility in at least some cases {1562}. It has also

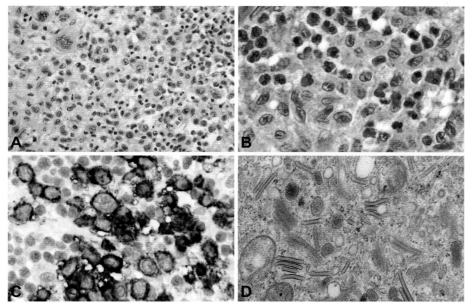

Fig. 14.02 Langerhans cell histiocytosis. **A** Mixed infiltrate composed of histiocytes, lymphocytes, eosinophils, and multinucleated cells. **B** The nuclei of Langerhans cells are typically slightly eccentric, ovoid, and reniform or convoluted, with linear grooves and inconspicuous nucleoli. **C** CD1a expression by neoplastic Langerhans cells. **D** Electron microscopy showing characteristic rod-shaped structures (Birbeck granules).

been suggested that interferon gamma and IL4 polymorphisms affect susceptibility to Langerhans cell histiocytosis and might be responsible for some of the clinical variation {541}.

Prognosis and predictive factors

The overall survival rates of patients with Langerhans cell histiocytosis at 5, 15, and 20 years are 88%, 88%, and 77%, respectively, with an event-free survival rate of only 30% at 15 years {2758}. Unifocal Langerhans cell histiocytosis may spontaneously recover or requires only minimal treatment (e.g. surgical resection), whereas multisystemic disease with organ dysfunction may require systemic chemotherapy. The mortality rate for multisystemic Langerhans cell histiocytosis with organ dysfunction is 20%. Late sequelae are seen in 64% of all patients with Langerhans cell histiocytosis, including skeletal defects (in 42%), diabetes insipidus (in 25%), growth failure (in 20%), hearing loss (in 16%), and other CNS dysfunction (in 14%) {2758}. No prognostic significance of histopathological features such as cytological atypia and mitotic activity was found in most studies. However, malignant Langerhans cell histiocytosis does exist, characterized morphologically by malignant-appearing Langerhans cells and clinically by atypical organ involvement and an aggressive clinical course {1051}; this form is very rare, and the frequency of CNS involvement is unknown. Neurodegenerative Langerhans cell histiocytosis seems to be progressive, with neurocognitive symptoms present in about 25% of patients after 6 years {889}.

Erdheim–Chester disease

Definition

Erdheim–Chester disease manifesting in the brain or the meninges.

Erdheim–Chester disease of the CNS corresponds histologically and immunohistochemically to its counterparts occurring elsewhere. Systemic lesions may be present or absent.

ICD-O code   9750/1

Epidemiology

The mean patient age is 53 years {383}.

Localization

Erdheim–Chester disease may involve the brain (preferentially the cerebellum and brain stem), spinal cord, cerebellopontine angle, choroid plexus, pituitary, meninges, and orbit {1411}.

Clinical features

Patients with Erdheim–Chester disease most commonly present with cerebellar signs (41%), pyramidal syndromes (45%), and/or diabetes insipidus (47%). Seizures, headaches, neuropsychiatric/cognitive impairments, sensory deficits, cranial neuropathies, and asymptomatic imaging lesions have also been reported {1411}.

Imaging

Extra-axial Erdheim–Chester disease may resemble meningioma on imaging {2848}. Erdheim–Chester disease lesions have been reported to demonstrate delayed gadolinium enhancement {2554}.

Macroscopy

Erdheim–Chester disease manifests as widespread infiltrative parenchymal lesions (44%), dural thickening / a meningioma-like mass (37%), or a combination (19%) {1411}.

Microscopy

Erdheim–Chester disease is composed of lipid-laden histiocytes with small nuclei, Touton-type multinucleated giant cells, scant lymphocytes, rare eosinophils, and variable fibrosis or gliosis. The histiocytic tumour cells can show a broad morphological spectrum, with round or elongated, foamy or eosinophilic cytoplasm.

Immunophenotype

The neoplastic histiocytes are positive for CD68 and negative for CD1a and S100 protein.

Genetic profile

Erdheim–Chester disease carries *BRAF* V600E mutations in at least 50% of cases and *NRAS* and *PIK3CA* mutations in 17% and 12% of cases, respectively. Expression of mutant BRAF protein has been reported to be limited to histiocytes {946}.

Prognosis and predictive factors

For tumours with *BRAF* V600E mutation, therapy with vemurafenib may lead to complete clinical remission of CNS lesions and systemic disease {655,947}.

Rosai–Dorfman disease

Definition
Rosai–Dorfman disease manifesting in the brain or the meninges.

Rosai–Dorfman disease of the CNS corresponds histologically and immuno-histochemically to its counterparts occurring elsewhere.

Epidemiology
The mean patient age is 21 years {1568}.

Localization
Rosai–Dorfman disease of the CNS forms solitary or multiple dural masses, especially in the cerebral convexity, cranial base, and cavernous sinuses, as well as parasagittal, suprasellar and petroclival regions {2551}. Parenchymal or intrasellar lesions may also occur.

Clinical features
Patients with Rosai–Dorfman disease present with headache, nausea and

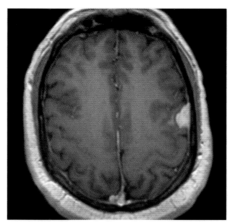

Fig. 14.03 MRI of a case of dural-based Rosai–Dorfman disease mimicking a meningioma.

vomiting, dizziness, epilepsy, fever, malaise, weight loss, night sweats, and/ or specific localized symptoms {2551}. Patients with sellar lesions present with signs of hypopituitarism and diabetes insipidus. The classic systemic signs of cervical lymphadenopathy, fever, and

weight loss are absent in 70% of patients, and 52% have no associated systemic disease {2045}.

Imaging
Rosai–Dorfman disease of the CNS often resembles meningioma on imaging. However, a lower T2 signal in Rosai–Dorfman disease may help to differentiate it from meningioma {1330}.

Macroscopy
Rosai–Dorfman disease of the CNS is typically a firm, vaguely lobulated, yellow to greyish-white dural mass.

Microscopy
Rosai–Dorfman disease presents as a multinodular mass composed of a mixed inflammatory infiltrate including large pale histiocytes, numerous lymphocytes and plasma cells, and variable fibrosis. Emperipolesis with histiocytic engulfment of intact lymphocytes, plasma cells, neutrophils, and occasionally eosinophils is typical, but may be inconspicuous on H&E staining. However, emperipolesis is not pathognomonic for Rosai–Dorfman disease and may occasionally be encountered in other neoplastic or non-neoplastic histiocytes and even in astrocytes.

Immunophenotype
The neoplastic histiocytes are positive for CD11c, CD68, L1 antigen (clone MAC387), and S100 protein; variably positive for lysozyme; and negative for CD1a and langerin.

Genetic profile
No recurrent genetic aberrations have been identified in Rosai–Dorfman disease to date. Clonality studies have demonstrated polyclonality of the infiltrates in two cases of Rosai–Dorfman disease {1912}.

Juvenile xanthogranuloma

Definition
Juvenile xanthogranuloma arising in the brain or the meninges, either with or without cutaneous lesions.

Juvenile xanthogranuloma of the CNS corresponds histologically and immunohistochemically to its cutaneous counterpart.

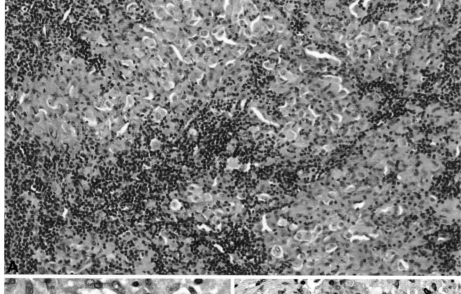

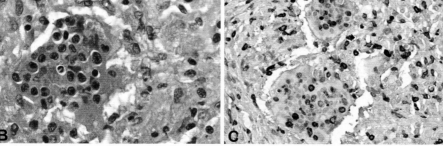

Fig. 14.04 Rosai–Dorfman disease. **A** Multinodular mass composed of a mixed inflammatory infiltrate, including large pale histiocytes, numerous lymphocytes, and plasma cells. **B** Emperipolesis with histiocytic engulfment of intact lymphocytes, plasma cells, neutrophils, and eosinophils. **C** CD45 expression by phagocytosed haematopoietic cells.

Epidemiology

The mean patient age is 22 months {1134}.

Localization

Juvenile xanthogranuloma of the CNS localizes to the brain (53%), intradural extramedullary spine (13%), or nerve roots (15%), with meningeal involvement also being common {568}.

Clinical features

The signs and symptoms of juvenile xanthogranuloma depend on the sites of involvement, but often include seizures, diabetes insipidus, and visual disturbances.

Macroscopy

Juvenile xanthogranuloma lesions are often received as fragmented, soft, yellow to tan-pink biopsy specimens.

Microscopy

Juvenile xanthogranuloma is composed of rounded to spindled, variably vacuolated histiocytes, scattered Touton and foreign body–type giant cells, lymphocytes, and occasional eosinophils {1411}.

Immunophenotype

The neoplastic histiocytes of juvenile xanthogranuloma are CD1a-negative, CD11c-positive, CD68-positive, factor XIIIa–positive, negative or positive for MAC387, lysozyme-negative, and S100-negative.

Histiocytic sarcoma

Definition

A rare, aggressive, malignant neoplasm with the histological and immunophenotypic characteristics of mature histiocytes. Most cases of histiocytic sarcoma occur in adults.

ICD-O code 9755/3

Epidemiology

The mean reported patient age in case series is 52 years {1043}.

Etiology

Isolated cases of radiation-associated histiocytic sarcoma of the CNS have been reported {399,2795}.

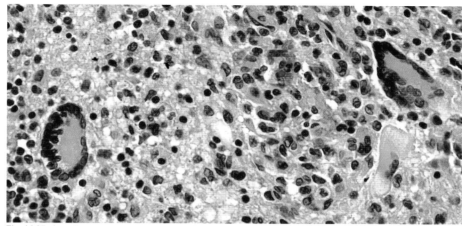

Fig. 14.05 Juvenile xanthogranuloma. Note numerous histiocytic cells and two large multinucleated Touton cells.

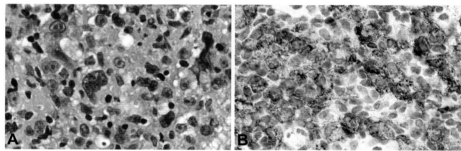

Fig. 14.06 Histiocytic sarcoma. **A** Large, highly pleomorphic histiocytic tumour cells with irregular nuclei and prominent nucleoli. **B** The lineage-specific marker CD163 was diagnostic in this high-grade neoplasm.

Localization

Reported cases of histiocytic sarcoma in the CNS have involved the brain parenchyma, meninges, and cavernous sinus {421}.

Clinical features

Patients with histiocytic sarcoma present with variable initial signs and symptoms, which tend to progress rapidly due to disseminated disease {421}.

Macroscopy

Histiocytic sarcomas are destructive, soft, fleshy white masses with occasional yellow necrotic foci.

Microscopy

Histiocytic sarcoma is characterized by highly cellular, non-cohesive infiltrates of large, moderately pleomorphic, mitotically active histiocytes with abundant eosinophilic cytoplasm, variably indented to irregular nuclei, and often prominent nucleoli. Occasional multinucleated or spindled forms are also common, as is background reactive inflammation {421}.

Immunophenotype

The tumour cells are typically positive for histiocytic markers (e.g. CD68, CD163, lysozyme, CD11c, and CD14), variably positive for CD34, and negative for myeloid antigens, dendritic antigens, CD30, ALK, and other lymphoid markers, as well as for glial, epithelial, and melanocytic antigens. The tumour cells are negative for the follicular dendritic cell antigens CD23 and CD35. However, follicular dendritic cell sarcoma expressing these antigens may primarily arise in the brain and must be differentiated from histiocytic sarcoma {966}.

Genetic profile

Histiocytic sarcoma is not defined by a certain genetic profile, although a single case with *BRAF* V600E mutation has been described {1085}. They usually lack *IGH* or T-cell receptor gene clonality {497}. Cases with evidence of clonal rearrangement are attributed to transdifferentiation from neoplastic T- or B-cell precursor lesions {2493}.

CHAPTER 15

Germ cell tumours
Germinoma
Embryonal carcinoma
Yolk sac tumour
Choriocarcinoma
Teratoma
Mixed germ cell tumour

Germm cell tumours

Rosenblum M.K.   Ichimura K.
Nakazato Y.   Leuschner I.
Matsutani M.   Huse J.T.

Definition

In the CNS, the morphological, immuno-phenotypic, and (in some respects) ge-netic homologues of gonadal and other extraneuraxial germ cell neoplasms.

The major germ cell tumour types are germinoma, teratoma, yolk sac tumour, embryonal carcinoma, and choriocarci-noma. Neoplasms harbouring multiple types are called mixed germ cell tumours. Otherwise pure germinomas containing syncytiotrophoblastic giant cells are rec-ognized as a distinct variant. Teratomas are subclassified as mature, immature, or exhibiting malignant transformation.

Epidemiology

CNS germ cell tumours principally affect children and adolescents and seem to be more prevalent in eastern Asia than in the Europe and the USA. These tumours ac-count for 2–3% of all primary intracranial neoplasms and for 8–15% of paediatric examples in series from Japan; Taiwan, China; and the Republic of Korea {485A, 1017,1192A,1612,2452}, but for only 0.3–0.6% of primary intracranial tumours and 3–4% of those affecting children in se-ries in Europe and North America {210, 506A,558,596,1025,1154,1862A,1863}. The highest reported incidence statis-tics come from Japan, where a recent survey of Kumamoto Prefecture revealed an annual age-adjusted incidence rate of 0.45 cases per 100 000 population aged < 15 years, more than double the rates in the USA and Germany {1573}.

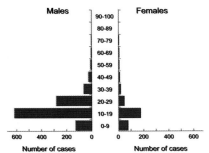

Fig. 15.01 Age and sex distribution of CNS germ cell tumours, based on 1463 cases; data from a report published by the Brain Tumor Registry of Japan (1969–1996).

Peak incidence occurs in patients aged 10–14 years, and a clear majority of cas-es of all histological types involve males {210,485,1017,2251}. Analysis of a regis-try containing 1463 Japanese patients found that 70% were aged 10–24 years and 73% were male {485}. Congenital examples (typically teratomas) are well recognized, but only 2.9% of patients in this series were aged < 5 years, and only 6.2% were aged > 35 years. The great majority of pineal region cases affect boys, whereas an excess of suprasellar lesions occur in girls. In the Japanese registry cited above, 89% of teratomas, 78% of germinomas, and 75% of other germ cell tumour types arose in males. Pure germinomas outnumber other types, followed by mixed lesions and teratomas. In a series of 153 histologically verified cases {1612}, 41.1% were germinomas (including examples with syncytiotropho-blastic elements, which accounted for 5.2% of all cases), 32% were mixed germ cell tumours, 19.6% were teratomas (of which 63.3% were mature, 23.3% were immature, and 13.3% exhibited malig-nant elements), 3.3% were embryonal carcinomas, 2% were yolk sac tumours, and 2% were choriocarcinomas. How-ever, the relative incidence rates of the specific tumour types vary according to location.

Etiology

CNS germ cell tumours' predilection to occur in peripubertal patients, their local-ization in diencephalic centres regulating gonadal activity, and their increased inci-dence in Klinefelter syndrome have been regarded as evidence that elevated cir-culating gonadotropin levels play a role in their pathogenesis. The association with Klinefelter syndrome could also reflect X chromosome overdosage, a common genetic feature of these neoplasms.

Localization

About 80% of CNS germ cell tumours arise along a midline axis extending from the pineal gland (their most common site) to the suprasellar compartment (their next

most common site) {1025,2251,2278}. Suprasellar examples originate in the neurohypophyseal / infundibular stalk. Intraventricular, diffuse periventricular, thalamostriate, cerebral hemispheric, cerebellar, bulbar, intramedullary, and intrasellar variants can be encountered, as can congenital holocranial examples (usually teratomas). Germinomas prevail in the suprasellar compartment and ba-sal ganglionic / thalamic regions, and non-germinomatous subtypes predomi-nate at other sites. Multifocal CNS germ cell tumours usually involve the pineal re-gion and suprasellar compartment, either simultaneously or sequentially. Bilateral basal ganglionic and thalamic lesions are also well recognized.

Clinical features

The clinical manifestations and their du-ration vary with histological type and location. Germinomas are generally as-sociated with a more protracted symp-tomatic interval than are other types. Le-sions in the pineal region compress and obstruct the cerebral aqueduct, resulting in progressive hydrocephalus with intra-cranial hypertension. These lesions are also prone to compressing and invading the tectal plate, producing a paralysis of upwards gaze and convergence called Parinaud syndrome. Neurohypophyseal/suprasellar germ cell tumours impinge on the optic chiasm, causing visual field defects, and often disrupt the hypo-thalamohypophyseal axis, precipitating diabetes insipidus and manifestations of pituitary failure such as delayed growth and sexual maturation. The secretion by neoplastic syncytiotrophoblasts of hCG, a stimulant of testosterone production, can cause precocious puberty (isosex-ual pseudoprecocity) in boys. The ad-ditional expression of cytochrome P450 aromatase, which catalyses the conver-sion of C19 steroids to estrogen, may explain the rare instances of precocious puberty in girls with hCG-producing tu-mours {1814}. In this setting, hCG may also have some intrinsic follicle stimulat-ing hormone–like activity {2415}.

Imaging

Germ cell tumours other than teratomas tend to present as solid and contrast-enhancing on CT and MRI, with germinomas often enhancing more homogeneously than other subtypes {748,1497}. Tumour tissue is usually hypointense/isointense on T1-weighted images and isointense/hyperintense on T2-weighted images. Thalamic and basal ganglia germinomas may be more prone to calcification and cystic change than those in the pineal or suprasellar regions and can exhibit little T1-weighted signal abnormality and only poorly defined T2-hyperintensity, with minimal or no enhancement. Intratumoural cysts, calcified regions, and components with the low-signal-attenuation characteristics of fat suggest teratoma, whereas haemorrhage is commonly associated with tumours composed (at least in part) of choriocarcinoma. Neuroendoscopic evaluation can reveal tumour spread along or beneath the ependymal lining of a ventricle that is not evident on MRI {2732}. Congenital germ cell neoplasms (typically teratomas) can be detected in utero by ultrasonography or fast MRI {1583}.

Cell of origin

Although the histological, immunophenotypic, and genetic attributes shared by gonadal and neuraxial germ cell tumours are compatible with the traditional assumption that neuraxial germ cell tumours derive from primordial germ cells that either aberrantly migrate to or purposefully target developing CNS, the issue of histogenesis remains controversial. Studies of the human CNS, including immunohistochemical analysis of fetal pineal glands with antibodies to the primordial germ cell marker PLAP, have never shown it to harbour primitive germ cell elements {684}. However, it has been argued that germ cells might differentiate into divergent forms upon entering the CNS. Specifically, an enigmatic population of skeletal muscle–like cells native to the developing pineal gland has been suggested to descend from primitive germinal elements migrating during neuroembryogenesis {2173}. Cited in support of this seemingly far-fetched idea is the fact that striated muscle–type cells of unknown function also populate the thymus, another organ ostensibly devoid of germ cells and yet a favoured site of extragonadal germ cell tumorigenesis.

Alternative hypotheses instead implicate native stem cells of embryonic (i.e. pluripotent) or neural type {1850,2502}. These formulations require the selective genetic programming of such precursors along the germ cell differentiation pathway, as well as their neoplastic transformation. Supporting the neural stem cell hypothesis is evidence that such cells share hypomethylation of the imprinted SNRPN gene with primordial germ cell elements and intracranial germ cell tumours (as well as with gonadal and other extraneuraxial germ cell tumours) {1459}. Experimental data suggest that overexpression of OCT4 in such cells induces teratoma formation {2502}. Some authors consider the characteristically pure teratomas of the spinal cord to be bona fide neoplasms of germ cell origin {37}, but others contend that they are in fact complex malformations {1319}.

Genetic profile

At the genetic level, pure intracranial teratomas presenting as congenital or infantile growths differ fundamentally from CNS germ cell tumours arising after early childhood. Whereas pure intracranial teratomas presenting as congenital or infantile growths resemble teratomas of the infant testis in their typically diploid status and general chromosomal integrity {2119}, CNS germ cell tumours arising after early childhood, irrespective of their histological composition, share with their testicular counterparts in young men characteristically aneuploid profiles, complex chromosomal anomalies, and overlapping patterns of net genetic imbalance {1833,2121,2292,2453,2536}. These imbalances are primarily gains of 12p, 8q, 1q, 2p, 7q, 10q, and X, as well as losses of 11q, 13, 5q, 10q, and 18q. Whether 12p gain and isochromosome 12p formation, which are especially characteristic of testicular and mediastinal germ cell tumours, also occur at relatively high frequencies in the CNS setting has been debated, as has the prevalence of X duplication in this locale. The weight of data suggests that fewer CNS germ cell tumours exhibit isochromosome 12p {1833,2121,2292,2453,2536}. Regions of particular gain have been reported to encompass CCND2 and PRDM14, a regulator of primordial germ cell specification, and losses of the RB1 locus have been suggested to implicate the cyclin /

CDK / retinoblastoma protein / E2F pathway {2536}.

Upregulated KIT/RAS signalling, which is a feature of gonadal and mediastinal seminomas, is also evident in most intracranial germinomas; most manifest mutually exclusive activating KIT or RAS family member mutations that are associated with severe chromosomal instability {758,2689}. These alterations are only infrequently found in other germ cell tumour types. Inactivating mutation of CBL, which encodes a negative KIT regulator, has also been described in CNS germinoma {2689}. Less prevalent abnormalities manifested by a variety of intracranial germ cell tumour types include inactivating mutations of BCORL1 (a tumour suppressor gene) and activating AKT/mTOR lesions {2689}. Epigenetic alterations shared by gonadal and some intracranial germ cell tumours include hypomethylation of the imprinted SNRPN gene {1459} and of the IGF2/H19 imprinting control region {2359}. Finally, as a pertinent negative, amplification of the chromosome 19 microRNA cluster (C19MC) has not been identified in immature teratoma, despite the frequent occurrence of neural tube–like rosettes in this tumour type {1798}.

Genetic susceptibility

CNS germ cell tumours typically occur sporadically. An increased risk of intracranial (and mediastinal) germ cell tumorigenesis is associated with Klinefelter syndrome, which is characterized by a 47 XXY genotype {1202}. This association may reflect an increased dosage of an X chromosome–associated gene, given that CNS (and other) germ cell tumours commonly exhibit additional X chromosomes, as well as the potentiating effects of chronically elevated gonadotropin levels. Down syndrome, which is associated with an increased risk of testicular germ cell tumorigenesis, may also be complicated by intracranial germ cell neoplasia {436,956}. CNS germ cell tumours have also been described in the setting of neurofibromatosis type 1 {2784} in siblings {84,2675}, in a parent and child {84}, and in the fetus (an intracranial teratoma) of a woman with independent ovarian teratoma {2009}. Rarely, patients with CNS germ cell tumours have been reported to develop second gonadal or mediastinal germ cell neoplasms {956,1109,2707}. One such patient had Down syndrome {956}. It has

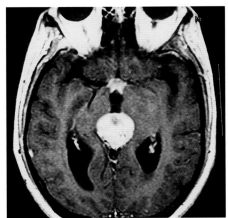

Fig. 15.02 MRI of a solid, contrast-enhancing germinoma of the pineal region, with a smaller cerebrospinal fluid–borne metastasis in the suprachiasmatic cistern.

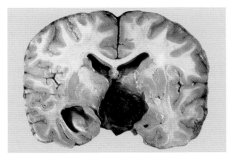

Fig. 15.03 Germinoma of the suprasellar region in a 7-year-old girl.

been suggested that germline variants of a chromatin-modifying gene, *JMJD1C*, may be associated with an increased risk of intracranial germ cell tumours in Japanese {2689}.

Prognosis and predictive factors

The factor that bears most heavily on outcome is histological subtype {1025, 1611,1612,2278}. Mature teratomas are potentially curable by surgical excision. Pure germinomas are remarkably radio-sensitive, with long-term survival rates of > 90% after craniospinal irradiation alone {1665}. The addition of chemotherapy to treatment regimens may provide comparable germinoma control at lower radiation doses and field volumes {1210,1449, 1611,1665,2251}. Whether germinomas harbouring syncytiotrophoblastic cells or associated with elevated beta-hCG levels carry an increased risk of recurrence and require intensified therapy has been controversial {1665}. A recent study demonstrating beta-hCG mRNA expression across CNS germ cell tumour types did not find that mRNA levels correlated with recurrence in the setting of

pure germinoma {2495}. The most virulent CNS germ cell tumours are yolk sac tumours, embryonal carcinomas, choriocarcinomas, and mixed lesions in which these types are prominent. In contrast, immature teratomas and mixed tumours dominated by teratoma or germinoma with only minor high-grade, non-germinomatous components seem to occupy an intermediate position in terms of biological behaviour {1611,2251}. Survival rates as high as 60–70% have been achieved through treatment of these more aggressive tumours with combined chemotherapy and irradiation {1665}. Local recurrence and cerebrospinal fluid–borne dissemination are the usual patterns of progression, but abdominal contamination via ventriculoperitoneal shunts and haematogenous spread (principally to lung and bone) can also occur.

Germinoma

Definition

A malignant germ cell tumour histologically characterized by the presence of large primordial germ cells with prominent nucleoli and variable cytoplasmic clearing.

Nearly all germinomas contain a substantial population of reactive lymphoid cells. Germinoma is the most common CNS germ cell tumour, and it can also occur as a component of a mixed germ cell tumour, in combination with other germ cell tumours. Germinoma is extremely sensitive to radiotherapy, and cure rates are high.

ICD-O code   9064/3

Macroscopy

Germinomas are composed of soft and friable tan-white tissue. They are generally solid, but may exhibit focal cystic change. Haemorrhage and necrosis are rare.

Microscopy

Germinomas contain large, undifferentiated cells that resemble primordial germinal elements. These are arranged in sheets, lobules, or (in examples manifesting stromal desmoplasia) regimented cords and trabeculae. The cytological features include round, vesicular, and centrally positioned nuclei; prominent nucleoli; discrete cell membranes; and relatively abundant cytoplasm, which is often clear due to glycogen accumulation. Mitotic activity is apparent and may be conspicuous, but necrosis is uncommon. Delicate fibrovascular septa (variably infiltrated by small lymphocytes) are a typical feature; some germinomas show a lymphoplasmacellular reaction so florid

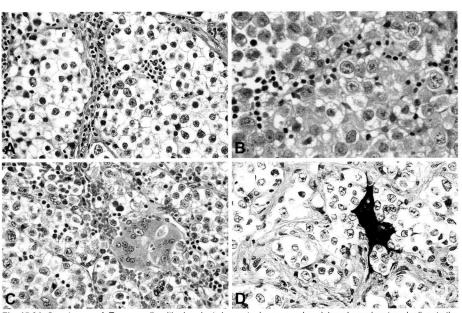

Fig. 15.04 Germinoma. **A** Tumour cells with abundant clear cytoplasm, round nuclei, and prominent nucleoli; note the lymphocytic infiltrates along fibrovascular septa. **B** Large tumour cells with round vesicular nuclei, prominent nucleoli, and clear cytoplasm. **C** Syncytiotrophoblastic giant cell in an otherwise typical germinoma. **D** Immunostaining for hCG.

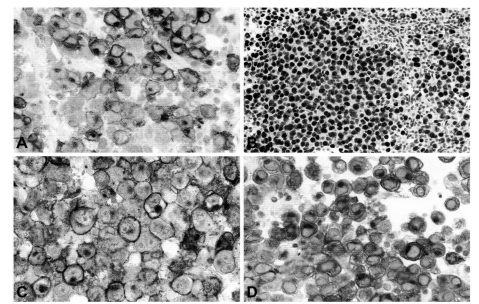

Fig. 15.05 Germinoma. **A** Membranous and Golgi region immunolabelling for KIT. **B** Immunoreactivity for OCT4. **C** Cytoplasmic and membranous reactivity for PLAP. **D** Expression of KIT protein in tumour cells.

that it obscures the neoplastic elements. Germinomas that provoke an intense granulomatous response can resemble sarcoidosis or tuberculosis {1331}.

Immunophenotype
Consistent cell membrane and Golgi region immunoreactivity for KIT and membranous D2-40 labelling distinguish germinomas from solid variants of embryonal carcinoma and yolk sac tumour {1080}. Less consistent (and non-specific) is cytoplasmic or membranous PLAP expression {210,1017,2196}. Germinomas regularly display immunoreactivity for the RNA-binding LIN28A protein {353} and nuclear expression of the transcription factors NANOG {2239}, OCT4 {1080}, ESRG {2695}, UTF1 {1885}, and SALL4 {1631}, but are typically non-reactive for CD30 and alpha-fetoprotein {210,684,1017,2196}. A minority display cytoplasmic labelling by the CAM5.2 and AE1/AE3 cytokeratin antibodies, a phenomenon which may, along with ultrastructural evidence of intercellular junction and lumen formation {1672}, indicate a capacity to differentiate along epithelial lines or towards embryonal carcinoma, but one that is without demonstrated clinical importance. Otherwise pure germinomas may harbour syncytiotrophoblastic elements that express beta-hCG and human placental lactogen.

Their biological significance has been controversial {1665}, but the presence of such cells should not prompt a diagnosis of choriocarcinoma.

The reactive lymphoid elements within germinomas are usually dominated by T cells, including both CD4-expressing helper/inducer and CD8-expressing cytotoxic/suppressor elements {2250, 2719}, but CD20-labelling B cells and CD138-labelling plasma cells may be conspicuous, and constitute evidence of humoral immune responses to tumour {2759}.

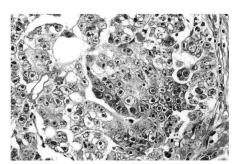

Fig. 15.06 Embryonal carcinoma composed of large epithelial cells forming abortive papillae and glandular structures with macronuclei.

Embryonal carcinoma

Definition
An aggressive non-germinomatous malignant germ cell tumour characterized by large epithelioid cells resembling those of the embryonic germ disc.

Other common features of embryonal carcinoma are geographical necrosis, a high mitotic count, and pseudoglandular or pseudopapillary structures. Embryonal carcinoma can also occur as a component of a mixed germ cell tumour, in combination with other germ cell tumours.

ICD-O code   9070/3

Macroscopy
Embryonal carcinomas are solid lesions composed of friable greyish-white tissue that may exhibit focal haemorrhage and necrosis.

Microscopy
Embryonal carcinomas are composed of large cells that proliferate in nests and sheets, form abortive papillae, or line gland-like spaces. Tumour cells exceptionally form so-called embryoid bodies replete with germ discs and miniature amniotic cavities. Other typical histological features include macronucleoli, abundant clear to violet-hued cytoplasm, a high mitotic count, and zones of coagulative necrosis.

Immunophenotype
Cytoplasmic immunoreactivity for CD30, although potentially shared by the epithelial and mesenchymal components of teratomas, distinguishes embryonal carcinomas from other germ cell tumours {1080}. Uniformly and strongly reactive for cytokeratins and often positive for PLAP {210,684,1017,2196}, these tumours also display labelling for LIN28A {353} and nuclear expression of OCT4 {1080}, ESRG {2695}, UTF1 {1885}, SALL4 {1080}, and SOX2 {2240}. KIT expression may be seen and is generally focal and non-membranous {1080}, but embryonal carcinomas are typically negative for alpha-fetoprotein, beta-hCG, and human placental lactogen {210,684, 1017,2196}.

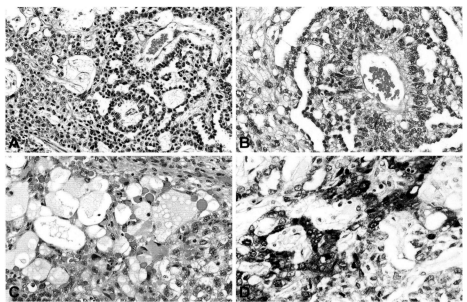

Fig. 15.07 Yolk sac tumour. **A** Typical sinusoidal growth pattern. **B** Schiller–Duval body and numerous mitoses. **C** Reticular growth pattern with numerous hyaline globules. **D** Alpha-fetoprotein immunolabelling.

Yolk sac tumour

Definition

An aggressive non-germinomatous malignant germ cell tumour composed of primitive germ cells arranged in various patterns, which can recapitulate the yolk sac, allantois, and extra-embryonic mesenchyme and produce alpha-fetoprotein. Yolk sac tumour can also occur as a component of a mixed germ cell tumour, in combination with other germ cell tumours.

ICD-O code 9071/3

Macroscopy

Yolk sac tumours are typically solid and greyish tan. They are usually friable or (due to extensive myxoid change) gelatinous in consistency. Focal haemorrhage may be apparent.

Microscopy

This neoplasm is composed of primitive-looking epithelial cells (which putatively differentiate towards yolk sac endoderm) set in a loose, variably cellular, and often myxoid matrix resembling extraembryonic mesoblast. The epithelial elements may form solid sheets, but are more commonly arranged in a loose network of irregular tissue spaces (termed 'reticular pattern') or around anastomosing sinusoidal channels as a cuboidal epithelium, in some cases draped over fibrovascular projections to form papillae called Schiller–Duval bodies. Yolk sac tumours can also contain eccentrically constricted cysts delimited by flattened epithelial elements (termed 'polyvesicular vitelline pattern'), enteric-type glands with goblet cells, and foci of hepatocellular differentiation (termed 'hepatoid variant'). Brightly eosinophilic, periodic acid–Schiff–positive, and diastase-resistant hyaline globules are characteristic, although variable; they may occupy the cytoplasm of epithelial cells or lie in extracellular spaces. Mitotic activity varies considerably, and necrosis is uncommon.

Immunophenotype

Cytoplasmic immunoreactivity of epithelial elements for alpha-fetoprotein, although potentially shared by the enteric glandular components of teratomas, distinguishes yolk sac tumours from other germ cell neoplasms {210,684,1017, 2196}. Hyaline globules are also reactive. Epithelial components consistently label for cytokeratins, are frequently positive for glypican-3 {1631}, and may also be positive for PLAP. Yolk sac tumours exhibit labelling for LIN28A {353} and nuclear expression of SALL4 {1631}. OCT4 expression is exceptional. KIT reactivity is also rare; when present, it is typically focal, cytoplasmic rather than membranous, and without Golgi area accentuation {1080}. Human placental lactogen and beta-hCG are not expressed.

Choriocarcinoma

Definition

An aggressive non-germinomatous malignant germ cell tumour composed of syncytiotrophoblasts, cytotrophoblasts, and occasionally intermediate trophoblasts. Necrosis and haemorrhage are often present in choriocarcinoma. There is usually a marked elevation of hCG in the blood or cerebrospinal fluid. Choriocarcinoma can also occur as a component of a mixed germ cell tumour, in combination with other germ cell tumours.

ICD-O code 9100/3

Macroscopy

Choriocarcinomas are solid, typically haemorrhagic, and often extensively necrotic.

Microscopy

Histological diagnosis requires the presence of both cytotrophoblastic elements and syncytiotrophoblastic giant cells. The giant cells typically contain multiple hyperchromatic or vesicular nuclei, often clustered in a knot-like fashion, within a large expanse of basophilic or violaceous cytoplasm. Neoplastic syncytiotrophoblast surrounds or partially drapes cytotrophoblastic components, which consist of cohesive masses of large mononucleated cells with vesicular nuclei and clear or acidophilic cytoplasm. Ectatic vascular channels, blood lakes, and extensive haemorrhagic necrosis are characteristic.

Immunophenotype

Syncytiotrophoblasts are characterized by diffuse cytoplasmic immunoreactivity for beta-hCG and human placental lactogen {210,684,1017,2196}. Cytokeratin

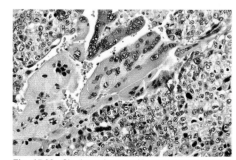

Fig. 15.08 Choriocarcinoma with syncytiotrophoblastic giant cells and cytotrophoblasts.

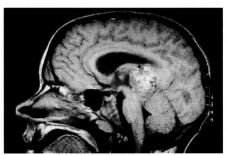

Fig. 15.09 Sagittal T1-weighted MRI of a teratoma in the pineal region, occupying the dorsal aspect of the third ventricle.

labelling is also demonstrable, with some choriocarcinomas also expressing PLAP, but KIT and OCT4 labelling are not seen {1080}.

Teratoma

Definition

A germ cell tumour composed of somatic tissues derived from two or three of the germ layers (i.e. the ectoderm, endoderm, and mesoderm).

Teratomas can be further subclassified as mature teratomas, which are composed exclusively of mature, adult-type tissues (e.g. mature skin, skin appendages, adipose tissue, neural tissue, smooth muscle, cartilage, bone, minor salivary glands, respiratory epithelium, and gastrointestinal epithelium) and immature teratomas, which contain immature, embryonic, or fetal tissues either exclusively or in addition to mature tissues. Rare teratomas contain a component resulting from the malignant transformation of a somatic tissue, usually a carcinoma or sarcoma, but embryonal tumours with the features of a primitive neuroectodermal tumour can also arise in this setting in the CNS, a fact prompting careful evaluation in certain clinicopathological settings, such as a pineal tumour of childhood. Pathologists should specify the type of secondary cancer present and avoid the non-specific designation "malignant teratoma".

ICD-O code   9080/1

Mature teratoma

ICD-O code   9080/0

Microscopy

Mature teratomas consist entirely of fully differentiated, adult-type tissue elements that exhibit little or no mitotic activity. Ectodermal components commonly include epidermis and skin appendages, central nervous tissue, and choroid plexus. Smooth and striated muscle, bone, cartilage, and adipose tissue are typical mesodermal components. Glands, often cystically dilated and lined by respiratory or enteric-type epithelia, are the usual endodermal components, but hepatic and pancreatic tissue may also be encountered. Gut- and bronchus-like structures replete with muscular coats or cartilaginous rings, respectively, as well as mucosa may also be formed.

Immature teratoma

ICD-O code   9080/3

Microscopy

Immature teratomas consist of incompletely differentiated elements resembling fetal tissues. When admixed with mature tissues, the presence of any immature teratoma component mandates classification of the tumour as immature teratoma, even if the incompletely differentiated elements constitute only a small part of the neoplastic process. Common features are compact and mitotically active stroma reminiscent of embryonic mesenchyme, as well as primitive neuroectodermal elements that may form neuroepithelial multilayered rosettes with a central lumen or canalicular arrays that resemble developing neural tube. Clefts lined by melanotic neuroepithelium are often seen; these result from abortive differentiation of the retinal pigment epithelium.

Teratoma with malignant transformation

ICD-O code   9084/3

Microscopy

Teratoma-containing intracranial germ cell tumours can include a variety of somatic-type cancers; the most commonly

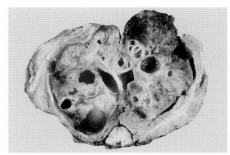

Fig. 15.10 Large immature teratoma of the cerebellum in a 4-week-old infant, with characteristic cysts and chondroid nodules.

encountered are rhabdomyosarcomas and undifferentiated sarcomas {210, 1612,2196}, followed by enteric-type adenocarcinomas {737,1275}, squamous carcinomas {1612}, and primitive neuroectodermal tumours {2595}. Erythroleukaemia {987} and leiomyosarcoma {2369} have also been reported to arise in this setting, as has a carcinoid tumour associated with an intradural spinal teratoma {1096}. The pathogenesis of an intrasellar tumour containing elements of germinoma and Burkitt-like B-cell lymphoma is unclear {2609}. Yolk sac tumour components (rather than teratomatous components) have been speculated to be the progenitors of select enteric-type adenocarcinomas originating in intracranial germ cell tumours {737}.

Mixed germ cell tumour

ICD-O code   9085/3

Macroscopy

The appearance of a mixed germ cell tumour reflects the macroscopic features of the constituent germ cell tumour components, as have been described for the pure forms.

Microscopy

Any combination of germ cell tumour variants can be encountered. Pathologists reporting such lesions must specify the subtypes present and state the relative proportions of each.

Immunophenotype
Individual components have the same antigenic profiles described for the pure forms of these tumour variants.

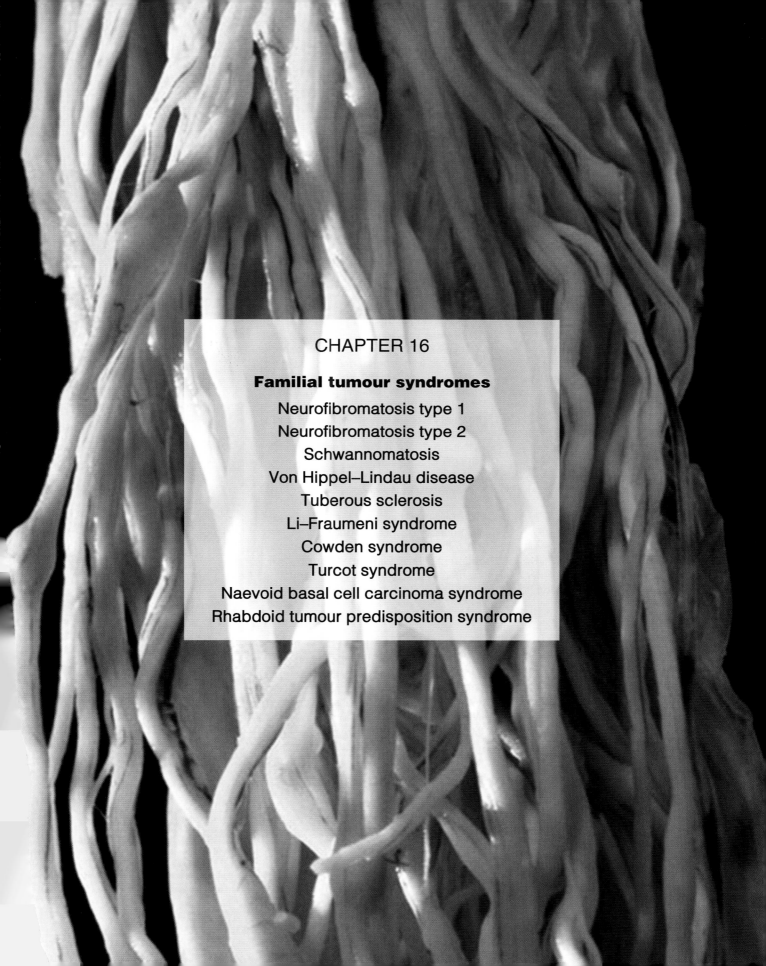

CHAPTER 16

Familial tumour syndromes

Neurofibromatosis type 1

Neurofibromatosis type 2

Schwannomatosis

Von Hippel–Lindau disease

Tuberous sclerosis

Li–Fraumeni syndrome

Cowden syndrome

Turcot syndrome

Naevoid basal cell carcinoma syndrome

Rhabdoid tumour predisposition syndrome

Neurofibromatosis type 1

Reuss D.E.
von Deimling A.
Perry A.

Definition

An autosomal dominant disorder characterized by neurofibromas, multiple café-au-lait spots, axillary and inguinal freckling, optic gliomas, osseous lesions and iris hamartomas (Lisch nodules). Patients with neurofibromatosis type 1 (NF1) have an increased risk for malignant peripheral nerve sheath tumour (MPNST), gastrointestinal stromal tumour, rhabdomyosarcoma, juvenile chronic myeloid leukaemia, duodenal carcinoids, C-cell hyperplasia / medullary thyroid carcinomas, other carcinomas, and phaeochromocytoma. The disorder is caused by mutations of the *NF1* gene on chromosome 17q11.2.

OMIM number {1624}   162200

Incidence/epidemiology

The birth frequency of NF1 has been estimated to be about 1 case per 3000 births {658,2680}.

Sites of involvement

Multiple sites and organ systems may be involved. The most commonly involved are the central and peripheral nervous system, the skin, the eyes, and the bones (see Table 16.01).

Table 16.01 National Institutes of Health (NIH) diagnostic criteria for neurofibromatosis type 1 (NF1) {739A}

The presence of ≥ 2 of the following features is diagnostic:
Six or more café-au-lait macules more than 5 mm in greatest diameter in prepubertal individuals and more than 15 mm in greatest diameter in postpubertal individuals
Two or more neurofibromas of any type or one plexiform neurofibroma
Freckling in the axillary or inguinal regions
Optic glioma
Two or more Lisch nodules (iris hamartomas)
A distinctive osseous lesion such as sphenoid dysplasia or tibial pseudarthrosis
A first-degree relative (parent, sib, or offspring) with NF1 as defined by the above criteria

Neurofibromas

Among the major subtypes of neurofibroma, the dermal and plexiform variants are characteristic of NF1. Deep-seated localized intraneural neurofibromas arise less commonly, and may cause neurological symptoms. Plexiform neurofibromas produce diffuse enlargement of major nerve trunks and their branches, sometimes yielding a rope-like mass, and are almost pathognomonic of NF1. Plexiform neurofibromas may develop during the first 1–2 years of life, as single subcutaneous swellings with poorly defined margins. They may also cause severe disfigurement later in life, affecting large areas of the body. If these tumours arise in the head or neck region, they can impair vital functions. Plexiform neurofibromas have a lifetime risk of malignant progression to MPNST of about 10% {1006}.

Malignant peripheral nerve sheath tumours

The MPNSTs that arise in patients with NF1 usually occur at a younger age, may be multiple, and may include divergent differentiations with rhabdomyoblastic elements (malignant triton tumour) or glandular elements (glandular MPNST). MPNSTs reduce life expectancy significantly {663}.

Gliomas

Most gliomas in patients with NF1 are pilocytic astrocytomas within the optic nerve. Bilateral growth is characteristic of NF1. Optic nerve gliomas in patients with NF1 may remain static for many years, and some may regress {1516}. Other gliomas observed at an increased frequency in NF1 include diffuse astrocytomas and glioblastomas {908,1470}.

Other CNS manifestations

The following features are more frequent in NF1: macrocephaly {2476}, learning disabilities and attention deficit hyperactivity disorder {1075}, epilepsy {1859}, aqueductal stenosis, hydrocephalus {587}, and symmetrical axonal neuropathy {691}.

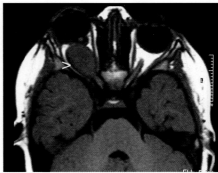

Fig. 16.01 Pilocytic astrocytoma of the optic nerve (optic nerve glioma; arrowhead) in a patient with neurofibromatosis type 1.

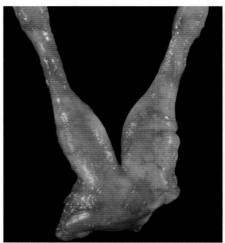

Fig. 16.02 Macroscopic preparation of a bilateral optic nerve glioma in a patient with neurofibromatosis type 1.

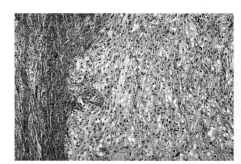

Fig. 16.03 Bilateral optic nerve glioma in a patient with neurofibromatosis type 1. Note the enlargement of the compartments of the optic nerves and collar-like extension into the subarachnoid space. Masson stain.

Extraneural manifestations
Abnormalities of pigmentation
Café-au-lait spots, freckling, and Lisch nodules all involve alterations of melanocytes. Café-au-lait spots are often the first manifestation of NF1 in the newborn. Their number and size increase during infancy, but may remain stable or even decrease in adulthood. Histopathologically, the ratio of melanocytes to keratinocytes is higher in the unaffected skin of patients with NF1, and this is more marked in the café-au-lait spots {738}. Melanocytes in café-au-lait spots have been shown to harbour somatic *NF1* mutations in addition to the germline mutation {552}. Axillary and/or inguinal freckling occurs in the vast majority of patients with NF1 {2476}. The histopathological features of these freckles are indistinguishable from those of café-au-lait spots. Lisch nodules are small, elevated, pigmented hamartomas on the surface of the iris. The presence of Lisch nodules is a particularly useful diagnostic criterion, because they occur in nearly all adults with NF1 {1544}.

Osseous and vascular lesions
In NF1, the orbits are often affected by sphenoid wing dysplasia. In addition, spinal deformities often result in severe scoliosis, which may require surgical intervention. Thinning, bending, and pseudarthrosis may affect the long bones (predominantly the tibia). Osteopenia/ osteoporosis and short stature may also be a component of NF1 {628,683}. Fibromuscular dysplasia of the renal and other arteries, cerebral aneurysm, and stenosis of the internal carotid, or cerebral arteries have also been reported {740,1815}.

Tumours
Patients with NF1 have increased risks of developing rhabdomyosarcomas, juvenile chronic myeloid leukaemia, juvenile xanthogranulomas, gastrointestinal stromal tumours, duodenal carcinoids, C-cell hyperplasia / medullary thyroid carcinomas, other carcinomas, and phaeochromocytomas {2879}.

Gene structure
The *NF1* locus is on chromosome 17q11.2 {2315}. The *NF1* gene is large, containing 59 exons and spanning about 350 kb {2194}. One of the two extensive introns, 27b, includes coding sequences for three embedded genes that are transcribed in a reverse direction: *EVI2A*, *EVI2B*, and

Table 16.02 Manifestations of neurofibromatosis type 1

Tumours
Neurofibromas
Dermal neurofibroma
Localized intraneural neurofibroma
Plexiform neurofibroma
Gliomas
Pilocytic astrocytoma, especially in the optic pathway (optic glioma)
Diffuse astrocytoma
Anaplastic astrocytoma
Glioblastoma
Sarcomas and stromal tumours
Malignant peripheral nerve sheath tumour (including malignant triton tumour)
Rhabdomyosarcoma
Gastrointestinal stromal tumour
Neuroendocrine/neuroectodermal tumours
Phaeochromocytoma
Carcinoid tumour
Medullary thyroid carcinoma
C-cell hyperplasia
Haematopoietic tumours
Juvenile chronic myeloid leukaemia
Juvenile xanthogranuloma
Other features
Osseous lesions
Scoliosis
Short stature
Macrocephaly
Pseudarthrosis
Sphenoid wing dysplasia
Eyes
Lisch nodules
Nervous system
Learning disabilities and attention deficit hyperactivity disorder
Epilepsy
Peripheral neuropathy
Hydrocephalus (aqueductal stenosis)
Vascular lesions
Fibromuscular dysplasia/hyperplasia of renal artery and other arteries
Skin
Café-au-lait spots
Freckling (axillary and/or inguinal)

OMG. There are 12 non-processed *NF1* pseudogenes localized on eight chromosomes. None of these pseudogenes extends beyond exon 29.

Gene expression
The *NF1* transcript is approximately 13 kb long and includes three alternatively spliced isoforms (exons 9a, 23a, and 48a), which are variably expressed depending on tissue type and differentiation {2194}. The product of the gene, neurofibromin, is a cytoplasmic protein that

can be found in two major isoforms, of 2818 amino acids (type 1) and 2839 amino acids (type 2), respectively. Neurofibromin has a predicted molecular weight of 320 kDa but runs in western blots at 220–250 kDa, most likely due to protein folding in denaturing gels {906}. Although neurofibromin is expressed almost ubiquitously in most mammalian tissues, the highest levels have been found in the CNS and peripheral nervous system and in the adrenal gland {911}.

Gene function
Neurofibromin harbours a small central GAP-related domain, and thus belongs to the group of mammalian RAS-GAPs. GAPs strongly accelerate the intrinsic GTPase activity of RAS, thereby promoting the conversion of active GTP-bound RAS to the inactive GDP-bound form {234}. In vitro, neurofibromin acts as the GAP for the classic RAS proteins (HRAS, NRAS, and KRAS) and related subfamily members (RRAS, RRAS2, and MRAS {1821}.

Of the several potential effector pathways of active RAS proteins, the best-studied and probably most important in the context of NF1 are the MAPK and the RAS/PI3K/AKT/mTOR pathways {910}. Both pathways have numerous and often synergistic effects in tumour cells, regulating proliferation, differentiation, migration, apoptosis, and angiogenesis {1620}. There is also some evidence of growth regulatory functions outside of the neurofibromin GAP-related domain. Mice with a constitutional homozygous *Nf1* knockout (*Nf1–/–*) die in utero at day 13.5 of embryogenesis, due to abnormal cardiac development {261,1110}. Isolated reconstitution of the GAP-related domain in these *Nf1–/–* mice rescues cardiovascular development, but is insufficient to inhibit overgrowth of neural crest–derived tissues, leading to perinatal lethality {1103}.Neurofibromin also controls adenylyl cyclase activity and intracellular cAMP levels {529,2568}. The mechanism for neurofibromin-mediated cAMP regulation remains unclear, but both RAS-dependent and RAS-independent models have been reported {289,940}.

Genotype/phenotype
Genotype–phenotype correlations are complicated by the unusually high degree of variable expressivity within families with NF1. The correlation between

clinical manifestations and the degree of relatedness of patients suggests a role for modifying non-allelic genes {2477}. Only two clear genotype–phenotype correlations have been established to date. About 5–10% of patients have the *NF1* microdeletion syndrome, caused by unequal homologous recombination of *NF1* repeats resulting in the loss of approximately 1.5 Mb of DNA on 17q, including the entire *NF1* gene and 13 surrounding genes {549}. Patients with this syndrome tend to have a more severe phenotype, including facial dysmorphism, mental retardation, developmental delay, increased burden of neurofibromas, and increased risk of MPNST development {550}, suggesting involvement of additional genes {1899}. *SUZ12* is one of the codeleted genes in patients with *NF1* microdeletion syndrome, and loss of this gene has been shown to play an important role in MPNST development {548}.

A specific 3 bp in-frame deletion in exon 17 of the *NF1* gene (c.2970–2972 delAAT) is associated with the absence of cutaneous neurofibromas and clinically obvious plexiform tumours {2600}.

There are several additional reports suggesting potential less-established genotype–phenotype correlations. *NF1* mutations in patients with optic pathway glioma appear to cluster at the 5′ end of the gene encompassing exons 1–15 {235,2332}. The heterozygous c.5425C→T missense variant (p.Arg1809Cys) has been associated with a mild phenotype with multiple café-au-lait spots and skinfold freckling only {1978}. *NF1* splice-site mutations have been putatively associated with an increased tendency to develop MPNSTs and gliomas {54}. A 1.4 Mb microduplication encompassing the *NF1* gene is reported not to be associated with a typical NF1 phenotype, but with learning difficulties and dysmorphic features {1698}.

Mosaicism

The occurrence of a segmental or regional form of NF1, caused by somatic mosaicism at the *NF1* gene locus, further extends the range of variability {1242,1517}. Patients with this form of NF1 often have only pigmentary manifestations within the affected limb or region; however, some patients develop classic tumours, such

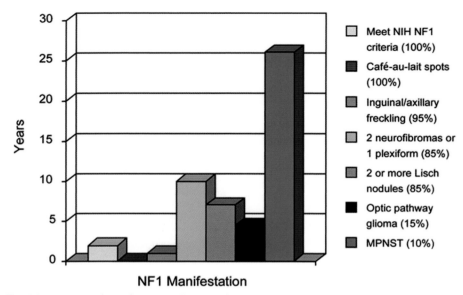

Fig. 16.04 Mean ages of onset for common clinical manifestations in patients with neurofibromatosis type 1 (NF1). The estimated frequencies for each manifestation within the patient population are given in parentheses. MPNST, malignant peripheral nerve sheath tumour; NIH, National Institutes of Health.

as plexiform neurofibromas or optic pathway gliomas.

Spinal neurofibromatosis

Spinal neurofibromatosis is a condition in which multiple bilateral spinal neurofibromas occur, but there are few or no cutaneous manifestations of NF1. Missense mutations are found more often in patients with spinal neurofibromatosis than in those with a classic NF1 phenotype, but no clear genotype–phenotype association has been established {2197}. Both familial and sporadic cases occur {326,1897,1985,2601}.

Differential diagnosis

NF1 belongs to a heterogeneous group of developmental syndromes known as RASopathies {2073}. All RASopathies are caused by germline mutations in genes encoding for members or regulators of the RAS/MAPK pathway. RASopathies also show some phenotypic overlap; for example, NF1 without neurofibromas and Legius syndrome (caused by *SPRED1* mutation) may be clinically indistinguishable {275}.

Genetic counselling

NF1 is inherited in an autosomal dominant manner, but about half of all patients have a sporadic, de novo *NF1* mutation. For each offspring of a person with NF1, the chance of inheriting the pathogenic *NF1* gene is 50%. The disease penetrance is 100%. Prenatal and preimplantation mutation testing are available. Genetic testing can be diagnostic in children who fulfil some but not all of the National Institutes of Health (NIH) criteria, and may be helpful in certain cases for distinguishing NF1 phenotypes from other conditions, such as Legius syndrome. Mutation screening of the *NF1* gene is difficult due to its large size, the presence of pseudogenes, and the diversity of mutations {1652}. More than 1000 different mutations have been reported at [https://grenada.lumc.nl/LOVD2/mendelian_genes/home.php?select_db=NF1] and [http://www.hgmd.org]. Using comprehensive screening techniques that may include various strategies such as long-range RT-PCR, protein truncation testing, cDNA sequencing, FISH, next-generation sequencing, and/or multiplex ligation-dependent probe amplification, as many as 95% of mutations may be detected in individuals fulfilling the NIH criteria for NF1 {1601,1652}. More than 80% of mutations are predicted to either encode a truncated protein or result in no protein production.

Neurofibromatosis type 2

Stemmer-Rachamimov A.O.
Wiestler O.D.
Louis D.N.

Definition

An autosomal dominant disorder characterized by neoplastic and dysplastic lesions that primarily affect the nervous system, with bilateral vestibular schwannomas as a diagnostic hallmark. Other manifestations include schwannomas of other cranial nerves, spinal and peripheral nerves, and the skin; intracranial and spinal meningiomas; gliomas, in particular spinal ependymomas; and a variety of non-tumoural and dysplastic/developmental lesions, including meningioangiomatosis, glial hamartomas, ocular abnormalities (e.g. posterior subcapsular cataracts, retinal hamartomas, and epiretinal membranes), and neuropathies. NF2 is caused by mutations of the *NF2* gene on chromosome 22q12.

OMIM number {1624}   101000

Incidence/epidemiology

The disorder affects between 1 in 25 000 and 1 in 40 000 individuals {662}. About half of all cases are sporadic, occurring in individuals with no family history of NF2 and caused by newly acquired germline mutations. In the past, the considerable variability of the clinical manifestations of NF2 resulted in underdiagnosis of the syndrome.

Table 16.03 National Institutes of Health (NIH) / Manchester criteria for neurofibromatosis type 2 (NF2) {655A}

The presence of one or more of the following features is diagnostic:
Bilateral vestibular schwannomas
A first-degree relative with NF2 AND unilateral vestibular schwannoma OR any two of: meningioma, schwannoma, glioma, neurofibroma, posterior subcapsular lenticular opacities*
Unilateral vestibular schwannoma AND any two of: meningioma, schwannoma, glioma, neurofibroma, posterior subcapsular lenticular opacities*
Multiple meningiomas AND unilateral vestibular schwannoma OR any two of: schwannoma, glioma, neurofibroma, cataract*

*Any two of = two individual tumours or cataracts.

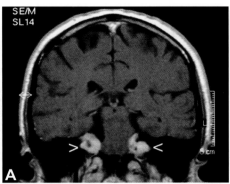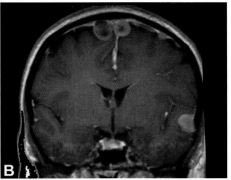

Fig. 16.05 T1-weighted, contrast-enhanced MRI from a patient with neurofibromatosis type 2. **A** Bilateral vestibular schwannomas (arrowheads), the diagnostic hallmark of neurofibromatosis type 2. **B** Multiple meningiomas presenting as contrast-enhanced masses.

Diagnostic criteria

The diagnosis of NF2 is based on clinical features and may be challenging because of the wide variability of symptoms and time of onset. Particularly difficult to diagnose are genetic mosaics (accounting for 30% of sporadic cases), in which segmental involvement or milder disease may occur {1307}, and paediatric cases in which the full manifestation of the disease has not yet developed. The distinction from other forms of neurofibromatosis (neurofibromatosis type 1 and schwannomatosis) is difficult in some cases. There is clinical phenotypic overlap between NF2 mosaic, early NF2, and schwannomatosis; some cases that fulfil the clinical diagnostic criteria for schwannomatosis have later proven to be NF2 {1990}.

The original clinical diagnostic criteria for NF2 were established at the National Institutes of Health (NIH) Consensus Development Conference on Neurofibromatosis in 1987 {1758}. Several revisions of these criteria have since been proposed: the NIH 1991 criteria, the Manchester criteria (see Table 16.03), the National Neurofibromatosis Foundation (NNFF) criteria, and the Baser criteria. Each of these revisions expanded the original criteria, aiming to also identify patients with multiple NF2 features who do not present with bilateral vestibular schwannomas and have no family history of NF2 {137, 659,905}.

Confirmatory testing for *NF2* mutations may be helpful when a patient does not meet the clinical criteria for a definite diagnosis but the phenotype is suggestive.

Nervous system neoplasms

Schwannomas

Schwannomas associated with NF2 are WHO grade I tumours composed of neoplastic Schwann cells, but differing from sporadic schwannomas in several ways. NF2 schwannomas present in younger patients (in the third decade of life) than do sporadic tumours (in the sixth decade), and many patients with NF2 develop the diagnostic hallmark of the disease, bilateral vestibular schwannomas, by their fourth decade of life {659,1599}. NF2 vestibular schwannomas may entrap seventh cranial nerve fibres {1198} and have higher proliferative activity {75}, although these features do

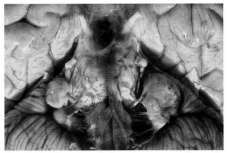

Fig. 16.06 Bilateral vestibular schwannomas, diagnostic for neurofibromatosis type 2.

not necessarily connote more aggressive behaviour. In addition to the vestibular division of the eighth cranial nerve, other sensory nerves may be affected, including the fifth cranial nerve and spinal dorsal roots. However, motor nerves such as the twelfth cranial nerve may also be involved {659,1536}. Cutaneous schwannomas are common and may be plexiform {659,1599}.

NF2 schwannomas may have a multilobular (cluster-of-grapes) appearance on both gross and microscopic examination {2738}, and multiple schwannomatous tumourlets may develop along individual nerves, particularly on spinal roots {1536, 2424}. A mosaic pattern of immunostaining for SMARCB1 expression (indicating patchy loss) has been reported in most syndrome-associated schwannomas, including both NF2 and schwannomatosis {1909}.

Meningiomas

Multiple meningiomas are the second hallmark of NF2 and occur in half of all patients with the disorder {1536}. NF2-associated meningiomas occur earlier in life than sporadic meningiomas, and may be the presenting feature of the disorder, especially in the paediatric population {656,659,1599}. Although most NF2-associated meningiomas are WHO grade I tumours, several studies have suggested

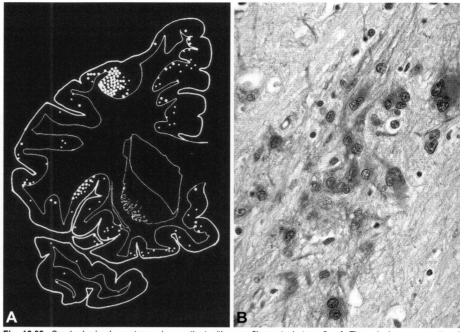

Fig. 16.08 Cerebral microhamartomas in a patient with neurofibromatosis type 2. **A** These lesions are scattered throughout the cortex and (**B**) show strong immunoreactivity for S100.

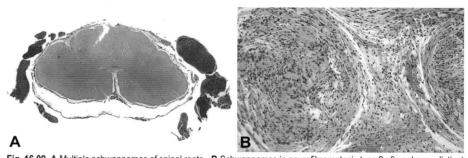

Fig. 16.09 **A** Multiple schwannomas of spinal roots. **B** Schwannomas in neurofibromatosis type 2 often show a distinct nodular pattern.

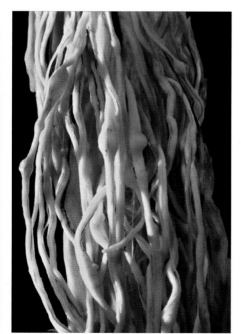

Fig. 16.07 Numerous schwannomas of the cauda equina in a patient with neurofibromatosis type 2.

that NF2-associated meningiomas have a higher mitotic index than sporadic meningiomas {74,1942}. All major subtypes of meningioma can occur in patients with NF2, but the most common subtype is fibroblastic {74,1536}. NF2-associated meningiomas can occur throughout the cranial and spinal meninges, and may affect sites such as the cerebral ventricles.

Gliomas

Approximately 80% of gliomas in patients with NF2 are spinal intramedullary or cauda equina tumours, with an additional 10% of gliomas occurring in the medulla {2158}. Ependymomas account for most of the histologically diagnosed gliomas in NF2, and for almost all spinal gliomas {2158,2204}. In most cases, NF2 spinal ependymomas are multiple, intramedullary, slow-growing, asymptomatic

masses {2158,2204}. Diffuse and pilocytic astrocytomas have been reported in NF2, but many probably constitute misdiagnosed tanycytic ependymomas {923}.

Neurofibromas

Cutaneous neurofibromas have been reported in NF2. However, on histological review, many such neurofibromas prove to be schwannomas, including plexiform schwannomas misdiagnosed as plexiform neurofibromas.

Other nervous system lesions

Schwannosis is a proliferation of Schwann cells, sometimes with entangled axons, but without frank tumour formation. In patients with NF2, schwannosis is often found in the spinal dorsal root entry zones (sometimes associated with a schwannoma of the dorsal root) or in the perivascular spaces of the central spinal cord, where the nodules look more like small traumatic neuromas {2195, 2204}. Less robust but otherwise identical schwannosis has been reported in reactive conditions.

Meningioangiomatosis is a cortical lesion characterized by a plaque-like proliferation of meningothelial and fibroblast-like cells surrounding small vessels. It occurs both sporadically and in NF2. Meningioangiomatosis is usually a single, intracortical lesion, although multifocal examples occur as well, as do non-cortical lesions {2195,2204}. Meningioangiomatosis may be predominantly vascular (resembling a vascular malformation) or predominantly meningothelial, sometimes with an associated meningioma. Sporadic meningioangiomatosis is a single lesion that usually occurs in young adults or children, who present with seizures or persistent headaches. In contrast, NF2-associated meningioangiomatosis may be multifocal and is often asymptomatic and diagnosed only at autopsy {2423}.

Glial hamartias (also called microhamartomas) of the cerebral cortex are circumscribed clusters of cells with medium to large atypical nuclei. These lesions are scattered throughout the cortex and basal ganglia and show strong immunoreactivity for S100, but are only focally positive for GFAP. Glial hamartias are common in and pathognomonic of NF2 {2195,2752}, and are not associated with mental retardation or astrocytomas. The hamartias are usually intracortical, with a predilection for the molecular and deeper cortical layers, but have also been observed in the basal ganglia, thalamus, cerebellum, and spinal cord {2752}. The fact that merlin expression is retained in glial hamartias suggests the possibility that haploinsufficiency during development underlies these malformations {2422}.

Intracranial calcifications are frequently noted in neuroimaging studies of patients with NF2. The most common locations are the cerebral and cerebellar cortices, periventricular areas, and choroid plexus.

Peripheral neuropathies not related to tumour mass are increasingly recognized as a common feature of NF2 {500,1536}. Mononeuropathies may be the presenting symptom in children {656}, whereas progressive polyneuropathies are more common in adults. Sural nerve biopsies from patients with NF2 suggest that NF2 neuropathies are mostly axonal and may be secondary to focal nerve compression by tumourlets or onion-bulb–like Schwann cell or perineurial cell proliferations without associated axons {2405, 2546}.

Extraneural manifestations can also occur. Posterior lens opacities are common and highly characteristic of NF2. A variety of retinal abnormalities (including hamartomas, tufts, and dysplasias) may also be found {403}. Ocular abnormalities may be helpful in the diagnosis of paediatric patients. Skin lesions other than cutaneous nerve sheath tumours, primarily café-au-lait spots, have been reported.

Gene structure

The *NF2* gene {2190,2575} spans 110 kb and consists of 17 exons. *NF2* mRNA transcripts encode at least two major protein forms generated by alternative splicing at the C-terminus. Isoform 1, encoded by exons 1–15 and 17, has intramolecular interactions similar to the ERM proteins – ezrin, radixin, and moesin (see *Gene function*). Isoform 2, encoded by exons 1–16, exists only in an unfolded state {901,2802}.

Gene mutations

Numerous germline and somatic *NF2* mutations have been detected, supporting the hypothesis that *NF2* functions as a tumour suppressor gene {900,1536}. Germline *NF2* mutations differ somewhat from the somatic mutations identified in sporadic schwannomas and meningiomas. The most frequent germline mutations are point mutations that alter splice junctions or create new stop codons {252,1536,1556,1647,2190,2221,2575}. Germline mutations are found in all parts of the gene (with the exception of the alternatively spliced exons), but they occur preferentially in exons 1–8 {1647}. One possible hotspot for mutations is position 169 in exon 2, in which a C→T transition at a CpG dinucleotide results in a stop at codon 57 {252,1647}; other CpG dinucleotides are also common targets for C→T transitions {2221}.

Gene expression

The *NF2* gene is expressed in most normal human tissues, including brain {2190,2575}.

Gene function

The predicted protein product shows a strong similarity with the highly conserved protein 4.1 family of cytoskeleton-associated proteins, which includes protein 4.1, talin, moesin, ezrin, radixin, and protein tyrosine phosphatases. The similarity of the *NF2*-encoded protein to the ERM proteins (moesin, ezrin, and radixin) resulted in the name "merlin" {2575}; the alternative name "schwannomin" has also been suggested {2190}. Members of the protein 4.1 family link the cell membrane to the actin cytoskeleton. These

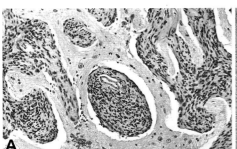 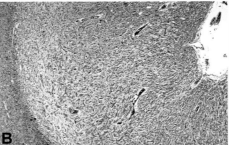 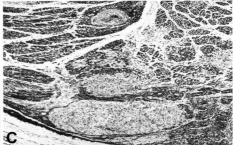

Fig. 16.10 A Meningioangiomatosis associated with neurofibromatosis type 2. An intracortical lesion composed of a perivascular proliferation of cells (predominantly meningothelial) in Virchow–Robin spaces. **B** Diffuse cortical meningioangiomatosis associated with neurofibromatosis type 2. Trichrome stain. **C** Multiple Schwann cell tumourlets arising in the cauda equina of a patient with neurofibromatosis type 2 (Luxol fast blue, H&E).

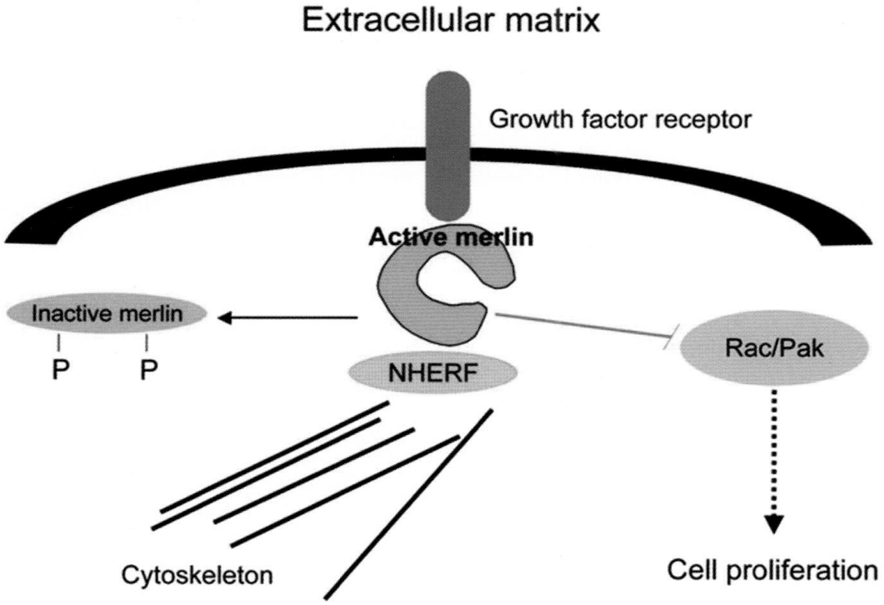

Fig. 16.11 In its active (hypophosphorylated) state, merlin suppresses cell proliferation and motility by inhibiting the transmission of growth signals from the extracellular environment to the Rac/PAK signalling system. Inactivated (phosphorylated) merlin dissociates from its protein scaffold, thus disinhibiting Rac/PAK signalling as well as cell proliferation and motility.

proteins consist of a globular N-terminal FERM domain, an alpha-helical domain containing a praline-rich region, and a C-terminal domain. The N-terminal domain interacts with cell membrane proteins such as CD44, CD43, ICAM1, and ICAM2; the C-terminal domain contains the actin-binding site. Merlin lacks the actin-binding site in the C-terminus but may have an alternative actin-binding site {2802}. The ERM proteins and merlin may be self-regulated by head-to-tail intramolecular associations that result in folded and unfolded states. The folded state of merlin is the functionally active molecule, which is inhibited by phosphorylation of the C-terminus on serine residues {2339}. Although the precise mechanism of tumour suppression by merlin is still unknown, the structural similarity of merlin to the ERM proteins suggests that merlin provides regulated linkage between membrane-associated proteins and the actin cytoskeleton; the tumour suppressor activity is thought to be exerted by regulation of signal transmission from the extracellular environment to the cell {1619} and activation of downstream pathways including the MAPK, FAK/SRC, PI3K/AKT, Rac/PAK/JNK, mTORC1, and WNT/beta-catenin pathways. Many merlin binding partners have been identified, including integrins and tyrosine receptor kinases {1288,1726}. Recent data suggest that merlin also suppresses signalling at the nucleus, where it suppresses the E3 ubiquitin ligase IL17RB {1493}.

Genotype/phenotype
The clinical course in patients with NF2 varies widely between and (to a lesser extent) within families {659,1599}. Some families feature early onset with diverse tumours and high tumour load (Wishart type), whereas others present later, with only vestibular schwannomas (Gardner type). An effect of maternal inheritance on severity has been noted, as have families with genetic anticipation. All families with NF2 show linkage of the disease to chromosome 22 {1757}, implying a single responsible gene. Correlations of genotype with phenotype have therefore been used to attempt to predict clinical course on the basis of the type of the underlying *NF2* mutation. Nonsense and frameshift mutations are often associated with a more severe phenotype, whereas missense mutations, large deletions, and somatic mosaicism have been associated with milder disease {138,664,1308, 1647}. Phenotypic variability is observed in splice-site mutations, with more severe phenotypes observed in mutations upstream from exon 7 {1306}.

Genetic counselling
The risk of transmission to offspring is 50%. Prenatal diagnosis by mutation analysis and testing of children of patients with NF2 is possible when the mutation is known.

Schwannomatosis

Stemmer-Rachamimov A.O.
Hulsebos T.J.M.
Wesseling P.

Definition

A usually sporadic and sometimes autosomal dominant disorder characterized by multiple schwannomas (spinal, cutaneous, and cranial) and multiple meningiomas (cranial and spinal), associated with inactivation of the *NF2* gene in tumours but not in the germline, and caused by mutations in *SMARCB1* on 22q or *LZTR1* on 22q.

For a diagnosis of schwannomatosis, it is important to exclude the other forms of neurofibromatosis by confirming the absence of vestibular schwannomas on MRI and the absence of other manifestations of neurofibromatosis type 2 (NF2) or neurofibromatosis type 1.

OMIM number {1624}   162091

Synonyms

The terms used to describe this disorder in the past include "neurilemmomatosis", "multiple schwannomas", and "multiple neurilemmomas".

Incidence/epidemiology

In several reports, schwannomatosis was found to be almost as common as NF2, with an estimated annual incidence of 1 case per 40 000–80 000 population {76,2322}. Familial schwannomatosis accounts for only 10–15% of all cases {1558,2322}.

Diagnostic criteria

Reports of patients with multiple non-vestibular schwannomas date back to 1984 {2350}, but it was long debated whether the condition constitutes a form of attenuated NF2 or a separate entity. Standardized clinical diagnostic criteria for schwannomatosis were first developed by a panel of experts in a consensus meeting in 2005 {1555} and later revised in 2012 to include molecular diagnosis {1990}. The exclusion of NF2 by clinical criteria and by imaging of the vestibular nerves is essential for the diagnosis of schwannomatosis. The distinction may be particularly challenging in paediatric patients, because vestibular

Table 16.04 The current proposed clinical and molecular diagnostic criteria for schwannomatosis {1990}

Molecular criteria for definite schwannomatosis:
Two or more schwannomas or meningiomas (pathology proven) AND genetic studies of at least two tumours with LOH for chromosome 22 and two different *NF2* mutations OR
One schwannoma or meningioma (pathology proven) AND *SMARCB1* germline mutation
Clinical criteria for definite schwannomatosis:
Two or more schwannomas (non-dermal, one pathology proven) AND no bilateral vestibular schwannomas (by thin-slice MRI) OR
One schwannoma or meningioma (pathology proven) AND first-degree relative affected by schwannomatosis
Clinical criteria for possible schwannomatosis:
Two or more schwannomas (no pathology) OR
Severe chronic pain associated with a schwannoma

schwannomas may develop only later in the course of the disease {661}. There can be overlap between the clinical features of early NF2 or NF2 mosaics and schwannomatosis {1990}.

Nervous system neoplasms

Schwannomas

Patients with schwannomatosis typically have multiple schwannomas. These tumours may develop in spinal roots, cranial nerves, skin, and (occasionally) unilaterally in the vestibular nerve. Cutaneous schwannomas may be plexiform. The tumours have a segmental distribution in about 30% of patients with schwannomatosis {1555,1649,2377,2378}. Severe pain associated with the tumours is characteristic of the disease. This is a distinguishing feature from NF2, in which pain is rare and neurological deficits and polyneuropathy are common {1649}. Histologically, schwannomatosis tumours may display prominent myxoid stroma and an intraneural growth pattern, and are sometimes misdiagnosed as neurofibromas or malignant peripheral nerve sheath tumours {1649}.

Many schwannomas of patients with familial schwannomatosis show mosaic immunohistochemical staining for SMARCB1 protein (i.e. an intimate mixture of positive and negative tumour cell nuclei), but with considerable inter- and intratumoural heterogeneity (with < 10% to > 50% immunonegative nuclei). Mosaic SMARCB1 staining is also often present in schwannomas of patients with sporadic schwannomatosis and NF2, corroborating an interaction between *NF2* and *SMARCB1* in the pathogenesis of these tumours {1064,1909}. In contrast, sporadic schwannomas rarely show mosaic SMARCB1 staining.

Meningiomas

Various studies have shown that *SMARCB1* germline mutations also predispose individuals to the development of multiple meningiomas, with preferential location of cranial meningiomas at the falx cerebri {102,455,2622}. The reported proportion of schwannomatosis patients who develop a meningioma is 5% {2375}. Occasionally, patients present with multiple meningiomas.

Extraneural manifestations

Extraneural manifestations associated with schwannomatosis are rare, unlike those associated with neurofibromatosis types 1 and 2. One study reported

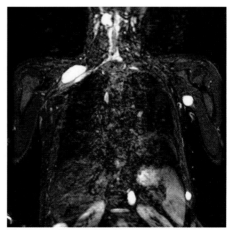

Fig. 16.12 Coronal MRI (short T1 inversion recovery sequence) showing multiple, bright, discrete tumours in a patient with schwannomatosis.

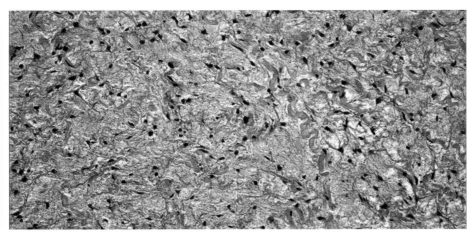

Fig. 16.13 Schwannomas in schwannomatosis are often myxoid, with an appearance that mimics that of neurofibromas.

a uterine leiomyoma in a patient with schwannomatosis; the tumour had a molecular profile similar to that of the schwannomas, as well as the corresponding mosaic staining for SMARCB1 protein, indicating that the SMARCB1 defect in schwannomatosis may occasionally contribute to the oncogenesis of extraneural neoplasms {1062}.

Inheritance and genetic heterogeneity

The great majority of schwannomatosis cases are sporadic, with only 15% of patients having a positive family history. In the familial form, the disease displays an autosomal dominant pattern of inheritance, with incomplete penetrance {1557}. In 2007, the *SMARCB1* gene on chromosome arm 22q was identified as a familial schwannomatosis-predisposing gene {1064}. In subsequent studies, the gene proved to be involved in about 50% of familial cases, but in ≤ 10% of sporadic cases {260,921,2191,2380}.

In 2014, the *LZTR1* gene, also on 22q, was identified as a second causative gene in schwannomatosis {1980}. In patients with schwannomatosis without *SMARCB1* germline mutations, *LZTR1* mutations were found in about 40% of familial and 25% of sporadic cases {1073, 1877,2377}. The fact that most schwannomatosis cases cannot be explained by the involvement of *SMARCB1* or *LZTR1* suggests the existence of additional causative genes {1073}.

Recently, a germline missense mutation was identified in the *COQ6* gene on chromosome arm 14q, which segregated with the disease in a large family affected by schwannomatosis {2856}. However, the oncogenic effect of the mutation has yet to be elucidated, and other families affected by schwannomatosis with *COQ6* involvement have not yet been reported. Germline mutations of the *NF2* gene have been excluded in schwannomatosis {1115,1237,1557}, but the presence of other, somatically acquired mutations in the *NF2* gene is characteristic in schwannomatosis-associated schwannomas.

One third of all patients with sporadic schwannomatosis have segmental distribution of their tumours, suggesting somatic mosaicism for the causative gene, but this has not yet been demonstrated for *SMARCB1* or *LZTR1*.

The *SMARCB1* gene

Gene structure and expression

The *SMARCB1* gene is located in chromosome region 22q11.23 and contains nine exons spanning 50 kb of genomic DNA {2649}. Alternative splicing of exon 2 results in two transcripts and two proteins with lengths of 385 and 376 amino acid residues, respectively. The so-called SNF5 homology domain in the second half of the protein harbours highly conserved structural motifs through which SMARCB1 interacts with other proteins {2430}. The SMARCB1 protein is a core subunit of mammalian SWI/SNF chromatin remodelling complexes, which regulate the expression of many genes by using ATP for sliding the nucleosomes along the DNA helix, facilitating or repressing transcription {2760}. The SMARCB1 protein functions as a tumour suppressor via repression of *CCND1* gene expression, induction of the *CDKN2A* gene, and hypophosphorylation of retinoblastoma protein, resulting in G0/G1 cell cycle arrest {185,2648}.

According to the tumour suppressor gene model, both copies of the *SMARCB1* gene are inactivated in these tumours. In schwannomas of patients with schwannomatosis with *SMARCB1* germline mutation in addition to loss of the second *SMARCB1* allele, there is also inactivation of both copies (by mutation and deletion) of the *NF2* gene, located 6 Mb distal to *SMARCB1* on chromosome 22 {260,921, 2325}. The deletion of *SMARCB1* and *NF2* is a consequence of the loss of one copy of chromosome 22 {922}.

Based on these observations, a four-hit, three-step model of tumorigenesis in schwannomatosis is proposed: (inherited) *SMARCB1* germline mutation occurs (hit 1), followed by loss of the other chromosome 22 with the wildtype copy of *SMARCB1* and one copy of *NF2* (hits 2 and 3), followed by a somatic mutation of the remaining copy of the *NF2* gene (hit 4). This model, with somatic mutations of the *NF2* gene as the last step, explains the observation of different *NF2* mutations in multiple schwannomas in a single patient with schwannomatosis {1990}. This four-hit model of genetic events also occurs in meningiomas in patients with *SMARCB1* germline mutation {102,455, 2622}.

In schwannomatosis, most germline mutations in *SMARCB1* are non-truncating missense mutations, splice-site mutations, or in-frame deletions, which are predicted to result in the synthesis of an altered SMARCB1 protein with modified activity {2380}. The mosaic staining pattern seen in many schwannomatosis-associated schwannomas suggests the absence of SMARCB1 protein in part of the tumour cells {1909}. Truncating nonsense and frameshift mutations, also reported in patients with schwannomatosis, generate a premature termination codon and are predicted to result in the absence of SMARCB1 protein expression. For the truncating mutations in exon 1 of *SMARCB1*, it was recently demonstrated that translational reinitiation at a downstream AUG codon occurs, resulting in the synthesis of an N-terminally truncated SMARCB1 protein {1063}. Other mechanisms, such as alternative splicing, may operate to overcome the deleterious effect of truncating mutations in the other exons of *SMARCB1*.

SMARCB1 mutations in rhabdoid tumours

SMARCB1 germline mutations may also predispose individuals to the development of rhabdoid tumours (very aggressive tumours of childhood), a disorder called rhabdoid tumour predisposition syndrome 1 (p. 321). In rhabdoid tumours, the two copies of the SMARCB1 gene are inactivated by a truncating mutation and deletion of the wildtype gene, resulting in total loss of SMARCB1 expression in tumour cells. This is in contrast to the presence of non-truncating SMARCB1 mutations and the mosaic SMARCB1 expression in the schwannomas of patients with schwannomatosis. Because children with a rhabdoid tumour usually die before the age of 3 years, familial inheritance of the predisposition is extremely rare, and most cases are sporadic {2327,2522}. However, 35% of patients with sporadic rhabdoid tumour carry a germline SMARCB1 alteration as the first hit {249,616}. A few families have been reported in which the affected individuals inherited a SMARCB1 mutation and developed schwannomatosis or a rhabdoid tumour {371,616,2472}. However, the schwannomas in these families (as well as the rhabdoid tumours) displayed total loss of SMARCB1 protein expression {371,2472}.

The LZTR1 gene

Gene structure and expression
The LZTR1 gene is situated proximal to SMARCB1 in chromosome region 22q11.21 and contains 21 exons, spanning 17 kb of genomic DNA {1980}. The wildtype gene codes for a protein with a length of 840 amino acid residues. LZTR1 may function as a substrate adaptor in cullin-3 ubiquitin ligase complexes, binding to cullin-3 and to substrates targeted for ubiquitination {735}. Somatically acquired NF2 mutations and deletions

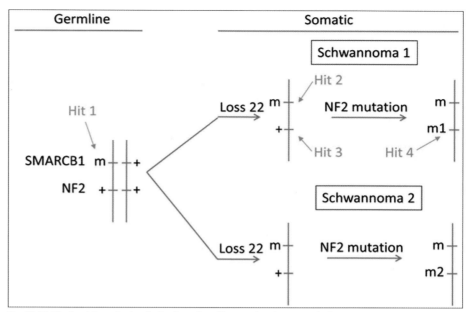

Fig. 16.14 The four-hit mechanism for the formation of tumours in schwannomatosis.

are also found in the schwannomas of patients with schwannomatosis with a germline LZTR1 mutation, suggesting that the four-hit, three-step model of tumorigenesis also applies to these tumours {1073,1877,1980,2377}. However, unlike in SMARCB1-associated schwannomas (in which LOH for chromosome 22 occurs by loss of chromosome), in LZTR1-associated schwannomas, mitotic recombination has been found in 30% of cases {2377}.

Gene mutations
The reported LZTR1 germline mutations in schwannomatosis include non-truncating (missense and splice-site) as well as truncating (nonsense and frameshift) mutations and are found along the entire coding sequence of the gene, affecting the functionally important domains of the LZTR1 protein {1073,1877,1980,2377}. Immunostaining of LZTR1-associated schwannomas with an LZTR1-specific

antibody demonstrates absent or reduced expression of the protein, consistent with its function as a tumour suppressor {1877}. Germline LZTR1 mutations (but no germline NF2 mutations) were also found in 3 of 39 patients with a unilateral vestibular schwannoma and at least one other schwannoma, suggesting that unilateral vestibular schwannoma may be present in schwannomatosis, especially in cases with a LZTR1 germline mutation {2377}.

Genetic counselling
The risk of transmission to offspring is assumed to be 50% for patients carrying a germline mutation of SMARCB1 or LZTR1 and in familial cases in which the germline is unidentified. The risk of transmission to the offspring of patients with sporadic cases with no SMARCB1 or LZTR1 mutation is unknown {1990}.

Von Hippel–Lindau disease

Plate K.H.
Vortmeyer A.O.
Zagzag D.
Neumann H.P.H.
Aldape K.D.

Definition

An autosomal dominant disorder characterized by the development of clear cell renal cell carcinoma (RCC), capillary haemangioblastoma of the CNS and retina, phaeochromocytoma, and pancreatic and inner ear tumours. Von Hippel–Lindau disease (VHL) is caused by germline mutations of the *VHL* tumour suppressor gene, located on chromosome 3p25–26. The von Hippel–Lindau disease tumour suppressor protein (VHL protein) plays a key role in cellular oxygen sensing.

OMIM number {1624}   193300

Historical annotation

Lindau described capillary haemangioblastoma and noted its association with retinal vascular tumours (previously described by von Hippel) and tumours of the visceral organs, including the kidney.

Incidence/epidemiology

VHL is estimated to have an annual incidence rate of 1 affected individual per 36 000–45 500 population.

Diagnostic criteria

The clinical diagnosis of VHL is based on the presence of capillary haemangioblastoma in the CNS or retina and the presence of one of the typical VHL-associated extraneural tumours or a pertinent family history. Germline *VHL* mutations can virtually always be identified in VHL.

Table 16.06 Sites of involvement in von Hippel–Lindau disease

Organ/ tissue	Tumours	Non- neoplastic lesions
CNS	Haemangioblastoma	
Eye (retina)	Haemangioblastoma	
Kidney	Clear cell renal cell carcinoma	Cysts
Adrenal gland	Phaeochromocytoma	
Pancreas	Neuroendocrine islet cell tumours	Cysts
Inner ear	Endolymphatic sac tumour	
Epididymis	Papillary cystadenoma	

Sites of involvement

Renal lesions in carriers of *VHL* germline mutations are either cysts or clear cell RCCs. They are typically multifocal and bilateral. The mean patient age at manifestation is 37 years (vs 61 years for sporadic clear cell RCC), with a patient age at onset of 16–67 years. There is a 70% chance of developing clear cell RCC by the age of 70 years. Metastatic RCC is the leading cause of death from VHL. The median life expectancy of patients with VHL is 49 years.

Eye

Retinal haemangioblastomas manifest earlier than kidney cancer (at a mean patient age of 25 years), and thus offer the possibility of an early diagnosis.

CNS

CNS haemangioblastomas develop mainly in young adults (at a mean patient age of 29 years). They are predominantly located in the cerebellum, followed by the brain stem and spinal cord. Approximately 25% of all cases are associated with VHL.

Adrenal gland

Phaeochromocytomas may constitute a major clinical challenge, particularly in families affected by VHL with predisposition to the development of these tumours. They are often associated with pancreatic cysts.

Other extrarenal manifestations

Other extrarenal manifestations include neuroendocrine tumours, endolymphatic sac tumours of the inner ear, and epididymal and broad ligament cystadenomas.

Gene structure

The *VHL* tumour suppressor gene is located at chromosome 3p25–26. It has three exons and a coding sequence of 639 nucleotides. Germline mutations of the *VHL* gene are spread over the three exons. Missense mutations are most common, but nonsense mutations, microdeletions/insertions, splice-site mutations, and large deletions also occur. In accordance with the function of *VHL* as a tumour suppressor gene, *VHL* gene

Table 16.05 Key characteristics of sporadic haemangioblastoma and haemangioblastoma associated with von Hippel–Lindau disease (VHL)

Criterion	Sporadic	VHL- associated
Female	41%	56%
Patient age	44 years (7–82)	23 years (7–64)
Intracranial	79%	73%
Spinal	11%	75%
Multiple	5%	65%

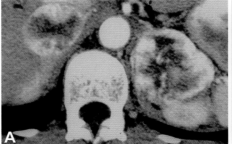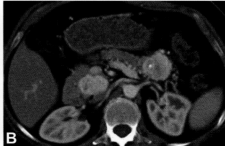

Fig. 16.15 Von Hippel–Lindau disease. **A** Bilateral adrenal phaeochromocytoma and (**B**) multiple pancreatic neuroendocrine tumours.

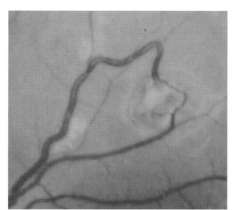

Fig. 16.16 Retinal angioma in von Hippel–Lindau disease.

mutations are also common in sporadic haemangioblastomas and RCCs.

Gene expression

The *VHL* gene is expressed in a variety of human tissues, in particular epithelial skin cells; the gastrointestinal, respiratory, and urogenital tracts; and endocrine and exocrine organs. In the CNS, immunoreactivity for the VHL protein is prominent in neurons, including Purkinje cells of the cerebellum {1526A}.

Gene function

The *VHL* tumour suppressor gene was identified in 1993. Mutational inactivation of the *VHL* gene in affected family members is responsible for their genetic susceptibility to tumour development at various organ sites, but the mechanisms by which the inactivation or loss of the suppressor gene product (the VHL protein) causes neoplastic transformation are only partly understood {873}.

Transcription elongation factor B binding
One signalling pathway points to a role of the VHL protein in protein degradation and angiogenesis. The alpha domain of the VHL protein forms a complex with TCEB2, TCEB1, cullin-2, and RBX1 that has ubiquitin ligase activity, thereby targeting cellular proteins for ubiquitination and proteasome-mediated degradation. The domain of the *VHL* gene involved in the binding to transcription elongation factor B (also called elongin) is frequently mutated in neoplasms associated with VHL.

HIF1
The VHL protein plays a key role in cellular oxygen sensing, by targeting hypoxia-inducible factors (which mediate

cellular responses to hypoxia) for ubiquitination and proteasomal degradation. The beta-domain of the VHL protein interacts with HIF1A. Binding of the hydroxylated subunit of the VHL protein causes polyubiquitination and thereby targets HIF1A for proteasome degradation. Under hypoxic conditions or in the absence of functional *VHL*, HIF1A accumulates and activates the transcription of hypoxia-inducible genes, including VEGF-A, *PDGFB*, *TGFA*, and *EPO*. Constitutive overexpression of VEGF explains the extraordinary capillary component of VHL-associated neoplasms. VEGF has been targeted as a novel therapeutic approach using neutralizing anti-VEGF antibody. Induction of *EPO* is responsible for the occasional paraneoplastic erythrocytosis in patients with kidney cancer and CNS haemangioblastoma.

Cell cycle exit
Recent studies in RCC cell lines suggest that the VHL protein is involved in the control of cell cycle exit, i.e. the transition from the G2 phase into the quiescent G0 phase, possibly by preventing accumulation of the cyclin-dependent kinase inhibitor CDKN1B.

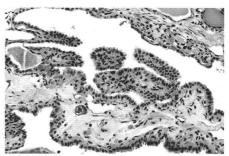

Fig. 16.17 Endolymphatic sac tumour. Papillary fronds and colloid secretions.

Invasion
Only wildtype (not tumour-derived) VHL protein binds to fibronectin. As a result, *VHL–/–* RCC cells show a defective assembly of an extracellular fibronectin matrix. Through down-regulation of the cellular response to hepatocyte growth factor / scatter factor and reduced levels of TIMP2, VHL protein–deficient tumour cells exhibit a significantly higher capacity for invasion.

Genotype/phenotype

Germline mutations of the *VHL* gene are spread over the three exons. Missense mutations are most common, but nonsense mutations, microdeletions/insertions, splice-site mutations, and large

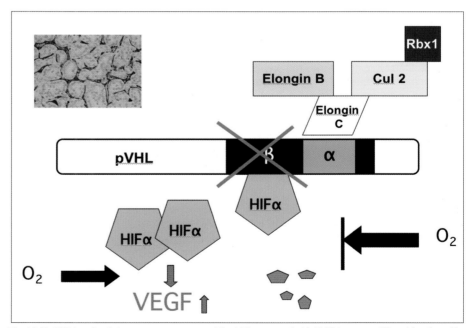

Fig. 16.18 *VHL* is a classic tumour suppressor gene. The *VHL* gene product (pVHL) has many different functions. The beta domain forms a complex with elongin and other proteins that regulate the function of hypoxia-inducible factors, including hypoxia-inducible factor protein (HIF) and VEGF. Under normoxic conditions, HIF degrades. Under hypoxic conditions, HIF accumulates. If pVHL is inactivated, there is no degradation of HIF, leading to an accumulation of VEGF, which explains why tumours associated with von Hippel–Lindau disease are highly vascularized.

deletions also occur. The spectrum of clinical manifestations of VHL reflects the type of germline mutation.

Type 1 is characterized by frequent haemangioblastomas and RCCs but rare or absent phaeochromocytomas, and is typically caused by deletions, truncations, and missense mutations.

Type 2A carries a high risk of developing haemangioblastomas and phaeochromocytomas, but rarely RCCs, and is caused by missense mutations.

Type 2B is characterized by a high frequency of haemangioblastomas, RCCs, and phaeochromocytomas, and is mainly caused by missense mutations.

Type 2C is characterized by frequent phaeochromocytomas but absence of haemangioblastomas and RCCs. It is caused by *VHL* missense mutations, but unlike the other types, shows no evidence of hypoxia-inducible factor dysregulation. In accordance with the function of *VHL* as a tumour suppressor gene, *VHL* gene mutations are common in sporadic haemangioblastomas (occurring in as many as 78% of cases) and are ubiquitous in clear cell RCCs.

Genetic counselling

Patients with *VHL* germline mutations require ongoing medical–genetic counselling. Analyses for germline mutations of the *VHL* gene are recommended for every patient with retinal or CNS haemangioblastoma, particularly for younger patients and those with multiple lesions, in order to promptly detect tumours associated with VHL. Periodic screening of patients with VHL is mandatory, beginning with retinoscopy at 5 years of age and by MRI of the CNS and abdomen at 10 years of age.

Tuberous sclerosis

Lopes M.B.S.
Wiestler O.D.
Stemmer-Rachamimov A.O.
Sharma M.C.
Santosh V.
Vinters H.V.

Definition

A group of autosomal dominant disorders characterized by hamartomas and benign neoplastic lesions that affect the CNS and various non-neural tissues. Major CNS manifestations of tuberous sclerosis include cortical hamartomas (tubers), subcortical glioneuronal hamartomas, subependymal glial nodules, and subependymal giant cell astrocytomas (SEGAs). Major extraneural manifestations include cutaneous angiofibromas (so-called adenoma sebaceum), peau chagrin, subungual fibromas, cardiac rhabdomyomas, intestinal polyps, visceral cysts, pulmonary lymphangioleiomyomatosis, and renal angiomyolipomas. Tuberous sclerosis is caused by a mutation of *TSC1* on 9q or *TSC2* on 16p.

OMIM numbers {1624}
Tuberous sclerosis 1	191100
Tuberous sclerosis 2	613254

Incidence/epidemiology

The variability of the clinical manifestations of tuberous sclerosis previously led to underdiagnosis. Recent data indicate that the disorder affects as many as 25 000–40 000 individuals in the USA and about 1–2 million individuals worldwide, with an estimated prevalence of 1 case per 6000–10 000 live births {1809}.

Diagnostic criteria

The diagnosis of tuberous sclerosis is based primarily on clinical features and may be challenging due to the considerable variability in phenotype, patient age at symptom onset, and penetrance among mutation carriers. The diagnostic criteria for tuberous sclerosis were

Table 16.07 Clinical diagnostic criteria for tuberous sclerosis; adapted from Northrup H et al. {1809}

Major features
≥ 3 hypomelanotic macules ≥ 5 mm in diameter
≥ 3 angiofibromas or fibrous cephalic plaque
≥ 2 ungual fibromas
Shagreen patch
Multiple retinal hamartomas
Cortical dysplasias (including tubers and cerebral white matter radial migration lines)
Subependymal nodules
Subependymal giant cell astrocytoma
Cardiac rhabdomyoma
Lymphangioleiomyomatosis
≥ 2 angiomyolipomas

Minor features
Confetti skin lesions
≥ 4 dental enamel pits
≥ 2 intraoral fibromas
Retinal achromic patch
Multiple renal cysts
Non-renal hamartomas

Definitive diagnosis: 2 major features or 1 major feature with ≥ 2 minor features

Possible diagnosis: 1 major feature or ≥ 2 minor features

revised in 2012 at the International Tuberous Sclerosis Complex Consensus Conference {1809}. These criteria are especially important because genetic testing is performed in relatively few centres, and therefore may not be accessible to many clinicians. Clinical manifestations are categorized as either major or minor features. The diagnostic categories, which are based on the number of major/minor manifestations present in a given individual, define disease likelihood as being definite or possible {1809} (see Table 16.07). Most patients have manifestations of tuberous sclerosis before the age of 10 years, although some cases may manifest much later in life {26}. Confirmatory testing for *TSC1* or *TSC2* mutations may be helpful when a patient does not meet the clinical criteria for a definite diagnosis but the phenotype is compelling. However, the TSC genes are large and complex, the genetic abnormalities vary substantially (from point mutations to deletions), and the testing is not widely available. Prenatal diagnosis by mutation analysis is possible when the mutation in other family members is known.

Sites of involvement

Clinical features

Tuberous sclerosis tends to shorten

lifespan (as compared with lifespan in a Caucasian control population), but often only slightly. The most common causes of death in the second decade of life are brain tumours and status epilepticus, followed by renal abnormalities {1809}. In patients aged > 40 years, mortality is most commonly associated with renal abnormalities (i.e. cystic disease or neoplasm) or an unusual proliferative lung condition, lymphangioleiomyomatosis. Cardiac rhabdomyomas are often a presenting feature of tuberous sclerosis in newborns and infants aged < 2 years, and more than half of all individuals found to have cardiac rhabdomyomas have tuberous sclerosis {2133}. Cutaneous manifestations include hypomelanotic nodules, facial angiofibromas, and shagreen patches. Ungual (or subungual) fibromas often only develop in childhood. Renal angiomyolipomas develop in as many as 80% of people with tuberous sclerosis by the age of 10 years. Renal cysts are present in as many as 20% of affected individuals, but polycystic kidney disease only occurs in 3–5%. Lymphangioleiomyomatosis is a condition of unknown pathogenesis that severely impairs lung function and may be fatal; it is present in as many as 40% of adult women with tuberous sclerosis. All the phenotypic features of tuberous sclerosis can also occur sporadically in individuals without the genetic condition {2133}. For example, about 50% of patients with lymphangioleiomyomatosis do not have tuberous sclerosis; sporadic angiomyolipomas can occur but are typically solitary, whereas tuberous sclerosis–associated angiomyolipomas are often multiple or bilateral. The proteins tuberin and hamartin (products of the *TSC2* and *TSC1* genes, respectively; see *Other CNS manifestations*) are identifiable by immunohistochemistry and western blotting in many organs and tissues throughout the body {1170}.

Neurological symptoms are among the most frequently observed and serious (sometimes life-threatening) manifestations of tuberous sclerosis {505,2538}. The most common initial signs of tuberous sclerosis are intractable epilepsy including infantile spasms (in 80–90% of cases), cognitive impairment (in 50%), autism spectrum disorder (in as many as 40%), and neurobehavioural disorders (in ≥ 60%) {863,2538}; these presentations may have any of several etiologies.

Table 16.08 Major manifestations of tuberous sclerosis

Manifestation	Frequency
CNS	
Cortical tuber	90–100%
Subependymal nodule	90–100%
White matter hamartoma and white matter heterotopia	90–100%
Subependymal giant cell astrocytoma	6–16%
Skin	
Facial angiofibroma (adenoma sebaceum)	80–90%
Hypomelanotic macule	80–90%
Shagreen patch	20–40%
Forehead plaque	20–30%
Peri- and subungual fibroma	20–30%
Eye	
Retinal hamartoma	50%
Retinal giant cell astrocytoma	20–30%
Hypopigmented iris spot	10–20%
Kidney	
Multiple, bilateral angiomyolipoma	50%
Renal cell carcinoma	1.2%
Polycystic kidney disease	2–3%
Isolated renal cyst	10–20%
Heart	
Cardiac rhabdomyoma	50%
Digestive system	
Microhamartomatous rectal polyp	70–80%
Liver hamartoma	40–50%
Hepatic cyst	24%
Adenomatous polyp of the duodenum and small intestine	Rare
Lung	
Lymphangioleiomyomatosis	1–2.3%
Pulmonary cyst	40%
Micronodular pulmonary hyperplasia of type II pneumocytes	Rare
Other	
Gingival fibroma	50–70%
Pitting of dental enamel	30%
Bone cyst	40%
Arterial aneurysm (intracranial arteries, aorta, and axillary artery)	Rare

In people with tuberous sclerosis, these manifestations are linked to the structural changes that involve cortex and subcortical white matter, usually as tubers (see *Other CNS manifestations*), although meticulous autopsy studies on small numbers of patients have also suggested that there may be more subtle degrees of cortical and white matter disorganization {1582}.

Subependymal giant cell astrocytoma
See p. 90.

Other CNS manifestations
CNS lesions include cerebral cortical tubers, white matter heterotopia, and subependymal hamartomatous nodules (i.e. candle guttering or dripping identified on neuroimaging studies). Cortical tubers in tuberous sclerosis may be detected by CT or MRI {2342}; structural abnormalities representative of tubers may be co-registered with metabolic brain studies, for example, using FDG-PET. These combined investigations, together with intraoperative electrocorticography can identify which of many tubers are most likely to be epileptogenic in a given individual, facilitating tuberectomy as a reasonable surgical approach to treating intractable seizures in patients with tuberous sclerosis. These malformative lesions have a strong association with the development of epilepsy, especially infantile spasms and generalized tonic–clonic seizures. They also resemble sporadic malformations of cortex not associated with tuberous sclerosis, classified as cortical dysplasia Type IIb according to the classification proposed by the International League Against Epilepsy (ILAE) {225}. Microscopically, they consist of giant cells (like those seen in SEGA) and dysmorphic neurons, disrupted cortical lamination, gliosis, calcification of blood vessel walls and/or parenchyma, and myelin loss. The surrounding cortex usually demonstrates a normal cytoarchitecture on cursory examination, although this conclusion is being questioned based on more detailed immunohistochemical and morphometric investigations {1072,1582}. Dysmorphic neurons and giant cells may be seen in all cortical layers and the underlying white matter. The dysmorphic neurons show altered radial orientation in the cortex, aberrant dendritic arborization, and accumulation of perikaryal fibrils. The perikaryal fibrils can be highlighted using silver impregnation techniques, which show many neurons with neurofibrillary tangle–like morphology. Another frequently observed element in tubers and adjacent brain (cortex and white matter) is the characteristic so-called balloon cell. Balloon cells resemble gemistocytic astrocytes in that they have eosinophilic glassy cytoplasm and may be clustered in small groups, but unlike gemistocytes, they often show prominently nucleolated nuclei {505,1009, 1072}. A spectrum of cellular elements with features of both neurons and astrocytes may be noted in the brains of people with tuberous sclerosis. Although the

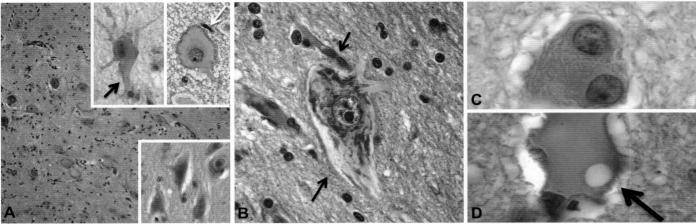

Fig. 16.19 Unusual cells within and adjacent to tuberous sclerosis cortical tubers. Panel **A** (inset, black arrow) shows a cell with eosinophilic cytoplasm and unusual dendritic arborization; a nearby cell (white arrow) shows neuronal morphology, with a nucleolated nucleus and amphophilic cytoplasm lacking obvious Nissl substance. Panel **B** shows a dysmorphic enlarged neuron (arrows). Panels **C** and **D** show balloon-like cells with eosinophilic cytoplasm; the cell in **C** is binucleated, whereas the cell in **D** shows a cytoplasmic vacuole (arrow). All panels are from H&E-stained sections.

neurons express neuronal-associated proteins, they display cytoarchitectural features of immature or poorly differentiated neurons, such as reduced axonal projections and spine density {1009, 1072}. Giant cells in cortical tubers show a cellular and molecular heterogeneity similar to that seen in SEGA, and immunohistochemical markers characteristic of glial and neuronal phenotypes suggest a mixed glioneuronal origin of these cells. Many giant cells in tubers express nestin mRNA and protein {506}. Some giant cells demonstrate immunoreactivity for GFAP {1009}, but others with an identical morphological phenotype express neuronal markers, including gap junction beta-2 protein and gap junction beta-1 protein (also called connexins 26 and 32), neurofilaments, class III beta-tubulin, MAP2, and alpha-internexin {506,1009}. However, formation of well-defined synapses between giant cells and adjacent neurons is not a consistent finding. Cortical hamartomas morphologically indistinguishable from tubers may occur in chronic focal epilepsies without clinical or genetic evidence of an underlying tuberous sclerosis condition {223,225, 2305}. The pathogenesis of these sporadic lesions is unclear. Subependymal hamartomas are elevated, often calcified nodules. They are composed of cells indistinguishable from those found in cortical tubers, but are smaller in size than cortical tubers.

Soon after the *TSC2* and *TSC1* genes were first cloned in the 1990s, probes for the gene transcripts and the translated proteins were developed. Immunostaining a given tuber with antihamartin or antituberin antibodies does not provide evidence of which mutation is present in a given subject, and therefore is not of great diagnostic value. Both proteins are widely expressed throughout the CNS of the normal developing brain {1169,2655}. Many approaches have been taken to studying tubers, especially surgically resected lesions, because DNA, mRNA, and proteins are better preserved within them than in autopsy specimens, and autopsies of patients with tuberous sclerosis are rare. Cell biology approaches have also been taken to examining the biology of hamartin and tuberin and how they may mediate cell adhesion through the ERM proteins (ezrin, radixin, and moesin) and the GTPase Rho {1423}. Deep sequencing of *TSC1*, *TSC2*, and *KRAS* demonstrates that small second-hit mutations in these genes are rare events within tubers {2048}. Insulin signalling pathways (normally impacted through inhibition by both tuberin and hamartin) show subtle but definite differences in tuberous sclerosis tubers versus foci of severe (i.e. ILAE Type IIb) cortical dysplasia {1690}. Electrophysiological approaches have also shown differences in neurophysiological and synaptic abnormalities in surgically resected brain tissue samples from patients with tuberous sclerosis versus patients with severe cortical dysplasia {390}. A mouse model of tuberous sclerosis, in which mosaic *Tsc1* loss was induced in neural progenitor cells, showed megalencephaly, marked cortical disorganization, and (cortical) giant cells with organellar dysfunction within the brains of affected animals {874}. This phenotype could be rescued by postnatal administration of sirolimus (also known as rapamycin), which resulted in abrogation of both seizures and premature death.

Extraneural manifestations
The extraneural manifestations of tuberous sclerosis and the frequencies at which they occur are summarized in Table 16.08.

Molecular genetics
Tuberous sclerosis is caused by inactivating mutations in one of two genes: *TSC1* at 9q or *TSC2* at 16p. The proteins encoded by the TSC genes, tuberin and hamartin, interact within the cell and form a complex {486,1212,1987}. Mutation of either gene results in disrupted function of the tuberin–hamartin complex, resulting in similar disease phenotypes. In sporadic tuberous sclerosis cases, mutations are 5 times as common in *TSC2* as in *TSC1* {51,516,1174}, whereas in families with multiple affected members the mutation ratio of the two genes is 1:1 {2231}. *TSC1* or *TSC2* mutations are identified in about 85% of patients with tuberous sclerosis. The remaining 15% of cases may be mosaics or have a mutation in an unanalysed non-coding gene area. Mosaicism has been reported for *TSC1* and *TSC2* mutations in some parents of patients with sporadic cases and in patients with tuberous sclerosis {2229,

2646}. Alternatively, there may be a third, unknown locus, although to date there is no evidence to support this possibility {2231}. Patients with tuberous sclerosis with no mutations identified have milder phenotype than do patients with TSC1 or TSC2 mutations {2231}.

The TSC1 gene
The TSC1 gene maps to chromosome 9q34 {486} and contains 23 exons {2625}, 21 of which carry coding information.

Gene expression
The TSC1-encoded protein, hamartin, has a molecular weight of 130 kDa. Hamartin is strongly expressed in brain, kidney, and heart, all of which are tissues frequently affected in tuberous sclerosis {1986}. Its pattern of expression overlaps with that of tuberin, the product of the TSC2 gene.

Gene mutations
Mutation analysis of large cohorts {418, 2626} showed that the most common mutations in the TSC1 gene are small deletions and nonsense mutations (each accounting for ~30% of all mutations in the gene). Virtually all mutations result in a truncated gene product, and more than half of the changes affect exons 15 and 17 {2626}.

The TSC2 gene
The TSC2 gene maps to chromosome 16p13.3 {1212} and contains 40 exons.

Gene expression
TSC2 encodes a large transcript of 5.5 kb, which shows widespread expression in many tissues, including the brain and other organs affected in tuberous sclerosis. Alternatively spliced mRNAs have been reported {2799}. A portion of the 180 kDa protein product tuberin bears significant homology with the catalytic domain of RAP1GAP, a member of the RAS family.

Gene mutations
The mutational spectrum of TSC2 is wider than that of TSC1; it includes large deletions and missense mutations, and less frequently, splice junction mutations {51, 516,1174}. Exons 16, 33, and 40 have the highest number of mutations. Large deletions in the TSC2 gene may extend into the adjacent PKD1 gene, with a resulting phenotype of tuberous sclerosis and polycystic kidney disease {231,2626}.

Multiple studies of genotype–phenotype correlations have demonstrated that TSC2 mutations are associated with a more severe phenotype overall: earlier seizure onset, higher number of tubers, and lower cognition index. However, within that spectrum, TSC2 missense mutations are associated with milder phenotypes {97,2231}.

Like in other tumour suppressor gene syndromes, somatic inactivation of the wildtype allele (i.e. LOH for the TSC1 or TSC2 locus) has been reported in kidney and cardiac lesions associated with tuberous sclerosis, as well as in SEGAs {406}. However, there is conflicting evidence of whether a so-called second hit is required for cortical tuber formation, raising the possibility that some lesions in tuberous sclerosis may be due to haploinsufficiency {1787,2762}. Furthermore, there is no evidence of inactivation of TSC1 or TSC2 in focal cortical dysplasias, which are histologically very similar to tuberous sclerosis tubers {2775}. In one recent study, loss of TSC1 in periventricular zone neuronal stem cells was sufficient to cause aberrant migration and giant cell phenotype, supportive of the two-hit hypothesis for tuber formation {683A,2862A}.

Signalling pathways involving tuberin and hamartin
The tuberin–hamartin complex is a signalling node that integrates growth factor and stress signals from the upstream PI3K/AKT pathway and transmits signals downstream to coordinate multiple cellular processes, including cell proliferation and cell size {486,1212,1987}. The complex negatively regulates the mTOR pathway {96,783,2528}. Disruption of the tuberin–hamartin complex causes upregulation of the mTOR pathway and increases proliferation and cell growth through two effector molecules: 4E-BP1 and S6K1 {96,2528}. The understanding of the basic mechanism of mTOR pathway activation in tuberous sclerosis lesions has led to the use of mTOR inhibitors in the treatment of manifestations of tuberous sclerosis. Several tuberous sclerosis–associated tumours, renal angiomyolipomas, SEGAs, and lymphangioleiomyomas show significant size reduction in response to treatment with mTOR inhibitors, and regrow when treatment is stopped. The effects of mTOR inhibitors are currently being evaluated for the clinical management of epilepsy and other neurological manifestations of tuberous sclerosis {509}.

Inheritance and genetic heterogeneity
Most tuberous sclerosis cases (~60%) are sporadic, with no family history, indicating a high rate of de novo mutations {2229A}. In affected kindreds, the disease follows an autosomal dominant pattern of inheritance, with high penetrance but considerable phenotypic variability {2354}.

Li–Fraumeni syndrome

Olivier M.
Kleihues P.
Ohgaki H.

Definition

An autosomal dominant disorder characterized by multiple primary neoplasms in children and young adults, with a predominance of soft tissue sarcomas, osteosarcomas, breast cancer, brain tumours, and adrenocortical carcinoma. Li–Fraumeni syndrome (LFS) is most commonly caused by a germline mutation in the *TP53* tumour suppressor gene on chromosome 17p13 {736,1575,2634}.

OMIM number {1624}   151623

Incidence/epidemiology

TP53 germline mutations have been estimated to occur at a rate of about 1 in 5000 to 1 in 20 000 births, and to account for as many as 17% of all familial cancer cases {864,1883}. Genetic and pedigree information on 767 families containing carriers of a *TP53* germline mutation is available in the International Agency for Research on Cancer (IARC) *TP53* Mutation Database [http://p53.iarc.fr].

Diagnostic criteria

Classic Li–Fraumeni syndrome clinical criteria

The classic LFS clinical criteria used to identify an affected individual in a family affected by LFS are: (1) occurrence of sarcoma before the age of 45 years, (2) at least one first-degree relative with any tumour before the age of 45 years, and (3) a second- or first-degree relative with cancer before the age of 45 years or a sarcoma at any age {1486}.

Criteria for diagnosis of Li–Fraumeni–like syndrome

Three main sets of criteria for the diagnosis of Li–Fraumeni–like syndrome (LFL), a variant of LFS, have been proposed to better identify *TP53* germline mutation carriers: the LFL-E2 definition, the LFL-B definition, and the Chompret criteria

The LFL-E2 definition

The criteria of the LFL-E2 definition (the second definition by Eeles) for the

Table 16.09 Frequency of tumour manifestation in various organ/tissue sites in *TP53* germline mutation carriers

Organ/tissue	Typical histological types	% of all tumours in *TP53* germline mutation carriers
Breast	Carcinoma	31%
Soft tissue	Soft tissue sarcoma	14%
CNS	Astrocytoma, glioblastoma, medulloblastoma, choroid plexus tumour	13%
Adrenal gland	Adrenal cortical carcinoma	12%
Bone	Osteosarcoma	9%

diagnosis of LFL are sarcoma at any age in the proband, plus any two of the following tumours within the family (including within a single individual): breast cancer at < 50 years, brain tumour, leukaemia, adrenocortical tumour, melanoma, prostate cancer, pancreatic cancer at < 60 years, or sarcoma at any age {1841}.

The LFL-B definition

The criteria of the LFL-B definition (the definition by Birch) for the diagnosis of LFL are any childhood cancer or sarcoma, brain tumour, or adrenocortical carcinoma at < 45 years in the proband, plus one first- or second-degree relative with a cancer typically associated with LFS (i.e. sarcoma, breast cancer, brain tumour, leukaemia, or adrenocortical carcinoma) at any age, plus one first- or second-degree relative in the same lineage with any cancer diagnosed at an age of < 60 years {208}.

The Chompret criteria

The 2009 version of the Chompret criteria for the diagnosis of LFL are (1) a tumour belonging to the LFS tumour spectrum (i.e. soft tissue sarcoma, osteosarcoma, premenopausal breast cancer, brain tumour, adrenocortical carcinoma, leukaemia, or lung adenocarcinoma in situ) at < 46 years in the proband and at least one first- or second-degree relative either with an LFS tumour (other than breast cancer if the proband is affected by breast cancer) at < 56 years or with multiple tumours; or (2) multiple tumours

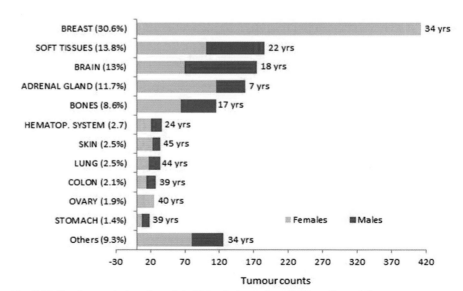

Fig. 16.20 Target organs for tumorigenesis in 1350 patients carrying a *TP53* germline mutation.

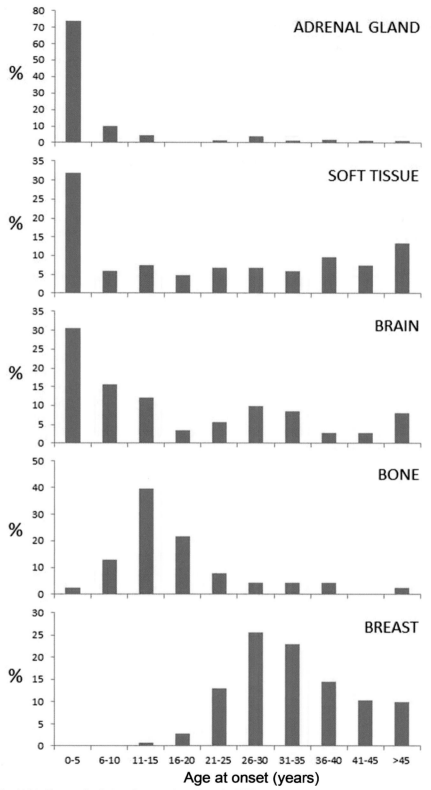

Fig. 16.21 The age distribution of tumours in carriers of a *TP53* germline mutation shows remarkable differences. Adrenocortical carcinomas occur almost exclusively in children aged ≤ 5 years. Soft tissue tumours (sarcomas) and brain tumours show an incidence peak in young children, whereas the remainder of the cases show a wide age distribution. Bone tumours have an incidence peak in the second decade of life, and breast carcinomas occur in young adults. Reprinted from Olivier M et al. {1294}.

(except multiple breast cancers) in the proband, the first of which occurs at < 46 years, and with at least two belonging to the LFS spectrum; or (3) adrenocortical carcinoma or choroid plexus carcinoma in the proband, regardless of family history {2559}.

Sites of involvement

Breast cancer, soft tissue sarcomas, CNS tumours, adrenal tumours, and bone tumours are the most frequent manifestations of LFS, accounting for about 80% of all tumours in patients carrying a *TP53* germline mutation. The sporadic counterparts of these tumours also show a high frequency of *TP53* mutations, suggesting that in these neoplasms, *TP53* mutations are capable of initiating the process of malignant transformation {1294}. In general, tumours associated with a *TP53* germline mutation develop earlier than their sporadic counterparts, but there are marked organ-specific differences. Adrenocortical carcinoma associated with a *TP53* germline mutation develops almost exclusively in children, in contrast to sporadic adrenocortical carcinoma, which has a broad age distribution with peak incidence in patients aged > 40 years {136}.

Nervous system neoplasms

In the 944 individuals carrying a *TP53* germline mutation who were included in the IARC *TP53* Database as of November 2013, a total of 1485 tumours were reported; 192 (13%) of which were located in the nervous system. The male-to-female ratio of patients with brain tumours associated with *TP53* germline mutation is 1.5:1 [http://p53.iarc.fr].

As with sporadic brain tumours, the age of patients with nervous system neoplasms associated with *TP53* germline mutations shows a bimodal distribution. The first incidence peak is in children (mainly medulloblastomas and related primitive neuroectodermal tumours, choroid plexus tumours, and ependymomas), and the second is in the third and fourth decades of life (mainly astrocytic brain tumours).

Gene structure

The *TP53* gene on chromosome 17p13 has 11 exons spanning 20 kb. Exon 1 is non-coding, and exons 5 to 8 are highly conserved among vertebrates.

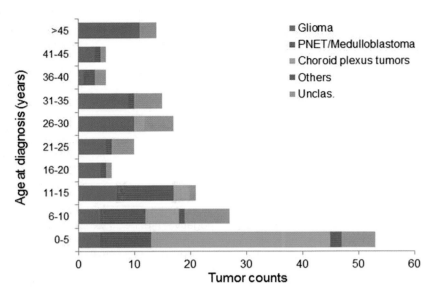

Fig. 16.22 Patient age at diagnosis and histological diagnosis of 173 brain tumours in carriers of a *TP53* germline mutation [http://p53.iarc.fr/SelectedStatistics.aspx]. PNET, primitive neuroectodermal tumour; Unclas., unclassified.

Distribution of *TP53* germline mutations

Most germline mutations of the *TP53* gene are spread over exons 5–8, with major hotspots at codons 133, 175, 245, 248, and 273 or 337. Missense mutations are most common, but nonsense mutations, deletions/insertions, and splice-site mutations also occur. Mutations observed at these codons are missense mutations that result in mutant proteins with complete loss of function, dominant negative phenotypes, and oncogenic activities.

Some codons (e.g. Cys176 and Arg249) that are commonly somatically mutated in sporadic tumours have never been reported as germline mutations {1841}. Residue 176 (Cys) is involved in the coordination of a zinc atom that forms a bridge between domain 1 and domain 3, and is crucial in stabilizing the architecture of the whole DNA-binding domain. Residue 249 (Arg) makes essential contacts with several residues of the scaffold through hydrogen bridges {447}. Two residues (codons 133 and 337) are hotspots for *TP53* germline mutations, but these are less frequent in sporadic cancers. A mutation at codon 133 (M133T) has been found in families with clustering of early-onset breast cancers (3–6 cases per family, with a mean patient age at onset of 34 years) [http://p53.iarc.fr], and a mutation at codon 337 (R337H) has been frequently found in Brazilian children affected by adrenocortical carcinomas {2111} and Brazilian families affected by LFL {5}.

Types of *TP53* mutations

The proportion of G:C→A:T transitions at CpG sites is higher in *TP53* germline mutations than in somatic mutations, but the proportions of G:C→A:T transitions at non-CpG sites and of G:C→T:A transversions are lower. G:C→A:T transitions at CpG sites are considered to be endogenous (e.g. resulting from deamination of 5-methylcytosine, which occurs spontaneously in almost all cell types but is usually corrected by DNA repair mechanisms). The difference observed may thus be explained by the fact that non-CpG G:C→A:T and G:C→T:A mutations are associated with exogenous carcinogen exposure, whereas germline mutations seem to result mainly from endogenous processes {1842,1843}.

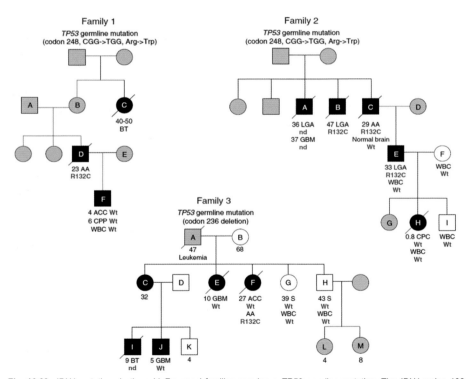

Fig. 16.23 *IDH1* mutations in three Li–Fraumeni families carrying a *TP53* germline mutation. The *IDH1* codon 132 status is indicated in blue letters. Wt, *IDH1*-wildtype; nd, not determined. DNA sequencing revealed identical *IDH1* R132C mutations in astrocytomas. All mutations were heterozygous. Round symbols, females; square symbols, males; black gender symbol, carrier of *TP53* germline mutation; white gender symbol, *TP53*-wildtype; grey gender symbol, no DNA available. Numbers below symbols indicate age at diagnosis or age at death (slash through symbol). All mutations were R132C mutations (CGT→TGT), which in sporadic astrocytomas account for < 5% of *IDH1* mutations. AA, anaplastic astrocytoma; LGA, low-grade diffuse astrocytoma; GBM, glioblastoma multiforme; ACC, adrenocortical carcinoma; CPP, choroid plexus papilloma; CPC, choroid plexus carcinoma; S, schwannoma; BT, brain tumour (no histological verification); WBC, white blood cells. No detailed medical history was available for family members without alphabetical letters. Reprinted from Watanabe T et al. {2710}.

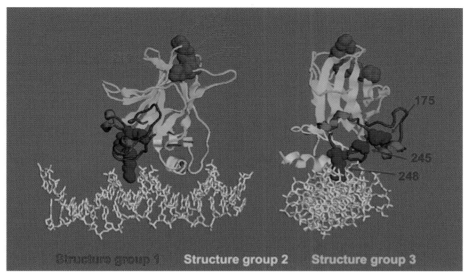

Fig. 16.24 Hotspot codon positions associated with adrenal gland carcinoma and brain tumours. A three-dimensional view of the central DNA-binding domain of the p53 protein in complex with DNA. Structural groups of residues are shown in different colours: group 1 residues, which correspond to L2 and L3 loops (binding in the minor groove of the DNA helix) are red; group 2 residues, which correspond to L1 loop and S2-S2'-H2 motifs (binding in the major groove of the DNA helix) are yellow; and group 3 residues, which correspond to the non–DNA-binding loops, the beta-sheet skeleton, or the oligomerization domain, are cyan. The codon positions of the mutations associated with adrenal gland carcinoma and brain tumours are indicated in violet and blue, respectively {1841}.

Multiple germline mutations

Recently, a family affected by LFS, with a *TP53* germline mutation (codon 236 deletion) and multiple nervous system tumours, was found to have additional germline mutations. Missense mutations in the *MSH4* DNA repair gene (c.2480T→A; p.I827N) were detected in 3 patients with gliomas (2 anaplastic astrocytomas, 2 glioblastomas). Another 2 family members, who developed peripheral schwannomas without a *TP53* germline mutation, also carried the *MSH4* germline mutation, as well as a germline mutation of the *LATS1* gene (c.286C→T; p.R96W), a downstream mediator of the *NF2* gene {1283}.

Gene expression

The *TP53* tumour suppressor gene encodes a 2.8 kb transcript encoding a 393 amino acid protein that is widely expressed at low levels. This protein is a multifunctional transcription factor involved in the control of cell cycle progression, DNA integrity, and the survival of cells exposed to DNA-damaging agents and non-genotoxic stimuli such as hypoxia. DNA damage or hypoxia induces a transient nuclear accumulation and activation of the p53 protein, with transcriptional activation of target genes that are responsible for the induction of cell cycle arrest or apoptosis {1311,1477}.

Gene function

The p53 protein is a multifunctional transcription factor involved in several pathways. Its best-characterized functions are in the control of cell cycle progression, DNA integrity, and the survival of cells exposed to DNA-damaging agents. However, accumulating evidence indicates that p53 also regulates other important processes, such as cell oxidative metabolism, the cellular response to nutrient deprivation, fertility, and the division and renewal of stem cells. The extent and consequences of the biological response elicited by p53 vary according to stress and cell type. *TP53* thus influences a wide range of biological and physiological processes {925}. The functions of p53 rely mainly on its transcriptional activity, but it can also act via interactions with various proteins. The roles of other protein isoforms in these activities remain largely unknown {1581}.

In most human cancers, *TP53* is inactivated through gene mutations that confer loss of the tumour suppressor role. p53-mutant proteins differ from each other in the extent to which they have lost suppressor function and in their capacity to inhibit wildtype p53 in a dominant negative manner {1232,1958}. In addition, some p53 mutants seem to exert an oncogenic activity of their own, but the molecular basis of this gain-of-function phenotype is still unclear {212}. The functional characteristics of each p53-mutant protein may depend, at least in part, on the degree of structural perturbation that the mutation imposes on the protein.

Genotype/phenotype

Among 139 families with at least one case of brain tumour, the mean number of CNS tumours per family was 1.55. Several reported families showed a remarkable clustering of brain tumours {155,1283, 2710}. This raises the question of whether some mutations carry an organ-specific or cell-specific risk.

An analysis of the IARC *TP53* Database [http://p53.iarc.fr] of germline mutations showed that brain tumours were more likely to be associated with missense mutations located in the DNA-binding surface of p53 protein that make contact with the minor groove of DNA {1841}. The type of mutation was also associated with the patient age at onset of brain tumours; truncating mutations were associated with early-onset brain tumours {1841}. Familial clustering may also be due to gene–environment interactions; for example, exposure of families to similar environmental carcinogens or lifestyle factors has been suggested in stomach and breast cancer {1294}.

Cowden syndrome

Eberhart C.G.
Wiestler O.D.
Eng C.

Definition

An autosomal dominant disorder characterized by multiple hamartomas involving tissues derived from all three germ cell layers and a high risk of breast, epithelial thyroid, endometrial, renal, and colon cancers. Facial trichilemmomas are highly characteristic of Cowden syndrome, which is caused mainly by germline mutations in *PTEN*. Adult-onset dysplastic cerebellar gangliocytoma (Lhermitte–Duclos disease) is also considered to be pathognomonic {245}. Recently, other Cowden syndrome predisposition genes have also been identified: the SDH genes, *PIK3CA*, and *KLLN*.

OMIM number {1624}   158350

Incidence/epidemiology

Before the identification of *PTEN*, the incidence of Cowden syndrome was estimated to be 1 case per 1 million population {2414}. After this gene for Cowden syndrome had been identified {1499}, a molecular-based estimate of prevalence in the same population was 1 case per 200 000 population {1764}. Due to difficulties in recognizing this syndrome, prevalence figures are likely to be underestimates. One recent study estimated de novo *PTEN* mutation frequency to be about 11% at minimum and 48% at maximum {1653}.

Diagnostic criteria

The National Comprehensive Cancer Network has established a set of operational clinical diagnostic criteria for identifying individuals with possible Cowden syndrome [http://www.nccn.org]. A recent prospective study subsequently led to the development of the Cleveland Clinic score – a semiquantitative scoring system that has shown greater adequacy than the National Comprehensive Cancer Network criteria [http://www.lerner.ccf.org/gmi/ccscore] {2503}. In response to the results of a study that found *PTEN* mutations in 15 of 18 unselected patients with a pathological diagnosis of dysplastic cerebellar gangliocytoma {2864},

Table 16.10 International Cowden Consortium operational diagnostic criteria

Pathognomonic criteria
Adult Lhermitte–Duclos disease (LDD)
Mucocutaneous lesions
Trichilemmomas (facial)
Acral keratoses
Papillomatous papules
Mucosal lesions
Major criteria
Breast cancer
Thyroid cancer (especially follicular)
Macrocephaly (> 97th percentile)
Endometrial carcinoma
Minor criteria
Other thyroid lesions (e.g. goitre or nodule)
Mental retardation
Hamartomatous intestinal polyps
Lipomas
Fibrocystic breast disease
Fibromas
Genitourinary tumours (e.g. uterine fibroids, renal cell carcinoma) or malformations
Requirements for diagnosis
Mucocutaneous lesions if:
- Six or more facial papules (of which three or more must be trichilemmoma), or
- Cutaneous facial papules and oral mucosal papillomatosis, or
- Oral mucosal papillomatosis and acral keratoses, or
- Six or more palmoplantar keratoses
- Two or more major criteria met (one must be macrocephaly or LDD)
One major criteria and three minor criteria
Four minor criteria
Requirements for diagnosis in individuals with a family member with Cowden syndrome
A pathognomonic criterion
Any one major criterion with or without minor criteria
Two minor criteria
History of Bannayan–Riley–Ruvalcaba syndrome

adult-onset Lhermitte–Duclos disease was revised from a major diagnostic criterion to a pathognomonic criterion and given the highest weight (of 10) in the *PTEN* Cleveland Clinic scoring system. Because of the variable and broad expression of Cowden syndrome and the lack of uniform diagnostic criteria prior to 1996, the International Cowden Consortium (ICC) {1765} compiled operational

diagnostic criteria for Cowden syndrome on the basis of the published literature and their own clinical experience {640, 2849}. Trichilemmomas and papillomatous papules are particularly important to recognize. Cowden syndrome usually presents within the third decade of life. It has variable and broad expression and an age-related penetrance. By the third decade of life, 99% of affected individuals have developed mucocutaneous stigmata, although any of the other features could already be present. The most commonly reported manifestations are mucocutaneous lesions, thyroid abnormalities, fibrocystic disease and carcinoma of the breast, gastrointestinal hamartomas, multiple early-onset uterine leiomyomas, macrocephaly (specifically, megalencephaly), and mental retardation {941,1525,2414,2849}.

Dysplastic cerebellar gangliocytoma (Lhermitte–Duclos disease)

This unusual tumour of the CNS is closely associated with Cowden syndrome {641, 1533,1873}. Adult-onset Lhermitte–Duclos disease, even in the absence of other features or family history, is highly predictive of a germline mutation in *PTEN* {2864}, and Lhermitte–Duclos disease is now considered pathognomonic for Cowden syndrome. Other malignancies and benign tumours have also been reported in patients or families with Cowden syndrome. Some authors believe that endometrial carcinoma could also be a component tumour of Cowden syndrome. It remains to be determined whether other tumours (e.g. sarcomas, lymphomas, leukaemias, and meningiomas) are true components of the syndrome. For details, see *Dysplastic cerebellar gangliocytoma (Lhermitte–Duclos disease)*, p. 142.

Intestinal hamartomatous polyps

In a small but systematic study of 9 well-documented cases of Cowden syndrome (7 of which had a germline mutation in *PTEN*), all 9 patients had hamartomatous polyps {2712}. Several varieties of hamartomatous polyps are seen in this syndrome, including hamartomas most similar to juvenile polyps composed of a mixture of connective tissues normally present in the mucosa (principally smooth muscle in continuity with the muscularis mucosae), lipomatous and ganglioneuromatous lesions, and lymphoid hyperplasia {364,2712}. These polyps are found in the stomach, duodenum, small bowel, and colon. Those in the colon and rectum usually measure 3–10 mm in diameter, but can reach 2 cm or more. Some of the polyps are no more than tags of mucosa, but others have a more definite structure. Examples containing adipose tissue have been described. The mucosal glands within the lesion are normal or elongated and irregularly formed, but the overlying epithelium is normal and includes goblet cells and columnar cells {364}. The presence of some ganglion tissue is not unusual in the juvenile-like polyps. Lesions in which autonomic nerves are predominant (resulting in a ganglioneuroma-like appearance) have also been described, but seem to be exceptional {1434}. The vast majority of Cowden syndrome hamartomatous polyps are asymptomatic, although adenomatous polyps and colon cancers have been observed in young patients with this condition {2850}. The association of gastrointestinal malignancy with Cowden syndrome is unknown, but appears to be likely. In a study of 9 individuals with Cowden syndrome, glycogenic acanthosis of the oesophagus was found in 6 of 7 individuals with PTEN mutation {2712}. It is likely that many more patients with Cowden syndrome will be identified in the future with ongoing screening for colon cancer, which should enable a more precise characterization of the phenotypic gastrointestinal features of this disease and the possible risk of gastrointestinal cancer. In an unselected series of 4 children with juvenile polyposis of infancy, this deletion also involved BMPR1A, upstream of PTEN. Subsequently, germline deletion involving both PTEN and BMPR1A was shown to characterize at least a subset of juvenile polyposis of infancy {571}.

Breast cancer

The two most commonly occurring cancers in Cowden syndrome are carcinomas of the breast and thyroid {2414, 2849}. In the general population, the lifetime risks of breast and thyroid cancers are approximately 11% (among women), and 1% (among both sexes), respectively. Breast cancer has also been rarely observed in men with Cowden syndrome {1589}. In women with Cowden syndrome, estimates of the lifetime risk of breast cancer range from 25% to 50% {640,941, 1525,2414,2849}. The mean patient age at diagnosis is probably about 10 years younger than for breast cancer occurring in the general population {1525,2414}. Although Rachel Cowden died of breast cancer at the age of 31 years {293,1521} and the youngest reported patient age at diagnosis of breast cancer is 14 years {2414}, the great majority of breast cancers are diagnosed in patients aged > 30–35 years (range: 14–65 years) {1525}. The predominant histology is ductal adenocarcinoma. Most Cowden syndrome breast carcinomas occur in the context of ductal carcinoma in situ, atypical ductal hyperplasia, adenosis, and sclerosis {2298}.

Thyroid cancer

The lifetime risk of epithelial thyroid cancer can be as high as 10% in patients with Cowden syndrome. Because of the small number of cases, it is unclear whether the average patient age at onset in this setting is truly younger than that in the general population. Histologically, thyroid cancer is predominantly follicular carcinoma, although papillary histology has also been rarely observed {941,1576, 2414,2849}. Medullary thyroid carcinoma has not been observed in patients with Cowden syndrome.

Skin tumours

The most important benign tumours in Cowden syndrome are trichilemmomas and papillomatous papules of the skin. Benign tumours and disorders of the breast and thyroid are the next most common, and probably constitute true component features of the syndrome. Fibroadenomas and fibrocystic disease of the breast are common signs of Cowden syndrome, as are follicular adenomas and multinodular goitre of the thyroid.

Prognosis and predictive factors

There have been no systematic studies to indicate whether the prognosis for patients with Cowden syndrome who have cancer is different from that of their counterparts with sporadic cancer.
When activated mTOR signalling was identified as an important downstream response to PTEN dysfunction or deficiency (see Gene expression), mTOR inhibition was shown to be effective in vitro and in animal models {2407}. The mTOR inhibitor sirolimus (also known as rapamycin) was shown to be effective in a child with Proteus syndrome who also carried a germline mutation in PTEN {1594}. An open-label phase II trial (NCI-08-C-0151) of sirolimus for the treatment of human Cowden syndrome and other syndromes characterized by germline PTEN mutations was recently completed, but the results have not yet been published [https://clinicaltrials.gov/ct2/show/study/NCT00971789].

Chromosomal location and mode of transmission

Cowden syndrome is an autosomal dominant disorder, with age-related penetrance and variable expression {641,1786,2504}. The major Cowden syndrome susceptibility gene, PTEN, is located on 10q23.3 {1489,1499,1765}. Other predisposition genes include the SDH genes, PIK3CA, AKT1, and KLLN {168,1781,1782,1852}.

Gene structure

PTEN, on 10q23, consists of nine exons spanning 120–150 kb of genomic distance and encodes a 1.2 kb transcript and a 403 amino acid lipid dual-specificity phosphatase (dephosphorylating both protein and lipid substrates), which is homologous to the focal adhesion molecules tensin and auxilin {1489,1589,2418}. The amino acid sequence that is homologous to tensin and auxilin is encoded by exons 1–6. A classic phosphatase core motif is encoded within exon 5, which is the largest exon, constituting 20% of the coding region {1485,1489,2418}. A longer isoform of PTEN has also been described, which apparently interacts with the mitochondrion, but its clinical impact is still unclear {2043}.

Gene expression

PTEN is virtually ubiquitously expressed {2418}. Detailed studies of expression in human development have not been performed, and only a single study has examined PTEN expression during human embryogenesis using a monoclonal antibody against the terminal 100 amino acids of PTEN {842}. The study revealed high levels of expression of PTEN protein in the skin, thyroid, and CNS – organs that are affected by the component neoplasias of Cowden syndrome. It also revealed prominent expression in the developing autonomic nervous system and gastrointestinal tract. Early embryonic death in *Pten–/–* mice also implies a crucial role for PTEN in early development {581,1992,2463}. PTEN is a tumour suppressor and a dual-specificity lipid phosphatase that plays multiple roles in the cell cycle, apoptosis, cell polarity, cell migration, and even genomic stability {1729,2340,2849}. The major substrate of PTEN is PIP_3, which is part of the PI3K pathway {517,767,1488,1563,2411}. When PTEN is ample and functional, PIP_3 is converted to PIP_2, which results in hypophosphorylated AKT, a known cell-survival factor. Hypophosphorylated AKT is apoptotic. When PTEN is in the cytoplasm, it predominantly signals via its lipid phosphatase activity down the PI3K/AKT pathways {1676}. In contrast, when PTEN is in the nucleus, it predominantly signals via protein phosphatase activity down the cyclin-D1/MAPK pathway, eliciting G1 arrest at least in breast and glioma cells {767,768,1488,1676}. It is also thought that PTEN can dephosphorylate FAK and inhibit integrin and MAPK signalling {892,2501}.

Genotype/phenotype

Gene mutations
Approximately 85% of Cowden syndrome cases, as strictly defined by the ICC criteria, have a germline mutation in *PTEN*, including intragenic mutations, promoter mutations, and large deletions/rearrangements {1499,1589,2865}. If the diagnostic criteria are relaxed, this mutation frequency drops to 10–50% {1554, 1766,2581}. A formal study that ascertained 64 unrelated Cowden syndrome–like cases found a mutation frequency of 2% if the criteria were not met, even if the diagnosis was made short of only one criterion {1590}. However, this study

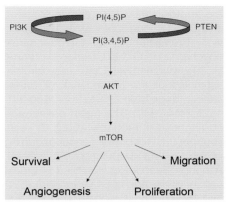

Fig. 16.25 Schematic representation of the PI3K/AKT/mTOR signalling pathway. When PTEN is downregulated, AKT is upregulated, leading to upregulation of mTOR. Reprinted from Blumenthal GM and Dennis PA {220}.

only looked at the nine exons of *PTEN*; presumably, further mutations would have been identified in the promoter or in *SDHB/SDHD*. A single-centre study involving 37 unrelated families affected by Cowden syndrome (as strictly defined by the ICC criteria) found a mutation frequency of 80% {1589}. Exploratory genotype–phenotype analyses showed that the presence of a germline mutation was associated with a familial risk of developing malignant breast disease {1589}. Additionally, missense mutations and/or mutations of the phosphatase core motif seem to be associated with a surrogate for disease severity (multiorgan involvement). A small study of 13 families with 8 *PTEN* mutation–positive members did not show any genotype–phenotype associations {1764}, but this may be due to the small sample size.

Bannayan–Riley–Ruvalcaba syndrome
Bannayan–Riley–Ruvalcaba syndrome, which is characterized by macrocephaly, lipomatosis, haemangiomatosis, and speckled penis, was previously thought to be clinically distinct, but is now considered likely to be allelic to Cowden syndrome {1591}. In a combined cohort of 16 sporadic and 27 familial cases of Bannayan–Riley–Ruvalcaba syndrome,

approximately 60% of the patients carried a germline mutation in *PTEN* {1592}. Of the 27 familial cases studied, 11 were classified as exhibiting true overlap of Cowden syndrome and Bannayan–Riley–Ruvalcaba syndrome, and 10 of those 11 had a *PTEN* mutation. Another 10% of patients with Bannayan–Riley–Ruvalcaba syndrome were subsequently found to harbour larger germline deletions of *PTEN* {2865}. The overlapping mutation spectrum, existence of true-overlap familial cases, and genotype–phenotype associations suggest that the presence of germline *PTEN* mutation is associated with cancer, and strongly suggest that Cowden syndrome and Bannayan–Riley–Ruvalcaba syndrome are allelic and part of a single spectrum at the molecular level. The aggregate term "*PTEN* hamartoma tumour syndrome" was first proposed in 1999 {1592} and has since become even more apt, now that germline *PTEN* mutations have been identified in autism spectrum disorder with macrocephaly, Proteus syndrome, and VATERL association (the co-occurrence of several birth defects) with macrocephaly {330,2081,2863}. In one case, the identification of a germline intragenic *PTEN* mutation in a patient thought to have juvenile polyposis {1844} was subsequently considered to exclude that specific clinical diagnosis; the finding instead suggests a molecular designation of *PTEN* hamartoma tumour syndrome {642,1052,1053,1396,1593,1851}. This conclusion has been further supported by the identification of germline *PTEN* mutations/deletions in individuals with juvenile polyps, and of large deletions involving both *PTEN* and *BMPR1A* in juvenile polyposis of infancy {571,2469}. An important finding of the polyp-ascertainment study was that the reasons for referral listed in the original pathology reports were often incorrect, suggesting that re-review of all polyp histologies by gastrointestinal pathologists based in major academic medical centres is a vital step for determining correct genetic etiology {2469}.

Turcot syndrome

Cavenee W.K.
Hawkins C.
Burger P.C.
Leung S.Y.
Van Meir E.G.
Tabori U.

Definition

When the association of brain tumours with gastrointestinal polyps and cancers was originally described, it was called Turcot syndrome {2590}. Now, these associations are considered to constitute two very distinct cancer syndromes with distinct inheritance and cancer spectrums {1886A}.

Early-onset colon cancer and gliomas have also been reported in Li–Fraumeni syndrome (see p. 310).

Brain tumour–polyposis syndrome 1 (BTP1) / Mismatch repair cancer syndrome

An autosomal dominant cancer syndrome with reduced penetrance, caused by biallelic mutations in one of four mismatch repair genes (MLH1, PMS2, MSH2, and MSH6) and hence also called mismatch repair cancer syndrome.

Unlike heterozygous carriers (i.e. patients with Lynch syndrome 1), who develop mostly colon and genitourinary cancers as adults, individuals with mismatch repair cancer syndrome develop multiple brain tumours and other malignancies during childhood {615}. Importantly, family history is often uninformative for these and Lynch-related cancers.

OMIM number {1624}   276300

Incidence/epidemiology

More than 200 cases of mismatch repair cancer syndrome have been reported {113,2763}. However, this syndrome is underdiagnosed and highly prevalent in South Asian and Middle Eastern countries, where consanguinity is high.

Diagnostic criteria

The combination of café-au-lait macules; consanguinity; and specific brain, haematological, and gastrointestinal cancers, in particular during childhood, should raise suspicion for mismatch repair cancer syndrome. Recently, a scoring system was developed for proceeding to genetic

testing for mismatch repair cancer syndrome {2763}. Detection of germline biallelic mutation in one of the four main mismatch repair genes is required for the diagnosis of mismatch repair cancer syndrome, but the abundance of variants of unknown significance and the technical problems with sequencing PMS2, which has multiple pseudogenes, has led to the development of several functional assays that can aid in rapid detection of mismatch repair deficiency in urgent cases. Unlike in Lynch syndrome, microsatellite instability is not a reliable test for mismatch repair cancer syndrome. Most mutations cause loss of gene expression; correspondingly, immunohistochemical staining demonstrates loss of expression of the protein encoded by the gene in both tumour and normal tissue in > 90% of cases {113}. Cell-based assays on normal fibroblasts and lymphoblasts can detect microsatellite instability, resistance to several compounds {230}, and failure to repair G–T mismatches {2353}.

Sites of involvement

Nervous system neoplasms

Brain tumours (most commonly malignant gliomas) occur in the first two decades of life and account for 25–40% of all mismatch repair cancer syndrome cancers {113,2763}. Many of these brain tumours have prominent nuclear pleomorphism and multinucleation reminiscent of pleomorphic xanthoastrocytoma or giant cell glioblastoma {652}. Recognition of these features may prompt immunohistochemical testing for loss of the mismatch repair proteins. Oligodendrogliomas, pleomorphic astrocytomas, and other low-grade gliomas have also been reported. Medulloblastoma and primitive neuroectodermal tumour have also been described and can include some glial features. Molecularly, these cancers have a unique ultra-hypermutation phenotype, which distinguishes them from other childhood tumours {2353}.

Extraneural manifestations

More than 90% of patients present with café-au-lait macules and other dermatological abnormalities {113}. These must be distinguished from neurofibromatosis type 1–related skin lesions. Haematological malignancies, predominantly T-cell lymphoma, occur mostly in the first decade, in as many as 30% of patients, whereas gastrointestinal polyposis and cancers are present in virtually all patients by the second decade of life. Other cancers (e.g. urinary tract cancers and sarcomas) have also been reported {113, 2763}.

Gene structure

The genetic defect underlying mismatch repair cancer syndrome is the inability to recognize and repair DNA mismatches during replication. Of the components of the mismatch repair apparatus, the human genes causing mismatch repair cancer syndrome are MLH1 at chromosome 3p21.3, MSH2 at 2p16, MSH3 at 5q11-q13, MSH6 at 2p16, PMS1 at 2q32, and PMS2 at 7p22. Recognition and repair of base-pair mismatches in human DNA is mediated by heterodimers of MSH2 and MSH6, which form a sliding clamp on DNA. The C-terminus of PMS2 interacts with MLH1, and this complex binds to MSH2/MSH6 heterodimers to form a functional strand-specific mismatch recognition complex {2366}. Cells that are deficient in any of the above genes are defective in repair of mismatched bases and insertions/deletions of single nucleotides, resulting in high mutation rates and microsatellite instability. Unlike in heterozygous carriers (in whom microsatellite instability is observed in all cancers), cancers originating in patients with biallelic mismatch repair cancer syndrome often lack microsatellite instability and are characterized instead by extremely high rates of single-nucleotide mutations {113,2353}.

Genotype/phenotype

In BTP1, the genotype/phenotype is difficult to ascertain due to the rarity of the syndrome. Whereas in Lynch syndrome germline mutations in *MLH1* and *MSH2* are the most prevalent, in BTP1 mutations in *PMS2* and *MSH6* predominate and germline mutations in *MSH2* are rarely observed. Heterozygous carriers are usually unaffected.

In one study, the median patient age at occurrence of glioblastoma in BTP1 / mismatch repair cancer syndrome was found to be 18 years (whereas the peak incidence in the general population occurs in patients aged 40–70 years) {2624}. These patients had an average survival of > 27 months, which is substantially longer than that of patients with sporadic cases (12 month). Many of the long-term survivors belong to the group of patients with biallelic germline *PMS2* mutation, some of whom were still alive > 10 years after treatment of their gliomas {554,937,2574}.

Genetic counselling

Patients with mismatch repair cancer syndrome and their family members may benefit from genetic counselling, because surveillance protocols exist and early detection may result in increased survival for both biallelic and heterozygous carriers {614,2635}. The inherent resistance of mismatch repair–deficient cells to several common chemotherapies, including temozolomide, should be considered in the management of gliomas in the setting of mismatch repair cancer syndrome. In contrast, the ultra-hypermutation phenotype of mismatch repair cancer syndrome–related cancers {2353} can be exploited by potential therapies such as immune checkpoint blockade {1441}.

Brain tumour–polyposis syndrome 2 (BTP2) / Familial adenomatous polyposis

An autosomal dominant cancer syndrome caused by heterozygous mutations in the tumour suppressor gene *APC*.

The prominent cancers associated with BTP2 are tumours of the gastrointestinal tract. The main brain tumour reported in association with BTP2 is medulloblastoma (rather than gliomas, which are associated with BTP1).

OMIM number {1624}   276300

Incidence/epidemiology

BTP2 is responsible for approximately 1% of all colon cancers. However, brain tumours, specifically medulloblastoma, are rare in BTP2, accounting for < 1% of all malignancies in this patient population {1472,2429}.

Diagnostic criteria

The hallmark of BTP2 is the emergence of hundreds to thousands of colonic polyps at a young age {2636}.

Sites of involvement

Nervous system neoplasms
Medulloblastoma is the only brain tumour clearly associated with BTP2. However, although the risk of developing medulloblastoma is 90 times as high among individuals with BTP2 as in the general population, this tumour is still rarely observed in BTP2, accounting for < 1% of all malignancies in this patient population {1472}.

Extraneural manifestations
Individuals with BTP2 are at high risk of developing colorectal cancers as well as additional cancers, such as osteomas (in 50–90% of cases), aggressive fibromatosis (in 10–15%), thyroid cancers (in 2–3%), and hepatoblastoma (in 1%) {1472}.

Gene structure

BTP2 results from germline heterozygous mutations in the tumour suppressor gene *APC* {1879}. *APC* is located on chromosome 5q21 and is a major tumour suppressor in the WNT pathway. Activation of the pathway, most commonly through alterations in beta-catenin, is observed in 10–15% of all medulloblastomas {2524}, but the association between WNT activation and BTP2-associated medulloblastoma is not clear.

Genotype/phenotype

In BTP2, the median patient age for occurrence of medulloblastomas was 15 years, which matches the patient age for the WNT-activated subtype of sporadic medulloblastoma, although whether these tumours carry the same favourable prognosis as WNT-activated medulloblastoma is unclear. Although the numbers are small, in families affected by familial adenomatous polyposis, the appearance of medulloblastoma at a young age in patients with no evidence of polyps may indicate a poor prognosis {2624}.

Genetic counselling

BTP2 is a well-characterized syndrome with clinical and molecular diagnostic criteria {2636}. Surveillance protocols exist and preventive colectomy is required in most patients. Due to the rarity of brain tumours in BTP2, surveillance does not include brain MRI, and no specific therapies are recommended for BTP2-related medulloblastoma {1472,2636}.

Naevoid basal cell carcinoma syndrome

Eberhart C.G.
Cavenee W.K.
Pietsch T.

Definition

An autosomal dominant disease associated with developmental disorders and predisposition to benign and malignant tumours, including basal cell carcinomas of the skin, odontogenic keratocysts, palmar and plantar dyskeratotic pits, intracranial calcifications, macrocephaly, and medulloblastomas of the desmoplastic/nodular subtypes; caused by germline mutations of genes encoding members of the hedgehog signalling pathway, including the *PTCH1* gene on 9q22, its homologue *PTCH2* on 1p34, and the *SUFU* gene on 10q24.

OMIM number {1624}   109400

Synonyms

Naevoid basal cell carcinoma syndrome is also known as Gorlin syndrome, Gorlin–Goltz syndrome, basal cell naevus syndrome, and fifth phacomatosis.

Incidence/epidemiology

A prevalence of 1 case per 57 000 population has been reported {657}. About 1–2% of patients with medulloblastoma carry a *PTCH1* germline mutation {657}. Of 131 children with medulloblastomas, 6% had germline *SUFU* mutations {294}. About 2% of patients with naevoid basal cell carcinoma syndrome with germline *PTCH1* mutations develop medulloblastoma, and the risk is as much as 20% higher in patients with germline *SUFU* mutations {2376}. Naevoid basal cell carcinoma syndrome caused by *PTCH2* mutations is rare; only two families have been described {667,747}.

Diagnostic criteria

The most common manifestations of naevoid basal cell carcinoma syndrome are multiple basal cell carcinomas, as well as odontogenic keratocysts of the jaw. In one study, basal cell carcinomas and odontogenic keratocysts were found together in > 90% of affected individuals by the age of 40 years {660}. Other major criteria include calcification of the falx cerebri, palmar and plantar pits, bifid or fused ribs, and first-degree relatives with the syndrome {1284,2331}. The minor criteria include medulloblastoma (mainly of the desmoplastic/nodular subtypes {67}), ovarian fibroma, macrocephaly, congenital facial abnormalities (e.g. cleft lip or palate, frontal bossing, and hypertelorism), skeletal abnormalities (e.g. digit syndactyly), and radiological bone abnormalities (e.g. bridging of the sella turcica) {67,1284}. The diagnosis of naevoid basal cell carcinoma syndrome is made when two or more major or one major and two or more minor criteria are present {67}. The clinical features manifest at different points in life. Macrocephaly and rib anomalies can be detected at birth, and medulloblastoma typically develops within the first 3 years of life. Jaw cysts do not become evident before the age of about 10 years, and basal cell carcinomas can be detected 10 years later {746A}. Several other tumour types have also been reported in individual patients with naevoid basal cell carcinoma syndrome, including meningioma, melanoma, chronic lymphocytic leukaemia, non-Hodgkin lymphoma, ovarian dermoid cyst, and breast and lung carcinoma. However, the statistical significance of the association between these neoplasms and naevoid basal cell carcinoma syndrome has yet to be demonstrated {2331}. Radiation treatment of patients with naevoid basal cell carcinoma syndrome, for example, craniospinal irradiation for the treatment of cerebellar medulloblastoma, induces multiple basal cell carcinomas of the skin as well as various other tumour types within the radiation field {405,1813,2416}.

Sites of involvement

Naevoid basal cell carcinoma syndrome–associated medulloblastoma

In a recent review of 33 reported medulloblastoma cases associated with naevoid basal cell carcinoma syndrome, all but one tumour had developed in children aged < 5 years, and 22 cases (66%) had presented in patients aged < 2 years {67}. Medulloblastomas associated with naevoid basal cell carcinoma syndrome seem to be exclusively of the desmoplastic/nodular variants (see *Desmoplastic/nodular medulloblastoma*, p. 195, and *Medulloblastoma with extensive nodularity*, p. 198) {67,787,2296,2376}. It has therefore been proposed that desmoplastic medulloblastomas in children aged < 2 years serve as a major criterion for the diagnosis of naevoid basal cell carcinoma syndrome {67,787}. The prognosis of naevoid basal cell carcinoma syndrome–associated medulloblastomas seems to be better than that of sporadic cases, and it has been suggested that radiation therapy protocols be adjusted in patients aged < 5 years with naevoid basal cell carcinoma syndrome, to prevent the formation of secondary tumours {67,2416}.

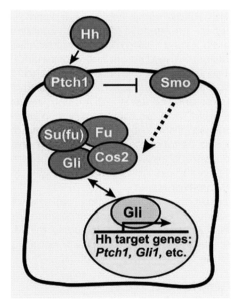

Fig. 16.26 The SHH pathway. In normal development, hedgehog signalling is activated by interaction of a secreted hedgehog ligand (Hh) with the multipass transmembrane receptor PTCH. Ligand binding relieves the repressive effects of PTCH on SMO and permits the activation and nuclear translocation of GLI transcription factors. GLI activation is also promoted by FU, and suppressed by SU(FU). COS2 proteins are thought to serve as a scaffold for these interactions. Once in the nucleus, GLI factors induce the transcription of various pathway targets, including feedback loops involving *PTCH1* and *GLI1*.

Other CNS manifestations

There is no statistically proven evidence of an increased risk of other CNS neoplasms in naevoid basal cell carcinoma syndrome. Nevertheless, several instances of meningioma arising in patients with naevoid basal cell carcinoma syndrome have been reported {40,2331}. Various malformative changes of the brain and skull, including calcification of the falx cerebri and/or tentorium cerebelli at a young age, dysgenesis of the corpus callosum, congenital hydrocephalus, and macrocephaly, may occur in affected family members.

Gene structure

Naevoid basal cell carcinoma syndrome results from inactivating germline mutations in the human homologue of the *Drosophila* segment polarity patched gene (*PTCH1*) on 9q22 {924,1172}, its homologue *PTCH2* on 1p34 {667,747}, or *SUFU* on 10q {2376}. The detection rate of specific mutations has increased significantly (with as many as 93% of cases found positive in recent years), due to the development of improved methods of detection {746A}.

The *PTCH1* gene spans approximately 50 kb of genomic DNA and contains ≥ 23 exons {924,1172}, with alternative usage of five different first exons {1740}. The *PTCH2* gene on chromosome 1p34 spans approximately 15 kb of genomic DNA and contains 22 coding exons {2384}. The *SUFU* gene is a human homologue of the *Drosophila* suppressor of fused (*Sufu*) gene. It maps to 10q24 and contains 12 exons {888A,1320A}.

Gene expression

Tissue-specific expression patterns of various PTC1 isoforms occur through extensive splicing events, including mRNA species encoding dominant negative forms of PTC1 {1739,1740,2591}.

Gene function

The *PTCH1* gene codes for a 12-transmembrane protein (PTC1) expressed on many progenitor cell types. PTC1 functions as a receptor for members of the secreted hedgehog protein family of signalling molecules {1585,2433}. In humans, this family consists of three members: SHH, IHH, and DHH. The *PTCH1* gene product has homology to bacterial transporter proteins {2491} and controls another transmembrane protein, SMO

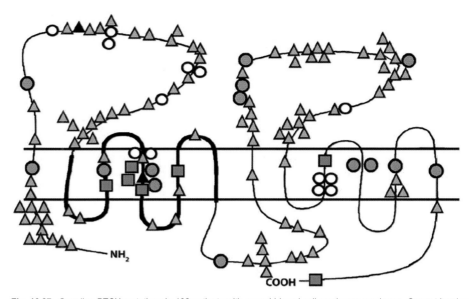

Fig. 16.27 Germline PTCH mutations in 132 patients with naevoid basal cell carcinoma syndrome. Green triangles represent nonsense mutations; open circles, splice mutations; purple circles, familial missense mutations; black triangles, de novo missense mutations; and blue squares, germline conserved missense mutations. The thick black line indicates the location of the sterol-sensing domain. Adapted from Lindström E et al. {1510}.

{44,2433}. In the absence of ligand, PTC1 inhibits the activity of SMO {44,2433}. Hedgehog signalling takes place in the primary cilium {96A}. Binding of hedgehog proteins to PTC1 can relieve this inhibition of SMO, allowing its translocation to the tip of the primary cilium, which results in the activation and translocation of GLI transcription factors into the cell nucleus and transcription of a set of specific target genes controlling the survival, differentiation, and proliferation of progenitor cells. In vertebrates, this pathway is critically involved in the development of various tissues and organ systems, such as limbs, gonads, bone, and the CNS {868,1092}. Germline mutations in the *SHH* and PTCH genes have been found to cause holoprosencephaly {163,1678A, 2161}. *PTCH2* encodes a homologue of *PTCH1*, whereas *SUFU* is located downstream in the hedgehog pathway. SUFU has been found to directly interact with GLI proteins and is a negative regulator of hedgehog signalling {2433A}.

Genotype/phenotype

To date, numerous different *PTCH1* germline mutations associated with naevoid basal cell carcinoma syndrome have been reported {746A,1510}, although mutations are not detected in all cases {1588}. However, the detection rate of specific mutations has increased significantly (with as many as 93% of cases

found positive in recent years), due to the development of improved methods of detection {746A}. The mutations are distributed over the entire *PTCH1* coding region, with no mutational hotspots, and there seems to be no clear genotype–phenotype correlation {2745}. Missense mutations cluster in a highly conserved region (the sterol-sensing domain), and particularly in transmembrane domain 4. Somatic *PTCH1* mutations have been demonstrated in various sporadic human tumours (for review, see {1510}), including basal cell carcinoma {774,924,1172}, trichoepithelioma {2668}, oesophageal squamous cell carcinoma {1565}, invasive transitional cell carcinoma of the bladder {1621}, and medulloblastoma {1510,1973,2055,2667}. Like germline mutations, the vast majority of mutations detected in sporadic tumours result in truncations at the protein level. There is no obvious clustering of mutation sites. In a study of 68 sporadic medulloblastomas, *PTCH1* mutations were exclusively detected in the desmoplastic variant, and not in the 57 tumours with classic morphology {1973}. Consistent with these data, LOH analyses of sporadic medulloblastomas have demonstrated frequent allelic loss at 9q22.3–q31 in desmoplastic medulloblastomas (in as many as 50% of cases), but not in classic medulloblastomas {42,2296}. These data are consistent with the observation that most medulloblastomas associated with naevoid basal cell carcinoma syndrome are of the desmoplastic/nodular variant types, indicating a strong association between desmoplastic phenotype and pathological hedgehog pathway activation {67}. PTCH2, a PTCH1 homologue located at chromosome band 1p34, has also been found to contain somatic mutations in isolated cases of medulloblastoma and basal cell carcinoma {2384}. This gene has been found to have caused naevoid basal cell carcinoma syndrome in two families; one mutation was a truncating frameshift mutation and the other was a missense mutation encoding a protein that could not inhibit cell proliferation

{667,747}. The SUFU mutations found to be associated with naevoid basal cell carcinoma syndrome are missense mutations, splice site mutations, or deletions {1905A,2376}. In 6% of patients with medulloblastoma, germline SUFU mutations were identified, including missense, nonsense, and splice site mutations leading to a frameshift. Large duplications and deletions were also found, although these patients do not fulfil the criteria of naevoid basal cell carcinoma syndrome {294,2523}. Several somatic SUFU mutations have also been identified in some hedgehog-activated medulloblastomas {1333}.

Genetic counselling
The condition follows an autosomal dominant pattern of inheritance, with full penetrance but variable clinical phenotypes. The rate of new PTCH1 mutations has not been precisely determined. It has been estimated that a high proportion (14–81%) of cases are the result of new mutations {660,869,2331,2744}. In 4 of 6 cases of naevoid basal cell carcinoma syndrome with a germline SUFU mutation, the mutation was inherited from an unaffected, healthy parent. In the other 2 cases, the mutation was new {2376}.

Rhabdoid tumour predisposition syndrome

Wesseling P.
Biegel J.A.
Eberhart C.G.
Judkins A.R.

Definition
A disorder characterized by a markedly increased risk of developing malignant rhabdoid tumours (MRTs), generally due to constitutional loss or inactivation of one allele of the SMARCB1 gene – rhabdoid tumour predisposition syndrome 1 (RTPS1) – or (extremely rarely) of the SMARCA4 gene – rhabdoid tumour predisposition syndrome 2 (RTPS2).
SMARCB1 has also been identified as a predisposing gene in familial schwannomatosis, and germline mutations in both SMARCB1 and SMARCA4 contribute to Coffin–Siris syndrome (a rare congenital malformation syndrome characterized by developmental delay or intellectual disability, coarse facial appearance, feeding difficulties, frequent infections, and hypoplasia/aplasia of the fifth fingernails and fifth distal phalanges).

OMIM numbers {1624}
RTPS1   609322
RTPS2   613325

Synonyms
Rhabdoid tumour predisposition syndrome (RTPS) is also known as rhabdoid predisposition syndrome and familial posterior fossa brain tumour syndrome of infancy.

Incidence/epidemiology
Germline SMARCB1 mutations are estimated to occur in more than one third of all patients with atypical teratoid/rhabdoid tumours (AT/RTs) (i.e. the CNS representative of MRTs) {192,616}. Given this risk, it is important to investigate the SMARCB1 status in all newly diagnosed cases by molecular genetic analysis. Individuals with a germline mutation are more likely to present with a tumour in the first year of life.

Diagnostic criteria
Demonstration of a germline SMARCB1 or SMARCA4 mutation in a patient with MRT is sufficient for the diagnosis of RTPS1 or RTPS2, respectively {2293, 2409}. Children with multiple MRTs or with affected siblings or other relatives are almost certain to be affected by RTPS themselves.

Sites of involvement

Nervous system neoplasms
Individuals with RTPS1 often present with AT/RT (p. 209). Patients with germline mutations or deletions of SMARCB1 may develop isolated AT/RTs or an AT/RT with a synchronous renal or extrarenal MRT {1454}. AT/RTs generally occur in early

childhood, but are occasionally found in adults {2063}.
Other CNS tumours that have been reported to be associated with RTPS include choroid plexus carcinoma {802}, medulloblastoma, and supratentorial primitive neuroectodermal tumour {2327}. However, because the histopathological distinction of these tumours from AT/RTs can be challenging, and because the rhabdoid component may be missed due to sampling effects, the occurrence of such tumours in the context of RTPS is controversial {918,1190,1192,2599}.
SMARCB1 has also been identified as a gene predisposing individuals to familial schwannomatosis. This gene seems to be involved in about 50% of familial cases (but ≤ 10% of sporadic cases) {260, 921,2191}. SMARCB1 germline mutations are also reported to predispose individuals to the development of multiple meningiomas, with preferential location of the cranial meningiomas at the falx cerebri {102,455,2622}.
A spectrum of CNS tumours, including meningiomas, gliomas, melanomas, and carcinomas, may show rhabdoid features. Generally, such so-called composite rhabdoid tumours retain nuclear SMARCB1 staining {1941}, strongly suggesting that they do not contain the same

genetic alterations as classic MRT and are therefore unlikely to be part of RTPS.

Extraneural manifestations
By far the most frequent extra-CNS location of MRT is the kidney. Bilateral renal MRTs are almost always associated with a germline *SMARCB1* mutation, but infants with an isolated MRT may carry germline mutations as well. Occasionally, MRTs have been reported to originate in the head and neck region, paraspinal soft tissues, heart, mediastinum, and liver {2737}. In a child surviving a thoracic MRT, a conventional chondrosarcoma developed in the mandibula. The chondrosarcoma showed deletion of one *SMARCB1* allele and a premature stop codon in the remaining allele {723}. In a patient with schwannomatosis, a leiomyoma of the cervix uteri was reported to display the genetic features that are characteristic of germline *SMARCB1* mutation–associated tumours {1062}. *SMARCB1* mutations may occasionally underlie the oncogenesis of other neoplasms, such as the proximal type of epithelioid sarcoma {1697}, but to date, these sarcomas have not been described in association with RTPS.

In a family with a *SMARCA4* germline mutation, AT/RT and ovarian cancer were diagnosed in a newborn and his mother, respectively, providing a link between AT/RT and small cell carcinoma of the ovary of hypercalcaemic type {2766}. After a subsequent study of three families with small cell carcinoma of the ovary of hypercalcaemic type revealed deleterious *SMARCA4* mutations in all cases, it was suggested that these tumours should be renamed "MRT of the ovary" {728}.

Gene structure and expression

The *SMARCB1* gene was the first subunit of the SWI/SNF complex found to be mutated in cancer. This gene is located in chromosome region 22q11.23 and contains nine exons spanning 50 kb of genomic DNA {2649}. Alternative splicing of exon 2 results in two transcripts and two proteins with lengths of 385 and 376 amino acid residues, respectively. The so-called SNF5 homology domain in the second half of the protein harbours highly conserved structural motifs through which SMARCB1 interacts with other proteins {2430}. The SMARCB1 protein is a core subunit of mammalian SWI/SNF chromatin remodelling complexes, which regulate the expression of many genes by using ATP for sliding the nucleosomes along the DNA helix, facilitating or repressing transcription {2760}. The SMARCB1 protein functions as a tumour suppressor via repression of *CCND1* gene expression, induction of the *CDKN2A* gene, and hypophosphorylation of retinoblastoma protein, resulting in G0/G1 cell cycle arrest {185,2136}. Loss of SMARCB1 leads to transcriptional activation of EZH2 and to repression and increased H3K27me3 of polycomb gene targets as part of the broader SWI/SNF modulation of the polycomb complex to maintain the epigenome. The Hippo signalling pathway is involved in the detrimental effects of SMARCB1 deficiency, and its main effector (YAP1) is overexpressed in AT/RT {1145,2761}. According to the tumour suppressor gene model, both copies of the *SMARCB1* gene are inactivated in these tumours.

The *SMARCA4* gene, located on chromosome 19p13.2 and encoding a cata-lytic subunit of the SWI/SNF complex, was the second member of this complex reported to be involved in a cancer predisposition syndrome {193,2293}. More recently, other genes encoding SWI/SNF subunits have also been identified as recurrently mutated in cancer. Collectively, 20% of all human cancers contain a SWI/SNF mutation, and because most of these tumours are not classic MRTs, it can be expected that the definition of RTPS will need adjustment in the near future {1276}.

Gene mutations

The types of *SMARCB1* mutations observed in sporadic MRTs are similar to the spectrum of germline mutations reported to date. However, single base deletions in exon 9 occur most often in AT/RTs in patients without detectable germline alterations {192,616}. The second inactivating event is most frequently a deletion of the wildtype allele, often due to monosomy 22. In familial cases of RTPS, unaffected adult carriers have been identified. Alternatively, new mutations can occur during oogenesis/spermatogenesis (gonadal mosaicism), or postzygotically during the early stages of embryogenesis {616,962,1133,2327}. Compared with germline *SMARCB1* mutations in patients with rhabdoid tumours, schwannomatosis mutations are significantly more likely to occur at either end of the gene and to be non-truncating mutations {2380}. One study reported a family in which the affected individuals inherited a *SMARCB1* mutation and developed schwannomatosis or rhabdoid tumour {2472}.

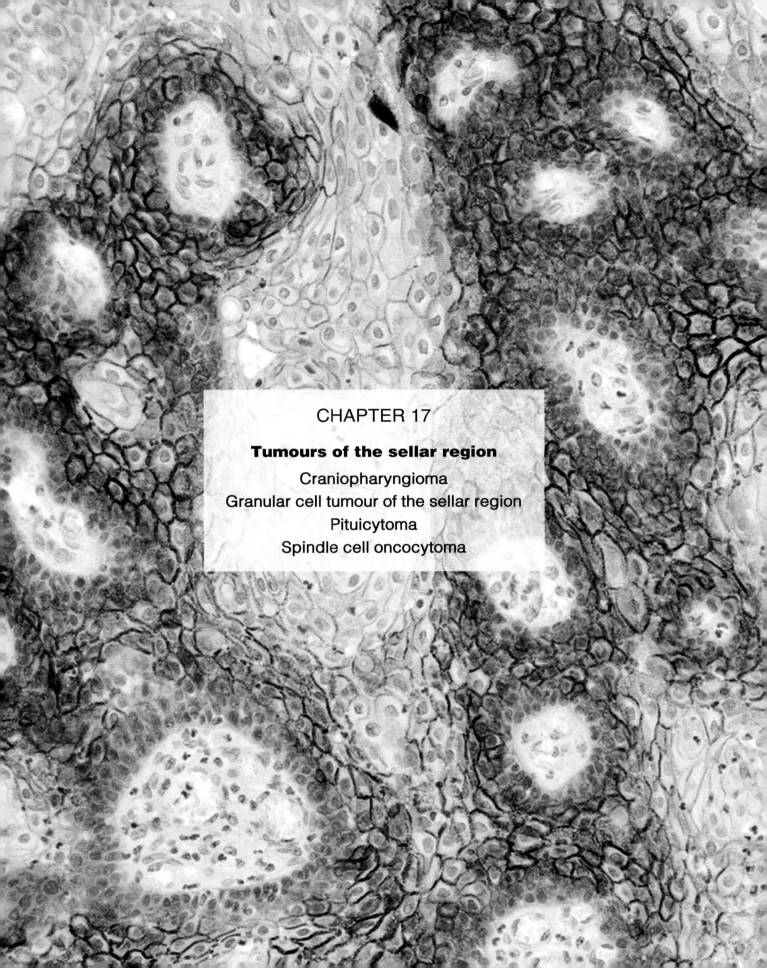

CHAPTER 17

Tumours of the sellar region

Craniopharyngioma
Granular cell tumour of the sellar region
Pituicytoma
Spindle cell oncocytoma

Craniopharyngioma

Buslei R.
Rushing E.J.
Giangaspero F.

Paulus W.
Burger P.C.
Santagata S.

Definition

A histologically benign, partly cystic epithelial tumour of the sellar region presumably derived from embryonic remnants of the Rathke pouch epithelium, with two clinicopathological variants (adamantinomatous and papillary) that have distinct phenotypes and characteristic mutations.
Adamantinomatous craniopharyngiomas show *CTNNB1* mutations and aberrant nuclear expression of beta-catenin in as many as 95% of cases. Papillary craniopharyngiomas show *BRAF* V600E mutations in 81–95% of cases, which can be detected by immunohistochemistry. Craniopharyngiomas may be infiltrative and therefore clinically difficult to manage.

Xanthogranuloma of the sellar region is a related but distinct clinicopathological entity.

ICD-O code   9350/1

Grading

Craniopharyngiomas correspond histologically to WHO grade I.

Epidemiology

Incidence

Craniopharyngiomas constitute 1.2–4.6% of all intracranial tumours, accounting for 0.5–2.5 new cases per 1 million population per year {310}. They are more frequent in Japan, with an annual

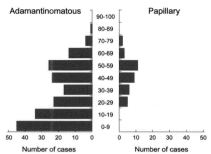

Fig. 17.01 Age distribution of adamantinomatous and papillary craniopharyngioma, based on 224 cases.

incidence of 3.8 cases per 1 million children {1572}. They are the most common non-neuroepithelial intracerebral neoplasm in children, accounting for 5–11% of intracranial tumours in this age group {846,2174}.

Age and sex distribution

Adamantinomatous craniopharyngioma has a bimodal age distribution {1784, 2836}, with incidence peaks in children aged 5–15 years and adults aged 45–60 years. Rare neonatal and fetal cases have been reported {431}. Papillary craniopharyngiomas occur almost exclusively in adults, at a mean patient age of 40–55 years {507}. Craniopharyngiomas show no obvious sex predilection.

Localization

The most common site for both subtypes is the suprasellar cistern, with a minor intrasellar component. Unusual locations

such as the sphenoid sinus {1338} and cerebellopontine angle {1277} have also been reported. Craniopharyngiomas, mainly the papillary variant, are also found in the third ventricle {507}.

Clinical features

The clinical features are non-specific and include visual deficits (observed in 62–84% of patients; more frequently in adults than in children) and endocrine deficiencies (observed in 52–87% of patients; more frequently in children) {13}. The endocrine disturbances observed include deficiencies of growth hormone (occurring in 75% of cases), luteinizing hormone / follicle-stimulating hormone (in 40%), adrenocorticotropic hormone (in 25%), and thyroid-stimulating hormone (in 25%). Diabetes insipidus is noted in as many as 17% of children and 30% of adults. Cognitive impairment and personality changes are observed in about half of all patients {13}. Obesity and hyperphagia (signs of hypothalamic dysfunction) have been described {1730, 2362}, although the occurrence of severe obesity can be reduced with resections that spare the hypothalamus {636}. Signs of increased intracranial pressure are frequent, especially in cases with compression or invasion of the third ventricle.

Imaging

Adamantinomatous craniopharyngiomas present as lobulated, multicystic masses.

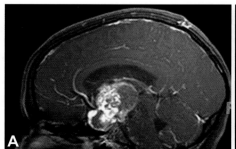
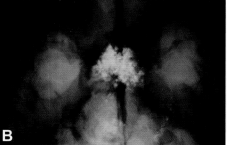

Fig. 17.02 Adamantinomatous craniopharyngioma. **A** Sagittal postcontrast T1-weighted MRI shows a large, enhancing, partially cystic suprasellar and sellar mass, characteristic of adamantinomatous craniopharyngioma. **B** Large adamantinomatous craniopharyngioma extending into the third ventricle. Postmortem X-ray showed extensive calcification, which is typical for this craniopharyngioma variant.

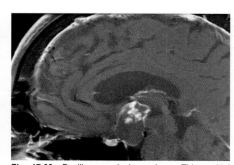

Fig. 17.03 Papillary craniopharyngioma. This sagittal postcontrast T1-weighted MRI shows an enhancing cystic mass involving the anterior third ventricle; the solid component shows papillary fronds.

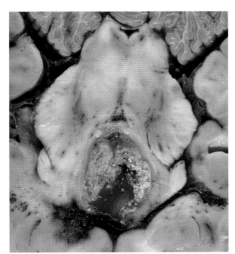

Fig. 17.04 Adamantinomatous craniopharyngioma extending towards the cerebral peduncles; note the so-called machine-oil appearance of the dorsal portion and calcifications.

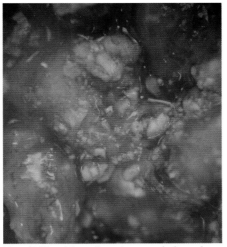

Fig. 17.05 Adamantinomatous craniopharyngioma. Fresh tumour material showing an uneven surface with small calcifications and flakes of wet keratin (white deposits).

CT shows contrast enhancement of the solid portions and of the cyst capsule, as well as typical calcifications. On MRI, the cystic areas are T1-hyperintense, whereas the solid components and the mural nodules are T1-isointense, with a slightly heterogeneous quality. On enhanced MRI images, the cystic portion is isointense with ring enhancement, whereas the solid components are hyperintense {2183}. Adamantinomatous tumours may superficially infiltrate neighbouring brain and adhere to adjacent blood vessels and nerves.

Papillary craniopharyngiomas are typically non-calcified, solid lesions with a more uniform appearance on CT and MRI {507,2245}.

Spread
Dissemination in the subarachnoid space or implantation along the surgical track or path of needle aspiration is a rare complication {190,1450,1473,2165,2287}.

Immunophenotype
The tumour cells immunolabel with antibodies against pancytokeratin, CK5/6, CK7, CK14, CK17, CK19, EMA, claudin-1 and beta-catenin. Only the adamantinomatous variant shows aberrant nuclear accumulation of beta-catenin, especially in the whorl-like cell clusters along the tumour margin and in finger-like tumour protrusions {1028}. Papillary craniopharyngiomas harbour *BRAF* V600E mutations that can be detected by immunohistochemistry, with uniform staining throughout the tumour epithelial cells {2307}. Papillary craniopharyngiomas show more robust membranous expression of claudin-1 than do either their adamantinomatous counterparts or Rathke cleft cysts {2410}.

Proliferation
Ki-67 immunoreactivity is concentrated along the peripherally palisading cells in the adamantinomatous type, and is more randomly distributed in papillary lesions {613,2058}. The reported Ki-67 proliferation index varies considerably from case to case, and is higher than might be expected given the relative indolence of the neoplasms {613,2058}. No consistent relationship between proliferation index and recurrence has been established.

Ultrastructure
Electron microscopy is seldom needed, given the relatively typical features in most cases. In addition to glycogen and the usual organelles, the constituent epithelial cells contain tonofilaments joined by desmosomes. Fenestrated capillary endothelium, amorphous ground matrix, and collagen fibrils characterize the connective tissue stroma. Mineral precipitates appear to arise in membrane-bound vesicles {24}.

Differential diagnosis
Xanthogranulomas of the sellar region are histologically composed of cholesterol clefts, macrophages (xanthoma cells), multinucleated giant cells, chronic inflammation, necrotic debris, and haemosiderin deposits {1914}. Xanthogranuloma of the sellar region is considered to be a

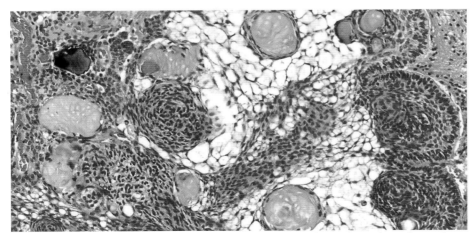

Fig. 17.06 Adamantinomatous craniopharyngioma. The distinctive epithelium features loose microcystic areas known as stellate reticulum, whorls, basal palisading, and anucleate nests of pale, squamous ghost cells known as wet keratin.

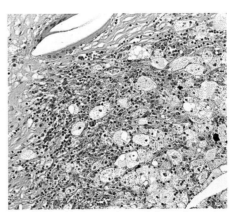

Fig. 17.07 Xanthogranuloma of the sellar region, showing xanthoma cells, lymphocytic infiltrates, haemosiderin deposits, cholesterol clefts, and occasional multinucleated giant cells.

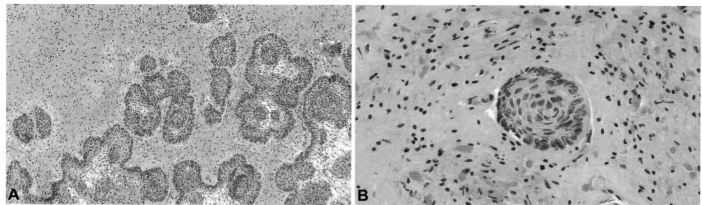

Fig. 17.08 Adamantinomatous craniopharyngioma. **A** Finger-like tumour protrusions in the surrounding brain tissue. **B** Cell groups of an adamantinomatous craniopharyngioma in the surrounding brain tissue, in which a distinct piloid gliosis with abundant Rosenthal fibres is evident.

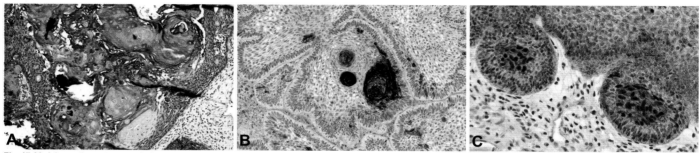

Fig. 17.09 Adamantinomatous craniopharyngioma. **A** Immunostaining for CK5/6 highlights foci of squamous differentiation, including foci of wet keratin. **B** Only focal immunoreactivity for claudin-1. **C** Finger-like protrusions in the surrounding brain tissue harbouring cell clusters with aberrant nuclear accumulation of beta-catenin.

reactive lesion, most often to remnants of Rathke cleft cyst {64}. Foci of squamous or cuboidal epithelium as well as small tubules may be encountered, whereas typical areas of adamantinomatous epithelium are usually absent or amount to < 10% of the tissue {1914}. Epithelial cells in xanthogranulomas do not exhibit nuclear accumulation of beta-catenin {329}. Epidermoid and Rathke cleft cysts are sometimes raised in the differential diagnosis, especially in small tissue fragments. Epidermoid cysts are distinguished by the presence of a uniloculated cavity lined by squamous epithelium and filled with flaky, dry keratin. Rathke cleft cysts enter into the differential diagnosis in particular when they show extensive squamous metaplasia {2307}. More commonly, the cyst wall is lined by simple columnar or cuboidal epithelium, which often is ciliated, with mucinous goblet cells. A respiratory-type epithelium may occasionally be present, accompanied by a xanthogranulomatous reaction after rupture of the cyst wall {932,2573, 2837}. Unlike papillary craniopharyngiomas, Rathke cleft cysts lack *BRAF* V600E mutations, although cross-reactive staining of cilia can be seen {1180,2307}. In

Rathke cleft cysts, beta-catenin localizes to the cell membrane, whereas the nuclear accumulation described in adamantinomatous craniopharyngiomas is typically absent {1028}.

Cell of origin

Several observations, including cytokeratin expression profiles, indicate that craniopharyngiomas arise from neoplastic transformation of ectodermal-derived epithelial cell remnants of Rathke pouch and the craniopharyngeal duct. Epithelial cell rests have been reported to occur between the roof of the pharynx and the floor of the third ventricle, most frequently along the anterior infundibulum and the anterior superior surface of the adenohypophysis – sites of the previous Rathke pouch and involuted duct that links these structures. Metaplasia of cells derived from the tooth primordia determine the adamantinomatous subtype, whereas metaplastic changes in cells derived from buccal mucosa primordia give rise to the squamous papillary variant {2014}. Further support for the origin of craniopharyngiomas from Rathke pouch epithelium is the occasional occurrence of mixed tumours with characteristics of

craniopharyngiomas and Rathke cleft cysts, as well as reports of unique congenital craniopharyngiomas with ameloblastic, tooth bud, and adenohypophyseal primordia components {60,1721, 2317,2807}. Additional evidence is the report of a tumour arising from a Rathke cleft cyst that contained cells that were transitional between squamous, mucus-producing, and anterior pituitary lobe secretory cells {1246}.

The hypothesis that craniopharyngiomas are of neuroendocrine lineage is supported by the finding that scattered tumour cells can (rarely) express pituitary hormones {2475}, chromogranin-A {2807}, and hCG {2486}. The finding that craniopharyngiomas share stem cell markers (e.g. SOX2, OCT4, KLF4, and SOX9) with the normal pituitary gland further supports a common origin {70,785}.

Genetic profile

The WNT signalling pathway is strongly implicated in the pathogenesis of adamantinomatous craniopharyngiomas. Genetic analyses have confirmed that as many as 95% of the tumours show mutations in exon 3 of the beta-catenin gene (*CTNNB1*) {263,329,1231,2316}. These mutations within the degradation targeting box of beta-catenin lead to activation of the WNT signalling pathway, indicated by aberrant cytoplasmic and nuclear accumulation of beta-catenin protein and respective target gene activation {1077}. Mouse models confirm the tumour-initiating strength of these alterations {790}.

In contrast, papillary craniopharyngiomas harbour the *BRAF* V600E mutation in nearly all cases {263,1432,2307}. The apparent mutual exclusivity of *CTNNB1* and *BRAF* V600E mutations in both craniopharyngioma variants demonstrates that these histological categories can be defined by their underlying molecular genetics.

Comparative genomic hybridization studies on two large series of craniopharyngiomas have failed to show significant recurrent chromosomal imbalances in either adamantinomatous or papillary variants {2120,2829}. In contrast, a comparative genomic hybridization–based study of nine adamantinomatous craniopharyngiomas revealed at least one genomic alteration in 67% of cases {2129}. Similarly, cytogenetic analysis of two cases revealed multiple chromosomal abnormalities on chromosomes 2 and 12 {871, 1224}.

Prognosis and predictive factors

In several large series, at 10 years of follow-up, 60–93% of patients were recurrence free and 64–96% were alive {507,2065,2806}. The most significant factor associated with recurrence is the extent of surgical resection {1922,2721, 2806}, with lesions > 5 cm in diameter carrying a markedly worse prognosis in an earlier series {2806}. After incomplete surgical resection, the recurrence rate

is significantly higher {1922,2806}; however, there is a trend towards less radical extirpation in order to avoid hypothalamic injury {1730}.

Radiotherapy is widely used in incompletely resected tumours. Histological evidence of brain invasion, which is more frequently documented in the adamantinomatous type than in the papillary type, does not correlate with a higher recurrence rate in cases with gross surgical resection {2721}. Some authors have documented a better prognosis for the papillary variant {13,2520}, whereas others found no significant differences {507, 2721}. Malignant transformation of craniopharyngioma to squamous carcinoma after multiple recurrences and irradiation is exceptional {2155,2388}.

Adamantinomatous craniopharyngioma

Definition

A craniopharyngioma characterized by a distinctive epithelium that forms stellate reticulum, wet keratin, and basal palisades, showing CTNNB1 *mutations and aberrant nuclear expression of beta-catenin in as many as 95% of cases.*

ICD-O code   9351/1

Epidemiology

Adamantinomatous craniopharyngioma has a bimodal age distribution {1784, 2836}, with incidence peaks in children aged 5–15 years and adults aged 45–60 years. Rare neonatal and fetal cases have been reported {431}.

Macroscopy

Adamantinomatous craniopharyngioma typically presents as a lobulated solid mass, but on closer inspection often demonstrates a spongy quality as a result of a variable cystic component. On sectioning, the yellowish-white cysts may contain dark greenish-brown liquid resembling machinery oil. The gross appearance also reflects secondary changes such as fibrosis, calcifications, ossification, and the presence of cholesterol-rich deposits.

Microscopy

Adamantinomatous craniopharyngiomas can be recognized by the presence of well-differentiated epithelium disposed in cords, lobules, nodular whorls, and irregular trabeculae bordered by palisading columnar epithelium. These islands of densely packed cells merge with loosely knit epithelium known as stellate reticulum. Pale nodules of wet keratin constituting anucleate ghost-like remnants of squamous cells may be found in both the compact and looser areas. Cystic cavities containing cell debris and fibrosis are lined by flattened epithelium. Lymphocytic infiltrates are frequent and giant cell–rich granulomatous inflammation may be associated with cholesterol clefts, although this is more typical of xanthogranuloma. Piloid gliosis with abundant Rosenthal fibres is often seen in the surrounding brain and should not be mistaken for pilocytic astrocytoma. Rare examples of malignant transformation, especially after multiple recurrences and radiotherapy, have been reported {1097,2155,2388}, but are extremely rare. Therefore, other diagnoses (e.g.

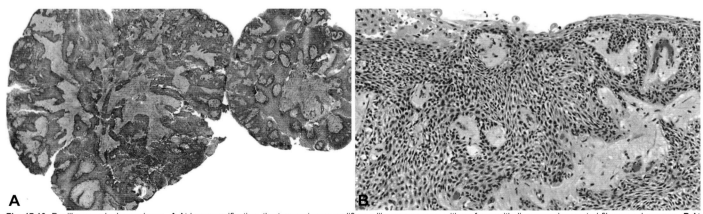

Fig. 17.10 Papillary craniopharyngioma. **A** At low magnification, the tumour has a cauliflower-like appearance, with surface epithelium covering central fibrovascular cores. **B** At higher magnification, the lining is consistent with non-keratinizing squamous epithelium.

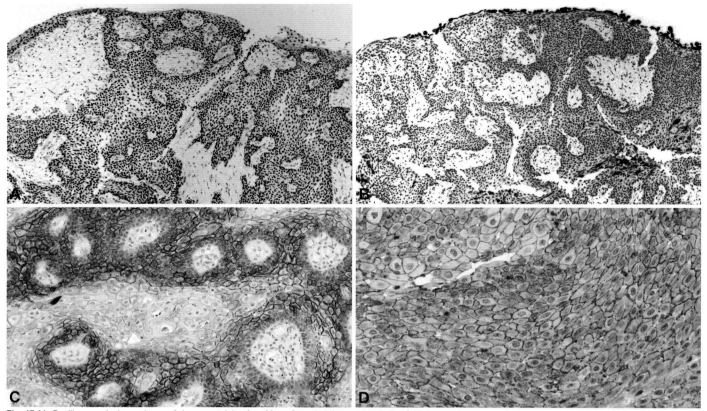

Fig. 17.11 Papillary craniopharyngioma. **A** Immunostaining for p63 confirms that the great majority of this tumour is composed of squamous epithelium. **B** Small component of surface respiratory epithelium is highlighted with CK7 staining; this feature overlaps with the lining of Rathke cleft cyst, which can also show squamous metaplasia, mimicking papillary craniopharyngioma. **C** Robust immunoreactivity for claudin-1. **D** Physiological expression of beta-catenin at the tumour cell membranes.

sinonasal carcinoma) should be carefully excluded.

Papillary craniopharyngioma

Definition
A papillary, mostly supratentorial or third ventricular craniopharyngioma characterized by fibrovascular cores lined by non-keratinizing squamous epithelium.
Papillary craniopharyngiomas occur almost exclusively in adults and frequently show *BRAF* V600E mutations (in 81–95%

of cases), which can be detected by immunohistochemistry.

ICD-O code   9352/1

Epidemiology
Papillary craniopharyngiomas occur almost exclusively in adults, with a mean patient age of 40–55 years {507}, and show no obvious sex predilection.

Macroscopy
Papillary craniopharyngiomas are solid or rarely cystic tumours, without

cholesterol-rich machinery oil–like fluid or calcifications. The surface of papillary craniopharyngioma, like that of other papillary tumours, may appear corrugated or cauliflower-like.

Microscopy
The essential features of papillary craniopharyngioma include compact, monomorphic sheets of well-differentiated squamous epithelium without surface keratinization. This variant typically lacks calcifications, picket fence–like palisades, whorl-like cell nodules, and wet keratin. T cells, macrophages, and neutrophils are scattered throughout the fibrovascular cores and tumour epithelium. Rudimentary papillae may surround the fibrovascular cores. Rarely, ciliated epithelium and periodic acid–Schiff–positive goblet cells are encountered.

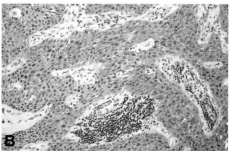

Fig. 17.12 Papillary craniopharyngioma. **A** Typical non-keratinizing squamous epithelium and focal lymphocytic infiltrate. **B** V600E-mutant BRAF is consistently expressed.

Granular cell tumour of the sellar region

Fuller G.N.
Brat D.J.
Wesseling P.
Roncaroli F.

Definition

A circumscribed tumour that is composed of large epithelioid to spindled cells with distinctively granular, eosinophilic cytoplasm (due to an abundance of intracytoplasmic lysosomes) and that arises from the neurohypophysis or infundibulum.

Granular cell tumour of the sellar region generally exhibits slow progression and a benign clinical course. Like pituicytomas and spindle cell oncocytomas, granular cell tumours show nuclear expression of TTF1, suggesting that these three tumours may constitute a spectrum of a single nosological entity.

ICD-O code   9582/0

Grading

Granular cell tumours correspond histologically to WHO grade I.

Synonyms

Synonyms previously applied to granular cell tumour include: Abrikossoff tumour, choristoma, granular cell myoblastoma, and granular cell neuroma.

Epidemiology

Symptomatic granular cell tumours are relatively rare and typically present in adulthood, with only exceptionally rare childhood cases {166}. There is a clear female predominance, with a female-to-male ratio of > 2:1. Peak incidence occurs in the sixth decade of life in men and in the fifth decade of life in women.

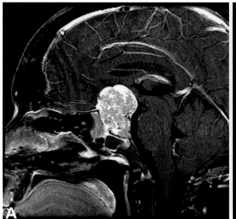 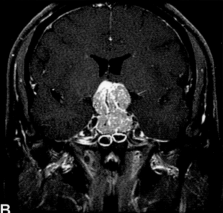

Fig. 17.14 Granular cell tumour of the sellar region. Postcontrast T1-weighted MRI. The sagittal plane (**A**) and coronal plane (**B**) show prominent contrast enhancement. Note the characteristic sellar/suprasellar anatomical location.

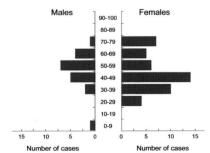

Fig. 17.13 Age and sex distribution of neurohypophyseal granular cell tumours, based on 66 symptomatic cases published in the literature; with a 1:2.3 male-to-female ratio.

Asymptomatic microscopic clusters of granular cells, called granular cell tumourettes {2330} or tumourlets {1547}, are more common than larger, symptomatic tumours, and have been documented at incidence rates as high as 17% in postmortem series {1547,2330,2564}.

Localization

Granular cell tumours arise along the anatomical distribution of the neurohypophysis, including the posterior pituitary and pituitary stalk / infundibulum. The tumours exhibit a preference for the pituitary stalk and thus most frequently arise in the suprasellar region, but may also arise from the posterior pituitary and present as an intrasellar mass; some examples occupy both the intrasellar and suprasellar compartments, mimicking pituitary macroadenoma. Granular cell tumours with morphological and immunophenotypic features identical to those of neurohypophyseal tumours have rarely been reported in other anatomical locations within the CNS, including the spinal meninges {1586}, cranial meninges {2631}, and third ventricle {2597}.

Clinical features

The most common presenting symptom of granular cell tumour of the sellar region is visual field deficit secondary to compression of the optic chiasm {479}.

Other presenting signs and symptoms include panhypopituitarism, galactorrhoea, amenorrhoea, decreased libido, and neuropsychological changes. Diabetes insipidus has been reported but is relatively uncommon {479}. Symptoms usually develop slowly over a period of years, although acute presentation with sudden-onset diplopia, confusion, headache, and vomiting can occur {479}. There are no disease-specific signs or symptoms that reliably distinguish granular cell tumours from other suprasellar mass lesions. Several cases have been found in association with pituitary adenoma {131,479,1527,2564}.

Imaging

MRI typically shows a well-circumscribed suprasellar mass that most commonly displays homogeneous or heterogeneous contrast enhancement. Tumour size most often ranges from 1.5 to 6.0 cm {479}. Calcification is unusual and thus helps to distinguish granular cell tumours from craniopharyngiomas. Similarly, a lack of a dural attachment (dural tail) and the anatomical location centred on the pituitary stalk help to distinguish granular cell tumours from most regional meningiomas. In addition to suprasellar presentations, intrasellar and intrasellar/suprasellar presentations are also recognized. Although there are no pathognomonic

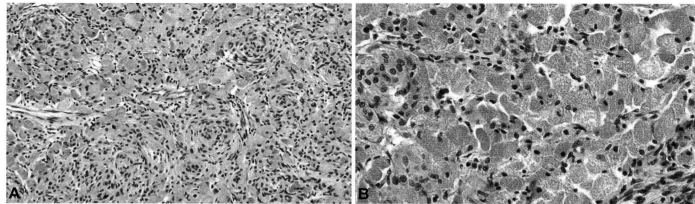

Fig. 17.15 Granular cell tumour of the neurohypophysis. **A** Spindled and whorled cellular architecture. **B** Characteristic abundant eosinophilic cytoplasm with prominent granularity.

imaging features, cases in which the tumour can be clearly seen to be separated from the pituitary by the inferior end of the pituitary stalk are suggestive of granular cell tumour {86}. Nevertheless, due to the relative rarity of the tumour, the diagnosis is rarely anticipated prior to surgical resection, which is also the case for suprasellar pituicytomas.

Macroscopy

The tumours are usually lobulated and well circumscribed, with a soft but rubbery consistency firmer than that of pituitary adenoma. The cut surface is typically grey to yellow. Necrosis, cystic degeneration, and haemorrhage are uncommon. The tumour may infiltrate surrounding structures, such as the optic chiasm and cavernous sinus; these features may prevent gross total surgical resection.

Microscopy

Granular cell tumours consist of densely packed polygonal cells with abundant granular eosinophilic cytoplasm. The architecture is typically nodular; sheets and/or spindled/fascicular patterns can also be seen, occasionally in a whorling pattern. Periodic acid–Schiff staining of cytoplasmic granules is resistant to diastase digestion. Small foci of foamy cells may be observed. The tumour cell nuclei are small, with inconspicuous nucleoli and evenly distributed chromatin. Perivascular lymphocytic aggregates are common. Mitotic activity is usually inconspicuous, and proliferative activity is usually very low. Some lesions are characterized by nuclear pleomorphism, prominent nucleoli, multinucleated cells, and increased mitotic activity (with as many as 5 mitoses per 10 high-power fields and a Ki-67 proliferation index of 7%). Such tumours have been referred to as atypical granular cell tumours by some authors, although the clinical and biological significance is uncertain {1230,2659}. By electron microscopy, the cytoplasm of the granular tumour cells is filled with phagolysosomes containing unevenly distributed electron-dense material and membranous debris. A few other organelles and intracytoplasmic filaments may be observed, but neurosecretory granules are absent {152}.

Immunophenotype

Granular cell tumours are variably positive for CD68 (by KP1 staining), S100 protein, alpha-1-antitrypsin, alpha-1-antichymotrypsin, and cathepsin B, and are negative for NFPs, cytokeratins, chromogranin-A, synaptophysin, desmin, SMA, and the pituitary hormones. Most tumours are negative for GFAP, although variable immunoreactivity has been noted in a subset of granular cell tumours. Granular cell tumours show nuclear staining for TTF1 {1452}.

Cell of origin

The finding that granular cell tumours strongly express the nuclear transcription factor TTF1, like pituicytes of the developing and mature neurohypophysis, suggests a pituicyte derivation {1452, 1654}. Both pituicytomas and spindle

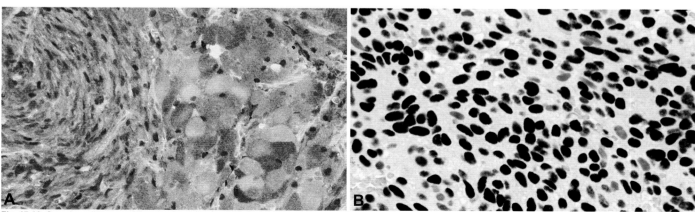

Fig. 17.16 Granular cell tumour of the neurohypophysis. **A** Marked S100 protein expression. **B** TTF1 nuclear immunoreactivity.

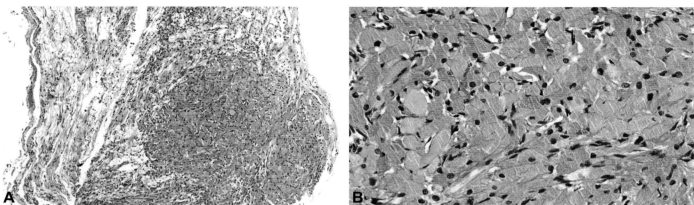

Fig. 17.17 Granular cell tumourlet (tumourette) of the infundibulum. **A** Whole-mount section. **B** High-power magnification showing discrete cellular borders and granular cytoplasm.

cell oncocytomas of the hypophysis also express nuclear TTF1, suggesting a histogenesis from pituicytes for these tumours as well. It has been speculated that granular cell tumours and spindle cell oncocytomas constitute pituicytomas that are composed of tumour cells with lysosome-rich and mitochondrion-rich cytoplasm, respectively, giving rise to distinct morphologies {1301,1452,1654}. The derivation of three morphologically distinct tumours from pituicytes might be explained by the existence of multiple subtypes of pituicytes in the normal neurohypophysis {1654,2499}. Granular cell tumours occasionally occur in the CNS outside the pituitary gland (e.g. in the meninges, cerebral hemispheres, third ventricle, or cranial nerves); these tumours may be derived from glial cells, Schwann cells, or macrophages {479, 2118,2631}.

Genetic profile
A unique genetic signature for granular cell tumour has not been defined. The limited number of cases that have been tested to date have not shown R132H-mutant IDH1, V600E-mutant BRAF, or *KIAA1549-BRAF* fusion {1654}.

Prognosis and predictive factors
Most granular cell tumours are clinically benign, with slow progression and lack of invasive growth. Surgical removal is the preferred therapy for larger tumours, but the firm and vascular nature of pituitary granular cell tumours, sometimes combined with the lack of an obvious dissection plane from the adjacent brain, may hamper gross total resection.

Pituicytoma

Brat D.J.
Wesseling P.
Fuller G.N.
Roncaroli F.

Definition
A circumscribed and generally solid low-grade glial neoplasm that originates in the neurohypophysis or infundibulum and is composed of bipolar spindled cells arranged in a fascicular or storiform pattern.

Like spindle cell oncocytomas and granular cell tumours of the sellar region, pituicytomas show nuclear expression of TTF1, suggesting that these three tumours may constitute a spectrum of a single nosological entity.

ICD-O code   9432/1

Grading
Pituicytomas correspond histologically to WHO grade I.

Synonyms and historical annotation
In the past, the term "pituicytoma" was used loosely for several histologically distinct tumours of the sellar and suprasellar region (e.g. granular cell tumours and pilocytic astrocytomas). Since the publication of the more restricted definition of pituicytoma by Brat et al. {273} in 2000 and its inclusion in the 2007 WHO classification, the term has instead been reserved for low-grade glial neoplasms that originate in the neurohypophysis or infundibulum and are histologically distinct {270,273}. Synonyms that were used in the past for pituicytoma include "posterior pituitary astrocytoma" and "infundibuloma".

Epidemiology
Pituicytomas are rare. Since 2000, approximately 70 examples have been described in the literature, often in case reports and small series {504,687,2877}. The largest series reported to date contains 9 tumours pooled from the consultation cases of two large institutions {273}. Nearly all reported pituicytomas have occurred in adult patients, with an average patient age at diagnosis of 50 years (range: 7–83 years) {504}. Nearly two thirds of all patients present between the

ages of 40 and 60 years. The male-to-female ratio is 1.5:1 {504}.

Localization
Pituicytomas arise along the distribution of the neurohypophysis, including the infundibulum / pituitary stalk and posterior pituitary. Accordingly, they may be located in the sella, in the suprasellar region, or in both the intrasellar and suprasellar compartments. Of these possibilities, purely intrasellar localization is the least common {504}.

Clinical features
The most common presenting signs and symptoms of pituicytoma are similar to those of other slowly expansive non–hormonally active tumours of the sellar/suprasellar region that compress the optic chiasm, infundibulum, and/or pituitary gland. These include visual disturbance; headache; and features of hypopituitarism such as fatigue, amenorrhoea, decreased libido, and mildly elevated serum prolactin (the stalk effect) {504,687, 2877}. Rarely, asymptomatic cases are found only at autopsy.

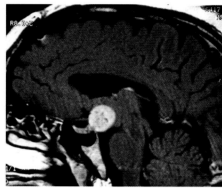

Fig. 17.18 Pituicytoma showing solid, circumscribed growth and diffuse contrast enhancement on T1-weighted MRI.

Imaging
Pituicytomas are typically solid and circumscribed mass lesions of the sellar and suprasellar spaces. Most often, they are isointense to grey matter on T1-weighted images, hyperintense on T2-weighted images, and uniformly contrast-enhancing {504}. Occasional tumours show heterogeneous contrast enhancement, and rare examples have a cystic component {273}.

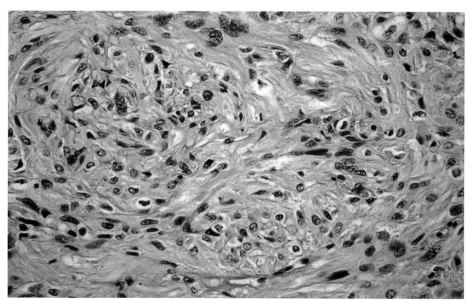

Fig. 17.19 Pituicytoma. Elongate and plump tumours cells arranged in a fascicular pattern.

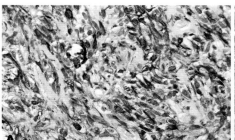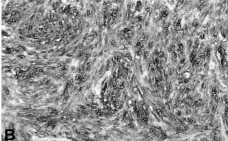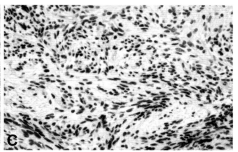

Fig. 17.20 Pituicytoma. **A** Patchy staining for GFAP. **B** Diffuse staining for S100 protein. **C** Strong nuclear TTF1 immunoreactivity.

Macroscopy

Pituicytomas are solid and circumscribed masses that can measure up to several centimetres and have a firm, rubbery texture. Only rarely has a cystic component been reported {273,2596}. Radiographical studies may give the impression of a smoothly contoured tumour, but pituicytomas can be firmly adherent to adjacent structures in the suprasellar space.

Microscopy

Pituicytomas have a solid, compact architecture and consist almost entirely of elongate, bipolar spindle cells arranged in a fascicular or storiform pattern {273,1452,1654,1966}. Although the tumours can show stubborn adherence to adjacent structures in the suprasellar space, an infiltrative pattern is generally not seen under the microscope. Individual tumour cells contain abundant eosinophilic cytoplasm, and cell shapes range from short and plump to elongate and angulated. Cell borders are readily apparent, especially on cross sections of fascicles. In strictly defined pituicytomas, there is not a significant amount of cytoplasmic granularity or vacuolization, and periodic acid–Schiff staining shows only minimal reaction. Similarly, substantial oncocytic change is not a recognized feature of pituicytoma. The nuclei are moderately sized and oval to elongate, with only mild irregularity of nuclear borders. Mitotic figures are rare. Reticulin fibres show a perivascular distribution, and intercellular reticulin is sparse. Importantly for the differential diagnosis with pilocytic astrocytoma and normal neurohypophysis, pituicytomas show no Rosenthal fibres, eosinophilic granular bodies, or Herring bodies (axonal dilatations for neuropeptide storage in the neurohypophysis).

Immunophenotype

Pituicytomas are low-grade gliomas that are positive by immunohistochemistry for vimentin and S100 protein and show nuclear staining for TTF1 {273,1452,1654, 1966}. GFAP staining is highly variable, ranging from faint and focal to moderate and patchy, and is only rarely strongly positive. Strong, diffuse staining is more typical for S100 protein and vimentin. BCL2 staining is variable, but can be intense {1654,1966}. Stains for cytokeratins are negative, and those for EMA may show a patchy pattern that is cytoplasmic rather than membranous. Pituicytomas do not demonstrate immunostaining for pituitary hormones or for neuronal or neuroendocrine markers such as synaptophysin and chromogranin. NFP immunoreactivity is limited to axons in peritumoural neurohypophyseal tissue and is not present within the tumour. The proliferation of these tumours is low as measured by immunoreactivity for MIB1, with the reported Ki-67 proliferation index ranging from 0.5% to 2.0% {273,1355}.

Cell of origin

Pituicytomas presumptively arise from specialized glial cells of the neurohypophysis, called pituicytes {1150,1514, 2261}. Such an origin accounts for the anatomical distribution of pituicytomas and is consistent with the tumour's morphological and immunophenotypic characteristics. The finding that pituicytomas strongly express the nuclear transcription factor TTF1, like pituicytes of the developing and mature neurohypophysis, supports a pituicyte derivation {1452, 1654}. Both granular cell tumours of the sellar region and spindle cell oncocytomas also express nuclear TTF1, suggesting a histogenesis from pituicytes for these tumours as well. It has been speculated that these granular cell tumours and spindle cell oncocytomas constitute pituicytomas that are composed of tumour cells with lysosome-rich and mitochondrion-rich cytoplasm, respectively, giving rise to distinct morphologies {1452,1654}. The derivation of three morphologically distinct tumours from pituicytes might be explained by the existence of multiple subtypes of pituicytes in the normal neurohypophysis {1654,2499}.

Genetic profile

A genetic signature for pituicytoma has not been defined. The limited number of cases that have been tested to date have not shown R132H-mutant IDH1, V600E-mutant BRAF, or *KIAA1549-BRAF* fusion {1654}. Microarray-based comparative genomic hybridization analysis of a single case demonstrated losses of chromosome arms 1p, 14q, and 22q, with gains on 5p {1966}.

Prognosis and predictive factors

Pituicytomas are slowly enlarging, localized tumours for which the current treatment is surgical resection {687,2877}. Local adherence of pituicytomas to regional structures may preclude complete resection, and residual disease may gradually regrow over a period of several years. There has been no correlation of proliferation with clinical outcome. No instances of malignant transformation or distant metastasis have been reported to date.

Spindle cell oncocytoma

Lopes M.B.S.
Fuller G.N.
Roncaroli F.
Wesseling P.

Definition

A spindled to epithelioid, oncocytic, non-neuroendocrine neoplasm of the pituitary gland.

Spindle cell oncocytomas manifest in adults and tend to follow a benign clinical course. Like pituicytomas and granular cell tumours of the sellar region, spindle cell oncocytomas show nuclear expression of TTF1, suggesting that these three tumours may constitute a spectrum of a single nosological entity.

ICD-O code   8290/0

Grading

Spindle cell oncocytoma corresponds histologically to WHO grade I.

Synonyms and historical annotation

In the initial report of the entity in 2002, Roncaroli et al. {2169} described spindle cell oncocytoma as spindle cell oncocytoma of the adenohypophysis. On the basis of the similar ultrastructural and immunohistochemical features of these neoplasms, derivation from folliculostellate cells of the anterior pituitary was suspected {2169}. However, more recent data on the shared TTF1 immunoreactivity of non-neoplastic pituicytes, pituicytomas, granular cell tumours, and spindle cell oncocytomas may suggest a similar origin of these tumours and a shared link to the posterior pituitary {1452,1654}.

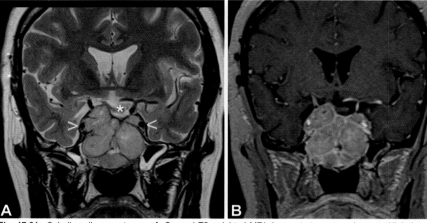

Fig. 17.21 Spindle cell oncocytoma. **A** Coronal T2-weighted MRI demonstrates a very large multilobulated sellar mass with osseous remodelling and suprasellar extension; the mass laterally displaces the internal carotid arteries (arrowheads) and exerts mass effect on the right aspect of the optic chiasm (asterisk). **B** Coronal postcontrast volumetric interpolated brain examination sequence demonstrates mildly heterogeneous enhancement with a small central non-enhancing component.

Epidemiology

Spindle cell oncocytoma is a rare tumour, but its true incidence is difficult to determine. In the experience of one institution, spindle cell oncocytomas accounted for 0.4% of all sellar tumours {2169}. About 25 cases have been reported in the literature {1719}. Based on the limited number of cases reported, spindle cell oncocytoma is assumed to be a tumour of adults, with reported patient ages of 24–76 years and a mean age of 56 years. The distribution is equal between the sexes {1719}.

Localization

Spindle cell oncocytoma is a pituitary tumour that may have a mixed intrasellar and suprasellar location. Clinical manifestation with a purely intrasellar tumour is relatively rare {504}. Extension into the cavernous sinus {243,519} and invasion of the sellar floor have been reported {1305}.

Clinical features

The clinical presentation and neuroimaging characteristics of spindle cell oncocytoma are indistinguishable from those

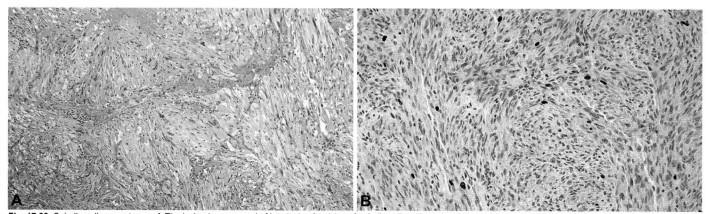

Fig. 17.22 Spindle cell oncocytoma. **A** The lesion is composed of interlacing fascicles of spindle cells with eosinophilic cytoplasm and mildly to moderately atypical nuclei. **B** The Ki-67 proliferation index is usually low.

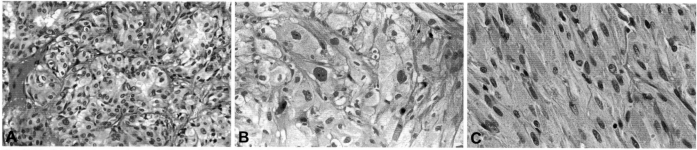

Fig. 17.23 Spindle cell oncocytoma. **A** Clear-cell appearance of the tumour cells arranged within a nested pattern. **B** Some examples have pleomorphic nuclei. **C** Oncocytic changes may be variable within a given tumour.

of a non-functioning pituitary adenoma. Visual disturbances have been found to be the most common presenting symptom, followed by pituitary hypofunction and (less frequently) headache, nausea, and vomiting {504,171,2169}. Decreased libido, sexual dysfunction, and oligomenorrhoea or amenorrhoea secondary to pituitary stalk effect, with mild hyperprolactinaemia, have been documented {1719}. None of the patients reported to date had diabetes insipidus at onset {504}. One patient with aggressive spindle cell oncocytoma and involvement of the skull base presented with epistaxis {1305}.

Imaging
The neuroimaging features of spindle cell oncocytoma are similar to those of pituitary adenoma, but spindle cell oncocytomas often avidly enhance following administration of paramagnetic contrast, because of their greater vascular supply relative to adenomas. Enhancement

can be heterogeneous {504}. Calcification may be seen on CT imaging {239}. Recurrent intratumoural bleeding has been reported, leading to an erroneous preoperative diagnosis of craniopharyngioma {239}. The rich tumoural blood supply can be seen on MR angiography; one study reported predominant feeding from the bilateral internal carotid arteries {753}.

Macroscopy
On gross inspection, spindle cell oncocytoma is often indistinguishable from pituitary adenoma. Most are large tumours, with an average craniocaudal dimension of 2.5–3 cm and a maximum reported size of 6.5 cm {519}. They vary from soft, creamy, and easily resectable lesions to firm tumours that adhere to surrounding structures, and infrequently show destruction of the sellar floor {519,1305}. Intratumoural haemorrhage can occur, and severe intraoperative bleeding has been

described {753}. A clear margin or a pseudocapsule, as can be seen in some pituitary adenomas, is usually absent.

Microscopy
Spindle cell oncocytomas are typically composed of interlacing fascicles and poorly defined lobules of spindle to epithelioid cells with eosinophilic and variably oncocytic cytoplasm. Oncocytic changes can be focal or widespread. The spectrum of morphological features that can be seen in spindle cell oncocytoma is broad. Formations of whorls, focal stromal myxoid changes {2189}, clear cells, osteoclastic-like giant cells, and follicle-like structures {2605,2830} have all been reported in individual cases, in addition to the more typical features. Mild to moderate nuclear atypia and even marked pleomorphism may be seen. Focal infiltrates of mature lymphocytes are seen in many lesions. The mitotic count is typically low, often with an average

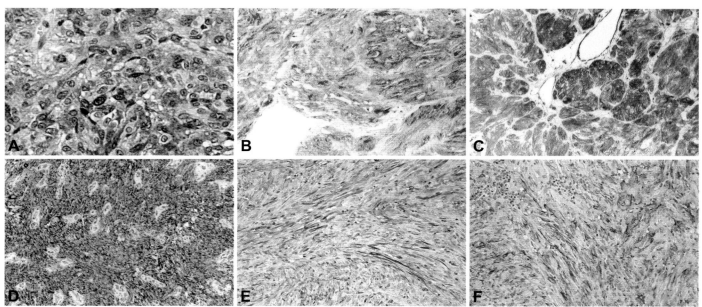

Fig. 17.24 Immunophenotype of spindle cell oncocytoma. **A** S100 protein. **B** Annexin. **C** Galectin-1. **D** Antimitochondrial antigen. **E** Vimentin. **F** EMA.

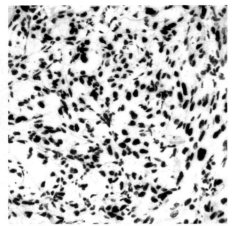

Fig. 17.25 Spindle cell oncocytoma. Positivity for TTF1 is characteristic.

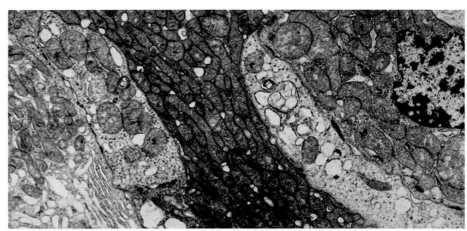

Fig. 17.26 Spindle cell oncocytoma. At the ultrastructural level, the tumour cells show numerous mitochondria (oncocytic change) as well as several cell–cell junctions, mainly short desmosomes.

of < 1 mitotic figure per 10 high-power fields. Recurrent lesions may or may not show increased mitotic activity {1305, 1719}.

Electron microscopy

Ultrastructural examination is useful in the diagnosis of spindle cell oncocytoma {1305,2169}. Neoplastic cells appear spindled or polygonal in configuration and are often filled with mitochondria, which may appear abnormal. The tumour cells lack secretory granules, a key distinction from pituitary adenomas. Well-formed desmosomes and intermediate-type junctions are encountered. Intracytoplasmic lumina with microvillous projections have been reported {2605}.

Immunophenotype

Unlike pituitary adenomas, spindle cell oncocytomas lack immunoreactivity for neuroendocrine markers and pituitary hormones. Typically, spindle cell oncocytomas express vimentin, S100 protein, BCL2, and EMA, and show staining with the antimitochondrial antibody MU213-UC clone 131-1, as well as nuclear staining for TTF1 {1305,1452,1654,2167, 2169}. EMA expression can vary from weak and focal to diffuse. The tumours are only focally positive for GFAP. CD44 and nestin have been reported in a single case, suggesting a possible neuronal precursor component {47}, and alpha-crystallin B chain was seen in another

case {2605}. Galectin-3 and annexin A1 are also commonly expressed; although these markers are non-specific, they initially suggested a link to the folliculostellate cell {2169}.

Proliferation

The Ki-67 proliferation index is usually low, with a reported range of 1–8% and an average value of 3%. One recurrent example had a Ki-67 proliferation index of 20%, but no data were available on the proliferation rate of the primary tumour {1305}.

Cell of origin

The histogenesis of spindle cell oncocytoma remains unresolved. Initially, a derivation from folliculostellate cells of the adenohypophysis was postulated on the basis of the immunoprofile (in particular galectin-3 and annexin A1 expression) and ultrastructural features {2169}. However, the finding that not only pituicytomas, but also granular cell tumours of the sellar region and spindle cell oncocytomas express the nuclear transcription factor TTF1, like pituicytes of the developing and mature neurohypophysis, suggests a pituicyte derivation {1452,1654}. It has been speculated that granular cell tumours of the sellar region and spindle cell oncocytomas constitute variants of pituicytoma in which the tumour cells display lysosome-rich and mitochondrion-rich cytoplasm, respectively, giving rise

to distinct morphologies {1452,1654}. The derivation of three morphologically distinct tumours from pituicytes might be explained by the existence of multiple subtypes of pituicytes in the normal neurohypophysis {1654,2499}.

Genetic profile

In a study that included 7 spindle cell oncocytomas, none of the neoplasms showed positive immunostaining for R132H-mutant IDH1 or any evidence of *BRAF* V600E mutation or KIAA-*BRAF* fusion {1654}.

Prognosis and predictive factors

Most spindle cell oncocytomas follow a benign clinical course, but about one third of reported cases have recurred, after 3–15 years {1719}. In only a small number of cases with recurrence did the original neoplasm show an increased Ki-67 proliferation index (ranging from 10% to 20%) or marked cytological atypia {243, 1719}. Additional follow-up is needed to definitively determine the prognostic significance of such features. Incomplete resection is a risk factor for recurrence. Moderate tumour volume and absence of invasion into surrounding structures facilitate complete resection, whereas hypervascularity may hamper the procedure {1816}. Recurrent tumours can follow a more aggressive course, with an increased Ki-67 proliferation index and necrosis {1305}.

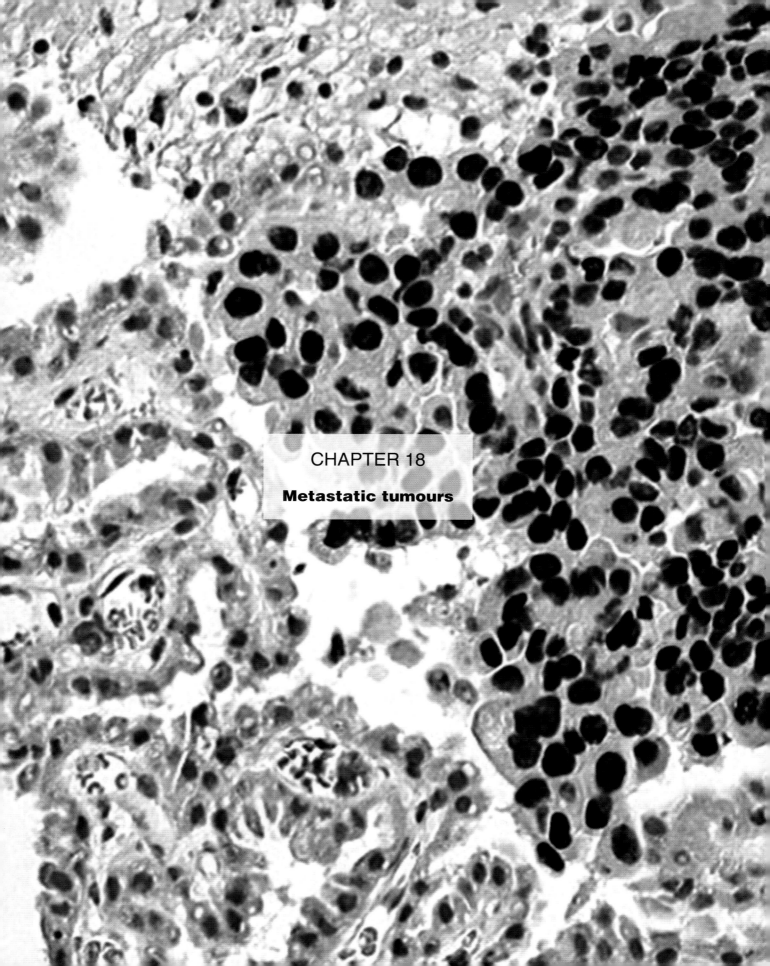

CHAPTER 18

Metastatic tumours

Metastatic tumours of the CNS

Wesseling P.
von Deimling A.
Aldape K.D.
Preusser M.

Rosenblum M.K.
Mittelbronn M.
Tanaka S.

Definition

Tumours that originate outside the CNS and spread via the haematogenous route to the CNS or (less frequently) directly invade the CNS from adjacent anatomical structures.

Epidemiology

Incidence

Due to underdiagnosis and inaccurate reporting, the incidence rates for brain metastases reported in the literature probably underestimate the true incidence {731,2484}. In a large, population-based study in Sweden, the incidence of patients admitted to hospital with brain metastases doubled to 14 cases per 100 000 population between 1987 and 2006. More efficient control of disease spread outside the CNS and the use of more advanced neuroimaging techniques may have contributed to this increase {2371}. Autopsy studies have reported that CNS metastases occur in about 25% of patients who die of cancer {792}. Leptomeningeal metastases occur in 4–15% of patients with solid tumours {400,2490} and dural metastases in 8–9% of patients with advanced cancer {1419}. Spinal epidural metastases are found in 5–10% and are much more frequent than spinal leptomeningeal or intramedullary metastases {1728}.

Age and sex distribution

CNS metastases are the most common CNS neoplasms in adults, but metastases account for only about 2% of all paediatric CNS tumours. As many as 30% of adults and 6–10% of children with cancer develop brain metastases. The relative proportions of various primary tumours are different between the two sexes, but sex has no significant independent effect on the occurrence of CNS metastasis for most tumour types {130,731,2749}. The incidence of brain metastases has been reported to be highest among patients diagnosed with primary lung cancer at an age of 40–49 years; with primary melanoma, renal cancer, or colorectal cancer

at an age of 50–59 years; and with breast cancer at an age of 20–39 years {2484}. The incidence of CNS metastases may be increasing, in part due to increased detection with improved imaging, an increase in the incidence of tumours with

a predilection for brain involvement (e.g. lung cancer), and the introduction of new therapeutic agents that prolong life and are relatively efficacious overall but ineffective at preventing or treating metastatic disease within the CNS {1868,2484}.

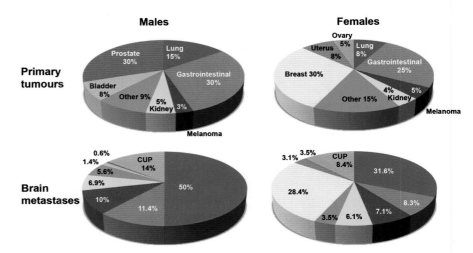

Fig. 18.01 Relative frequencies of primary tumours and of brain metastases derived thereof {354,2032}. Tumours with a high propensity to metastasize to the brain are lung cancer, breast cancer, renal cell carcinoma, and melanoma. In this series of brain metastases, about 14% of cases in males and 8% of cases in females were diagnosed as carcinoma of unknown primary (CUP). Based on the histology of archival tissue samples (874 cases collected in 1990–2011 at the Institute of Neurology/Neuropathology in Vienna); metastases for which surgery was not performed are not represented. The relative frequency of brain metastases may differ substantially in other regions of the world.

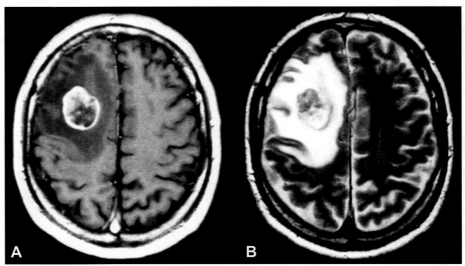

Fig. 18.02 Metastasis of an adenocarcinoma in the right frontal lobe. **A** Gadolinium-enhanced T1-weighted MRI showing a contrast-enhancing tumour surrounded by a large hypointense area corresponding to perifocal oedema. **B** Both the tumour and perifocal oedema show bright T2-hyperintensity.

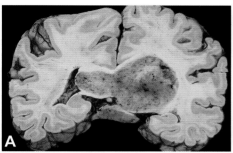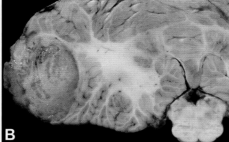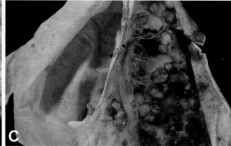

Fig. 18.03 Patterns of CNS metastases. **A** Intraparenchymal metastasis of a lung carcinoma extending into the left hemisphere via the splenium of the corpus callosum. **B** Cerebellar, intraparenchymal metastasis of a ductal carcinoma of the pancreas extending to the leptomeningeal compartment. **C** Multiple dural metastases of a carcinoma of the gastric cardia.

Origin of CNS metastases

The most common source of brain metastasis in adults is lung cancer (especially adenocarcinoma and small cell carcinoma), followed by breast cancer, melanoma, renal cell carcinoma, and colorectal cancer {354,1783,2032}. Prostate, breast, and lung cancer are the most common origins of spinal epidural metastasis, followed by non-Hodgkin lymphoma, multiple myeloma, and renal cancer {1728}. Tumours and their molecular subtypes vary in their propensity to metastasize to the CNS {130,510,2297}. In as many as 10% of patients with brain metastases, no primary tumour is found at presentation {2032}. In children, the most common sources of CNS metastases are leukaemias and lymphomas, followed by non-haematopoietic CNS neoplasms such as germ cell tumours, osteosarcoma, neuroblastoma, Ewing sarcoma, and rhabdomyosarcoma {510,2749}. Occasionally, primary neoplasms in the head and neck region extend intracranially by direct invasion (per continuitatem), sometimes along cranial nerves, and present as intracranial tumours {2323}.

Localization

Approximately 80% of all brain metastases are located in the cerebral hemispheres (particularly in arterial border zones and at the junction of cerebral cortex and white matter), 15% in the cerebellum, and 5% in the brain stem. Fewer than half of all brain metastases are single (i.e. the only metastatic lesion in the brain), and very few are solitary (i.e. the only metastasis in the body) {792,1923}. Other intracranial sites include the dura and leptomeninges; in these sites, extension from or to other compartments is more common {1419,1760}. The vast majority of metastases affecting the spinal cord expand from the vertebral body or paravertebral tissues into the epidural space {1728}. Occasionally, metastatic CNS tumours seed along the walls of the ventricles or are located in the pituitary gland or choroid plexus. Rarely, tumour-to-tumour metastasis occurs, with lung and breast cancer being the most common donor tumours and meningioma the most common recipient {1711}. Of particular diagnostic challenge is metastasis of renal cell carcinoma to haemangioblastoma in the setting of von Hippel–Lindau disease {62,1138}. Dural metastases are relatively common in cancer of the prostate, breast, and lung, and in haematological malignancies {1419,1760}. Leptomeningeal metastases are more common in lung and breast cancer,

melanoma, and haematopoietic tumours {2490}. Spinal epidural metastases are more common in cancer of the prostate, breast, lung, and kidney, non-Hodgkin lymphoma, and multiple myeloma. Intramedullary spinal cord metastases are more common in small cell lung carcinoma {1728}.

Clinical features

Symptoms and signs

The neurological signs and symptoms of intracranial metastases are generally caused by increased intracranial pressure or local effect of the tumour on the adjacent brain tissue. The signs and symptoms may progress gradually and include headache, altered mental status, paresis, ataxia, visual changes, nausea, and sensory disturbances. Some patients present acutely with seizure, infarct, or haemorrhage {1453}. The interval between diagnosis of the primary tumour and the CNS metastasis is generally < 1 year for lung carcinoma, but can be multiple years for breast cancer and melanoma {2297}. Many patients with leptomeningeal metastasis have multiple, varied neurological symptoms and signs at presentation, including headache, mental alteration, ataxia, cranial

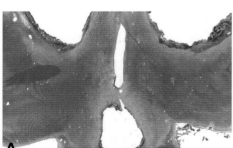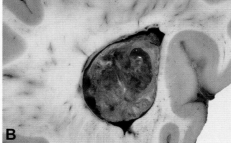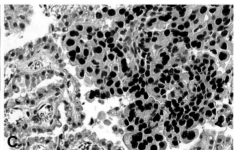

Fig. 18.04 Patterns of CNS metastasis. **A** Extensive CSF spread of small cell lung carcinoma cells along the walls of both lateral ventricles and the third ventricle. **B** Intraventricular metastasis of a lung adenocarcinoma infiltrating the choroid plexus with (**C**) TTF1 staining of tumour cell nuclei.

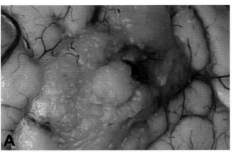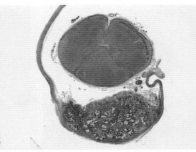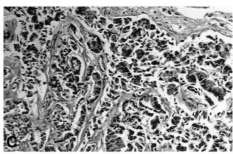

Fig. 18.05 Patterns of CNS metastasis. **A** Leptomeningeal metastasis of a non-Hodgkin lymphoma. **B,C** Intraspinal dural metastasis of lung adenocarcinoma.

nerve dysfunction, and radiculopathy. Cytological examination reveals malignant cells in the initial cerebrospinal fluid sample in about 50% of such patients; this proportion may increase to ≥ 80% when cerebrospinal fluid sampling is repeated and adequate volumes (≥ 10 mL) are available for cytological analysis {400,1453}. Spinal metastases generally result in compression of the spinal cord or nerve roots and may cause back pain, weakness of the extremities, sensory disturbances, and incontinence over the course of hours, days, or weeks {1453}.

Imaging
On MRI, intraparenchymal metastases are generally circumscribed and show mild T1-hypointensity, T2-hyperintensity, and diffuse or ring-like contrast enhancement with a surrounding zone of parenchymal oedema. Haemorrhagic metastases and metastatic melanomas containing melanin pigment may demonstrate hyperintensity on non-contrast MRI or CT {2833}. In patients with leptomeningeal metastasis, MRI can show focal or diffuse leptomeningeal thickening and contrast enhancement (sometimes with dispersed tumour nodules in the subarachnoid space). Enhancement and enlargement of the cranial nerves and communicating hydrocephalus may also be found {848,1728}. MRI can depict dural metastases as nodular masses or dural thickening along the bone structures, whereas metastases in vertebral bodies are visualized as discrete, confluent or diffuse areas of low signal intensity. CT scan may be useful for detection of bone involvement {1419}.

Macroscopy
Metastases in the brain and spinal cord parenchyma often form grossly circumscribed and rounded, greyish-white or tan masses with variable central necrosis and peritumoural oedema. Metastases of adenocarcinomas may contain collections of mucoid material. Haemorrhage is relatively frequent in metastases of choriocarcinoma, melanoma, and clear cell renal cell carcinoma. Melanoma metastases with abundant melanin pigment have a brown to black colour. Leptomeningeal metastasis may produce diffuse opacification of the membranes or present as multiple nodules {1923}. Dural metastases can grow as localized plaques or nodules and as diffuse lesions. Primary neoplasms in the head and neck region that extend intracranially by direct invasion generally cause significant destruction of the skull bones. However, in some cases, the skull is penetrated by relatively subtle, perivascular or perineural invasion, without major bone destruction {2323}.

Microscopy
The histological and immunohistochemical features of secondary CNS tumours are as diverse as those of the primary tumours from which they arise. Most brain metastases are fairly well demarcated, with variable perivascular growth (so-called vascular cooption) in the adjacent CNS tissue {172}. On occasion, small cell carcinomas and lymphomas may show more diffuse infiltration (pseudogliomatous growth) in the adjacent brain parenchyma {145,1770}. Tumour necrosis may be extensive, leaving recognizable tumour tissue only at the periphery of the lesion and around blood vessels {1923}. In leptomeningeal metastasis, the tumour cells are dispersed in the subarachnoid and Virchow–Robin spaces and may invade the adjacent CNS parenchyma and nerve roots {2490}. Although the pattern of infiltration is often helpful in distinguishing a metastatic tumour from a primary CNS tumour (e.g. a diffuse glioma), occasional cases of glioblastoma can demonstrate a pushing margin and/or invasion via Virchow–Robin spaces rather than a single-cell infiltration pattern (especially in focal areas) and can therefore occasionally be confused for metastatic tumours on a morphological basis.

Immunophenotype
The immunohistochemical characteristics of secondary CNS tumours are generally similar to those of the tumours from which they originate. Immunohistochemical analysis is often very helpful for distinguishing primary from secondary CNS tumours and for assessment of the exact nature and origin of the metastatic neoplasm (particularly in cases with an unknown primary tumour) {149,1923}.

Proliferation
Metastatic CNS tumours show variable and often marked mitotic activity. The proliferation index may be significantly higher than in the primary neoplasm {171}.

Pathogenesis
Before they present as haematogenous metastases in the CNS, tumour cells must successfully complete a series of steps: escape from the primary tumour, entry into and survival in the blood stream, arrest and extravasation in the CNS, and survival and growth in the CNS microenvironment {1264,2032}. The molecular basis of CNS spread in the various tumour types is poorly elucidated and requires further study. Secondary CNS tumours may also develop by direct extension from primary tumours in adjacent anatomical structures (e.g. paranasal sinuses and bone) {2323}. Such tumours are not formally considered metastases, because they remain in continuity with the primary neoplasm. Once in contact with the cerebrospinal fluid–containing compartments, cells of those tumours

Table 18.01 Immunohistochemical profiles of metastatic carcinomas and melanoma; adapted from Pekmezci M and Perry A {1923}

	CK5/6	NCAM1 (CD56)	CK7	CK20	TTF1	NapA	GCDFP15	CDX2	RCCm	PSA	EMA	PAX8	Vim	Melan-A
Squamous cell carcinoma	+	−	+	−	−	−	−	−	−	−	+	−	−	−
Lung small cell carcinoma	−	+	+	−	+	−	−	−	−	−	+	−	−	−
Lung adenocarcinoma	−	−	+	−	+	+	−	−	+/−	−	+	−	−	−
Breast adenocarcinoma	+/−	−	+	−	−	−	+	−	−	−	+	−	−	−
Colorectal adenocarcinoma	−	−	−	+	−	−	−	+	−	−	+	−	−	−
Stomach adenocarcinoma	−	−	+	+	−	−	−	+	−	−	+	−	−	−
Renal cell carcinoma	−	−	−	−	−	−	−	−	+	−	+	+	+	−
Prostate adenocarcinoma	−	−	−	−	−	−	−	−	−	+	+	−	−	−
Urothelial carcinoma	+	−	+	+	−	−	−	−	−	−	+	−	−	−
Melanoma	−	−	−	−	−	−	−	−	−	−	−	−	+	+

−: usually negative; +/−: positive in a significant subset; +: usually positive.
Abbreviations: NapA, napsin-A; PSA, prostate-specific antigen; RCCm, renal cell carcinoma marker; Vim, vimentin.
Note: This table lists the most common patterns of expression, but many exceptions exist. The list in this table is not complete; other markers may also be useful, such as HMB45 and microphthalmia-associated transcription factor (MITF) for melanocytic tumours. If the primary versus metastatic nature of the CNS neoplasm is uncertain, other immunohistochemical markers are useful, such as GFAP and OLIG2 for gliomas; inhibin and D2-40 for haemangioblastomas; and GFAP, transthyretin, and KIR7.1 for choroid plexus tumours.

may disseminate (seed) throughout the CNS.

Molecular genetics and predictive factors

A wide range of tumour types cause brain metastases, and some molecularly defined tumour subtypes have higher propensity to metastasize to the CNS (e.g. ERBB2-positive and triple-negative breast cancer) {1505}. Systemic therapy with novel targeted agents is increasingly being used for patients with CNS metastases. Biomarker tests to be considered for such therapies include *EGFR* mutation and *ALK* rearrangement in non-small cell lung cancer, *ERBB2* amplification and estrogen and progesterone receptor expression in breast cancer, *BRAF* mutation in melanoma, RAS mutation in colorectal cancer, and *ERBB2* amplification in gastro-oesophageal cancer {170}. For some markers, there are significant discordance rates between primary tumours and brain metastases, which may influence the necessity of performing biomarker analyses on brain metastasis tissue samples for therapy planning {170, 1024}.

Prognostic factors

The main established prognostic factors for patients with brain metastases are patient age, Karnofsky performance status, number of brain metastases, and status of extracranial disease. Several prognostic scores taking these parameters into account have been described, but require validation in independent and prospective studies {1328,2404}. Other factors of prognostic significance include the specific tumour type and the molecular drivers involved (e.g. ERBB2 in breast cancer) {1505}. Neuroradiological parameters such as peritumoural brain oedema may also provide prognostic information {2401}. In more recent studies, the reported improvement in overall survival of patients with CNS metastases may be attributable to improvements in focal and systemic therapies in combination with earlier detection of such metastases {1783}.

Contributors

Dr Kenneth D. ALDAPE*
Ontario Cancer Institute
Brain Tumor Biology Program
Princess Margaret Cancer Centre
Toronto Medical Discovery Tower
101 College Street, Room 14-601
Toronto ON M5G 1L7
CANADA
Tel. +1 416 634 8793
kadalpe@gmail.com

Dr Cristina R. ANTONESCU*
Department of Pathology
Memorial Sloan Kettering Cancer Center
1275 York Avenue
New York NY 10021
USA
Tel. +1 212 639 5905
Fax +1 212 717 3203
antonesc@mskcc.org

Dr Jill BARNHOLTZ-SLOAN
Case Comprehensive Cancer Center
Case Western Reserve University
2-526 Wolstein Research Building
2103 Cornell Road
Cleveland OH 44106-7295
USA
Tel. +1 216 368 1506
Fax +1 216 368 2606
jill.barnholtz-sloan@case.edu

Dr Boris C. BASTIAN
Department of Pathology and Dermatology
University of California
San Francisco Helen Diller
Family Comprehensive Cancer Center
1450 Third Street, Box 3116
San Francisco CA 94158-9001
USA
Tel. +1 415 502 0267
boris.bastian@ucsf.edu

Dr Albert J. BECKER
Department of Neuropathology
University of Bonn Medical Center
Sigmund-Freud-Strasse 25
53105 Bonn
GERMANY
Tel. +49 228 287 11352
Fax +49 228 287 14331
albert_becker@uni-bonn.de

Dr Mitchel S. BERGER*
Department of Neurological Surgery
University of California, San Francisco
505 Parnassus Avenue, Room M786
San Francisco CA 94143-0112
USA
Tel. +1 415 353 3933; +1 415 353 2637
Fax +1 415 353 3910
bergerm@neurosurg.ucsf.edu

Dr Jaclyn A. BIEGEL
Pathology and Laboratory Medicine
Children's Hospital Los Angeles and
Keck School of Medicine of USC
4650 Sunset Boulevard, Mail Stop #173
Los Angeles CA 90027
USA
Tel. +1 323 361 8674
Fax +1 323 644 8580
jbiegel@chla.usc.edu

Dr Wojciech BIERNAT
Department of Pathomorphology
Medical University of Gdańsk
ulica Smoluchowskiego 17
80-214 Gdansk
POLAND
Tel. +48 58 349 3750
Fax +48 58 349 3750
biernat@gumed.edu.pl

Dr Darell D. BIGNER
Department of Pathology
Duke University Medical Center
Box 3156, Research Drive, 177 MSRB
Durham NC 27710
USA
Tel. +1 919 684 5018; +1 919 684 6790
Fax +1 919 684 6458
darell.bigner@duke.edu

Dr Ingmar BLÜMCKE
University of Erlangen
Institute of Neuropathology
Schwabachanlage 6
91054 Erlangen
GERMANY
bluemcke@uk-erlangen.de

Dr Corinne BOUVIER
Service d'Anatomie Pathologique et
de Neuropathologie
Hôpital de la Timone 2
265 rue Saint-Pierre
13385 Marseille Cedex 05
FRANCE
Tel. +33 4 13 42 90 13
Fax +33 4 13 42 90 42
corinne.labit@ap-hm.fr

Dr Michael BRADA*
Department of Molecular and
Clinical Cancer Medicine
University of Liverpool
Clatterbridge Cancer Centre
Bebington, Wirral CH63 4JY
UNITED KINGDOM
Tel. +44 15 148 277 93
Fax +44 15 148 276 21
michael.brada@liverpool.ac.uk

Dr Sebastian BRANDNER
Division of Neuropathology
UCL Institute of Neurology and National
Hospital for Neurology and Neurosurgery
Mailbox 126, Queen Square
London WC1N 3BG
UNITED KINGDOM
Tel. +44 20 344 844 35
Fax +44 20 344 844 86
s.brandner@ucl.ac.uk

Dr Daniel J. BRAT*
Department of Pathology and
Laboratory Medicine
Emory University Hospital
H-176, 1364 Clifton Road NE
Atlanta GA 30322
USA
Tel. +1 404 712 1266
Fax +1 404 712 0148
dbrat@emory.edu

Dr Herbert BUDKA
Institute of Neuropathology
University Hospital Zurich
Schmelzbergstrasse 12
8091 Zurich
SWITZERLAND
Tel. +41 44 255 25 02
Fax +41 44 255 44 02
herbert.budka@usz.ch

*Indicates participation in the Working Group Meeting on the *WHO Classification of Tumours of the Central Nervous System* that was held in Heidelberg, Germany, 21–24 June 2015.
# Indicates disclosure of interests.

Dr Peter C. BURGER*
Department of Pathology
Johns Hopkins Medical Institutions
Pathology Building, Zayed Tower
Room 2101, 1800 Orleans Street
Baltimore MD 21231
USA
Tel. +1 410 955 8378
Fax +1 410 614 9310
pburger@jhmi.edu

Dr Rolf BUSLEI
University of Erlangen
Institute of Neuropathology
Schwabachanlage 6
91054 Erlangen
GERMANY
Tel. +49 9131 852 60 31
Fax +49 9131 852 60 33
rolf.buslei@uk-erlangen.de

Dr J. Gregory CAIRNCROSS
Department of Clinical Neurosciences
University of Calgary and
Foothills Medical Centre
HRIC 2AA-19 3280 Hospital Drive NW
Calgary AB T2N 4Z6
CANADA
Tel. +1 403 210 3934
Fax +1 403 210 8135
jgcairnx@ucalgary.ca

Dr David CAPPER*#
Institute of Pathology
Department of Neuropathology
Heidelberg University
Im Neuenheimer Feld 224
69120 Heidelberg
GERMANY
Tel. +49 6221 56 37 254
Fax +49 6221 56 45 66
david.capper@med.uni-heidelberg.de

Dr Webster K. CAVENEE*
Cellular and Molecular Medicine East
University of California, San Diego
9500 Gilman Drive, #0660, Room 3080
La Jolla, San Diego CA 92093-0660
USA
Tel. +1 858 534 7805
Fax +1 858 534 7750
wcavenee@ucsd.edu

Dr Leila CHIMELLI
Department of Pathology
University Hospital CFF - UFRJ
Avenida Epitacio Pessoa 4720/501
Rio de Janeiro 22471-003
BRAZIL
Tel. +55 21 99604 4880; +55 21 2226 9998
Fax +55 21 3207 6548
leila.chimelli@gmail.com

Dr Elizabeth B. CLAUS
Department of Biostatistics/
Epidemiology/Neurosurgery
Yale University School of Medicine
60 College Street, Box 208034
New Haven CT 06520-8034
USA
Tel. +1 203 785 2838
Fax +1 203 785 6912
elizabeth.claus@yale.edu

Dr V. Peter COLLINS*
Department of Pathology
University of Cambridge
Tennis Court Road
Cambridge CB2 1QP
UNITED KINGDOM
Tel. +44 1223 336 072; +44 1223 217 164
Fax +44 1223 216 980
vpc20@cam.ac.uk

Dr Martina DECKERT
Department of Neuropathology
University of Cologne
Kerpener Strasse 62
50931 Cologne
GERMANY
Tel. +49 221 478 52 65
Fax +49 221 478 72 37
martina.deckert@uni-koeln.de

Dr Charles G. EBERHART*
Department of Pathology
Johns Hopkins University
720 Rutland Avenue, Ross Building 558
Baltimore MD 21205
USA
Tel. +1 410 502 5185
Fax +1 410 959 9777
ceberha@jhmi.edu

Dr David W. ELLISON*
Department of Pathology
St. Jude Children's Research Hospital
262 Danny Thomas Place, MS 250
Room C-5001
Memphis TN 38105-3678
USA
Tel. +1 901 595 5438
Fax +1 901 595 3100
david.ellison@stjude.org

Dr Charis ENG
Genomic Medicine Institute
Cleveland Clinic Lerner Research Institute
9500 Euclid Avenue, NE-50
Cleveland OH 44195
USA
Tel. +1 216 444 3440
Fax +1 216 636 0655
engc@ccf.org

Dr Judith A. FERRY
Department of Pathology
Massachusetts General Hospital
55 Fruit Street
Boston MA 02114
USA
Tel. +1 617 726 4826
Fax +1 617 726 7474
jferry@mgh.harvard.edu

Dr Dominique FIGARELLA-BRANGER*
Laboratoire d'anatomie
pathologique-neuropathologique
Hôpital de la Timone
264 rue Saint-Pierre
13385 Marseille Cedex 05
FRANCE
Tel. +33 4 13 42 90 38
Fax +33 4 91 38 44 11
dominique.figarella-branger@univ-amu.fr

Dr Gregory N. FULLER*
Department of Pathology
University of Texas
MD Anderson Cancer Center
1515 Holcombe Boulevard, Unit 085
Houston TX 77030
USA
Tel. +1 713 792 2042
Fax +1 713 792 3696
gfuller@mdanderson.org

Dr Marco GESSI
Department of Neuropathology
University of Bonn Medical Center
Sigmund-Freud-Strasse 25
53105 Bonn
GERMANY
Tel. +49 228 287 166 42
Fax +49 228 287 143 31
marco.gessi@ukb.uni-bonn.de
mgessimd@yahoo.com

Dr Felice GIANGASPERO*
Department of Radiological, Oncological and
Anatomopathological Sciences
Policlinico Umberto I, Sapienza University
Viale Regina Elena, 324
00161 Rome
ITALY
Tel. +39 06 49 73 710; +39 06 44 46 86 06
Fax +39 06 48 97 91 75
felice.giangaspero@uniroma1.it

Dr Caterina GIANNINI*
Anatomic Pathology
Mayo Clinic College of Medicine
200 First Street SW
Rochester MN 55905
USA
Tel. +1 507 538 1181
Fax +1 507 284 1599
giannini.caterina@mayo.edu

Dr Hannu HAAPASALO
Department of Pathology
University of Tampere / Finlab Laboratories
POB 66
SF-335101 Tampere
FINLAND
Tel. +358 3 247 65 60
Fax +358 3 247 55 03
hannu.haapasalo@pshp.fi

Dr Johannes A. HAINFELLNER#
Institute of Neurology
Medical University of Vienna
Währinger Gürtel 18–20
1090 Vienna
AUSTRIA
Tel. +43 1 404 00 55 000
Fax +43 1 404 00 55 110
johannes.hainfellner@meduniwien.ac.at

Dr Christian HARTMANN#
Department of Neuropathology
Institute of Pathology
Hannover Medical School
Carl-Neubert-Strasse 1
30625 Hannover
GERMANY
Tel. +49 511 532 52 37
Fax +49 511 532 18 512
hartmann.christian@mh-hannover.de

Dr Martin HASSELBLATT
Institute of Neuropathology
University of Münster
Pottkamp 2
48149 Muenster
GERMANY
Tel. +49 251 83 569 69
Fax +49 251 83 569 71
martin.hasselblatt@ukmuenster.de

Dr Cynthia HAWKINS*
Division of Pathology, Department of
Paediatric Laboratory Medicine
Hospital for Sick Children
555 University Avenue
Toronto ON M5G 1X8
CANADA
Tel. +1 416 813 5938
Fax +1 416 813 5974
cynthia.hawkins@sickkids.ca

Dr Monika HEGI#
Department of Clinical Neurosciences
University of Lausanne Hospital
Chemin des Boveresses
1066 Epalinges
SWITZERLAND
Tel. +41 21 314 25 82
Fax +41 21 314 25 87
monika.hegi@chuv.ch

Dr Takanori HIROSE*
Department of Pathology
Kobe University Hospital
7-5-2 Kusunoki-cho, Chuo-ku
Hyogo Prefecture
Kobe City 650-0017
JAPAN
thirose@hp.pref.hyogo.jp

Dr Mrinalini HONAVAR
Department of Anatomical Pathology
Pedro Hispano Hospital
Rua de Alfredo Cunha 365
Matosinhos
PORTUGAL
minalhonavar@gmail.com
mrinalini.honavar@ulsm.min-saude.pt

Dr Annie HUANG
Department of Paediatric Oncology
Hospital for Sick Children
555 University Avenue
Toronto ON M5G 1X8
CANADA
Tel. +1 416 813 8221
Fax +1 416 813 5327
annie.huang@sickkids.ca

Dr Theo J.M. HULSEBOS
Department of Genome Analysis
Academic Medical Center
Meibergdreef 9
1105 AZ Amsterdam
THE NETHERLANDS
Tel. +31 20 566 30 24
Fax +31 20 566 93 12
t.j.hulsebos@amc.uva.nl

Dr Stephen HUNTER
Department of Pathology
Emory University School of Medicine
1364 Clifton Road NE
Atlanta GA 30322
USA
Tel. +1 404 712 4278
Fax +1 404 712 0714
stephen_hunter@emory.org

Dr Jason T. HUSE
Department of Pathology
Memorial Sloan Kettering Cancer Center
1275 York Avenue
New York NY 10065
USA
Tel. +1 646 888 2642
Fax +1 646 422 0856
husej@mskcc.org

Dr Koichi ICHIMURA#
Division of Brain Tumor
Translational Research
National Cancer Center Research Institute
5-1-1 Tsukiji, Chuo-ku
Tokyo 104-0045
JAPAN
Tel. +81 3 3547 52 01 ext. 28 26
Fax +81 3 3542 25 30
kichimur@ncc.go.jp

Dr David JONES#
Division of Pediatric Neurooncology
German Cancer Research Center
Im Neuenheimer Feld 280
69120 Heidelberg
GERMANY
Tel. +49 6221 42 45 94
Fax +49 6221 42 46 39
david.jones@dkfz.de

Dr Anne JOUVET*
Centre de Pathologie et de
Neuropathologie Est
Groupement Hospitalier Est
59 boulevard Pinel
69677 Bron Cedex
FRANCE
Tel. +33 4 72 35 76 34
Fax +33 4 72 35 70 67
anne.jouvet@chu-lyon.fr

Dr Alexander R. JUDKINS
Pathology and Laboratory Medicine
Children's Hospital Los Angeles and
Keck School of Medicine of USC
4650 Sunset Boulevard, Mail Stop #43
Los Angeles CA 90027
USA
Tel. +1 323 361 4516
Fax +1 323 361 8005
ajudkins@chla.usc.edu

Dr Paul KLEIHUES*
Faculty of Medicine
University of Zurich
Pestalozzistrasse 5
8032 Zurich
SWITZERLAND
Tel. +41 44 362 21 10
kleihues@pathol.uzh.ch

Dr Bette K. KLEINSCHMIDT-DeMASTERS
Department of Neuropathology
University of Colorado
Anschutz Medical Campus
12605 East 16th Avenue, Room 3017
Aurora CO 80045
USA
bk.demasters@ucdenver.edu

Dr Philip M. KLUIN
Department of Pathology and Medical Biology
University of Groningen
Hanzeplein 1
9713 GZ Groningen
THE NETHERLANDS
Tel. +31 50 361 46 84
p.m.kluin@umcg.nl

Dr Takashi KOMORI*
Department of Laboratory Medicine and
Pathology, Neuropathology
Tokyo Metropolitan Neurological Hospital
2-6-1 Musashidai, Fuchu
Tokyo 183-0042
JAPAN
Tel. +81 42 323 51 10
Fax +81 42 322 62 19
komori-tk@igakuken.or.jp

Dr Marcel KOOL
Division of Pediatric Neurooncology
German Cancer Research Center
Im Neuenheimer Feld 280
69120 Heidelberg
GERMANY
Tel. +49 6221 42 46 36
Fax +49 6221 42 46 39
m.kool@dkfz.de

Dr Andrey KORSHUNOV
Clinical Cooperation Unit Neuropathology
German Cancer Research Center
Im Neuenheimer Feld 280
69120 Heidelberg
GERMANY
Tel. +49 6221 56 41 45
a.korshunov@dkfz-heidelberg.de

Dr Johan M. KROS*
Division of Pathology/Neuropathology
Erasmus Medical Center
Dr. Molewaterplein 50
3015 GE Rotterdam
THE NETHERLANDS
Tel. +31 61 884 57 51
Fax +31 10 408 79 05
j.m.kros@erasmusmc.nl

Dr Suet Yi LEUNG#
Department of Pathology
Li Ka Shing Faculty of Medicine
University of Hong Kong Queen Mary Hospital
Pokfulam Road
Hong Kong SAR
CHINA
Tel. +852 225 54 401
Fax +852 287 25 197
suetyi@hku.hk

Dr Ivo LEUSCHNER
Kiel Pediatric Tumor Registry
Department of Pediatric Pathology
University of Kiel
Arnold-Heller-Strasse 3, House 14
24105 Kiel
GERMANY
Tel. +49 431 597 34 44
Fax +49 431 597 34 86
ileuschner@path.uni-kiel.de

Dr Pawel P. LIBERSKI
Department of Molecular Pathology and
Neuropathology
Medical University of Lodz
ulica Kosciuszki 4
90-419 Lodz
POLAND
Fax +48 42 679 14 77
ppliber@csk.am.lodz.pl

Dr Jay LOEFFLER
Department of Radiation Oncology
Massachusetts General Hospital
Clark Center for Radiation Oncology
100 Blossom Street
Boston MA 02114-2606
USA
Tel. +1 617 724 1548
Fax +1 617 724 8334
jloeffler@partners.org

Dr M. Beatriz S. LOPES
Department of Pathology (Neuropathology)
University of Virginia Health System
Box 800214 - HSC
Charlottesville VA 22908-0214
USA
Tel. +1 434 924 9175
Fax +1 434 924 9177
msl2e@virginia.edu

Dr David N. LOUIS*
James Homer Wright Pathology Laboratories
Massachusetts General Hospital
55 Fruit Street, Warren 225
Boston MA 02114
USA
Tel. +1 617 726 2966
Fax +1 617 726 7533
dlouis@mgh.harvard.edu

Dr Masao MATSUTANI
Department of Neuro-Oncology/Neurosurgery
Saitama Medical University International
Medical Center
Yamane 1397, Hidaka-shi
Saitama 350-1298
JAPAN
Tel. +81 492 76 15 51
Fax +81 492 76 15 51
matutani@saitama-med.ac.jp

Dr Christian MAWRIN
Department of Neuropathology
Otto-von-Guericke University
Leipziger Strasse 44
39120 Magdeburg
GERMANY
christian.mawrin@med.ovgu.de

Dr Roger McLENDON*#
Department of Pathology
Duke University Medical Center
DUMC Box 3712
Durham NC 27710
USA
Tel. +1 919 684 6940
Fax +1 919 681 7634
mclen001@mc.duke.edu

Dr Michel MITTELBRONN
Institute of Neurology (Edinger Institute)
Goethe University Frankfurt
Heinrich-Hoffmann-Strasse 7
60528 Frankfurt am Main
GERMANY
Tel. +49 69 6301 841 69
Fax +49 69 9301 841 50
michel.mittelbronn@kgu.de

Dr Yoichi NAKAZATO
Department of Pathology
Hidaka Hospital
886 Nakaomachi, Takasaki
Gunma 370-0001
JAPAN
Tel. +81 27 362 62 01
Fax +81 27 362 89 01
nakazato_yoichi@gunma-u.ac.jp

Dr Hartmut P.H. NEUMANN
Department of Nephrology and Hypertension
Albert Ludwigs University of Freiburg
Hugstetterstrasse 55
79106 Freiburg
GERMANY
Tel. +49 761 270 35 78
Fax +49 761 270 37 78
hartmut.neumann@uniklinik-freiburg.de

Dr Ho-Keung NG*
Anatomical and Cellular Pathology
Prince of Wales Hospital
Chinese University of Hong Kong
Shatin
Hong Kong SAR
CHINA
Tel. +852 2632 33 37
Fax +852 2637 62 74
hkng@cuhk.edu.hk

Dr Hiroko OHGAKI*
Section of Molecular Pathology
International Agency for Research on Cancer
150 Cours Albert Thomas
69372 Lyon Cedex 08
FRANCE
Tel. +33 4 72 73 85 34
Fax +33 4 72 73 86 98
ohgakih@iarc.fr

Dr Magali OLIVIER
Molecular Mechanisms and
Biomarkers Group
International Agency for Research on Cancer
150 Cours Albert Thomas
69372 Lyon Cedex 08
FRANCE
Tel. +33 4 72 73 86 69
Fax +33 4 72 73 83 45
olivierm@iarc.fr

Dr Anne OSBORN#
Department of Radiology
University of Utah
30 N 1900 E, #1A71
Salt Lake City UT 84132
USA
Tel. +1 801 581 7553
anne.osborn@hsc.utah.edu

Dr Sung-Hye PARK
Department of Pathology
Seoul National University College of Medicine
Seoul National University Hospital
101 Daehak-ro, Jongno-gu
Seoul 110-744
REPUBLIC OF KOREA
Tel. +82 2 2072 30 90
Fax +82 2 7435 530
shparknp@snu.ac.kr

Dr Werner PAULUS*
Institute of Neuropathology
University Hospital Münster
Pottkamp 2
48149 Muenster
GERMANY
Tel. +49 251 83 569 66
Fax +49 251 83 569 71
werner.paulus@uni-muenster.de

Dr Arie PERRY*
Department of Pathology
Division of Neuropathology
University of California, San Francisco
505 Parnassus Avenue, M551, Box 0102
San Francisco CA 94143
USA
Tel. +1 415 476 5236
Fax +1 415 476 7963
arie.perry@ucsf.edu

Dr Stefan PFISTER*#
Division of Pediatric Neurooncology and
Pediatrics Clinic III
German Cancer Research Center
Im Neuenheimer Feld 280 and 430
69120 Heidelberg
GERMANY
Tel. +49 6221 42 46 18
Fax +49 6221 42 46 39
stefan.pfister@med.uni-heidelberg.de

Dr Torsten PIETSCH*#
Department of Neuropathology
University of Bonn Medical Center
Sigmund-Freud-Strasse 25
53105 Bonn
GERMANY
Tel. +49 228 287 166 06
Fax +49 228 287 143 31
t.pietsch@uni-bonn.de

Dr Karl H. PLATE
Institute of Neurology (Edinger Institute)
Goethe University Medical School
NeuroScienceCenter
Heinrich-Hoffmann-Strasse 7
60528 Frankfurt am Main
GERMANY
Tel. +49 69 6301 60 42
Fax +49 69 6301 84 150
karl-heinz.plate@kgu.de

Dr Matthias PREUSSER
Department of Internal Medicine I and
Comprehensive Cancer Center Vienna
Medical University of Vienna
Währinger Gürtel 18–20
1097 Vienna
AUSTRIA
Tel. +43 1 40400 44 570
Fax +43 1 40400 60 880
matthias.preusser@meduniwien.ac.at

Dr Guido REIFENBERGER*#
Institute of Neuropathology
University Hospital Düsseldorf
Moorenstrasse 5, Building 14.79, Floor III
40225 Düsseldorf
GERMANY
Tel. +49 211 811 86 60
Fax +49 211 811 78 04
reifenberger@med.uni-duesseldorf.de

Dr David E. REUSS
Institute of Pathology
Department of Neuropathology
Heidelberg University
Im Neuenheimer Feld 224
69120 Heidelberg
GERMANY
Tel. +49 6221 56 37 885
david.reuss@med.uni-heidelberg.de

Dr Fausto RODRIGUEZ
Department of Pathology
Division of Neuropathology
Johns Hopkins Hospital
Sheikh Zayed Tower, Room M2101
1800 Orleans Street
Baltimore MD 21231
USA
Tel. +1 443 287 6646
Fax +1 410 614 9310
frodrig4@jhmi.edu

Dr Frederico RONCAROLI
Department of Pathology
Salford Royal Foundation Hospital
University of Manchester
Stott Lane
Salford, Manchester M68HD
UNITED KINGDOM
Tel: +44 161 206 5013
federico.roncaroli@manchester.ac.uk

Dr Marc K. ROSENBLUM
Department of Pathology
Memorial Sloan Kettering Cancer Center
1275 York Avenue
New York NY 10021
USA
Tel. +1 212 639 3844
Fax +1 212 717 3203
rosenbl1@mskcc.org

Dr Brian ROUS*
National Cancer Registration Service -
Eastern Office
Victoria House, Capital Park
Fulbourn, Cambridge CB21 5XB
UNITED KINGDOM
Tel. +44 122 321 3625
Fax +44 122 321 3571
brian.rous@phe.gov.uk

Dr Elisabeth J. RUSHING#
Institute of Neuropathology
University Hospital Zurich
Schmelzbergstrasse 12
8091 Zurich
SWITZERLAND
Tel. +41 44 255 43 81
elisabethjane.rushing@usz.ch

Dr Siegal SADETZKI
Cancer and Radiation Epidemiology Unit
Gertner Institute
Chaim Sheba Medical Center
5262000 Tel Hashomer
& Sackler Faculty of Medicine
Tel Aviv University, Tel Aviv
ISRAEL
Tel. +972 3 530 32 62
Fax +972 3 534 83 60
siegals@gertner.health.gov.il

Dr Felix SAHM#
Department of Neuropathology
Heidelberg University and Clinical
Cooperation Unit Neuropathology
German Cancer Research Center
Im Neuenheimer Feld 224
69120 Heidelberg
GERMANY
Tel. +49 6221 56 378 86
felix.sahm@med.uni-heidelberg.de

Dr Sandro SANTAGATA#
Department of Pathology
Division of Neuropathology
Brigham and Women's Hospital, Harvard
Medical School, Harvard Institute of Medicine
HIM-921, 77 Avenue Louis Pasteur
Boston MA 02115
USA
Tel. +1 617 525 5686
ssantagata@partners.org

Dr Mariarita SANTI
Division of Neuropathology
Children's Hospital of Philadelphia
34th Street and Civic Center Boulevard
Philadelphia PA 19104
USA
Tel. +1 215 590 3184
santim@chop.edu

Dr Vani SANTOSH
Department of Neuropathology
National Institute of Mental Health and
Neuroscience
Hosur Road
Bangalore 560029
INDIA
vani.santosh@gmail.com

Dr Chitra SARKAR
Department of Pathology
All India Institute of Medical Sciences
Ansari Nagar
New Delhi 110029
INDIA
Tel. +91 11 265 93 371
Fax +91 11 265 88 663
sarkar.chitra@gmail.com

Dr Davide SCHIFFER
Policlinico di Monza Foundation
University of Turin
Via Cherasco 15, Corso Massimo D'Azeglio 51
10126 Torino TO
ITALY
Tel. +39 011 696 44 79
Fax +39 016 136 91 09
davide.schiffer@unito.it

Dr M.C. SHARMA
Department of Pathology
All India Institute of Medical Sciences
Ansari Nagar
New Delhi 110029
INDIA
Tel. +91 11 659 33 71
Fax +91 11 686 26 63
sharmamehar@yahoo.co.in

Dr Dov SOFFER
Department of Pathology
Tel Aviv Sourasky Medical Center
6 Weizman Street
64239 Tel Aviv
ISRAEL
Tel. +972 3 694 75 72
Fax +972 3 697 46 48
soffer@cc.huji.ac.il

Dr Figen SÖYLEMEZOGLU
Department of Pathology
Hacettepe University
Tip Fakultesi, Patoloji Anabilim Dali
06100 Ankara
TURKEY
Tel. +90 312 241 99 51
Fax +90 312 305 26 21
figensoylemezoglu@gmail.com

Dr Anat O. STEMMER-RACHAMIMOV
Molecular Neuro-Oncology Laboratory
Massachusetts General Hospital
CNY6, Building 149, 149 13th Street
Charlestown MA 02129
USA
Tel. +1 617 726 5510
Fax +1 617 726 5079
astemmerrachamimov@partners.org

Dr Constantine A. STRATAKIS
Section on Endocrinology and Genetics
Eunice Kennedy Shriver National Institute of
Child Health and Human Development
Building 10, CRC, Room 1-3330
(East Laboratories), MSC 1103
Bethesda MD 20892, USA
Tel. +1 301 402 1998
Fax +1 301 402 0574
stratakc@exchange.nih.gov

Dr Roger STUPP
Department of Oncology
University Hospital Zurich
Rämistrasse 100
8091 Zurich
SWITZERLAND
Tel. +41 44 255 9779
Fax +41 44 255 9778
roger.stupp@usz.ch

Dr Dominik STURM
German Cancer Research Center and
Heidelberg University Medical Center for
Children and Adolescents
Im Neuenheimer Feld 580
69120 Heidelberg
GERMANY
Tel. +49 6221 42 46 76
Fax +49 6221 42 46 39
d.sturm@dkfz.de

Dr Mario L. SUVÀ
James Homer Wright Pathology Laboratories
Massachusetts General Hospital
149 13th Street, Office 6.010
Charlestown MA 02129
USA
Tel. +1 617 726 5695
Fax +1 617 724 1813
suva.mario@mgh.harvard.edu

Dr Uri TABORI
Paediatric Haematology/Oncology
Hospital for Sick Children
555 University Avenue
Toronto ON M5G 1X8
CANADA
Tel. +1 416 813 8221
Fax +1 416 813 5327
uri.tabori@sickkids.ca

Dr Shinya TANAKA
Department of Cancer Pathology
Hokkaido University
Graduate School of Medicine
N15, W7
Sapporo 060-8638
JAPAN
Tel. +81 11 706 50 52
Fax +81 11 706 59 02
tanaka@med.hokudai.ac.jp

Dr Tarik TIHAN
Department of Pathology
University of California, San Francisco Helen
Diller Family Comprehensive Cancer Center
505 Parnassus Avenue, Moffitt
San Francisco CA 94143-0511
USA
Tel. +1 415 476 5236
Fax +1 415 476 7963
tihan@itsa.ucsf.edu

Dr Scott R. VANDENBERG
Department of Pathology
University of California
San Diego School of Medicine
9500 Gilman Drive, La Jolla
San Diego CA 92093
USA
Tel. +1 858 534 0455
srvandenberg@mail.ucsd.edu

Dr Erwin G. VAN MEIR
Winship Cancer Institute
Emory University School of Medicine
1365-C Clifton Road NE, Suite C 5078
Atlanta GA 30322
USA
Tel. +1 404 778 5563
Fax +1 404 778 5550
evanmei@emory.edu

Dr Pascale VARLET#
Laboratoire d'anatomie pathologique
Centre hospitalier Sainte-Anne
1 rue Cabanis
75674 Paris Cedex 14
FRANCE
Tel. +33 1 45 65 86 56
Fax +33 1 45 65 87 28
p.varlet@ch-sainte-anne.fr

Dr Alexandre VASILJEVIC
Centre de Pathologie et de
Neuropathologie Est
Groupement Hospitalier Est
59 boulevard Pinel
69677 Bron Cedex
FRANCE
Tel. +33 4 72 12 96 04
Fax +33 4 72 35 70 67
alexandre.vasiljevic@chu-lyon.fr

Dr Roel G.W. VERHAAK
Department of Genomic Medicine
Department of Bioinformatics and
Computational Biology, University of Texas
MD Anderson Cancer Center
1400 Pressler Street, Unit #1410
Houston TX 77030
USA
Tel. +1 713 563 2293
Fax +1 713 563 4242
rverhaak@mdanderson.org

Dr Harry V. VINTERS#
UCLA Pathology & Laboratory Medicine
David Geffen School of Medicine at UCLA
Box 951732, 18-170B NPI
Los Angeles CA 90095-1732
USA
Tel. +1 310 825 6191
hvinters@mednet.ucla.edu

Dr Andreas VON DEIMLING*
Institute of Pathology, Division of
Neuropathology and Clinical Cooperation Unit
Neuropathology, Heidelberg University and
German Cancer Research Center
Im Neuenheimer Feld 224
69120 Heidelberg
GERMANY
Tel. +49 6221 56 46 50
andreas.vondeimling@med.uni-heidelberg.de

Dr Alexander O. VORTMEYER
Department of Pathology
Yale University School of Medicine
310 Cedar Street, LH416
New Haven CT 06520
USA
Tel. +1 203 785 6843
Fax +1 203 785 6899
alexander.vortmeyer@yale.edu

Dr Michael WELLER#
Department of Neurology
University Hospital Zurich
Frauenklinikstrasse 26
8091 Zurich
SWITZERLAND
Tel. +41 44 255 55 00
Fax +41 44 255 45 07
michael.weller@usz.ch

Dr Pieter WESSELING*
Department of Pathology
VU University Medical Center Amsterdam and
Radboud University Medical Center Nijmegen
Box 9101
6500 HB Nijmegen
THE NETHERLANDS
Tel. +31 24 361 43 23
Fax +31 24 366 87 50
pieter.wesseling@radboudumc.nl

Dr Wolfgang WICK*#
Neurology Clinic
Heidelberg University Hospital
Im Neuenheimer Feld 400
69120 Heidelberg
GERMANY
Tel. +49 6221 56 70 75
Fax +49 6221 56 75 54
wolfgang.wick@med.uni-heidelberg.de

Dr Otmar D. WIESTLER*
German Cancer Research Center
Im Neuenheimer Feld 280
69120 Heidelberg
GERMANY
Tel. +49 6221 42 26 53
Fax +49 6221 42 21 62
o.wiestler@dkfz.de

Dr Hendrik WITT
Department of Pediatric Oncology
Heidelberg University
Division of Pediatric Neurooncology
German Cancer Research Center
Im Neuenheimer Feld 430
69120 Heidelberg
GERMANY
Tel. +49 6221 56 357 02
Fax +49 6221 56 455 5
h.witt@dkfz.de

Dr Hai YAN#
Molecular Oncogenomics Laboratory
Duke University
199B MSRB, DUMC 3156
Durham NC 27710
USA
Tel. +1 919 668 7850
hai.yan@duke.edu

Dr Stephen YIP
Pathology and Laboratory Medicine
University of British Columbia
Vancouver General Hospital
855 West 12th Avenue
Vancouver BC V5Z 1M9
CANADA
Tel. +1 604 875 4111
Fax +1 604 875 4797
stephen.yip@vch.ca

Dr Hideaki YOKOO
Department of Human Pathology
Gunma University
3-39-22 Showa
Maebashi 371-8511
JAPAN
Tel. +81 27 220 71 11
Fax +81 27 220 79 78
hyokoo@gunma-u.ac.jp

Dr Tarek YOUSRY
Division of Neuroradiology and Neurophysics
UCL Institute of Neurology
Lysholm Department of Neuroradiology,
NHNN, University College London Hospitals
Queen Square
London WC1N 3BG
UNITED KINGDOM
t.yousry@ucl.ac.uk

Dr David ZAGZAG
Department of Pathology and Neurosurgery
NYU Medical Center and School of Medicine
550 First Avenue
New York NY 10016
USA
Tel. +1 212 263 2262
Fax +1 212 263 7916
dz4@nyu.edu

Declaration of interest statements

Dr Capper reports receiving income from two patents held by the German Cancer Research Center (DKFZ): one for an antibody to detect R132H-mutant IDH1 in fixed glioma samples, licensed to Dianova, and one for an antibody to detect V600E-mutant BRAF in formalin-fixed paraffin-embedded tumour samples, licensed to Ventana Medical Systems (a member of the Roche Group).

Dr Hainfellner reports that the Austrian Brain Tumour Registry at the Institute of Neurology, Medical University of Vienna, receives research support from Roche.

Dr Hartmann reports having received personal consultancy fees from Apogenix. Dr Hartmann reports receiving income from a patent held by DKFZ for an antibody to detect R132H-mutant IDH1, licensed to Dianova

Dr Hegi reports that her department at the Lausanne University Hospital has received non-financial research support from MDxHealth.

Dr Ichimura reports receiving research support from SRL. Dr Ichimura reports receiving travel support from MSD K.K. (a subsidiary of Merck & Co.). Dr Ichimura reports receiving personal speaker's fees from Eisai Co., Astellas Pharma, Otsuka Pharmaceutical, Sanofi K.K., Daiichi Sankyo, Chugai Pharmaceutical, and Teijin Pharma.

Dr Jones reports receiving non-financial research support from Illumina. Dr Jones reports having a patent pending for a brain tumour classification based on DNA methylation fingerprinting.

Dr Leung reports that the Department of Pathology at the University of Hong Kong has a collaborative research agreement with Merck, Pfizer, and Servier.

Dr McLendon reports being part of a pending patent application, with Duke University, for a technique to identify and measure FUBP1 and CIC in brain tumours.

Dr Osborn reports having been a founder and shareholder of Amirsys and Amirsys Publishing. Dr Osborn reports receiving personal consultancy fees from Elsevier. Dr Osborn reports having received personal speaker's fees from Mallinckrodt.

Dr Pfister reports receiving non-financial research support from Illumina. Dr Pfister reports having a patent pending for a brain tumour classification based on DNA methylation fingerprinting.

Dr Pietsch reports having received travel support from Affymetrix. Dr Pietsch reports having received personal speaker's fees from Roche.

Dr Reifenberger reports having received research funding from Roche and Merck and honoraria for advisory boards or lectures from Amgen, Roche and Celldex.

Dr Rushing reports having received research funding from Novartis.

Dr Sahm reports having a patent pending for a method for detecting the presence of antigens in situ.

Dr Santagata reports having cofounded Bayesian Diagnostics. Dr Santagata reports having received personal consultancy fees from Bayesian Diagnostics. Dr Santagata reports that a close relative receives royalties from BioReference Laboratories for intellectual property rights for a targeted genotyping platform for cancer diagnostics.

Dr Varlet reports receiving travel support from Hoffmann-La Roche and Boehringer Ingelheim. Dr Varlet reports that a close relative is employed by Novartis France.

Dr Vinters reports that the UCLA Department of Pathology and Laboratory Medicine conducts contract work for Neuroindex funded by an NIH grant. Dr Vinters reports receiving royalties from Mosby Elsevier. Dr Vinters reports holding shares in 3M Company; General Electric; Teva Pharmaceutical Industries; Pfizer; GlaxoSmithKline; and Becton, Dickinson and Company.

Dr Weller reports receiving personal consultancy fees from MagForce AG, Isarna Therapeutics, Celldex Therapeutics, ImmunoCellular Therapeutics, Roche, and Merck Serono. Dr Weller reports receiving personal speaker's fees from Isarna Therapeutics, MSD, Roche, and Merck Serono. Dr Weller reports that the University Hospital Zurich and University of Zurich receive research support from Roche, Merck Serono, Bayer, Isarna Therapeutics, Piqur Therapeutics, and Novocure.

Dr Wick reports holding patents related to CD95L as a diagnostic marker, IDH1 immunotherapy, and IDH1 antibody.

Dr Yan reports being the chief security officer of Genentron Health and having substantial shareholding in the company. Dr Yan reports receiving personal consultancy fees from Sanofi and Blueprint Medicines and reports receiving royalties for IDH-targeted therapy and diagnosis from Agios and Personal Genome Diagnostics. Dr Yan reports having received royalties from Blueprint Medicines. Dr Yan reports having a patent pending for *IDH1* and *TERT* mutations in gliomas. Dr Yan reports that his laboratory at the Duke University Medical Center received research support from Gilead Sciences and Sanofi.

IARC/WHO Committee for the International Classification of Diseases for Oncology (ICD-O)

Dr Freddie BRAY
Section of Cancer Surveillance
International Agency for Research on Cancer
150 Cours Albert Thomas
69372 Lyon Cedex 08
FRANCE
Tel. +33 4 72 73 84 53
Fax +33 4 72 73 86 96
brayf@iarc.fr

Dr David W. ELLISON
Department of Pathology
St. Jude Children's Research Hospital
262 Danny Thomas Place, MS 250
Room C-5001
Memphis TN 38105-3678
USA
Tel. +1 901 595 5438
Fax +1 901 595 3100
david.ellison@stjude.org

Mrs April FRITZ
A. Fritz and Associates, LLC
21361 Crestview Road
Reno NV 89521
USA
Tel. +1 775 636 7243
Fax +1 888 891 3012
april@afritz.org

Dr Robert JAKOB
Data Standards and Informatics
Information, Evidence and Research
World Health Organization (WHO)
20 Avenue Appia
1211 Geneva 27
SWITZERLAND
Tel. +41 22 791 58 77
Fax +41 22 791 48 94
jakobr@who.int

Dr Paul KLEIHUES
Faculty of Medicine
University of Zurich
Pestalozzistrasse 5
8032 Zurich
SWITZERLAND
Tel. +41 44 362 21 10
kleihues@pathol.uzh.ch

Dr David N. LOUIS
James Homer Wright Pathology Laboratories
Massachusetts General Hospital
55 Fruit Street, Warren 225
Boston MA 02114
USA
Tel. +1 617 726 2966
Fax +1 617 726 7533
dlouis@mgh.harvard.edu

Dr Hiroko OHGAKI
Section of Molecular Pathology
International Agency for Research on Cancer
150 Cours Albert Thomas
69372 Lyon Cedex 08
FRANCE
Tel. +33 4 72 73 85 34
Fax +33 4 72 73 86 98
ohgakih@iarc.fr

Dr Marion PIÑEROS
Section of Cancer Surveillance
International Agency for Research on Cancer
150 Cours Albert Thomas
69372 Lyon Cedex 08
FRANCE
Tel. +33 4 72 73 84 18
Fax +33 4 72 73 80 22
pinerosm@iarc.fr

Dr Brian ROUS
National Cancer Registration Service -
Eastern Office
Victoria House, Capital Park
Fulbourn, Cambridge CB21 5XB
UNITED KINGDOM
Tel. +44 122 321 3625
Fax +44 122 321 3571
brian.rous@phe.gov.uk

Dr Leslie H. SOBIN
Frederick National Laboratory for
Cancer Research
The Cancer Human Biobank
National Cancer Institute
6110 Executive Boulevard, Suite 250
Rockville MD 20852, USA
Tel. +1 301 443 7947
Fax +1 301 402 9325
leslie.sobin@nih.gov

Sources of figures and tables

Sources of figures

1.01	Louis DN
1.02	From N Engl J Med, Yan H, Parsons DW, Jin G, et al., IDH1 and IDH2 mutations in gliomas, 360, 765–73. Copyright © 2009 Massachusetts Medical Society. Reprinted with permission from Massachusetts Medical Society.
1.03	Reuss DE
1.04A,B	Kleihues P
1.05A	Nakazato Y
1.05B	Rushing EJ
1.06	Perry A
1.07	Kros JM
1.08A,B	Nakazato Y
1.09A,B	Fuller GN
1.10A	Nobusawa S Department of Human Pathology, Gunma University Graduate School of Medicine, Gunma, Japan
1.10B	Kleihues P
1.10C	Ohgaki H
1.11A–C	Kleihues P
1.12	Burger PC
1.13	Rushing EJ
1.14A	Burger PC
1.14B	Perry A
1.15A	Ohgaki H
1.15B	Perry A
1.15C	Kleihues P
1.16	From N Engl J Med, Cancer Genome Atlas Research Network, Brat DJ, Verhaak RG, et al., Comprehensive, integrative genomic analysis of diffuse lower-grade gliomas, 372, 2481–98. Copyright © 2015 Massachusetts Medical Society. Reprinted with permission from Massachusetts Medical Society.
1.17	IARC; based on data from Nobusawa S et al. {1797}
1.18A–C	Perry A
1.19	Burger PC
1.20A,B	Kleihues P
1.21A–D	Kleihues P
1.22	Burger PC
1.23	Kleihues P
1.24A,B	Louis DN
1.25A–C	Perry A
1.26A–C	Perry A
1.27A–D	Perry A
1.28A	Nakazato Y
1.28B	Reifenberger G
1.29A,B	Perry A
1.29C	Iwasaki Y (deceased)
1.30A,B	Perry A
1.31	Louis DN
1.32	Perry A
1.33A–D	Reprinted from Rong Y, Durden DL, Van Meir EG, et al., 'Pseudopalisading' necrosis in glioblastoma: a familiar morphologic feature that links vascular pathology, hypoxia, and angiogenesis, J Neuropathol Exp Neurol, 2006, 65, 6, 529–39, by permission of Oxford University Press / the American Association of Neuropathologists, Inc.
1.34	© 2005 Mica Duran, http://www.micaduran.com, info@micaduran.com. Adapted from Rong Y, Durden DL, Van Meir EG, et al., 'Pseudopalisading' necrosis in glioblastoma: a familiar morphologic feature that links vascular pathology, hypoxia, and angiogenesis, J Neuropathol Exp Neurol, 2006, 65, 6, 529–39, by permission of Oxford University Press / the American Association of Neuropathologists, Inc.
1.35	Kleihues P
1.36A	Kleihues P
1.36B	Iwasaki Y (deceased)
1.37	Adapted from Suvà ML, Riggi N, Bernstein BE (2013). Epigenetic reprogramming in cancer. Science. 339(6127):1567–70. Reprinted with permission from AAAS.
1.38	From N Engl J Med, Hegi ME, Diserens AC, Gorlia T, et al., MGMT gene silencing and benefit from temozolomide in glioblastoma, 352, 997–1003. Copyright © 2005 Massachusetts Medical Society. Reprinted with permission from Massachusetts Medical Society.
1.39	Reprinted from Taylor TE, Furnari FB, Cavenee WK (2012). Targeting EGFR for treatment of glioblastoma: molecular basis to overcome resistance. Curr Cancer Drug Targets. 12(3):197–209. Reprinted by permission of Eureka Science Ltd. © 2012 Bentham Science Publishers.
1.40	Nakazato Y
1.41	Burger PC
1.42	Nakazato Y
1.43A–C	Nakazato Y
1.43D	Kleihues P
1.44	Reprinted from Burger PC (2009). Smears and frozen sections in surgical neuropathology. PB Medical Publishing: Baltimore.
1.45A,B	Kleihues P
1.46A,B	Kleihues P
1.46C	Nakazato Y
1.47	Kleinschmidt-DeMasters BK
1.48A,B	Kleinschmidt-DeMasters BK
1.49A,B	Ellison DW
1.49C	Kleinschmidt-DeMasters BK
1.50	Adapted from Ohgaki H, Kleihues P (2013). The definition of primary and secondary glioblastoma. Clin Cancer Res. 15;19:764–72.
1.51	IARC; based on combined data from Nobusawa S et al. {1797} and The Cancer Genome Atlas Research Network {350}
1.52	Kleihues P
1.53	Capper D
1.54A	Reprinted from Nobusawa S, Watanabe T, Kleihues P, et al. (2009). IDH1 mutations as molecular signature and predictive factor of secondary glioblastomas. Clin Cancer Res. 15:6002–7.
1.54B	From N Engl J Med, Yan H, Parsons DW, Jin G, et al., IDH1 and IDH2 mutations in gliomas, 360, 765–73. Copyright © 2009 Massachusetts Medical Society. Reprinted with permission from Massachusetts Medical Society.
1.55A–D	Laughlin S Department of Diagnostic Imaging Hospital for Sick Children Toronto (ON), Canada
1.56	Reprinted from Solomon DA, Wood MD, Tihan T, et al. (2015). Diffuse midline gliomas with histone H3-K27M mutation: a series of 47 cases assessing the spectrum of morphologic variation and associated genetic alterations. Brain Pathol. doi: 10.1111/bpa.12336. [Epub ahead of print] © 2015 International Society of Neuropathology; with permission of John Wiley & Sons.
1.57	Hawkins C
1.58A	Ellison DW
1.58B	Hawkins C
1.59	Perry A
1.60	IARC, based on combined data from the German Glioma Network (Reifenberger G) and the University of Heidelberg (Capper D, von Deimling A)
1.61A,B	Kleihues P

1.62	Kleihues P
1.63A,C	Nakazato Y
1.63B	Yip S
1.63D	Nobusawa S
	Department of Human Pathology, Gunma University Graduate School of Medicine, Gunma, Japan
1.64A	Reifenberger G
1.64B,C	Nakazato Y
1.65A,B	Nakazato Y
1.66A,C	Yip S
1.66B	Nakazato Y
1.67	Reifenberger G
1.68	Kleihues P
1.69A,D	Reifenberger G
1.69B	Nakazato Y
1.69C	VandenBerg SR
1.70	Reifenberger G
1.71A,B	Reifenberger G
1.72	Kleihues P
1.73	Reprinted from Acta Neuropathol, ATRX and IDH1-R132H immunohistochemistry with subsequent copy number analysis and IDH sequencing as a basis for an "integrated" diagnostic approach for adult astrocytoma, oligodendroglioma and glioblastoma, 129, 2015, 133–46, Reuss DE, Sahm F, Schrimpf D, et al., © Springer-Verlag Berlin Heidelberg 2014; With permission of Springer.
2.01	Kleihues P
2.02A–F	Giannini C
2.03A–C	Koeller K
	Department of Radiology Mayo Clinic Rochester (MN), USA
2.04A,B	Kleihues P
2.04C	Paulus W
2.05A–F	Giannini C
2.06A	Perry A
2.06B	Figarella-Branger D
2.07A,B	Figarella-Branger D
2.08	Adapted by permission from Macmillan Publishers Ltd: Nat Genet. Jones DTW, Hutter B, Jäger N, et al. (2013). Recurrent somatic alterations of FGFR1 and NTRK2 in pilocytic astrocytoma. 45(8):927–32, copyright 2013; Reprinted from Collins VP, Jones DTW, Giannini C (2015). Pilocytic astrocytoma: pathology, molecular mechanisms and markers. Acta Neuropathol. 129(6):775–88.
2.09	Reprinted from Collins VP, Jones DTW, Giannini C (2015). Pilocytic astrocytoma: pathology, molecular mechanisms and markers. Acta Neuropathol. 129(6):775–88.
2.10	See 2.09
2.11	Tihan T
2.12	Tihan T
2.13A,B	Tihan T
2.14	Giannini C

2.15A,B	Ornan DA
	Department of Radiology and Medical Imaging University of Virginia School of Medicine, Charlottesville (VA), USA
2.16A	Vonsattel J-P
	Columbia University New York (NY), USA
2.16B	Paulus W
2.17A,B	Santosh V
2.17C	Lopes MBS
2.18A	Lopes MBS
2.18B	Perry A
2.19A,B	Sharma MC
2.19C–F	Lopes MBS
2.20	Giannini C
2.21A,B	Giannini C
2.22A–C	Giannini C
2.22D	Reprinted from Hum Pathol, 22(11), Kros JM, Vecht CJ, Stefanko SZ, The pleomorphic xanthoastrocytoma and its differential diagnosis: a study of five cases, 1128–35, Copyright (1991), with permission from Elsevier.
2.23A,B	Giannini C
2.24A–D	Giannini C
2.25	Giannini C
2.26A–D	Giannini C
3.01	McLendon R
3.02A–D	Kleihues P
3.03A	Rushing EJ
3.03B,C	Ellison DW
3.04	McLendon R
3.05	McLendon R
3.06A,C	McLendon R
3.06B	Santi M
3.06D	Wiestler OD
3.07	Schiffer D
3.08A	Santi M
3.08B	Westphal MM
	Department of Neurosurgery University Cancer Center Hamburg Hamburg, Germany
3.09	Kleihues P
3.10A	Louis DN
3.10B,C	Perry A
3.10D	Kleihues P
3.11A	Kleihues P
3.11B,C	McLendon R
3.12A	Perry A
3.12B	Nakazato Y
3.12C	Kleihues P
3.13	Nakazato Y
3.14A	Ellison DW
3.14B	Rosenblum MK
3.15	Ellison DW
3.16	Ellison DW
3.17	Westphal MM
	Department of Neurosurgery University Cancer Center Hamburg Hamburg, Germany
3.18	Jellinger K
	Institute of Clinical Neurobiology Vienna, Austria
3.19A	Rosenblum MK
3.19B	Schiffer D

3.19C	Nakazato Y
3.20A,B	Ellison DW
4.01	Brat DJ
4.02	Brat DJ
4.03A–F	Brat DJ
4.04	Brat DJ
4.05A	Tihan T
4.05B	Burger PC
4.06A	Figarella-Branger D
4.06B	Fuller GN
4.07A,C,D	Burger PC
4.07B	Figarella-Branger D
4.08A,B	Brat DJ
4.09A–C	Brat DJ
4.09D	Rushing EJ
5.01	Paulus W
5.02	Figarella-Branger D
5.03A	Rosenblum MK
5.03B	Rorke-Adams LB
5.04A	Paulus W
5.04B	Figarella-Branger D
5.05A,B	Paulus W
5.06	Fuller GN
5.07	Vital A
	Service de Pathologie Centre Hospitalier Universitaire de Bordeaux Bordeaux, France
5.08	Louis DN
5.09A	Brandner S
5.09B	Nakazato Y
5.10A,C	Paulus W
5.10B	Fuller GN
5.10D	Kleihues P
6.01	Pietsch T
6.02A	Blümcke I
6.02B	Hattingen E
	Institute of Neuropathology University of Bonn Medical Center, Bonn, Germany
6.03	Blümcke I
6.04	Blümcke I
6.05A,B	Perry A
6.06A,B	Varlet P
6.07	Varlet P
6.08A	Kleihues P
6.08B,C	Blümcke I
6.09A,B	Giannini C
6.09C,D	Blümcke I
6.10	Blümcke I
6.11A	Osborn A
6.11B	Urbach H
	Department of Neuroradiology University Medical Center Freiburg, Freiburg im Breisgau, Germany
6.12	Kleihues P
6.13	Blümcke I
6.14A,C	Blümcke I
6.14B,D	Varlet P
6.15A	Kleihues P
6.15B	Perry A
6.15C	Capper D
6.16A,B	Perry A
6.17	Eberhart CG
6.18	Allen SH
	Carolina Radiology Associates, McLeod Regional Medical Center Florence (SC), USA

6.19A	Reifenberger G	6.53A	Zrinzo L	8.10	Ellison DW
6.19B	Nakazato Y		National Hospital for Neurology	8.11A,B	Giangaspero F
6.20A–C	Eberhart CG		and Neurosurgery	8.11C	Kleihues P
6.21	Brat DJ		London, United Kingdom	8.12A,B	Kleihues P
6.22A	Osborn A	6.53B	Jaunmuktane Z	8.12C	Rorke-Adams LB
6.22B	Taratuto AL		Department of Neuropathology	8.13A,B	Ellison DW
6.23A	Taratuto AL		UCL Institute of Neurology	8.14	Eberhart CG
6.23B,C	Nakazato Y		London, United Kingdom	8.15	Pietsch T
6.23D	Brat DJ	6.54	Yousry T	8.16A,B	Warmuth-Metz M
6.24A	Brat DJ	6.55	Yousry T		Department of Neuroradiology
6.24B	Taratuto AL	6.56	Brandner S		University Hospital Würzburg
6.24C	Rorke-Adams LB	6.57A–C	Yousry T		Wurzburg, Germany
6.25A–D	Park S-H	6.57D	Perry A	8.16C	Perry A
6.26A	Figarella-Branger D			8.17A,C,D	Pietsch T
6.26B	Nakazato Y	7.01	Jouvet A	8.17B	Perry A
6.27A–D	Nakazato Y	7.02	Sasajima T	8.18A	Giangaspero F
6.28A–C	Nakazato Y		Department of Neurosurgery	8.18B	Pietsch T
6.29A,B	Hainfellner JA		Akita University Graduate	8.19	Pietsch T
6.30	Hainfellner JA		School of Medicine, Hondo,	8.20A,B	Doz F
6.31A–C	Hainfellner JA		Akita, Japan		Department of Paediatric
6.32	Gessi M	7.03	Nakazato Y		Oncology, Institut Curie
6.33	Rodriguez F	7.04A	Vasiljevic A		Paris, France
6.34A	Krawitz S	7.04B	Nakazato Y	8.20C	Garrè ML
	Department of Pathology	7.05A,B	Nakazato Y		Neuroncology Unit
	University of Manitoba	7.06A	Vasiljevic A		Istituto Giannina Gaslini
	Winnipeg (MB), Canada	7.06B,C	Nakazato Y		Genoa, Italy
6.34B,C	Perry A	7.07A–C	Nakazato Y	8.21A,B	Giangaspero F
6.35A	Perry A	7.08	Vasiljevic A	8.21C,D	Ellison DW
6.35B–D	Rodriguez F	7.09A	Jouvet A	8.22A,B	Ellison DW
6.36A–C	Perry A	7.09B	Fèvre Montange M	8.23	Eberhart CG
6.37A–C	Perry A	7.10A	Fèvre Montange M	8.24	Korshunov A
6.38	Capper D	7.10B	Vasiljevic A	8.25	Korshunov A
6.39	Söylemezoglu F	7.11A	Fèvre Montange M	8.26A–C	Korshunov A
6.40A,B	Figarella-Branger D	7.11B	Vasiljevic A	8.27A–C	Korshunov A
6.41	Soffer D	7.11C	Nakazato Y	8.28	Korshunov A
6.42A	Vasiljevic A	7.12	Vasiljevic A	8.29	Korshunov A
6.42B	Kleihues P	7.13	Osborn A	8.30	Korshunov A
6.43A	Kleihues P	7.14	Taratuto AL	8.31	Korshunov A
6.43B,E,F	Figarella-Branger D	7.15A	Vasiljevic A	8.32	Korshunov A
6.43C	Burger PC	7.15B	Rosenblum MK	8.33	Ellison DW
6.43D	Vasiljevic A	7.15C	Ellison DW	8.34A,B	Perry A
6.44A,B	Honavar M	7.15D	Kros JM	8.35	Judkins AR
6.45A	Furtado A	7.16A–C	Vasiljevic A	8.36	Tamrazi B
	Anatomic Pathology Service	7.17A–D	Fèvre Montange M		Department of Radiology
	Vila Nova de Gaia-Espinho	7.18	Vasiljevic A		Children's Hospital Los Angeles
	Medical Center	7.19	Figarella-Branger D		Los Angeles (CA), USA
	Vila Nova de Gaia, Portugal	7.20A–C	Vasiljevic A	8.37	Rorke-Adams LB
6.45B–F	Honavar M	7.21A–C	Vasiljevic A	8.38A	Judkins AR
6.46	Ohgaki H			8.38B	Wesseling P
6.47A	Reprinted from Jenkinson	8.01	Pietsch T	8.39A–C	Judkins AR
	MD, Bosma JJ, Du Plessis	8.02A–C	Kleihues P	8.40A	Wesseling P
	D, et al. (2003). Cerebellar	8.03A,B	Kleihues P	8.40B–D	Judkins AR
	liponeurocytoma with	8.04	Kleihues P	8.41A,B	Ellison DW
	an unusually aggressive	8.05A	Nakazato Y	8.41C	Hasselblatt M
	clinical course: case report.	8.05B	Kalimo H		
	Neurosurgery. 53(6):1425–7;	8.05C	Wiestler OD	9.01	Kleihues P
	discussion 1428.	8.05D	García-Bragado F	9.02A,B	Perry A
6.47B	Kollias S		J. Servicio Anatomía Patológica	9.03A,B	Perry A
	Department of Neuroradiology		Complejo Hospitalario de	9.04A,B	Kleihues P
	University Hospital Zurich		Navarra	9.05A,B	Perry A
	Zurich, Switzerland		Pamplona, Spain	9.06A–C	Perry A
6.48A	Ohgaki H	8.06	Patay Z	9.07	Perry A
6.48B	Kleihues P		Department of Diagnostic	9.08A–D	Perry A
6.49A	Giangaspero F		Imaging, St. Jude Children's	9.09A	Stemmer-Rachamimov AO
6.49B,C	Ohgaki H		Research Hospital	9.09B	Perry A
6.50	Cenacchi G		Memphis (TN), USA	9.10	Woodruff JM (deceased)
	Department of Biomedical and	8.07A–C	Ellison DW	9.11A–C	Perry A
	Neuromotor Sciences	8.08	Patay Z	9.12	Perry A
	University of Bologna		Department of Diagnostic	9.13	Budka H
	Bologna, Italy		Imaging, St. Jude Children's	9.14A,B	Perry A
6.51	Ohgaki H		Research Hospital	9.15A,B	Perry A
6.52	Soffer D		Memphis (TN), USA	9.16A,B	Perry A
		8.09A,B	Hawkins C	9.17A,B	Perry A

17.14A,B	Fuller GN
17.15A,B	Fuller GN
17.16A,B	Fuller GN
17.17A,B	Fuller GN
17.18	Brat DJ
17.19	Brat DJ
17.20A,B	Brat DJ
17.20C	Lopes MBS
17.21A,B	Ornan DA
	Department of Radiology and Medical Imaging
	University of Virginia
	Charlottesville (VA), USA
17.22A,B	Roncaroli F
17.23A,C	Lopes MBS
17.23B	Roncaroli F
17.24A	Lopes MBS
17.24B,C,E,F	Roncaroli F
17.24D	Perry A
17.25	Lopes MBS
17.26	Roncaroli F
18.01	Wesseling P
18.02A,B	Westphal MM
	Department of Neurosurgery
	University Cancer Center Hamburg
	Hamburg, Germany
18.03A–C	Kleihues P
18.04A	Wesseling P
18.04B	Kleihues P
18.04C	Wesseling P
18.05A	Wesseling P
18.05B	Wesseling P
18.05C	Wesseling P

Sources of figures on front cover

Top left	Kleihues P
Top centre	Perry A
Top right	Wiestler OD
Middle left	Perry A
Middle centre	Perry A
Middle right	Rorke-Adams LB
Bottom left	Adapted by permission from Macmillan Publishers Ltd: Nat Genet. Jones DTW, Hutter B, Jäger N, et al. (2013). Recurrent somatic alterations of FGFR1 and NTRK2 in pilocytic astrocytoma. 45(8):927–32, copyright 2013; Reprinted from Collins VP, Jones DTW, Giannini C (2015). Pilocytic astrocytoma: pathology, molecular mechanisms and markers. Acta Neuropathol. 129(6):775–88.
Bottom centre	Perry A
Bottom right	Adapted from Suvà ML, Riggi N, Bernstein BE (2013). Epigenetic reprogramming in cancer. Science. 339(6127):1567–70. Reprinted with permission from AAAS.

Sources of tables

1.01	Kleihues P
1.02	Ellison DW
1.03	Cavenee WK
1.04	Adapted from Oh JE, Ohta T, Nonoguchi N, et al. (2015). Genetic alterations in gliosarcoma and giant cell glioblastoma. Brain Pathol. PMID:26443480.
1.05	Ohgaki H, Kleihues P, von Deimling A, Louis DN, Reifenberger G, Yan H, Weller M
1.06	Hawkins C, Ellison DW, Sturm D
1.07	Kleihues P, Reifenberger G
2.01	Adapted from Collins VP, Jones DTW, Giannini C (2015). Pilocytic astrocytoma: pathology, molecular mechanisms and markers. Acta Neuropathol. 129(6):775–88.
3.01	Ellison DW
6.01	Blümcke I
8.01	Ellison DW
8.02	Ellison DW
8.03	McLendon R
10.01	Louis DN, Perry A
11.01	Plate KH, Aldape KD, Vortmeyer AO, Zagzag D, Neumann HPH
16.01	Kleihues P
16.02	von Deimling A
16.03	Kleihues P
16.04	Stemmer-Rachamimov AO, Hulsebos TJM, Wesseling P
16.05	Plate KH, Vortmeyer AO, Zagzag D, Neumann HPH, Aldape KD
16.06	Plate KH, Vortmeyer AO, Zagzag D, Neumann HPH, Aldape KD
16.07	Adapted from Pediatr Neurol, 49(4), Northrup H, Krueger DA, International Tuberous Sclerosis Complex Consensus Group, Tuberous sclerosis complex diagnostic criteria update: recommendations of the 2012 International Tuberous Sclerosis Complex Consensus Conference, 243–54, Copyright 2013, with permission from Elsevier.
16.08	Sharma MC
16.09	Olivier M; based on data from the IARC TP53 Database (R17, November 2013)
16.10	Eng C
18.01	Adapted from Pekmezci M, Perry A (2013). Neuropathology of brain metastases. Surg Neurol Int. 4(Suppl 4):S245–55.

References

1. Abe M, Tabuchi K, Tanaka S, Hodozuka A, Kunishio K, Kubo N, et al. (2004). Capillary hemangioma of the central nervous system. J Neurosurg. 101(1):73–81. PMID:15255254
2. Abedalthagafi MS, Merrill PH, Bi WL, Jones RT, Listewnik ML, Ramkissoon SH, et al. (2014). Angiomatous meningiomas have a distinct genetic profile with multiple chromosomal polysomies including polysomy of chromosome 5. Oncotarget. 5(21):10596–606. PMID:25347344
3. Abel TW, Baker SJ, Fraser MM, Tihan T, Nelson JS, Yachnis AT, et al. (2005). Lhermitte-Duclos disease: a report of 31 cases with immunohistochemical analysis of the PTEN/AKT/mTOR pathway. J Neuropathol Exp Neurol. 64(4):341–9. PMID:15835270
4. Abrey LE, DeAngelis LM, Yahalom J (1998). Long-term survival in primary CNS lymphoma. J Clin Oncol. 16(3):859–63. PMID:9508166
5. Achatz MI, Olivier M, Le Calvez F, Martel-Planche G, Lopes A, Rossi BM, et al. (2007). The TP53 mutation, R337H, is associated with Li-Fraumeni and Li-Fraumeni-like syndromes in Brazilian families. Cancer Lett. 245(1-2):96–102. PMID:16494995
6. Acker T, Plate KH (2004). Hypoxia and hypoxia inducible factors (HIF) as important regulators of tumor physiology. Cancer Treat Res. 117:219–48. PMID:15015563
7. Actor B, Cobbers JM, Büschges R, Wolter M, Knobbe CB, Lichter P, et al. (2002). Comprehensive analysis of genomic alterations in gliosarcoma and its two tissue components. Genes Chromosomes Cancer. 34(4):416–27. PMID:12112531
8. Adair JE, Johnston SK, Mrugala MM, Beard BC, Guyman LA, Baldock AL, et al. (2014). Gene therapy enhances chemotherapy tolerance and efficacy in glioblastoma patients. J Clin Invest. 124(9):4082–92. PMID:25105369
9. Adam C, Polivka M, Carpentier A, George B, Gray F (2007). Papillary glioneuronal tumor: not always a benign tumor? Clin Neuropathol. 26(3):119–24. PMID:19157003
10. Adamek D, Sofowora KD, Cwiklinska M, Herman-Sucharska I, Kwiatkowski S (2013). Embryonal tumor with abundant neuropil and true rosettes: an autopsy case-based update and review of the literature. Childs Nerv Syst. 29(5):849–54. PMID:23358909
11. Adams S, Teo C, McDonald KL, Zinger A, Bustamante S, Lim CK, et al. (2014). Involvement of the kynurenine pathway in human glioma pathophysiology. PLoS One. 9(11):e112945. PMID:25415278
12. Adams SA, Hilton DA (2002). Recurrent haemangioblastoma with glial differentiation. Neuropathol Appl Neurobiol. 28(2):142–6. PMID:11972801
13. Adamson TE, Wiestler OD, Kleihues P, Yaşargil MG (1990). Correlation of clinical and pathological features in surgically treated craniopharyngiomas. J Neurosurg. 73(1):12–7. PMID:2352012
14. Adeleye AO, Okolo CA, Akang EE, Adesina AM (2012). Cerebral pleomorphic xanthoastrocytoma associated with NF1: an updated review with a rare atypical case from Africa. Neurosurg Rev. 35(3):313–9, discussion 319. PMID:22020543
15. Adriani KS, Stenvers DJ, Imanse JG (2012). Pearls & oy-sters: Lumbar paraganglioma: can you see it in the eyes? Neurology. 78(4):e27–8. PMID:22271522
16. Aerts I, Pacquement H, Doz F, Mosseri V, Desjardins L, Sastre X, et al. (2004). Outcome of second malignancies after retinoblastoma: a retrospective analysis of 25 patients treated at the Institut Curie. Eur J Cancer. 40(10):1522–9. PMID:15196536
17. Agaimy A (2014). Microscopic intraneural perineurial cell proliferations in patients with neurofibromatosis type 1. Ann Diagn Pathol. 18(2):95–8. PMID:24461704
18. Agaimy A, Barthelmeß S, Geddert H, Boltze C, Moskalev EA, Koch M, et al. (2014). Phenotypical and molecular distinctness of sinonasal haemangiopericytoma compared to solitary fibrous tumour of the sinonasal tract. Histopathology. 65(5):667–73. PMID:24807787
19. Agamanolis DP, Katsetos CD, Klonk CJ, Bartkowski HM, Ganapathy S, Staugaitis SM, et al. (2012). An unusual form of superficially disseminated glioma in children: report of 3 cases. J Child Neurol. 27(6):727–33. PMID:22596013
20. Agaram NP, Prakash S, Antonescu CR (2005). Deep-seated plexiform schwannoma: a pathologic study of 16 cases and comparative analysis with the superficial variety. Am J Surg Pathol. 29(8):1042–8. PMID:16006798
21. Agarwal S, Sharma MC, Sarkar C, Suri V, Jain A, Sharma MS, et al. (2011). Extraventricular neurocytomas: a morphological and histogenetic consideration. A study of six cases. Pathology. 43(4):327–34. PMID:21532524
22. Agarwal S, Sharma MC, Singh G, Suri V, Sarkar C, Garg A, et al. (2012). Papillary glioneuronal tumor–a rare entity: report of four cases and brief review of literature. Childs Nerv Syst. 28(11):1897–904. PMID:22868530
23. Aghi MK, Carter BS, Cosgrove GR, Ojemann RG, Amin-Hanjani S, Martuza RL, et al. (2009). Long-term recurrence rates of atypical meningiomas after gross total resection with or without postoperative adjuvant radiation. Neurosurgery. 64(1):56–60, discussion 60. PMID:19145156
24. Agozzino L, Ferraraccio F, Accardo M, Esposito S, Agozzino M, Cuccurullo L (2006). Morphological and ultrastructural findings of prognostic impact in craniopharyngiomas. Ultrastruct Pathol. 30(3):143–50. PMID:16825115
25. Agrawal D, Singhal A, Hendson G, Durity FA (2007). Gyriform differentiation in medulloblastoma - a radiological predictor of histology. Pediatr Neurosurg. 43(2):142–5. PMID:17337929
26. Ahlsén G, Gillberg IC, Lindblom R, Gillberg C (1994). Tuberous sclerosis in Western Sweden. A population study of cases with early childhood onset. Arch Neurol. 51(1):76–81. PMID:8274113
27. Ahmadi R, Stockhammer F, Becker N, Hohlen K, Misch M, Christians A, et al. (2012). No prognostic value of IDH1 mutations in a series of 100 WHO grade II astrocytomas. J Neurooncol. 109(1):15–22. PMID:22528790
28. Ahmed KA, Allen PK, Mahajan A, Brown PD, Ghia AJ (2014). Astroblastomas: a Surveillance, Epidemiology, and End Results (SEER)-based patterns of care analysis. World Neurosurg. 82(1-2):e291–7. PMID:24141003
29. Ahuja A, Sharma MC, Suri V, Sarkar C, Sharma BS, Garg A (2011). Pineal anlage tumour - a rare entity with divergent histology. J Clin Neurosci. 18(6):811–3. PMID:21435885
30. Aicardi J (2005). Aicardi syndrome. Brain Dev. 27(3):164–71. PMID:15737696
30A. Aizer AA, Bi WL, Kandola MS, Lee EQ, Nayak L, Rinne ML, et al. (2015). Extent of resection and overall survival for patients with atypical and malignant meningioma. Cancer. 121(24):4376–81. PMID:26308667
31. Akamatsu Y, Utsunomiya A, Suzuki S, Endo T, Suzuki I, Nishimura S, et al. (2010). Subependymoma in the lateral ventricle manifesting as intraventricular hemorrhage. Neurol Med Chir (Tokyo). 50(11):1020–3. PMID:21123990
32. Aker FV, Ozkara S, Eren P, Peker O, Armağan S, Hakan T (2005). Cerebellar liponeurocytoma/lipidized medulloblastoma. J Neurooncol. 71(1):53–9. PMID:15719276
33. Akers AL, Johnson E, Steinberg GK, Zabramski JM, Marchuk DA (2009). Biallelic somatic and germline mutations in cerebral cavernous malformations (CCMs): evidence for a two-hit mechanism of CCM pathogenesis. Hum Mol Genet. 18(5):919–30. PMID:19088123
34. Akhaddar A, Zrara I, Gazzaz M, El Moustarchid B, Benomar S, Boucetta M (2003). Cerebellar liponeurocytoma (lipomatous medulloblastoma). J Neuroradiol. 30(2):121–6. PMID:12717299
35. Akyurek S, Chang EL, Yu TK, Little D, Allen PK, McCutcheon I, et al. (2006). Spinal myxopapillary ependymoma outcomes in patients treated with surgery and radiotherapy at M.D. Anderson Cancer Center. J Neurooncol. 80(2):177–83. PMID:16648988
36. Al-Hussaini M, Abuirmeileh N, Swaidan M, Al-Jumaily U, Rajjal H, Musharbash A, et al. (2011). Embryonal tumor with abundant neuropil and true rosettes: a report of three cases of a rare tumor, with an unusual case showing rhabdomyoblastic and melanocytic differentiation. Neuropathology. 31(6):620–5. PMID:22103481
37. al-Sarraj ST, Parmar D, Dean AF, Phookun G, Bridges LR (1998). Clinicopathological study of seven cases of spinal cord teratoma: a possible germ cell origin. Histopathology. 32(1):51–6. PMID:9522216
38. Alameda F, Lloreta J, Galitó E, Roquer J, Serrano S (1998). Meningeal melanocytoma: a case report and literature review. Ultrastruct Pathol. 22(4):349–56. PMID:9805360
39. Albrecht S, Connelly JH, Bruner JM (1993). Distribution of p53 protein expression in gliosarcomas: an immunohistochemical study. Acta Neuropathol. 85(2):222–6. PMID:8382897
40. Albrecht S, Goodman JC, Rajagopolan S, Levy M, Cech DA, Cooley LD (1994). Malignant meningioma in Gorlin's syndrome: cytogenetic and p53 gene analysis. Case report. J Neurosurg. 81(3):466–71. PMID:8057157
41. Albrecht S, Rouah E, Becker LE, Bruner J (1991). Transthyretin immunoreactivity in choroid plexus neoplasms and brain metastases. Mod Pathol. 4(5):610–4. PMID:1758873
42. Albrecht S, von Deimling A, Pietsch T, Giangaspero F, Brandner S, Kleihues P, et al. (1994). Microsatellite analysis of loss of heterozygosity on chromosomes 9q, 11p and 17p in medulloblastomas. Neuropathol Appl Neurobiol. 20(1):74–81. PMID:8208343
43. Albright AL, Wisoff JH, Zeltzer P, Boyett J, Rorke LB, Stanley P, et al. (1995). Prognostic factors in children with supratentorial (nonpineal) primitive neuroectodermal tumors. A neurosurgical perspective from the Children's Cancer Group. Pediatr Neurosurg. 22(1):1–7. PMID:7888387
44. Alcedo J, Noll M (1997). Hedgehog and its patched-smoothened receptor complex: a novel signalling mechanism at the cell surface. Biol Chem. 378(7):583–90. PMID:9278137
45. Alderson L, Fetell MR, Sisti M, Hochberg F, Cohen M, Louis DN (1996). Sentinel lesions of primary CNS lymphoma. J Neurol Neurosurg Psychiatry. 60(1):102–5. PMID:8558135
45A. Alentorn A, Dehais C, Ducray F, Carpentier C, Mokhtari K, Figarella-Branger D, et al. (2015). Allelic loss of 9p21.3 is a prognostic factor in 1p/19q codeleted anaplastic gliomas. Neurology. 85(15):1325–31. PMID:26385879
46. Alexander RT, McLendon RE, Cummings TJ (2004). Meningioma with eosinophilic granular inclusions. Clin Neuropathol. 23(6):292–7. PMID:15584214
47. Alexandrescu S, Brown RE, Tandon N, Bhattacharjee MB (2012). Neuron precursor features of spindle cell oncocytoma of adenohypophysis. Ann Clin Lab Sci. 42(2):123–9. PMID:22585606
48. Alexandrescu S, Korshunov A, Lai SH, Dabiri S, Patil S, Li R, et al. (2015). Epithelioid Glioblastomas and Anaplastic Epithelioid Pleomorphic Xanthoastrocytomas-Same Entity or First Cousins? Brain Pathol. PMID:26238627
49. Alexiou GA, Moschovi M, Georgoulis G, Neroutsou R, Stefanaki K, Sfakianos G, et al. (2010). Anaplastic oligodendrogliomas after treatment of acute lymphoblastic leukemia in children: report of 2 cases. J Neurosurg Pediatr. 5(2):179–83. PMID:20121367
50. Alexiou GA, Stefanaki K, Vartholomatos G, Sfakianos G, Prodromou N, Moschovi M (2013). Embryonal tumor with abundant neuropil and true rosettes: a systematic literature review and report of 2 new cases. J Child Neurol. 28(12):1709–15. PMID:23334078
51. Ali JB, Sepp T, Ward S, Green AJ, Yates JR (1998). Mutations in the TSC1 gene account for a minority of patients with tuberous sclerosis. J Med Genet. 35(12):969–72. PMID:9863590
52. Alimova I, Birks DK, Harris PS, Knipstein JA, Venkataraman S, Marquez VE, et al. (2013). Inhibition of EZH2 suppresses self-renewal and induces radiation sensitivity in atypical rhabdoid teratoid tumor cells. Neuro Oncol. 15(2):149–60. PMID:23190500
53. Alkadhi H, Keller M, Brandner S, Yonekawa Y, Kollias SS (2001). Neuroimaging of cerebellar liponeurocytoma. Case report. J Neurosurg. 95(2):324–31. PMID:11780904
54. Alkindy A, Chuzhanova N, Kini U, Cooper DN, Upadhyaya M (2012). Genotype-phenotype associations in neurofibromatosis type 1 (NF1): an increased risk of tumor complications in patients with NF1 splice-site mutations? Hum Genomics. 6:12. PMID:23244495
55. Allen JC, Judkins AR, Rosenblum MK, Biegel JA (2006). Atypical teratoid/rhabdoid tumor evolving from an optic pathway ganglioglioma: case study. Neuro Oncol. 8(1):79–82. PMID:16443951
56. Alles JU, Bosslet K, Schachenmayr W (1986). Hemangioblastoma of the cerebellum–an immunocytochemical study. Clin Neuropathol. 5(6):238–41. PMID:3815934
57. Alleyne CH Jr, Hunter S, Olson JJ, Barrow DL (1998). Lipomatous glioneurocytoma of the posterior fossa with divergent differentiation: case report. Neurosurgery. 42(3):639–43. PMID:9526999
58. Allinson KS, O'Donovan DG, Jena R, Cross

JJ, Santarius TS (2015). Rosette-forming glioneuronal tumor with dissemination throughout the ventricular system: a case report. Clin Neuropathol. 34(2):64–9. PMID:25373141
59. Almefty R, Webber BL, Arnautovic KI (2006). Intraneural perineurioma of the third cranial nerve: occurrence and identification. Case report. J Neurosurg. 104(5):824–7. PMID:16703891
60. Alomari AK, Kelley BJ, Damisah E, Marks A, Hui P, DiLuna M, et al. (2015). Craniopharyngioma arising in a Rathke's cleft cyst: case report. J Neurosurg Pediatr. 15(3):250–4. PMID:25555112
61. Alpers CE, Davis RL, Wilson CB (1982). Persistence and late malignant transformation of childhood cerebellar astrocytoma. Case report. J Neurosurg. 57(4):548–51. PMID:7108605
62. Altinoz MA, Santaguida C, Guiot MC, Del Maestro RF (2005). Spinal hemangioblastoma containing metastatic renal cell carcinoma in von Hippel-Lindau disease. Case report and review of the literature. J Neurosurg Spine. 3(6):495–500. PMID:16381215
63. Altundag MK, Ozişik Y, Yalcin S, Akyol F, Uner A (2000). Primary low grade B-cell lymphoma of the dura in an immunocompetent patient. J Exp Clin Cancer Res. 19(2):249–51. PMID:10965827
64. Amano K, Kubo O, Komori T, Tanaka M, Kawamata T, Hori T, et al. (2013). Clinicopathological features of sellar region xanthogranuloma: correlation with Rathke's cleft cyst. Brain Tumor Pathol. 30(4):233–41. PMID:23322180
65. Amemiya S, Shibahara J, Aoki S, Takao H, Ohtomo K (2008). Recently established entities of central nervous system tumors: review of radiological findings. J Comput Assist Tomogr. 32(2):279–85. PMID:18379318
66. Amirian ES, Goodman JC, New P, Scheurer ME (2014). Pediatric and adult malignant peripheral nerve sheath tumors: an analysis of data from the surveillance, epidemiology, and end results program. J Neurooncol. 116(3):609–16. PMID:24390465
67. Amlashi SF, Riffaud L, Brassier G, Morandi X (2003). Nevoid basal cell carcinoma syndrome: relation with desmoplastic medulloblastoma in infancy. A population-based study and review of the literature. Cancer. 98(3):618–24. PMID:12879481
68. Anan M, Inoue R, Ishii K, Abe T, Fujiki M, Kobayashi H, et al. (2009). A rosette-forming glioneuronal tumor of the spinal cord: the first case of a rosette-forming glioneuronal tumor originating from the spinal cord. Hum Pathol. 40(6):898–901. PMID:19269010
69. Anan M, Ishii K, Nakamura T, Yamashita M, Katayama S, Sainoo M, et al. (2006). Postoperative adjuvant treatment for pineal parenchymal tumour of intermediate differentiation. J Clin Neurosci. 13(9):965–8. PMID:16904896
70. Andoniadou CL, Gaston-Massuet C, Reddy R, Schneider RP, Blasco MA, Le Tissier P, et al. (2012). Identification of novel pathways involved in the pathogenesis of human adamantinomatous craniopharyngioma. Acta Neuropathol. 124(2):259–71. PMID:22349813
71. Andreasson A, Kiss NB, Caramuta S, Sulaiman L, Svahn F, Bäckdahl M, et al. (2013). The VHL gene is epigenetically inactivated in pheochromocytomas and abdominal paragangliomas. Epigenetics. 8(12):1347–54. PMID:24149047
72. Andreiuolo F, Puget S, Peyre M, Dantas-Barbosa C, Boddaert N, Philippe C, et al. (2010). Neuronal differentiation distinguishes supratentorial and infratentorial childhood ependymomas. Neuro Oncol. 12(11):1126–34. PMID:20615923
73. Anghileri E, Eoli M, Paterra R, Ferroli P, Pollo B, Cuccarini V, et al. (2012). FABP4 is a candidate marker of cerebellar liponeurocytomas. J Neurooncol. 108(3):513–9. PMID:22476608
74. Antinheimo J, Haapasalo H, Haltia M, Tatagiba M, Thomas S, Brandis A, et al. (1997). Proliferation potential and histological features in neurofibromatosis 2-associated and sporadic meningiomas. J Neurosurg. 87(4):610–4. PMID:9322850
75. Antinheimo J, Haapasalo H, Seppälä M, Sainio M, Carpen O, Jääskeläinen J (1995). Proliferative potential of sporadic and neurofibromatosis 2-associated schwannomas as studied by MIB-1 (Ki-67) and PCNA labeling. J Neuropathol Exp Neurol. 54(6):776–82. PMID:7595650
76. Antinheimo J, Sankila R, Carpén O, Pukkala E, Sainio M, Jääskeläinen J (2000). Population-based analysis of sporadic and type 2 neurofibromatosis-associated meningiomas and schwannomas. Neurology. 54(1):71–6. PMID:10636128
77. Anton T, Guttierez J, Rock J (2006). Tentorial schwannoma: a case report and review of the literature. J Neurooncol. 76(3):307–11. PMID:16200344
78. Antonelli M, Korshunov A, Mastronuzzi A, Diomedi Camassei F, Carai A, Colafati GS, et al. (2015). Long-term survival in a case of ETANTR with histological features of neuronal maturation after therapy. Virchows Arch. 466(5):603–7. PMID:25697539
79. Antonescu CR (2006). The role of genetic testing in soft tissue sarcoma. Histopathology. 48(1):13–21. PMID:16359533
80. Antonescu CR, Le Loarer F, Mosquera JM, Sboner A, Zhang L, Chen CL, et al. (2013). Novel YAP1-TFE3 fusion defines a distinct subset of epithelioid hemangioendothelioma. Genes Chromosomes Cancer. 52(8):775–84. PMID:23737213
81. Antonescu CR, Suurmeijer AJ, Zhang L, Sung YS, Jungbluth AA, Travis WD, et al. (2015). Molecular characterization of inflammatory myofibroblastic tumors with frequent ALK and ROS1 gene fusions and rare novel RET rearrangement. Am J Surg Pathol. 39(7):957–67. PMID:25723109
82. Antonescu CR, Woodruff JM (2006). Primary Tumors and Cranial, Spinal and Peripheral Nerves. In: McLendon RE, Rosenblum MK, Bigner DD, editors. Russel and Rubinstein's Pathology of the Nervous System. Hoder Arnold; pp. 787–835.
83. Aoki Y, Niihori T, Narumi Y, Kure S, Matsubara Y (2008). The RAS/MAPK syndromes: novel roles of the RAS pathway in human genetic disorders. Hum Mutat. 29(8):992–1006. PMID:18470943
84. Aoyama I, Kondo A, Ogawa H, Ikai Y (1994). Germinoma in siblings: case reports. Surg Neurol. 41(4):313–7. PMID:8165502
85. Appin CL, Gao J, Chisolm C, Torian M, Alexis D, Vincentelli C, et al. (2013). Glioblastoma with oligodendroglioma component (GBM-O): molecular genetic and clinical characteristics. Brain Pathol. 23(4):454–61. PMID:23289977
86. Aquilina K, Kamel M, Kalimuthu SG, Marks JC, Keohane C (2006). Granular cell tumour of the neurohypophysis: a rare sellar tumour with specific radiological and operative features. Br J Neurosurg. 20(1):51–4. PMID:16698612
87. Aquilina K, Nanra JS, Allcutt DA, Farrell M (2005). Choroid plexus adenoma: case report and review of the literature. Childs Nerv Syst. 21(5):410–5. PMID:15565450
88. Arai H, Ikota H, Sugawara K, Nobusawa S, Hirato J, Nakazato Y (2012). Nestin expression in brain tumors: its utility for pathological diagnosis and correlation with the prognosis of high-grade gliomas. Brain Tumor Pathol. 29(3):160–7. PMID:22350668
89. Arita H, Narita Y, Fukushima S, Tateishi K, Matsushita Y, Yoshida A, et al. (2013). Upregulating mutations in the TERT promoter commonly occur in adult malignant gliomas and are strongly associated with total 1p19q loss. Acta Neuropathol. 126(2):267–76. PMID:23764841
90. Arita N, Taneda M, Hayakawa T (1994). Leptomeningeal dissemination of malignant gliomas. Incidence, diagnosis and outcome. Acta Neurochir (Wien). 126(2-4):84–92. PMID:8042560
91. Arivazhagan A, Anandh B, Santosh V, Chandramouli BA (2008). Pineal parenchymal tumors–utility of immunohistochemical markers in prognostication. Clin Neuropathol. 27(5):325–33. PMID:18808064
92. Arnold MA, Stallings-Archer K, Marlin E, Grondin R, Olshefski R, Biegel JA, et al. (2013). Cribriform neuroepithelial tumor arising in the lateral ventricle. Pediatr Dev Pathol. 16(4):301–7. PMID:23495723
93. Aronica E, Boer K, Becker A, Redeker S, Spliet WG, van Rijen PC, et al. (2008). Gene expression profile analysis of epilepsy-associated gangliogliomas. Neuroscience. 151(1):272–92. PMID:18093740
94. Aronica E, Leenstra S, van Veelen CW, van Rijen PC, Hulsebos TJ, Tersmette AC, et al. (2001). Glioneuronal tumors and medically intractable epilepsy: a clinical study with long-term follow-up of seizure outcome after surgery. Epilepsy Res. 43(3):179–91. PMID:11248530
94A. Arvela E, Söderström M, Korhonen M, Halmesmäki K, Albäck A, Lepäntalo M, et al. (2010). Finnvasc score and modified Prevent III score predict long-term outcome after infrainguinal surgical and endovascular revascularization for critical limb ischemia.J Vasc Surg52(5):1218–25. PMID:20709482
95. Asha U, Mahadevan A, Sathiyabama D, Ravindra T, Sagar BK, Bhat DI, et al. (2015). Lack of IDH1 mutation in astroblastomas suggests putative origin from ependymoglial cells? Neuropathology. 35(4):303–11. PMID:25786545
96. Astrinidis A, Henske EP (2005). Tuberous sclerosis complex: linking growth and energy signaling pathways with human disease. Oncogene. 24(50):7475–81. PMID:16288294
96A. Athar M, Li C, Kim AL, Spiegelman VS, Bickers DR (2014). Sonic hedgehog signaling in basal cell nevus syndrome. Cancer Res. 74(18):4967–75. PMID:25172843
97. Au KS, Williams AT, Roach ES, Batchelor L, Sparagana SP, Delgado MR, et al. (2007). Genotype/phenotype correlation in 325 individuals referred for a diagnosis of tuberous sclerosis complex in the United States. Genet Med. 9(2):88–100. PMID:17304050
98. Awaya H, Kaneko M, Amatya VJ, Takeshima Y, Oka S, Inai K (2003). Myxopapillary ependymoma with anaplastic features. Pathol Int. 53(10):700–3. PMID:14516321
99. Aydin F, Ghatak NR, Salvant J, Muizelaar P (1993). Desmoplastic cerebral astrocytoma of infancy. A case report with immunohistochemical, ultrastructural and proliferation studies. Acta Neuropathol. 86(6):666–70. PMID:7906073
100. Aziz M, Chaurasia JK, Khan R, Afroz N (2014). Primary low-grade diffuse small lymphocytic lymphoma of the central nervous system. BMJ Case Rep. 2014:2014. PMID:24729110
101. Azzarelli B, Rekate HL, Roessmann U (1977). Subependymoma: a case report with ultrastructural study. Acta Neuropathol. 40(3):279–82. PMID:203160
102. Bacci C, Sestini R, Provenzano A, Paganini I, Mancini I, Porfirio B, et al. (2010). Schwannomatosis associated with multiple meningiomas due to a familial SMARCB1 mutation. Neurogenetics. 11(1):73–80. PMID:19582488
103. Badalian-Very G, Vergilio JA, Degar BA, MacConaill LE, Brandner B, Calicchio ML, et al. (2010). Recurrent BRAF mutations in Langerhans cell histiocytosis. Blood. 116(11):1919–23. PMID:20519626
104. Badiali M, Gleize V, Paris S, Moi L, Elhouadani S, Arcella A, et al. (2012). KIAA1549-BRAF fusions and IDH mutations can coexist in diffuse gliomas of adults. Brain Pathol. 22(6):841–7. PMID:22591444
105. Bady P, Sciuscio D, Diserens AC, Bloch J, van den Bent MJ, Marosi C, et al. (2012). MGMT methylation analysis of glioblastoma on the Infinium methylation BeadChip identifies two distinct CpG regions associated with gene silencing and outcome, yielding a prediction model for comparisons across datasets, tumor grades, and CIMP-status. Acta Neuropathol. 124(4):547–60. PMID:22810491
106. Baehring JM, Dickey PS, Bannykh SI (2004). Epithelioid hemangioendothelioma of the suprasellar area: a case report and review of the literature. Arch Pathol Lab Med. 128(11):1289–93. PMID:15504067
107. Bailey P, Bucy PC (1929). Oligodendrogliomas of the brain. J Path Bact. 32:735–51.
108. Bailey P, Cushing H (1926). A classification of tumors of the glioma group on a histogenetic basis with a correlation study of prognosis. Philadelphia: Lippincott.
109. Bailey P, Cushing H (1926). Classification of the Tumors of the Glioma Group. Philadelphia: Lippincott.
110. Bainbridge MN, Armstrong GN, Gramatges MM, Bertuch AA, Jhangiani SN, Doddapaneni H, et al.; Gliogene Consortium (2015). Germline mutations in shelterin complex genes are associated with familial glioma. J Natl Cancer Inst. 107(1):384. PMID:25482530
111. Baisden BL, Brat DJ, Melhem ER, Rosenblum MK, King AP, Burger PC (2001). Dysembryoplastic neuroepithelial tumor-like neoplasm of the septum pellucidum: a lesion often misdiagnosed as glioma: report of 10 cases. Am J Surg Pathol. 25(4):494–9. PMID:11257624
112. Baker KB, Moran CJ, Wippold FJ 2nd, Smirniotopoulos JG, Rodriguez FJ, Meyers SP, et al. (2000). MR imaging of spinal hemangioblastoma. AJR Am J Roentgenol. 174(2):377–82. PMID:10658709
113. Bakry D, Aronson M, Durno C, Rimawi H, Farah R, Alharbi QK, et al. (2014). Genetic and clinical determinants of constitutional mismatch repair deficiency syndrome: report from the constitutional mismatch repair deficiency consortium. Eur J Cancer. 50(5):987–96. PMID:24440087
114. Bakshi R, Shaikh ZA, Kamran S, Kinkel PR (1999). MRI findings in 32 consecutive lipomas using conventional and advanced sequences. J Neuroimaging. 9(3):134–40. PMID:10436754
115. Baldini F, Baiocchini A, Schininà V, Agrati C, Giancola ML, Alba L, et al. (2013). Brain localization of Kaposi's sarcoma in a patient treated by combination antiretroviral therapy. BMC Infect Dis. 13:600. PMID:24359263
116. Balik V, Srovnal J, Sulla I, Kalita O, Foltanova T, Vaverka M, et al. (2013). MEG3: a novel long noncoding potentially tumour-suppressing RNA in meningiomas. J Neurooncol. 112(1):1–8. PMID:23307326
117. Balmaceda CM, Fetell MR, O'Brien JL, Housepian EH (1993). Nevus of Ota and leptomeningeal melanocytic lesions. Neurology. 43(2):381–6. PMID:8437707
118. Balss J, Meyer J, Mueller W, Korshunov A, Hartmann C, von Deimling A (2008). Analysis of the IDH1 codon 132 mutation in brain tumors. Acta Neuropathol. 116(6):597–602. PMID:18985363
118A. Bandopadhayay P, Ramkissoon LA, Jain P, Bergthold G, Wala J, Zeid R, et al. (2016). MYB-QKI rearrangements in angiocentric glioma drive tumorigenicity through a tripartite mechanism. Nat Genet. 48(3): 273-82. PMID:26829751
119. Banerjee AK, Sharma BS, Kak VK, Ghatak NR (1989). Gliosarcoma with cartilage formation. Cancer. 63(3):518–23. PMID:2643455
120. Bannykh S, Strugar J, Baehring J (2005). Paraganglioma of the lumbar spinal canal. J Neurooncol. 75(2):119. PMID:16283440
121. Bannykh SI, Stolt CC, Kim J, Perry A, Wegner M (2006). Oligodendroglial-specific transcriptional factor SOX10 is ubiquitously expressed in human gliomas. J Neurooncol. 76(2):115–27. PMID:16205963
122. Bao S, Wu Q, McLendon RE, Hao Y, Shi Q,

Hjelmeland AB, et al. (2006). Glioma stem cells promote radioresistance by preferential activation of the DNA damage response. Nature. 444(7120):756–60. PMID:17051156
123. Bar EE, Lin A, Tihan T, Burger PC, Eberhart CG (2008). Frequent gains at chromosome 7q34 involving BRAF in pilocytic astrocytoma. J Neuropathol Exp Neurol. 67(9):878–87. PMID:18716556
124. Baraniskin A, Kuhnhenn J, Schlegel U, Chan A, Deckert M, Gold R, et al. (2011). Identification of microRNAs in the cerebrospinal fluid as marker for primary diffuse large B-cell lymphoma of the central nervous system. Blood. 117(11):3140–6. PMID:21200023
125. Baraniskin A, Kuhnhenn J, Schlegel U, Schmiegel W, Hahn S, Schroers R (2012). MicroRNAs in cerebrospinal fluid as biomarker for disease course monitoring in primary central nervous system lymphoma. J Neurooncol. 109(2):239–44. PMID:22729947
126. Barker FG 2nd, Davis RL, Chang SM, Prados MD (1996). Necrosis as a prognostic factor in glioblastoma multiforme. Cancer. 77(6):1161–6. PMID:8635139
127. Barkovich AJ, Guerrini R, Kuzniecky RI, Jackson GD, Dobyns WB (2012). A developmental and genetic classification for malformations of cortical development: update 2012. Brain. 135(Pt 5):1348–69. PMID:22427329
128. Barnard RO, Geddes JF (1987). The incidence of multifocal cerebral gliomas. A histologic study of large hemisphere sections. Cancer. 60(7):1519–31. PMID:3113716
129. Barnard ZR, Agarwalla PK, Jeyaretna DS, Farrell CJ, Gerstner ER, Tian D, et al. (2011). Sporadic primary malignant intracerebral nerve sheath tumors: case report and literature review. J Neurooncol. 104(2):605–10. PMID:21327709
130. Barnholtz-Sloan JS, Sloan AE, Davis FG, Vigneau FD, Lai P, Sawaya RE (2004). Incidence proportions of brain metastases in patients diagnosed (1973 to 2001) in the Metropolitan Detroit Cancer Surveillance System. J Clin Oncol. 22(14):2865–72. PMID:15254054
131. Barrande G, Kujas M, Gancel A, Turpin G, Bruckert E, Kuhn JM, et al. (1995). [Granular cell tumors. Rare tumors of the neurohypophysis]. Presse Med. 24(30):1376–80. PMID:8545314
132. Barresi V, Cerasoli S, Morigi F, Cremonini AM, Volpini M, Tuccari G (2006). Gliosarcoma with features of osteoblastic osteosarcoma: a review. Arch Pathol Lab Med. 130(8):1208–11. PMID:16879025
133. Barresi V, Vitarelli E, Branca G, Antonelli M, Giangaspero F, Barresi G (2012). Expression of brachyury in hemangioblastoma: potential use in differential diagnosis. Am J Surg Pathol. 36(7):1052–7. PMID:22446946
134. Barrett AW, Hopper C, Landon G (2002). Intra-osseous soft tissue perineurioma of the inferior alveolar nerve. Oral Oncol. 38(8):793–6. PMID:12570059
135. Bartels U, Hawkins C, Vézina G, Kun L, Souweidane M, Bouffet E (2011). Proceedings of the diffuse intrinsic pontine glioma (DIPG) Toronto Think Tank: advancing basic and translational research and cooperation in DIPG. J Neurooncol. 105(1):119–25. PMID:21901544
136. Barzilay JI, Pazianos AG (1989). Adrenocortical carcinoma. Urol Clin North Am. 16(3):457–68. PMID:2665272
137. Baser ME, Friedman JM, Joe H, Shenton A, Wallace AJ, Ramsden RT, et al. (2011). Empirical development of improved diagnostic criteria for neurofibromatosis 2. Genet Med. 13(6):576–81. PMID:21451418
138. Baser ME, Kuramoto L, Joe H, Friedman JM, Wallace AJ, Gillespie JE, et al. (2004). Genotype-phenotype correlations for nervous system tumors in neurofibromatosis 2: a population-based study. Am J Hum Genet. 75(2):231–9. PMID:15190457
139. Bastian BC (2014). The molecular pathology of melanoma: an integrated taxonomy of melanocytic neoplasia. Annu Rev Pathol. 9:239–71. PMID:24460190
140. Batchelor T, Loeffler JS (2006). Primary CNS lymphoma. J Clin Oncol. 24(8):1281–8. PMID:16525183
141. Batchelor TT, Reardon DA, de Groot JF, Wick W, Weller M (2014). Antiangiogenic therapy for glioblastoma: current status and future prospects. Clin Cancer Res. 20(22):5612–9. PMID:25398844
142. Batora NV, Sturm D, Jones DT, Kool M, Pfister SM, Northcott PA (2014). Transitioning from genotypes to epigenotypes: why the time has come for medulloblastoma epigenomics. Neuroscience. 264:171–85. PMID:23876321
143. Batzdorf U, Malamud N (1963). The problem of multicentric gliomas. J Neurosurg. 20:122–36. PMID:14192080
144. Bauman GS, Wara WM, Ciricillo SF, Davis RL, Zoger S, Edwards MS (1997). Primary intracerebral osteosarcoma: a case report. J Neurooncol. 32(3):209–13. PMID:9049882
145. Baumert BG, Rutten I, Dehing-Oberije C, Twijnstra A, Dirx MJ, Debougnoux-Huppertz RM, et al. (2006). A pathology-based substrate for target definition in radiosurgery of brain metastases. Int J Radiat Oncol Biol Phys. 66(1):187–94. PMID:16814946
146. Baumgarten P, Harter PN, Tönjes M, Capper D, Blank AE, Sahm F, et al. (2014). Loss of FUBP1 expression in gliomas predicts FUBP1 mutation and is associated with oligodendroglial differentiation, IDH1 mutation and 1p/19q loss of heterozygosity. Neuropathol Appl Neurobiol. 40(2):205–16. PMID:24117486
147. Baysal BE (2002). Hereditary paraganglioma targets diverse paraganglia. J Med Genet. 39(9):617–22. PMID:12205103
148. Beaumont TL, Kupsky WJ, Barger GR, Sloan AE (2007). Gliosarcoma with multiple extracranial metastases: case report and review of the literature. J Neurooncol. 83(1):39–46. PMID:17171442
149. Becher MW, Abel TW, Thompson RC, Weaver KD, Davis LE (2006). Immunohistochemical analysis of metastatic neoplasms of the central nervous system. J Neuropathol Exp Neurol. 65(10):935–44. PMID:17021398
150. Bechet D, Gielen GG, Korshunov A, Pfister SM, Rousso C, Faury D, et al. (2014). Specific detection of methionine 27 mutation in histone 3 variants (H3K27M) in fixed tissue from high-grade astrocytomas. Acta Neuropathol. 128(5):733–41. PMID:25200321
151. Beck DJK, Russell DS (1942). Oligodendrogliomatosis of the cerebrospinal pathway. Brain. 352–72.
152. Becker DH, Wilson CB (1981). Symptomatic parasellar granular cell tumors. Neurosurgery. 8(2):173–80. PMID:6259552
153. Becker I, Paulus W, Roggendorf W (1989). Histogenesis of stromal cells in cerebellar hemangioblastomas. An immunohistochemical study. Am J Pathol. 134(2):271–5. PMID:2916647
154. Becker RL, Becker AD, Sobel DF (1995). Adult medulloblastoma: review of 13 cases with emphasis on MRI. Neuroradiology. 37(2):104–8. PMID:7760992
155. Beert E, Brems H, Daniëls B, De Wever I, Van Calenbergh F, Schoenaers J, et al. (2011). Atypical neurofibromas in neurofibromatosis type 1 are premalignant tumors. Genes Chromosomes Cancer. 50(12):1021–32. PMID:21987445
156. Beert E, Brems H, Renard M, Ferreiro JF, Melotte C, Thoelen R, et al. (2012). Biallelic inactivation of NF1 in a sporadic plexiform neurofibroma. Genes Chromosomes Cancer. 51(9):852–7. PMID:22585738
157. Behdad A, Perry A (2010). Central nervous system primitive neuroectodermal tumors: a clinicopathologic and genetic study of 33 cases. Brain Pathol. 20(2):441–50. PMID:19725831
158. Beier D, Hau P, Proescholdt M, Lohmeier A, Wischhusen J, Oefner PJ, et al. (2007). CD133(+) and CD133(-) glioblastoma-derived cancer stem cells show differential growth characteristics and molecular profiles. Cancer Res. 67(9):4010–5. PMID:17483311
159. Bell DA, Woodruff JM, Scully RE (1984). Ependymoma of the broad ligament. A report of two cases. Am J Surg Pathol. 8(3):203–9. PMID:6703196
159A. Bell RJ, Rube HT, Kreig A, Mancini A, Fouse SD, Nagarajan RP, et al. (2015). Cancer. The transcription factor GABP selectively binds and activates the mutant TERT promoter in cancer. Science. 348(6238):1036–9. PMID:25977370
160. Bellail AC, Hunter SB, Brat DJ, Tan C, Van Meir EG (2004). Microregional extracellular matrix heterogeneity in brain modulates glioma cell invasion. Int J Biochem Cell Biol. 36(6):1046–69. PMID:15094120
161. Bello MJ, Leone PE, Vaquero J, de Campos JM, Kusak ME, Sarasa JL, et al. (1995). Allelic loss at 1p and 19q frequently occurs in association and may represent early oncogenic events in oligodendroglial tumors. Int J Cancer. 64(3):207–10. PMID:7622310
162. Bello MJ, Rey JA, de Campos JM, Kusak ME (1993). Chromosomal abnormalities in a pineocytoma. Cancer Genet Cytogenet. 71(2):185–6. PMID:8281527
163. Belloni E, Muenke M, Roessler E, Traverso G, Siegel-Bartelt J, Frumkin A, et al. (1996). Identification of Sonic hedgehog as a candidate gene responsible for holoprosencephaly. Nat Genet. 14(3):353–6. PMID:8896571
164. Benesch M, Frappaz D, Massimino M (2012). Spinal cord ependymomas in children and adolescents. Childs Nerv Syst. 28(12):2017–28. PMID:22961356
165. Beni-Adani L, Gomori M, Spektor S, Constantini S (2000). Cyst wall enhancement in pilocytic astrocytoma: neoplastic or reactive phenomena. Pediatr Neurosurg. 32(5):234–9. PMID:10965269
166. Benites Filho PR, Sakamoto D, Machuca TN, Serapião MJ, Ditzel L, Bleggi Torres LF (2005). Granular cell tumor of the neurohypophysis: report of a case with unusual age presentation. Virchows Arch. 447(3):649–52. PMID:16133355
167. Bennett JP Jr, Rubinstein LJ (1984). The biological behavior of primary cerebral neuroblastoma: a reappraisal of the clinical course in a series of 70 cases. Ann Neurol. 16(1):21–7. PMID:6431897
168. Bennett KL, Mester J, Eng C (2010). Germline epigenetic regulation of KILLIN in Cowden and Cowden-like syndrome. JAMA. 304(24):2724–31. PMID:21177507
169. Benzagmout M, Karachi C, Mokhtari K, Capelle L (2013). Hemorrhagic papillary glioneuronal tumor mimicking cavernoma: two case reports. Clin Neurol Neurosurg. 115(2):200–3. PMID:22717600
170. Berghoff AS, Bartsch R, Wöhrer A, Streubel B, Birner P, Kros JM, et al. (2014). Predictive molecular markers in metastases to the central nervous system: recent advances and future avenues. Acta Neuropathol. 128(6):879–91. PMID:25287912
171. Berghoff AS, Ilhan-Mutlu A, Dinhof C, Magerle M, Hackl M, Widhalm G, et al. (2015). Differential role of angiogenesis and tumour cell proliferation in brain metastases according to primary tumour type: analysis of 639 cases. Neuropathol Appl Neurobiol. 41(2):e41–55. PMID:25256708
171A. Berghoff AS, Preusser M (2014). BRAF alterations in brain tumours: molecular pathology and therapeutic opportunities. Curr Opin Neurol. 27(6):689–96. PMID:25268071
172. Berghoff AS, Rajky O, Winkler F, Bartsch R, Furtner J, Hainfellner JA, et al. (2013). Invasion patterns in brain metastases of solid cancers. Neuro Oncol. 15(12):1664–72. PMID:24084410
173. Berho M, Suster S (1994). Mucinous meningioma. Report of an unusual variant of meningioma that may mimic metastatic mucin-producing carcinoma. Am J Surg Pathol. 18(1):100–6. PMID:8279622
174. Beristain X, Azzarelli B (2002). The neurological masquerade of intravascular lymphomatosis. Arch Neurol. 59(3):439–43. PMID:11890850
175. Berkman RA, Clark WC, Saxena A, Robertson JT, Oldfield EH, Ali IU (1992). Clonal composition of glioblastoma multiforme. J Neurosurg. 77(3):432–7. PMID:1324297
176. Bernell WR, Kepes JJ, Seitz EP (1972). Late malignant recurrence of childhood cerebellar astrocytoma. Report of two cases. J Neurosurg. 37(4):470–4. PMID:5070873
177. Berns S, Pearl G (2006). Review of pineal anlage tumor with divergent histology. Arch Pathol Lab Med. 130(8):1233–5. PMID:16879032
178. Bernthal NM, Jones KB, Monument MJ, Liu T, Viskochil D, Randall RL (2013). Lost in translation: ambiguity in nerve sheath tumor nomenclature and its resultant treatment effect. Cancers (Basel). 5(2):519–28. PMID:24216989
179. Bernthal NM, Putnam A, Jones KB, Viskochil D, Randall RL (2014). The effect of surgical margins on outcomes for low grade MPNSTs and atypical neurofibroma. J Surg Oncol. 110(7):813–6. PMID:25111615
180. Beschorner R, Pantazis G, Jeibmann A, Boy J, Meyermann R, Mittelbronn M, et al. (2009). Expression of EAAT-1 distinguishes choroid plexus tumors from normal and reactive choroid plexus epithelium. Acta Neuropathol. 117(6):667–75. PMID:19283393
181. Bethke L, Murray A, Webb E, Schoemaker M, Muir K, McKinney P, et al. (2008). Comprehensive analysis of DNA repair gene variants and risk of meningioma. J Natl Cancer Inst. 100(4):270–6. PMID:18270339
182. Bettegowda C, Adogwa O, Mehta V, Chaichana KL, Weingart J, Carson BS, et al. (2012). Treatment of choroid plexus tumors: a 20-year single institutional experience. J Neurosurg Pediatr. 10(5):398–405. PMID:22938081
183. Bettegowda C, Agrawal N, Jiao Y, Sausen M, Wood LD, Hruban RH, et al. (2011). Mutations in CIC and FUBP1 contribute to human oligodendroglioma. Science. 333(6048):1453–5. PMID:21817013
184. Bettegowda C, Agrawal N, Jiao Y, Wang Y, Wood LD, Rodriguez FJ, et al. (2013). Exomic sequencing of four rare central nervous system tumor types. Oncotarget. 4(4):572–83. PMID:23592488
185. Betz BL, Strobeck MW, Reisman DN, Knudsen ES, Weissman BE (2002). Re-expression of hSNF5/INI1/BAF47 in pediatric tumor cells leads to G1 arrest associated with induction of p16ink4a and activation of RB. Oncogene. 21(34):5193–203. PMID:12149641
186. Bhagavathi S, Greiner TC, Kazmi SA, Fu K, Sanger WG, Chan WC (2008). Extranodal marginal zone lymphoma of the dura mater with IgH/MALT1 translocation and review of literature. J Hematop. 1(2):131–7. PMID:19669212
187. Bhargava D, Sinha P, Chumas P, Al-Tamimi Y, Shivane A, Chakrabarty A, et al. (2013). Occurrence and distribution of pilomyxoid astrocytoma. Br J Neurosurg. 27(4):413–8. PMID:23281683
188. Bhattacharjee MB, Armstrong DD, Vogel H, Cooley LD (1997). Cytogenetic analysis of 120 primary pediatric brain tumors and literature review. Cancer Genet Cytogenet. 97(1):39–53. PMID:9242217
189. Bhatti P, Veiga LH, Ronckers CM, Sigurdson AJ, Stovall M, Smith SA, et al. (2010). Risk of second primary thyroid cancer after radiotherapy for a childhood cancer in a large cohort study: an update from the childhood cancer

survivor study. Radiat Res. 174(6):741–52. PMID:21128798
190. Bianco AdeM, Madeira LV, Rosemberg S, Shibata MK (2006). Cortical seeding of a craniopharyngioma after craniotomy: Case report. Surg Neurol. 66(4):437–40, discussion 440. PMID:17015135
191. Biegel JA (1999). Cytogenetics and molecular genetics of childhood brain tumors. Neuro Oncol. 1(2):139–51. PMID:11550309
192. Biegel JA (2006). Molecular genetics of atypical teratoid/rhabdoid tumor. Neurosurg Focus. 20(1):E11. PMID:16459991
193. Biegel JA, Busse TM, Weissman BE (2014). SWI/SNF chromatin remodeling complexes and cancer. Am J Med Genet C Semin Med Genet. 166C(3):350–66. PMID:25169151
194. Biegel JA, Zhou JY, Rorke LB, Stenstrom C, Wainwright LM, Fogelgren B (1999). Germline and acquired mutations of INI1 in atypical teratoid and rhabdoid tumors. Cancer Res. 59(1):74–9. PMID:9892189
195. Bielle F, Navarro S, Bertrand A, Cornu P, Mazeron JJ, Jouvet A, et al. (2014). Late dural relapse of a resected and irradiated pineal parenchymal tumor of intermediate differentiation. Clin Neuropathol. 33(6):424–7. PMID:24887399
196. Bielle F, Villa C, Giry M, Bergemer-Fouquet AM, Polivka M, Vasiljevic A, et al.; RENOP (2015). Chordoid gliomas of the third ventricle share TTF-1 expression with organum vasculosum of the lamina terminalis. Am J Surg Pathol. 39(7):948–56. PMID:25786084
197. Biernat W, Aguzzi A, Sure U, Grant JW, Kleihues P, Hegi ME (1995). Identical mutations of the p53 tumor suppressor gene in the gliomatous and the sarcomatous components of gliosarcomas suggest a common origin from glial cells. J Neuropathol Exp Neurol. 54(5):651–6. PMID:7666053
198. Biernat W, Huang H, Yokoo H, Kleihues P, Ohgaki H (2004). Predominant expression of mutant EGFR (EGFRvIII) is rare in primary glioblastomas. Brain Pathol. 14(2):131–6. PMID:15193025
199. Biernat W, Kleihues P, Yonekawa Y, Ohgaki H (1997). Amplification and overexpression of MDM2 in primary (de novo) glioblastomas. J Neuropathol Exp Neurol. 56(2):180–5. PMID:9034372
200. Biernat W, Tohma Y, Yonekawa Y, Kleihues P, Ohgaki H (1997). Alterations of cell cycle regulatory genes in primary (de novo) and secondary glioblastomas. Acta Neuropathol. 94(4):303–9. PMID:9341929
201. Bigelow DC, Eisen MD, Smith PG, Yousem DM, Levine RS, Jackler RK, et al. (1998). Lipomas of the internal auditory canal and cerebellopontine angle. Laryngoscope. 108(10):1459–69. PMID:9778284
202. Biggs PJ, Garen PD, Powers JM, Garvin AJ (1987). Malignant rhabdoid tumor of the central nervous system. Hum Pathol. 18(4):332–7. PMID:3030922
203. Bigner SH, McLendon RE, Fuchs H, McKeever PE, Friedman HS (1997). Chromosomal characteristics of childhood brain tumors. Cancer Genet Cytogenet. 97(2):125–34. PMID:9283596
204. Bijlsma EK, Merel P, Bosch DA, Westerveld A, Delattre O, Thomas G, et al. (1994). Analysis of mutations in the SCH gene in schwannomas. Genes Chromosomes Cancer. 11(1):7–14. PMID:7529050
205. Bilsky MH, Schefler AC, Sandberg DI, Dunkel IJ, Rosenblum MK (2000). Sclerosing epithelioid fibrosarcomas involving the neuraxis: report of three cases. Neurosurgery. 47(4):956–9, discussion 959–60. PMID:11014436
206. Binning MJ, Niazi T, Pedone CA, Lal B, Eberhart CG, Kim KJ, et al. (2008). Hepatocyte growth factor and sonic Hedgehog expression in cerebellar neural progenitor cells costimulate medulloblastoma initiation and growth. Cancer Res. 68(19):7838–45. PMID:18829539
207. Birch BD, Johnson JP, Parsa A, Desai RD, Yoon JT, Lycette CA, et al. (1996). Frequent type 2 neurofibromatosis gene transcript mutations in sporadic intramedullary spinal cord ependymomas. Neurosurgery. 39(1):135–40. PMID:8805149
208. Birch JM, Blair V, Kelsey AM, Evans DG, Harris M, Tricker KJ, et al. (1998). Cancer phenotype correlates with constitutional TP53 genotype in families with the Li-Fraumeni syndrome. Oncogene. 17(9):1061–8. PMID:9764816
209. Bisceglia M, Galliani C, Giannatempo G, Lauriola W, Bianco M, D'angelo V, et al. (2011). Solitary fibrous tumor of the central nervous system: a 15-year literature survey of 220 cases (August 1996-July 2011). Adv Anat Pathol. 18(5):356–92. PMID:21841406
210. Bjornsson J, Scheithauer BW, Okazaki H, Leech RW (1985). Intracranial germ cell tumors: pathobiological and immunohistochemical aspects of 70 cases. J Neuropathol Exp Neurol. 44(1):32–46. PMID:4038412
211. Blades DA, Hardy RW, Cohen M (1991). Cervical paraganglioma with subsequent intracranial and intraspinal metastases. Case report. J Neurosurg. 75(2):320–3. PMID:2072174
212. Blandino G, Levine AJ, Oren M (1999). Mutant p53 gain of function: differential effects of different p53 mutants on resistance of cultured cells to chemotherapy. Oncogene. 18(2):477–85. PMID:9927204
213. Blaser SI, Harwood-Nash DC (1996). Neuroradiology of pediatric posterior fossa medulloblastoma. J Neurooncol. 29(1):23–34. PMID:8817413
214. Bleeker FE, Atai NA, Lamba S, Jonker A, Rijkeboer D, Bosch KS, et al. (2010). The prognostic IDH1(R132) mutation is associated with reduced NADP+-dependent IDH activity in glioblastoma. Acta Neuropathol. 119(4):487–94. PMID:20127344
215. Bleistein M, Geiger K, Franz K, Stoldt P, Schlote W (2000). Transthyretin and transferrin in hemangioblastoma stromal cells. Pathol Res Pract. 196(10):675–81. PMID:11087054
216. Blesa D, Mollejo M, Ruano Y, de Lope AR, Fiaño C, Ribalta T, et al. (2009). Novel genomic alterations and mechanisms associated with tumor progression in oligodendroglioma and mixed oligoastrocytoma. J Neuropathol Exp Neurol. 68(3):274–85. PMID:19225409
216A. Blitshteyn S, Crook JE, Jaeckle KA (2008). Is there an association between meningioma and hormone replacement therapy? J Clin Oncol. 26(2):279–82. PMID:18182668
217. Blough MD, Al-Najjar M, Chesnelong C, Binding CE, Rogers AD, Luchman HA, et al. (2012). DNA hypermethylation and 1p Loss silence NHE-1 in oligodendroglioma. Ann Neurol. 71(6):845–9. PMID:22718548
218. Blount JP, Elton S (2001). Spinal lipomas. Neurosurg Focus. 10(1):e3. PMID:16749755
219. Blumcke I, Aronica E, Urbach H, Alexopoulos A, Gonzalez-Martinez JA (2014). A neuropathology-based approach to epilepsy surgery in brain tumors and proposal for a new terminology use for long-term epilepsy-associated brain tumors. Acta Neuropathol. 128(1):39–54. PMID:24858213
220. Blumenthal GM, Dennis PA (2008). PTEN hamartoma tumor syndromes. Eur J Hum Genet. 16(11):1289–300. PMID:18781191
221. Blümcke I, Becker AJ, Normann S, Hans V, Riederer BM, Krajewski S, et al. (2001). Distinct expression pattern of microtubule-associated protein-2 in human oligodendrogliomas and glial precursor cells. J Neuropathol Exp Neurol. 60(10):984–93. PMID:11589429
222. Blümcke I, Giencke K, Wardelmann E, Beyenburg S, Kral T, Sarioglu N, et al. (1999). The CD34 epitope is expressed in neoplastic and malformative lesions associated with chronic, focal epilepsies. Acta Neuropathol. 97(5):481–90. PMID:10334485
223. Blümcke I, Löbach M, Wolf HK, Wiestler OD (1999). Evidence for developmental precursor lesions in epilepsy-associated glioneuronal tumors. Microsc Res Tech. 46(1):53–8. PMID:10402272
224. Blümcke I, Müller S, Buslei R, Riederer BM, Wiestler OD (2004). Microtubule-associated protein-2 immunoreactivity: a useful tool in the differential diagnosis of low-grade neuroepithelial tumors. Acta Neuropathol. 108(2):89–96. PMID:15146346
225. Blümcke I, Thom M, Aronica E, Armstrong DD, Vinters HV, Palmini A, et al. (2011). The clinicopathologic spectrum of focal cortical dysplasias: a consensus classification proposed by an ad hoc Task Force of the ILAE Diagnostic Methods Commission. Epilepsia. 52(1):158–74. PMID:21219302
226. Blümcke I, Wiestler OD (2002). Gangliogliomas: an intriguing tumor entity associated with focal epilepsies. J Neuropathol Exp Neurol. 61(7):575–84. PMID:12125736
227. Bodey B, Bodey B Jr, Siegel SE (1995). Immunophenotypic characterization of infiltrating polynuclear and mononuclear cells in childhood brain tumors. Mod Pathol. 8(3):333–8. PMID:7617661
228. Bodi I, Curran O, Selway R, Elwes R, Burrone J, Laxton R, et al. (2014). Two cases of multinodular and vacuolating neuronal tumour. Acta Neuropathol Commun. 2:7. PMID:24444358
229. Bodi I, Selway R, Bannister P, Doey L, Mullatti N, Elwes R, et al. (2012). Diffuse form of dysembryoplastic neuroepithelial tumour: the histological and immunohistochemical features of a distinct entity showing transition to dysembryoplastic neuroepithelial tumour and ganglioglioma. Neuropathol Appl Neurobiol. 38(5):411–25. PMID:21988102
230. Bodo S, Colas C, Buhard O, Collura A, Tinat J, Lavoine N, et al.; European Consortium "Care for CMMRD" (2015). Diagnosis of Constitutional Mismatch Repair-Deficiency Syndrome Based on Microsatellite Instability and Lymphocyte Tolerance to Methylating Agents. Gastroenterology. 149(4):1017–1029.e3. PMID:26116798
231. Boehm D, Bacher J, Neumann HP (2007). Gross genomic rearrangement involving the TSC2-PKD1 contiguous deletion syndrome: characterization of the deletion event by quantitative polymerase chain reaction deletion assay. Am J Kidney Dis. 49(1):e11–21. PMID:17185137
232. Boerman RH, Anderl K, Herath J, Borell T, Johnson N, Schaeffer-Klein J, et al. (1996). The glial and mesenchymal elements of gliosarcomas share similar genetic alterations. J Neuropathol Exp Neurol. 55(9):973–81. PMID:8800093
233. Bognár L, Bálint K, Bárdóczy Z (2002). Symptomatic osteolipoma of the tuber cinereum. Case report. J Neurosurg. 96(2):361–3. PMID:11838812
234. Boguski MS, McCormick F (1993). Proteins regulating Ras and its relatives. Nature. 366(6456):643–54. PMID:8259209
235. Bolcekova A, Nemethova M, Zatkova A, Hlinkova K, Pozgayova S, Hlavata A, et al. (2013). Clustering of mutations in the 5' tertile of the NF1 gene in Slovakia patients with optic pathway glioma. Neoplasma. 60(6):655–65. PMID:23906300
236. Bonnin JM, Rubinstein LJ (1989). Astroblastomas: a pathological study of 23 tumors, with a postoperative follow-up in 13 patients. Neurosurgery. 25(1):6–13. PMID:2755581
237. Booman M, Douwes J, Glas AM, Riemersma SA, Jordanova ES, Kok K, et al. (2006). Mechanisms and effects of loss of human leukocyte antigen class II expression in immune-privileged site-associated B-cell lymphoma. Clin Cancer Res. 12(9):2698–705. PMID:16675561
238. Boop FA (2011). Repeat surgery for residual ependymoma. J Neurosurg Pediatr. 8(3):244–5, discussion 245. PMID:21882913
239. Borges MT, Lillehei KO, Kleinschmidt-DeMasters BK (2011). Spindle cell oncocytoma with late recurrence and unique neuroimaging characteristics due to recurrent subclinical intratumoral bleeding. J Neurooncol. 101(1):145–54. PMID:20495848
240. Borit A, Blackwood W, Mair WG (1980). The separation of pineocytoma from pineoblastoma. Cancer. 45(6):1408–18. PMID:6986979
241. Borkowska J, Schwartz RA, Kotulska K, Jozwiak S (2011). Tuberous sclerosis complex: tumors and tumorigenesis. Int J Dermatol. 50(1):13–20. PMID:21182496
242. Borota OC, Scheie D, Bjerkhagen B, Jacobsen EA, Skullerud K (2006). Gliosarcoma with liposarcomatous component, bone infiltration and extracranial growth. Clin Neuropathol. 25(4):200–3. PMID:16866302
243. Borota OC, Scheithauer BW, Fougner SL, Hald JK, Ramm-Pettersen J, Bollerslev J (2009). Spindle cell oncocytoma of the adenohypophysis: report of a case with marked cellular atypia and recurrence despite adjuvant treatment. Clin Neuropathol. 28(2):91–5. PMID:19353839
244. Borovich B, Doron Y (1986). Recurrence of intracranial meningiomas: the role played by regional multicentricity. J Neurosurg. 64(1):58–63. PMID:3941351
245. Bosman FT, Carneiro F, Hruban RH, Theise ND, editors. (2010). WHO Classification of Tumours of the Digestive System. 4th ed. Lyon: International Agency for Research on Cancer.
246. Boström J, Meyer-Puttlitz B, Wolter M, Blaschke B, Weber RG, Lichter P, et al. (2001). Alterations of the tumor suppressor genes CDKN2A (p16(INK4a)), p14(ARF), CDKN2B (p15(INK4b)), and CDKN2C (p18(INK4c)) in atypical and anaplastic meningiomas. Am J Pathol. 159(2):661–9. PMID:11485924
247. Bouffard JP, Sandberg GD, Golden JA, Rorke LB (2004). Double immunolabeling of central nervous system atypical teratoid/rhabdoid tumors. Mod Pathol. 17(6):679–83. PMID:15105808
248. Bouffet E, Perilongo G, Canete A, Massimino M (1998). Intracranial ependymomas in children: a critical review of prognostic factors and a plea for cooperation. Med Pediatr Oncol. 30(6):319–29, discussion 329–31. PMID:9589080
249. Bourdeaut F, Lequin D, Brugières L, Reynaud S, Dufour C, Doz F, et al. (2011). Frequent hSNF5/INI1 germline mutations in patients with rhabdoid tumor. Clin Cancer Res. 17(1):31–8. PMID:21208904
249A. Bourdeaut F, Miquel C, Richer W, Grill J, Zerah M, Grison C, et al. (2014). Rubinstein-Taybi syndrome predisposing to non-WNT, non-SHH, group 3 medulloblastoma. Pediatr Blood Cancer. 61(2):383–6. PMID:24115570
250. Bourekas EC, Bell SD, Ladwig NR, Gandhe AR, Shilo K, McGregor JM, et al. (2014). Anaplastic papillary glioneuronal tumor with extraneural metastases. J Neuropathol Exp Neurol. 73(5):474–6. PMID:24709681
251. Bourgeois M, Sainte-Rose C, Lellouch-Tubiana A, Malucci C, Brunelle F, Maixner W, et al. (1999). Surgery of epilepsy associated with focal lesions in childhood. J Neurosurg. 90(5):833–42. PMID:10223448
252. Bourn D, Carter SA, Mason S, Gareth D, Evans R, Strachan T (1994). Germline mutations in the neurofibromatosis type 2 tumour suppressor gene. Hum Mol Genet. 3(5):813–6. PMID:8081368
253. Bourne TD, Mandell JW, Matsumoto JA, Jane JA Jr, Lopes MB (2006). Primary disseminated leptomeningeal oligodendroglioma with 1p deletion. Case report. J Neurosurg. 105(6) Suppl:465–9. PMID:17184079
254. Bourne TD, Schiff D (2010). Update on

molecular findings, management and outcome in low-grade gliomas. Nat Rev Neurol. 6(12):695–701. PMID:21045797
255. Bouvier C, Bertucci F, Métellus P, Finetti P, Maues de Paula A, Forest F, et al. (2013). ALDH1 is an immunohistochemical diagnostic marker for solitary fibrous tumours and haemangiopericytomas of the meninges emerging from gene profiling study. Acta Neuropathol Commun. 1:10. PMID:24252471
256. Bouvier C, Métellus P, de Paula AM, Vasiljevic A, Jouvet A, Guyotat J, et al. (2012). Solitary fibrous tumors and hemangiopericytomas of the meninges: overlapping pathological features and common prognostic factors suggest the same spectrum of tumors. Brain Pathol. 22(4):511–21. PMID:22082190
257. Bouvier-Labit C, Daniel L, Dufour H, Grisoli F, Figarella-Branger D (2000). Papillary glioneuronal tumour: clinicopathological and biochemical study of one case with 7-year follow up. Acta Neuropathol. 99(3):321–6. PMID:10663977
258. Bowers DC, Gargan L, Kapur P, Reisch JS, Mulne AF, Shapiro KN, et al. (2003). Study of the MIB-1 labeling index as a predictor of tumor progression in pilocytic astrocytomas in children and adolescents. J Clin Oncol. 21(15):2968–73. PMID:12885817
259. Bowers DC, Mulne AF, Weprin B, Bruce DA, Shapiro K, Margraf LR (2002). Prognostic factors in children and adolescents with low-grade oligodendrogliomas. Pediatr Neurosurg. 37(2):57–63. PMID:12145513
260. Boyd C, Smith MJ, Kluwe L, Balogh A, Maccollin M, Plotkin SR (2008). Alterations in the SMARCB1 (INI1) tumor suppressor gene in familial schwannomatosis. Clin Genet. 74(4):358–66. PMID:18647326
261. Brannan CI, Perkins AS, Vogel KS, Ratner N, Nordlund ML, Reid SW, et al. (1994). Targeted disruption of the neurofibromatosis type-1 gene leads to developmental abnormalities in heart and various neural crest-derived tissues. Genes Dev. 8(9):1019–29. PMID:7926784
262. Brastianos PK, Horowitz PM, Santagata S, Jones RT, McKenna A, Getz G, et al. (2013). Genomic sequencing of meningiomas identifies oncogenic SMO and AKT1 mutations. Nat Genet. 45(3):285–9. PMID:23334667
263. Brastianos PK, Taylor-Weiner A, Manley PE, Jones RT, Dias-Santagata D, Thorner AR, et al. (2014). Exome sequencing identifies BRAF mutations in papillary craniopharyngiomas. Nat Genet. 46(2):161–5. PMID:24413733
264. Brat DJ, Castellano-Sanchez AA, Hunter SB, Pecot M, Cohen C, Hammond EH, et al. (2004). Pseudopalisades in glioblastoma are hypoxic, express extracellular matrix proteases, and are formed by an actively migrating cell population. Cancer Res. 64(3):920–7. PMID:14871821
265. Brat DJ, Cohen KJ, Sanders JM, Feuerstein BG, Burger PC (1999). Clinicopathologic features of astroblastoma. J Neuropathol Exp Neurol. 58:509.
266. Brat DJ, Giannini C, Scheithauer BW, Burger PC (1999). Primary melanocytic neoplasms of the central nervous systems. Am J Surg Pathol. 23(7):745–54. PMID:10403296
267. Brat DJ, Hirose Y, Cohen KJ, Feuerstein BG, Burger PC (2000). Astroblastoma: clinicopathologic features and chromosomal abnormalities defined by comparative genomic hybridization. Brain Pathol. 10(3):342–52. PMID:10885653
268. Brat DJ, Ryken TC, Kalkanis SN, Olson JJ; AANS/CNS Joint Guidelines Committee (2014). The role of neuropathology in the management of progressive glioblastoma : a systematic review and evidence-based clinical practice guideline. J Neurooncol. 118(3):461–78. PMID:24733643
269. Brat DJ, Scheithauer BW, Eberhart CG, Burger PC (2001). Extraventricular neurocytomas: pathologic features and clinical outcome. Am J Surg Pathol. 25(10):1252–60. PMID:11688459
270. Brat DJ, Scheithauer BW, Fuller GN, Tihan T (2007). Newly codified glial neoplasms of the 2007 WHO Classification of Tumours of the Central Nervous System: angiocentric glioma, pilomyxoid astrocytoma and pituicytoma. Brain Pathol. 17(3):319–24. PMID:17598825
271. Brat DJ, Scheithauer BW, Medina-Flores R, Rosenblum MK, Burger PC (2002). Infiltrative astrocytomas with granular cell features (granular cell astrocytomas): a study of histopathologic features, grading, and outcome. Am J Surg Pathol. 26(6):750–7. PMID:12023579
272. Brat DJ, Scheithauer BW, Staugaitis SM, Cortez SC, Brecher K, Burger PC (1998). Third ventricular chordoid glioma: a distinct clinicopathologic entity. J Neuropathol Exp Neurol. 57(3):283–90. PMID:9600220
273. Brat DJ, Scheithauer BW, Staugaitis SM, Holtzman RN, Morgello S, Burger PC (2000). Pituicytoma: a distinctive low-grade glioma of the neurohypophysis. Am J Surg Pathol. 24(3):362–8. PMID:10716149
273A. Bredel M, Scholtens DM, Yadav AK, Alvarez AA, Renfrow JJ, Chandler JP, et al. (2011). NFKBIA deletion in glioblastomas. N Engl J Med. 364(7):627–37. PMID:21175304
274. Brekke HR, Ribeiro FR, Kolberg M, Agesen TH, Lind GE, Eknaes M, et al. (2010). Genomic changes in chromosomes 10, 16, and X in malignant peripheral nerve sheath tumors identify a high-risk patient group. J Clin Oncol. 28(9):1573–82. PMID:20159821
275. Brems H, Chmara M, Sahbatou M, Denayer E, Taniguchi K, Kato R, et al. (2007). Germline loss-of-function mutations in SPRED1 cause a neurofibromatosis 1-like phenotype. Nat Genet. 39(9):1120–6. PMID:17704776
276. Brennan C (2011). Genomic profiles of glioma. Curr Neurol Neurosci Rep. 11(3):291–7. PMID:21465149
277. Brennan CW, Verhaak RG, McKenna A, Campos B, Noushmehr H, Salama SR, et al.; TCGA Research Network (2013). The somatic genomic landscape of glioblastoma. Cell. 155(2):462–77. PMID:24120142
278. Bridge JA, Liu XQ, Sumegi J, Nelson M, Reyes C, Bruch LA, et al. (2013). Identification of a novel, recurrent SLC44A1-PRKCA fusion in papillary glioneuronal tumor. Brain Pathol. 23(2):121–8. PMID:22725730
279. Bridge RS, Rajaram V, Dehner LP, Pfeifer JD, Perry A (2006). Molecular diagnosis of Ewing sarcoma/primitive neuroectodermal tumor in routinely processed tissue: a comparison of two FISH strategies and RT-PCR in malignant round cell tumors. Mod Pathol. 19(1):1–8. PMID:16258512
280. Briscoe J, Thérond PP (2013). The mechanisms of Hedgehog signalling and its roles in development and disease. Nat Rev Mol Cell Biol. 14(7):416–29. PMID:23719536
281. Brock JE, Perez-Atayde AR, Kozakewich HP, Richkind KE, Fletcher JA, Vargas SO (2005). Cytogenetic aberrations in perineurioma: variation with subtype. Am J Surg Pathol. 29(9):1164–9. PMID:16096405
282. Brodbelt A, Greenberg D, Winters T, Williams M, Vernon S, Collins VP; (UK) National Cancer Information Network Brain Tumour Group (2015). Glioblastoma in England: 2007–2011. Eur J Cancer. 51(4):533–42. PMID:25661102
282A. Broderick DK, Di C, Parrett TJ, Samuels YR, Cummins JM, McLendon RE, et al. (2004). Mutations of PIK3CA in anaplastic oligodendrogliomas, high-grade astrocytomas, and medulloblastomas. Cancer Res. 64(15):5048–50. PMID:15289301
283. Broholm H, Madsen FF, Wagner AA, Laursen H (2002). Papillary glioneuronal tumor–a new tumor entity. Clin Neuropathol. 21(1):1–4. PMID:11846038
284. Broniscer A, Baker SJ, West AN, Fraser MM, Proko E, Kocak M, et al. (2007). Clinical and molecular characteristics of malignant transformation of low-grade glioma in children. J Clin Oncol. 25(6):682–9. PMID:17308273
285. Broniscer A, Tatevossian RG, Sabin ND, Klimo P Jr, Dalton J, Lee R, et al. (2014). Clinical, radiological, histological and molecular characteristics of paediatric epithelioid glioblastoma. Neuropathol Appl Neurobiol. 40(3):327–36. PMID:24127995
286. Brown AE, Leibundgut K, Niggli FK, Betts DR (2006). Cytogenetics of pineoblastoma: four new cases and a literature review. Cancer Genet Cytogenet. 170(2):175–9. PMID:17011992
287. Brown HG, Burger PC, Olivi A, Sills AK, Barditch-Crovo PA, Lee RR (1999). Intracranial leiomyosarcoma in a patient with AIDS. Neuroradiology. 41(1):35–9. PMID:9987766
288. Brown HG, Kepner JL, Perlman EJ, Friedman HS, Strother DR, Duffner PK, et al. (2000). "Large cell/anaplastic" medulloblastomas: a Pediatric Oncology Group Study. J Neuropathol Exp Neurol. 59(10):857–65. PMID:11079775
289. Brown JA, Gianino SM, Gutmann DH (2010). Defective cAMP generation underlies the sensitivity of CNS neurons to neurofibromatosis-1 heterozygosity. J Neurosci. 30(16):5579–89. PMID:20410111
290. Brown NA, Furtado LV, Betz BL, Kiel MJ, Weigelin HC, Lim MS, et al. (2014). High prevalence of somatic MAP2K1 mutations in BRAF V600E-negative Langerhans cell histiocytosis. Blood. 124(10):1655–8. PMID:24982505
291. Brown PD, Buckner JC, O'Fallon JR, Iturria NL, Brown CA, O'Neill BP, et al.; North Central Cancer Treatment Group; Mayo Clinic (2004). Adult patients with supratentorial pilocytic astrocytomas: a prospective multicenter clinical trial. Int J Radiat Oncol Biol Phys. 58(4):1153–60. PMID:15001258
292. Brown R, Zlatescu M, Sijben A, Roldan G, Easaw J, Forsyth P, et al. (2008). The use of magnetic resonance imaging to noninvasively detect genetic signatures in oligodendroglioma. Clin Cancer Res. 14(8):2357–62. PMID:18413825
293. Brownstein MH, Wolf M, Bikowski JB (1978). Cowden's disease: a cutaneous marker of breast cancer. Cancer. 41(6):2393–8. PMID:657103
294. Brugières L, Remenieras A, Pierron G, Varlet P, Forget S, Byrde V, et al. (2012). High frequency of germline SUFU mutations in children with desmoplastic/nodular medulloblastoma younger than 3 years of age. J Clin Oncol. 30(17):2087–93. PMID:22508808
295. Brunn A, Nagel I, Montesinos-Rongen M, Klapper W, Vater I, Paulus W, et al. (2013). Frequent triple-hit expression of MYC, BCL2, and BCL6 in primary lymphoma of the central nervous system and absence of a favorable MYC(low)BCL2 (low) subgroup may underlie the inferior prognosis as compared to systemic diffuse large B cell lymphomas. Acta Neuropathol. 126(4):603–5. PMID:24061549
297. Bruno A, Boisselier B, Labreche K, Marie Y, Polivka M, Jouvet A, et al. (2014). Mutational analysis of primary central nervous system lymphoma. Oncotarget. 5(13):5065–75. PMID:24970810
298. Brück W, Brunn A, Klapper W, Kuhlmann T, Metz I, Paulus W, et al.; Netzwerk Lymphome und Lymphomatoide Läsionen des Nervensystems (2013). [Differential diagnosis of lymphoid infiltrates in the central nervous system: experience of the Network Lymphomas and Lymphomatoid Lesions in the Nervous System]. Pathologe. 34(3):186–97. PMID:23471726
299. Buccoliero AM, Bacci S, Mennonna P, Taddei GL (2004). Pathologic quiz case: infratentorial tumor in a middle-aged woman. Oncocytic variant of choroid plexus papilloma. Arch Pathol Lab Med. 128(12):1448–50. PMID:15578895
300. Buccoliero AM, Castiglione F, Degl'innocenti DR, Moncini D, Spacca B, Giordano F, et al. (2013). Angiocentric glioma: clinical, morphological, immunohistochemical and molecular features in three pediatric cases. Clin Neuropathol. 32(2):107–13. PMID:23073165
301. Buccoliero AM, Castiglione F, Rossi Degl'Innocenti D, Franchi A, Paglierani M, Sanzo M, et al. (2010). Embryonal tumor with abundant neuropil and true rosettes: morphological, immunohistochemical, ultrastructural and molecular study of a case showing features of medulloepithelioma and areas of mesenchymal and epithelial differentiation. Neuropathology. 30(1):84–91. PMID:19563506
302. Buccoliero AM, Franchi A, Castiglione F, Gheri CF, Mussa F, Giordano F, et al. (2009). Subependymal giant cell astrocytoma (SEGA): Is it an astrocytoma? Morphological, immunohistochemical and ultrastructural study. Neuropathology. 29(1):25–30. PMID:18564101
303. Buccoliero AM, Giordano F, Mussa F, Taddei A, Genitori L, Taddei GL (2006). Papillary glioneuronal tumor radiologically mimicking a cavernous hemangioma with hemorrhagic onset. Neuropathology. 26(3):206–11. PMID:16771176
304. Buczkowicz P, Bartels U, Bouffet E, Becher O, Hawkins C (2014). Histopathological spectrum of paediatric diffuse intrinsic pontine glioma: diagnostic and therapeutic implications. Acta Neuropathol. 128(4):573–81. PMID:25047029
305. Buczkowicz P, Hoeman C, Rakopoulos P, Pajovic S, Letourneau L, Dzamba M, et al. (2014). Genomic analysis of diffuse intrinsic pontine gliomas identifies three molecular subgroups and recurrent activating ACVR1 mutations. Nat Genet. 46(5):451–6. PMID:24705254
306. Budka H (1974). Intracranial lipomatous hamartomas (intracranial "lipomas"). A study of 13 cases including combinations with medulloblastoma, colloid and epidermoid cysts, angiomatosis and other malformations. Acta Neuropathol. 28(3):205–22. PMID:4611131
307. Budka H (1975). Partially resected and irradiated cerebellar astrocytoma of childhood: malignant evolution after 28 years. Acta Neurochir (Wien). 32(1-2):139–46. PMID:1163315
308. Budka H, Chimelli L (1994). Lipomatous medulloblastoma in adults: a new tumor type with possible favorable prognosis. Hum Pathol. 25(7):730–1. PMID:8026834
309. Bukhtoiarov AP, Zil'berberg LB, Levitski? VA (1975). [Evacuation hospitals in Pyatigorsk during the Great Patriotic War] . Zdravookhr Ross Fed : 22-3. PMID:131445
310. Bunin GR, Surawicz TS, Witman PA, Preston-Martin S, Davis F, Bruner JM (1998). The descriptive epidemiology of craniopharyngioma. J Neurosurg. 89(4):547–51. PMID:9761047
311. Burger PC (1996). Pathology of brain stem astrocytomas. Pediatr Neurosurg. 24(1):35–40. PMID:8817613
312. Burger PC (2009). Smears and frozen sections in surgical neuropathology. PB Medical Publishing: Baltimore.
313. Burger PC (2012). Paraganglioma of the filum terminale. In: Burger PC, Scheithauer BW, Kleinschmidt-DeMaster BK, Ersen A, Rodriguez FJ, Tihan T, et al., editors. Diagnostic Pathology, Neuropathology. Salt Lake City: Amysys.
314. Burger PC, Grahmann FC, Bliestle A, Kleihues P (1987). Differentiation in the medulloblastoma. A histological and immunohistochemical study. Acta Neuropathol. 73(2):115–23. PMID:3604579
315. Burger PC, Green SB (1987). Patient age, histologic features, and length of survival in patients with glioblastoma multiforme. Cancer. 59(9):1617–25. PMID:3030531
316. Burger PC, Heinz ER, Shibata T, Kleihues P (1988). Topographic anatomy and CT correlations in the untreated glioblastoma multiforme. J Neurosurg. 68(5):698–704. PMID:2833587
317. Burger PC, Kleihues P (1989). Cytologic

composition of the untreated glioblastoma with implications for evaluation of needle biopsies. Cancer. 63(10):2014–23. PMID:2539242
318. Burger PC, Pearl DK, Aldape K, Yates AJ, Scheithauer BW, Passe SM, et al. (2001). Small cell architecture–a histological equivalent of EGFR amplification in glioblastoma multiforme? J Neuropathol Exp Neurol. 60(11):1099–104. PMID:11706939
319. Burger PC, Scheithauer B (2008).Tumors of the Central Nervous System. AFIP Atlas of Tumour Pathology, Series 4, Fascicle 7 Washington DC: American Registry of Pathology.
320. Burger PC, Scheithauer BW (1994). Tumors of the Central Nervous System. Washington: Armed Forces Institute of Pathology.
321. Burger PC, Scheithauer BW, Vogel FS (2002). Surgical Pathology of the Nervous System and Its Coverings. 4th ed. London: Churchill Livingston.
322. Burger PC, Vogel FS, Green SB, Strike TA (1985). Glioblastoma multiforme and anaplastic astrocytoma. Pathologic criteria and prognostic implications. Cancer. 56(5):1106–11. PMID:2990664
323. Burger PC, Vollmer RT (1980). Histologic factors of prognostic significance in the glioblastoma multiforme. Cancer. 46(5):1179–86. PMID:6260329
324. Burger PC, Yu IT, Tihan T, Friedman HS, Strother DR, Kepner JL, et al. (1998). Atypical teratoid/rhabdoid tumor of the central nervous system: a highly malignant tumor of infancy and childhood frequently mistaken for medulloblastoma: a Pediatric Oncology Group study. Am J Surg Pathol. 22(9):1083–92. PMID:9737241
325. Burkhard C, Di Patre PL, Schüler D, Schüler G, Yaşargil MG, Yonekawa Y, et al. (2003). A population-based study of the incidence and survival rates in patients with pilocytic astrocytoma. J Neurosurg. 98(6):1170–4. PMID:12816259
326. Burkitt Wright EM, Sach E, Sharif S, Quarrell O, Carroll T, Whitehouse RW, et al. (2013). Can the diagnosis of NF1 be excluded clinically? A lack of pigmentary findings in families with spinal neurofibromatosis demonstrates a limitation of clinical diagnosis. J Med Genet. 50(9):606–13. PMID:23812910
327. Burnett ME, White EC, Sih S, von Haken MS, Cogen PH (1997). Chromosome arm 17p deletion analysis reveals molecular genetic heterogeneity in supratentorial and infratentorial primitive neuroectodermal tumors of the central nervous system. Cancer Genet Cytogenet. 97(1):25–31. PMID:9242214
328. Bush K, Bateman DE (2014). Papilloedema secondary to a spinal paraganglioma. Pract Neurol. 14(3):179–81. PMID:23918468
329. Buslei R, Nolde M, Hofmann B, Meissner S, Eyupoglu IY, Siebzehnrübl F, et al. (2005). Common mutations of beta-catenin in adamantinomatous craniopharyngiomas but not in other tumours originating from the sellar region. Acta Neuropathol. 109(6):589–97. PMID:15891929
330. Butler MG, Dasouki MJ, Zhou XP, Talebizadeh Z, Brown M, Takahashi TN, et al. (2005). Subset of individuals with autism spectrum disorders and extreme macrocephaly associated with germline PTEN tumour suppressor gene mutations. J Med Genet. 42(4):318–21. PMID:15805158
331. Byeon SJ, Cho HJ, Baek HW, Park CK, Choi SH, Kim SH, et al. (2014). Rhabdoid glioblastoma is distinguishable from classical glioblastoma by cytogenetics and molecular genetics. Hum Pathol. 45(3):611–20. PMID:24457079
332. Bühren J, Christoph AH, Buslei R, Albrecht S, Wiestler OD, Pietsch T (2000). Expression of the neurotrophin receptor p75NTR in medulloblastomas is correlated with distinct histological and clinical features: evidence for a medulloblastoma subtype derived from the external granule cell layer. J Neuropathol Exp Neurol. 59(3):229–40. PMID:10744061
333. Büschges R, Ichimura K, Weber RG, Reifenberger G, Collins VP (2002). Allelic gain and amplification on the long arm of chromosome 17 in anaplastic meningiomas. Brain Pathol. 12(2):145–53. PMID:11958368
334. Büttner A, Marquart KH, Mehraein P, Weis S (1997). Kaposi's sarcoma in the cerebellum of a patient with AIDS. Clin Neuropathol. 16(4):185–9. PMID:9266142
335. Böhling T, Hatva E, Kujala M, Claesson-Welsh L, Alitalo K, Haltia M (1996). Expression of growth factors and growth factor receptors in capillary hemangioblastoma. J Neuropathol Exp Neurol. 55(5):522–7. PMID:8627342
336. Böhling T, Mäenpää A, Timonen T, Vantunen L, Paetau A, Haltia M (1996). Different expression of adhesion molecules on stromal cells and endothelial cells of capillary hemangioblastoma. Acta Neuropathol. 92(5):461–6. PMID:8922057
337. Böhling T, Turunen O, Jääskeläinen J, Carpen O, Sainio M, Wahlström T, et al. (1996). Ezrin expression in stromal cells of capillary hemangioblastoma. An immunohistochemical survey of brain tumors. Am J Pathol. 148(2):367–73. PMID:8579099
338. Cabello A, Madero S, Castresana A, Diaz-Lobato R (1991). Astroblastoma: electron microscopy and immunohistochemical findings: case report. Surg Neurol. 35(2):116–21. PMID:1990478
339. Caccamo DV, Ho KL, Garcia JH (1992). Cauda equina tumor with ependymal and paraganglionic differentiation. Hum Pathol. 23(7):835–8. PMID:1612583
340. Cachia D, Prado MP, Theeler B, Hamilton J, McCutcheon I, Fuller GN (2014). Synchronous rosette-forming glioneuronal tumor and diffuse astrocytoma with molecular characterization: a case report. Clin Neuropathol. 33(6):407–11. PMID:24986181
341. Cady FM, O'Neill BP, Law ME, Decker PA, Kurtz DM, Giannini C, et al. (2008). Del(6)(q22) and BCL6 rearrangements in primary CNS lymphoma are indicators of an aggressive clinical course. J Clin Oncol. 26(29):4814–9. PMID:18645192
342. Cahill DP, Levine KK, Betensky RA, Codd PJ, Romany CA, Reavie LB, et al. (2007). Loss of the mismatch repair protein MSH6 in human glioblastomas is associated with tumor progression during temozolomide treatment. Clin Cancer Res. 13(7):2038–45. PMID:17404084
343. Cai DX, James CD, Scheithauer BW, Couch FJ, Perry A (2001). PS6K amplification characterizes a small subset of anaplastic meningiomas. Am J Clin Pathol. 115(2):213–8. PMID:11211609
344. Cairncross G, Wang M, Shaw E, Jenkins R, Brachman D, Buckner J, et al. (2013). Phase III trial of chemoradiotherapy for anaplastic oligodendroglioma: long-term results of RTOG 9402. J Clin Oncol. 31(3):337–43. PMID:23071247
345. Cairncross JG, Ueki K, Zlatescu MC, Lisle DK, Finkelstein DM, Hammond RR, et al. (1998). Specific genetic predictors of chemotherapeutic response and survival in patients with anaplastic oligodendrogliomas. J Natl Cancer Inst. 90(19):1473–9. PMID:9776413
346. Cairncross JG, Wang M, Jenkins RB, Shaw EG, Giannini C, Brachman DG, et al. (2014). Benefit from procarbazine, lomustine, and vincristine in oligodendroglial tumors is associated with mutation of IDH. J Clin Oncol. 32(8):783–90. PMID:24516018
347. Camelo-Piragua S, Jansen M, Ganguly A, Kim JC, Cosper AK, Dias-Santagata D, et al. (2011). A sensitive and specific diagnostic panel to distinguish diffuse astrocytoma from astrocytosis: chromosome 7 gain with mutant isocitrate dehydrogenase 1 and p53. J Neuropathol Exp Neurol. 70(2):110–5. PMID:21343879
348. Campos AR, Clusmann H, von Lehe M, Niehusmann P, Becker AJ, Schramm J, et al. (2009). Simple and complex dysembryoplastic neuroepithelial tumors (DNT) variants: clinical profile, MRI, and histopathology. Neuroradiology. 51(7):433–43. PMID:19242688
349. Brat DJ, Verhaak RG, Aldape KD, Yung WK, Salama SR, Cooper LA, et al.; Cancer Genome Atlas Research Network (2015). Comprehensive, Integrative Genomic Analysis of Diffuse Lower-Grade Gliomas. N Engl J Med. 372(26):2481–98. PMID:26061751
350. Cancer Genome Atlas Research Network (2008). Comprehensive genomic characterization defines human glioblastoma genes and core pathways. Nature. 455(7216):1061–8. PMID:18772890
351. Cannon DM, Mohindra P, Gondi V, Kruser TJ, Kozak KR (2015). Choroid plexus tumor epidemiology and outcomes: implications for surgical and radiotherapeutic management. J Neurooncol. 121(1):151–7. PMID:25270349
352. Cannon TC, Bane BL, Kistler D, Schoenhals GW, Hahn M, Leech RW, et al. (1998). Primary intracerebellar osteosarcoma arising within an epidermoid cyst. Arch Pathol Lab Med. 122(8):737–9. PMID:9701337
353. Cao D, Liu A, Wang F, Allan RW, Mei K, Peng Y, et al. (2011). RNA-binding protein LIN28 is a marker for primary extragonadal germ cell tumors: an immunohistochemical study of 131 cases. Mod Pathol. 24(2):288–96. PMID:21057460
354. Capper D, Berghoff AS, Magerle M, Ilhan A, Wöhrer A, Hackl M, et al. (2012). Immunohistochemical testing of BRAF V600E status in 1,120 tumor tissue samples of patients with brain metastases. Acta Neuropathol. 123(2):223–33. PMID:22012135
355. Capper D, Preusser M, Habel A, Sahm F, Ackermann U, Schindler G, et al. (2011). Assessment of BRAF V600E mutation status by immunohistochemistry with a mutation-specific monoclonal antibody. Acta Neuropathol. 122(1):11–9. PMID:21638088
356. Capper D, Reuss D, Schittenhelm J, Hartmann C, Bremer J, Sahm F, et al. (2011). Mutation-specific IDH1 antibody differentiates oligodendrogliomas and oligoastrocytomas from other brain tumors with oligodendroglioma-like morphology. Acta Neuropathol. 121(2):241–52. PMID:21069360
357. Capper D, Sahm F, Hartmann C, Meyermann R, von Deimling A, Schittenhelm J (2010). Application of mutant IDH1 antibody to differentiate diffuse glioma from nonneoplastic central nervous system lesions and therapy-induced changes. Am J Surg Pathol. 34(8):1199–204. PMID:20661018
358. Capper D, Simon M, Langhans CD, Okun JG, Tonn JC, Weller M, et al.; German Glioma Network (2012). 2-Hydroxyglutarate concentration in serum from patients with gliomas does not correlate with IDH1/2 mutation status or tumor size. Int J Cancer. 131(3):766–8. PMID:21913188
359. Capper D, Weissert S, Balss J, Habel A, Meyer J, Jäger D, et al. (2010). Characterization of R132H mutation-specific IDH1 antibody binding in brain tumors. Brain Pathol. 20(1):245–54. PMID:19903171
360. Capper D, Zentgraf H, Balss J, Hartmann C, von Deimling A (2009). Monoclonal antibody specific for IDH1 R132H mutation. Acta Neuropathol. 118(5):599–601. PMID:19798509
361. Cardoso C, Lutz Y, Mignon C, Compe E, Depetris D, Mattei MG, et al. (2000). ATR-X mutations cause impaired nuclear location and altered DNA binding properties of the XNP/ATR-X protein. J Med Genet. 37(10):746–51. PMID:11015451
362. Caretti V, Bugiani M, Freret M, Schellen P, Jansen M, van Vuurden D, et al. (2014). Subventricular spread of diffuse intrinsic pontine glioma. Acta Neuropathol. 128(4):605–7. PMID:24929912
363. Carlotti CG Jr, Salhia B, Weitzman S, Greenberg M, Dirks PB, Mason W, et al. (2002). Evaluation of proliferative index and cell cycle protein expression in choroid plexus tumors in children. Acta Neuropathol. 103(1):1–10. PMID:11837741
364. Carlson GJ, Nivatvongs S, Snover DC (1984). Colorectal polyps in Cowden's disease (multiple hamartoma syndrome). Am J Surg Pathol. 8(10):763–70. PMID:6496844
365. Carneiro SS, Scheithauer BW, Nascimento AG, Hirose T, Davis DH (1996). Solitary fibrous tumor of the meninges: a lesion distinct from fibrous meningioma. A clinicopathologic and immunohistochemical study. Am J Clin Pathol. 106(2):217–24. PMID:8712177
366. Carney EM, Banerjee P, Ellis CL, Albadine R, Sharma R, Chaux AM, et al. (2011). PAX2(-)/PAX8(-)/inhibin A(+) immunoprofile in hemangioblastoma: A helpful combination in the differential diagnosis with metastatic clear cell renal cell carcinoma to the central nervous system. Am J Surg Pathol. 35(2):262–7. PMID:21263247
367. Carney JA (1990). Psammomatous melanotic schwannoma. A distinctive, heritable tumor with special associations, including cardiac myxoma and the Cushing syndrome. Am J Surg Pathol. 14(3):206–22. PMID:2305928
368. Carney JA, Gordon H, Carpenter PC, Shenoy BV, Go VL (1985). The complex of myxomas, spotty pigmentation, and endocrine overactivity. Medicine (Baltimore). 64(4):270–83. PMID:4010501
369. Carrasco R, Pascual JM, Navas M, Fraga J, Manzanares-Soler R, Sola RG (2010). Spontaneous acute hemorrhage within a subependymoma of the lateral ventricle: successful emergent surgical removal through a frontal transcortical approach. Neurocirugia (Astur). 21(6):478–83. PMID:21165545
370. Carstens PH, Johnson GS, Jelsma LF (1995). Spinal gliosarcoma: a light, immunohistochemical and ultrastructural study. Ann Clin Lab Sci. 25(3):241–6. PMID:7605106
371. Carter JM, O'Hara C, Dundas G, Gilchrist D, Collins MS, Eaton K, et al. (2012). Epithelioid malignant peripheral nerve sheath tumor arising in a schwannoma, in a patient with "neuroblastoma-like" schwannomatosis and a novel germline SMARCB1 mutation. Am J Surg Pathol. 36(1):154–60. PMID:22082606
372. Carter M, Nicholson J, Ross F, Crolla J, Allibone R, Balaji V, et al. (2002). Genetic abnormalities detected in ependymomas by comparative genomic hybridisation. Br J Cancer. 86(6):929–39. PMID:11953826
373. Carvalho AT, Linhares P, Castro L, Sá MJ (2014). Multiple sclerosis and oligodendroglioma: an exceptional association. Case Rep Neurol Med. 2014:546817. PMID:25180114
374. Casadei GP, Arrigoni GL, D'Angelo V, Bizzozero L (1990). Late malignant recurrence of childhood cerebellar astrocytoma. Clin Neuropathol. 9(6):295–8. PMID:2286021
375. Casadei GP, Komori T, Scheithauer BW, Miller GM, Parisi JE, Kelly PJ (1993). Intracranial parenchymal schwannoma. A clinicopathological and neuroimaging study of nine cases. J Neurosurg. 79(2):217–22. PMID:8331403
376. Casadei GP, Scheithauer BW, Hirose T, Manfrini M, Van Houton C, Wood MB (1995). Cellular schwannoma. A clinicopathologic, DNA flow cytometric, and proliferation marker study of 70 patients. Cancer. 75(5):1109–19. PMID:7850709
377. Cassarino DS, Auerbach A, Rushing EJ (2003). Widely invasive solitary fibrous tumor of the sphenoid sinus, cavernous sinus, and pituitary fossa. Ann Diagn Pathol. 7(3):169–73. PMID:12808569
378. Cassol CA, Winer D, Liu W, Guo M, Ezzat S, Asa SL (2014). Tyrosine kinase receptors as molecular targets in pheochromocytomas and

paragangliomas. Mod Pathol. 27(8):1050–62. PMID:24390213
379. Castellano-Sanchez AA, Schemankewitz E, Mazewski C, Brat DJ (2001). Pediatric chordoid glioma with chondroid metaplasia. Pediatr Dev Pathol. 4(6):564–7. PMID:11826363
380. Castro-Vega LJ, Buffet A, De Cubas AA, Cascón A, Menara M, Khalifa E, et al. (2014). Germline mutations in FH confer predisposition to malignant pheochromocytomas and paragangliomas. Hum Mol Genet. 23(9):2440–6. PMID:24334767
381. Castro-Vega LJ, Letouzé E, Burnichon N, Buffet A, Disderot PH, Khalifa E, et al. (2015). Multi-omics analysis defines core genomic alterations in pheochromocytomas and paragangliomas. Nat Commun. 6:6044. PMID:25625332
382. Cataltepe O, Turanli G, Yalnizoglu D, Topçu M, Akalan N (2005). Surgical management of temporal lobe tumor-related epilepsy in children. J Neurosurg. 102(3) Suppl:280–7. PMID:15881751
383. Cavalli G, Guglielmi B, Berti A, Campochiaro C, Sabbadini MG, Dagna L (2013). The multifaceted clinical presentations and manifestations of Erdheim-Chester disease: comprehensive review of the literature and of 10 new cases. Ann Rheum Dis. 72(10):1691–5. PMID:23396641
384. Ceccom J, Bourdeaut F, Loukh N, Rigau V, Milin S, Takin R, et al. (2014). Embryonal tumor with multilayered rosettes: diagnostic tools update and review of the literature. Clin Neuropathol. 33(1):15–22. PMID:23863344
385. Ceeraz S, Nowak EC, Noelle RJ (2013). B7 family checkpoint regulators in immune regulation and disease. Trends Immunol. 34(11):556–63. PMID:23954143
387. Cenacchi G, Giangaspero F (2004). Emerging tumor entities and variants of CNS neoplasms. J Neuropathol Exp Neurol. 63(3):185–92. PMID:15055442
388. Cenacchi G, Giangaspero F, Cerasoli S, Manetto V, Martinelli GN (1996). Ultrastructural characterization of oligodendroglial-like cells in central nervous system tumors. Ultrastruct Pathol. 20(6):537–47. PMID:8940761
389. Cenacchi G, Roncaroli F, Cerasoli S, Ficarra G, Merli GA, Giangaspero F (2001). Chordoid glioma of the third ventricle: an ultrastructural study of three cases with a histogenetic hypothesis. Am J Surg Pathol. 25(3):401–5. PMID:11224612
390. Cepeda C, André VM, Yamazaki I, Hauptman JS, Chen JY, Vinters HV, et al. (2010). Comparative study of cellular and synaptic abnormalities in brain tissue samples from pediatric tuberous sclerosis complex and cortical dysplasia type II. Epilepsia. 51 Suppl 3:160–5. PMID:20618424
391. Cerami E, Gao J, Dogrusoz U, Gross BE, Sumer SO, Aksoy BA, et al. (2012). The cBio cancer genomics portal: an open platform for exploring multidimensional cancer genomics data. Cancer Discov. 2(5):401–4. PMID:22588877
392. Cerase A, Vallone IM, Di Pietro G, Oliveri G, Miracco C, Venturi C (2009). Neuroradiological follow-up of the growth of papillary tumor of the pineal region: a case report. J Neurooncol. 95(3):433–5. PMID:19517065
393. Cerdá-Nicolás M, Lopez-Gines C, Gil-Benso R, Donat J, Fernandez-Delgado R, Pellin A, et al. (2006). Desmoplastic infantile ganglioglioma. Morphological, immunohistochemical and genetic features. Histopathology. 48(5):617–21. PMID:16623795
394. Cervera-Pierot P, Varlet P, Chodkiewicz JP, Daumas-Duport C (1997). Dysembryoplastic neuroepithelial tumors located in the caudate nucleus area: report of four cases. Neurosurgery. 40(5):1065–9, discussion 1069–70. PMID:9149266
395. Cervoni L, Celli P, Caruso R, Gagliardi FM, Cantore GP (1997). [Neurinomas and ependymomas of the cauda equina. A review of the clinical characteristics]. Minerva Chir. 52(5):629–33. PMID:9297152
396. Chacko G, Chacko AG, Dunham CP, Judkins AR, Biegel JA, Perry A (2007). Atypical teratoid/rhabdoid tumor arising in the setting of a pleomorphic xanthoastrocytoma. J Neurooncol. 84(2):217–22. PMID:17431546
397. Chacón-Quesada T, Rodriguez GJ, Maud A, Ramos-Duran L, Torabi A, Fitzgerald T, et al. (2015). Trans-arterial Onyx Embolization of a Functional Thoracic Paraganglioma. Neurointervention. 10(1):34–8. PMID:25763296
398. Chakraborty R, Hampton OA, Shen X, Simko SJ, Shih A, Abhyankar H, et al. (2014). Mutually exclusive recurrent somatic mutations in MAP2K1 and BRAF support a central role for ERK activation in LCH pathogenesis. Blood. 124(19):3007–15. PMID:25202140
399. Chalasani S, Hennick MR, Hocking WG, Shaw GR, Lawler B (2013). Unusual presentation of a rare cancer: histiocytic sarcoma in the brain 16 years after treatment for acute lymphoblastic leukemia. Clin Med Res. 11(1):31–5. PMID:22997353
400. Chamberlain M, Soffietti R, Raizer J, Rudà R, Brandsma D, Boogerd W, et al. (2014). Leptomeningeal metastasis: a Response Assessment in Neuro-Oncology critical review of endpoints and response criteria of published randomized clinical trials. Neuro Oncol. 16(9):1176–85. PMID:24867803
401. Chan AK, Pang JC, Chung NY, Li KK, Poon WS, Chan DT, et al. (2014). Loss of CIC and FUBP1 expressions are potential markers of shorter time to recurrence in oligodendroglial tumors. Mod Pathol. 27(3):332–42. PMID:24030748
402. Chan AS, Leung SY, Wong MP, Yuen ST, Cheung N, Fan YW, et al. (1998). Expression of vascular endothelial growth factor and its receptors in the anaplastic progression of astrocytoma, oligodendroglioma, and ependymoma. Am J Surg Pathol. 22(7):816–26. PMID:9669344
403. Chan CC, Koch CA, Kaiser-Kupfer MI, Parry DM, Gutmann DH, Zhuang Z, et al. (2002). Loss of heterozygosity for the NF2 gene in retinal and optic nerve lesions of patients with neurofibromatosis 2. J Pathol. 198(1):14–20. PMID:12210058
404. Chan CH, Bittar RG, Davis GA, Kalnins RM, Fabinyi GC (2006). Long-term seizure outcome following surgery for dysembryoplastic neuroepithelial tumor. J Neurosurg. 104(1):62–9. PMID:16509148
405. Chan GL, Little JB (1983). Cultured diploid fibroblasts from patients with the nevoid basal cell carcinoma syndrome are hypersensitive to killing by ionizing radiation. Am J Pathol. 111(1):50–5. PMID:6837723
406. Chan JA, Zhang H, Roberts PS, Jozwiak S, Wieslawa G, Lewin-Kowalik J, et al. (2004). Pathogenesis of tuberous sclerosis subependymal giant cell astrocytomas: biallelic inactivation of TSC1 or TSC2 leads to mTOR activation. J Neuropathol Exp Neurol. 63(12):1236–42. PMID:15624760
407. Chandler JP, Yashar P, Laskin WB, Russell EJ (2004). Intracranial chondrosarcoma: a case report and review of the literature. J Neurooncol. 68(1):33–9. PMID:15174519
408. Chang AH, Fuller GN, Debnam JM, Karis JP, Coons SW, Ross JS, et al. (2008). MR imaging of papillary tumor of the pineal region. AJNR Am J Neuroradiol. 29(1):187–9. PMID:17925365
409. Chang MW (2003). Updated classification of hemangiomas and other vascular anomalies. Lymphat Res Biol. 1(4):259–65. PMID:15624554
410. Chang Q, Pang JC, Li KK, Poon WS, Zhou L, Ng HK (2005). Promoter hypermethylation profile of RASSF1A, FHIT, and sFRP1 in intracranial primitive neuroectodermal tumors. Hum Pathol. 36(12):1265–72. PMID:16311119
411. Chang S, Prados MD (1994). Identical twins with Ollier's disease and intracranial gliomas: case report. Neurosurgery. 34(5):903–6, discussion 906. PMID:8052390
412. Chang SM, Lillis-Hearne PK, Larson DA, Wara WM, Bollen AW, Prados MD (1995). Pineoblastoma in adults. Neurosurgery. 37(3):383–90, discussion 390–1. PMID:7501100
413. Chao L, Tao XB, Jun YK, Xia HH, Wan WK, Tao QS (2013). Recurrence and histological evolution of dysembryoplastic neuroepithelial tumor: A case report and review of the literature. Oncol Lett. 6(4):907–14. PMID:24137435
414. Chappé C, Padovani L, Scavarda D, Forest F, Nanni-Metellus I, Loundou A, et al. (2013). Dysembryoplastic neuroepithelial tumors share with pleomorphic xanthoastrocytomas and gangliogliomas BRAF(V600E) mutation and expression. Brain Pathol. 23(5):574–83. PMID:23442159
415. Charles NA, Holland EC, Gilbertson R, Glass R, Kettenmann H (2012). The brain tumor microenvironment. Glia. 60(3):502–14. PMID:22379614
416. Chaskis C, Michotte A, Goossens A, Stadnik T, Koerts G, D'Haens J (2002). Primary intracerebral myxoid chondrosarcoma. Case illustration. J Neurosurg. 97(1):228. PMID:12134922
417. Chaudhry NS, Ahmad F, Blieden C, Morcos JJ (2013). Suprasellar and sellar paraganglioma presenting as a nonfunctioning pituitary macroadenoma. J Clin Neurosci. 20(11):1615–8. PMID:23876285
418. Cheadle JP, Reeve MP, Sampson JR, Kwiatkowski DJ (2000). Molecular genetic advances in tuberous sclerosis. Hum Genet. 107(2):97–114. PMID:11030407
419. Chelliah D, Mensah Sarfo-Poku C, Stea BD, Gardetto J, Zumwalt J (2010). Medulloblastoma with extensive nodularity undergoing post-therapeutic maturation to a gangliocytoma: a case report and literature review. Pediatr Neurosurg. 46(5):381–4. PMID:21389751
420. Chen BJ, Mariño-Enríquez A, Fletcher CD, Hornick JL (2012). Loss of retinoblastoma protein expression in spindle cell/pleomorphic lipomas and cytogenetically related tumors: an immunohistochemical study with diagnostic implications. Am J Surg Pathol. 36(8):1119–28. PMID:22790852
421. Chen CJ, Williams EA, McAneney TE, Williams BJ, Mandell JW, Shaffrey ME (2015). Histiocytic sarcoma of the cavernous sinus: case report and literature review. Brain Tumor Pathol. 32(1):66–71. PMID:24807104
422. Chen G, Luo Z, Liu T, Yang H (2011). Functioning paraganglioma of the cervical spine. Orthopedics. 34(10):e700–2. PMID:21956072
423. Chen J, McKay RM, Parada LF (2012). Malignant glioma: lessons from genomics, mouse models, and stem cells. Cell. 149(1):36–47. PMID:22464322
424. Chen L, Li Y, Lin JH (2005). Intraneural perineurioma in a child with Beckwith-Wiedemann syndrome. J Pediatr Surg. 40(2):E12–4. PMID:15750909
425. Chen L, Voronovich Z, Clark K, Hands I, Mannas J, Walsh M, et al. (2014). Predicting the likelihood of an isocitrate dehydrogenase 1 or 2 mutation in diagnoses of infiltrative glioma. Neuro Oncol. 16(11):1478–83. PMID:24860178
426. Chen SC, Lin DS, Lee CC, Hung SC, Chen YW, Hsu SP, et al. (2013). Rhabdoid glioblastoma: a recently recognized subtype of glioblastoma. Acta Neurochir (Wien). 155(8):1443–8, discussion 1448. PMID:23812963
427. Chen SM, Chuang CC, Toh CH, Jung SM, Lui TN (2013). Solitary intracranial osteoma with attachment to the falx: a case report. World J Surg Oncol. 11:221. PMID:24010982
428. Chen Y, Tachibana O, Oda M, Xu R, Hamada J, Yamashita J, et al. (2006). Increased expression of aquaporin 1 in human hemangioblastomas and its correlation with cyst formation. J Neurooncol. 80(3):219–25. PMID:17077939
429. Chen Z, Liu C, Patel AJ, Liao CP, Wang Y, Le LQ (2014). Cells of origin in the embryonic nerve roots for NF1-associated plexiform neurofibroma. Cancer Cell. 26(5):695–706. PMID:25446898
430. Cheng TM, Coffey RJ, Gelber BR, Scheithauer BW (1993). Simultaneous presentation of symptomatic subependymomas in siblings: case reports and review. Neurosurgery. 33(1):145–50. PMID:8355833
431. Chentli F, Belhimer F, Kessaci F, Mansouri B (2012). Congenital craniopharyngioma: a case report and literature review. J Pediatr Endocrinol Metab. 25(11-12):1181–3. PMID:23329768
432. Chetty R (1999). Cytokeratin expression in cauda equina paragangliomas. Am J Surg Pathol. 23(4):491. PMID:10199484
433. Chi SN, Zimmerman MA, Yao X, Cohen KJ, Burger P, Biegel JA, et al. (2009). Intensive multimodality treatment for children with newly diagnosed CNS atypical teratoid rhabdoid tumor. J Clin Oncol. 27(3):385–9. PMID:19064966
434. Chidambaram B, Santhosh V, Shankar SK (1998). Identical twins with medulloblastoma occurring in infancy. Childs Nerv Syst. 14(9):421–5. PMID:9808250
435. Chiechi MV, Smirniotopoulos JG, Mena H (1995). Pineal parenchymal tumors: CT and MR features. J Comput Assist Tomogr. 19(4):509–17. PMID:7622675
436. Chik K, Li C, Shing MM, Leung T, Yuen PM (1999). Intracranial germ cell tumors in children with and without Down syndrome. J Pediatr Hematol Oncol. 21(2):149–51. PMID:10206462
437. Chikai K, Ohnishi A, Kato T, Ikeda J, Sawamura Y, Iwasaki Y, et al. (2004). Clinico-pathological features of pilomyxoid astrocytoma of the optic pathway. Acta Neuropathol. 108(2):109–14. PMID:15168135
438. Chikwava K, Jaffe R (2004). Langerin (CD207) staining in normal pediatric tissues, reactive lymph nodes, and childhood histiocytic disorders. Pediatr Dev Pathol. 7(6):607–14. PMID:15630529
439. Chinot OL, Wick W, Mason W, Henriksson R, Saran F, Nishikawa R, et al. (2014). Bevacizumab plus radiotherapy-temozolomide for newly diagnosed glioblastoma. N Engl J Med. 370(8):709–22. PMID:24552318
440. Chintagumpala M, Hassall T, Palmer S, Ashley D, Wallace D, Kasow K, et al. (2009). A pilot study of risk-adapted radiotherapy and chemotherapy in patients with supratentorial PNET. Neuro Oncol. 11(1):33–40. PMID:18796696
441. Chirindel A, Chaudhry M, Blakeley JO, Wahl R (2015). 18F-FDG PET/CT qualitative and quantitative evaluation in neurofibromatosis type 1 patients for detection of malignant transformation: comparison of early to delayed imaging with and without liver activity normalization. J Nucl Med. 56(3):379–85. PMID:25655626
442. Chitoku S, Kawai S, Watabe Y, Nishitani M, Fujimoto K, Otsuka H, et al. (1998). Intradural spinal hibernoma: case report. Surg Neurol. 49(5):509–12, discussion 512–3. PMID:9586928
443. Chittaranjan S, Chan S, Yang C, Yang KC, Chen V, Moradian A, et al. (2014). Mutations in CIC and IDH1 cooperatively regulate 2-hydroxyglutarate levels and cell clonogenicity. Oncotarget. 5(17):7960–79. PMID:25277207
444. Chmielecki J, Crago AM, Rosenberg M, O'Connor R, Walker SR, Ambrogio L, et al. (2013). Whole-exome sequencing identifies a recurrent NAB2-STAT6 fusion in solitary fibrous tumors. Nat Genet. 45(2):131–2. PMID:23313954
445. Cho BK, Wang KC, Nam DH, Kim DG, Jung HW, Kim HJ, et al. (1998). Pineal tumors: experience with 48 cases over 10 years. Childs

Nerv Syst. 14(1-2):53–8. PMID:9548342
446. Cho HJ, Myung JK, Kim H, Park CK, Kim SK, Chung CK, et al. (2015). Primary diffuse leptomeningeal glioneuronal tumors. Brain Tumor Pathol. 32(1):49–55. PMID:24770606
447. Cho Y, Gorina S, Jeffrey PD, Pavletich NP (1994). Crystal structure of a p53 tumor suppressor-DNA complex: understanding tumorigenic mutations. Science. 265(5170):346–55. PMID:8023157
448. Cho YJ, Tsherniak A, Tamayo P, Santagata S, Ligon A, Greulich H, et al. (2011). Integrative genomic analysis of medulloblastoma identifies a molecular subgroup that drives poor clinical outcome. J Clin Oncol. 29(11):1424–30. PMID:21098324
449. Choi C, Ganji SK, DeBerardinis RJ, Hatanpaa KJ, Rakheja D, Kovacs Z, et al. (2012). 2-hydroxyglutarate detection by magnetic resonance spectroscopy in IDH-mutated patients with gliomas. Nat Med. 18(4):624–9. PMID:22281806
450. Choi JS, Nam DH, Ko YH, Seo JW, Choi YL, Suh YL, et al. (2003). Primary central nervous system lymphoma in Korea: comparison of B- and T-cell lymphomas. Am J Surg Pathol. 27(7):919–28. PMID:12826884
451. Chou SM, Anderson JS (1991). Primary CNS malignant rhabdoid tumor (MRT): report of two cases and review of literature. Clin Neuropathol. 10(1):1–10. PMID:2015720
452. Chow E, Jenkins JJ, Burger PC, Reardon DA, Langston JW, Sanford RA, et al. (1999). Malignant evolution of choroid plexus papilloma. Pediatr Neurosurg. 31(3):127–30. PMID:10708353
453. Chowdhary A, Spence AM, Sales L, Rostomily RC, Rockhill JK, Silbergeld DL (2012). Radiation associated tumors following therapeutic cranial radiation. Surg Neurol Int. 3:48. PMID:22629485
454. Christensen BC, Smith AA, Zheng S, Koestler DC, Houseman EA, Marsit CJ, et al. (2011). DNA methylation, isocitrate dehydrogenase mutation, and survival in glioma. J Natl Cancer Inst. 103(2):143–53. PMID:21163902
455. Christiaans I, Kenter SB, Brink HC, van Os TA, Baas F, van den Munckhof P, et al. (2011). Germline SMARCB1 mutation and somatic NF2 mutations in familial multiple meningiomas. J Med Genet. 48(2):93–7. PMID:20930055
456. Christov C, Adle-Biassette H, Le Guerinel C, Natchev S, Gherardi RK (1998). Immunohistochemical detection of vascular endothelial growth factor (VEGF) in the vasculature of oligodendrogliomas. Neuropathol Appl Neurobiol. 24(1):29–35. PMID:9549726
457. Chu LC, Eberhart CG, Grossman SA, Herman JG (2006). Epigenetic silencing of multiple genes in primary CNS lymphoma. Int J Cancer. 119(10):2487–91. PMID:16858686
458. Ciardiello F, Tortora G (2001). A novel approach in the treatment of cancer: targeting the epidermal growth factor receptor. Clin Cancer Res. 7(10):2958–70. PMID:11595683
459. Cimino PJ, Agarwal A, Dehner LP (2014). Myxopapillary ependymoma in children: a study of 11 cases and a comparison with the adult experience. Pediatr Blood Cancer. 61(11):1969–71. PMID:25066546
460. Cimino PJ, Gonzalez-Cuyar LF, Perry A, Dahiya S (2015). Lack of BRAF-V600E Mutation in Papillary Tumor of the Pineal Region. Neurosurgery. 77(4):621–8. PMID:26125673
461. Cinalli G, Zerah M, Carteret M, Doz F, Vinikoff L, Lellouch-Tubiana A, et al. (1997). Subdural sarcoma associated with chronic subdural hematoma. Report of two cases and review of the literature. J Neurosurg. 86(3):553–7. PMID:9046316
462. Ciriello G, Miller ML, Aksoy BA, Senbabaoglu Y, Schultz N, Sander C (2013). Emerging landscape of oncogenic signatures across human cancers. Nat Genet. 45(10):1127–33. PMID:24071851
463. Claes A, Idema AJ, Wesseling P (2007). Diffuse glioma growth: a guerilla war. Acta Neuropathol. 114(5):443–58. PMID:17805551
464. Clarenbach P, Kleihues P, Metzel E, Dichgans J (1979). Simultaneous clinical manifestation of subependymoma of the fourth ventricle in identical twins. Case report. J Neurosurg. 50(5):655–9. PMID:571009
465. Clark AJ, Sughrue ME, Ivan ME, Aranda D, Rutkowski MJ, Kane AJ, et al. (2010). Factors influencing overall survival rates for patients with pineocytoma. J Neurooncol. 100(2):255–60. PMID:20461445
466. Clark GB, Henry JM, McKeever PE (1985). Cerebral pilocytic astrocytoma. Cancer. 56(5):1128–33. PMID:4016701
467. Clark VE, Erson-Omay EZ, Serin A, Yin J, Cotney J, Ozduman K, et al. (2013). Genomic analysis of non-NF2 meningiomas reveals mutations in TRAF7, KLF4, AKT1, and SMO. Science. 339(6123):1077–80. PMID:23348505
468. Clarke MJ, Foy AB, Wetjen N, Raffel C (2006). Imaging characteristics and growth of subependymal giant cell astrocytomas. Neurosurg Focus. 20(1):E5. PMID:16459995
468A. Claus EB, Black PM, Bondy ML, Calvocoressi L, Schildkraut JM, Wiemels JL, et al. (2007). Exogenous hormone use and meningioma risk: what do we tell our patients? Cancer. 110(3):471–6. PMID:17580362
469. Claus EB, Calvocoressi L, Bondy ML, Schildkraut JM, Wiemels JL, Wrensch M (2011). Family and personal medical history and risk of meningioma. J Neurosurg. 115(6):1072–7. PMID:21780859
470. Claus EB, Calvocoressi L, Bondy ML, Schildkraut JM, Wiemels JL, Wrensch M (2012). Dental x-rays and risk of meningioma. Cancer. 118(18):4530–7. PMID:22492363
471. Claus EB, Calvocoressi L, Bondy ML, Wrensch M, Wiemels JL, Schildkraut JM (2013). Exogenous hormone use, reproductive factors, and risk of intracranial meningioma in females. J Neurosurg. 118(3):649–56. PMID:23101448
472. Clifford SC, Lusher ME, Lindsey JC, Langdon JA, Gilbertson RJ, Straughton D, et al. (2006). Wnt/Wingless pathway activation and chromosome 6 loss characterize a distinct molecular sub-group of medulloblastomas associated with a favorable prognosis. Cell Cycle. 5(22):2666–70. PMID:17172831
473. Clynes D, Higgs DR, Gibbons RJ (2013). The chromatin remodeller ATRX: a repeat offender in human disease. Trends Biochem Sci. 38(9):461–6. PMID:23916100
474. Coakley KJ, Huston J 3rd, Scheithauer BW, Forbes G, Kelly PJ (1995). Pilocytic astrocytomas: well-demarcated magnetic resonance appearance despite frequent infiltration histologically. Mayo Clin Proc. 70(8):747–51. PMID:7630212
475. Cobbers JM, Wolter M, Reifenberger J, Ring GU, Jessen F, An HX, et al. (1998). Frequent inactivation of CDKN2A and rare mutation of TP53 in PCNSL. Brain Pathol. 8(2):263–76. PMID:9546285
476. Coca S, Moreno M, Martos JA, Rodriguez J, Barcena A, Vaquero J (1994). Neurocytoma of spinal cord. Acta Neuropathol. 87(5):537–40. PMID:8059608
477. Coca S, Vaquero J, Escandon J, Moreno M, Peralba J, Rodriguez J (1992). Immunohistochemical characterization of pineocytomas. Clin Neuropathol. 11(6):298–303. PMID:1473313
478. Cohen BH, Zeltzer PM, Boyett JM, Geyer JR, Allen JC, Finlay JL, et al. (1995). Prognostic factors and treatment results for supratentorial primitive neuroectodermal tumors in children using radiation and chemotherapy: a Childrens Cancer Group randomized trial. J Clin Oncol. 13(7):1687–96. PMID:7602359
479. Cohen-Gadol AA, Pichelmann MA, Link MJ, Scheithauer BW, Krecke KN, Young WF Jr, et al. (2003). Granular cell tumor of the sellar and suprasellar region: clinicopathologic study of 11 cases and literature review. Mayo Clin Proc. 78(5):567–73. PMID:12744543
480. Colin C, Padovani L, Chappé C, Mercurio S, Scavarda D, Loundou A, et al. (2013). Outcome analysis of childhood pilocytic astrocytomas: a retrospective study of 148 cases at a single institution. Neuropathol Appl Neurobiol. 39(6):693–705. PMID:23278243
481. Colin C, Virard I, Baeza N, Tchoghandjian A, Fernandez C, Bouvier C, et al. (2007). Relevance of combinatorial profiles of intermediate filaments and transcription factors for glioma histogenesis. Neuropathol Appl Neurobiol. 33(4):431–9. PMID:17442061
482. Collins VP, Jones DT, Giannini C (2015). Pilocytic astrocytoma: pathology, molecular mechanisms and markers. Acta Neuropathol. 129(6):775–88. PMID:25792358
483. Colnat-Coulbois S, Kremer S, Weinbreck N, Pinelli C, Auque J (2008). Lipomatous meningioma: report of 2 cases and review of the literature. Surg Neurol. 69(4):398–402, discussion 402. PMID:17825370
483A. Combs SE, Schulz-Ertner D, Debus J, von Deimling A, Hartmann C (2011). Improved correlation of the neuropathologic classification according to adapted world health organization classification and outcome after radiotherapy in patients with atypical and anaplastic meningiomas. Int J Radiat Oncol Biol Phys. 81(5):1415–21. PMID:20932661
484. Comino-Méndez I, Gracia-Aznárez FJ, Schiavi F, Landa I, Leandro-García LJ, Letón R, et al. (2011). Exome sequencing identifies MAX mutations as a cause of hereditary pheochromocytoma. Nat Genet. 43(7):663–7. PMID:21685915
485. Committee of Brain Tumor Registry of Japan (2003). Report of Brain Tumor Registry of Japan (1969–1996). Neurol Med Chir (Tokyo). 43 Suppl:i-vii, 1–111. PMID:14705327
485A. Committee of Brain Tumor Registry of Japan (2014). Report of Brain Tumor Registry of Japan (2001–2004), Vol. 13. Neurol Med Chir (Tokyo) 54:1–102.
486. Connor JM, Pirrit LA, Yates JR, Fryer AE, Ferguson-Smith MA (1987). Linkage of the tuberous sclerosis locus to a DNA polymorphism detected by v-abl. J Med Genet. 24(9):544–6. PMID:2889832
487. Constantini S, Soffer D, Siegel T, Shalit MN (1989). Paraganglioma of the thoracic spinal cord with cerebrospinal fluid metastasis. Spine (Phila Pa 1976). 14(6):643–5. PMID:2749382
488. Conte D, Huh M, Goodall E, Delorme M, Parks RJ, Picketts DJ (2012). Loss of Atrx sensitizes cells to DNA damaging agents through p53-mediated death pathways. PLoS One. 7(12):e52167. PMID:23284920
489. Conti P, Mouchaty H, Spacca B, Buccoliero AM, Conti R (2006). Thoracic extradural paragangliomas: a case report and review of the literature. Spinal Cord. 44(2):120–5. PMID:16130022
490. Conway JE, Chou D, Clatterbuck RE, Brem H, Long DM, Rigamonti D (2001). Hemangioblastomas of the central nervous system in von Hippel-Lindau syndrome and sporadic disease. Neurosurgery. 48(1):55–62, discussion 62–3. PMID:11152361
491. Cook DJ, Christie SD, Macaulay RJ, Rheaume DE, Holness RO (2004). Fourth ventricular neurocytoma: case report and review of the literature. Can J Neurol Sci. 31(4):558–64. PMID:15595267
492. Coons SW, Johnson PC (1993). Regional heterogeneity in the proliferative activity of human gliomas as measured by the Ki-67 labeling index. J Neuropathol Exp Neurol. 52(6):609–18. PMID:8229080
493. Coons SW, Johnson PC, Pearl DK (1997). The prognostic significance of Ki-67 labeling indices for oligodendrogliomas. Neurosurgery. 41(4):878–84, discussion 884–5. PMID:9316050
494. Coons SW, Johnson PC, Scheithauer BW, Yates AJ, Pearl DK (1997). Improving diagnostic accuracy and interobserver concordance in the classification and grading of primary gliomas. Cancer. 79(7):1381–93. PMID:9083161
495. Cooper ERA (1935). The relation of oligodendrocytes and astrocytes in cerebral tumours. J Path Bact. 41:259–66.
496. Cooper LA, Gutman DA, Long Q, Johnson BA, Cholleti SR, Kurc T, et al. (2010). The proneural molecular signature is enriched in oligodendrogliomas and predicts improved survival among diffuse gliomas. PLoS One. 5(9):e12548. PMID:20838435
497. Copie-Bergman C, Wotherspoon AC, Norton AJ, Diss TC, Isaacson PG (1998). True histiocytic lymphoma: a morphologic, immunohistochemical, and molecular genetic study of 13 cases. Am J Surg Pathol. 22(11):1386–92. PMID:9808131
498. Cornejo KM, Hutchinson L, Cosar EF, Smith T, Tomaszewicz K, Dresser K, et al. (2013). Is it a primary or metastatic melanocytic neoplasm of the central nervous system?: A molecular based approach. Pathol Int. 63(11):559–64. PMID:24274719
499. Corti ME, Yampolsky C, Metta H, Valerga M, Sevlever G, Capizzano A (2004). Oligodendroglioma in a patient with AIDS: case report and review of the literature. Rev Inst Med Trop Sao Paulo. 46(4):195–7. PMID:15361970
500. Cosar M, Iplikcioglu AC, Bek S, Gokduman CA (2005). Intracranial falcine and convexity chondromas: two case reports. Br J Neurosurg. 19(3):241–3. PMID:16455525
501. Couce ME, Aker FV, Scheithauer BW (2000). Chordoid meningioma: a clinicopathologic study of 42 cases. Am J Surg Pathol. 24(7):899–905. PMID:10895812
502. Courts C, Montesinos-Rongen M, Brunn A, Bug S, Siemer D, Hans V, et al. (2008). Recurrent inactivation of the PRDM1 gene in primary central nervous system lymphoma. J Neuropathol Exp Neurol. 67(7):720–7. PMID:18596541
503. Courville CB, Broussalian SL (1961). Plastic ependymomas of the lateral recess. Report of eight verified cases. J Neurosurg. 18:792–9. PMID:13881784
504. Covington MF, Chin SS, Osborn AG (2011). Pituicytoma, spindle cell oncocytoma, and granular cell tumor: clarification and meta-analysis of the world literature since 1893. AJNR Am J Neuroradiol. 32(11):2067–72. PMID:21960498
505. Crino PB, Mehta R, Vinters HV (2010). Pathogenesis of TSC in the brain. In: Tuberous sclerosis complex. Genes, clinical features, and therapeutics. Kwiatkowski DJ, Whittemore VH, Thiele EA, eds. Wiley-Blackwell: Weinheim, Germany, pp. 161-185.
506. Crino PB, Trojanowski JQ, Dichter MA, Eberwine J (1996). Embryonic neuronal markers in tuberous sclerosis: single-cell molecular pathology. Proc Natl Acad Sci U S A. 93(24):14152–7. PMID:8943076
506A. Crocetti E, Trama A, Stiller C, Caldarella A, Soffietti R, Jaal J, et al. (2012). Epidemiology of glial and non-glial brain tumours in Europe. Eur J Cancer. 48(10):1532–42. PMID:22227039
507. Crotty TB, Scheithauer BW, Young WF Jr, Davis DH, Shaw EG, Miller GM, et al. (1995). Papillary craniopharyngioma: a clinicopathological study of 48 cases. J Neurosurg. 83(2):206–14. PMID:7616262
508. Cuccia V, Rodríguez F, Palma F, Zuccaro G (2006). Pinealoblastomas in children. Childs Nerv Syst. 22(6):577–85. PMID:16555075
509. Curatolo P, Moavero R (2012). mTOR Inhibitors in Tuberous Sclerosis Complex. Curr Neuropharmacol. 10(4):404–15. PMID:23730262
510. Curless RG, Toledano SR, Ragheb J, Cleveland WW, Falcone S (2002). Hematogenous brain metastasis in children. Pediatr Neurol. 26(3):219–21. PMID:11955930
511. Curran EK, Sainani KL, Le GM, Propp

JM, Fisher PG (2009). Gender affects survival for medulloblastoma only in older children and adults: a study from the Surveillance Epidemiology and End Results Registry. Pediatr Blood Cancer. 52(1):60–4. PMID:19006250
511A. Custer B, Longstreth WT, Phillips LE, Koepsell TD, Van Belle G (2006). Hormonal exposures and the risk of intracranial meningioma in women: a population-based case-control study. BMC Cancer. 6:152. PMID:16759391
512. Cykowski MD, Wartchow EP, Mierau GW, Stolzenberg ED, Gumerlock MK, Fung KM (2012). Papillary tumor of the pineal region: ultrastructural study of a case. Ultrastruct Pathol. 36(1):68–77. PMID:22292738
513. D'Ambrosio N, Soohoo S, Warshall C, Johnson A, Karimi S (2008). Craniofacial and intracranial manifestations of langerhans cell histiocytosis: report of findings in 100 patients. AJR Am J Roentgenol. 191(2):589–97. PMID:18647937
515. da Cruz Perez DE, Amanajás de Aguiar FC Jr, Leon JE, Graner E, Paes de Almeida O, Vargas PA (2006). Intraneural perineurioma of the tongue: a case report. J Oral Maxillofac Surg. 64(7):1140–2. PMID:16781350
516. Dabora SL, Jozwiak S, Franz DN, Roberts PS, Nieto A, Chung J, et al. (2001). Mutational analysis in a cohort of 224 tuberous sclerosis patients indicates increased severity of TSC2, compared with TSC1, disease in multiple organs. Am J Hum Genet. 68(1):64–80. PMID:11112665
517. Dahia PL, Aguiar RC, Alberta J, Kum JB, Caron S, Sill H, et al. (1999). PTEN is inversely correlated with the cell survival factor Akt/PKB and is inactivated via multiple mechanismsin haematological malignancies. Hum Mol Genet. 8(2):185–93. PMID:9931326
518. Dahiya S, Haydon DH, Alvarado D, Gurnett CA, Gutmann DH, Leonard JR (2013). BRAF(V600E) mutation is a negative prognosticator in pediatric ganglioglioma. Acta Neuropathol. 125(6):901–10. PMID:23609006
519. Dahiya S, Sarkar C, Hedley-Whyte ET, Sharma MC, Zervas NT, Sridhar E, et al. (2005). Spindle cell oncocytoma of the adenohypophysis: report of two cases. Acta Neuropathol. 110(1):97–9. PMID:15973544
520. Dahlback HS, Gorunova L, Micci F, Scheie D, Brandal P, Meling TR, et al. (2011). Molecular cytogenetic analysis of a gliosarcoma with osseous metaplasia. Cytogenet Genome Res. 134(2):88–95. PMID:21555877
521. Dai C, Celestino JC, Okada Y, Louis DN, Fuller GN, Holland EC (2001). PDGF autocrine stimulation dedifferentiates cultured astrocytes and induces oligodendrogliomas and oligoastrocytomas from neural progenitors and astrocytes in vivo. Genes Dev. 15(15):1913–25. PMID:11485986
522. Damodaran O, Robbins P, Knuckey N, Bynevelt M, Wong G, Lee G (2014). Primary intracranial haemangiopericytoma: comparison of survival outcomes and metastatic potential in WHO grade II and III variants. J Clin Neurosci. 21(8):1310–4. PMID:24726230
523. Dang L, White DW, Gross S, Bennett BD, Bittinger MA, Driggers EM, et al. (2009). Cancer-associated IDH1 mutations produce 2-hydroxyglutarate. Nature. 462(7274):739–44. PMID:19935646
524. Dardick I, Hammar SP, Scheithauer BW (1989). Ultrastructural spectrum of hemangiopericytoma: a comparative study of fetal, adult, and neoplastic pericytes. Ultrastruct Pathol. 13(2-3):111–54. PMID:2734855
525. Dario A, Cerati M, Taborelli M, Finzi G, Pozzi M, Dorizzi A (2000). Cytogenetic and ultrastructural study of a pineocytoma case report. J Neurooncol. 48(2):131–4. PMID:11083076
526. Darrouzet V, Martel J, Enée V, Bébéar JP, Guérin J (2004). Vestibular schwannoma surgery outcomes: our multidisciplinary experience in 400 cases over 17 years. Laryngoscope. 114(4):681–8. PMID:15064624
527. Darwish B, Arbuckle S, Kellie S, Besser M, Chaseling R (2007). Desmoplastic infantile ganglioglioma/astrocytoma with cerebrospinal metastasis. J Clin Neurosci. 14(5):498–501. PMID:17386372
528. Darwish BS, Balakrishnan V, Maitra R (2002). Intramedullary ancient schwannoma of the cervical spinal cord: case report and review of literature. J Clin Neurosci. 9(3):321–3. PMID:12093146
529. Dasgupta B, Dugan LL, Gutmann DH (2003). The neurofibromatosis 1 gene product neurofibromin regulates pituitary adenylate cyclase-activating polypeptide-mediated signaling in astrocytes. J Neurosci. 23(26):8949–54. PMID:14523097
530. Daumas Duport C (1995). Patterns of tumor growth and problems associated with histological typing of low-grade gliomas. In: Apuzzo LJ, editor. Benign Cerebral Gliomas. Park Ridge: AANS; pp. 125–47.
531. Daumas-Duport C (1993). Dysembryoplastic neuroepithelial tumours. Brain Pathol. 3(3):283–95. PMID:8293188
532. Daumas-Duport C (1995). Dysembryoplastic neuroepithelial tumours in epilepsy surgery. In: Guerrini R, editor. Dysplasia of Cerebral Cortex and Epilepsy. New York: Raven Press; pp. 125–47.
533. Daumas-Duport C, Scheithauer B, O'Fallon J, Kelly P (1988). Grading of astrocytomas. A simple and reproducible method. Cancer. 62(10):2152–65. PMID:3179928
534. Daumas-Duport C, Scheithauer BW, Chodkiewicz JP, Laws ER Jr, Vedrenne C (1988). Dysembryoplastic neuroepithelial tumor: a surgically curable tumor of young patients with intractable partial seizures. Report of thirty-nine cases. Neurosurgery. 23(5):545–56. PMID:3143922
535. Daumas-Duport C, Scheithauer BW, Kelly PJ (1987). A histologic and cytologic method for the spatial definition of gliomas. Mayo Clin Proc. 62(6):435–49. PMID:2437411
536. Daumas-Duport C, Varlet P (2003). [Dysembryoplastic neuroepithelial tumors]. Rev Neurol (Paris). 159(6-7 Pt 1):622–36. PMID:12910070
537. Daumas-Duport C, Varlet P, Bacha S, Beuvon F, Cervera-Pierot P, Chodkiewicz JP (1999). Dysembryoplastic neuroepithelial tumors: nonspecific histological forms – a study of 40 cases. J Neurooncol. 41(3):267–80. PMID:10359147
538. de Chadarévian JP, Montes JL, O'Gorman AM, Freeman CR (1987). Maturation of cerebellar neuroblastoma into ganglioneuroma with melanosis. A histologic, immunocytochemical, and ultrastructural study. Cancer. 59(1):69–76. PMID:3539310
539. de Chadarévian JP, Pattisapu JV, Faerber EN (1990). Desmoplastic cerebral astrocytoma of infancy. Light microscopy, immunocytochemistry, and ultrastructure. Cancer. 66(1):173–9. PMID:2354404
540. de Cubas AA, Leandro-García LJ, Schiavi F, Mancikova V, Comino-Méndez I, Inglada-Pérez L, et al. (2013). Integrative analysis of miRNA and mRNA expression profiles in pheochromocytoma and paraganglioma identifies genotype-specific markers and potentially regulated pathways. Endocr Relat Cancer. 20(4):477–93. PMID:23660872
541. De Filippi P, Badulli C, Cuccia M, De Silvestri A, Dametto E, Pasi A, et al. (2006). Specific polymorphisms of cytokine genes are associated with different risks to develop single-system or multi-system childhood Langerhans cell histiocytosis. Br J Haematol. 132(6):784–7. PMID:16487180
542. de Groot JF, Fuller G, Kumar AJ, Piao Y, Eterovic K, Ji Y, et al. (2010). Tumor invasion after treatment of glioblastoma with bevacizumab: radiographic and pathologic correlation in humans and mice. Neuro Oncol. 12(3):233–42. PMID:20167811
543. De Jesús O, Rifkinson N (1995). Pleomorphic xanthoastrocytoma with invasion of the tentorium and falx. Surg Neurol. 43(1):77–9. PMID:7701430
544. de Jong MC, Kors WA, de Graaf P, Castelijns JA, Kivelä T, Moll AC (2014). Trilateral retinoblastoma: a systematic review and meta-analysis. Lancet Oncol. 15(10):1157–67. PMID:25126964
545. de Kock L, Sabbaghian N, Druker H, Weber E, Hamel N, Miller S, et al. (2014). Germline and somatic DICER1 mutations in pineoblastoma. Acta Neuropathol. 128(4):583–95. PMID:25022261
546. de la Monte SM, Horowitz SA (1989). Hemangioblastomas: clinical and histopathological factors correlated with recurrence. Neurosurgery. 25(5):695–8. PMID:2586723
547. De Munnynck K, Van Gool S, Van Calenbergh F, Demaerel P, Uyttebroeck A, Buyse G, et al. (2002). Desmoplastic infantile ganglioglioma: a potentially malignant tumor? Am J Surg Pathol. 26(11):1515–22. PMID:12409729
548. De Raedt T, Beert E, Pasmant E, Luscan A, Brems H, Ortonne N, et al. (2014). PRC2 loss amplifies Ras-driven transcription and confers sensitivity to BRD4-based therapies. Nature. 514(7521):247–51. PMID:25119042
549. De Raedt T, Brems H, Lopez-Correa C, Vermeesch JR, Marynen P, Legius E (2004). Genomic organization and evolution of the NF1 microdeletion region. Genomics. 84(2):346–60. PMID:15233998
550. De Raedt T, Brems H, Wolkenstein P, Vidaud D, Pilotti S, Perrone F, et al. (2003). Elevated risk for MPNST in NF1 microdeletion patients. Am J Hum Genet. 72(5):1288–92. PMID:12660952
551. de Ribaupierre S, Dorfmüller G, Bulteau C, Fohlen M, Pinard JM, Chiron C, et al. (2007). Subependymal giant-cell astrocytomas in pediatric tuberous sclerosis disease: when should we operate? Neurosurgery. 60(1):83–9, discussion 89–90. PMID:17228255
552. De Schepper S, Maertens O, Callens T, Naeyaert JM, Lambert J, Messiaen L (2008). Somatic mutation analysis in NF1 café au lait spots reveals two NF1 hits in the melanocytes. J Invest Dermatol. 128(4):1050–3. PMID:17914445
553. De Tommasi A, Luzzi S, D'Urso PI, De Tommasi C, Resta N, Ciappetta P (2008). Molecular genetic analysis in a case of ganglioglioma: identification of a new mutation. Neurosurgery. 63(5):976–80, discussion 980. PMID:19005389
554. De Vos M, Hayward BE, Charlton R, Taylor GR, Glaser AW, Picton S, et al. (2006). PMS2 mutations in childhood cancer. J Natl Cancer Inst. 98(5):358–61. PMID:16507833
555. de Vries J, Scheremet R, Altmannsberger M, Michilli R, Lindemann A, Hinkelbein W (1994). Primary leiomyosarcoma of the spinal leptomeninges. J Neurooncol. 18(1):25–31. PMID:8057131
556. de Vries NA, Hulsman D, Akhtar W, de Jong J, Miles DC, Blom M, et al. (2015). Prolonged Ezh2 Depletion in Glioblastoma Causes a Robust Switch in Cell Fate Resulting in Tumor Progression. Cell Rep. PMID:25600873
557. DeAngelis LM (2001). Brain tumors. N Engl J Med. 344(2):114–23. PMID:11150363
558. Dearnaley DP, A'Hern RP, Whittaker S, Bloom HJ (1990). Pineal and CNS germ cell tumors: Royal Marsden Hospital experience 1962–1987. Int J Radiat Oncol Biol Phys. 18(4):773–81. PMID:2323968
559. Deb P, Sharma MC, Gaikwad S, Gupta A, Mehta VS, Sarkar C (2005). Cerebellopontine angle paraganglioma - report of a case and review of literature. J Neurooncol. 74(1):65–9. PMID:16078110
560. Debiec-Rychter M, Jesionek-Kupnicka D, Zakrzewski K, Liberski PP (1999). Cytogenetic changes in two cases of subependymal giant-cell astrocytoma. Cancer Genet Cytogenet. 109(1):29–33. PMID:9973956
561. Deckert M, Brunn A, Montesinos-Rongen M, Terreni MR, Ponzoni M (2014). Primary lymphoma of the central nervous system–a diagnostic challenge. Hematol Oncol. 32(2):57–67. PMID:23949943
562. Deckert M, Engert A, Brück W, Ferreri AJ, Finke J, Illerhaus G, et al. (2011). Modern concepts in the biology, diagnosis, differential diagnosis and treatment of primary central nervous system lymphoma. Leukemia. 25(12):1797–807. PMID:21818113
563. DeDavid M, Orlow SJ, Provost N, Marghoob AA, Rao BK, Huang CL, et al. (1997). A study of large congenital melanocytic nevi and associated malignant melanomas: review of cases in the New York University Registry and the world literature. J Am Acad Dermatol. 36(3 Pt 1):409–16. PMID:9091472
564. DeDavid M, Orlow SJ, Provost N, Marghoob AA, Rao BK, Wasti Q, et al. (1996). Neurocutaneous melanosis: clinical features of large congenital melanocytic nevi in patients with manifest central nervous system melanosis. J Am Acad Dermatol. 35(4):529–38. PMID:8859278
565. Dedeurwaerdere F, Giannini C, Sciot R, Rubin BP, Perilongo G, Borghi L, et al. (2002). Primary peripheral PNET/Ewing's sarcoma of the dura: a clinicopathologic entity distinct from central PNET. Mod Pathol. 15(6):673–8. PMID:12065782
566. Degen R, Ebner A, Lahl R, Leonhardt S, Pannek HW, Tuxhorn I (2002). Various findings in surgically treated epilepsy patients with dysembryoplastic neuroepithelial tumors in comparison with those of patients with other low-grade brain tumors and other neuronal migration disorders. Epilepsia. 43(11):1379–84. PMID:12423388
567. Dehghani F, Schachenmayr W, Laun A, Korf HW (1998). Prognostic implication of histopathological, immunohistochemical and clinical features of oligodendrogliomas: a study of 89 cases. Acta Neuropathol. 95(5):493–504. PMID:9600596
568. Deisch JK, Patel R, Koral K, Cope-Yokoyama SD (2013). Juvenile xanthogranulomas of the nervous system: A report of two cases and review of the literature. Neuropathology. 33(1):39–46. PMID:22640164
569. Del Bigio MR, Deck JH (1993). Rosenthal fibers producing a granular cell appearance in a glioblastoma. Acta Neuropathol. 86(1):100–4. PMID:8396834
570. Del Valle L, Enam S, Lara C, Ortiz-Hidalgo C, Katsetos CD, Khalili K (2002). Detection of JC polyomavirus DNA sequences and cellular localization of T-antigen and agnoprotein in oligodendrogliomas. Clin Cancer Res. 8(11):3332–40. PMID:12429619
571. Delnatte C, Sanlaville D, Mougenot JF, Vermeesch JR, Houdayer C, Blois MC, et al. (2006). Contiguous gene deletion within chromosome arm 10q is associated with juvenile polyposis of infancy, reflecting cooperation between the BMPR1A and PTEN tumor-suppressor genes. Am J Hum Genet. 78(6):1066–74. PMID:16685657
572. Demetriades AK, Al Hyassat S, Al-Sarraj S, Bhangoo RS, Ashkan K (2013). Papillary glioneuronal tumour: a review of the literature with two illustrative cases. Br J Neurosurg. 27(3):401–4. PMID:23173837
573. Demuth T, Berens ME (2004). Molecular mechanisms of glioma cell migration and invasion. J Neurooncol. 70(2):217–28. PMID:15674479
574. Derlin T, Tornquist K, Münster S, Apostolova I, Hagel C, Friedrich RE, et al. (2013). Comparative effectiveness of 18F-FDG PET/CT versus whole-body MRI for detection of

malignant peripheral nerve sheath tumors in neurofibromatosis type 1. Clin Nucl Med. 38(1):e19–25. PMID:23242059
575. Deshmukh H, Yu J, Shaik J, MacDonald TJ, Perry A, Payton JE, et al. (2011). Identification of transcriptional regulatory networks specific to pilocytic astrocytoma. BMC Med Genomics. 4:57. PMID:21745356
576. Desouza RM, Bodi I, Thomas N, Marsh H, Crocker M (2010). Chordoid glioma: ten years of a low-grade tumor with high morbidity. Skull Base. 20(2):125–38. PMID:20808539
577. Dessauvagie BF, Wong G, Robbins PD (2015). Renal cell carcinoma to haemangioblastoma metastasis: a rare manifestation of Von Hippel-Lindau syndrome. J Clin Neurosci. 22(1):215–8. PMID:25088480
578. Dewan R, Pemov A, Kim HJ, Morgan KL, Vasquez RA, Chittiboina P, et al. (2015). Evidence of polyclonality in neurofibromatosis type 2-associated multilobulated vestibular schwannomas. Neuro Oncol. 17(4):566–73. PMID:25452392
580. Dhimes P, Martinez-Gonzalez MA, Carabias E, Perez-Espejo G (1996). Ultrastructural study of a perineurioma with ribosome-lamella complexes. Ultrastruct Pathol. 20(2):167–72. PMID:8882362
581. Di Cristofano A, Pesce B, Cordon-Cardo C, Pandolfi PP (1998). Pten is essential for embryonic development and tumour suppression. Nat Genet. 19(4):348–55. PMID:9697695
582. Di Rocco F, Carroll RS, Zhang J, Black PM (1998). Platelet-derived growth factor and its receptor expression in human oligodendrogliomas. Neurosurgery. 42(2):341–6. PMID:9482185
583. Di Rocco F, Sabatino G, Koutzoglou M, Battaglia D, Caldarelli M, Tamburrini G (2004). Neurocutaneous melanosis. Childs Nerv Syst. 20(1):23–8. PMID:14576958
584. Dias-Santagata D, Lam Q, Vernovsky K, Vena N, Lennerz JK, Borger DR, et al. (2011). BRAF V600E mutations are common in pleomorphic xanthoastrocytoma: diagnostic and therapeutic implications. PLoS One. 6(3):e17948. PMID:21479234
585. Díaz-Flores L, Alvarez-Argüelles H, Madrid JF, Varela H, Gonzalez MP, Gutierrez R (1997). Perineurial cell tumor (perineurioma) with granular cells. J Cutan Pathol. 24(9):575–9. PMID:9404856
586. Dim DC, Lingamfelter DC, Taboada EM, Fiorella RM (2006). Papillary glioneuronal tumor: a case report and review of the literature. Hum Pathol. 37(7):914–8. PMID:16784993
587. Dinçer A, Yener U, Özek MM (2011). Hydrocephalus in patients with neurofibromatosis type 1: MR imaging findings and the outcome of endoscopic third ventriculostomy. AJNR Am J Neuroradiol. 32(4):643–6. PMID:21330395
588. Dinda AK, Sarkar C, Roy S (1990). Rosenthal fibres: an immunohistochemical, ultrastructural and immunoelectron microscopic study. Acta Neuropathol. 79(4):456–60. PMID:2339597
589. Ding H, Shannon P, Lau N, Wu X, Roncari L, Baldwin RL, et al. (2003). Oligodendrogliomas result from the expression of an activated mutant epidermal growth factor receptor in a RAS transgenic mouse astrocytoma model. Cancer Res. 63(5):1106–13. PMID:12615729
590. Dirks PB, Harris L, Hoffman HJ, Humphreys RP, Drake JM, Rutka JT (1996). Supratentorial primitive neuroectodermal tumors in children. J Neurooncol. 29(1):75–84. PMID:8817418
591. Dirks PB, Jay V, Becker LE, Drake JM, Humphreys RP, Hoffman HJ, et al. (1994). Development of anaplastic changes in low-grade astrocytomas of childhood. Neurosurgery. 34(1):68–78. PMID:8121571
592. do Nascimento A, Maranha LA, Corredato RA, Araújo JC, Bleggi-Torres LF (2012). 33 year-old woman with a large sellar tumor. Brain Pathol. 22(6):869–70. PMID:23050874
593. Dobbins SE, Broderick P, Melin B, Feychting M, Johansen C, Andersson U, et al. (2011). Common variation at 10p12.31 near MLLT10 influences meningioma risk. Nat Genet. 43(9):825–7. PMID:21804547
594. Doglioni C, Dell'Orto P, Coggi G, Iuzzolino P, Bontempini L, Viale G (1987). Choroid plexus tumors. An immunocytochemical study with particular reference to the coexpression of intermediate filament proteins. Am J Pathol. 127(3):519–29. PMID:2438940
595. Dohrmann GJ, Farwell JR, Flannery JT (1976). Glioblastoma multiforme in children. J Neurosurg. 44(4):442–8. PMID:176331
596. Dolecek TA, Propp JM, Stroup NE, Kruchko C (2012). CBTRUS statistical report: primary brain and central nervous system tumors diagnosed in the United States in 2005–2009. Neuro Oncol. 14 Suppl 5:v1–49. PMID:23095881
597. Donoho D, Zada G (2015). Imaging of central neurocytomas. Neurosurg Clin N Am. 26(1):11–9. PMID:25432179
598. Donovan MJ, Yunis EJ, DeGirolami U, Fletcher JA, Schofield DE (1994). Chromosome aberrations in choroid plexus papillomas. Genes Chromosomes Cancer. 11(4):267–70. PMID:7533531
599. Donson AM, Kleinschmidt-DeMasters BK, Aisner DL, Bemis LT, Birks DK, Levy JM, et al. (2014). Pediatric brainstem gangliogliomas show BRAF(V600E) mutation in a high percentage of cases. Brain Pathol. 24(2):173–83. PMID:24238153
600. Doskaliyev A, Yamasaki F, Kenjo M, Shrestha P, Saito T, Hanaya R, et al. (2008). Secondary anaplastic oligodendroglioma after cranial irradiation: a case report. J Neurooncol. 88(3):299–303. PMID:18373067
601. Dougherty MJ, Santi M, Brose MS, Ma C, Resnick AC, Sievert AJ, et al. (2010). Activating mutations in BRAF characterize a spectrum of pediatric low-grade gliomas. Neuro Oncol. 12(7):621–30. PMID:20156809
602. Douglas-Akinwande AC, Payner TD, Hattab EM (2009). Medulloblastoma mimicking Lhermitte-Duclos disease on MRI and CT. Clin Neurol Neurosurg. 111(6):536–9. PMID:19233547
603. Dragojević S, Mehraein P, Bock HJ (1973). [Lipoma of the temporal region with cortical malformation and epilepsy. Clinicopathological study (author's transl)]. Arch Psychiatr Nervenkr (1970). 217(4):335–42. PMID:4203636
604. Dratman MB (1979). Mechanism of thyroxine action. N Engl J Med. 300(23):1336. PMID:220535
605. Dropcho EJ, Soong SJ (1996). The prognostic impact of prior low grade histology in patients with anaplastic gliomas: a case-control study. Neurology. 47(3):684–90. PMID:8797465
606. Ducatman BS, Scheithauer BW, Piepgras DG, Reiman HM, Ilstrup DM (1986). Malignant peripheral nerve sheath tumors. A clinicopathologic study of 120 cases. Cancer. 57(10):2006–21. PMID:3082508
607. Ducray F, Crinière E, Idbaih A, Mokhtari K, Marie Y, Paris S, et al. (2009). alpha-Internexin expression identifies 1p19q codeleted gliomas. Neurology. 72(2):156–61. PMID:19139367
608. Ducray F, Idbaih A, de Reyniès A, Bièche I, Thillet J, Mokhtari K, et al. (2008). Anaplastic oligodendrogliomas with 1p19q codeletion have a proneural gene expression profile. Mol Cancer. 7:41. PMID:18492260
609. Duffell D, Farber L, Chou S, Hartmann JF, Nelson E (1963). Electron microscopic observations on astrocytomas. Am J Pathol. 43:539–45. PMID:14068386
610. Duffner PK, Horowitz ME, Krischer JP, Burger PC, Cohen ME, Sanford RA, et al. (1999). The treatment of malignant brain tumors in infants and very young children: an update of the Pediatric Oncology Group experience. Neuro Oncol. 1(2):152–61. PMID:11554387
611. Dunham C, Sugo E, Tobias V, Wills E, Perry A (2007). Embryonal tumor with abundant neuropil and true rosettes (ETANTR): report of a case with prominent neurocytic differentiation. J Neurooncol. 84(1):91–8. PMID:17332950
612. Dunham C, Yip S (2013). Cribriform neuroepithelial tumor or atypical teratoid/rhabdoid tumor? J Neurosurg Pediatr. 11(4):486–8. PMID:23394355
613. Duò D, Gasverde S, Benech F, Zenga F, Giordana MT (2003). MIB-1 immunoreactivity in craniopharyngiomas: a clinico-pathological analysis. Clin Neuropathol. 22(5):229–34. PMID:14531547
614. Durno CA, Aronson M, Tabori U, Malkin D, Gallinger S, Chan HS (2012). Oncologic surveillance for subjects with biallelic mismatch repair gene mutations: 10 year follow-up of a kindred. Pediatr Blood Cancer. 59(4):652–6. PMID:22180144
615. Durno CA, Sherman PM, Aronson M, Malkin D, Hawkins C, Bakry D, et al.; International BMMRD Consortium (2015). Phenotypic and genotypic characterisation of biallelic mismatch repair deficiency (BMMR-D) syndrome. Eur J Cancer. 51(8):977–83. PMID:25883011
616. Eaton KW, Tooke LS, Wainwright LM, Judkins AR, Biegel JA (2011). Spectrum of SMARCB1/INI1 mutations in familial and sporadic rhabdoid tumors. Pediatr Blood Cancer. 56(1):7–15. PMID:21108436
617. Eberhart CG (2007). In search of the medulloblast: neural stem cells and embryonal brain tumors . Neurosurg Clin N Am 18: 59-69, viii-ix. PMID:17244554
618. Eberhart CG, Brat DJ, Cohen KJ, Burger PC (2000). Pediatric neuroblastic brain tumors containing abundant neuropil and true rosettes. Pediatr Dev Pathol. 3(4):346–52. PMID:10890250
619. Eberhart CG, Kepner JL, Goldthwaite PT, Kun LE, Duffner PK, Friedman HS, et al. (2002). Histopathologic grading of medulloblastomas: a Pediatric Oncology Group study. Cancer. 94(2):552–60. PMID:11900240
620. Eberhart CG, Kratz J, Wang Y, Summers K, Stearns D, Cohen K, et al. (2004). Histopathological and molecular prognostic markers in medulloblastoma: c-myc, N-myc, TrkC, and anaplasia. J Neuropathol Exp Neurol. 63(5):441–9. PMID:15198123
621. Ebert C, von Haken M, Meyer-Puttlitz B, Wiestler OD, Reifenberger G, Pietsch T, et al. (1999). Molecular genetic analysis of ependymal tumors. NF2 mutations and chromosome 22q loss occur preferentially in intramedullary spinal ependymomas. Am J Pathol. 155(2):627–32. PMID:10433955
622. Eckel-Passow JE, Lachance DH, Molinaro AM, Walsh KM, Decker PA, Sicotte H, et al. (2015). Glioma Groups Based on 1p/19q, IDH, and TERT Promoter Mutations in Tumors. N Engl J Med. 372(26):2499–508. PMID:26061753
623. Eckhardt BP, Brandner S, Zollikofer CL, Wentz KU (2004). Primary cerebral leiomyosarcoma in a child. Pediatr Radiol. 34(6):495–8. PMID:15057493
624. Edwards A, Bermudez C, Piwonka G, Berr ML, Zamorano J, Larrain E, et al. (2002). Carney's syndrome: complex myxomas. Report of four cases and review of the literature. Cardiovasc Surg. 10(3):264–75. PMID:12044436
625. Eigenbrod S, Roeber S, Thon N, Giese A, Krieger A, Grasbon-Frodl E, et al. (2011). α-Internexin in the diagnosis of oligodendroglial tumors and association with 1p/19q status. J Neuropathol Exp Neurol. 70(11):970–8. PMID:22002423
626. Ekstrand AJ, James CD, Cavenee WK, Seliger B, Pettersson RF, Collins VP (1991). Genes for epidermal growth factor receptor, transforming growth factor alpha, and epidermal growth factor and their expression in human gliomas in vivo. Cancer Res. 51(8):2164–72. PMID:2009534
627. Ekstrand AJ, Sugawa N, James CD, Collins VP (1992). Amplified and rearranged epidermal growth factor receptor genes in human glioblastomas reveal deletions of sequences encoding portions of the N- and/or C-terminal tails. Proc Natl Acad Sci U S A. 89(10):4309–13. PMID:1584765
628. Elefteriou F, Kolanczyk M, Schindeler A, Viskochil DH, Hock JM, Schorry EK, et al. (2009). Skeletal abnormalities in neurofibromatosis type 1: approaches to therapeutic options. Am J Med Genet A. 149A(10):2327–38. PMID:19764036
629. Ellezam B, Theeler BJ, Luthra R, Adesina AM, Aldape KD, Gilbert MR (2012). Recurrent PIK3CA mutations in rosette-forming glioneuronal tumor. Acta Neuropathol. 123(2):285–7. PMID:21997360
630. Ellison DW (2010). Childhood medulloblastoma: novel approaches to the classification of a heterogeneous disease. Acta Neuropathol. 120(3):305–16. PMID:20652577
631. Ellison DW, Dalton J, Kocak M, Nicholson SL, Fraga C, Neale G, et al. (2011). Medulloblastoma: clinicopathological correlates of SHH, WNT, and non-SHH/WNT molecular subgroups. Acta Neuropathol. 121(3):381–96. PMID:21267586
632. Ellison DW, Kocak M, Dalton J, Megahed H, Lusher ME, Ryan SL, et al. (2011). Definition of disease-risk stratification groups in childhood medulloblastoma using combined clinical, pathologic, and molecular variables. J Clin Oncol. 29(11):1400–7. PMID:20921458
633. Ellison DW, Kocak M, Figarella-Branger D, Felice G, Catherine G, Pietsch T, et al. (2011). Histopathological grading of pediatric ependymoma: reproducibility and clinical relevance in European trial cohorts. J Negat Results Biomed. 10:7. PMID:21627842
634. Ellison DW, Onilude OE, Lindsey JC, Lusher ME, Weston CL, Taylor RE, et al.; United Kingdom Children's Cancer Study Group Brain Tumour Committee (2005). beta-Catenin status predicts a favorable outcome in childhood medulloblastoma: the United Kingdom Children's Cancer Study Group Brain Tumour Committee. J Clin Oncol. 23(31):7951–7. PMID:16258095
635. Ellison DW, Zygmunt SC, Weller RO (1993). Neurocytoma/lipoma (neurolipocytoma) of the cerebellum. Neuropathol Appl Neurobiol. 19(1):95–8. PMID:8474606
636. Elowe-Gruau E, Beltrand J, Brauner R, Pinto G, Samara-Boustani D, Thalassinos C, et al. (2013). Childhood craniopharyngioma: hypothalamus-sparing surgery decreases the risk of obesity. J Clin Endocrinol Metab. 98(6):2376–82. PMID:23633208
637. Emory TS, Scheithauer BW, Hirose T, Wood M, Onofrio BM, Jenkins RB (1995). Intraneural perineurioma. A clonal neoplasm associated with abnormalities of chromosome 22. Am J Clin Pathol. 103(6):696–704. PMID:7785653
638. En-Nafaa I, Latib R, Fikri M, Cisse A, El Kettani N, Chami I, et al. (2010). [Frontoparietal paraganglioma: a case report]. J Radiol. 91(12 Pt 1):1318–9. PMID:21242920
639. Ene CI, Morton RP, Ferreira M Jr, Sekhar LN, Kim LJ (2015). Spontaneous Hemorrhage from Central Nervous System Hemangioblastomas. World Neurosurg. 83(6):1180.e13–7. PMID:25727302
640. Eng C (1997). Cowden Syndrome. J Genet Couns. 6(2):181–92. PMID:26142096
641. Eng C, Murday V, Seal S, Mohammed S, Hodgson SV, Chaudary MA, et al. (1994). Cowden syndrome and Lhermitte-Duclos disease in a family: a single genetic syndrome with pleiotropy? J Med Genet. 31(6):458–61. PMID:8071972
642. Eng C, Peacocke M (1998). PTEN and inherited hamartoma-cancer syndromes. Nat Genet. 19(3):223. PMID:9662392
643. Eng DY, DeMonte F, Ginsberg L, Fuller GN,

Jaeckle K (1997). Craniospinal dissemination of central neurocytoma. Report of two cases. J Neurosurg. 86(3):547–52. PMID:9046315
644. Eoli M, Menghi F, Bruzzone MG, De Simone T, Valletta L, Pollo B, et al. (2007). Methylation of O6-methylguanine DNA methyltransferase and loss of heterozygosity on 19q and/or 17p are overlapping features of secondary glioblastomas with prolonged survival. Clin Cancer Res. 13(9):2606–13. PMID:17473190
645. Erdem-Eraslan L, Gravendeel LA, de Rooi J, Eilers PH, Idbaih A, Spliet WG, et al. (2013). Intrinsic molecular subtypes of glioma are prognostic and predict benefit from adjuvant procarbazine, lomustine, and vincristine chemotherapy in combination with other prognostic factors in anaplastic oligodendroglial brain tumors: a report from EORTC study 26951. J Clin Oncol. 31(3):328–36. PMID:23269986
646. Erickson ML, Johnson R, Bannykh SI, de Lotbiniere A, Kim JH (2005). Malignant rhabdoid tumor in a pregnant adult female: literature review of central nervous system rhabdoid tumors. J Neurooncol. 74(3):311–9. PMID:16132523
647. Erlandson RA (1994). Paragangliomas. Diagnostic Transmission Electron Microscopy of Tumors. Diagnostic Transmission Electron Microscopy of Tumors. New York: Raven Press; pp. 615–22.
648. Erlandson RA, Woodruff JM (1982). Peripheral nerve sheath tumors: an electron microscopic study of 43 cases. Cancer. 49(2):273–87. PMID:7053827
649. Ernestus RI, Schröder R, Stützer H, Klug N (1996). Prognostic relevance of localization and grading in intracranial ependymomas of childhood. Childs Nerv Syst. 12(9):522–6. PMID:8906366
650. Ernestus RI, Schröder R, Stützer H, Klug N (1997). The clinical and prognostic relevance of grading in intracranial ependymomas. Br J Neurosurg. 11(5):421–8. PMID:9474274
651. Errani C, Zhang L, Sung YS, Hajdu M, Singer S, Maki RG, et al. (2011). A novel WWTR1-CAMTA1 gene fusion is a consistent abnormality in epithelioid hemangioendothelioma of different anatomic sites. Genes Chromosomes Cancer. 50(8):644–53. PMID:21584898
652. Erson-Omay EZ, Çağlayan AO, Schultz N, Weinhold N, Omay SB, Özduman K, et al. (2015). Somatic POLE mutations cause an ultramutated giant cell high-grade glioma subtype with better prognosis. Neuro Oncol. 17(10):1356–64. PMID:25740784
653. Esteller M, Garcia-Foncillas J, Andion E, Goodman SN, Hidalgo OF, Vanaclocha V, et al. (2000). Inactivation of the DNA-repair gene MGMT and the clinical response of gliomas to alkylating agents. N Engl J Med. 343(19):1350–4. PMID:11070098
654. Esteller M, Hamilton SR, Burger PC, Baylin SB, Herman JG (1999). Inactivation of the DNA repair gene O6-methylguanine-DNA methyltransferase by promoter hypermethylation is a common event in primary human neoplasia. Cancer Res. 59(4):793–7. PMID:10029064
655. Euskirchen P, Haroche J, Emile JF, Buchert R, Vandersee S, Meisel A (2015). Complete remission of critical neurohistiocytosis by vemurafenib. Neurol Neuroimmunol Neuroinflamm. 2(2):e78. PMID:25745636
655A. Evans DG. Neurofibromatosis 2. 1998 [Updated 2011 Aug 18]. In: Pagon RA, Adam MP, Ardinger HH, et al., editors. GeneReviews® [Internet]. Seattle (WA): University of Washington, Seattle; 1993–2016. Available from: http://www.ncbi.nlm.nih.gov/books/NBK1201/
656. Evans DG, Birch JM, Ramsden RT (1999). Paediatric presentation of type 2 neurofibromatosis. Arch Dis Child. 81(6):496–9. PMID:10569966
657. Evans DG, Farndon PA, Burnell LD, Gattamaneni HR, Birch JM (1991). The incidence of Gorlin syndrome in 173 consecutive cases of medulloblastoma. Br J Cancer. 64(5):959–61. PMID:1931625
658. Evans DG, Howard E, Giblin C, Clancy T, Spencer H, Huson SM, et al. (2010). Birth incidence and prevalence of tumor-prone syndromes: estimates from a UK family genetic register service. Am J Med Genet A. 152A(2):327–32. PMID:20082463
659. Evans DG, Huson SM, Donnai D, Neary W, Blair V, Newton V, et al. (1992). A clinical study of type 2 neurofibromatosis. Q J Med. 84(304):603–18. PMID:1484939
660. Evans DG, Ladusans EJ, Rimmer S, Burnell LD, Thakker N, Farndon PA (1993). Complications of the naevoid basal cell carcinoma syndrome: results of a population based study. J Med Genet. 30(6):460–4. PMID:8326488
661. Evans DG, Mason S, Huson SM, Ponder M, Harding AE, Strachan T (1997). Spinal and cutaneous schwannomatosis is a variant form of type 2 neurofibromatosis: a clinical and molecular study. J Neurol Neurosurg Psychiatry. 62(4):361–6. PMID:9120449
662. Evans DG, Moran A, King A, Saeed S, Gurusinghe N, Ramsden R (2005). Incidence of vestibular schwannoma and neurofibromatosis 2 in the North West of England over a 10-year period: higher incidence than previously thought. Otol Neurotol. 26(1):93–7. PMID:15699726
663. Evans DG, O'Hara C, Wilding A, Ingham SL, Howard E, Dawson J, et al. (2011). Mortality in neurofibromatosis 1: in North West England: an assessment of actuarial survival in a region of the UK since 1989. Eur J Hum Genet. 19(11):1187–91. PMID:21694737
664. Evans DG, Wallace AJ, Wu CL, Trueman L, Ramsden RT, Strachan T (1998). Somatic mosaicism: a common cause of classic disease in tumor-prone syndromes? Lessons from type 2 neurofibromatosis. Am J Hum Genet. 63(3):727–36. PMID:9718334
665. Fakhran S, Escott EJ (2008). Pineocytoma mimicking a pineal cyst on imaging: true diagnostic dilemma or a case of incomplete imaging? AJNR Am J Neuroradiol. 29(1):159–63. PMID:17925371
666. Fallon KB, Palmer CA, Roth KA, Nabors LB, Wang W, Carpenter M, et al. (2004). Prognostic value of 1p, 19q, 9p, 10q, and EGFR-FISH analyses in recurrent oligodendrogliomas. J Neuropathol Exp Neurol. 63(4):314–22. PMID:15099021
667. Fan Z, Li J, Du J, Zhang H, Shen Y, Wang CY, et al. (2008). A missense mutation in PTCH2 underlies dominantly inherited NBCCS in a Chinese family. J Med Genet. 45(5):303–8. PMID:18285427
668. Fanburg-Smith JC, Auerbach A, Marwaha JS, Wang Z, Rushing EJ (2010). Reappraisal of mesenchymal chondrosarcoma: novel morphologic observations of the hyaline cartilage and endochondral ossification and beta-catenin, Sox9, and osteocalcin immunostaining of 22 cases. Hum Pathol. 41(5):653–62. PMID:20138330
669. Fargen KM, Opalach KJ, Wakefield D, Jacob RP, Yachnis AT, Lister JR (2011). The central nervous system solitary fibrous tumor: a review of clinical, imaging and pathologic findings among all reported cases from 1996 to 2010. Clin Neurol Neurosurg. 113(9):703–10. PMID:21872387
670. Faria C, Miguéns J, Antunes JL, Barroso C, Pimentel J, Martins MdoC, et al. (2008). Genetic alterations in a papillary glioneuronal tumor. J Neurosurg Pediatr. 1(1):99–102. PMID:18352813
671. Farnia B, Allen PK, Brown PD, Khatua S, Levine NB, Li J, et al. (2014). Clinical outcomes and patterns of failure in pineoblastoma: a 30-year, single-institution retrospective review. World Neurosurg. 82(6):1232–41. PMID:25045788
672. Faro SH, Turtz AR, Koenigsberg RA, Mohamed FB, Chen CY, Stein H (1997). Paraganglioma of the cauda equina with associated intramedullary cyst: MR findings. AJNR Am J Neuroradiol. 18(8):1588–90. PMID:9296205
673. Farwell JR, Dohrmann GJ, Flannery JT (1984). Medulloblastoma in childhood: an epidemiological study. J Neurosurg. 61(4):657–64. PMID:6470775
674. Fassett DR, Pingree J, Kestle JR (2005). The high incidence of tumor dissemination in myxopapillary ependymoma in pediatric patients. Report of five cases and review of the literature. J Neurosurg. 102(1) Suppl:59–64. PMID:16206735
675. Fassunke J, Majores M, Tresch A, Niehusmann P, Grote A, Schoch S, et al. (2008). Array analysis of epilepsy-associated gangliogliomas reveals expression patterns related to aberrant development of neuronal precursors. Brain. 131(Pt 11):3034–50. PMID:18819986
676. Fauchon F, Hasselblatt M, Jouvet A, Champier J, Popovic M, Kirollos R, et al. (2013). Role of surgery, radiotherapy and chemotherapy in papillary tumors of the pineal region: a multicenter study. J Neurooncol. 112(2):223–31. PMID:23314823
677. Fauchon F, Jouvet A, Paquis P, Saint-Pierre G, Mottolese C, Ben Hassel M, et al. (2000). Parenchymal pineal tumors: a clinicopathological study of 76 cases. Int J Radiat Oncol Biol Phys. 46(4):959–68. PMID:10705018
677A. Faulkner C, Ellis HP, Shaw A, Penman C, Palmer A, Wragg C, et al. (2015). BRAF Fusion Analysis in Pilocytic Astrocytomas: KIAA1549-BRAF 15-9 Fusions Are More Frequent in the Midline Than Within the Cerebellum. J Neuropathol Exp Neurol. 74(9):867–72. PMID:26222501
678. Faulkner C, Palmer A, Williams H, Wragg C, Haynes HR, White P, et al. (2014). EGFR and EGFRvIII analysis in glioblastoma as therapeutic biomarkers. Br J Neurosurg. 1–7. PMID:25141189
679. Fauria-Robinson C, Nguyen J, Palacios E, Castillo-Jorge S (2014). Dysplastic cerebellar gangliocytoma lhermitte-duclos disease imaging and magnetic resonance spectroscopy. J La State Med Soc. 166(5):193–6. PMID:25369219
680. Favier J, Gimenez-Roqueplo AP (2010). Pheochromocytomas: the (pseudo)-hypoxia hypothesis. Best Pract Res Clin Endocrinol Metab. 24(6):957–68. PMID:21115164
681. Feany MB, Anthony DC, Fletcher CD (1998). Nerve sheath tumours with hybrid features of neurofibroma and schwannoma: a conceptual challenge. Histopathology. 32(5):405–10. PMID:9639114
682. Feigin IH, Gross SW (1955). Sarcoma arising in glioblastoma of the brain. Am J Pathol. 31(4):633–53. PMID:14388124
683. Feldman DS, Jordan C, Fonseca L (2010). Orthopaedic manifestations of neurofibromatosis type 1. J Am Acad Orthop Surg. 18(6):346–57. PMID:20511440
683A. Feliciano DM, Quon JL, Su T, Taylor MM, Bordey A (2012). Postnatal neurogenesis generates heterotopias, olfactory micronodules and cortical infiltration following single-cell Tsc1 deletion. Hum Mol Genet. 21(4):799–810. PMID:22068588
684. Felix I, Becker LE (1990-1991). Intracranial germ cell tumors in children: an immunohistochemical and electron microscopic study. Pediatr Neurosurg. 16(3):156–62. PMID:1966857
685. Fellah S, Caudal D, De Paula AM, Dory-Lautrec P, Figarella-Branger D, Chinot O, et al. (2013). Multimodal MR imaging (diffusion, perfusion, and spectroscopy): is it possible to distinguish oligodendroglial tumor grade and 1p/19q codeletion in the pretherapeutic diagnosis? AJNR Am J Neuroradiol. 34(7):1326–33. PMID:23221948
686. Felsberg J, Erkwoh A, Sabel MC, Kirsch L, Fimmers R, Blaschke B, et al. (2004). Oligodendroglial tumors: refinement of candidate regions on chromosome arm 1p and correlation of 1p/19q status with survival. Brain Pathol. 14(2):121–30. PMID:15193024
687. Feng M, Carmichael JD, Bonert V, Bannykh S, Mamelak AN (2014). Surgical management of pituicytomas: case series and comprehensive literature review. Pituitary. 17(5):399–413. PMID:24037647
688. Fernandez C, Figarella-Branger D, Girard N, Bouvier-Labit C, Gouvernet J, Paz Paredes A, et al. (2003). Pilocytic astrocytomas in children: prognostic factors–a retrospective study of 80 cases. Neurosurgery. 53(3):544–53, discussion 554–5. PMID:12943571
689. Fernandez C, Girard N, Paz Paredes A, Bouvier-Labit C, Lena G, Figarella-Branger D (2003). The usefulness of MR imaging in the diagnosis of dysembryoplastic neuroepithelial tumor in children: a study of 14 cases. AJNR Am J Neuroradiol. 24(5):829–34. PMID:12748079
690. Fernandez-L A, Northcott PA, Dalton J, Fraga C, Ellison D, Angers S, et al. (2009). YAP1 is amplified and up-regulated in hedgehog-associated medulloblastomas and mediates Sonic hedgehog-driven neural precursor proliferation. Genes Dev. 23(23):2729–41. PMID:19952108
691. Ferner RE, Hughes RA, Hall SM, Upadhyaya M, Johnson MR (2004). Neurofibromatous neuropathy in neurofibromatosis 1 (NF1). J Med Genet. 41(11):837–41. PMID:15520408
692. Ferreri AJ, Dell'Oro S, Capello D, Ponzoni M, Iuzzolino P, Rossi D, et al. (2004). Aberrant methylation in the promoter region of the reduced folate carrier gene is a potential mechanism of resistance to methotrexate in primary central nervous system lymphomas. Br J Haematol. 126(5):657–64. PMID:15327516
693. Ferreri AJ, Reni M, Pasini F, Calderoni A, Tirelli U, Pivnik A, et al. (2002). A multicenter study of treatment of primary CNS lymphoma. Neurology. 58(10):1513–20. PMID:12034789
694. Ferry JA, Harris NL, Picker LJ, Weinberg DS, Rosales RK, Tapia J, et al. (1988). Intravascular lymphomatosis (malignant angioendotheliomatosis). A B-cell neoplasm expressing surface homing receptors. Mod Pathol. 1(6):444–52. PMID:3065781
695. Fetsch JF, Miettinen M (1997). Sclerosing perineurioma: a clinicopathologic study of 19 cases of a distinctive soft tissue lesion with a predilection for the fingers and palms of young adults. Am J Surg Pathol. 21(12):1433–42. PMID:9414186
696. Fèvre Montange M, Vasiljevic A, Bergemer Fouquet AM, Bernier M, Champier J, Chrétien F, et al. (2012). Histopathologic and ultrastructural features and claudin expression in papillary tumors of the pineal region: a multicenter analysis. Am J Surg Pathol. 36(6):916–28. PMID:22588068
697. Fèvre Montange M, Vasiljevic A, Champier J, Jouvet A (2015). Papillary tumor of the pineal region: Histopathological characterization and review of the literature. Neurochirurgie. 61(2-3):138–42 PMID:24556386
698. Fèvre-Montange M, Champier J, Szathmari A, Wierinckx A, Mottolese C, Guyotat J, et al. (2006). Microarray analysis reveals differential gene expression patterns in tumors of the pineal region. J Neuropathol Exp Neurol. 65(7):675–84. PMID:16825954
699. Fèvre-Montange M, Hasselblatt M, Figarella-Branger D, Chauveinc L, Champier J, Saint-Pierre G, et al. (2006). Prognosis and histopathologic features in papillary tumors of the pineal region: a retrospective multicenter study of 31 cases. J Neuropathol Exp Neurol. 65(10):1004–11. PMID:17021405
700. Fèvre-Montange M, Jouvet A, Privat K, Korf HW, Champier J, Reboul A, et al. (1998). Immunohistochemical, ultrastructural, biochemical and in vitro studies of a pineocytoma.

Acta Neuropathol. 95(5):532–9. PMID:9600600

701. Fèvre-Montange M, Szathmari A, Champier J, Mokhtari K, Chrétien F, Coulon A, et al. (2008). Pineocytoma and pineal parenchymal tumors of intermediate differentiation presenting cytologic pleomorphism: a multicenter study. Brain Pathol. 18(3):354–9. PMID:18371183

702. Fèvre-Montange M, Vasiljevic A, Frappaz D, Champier J, Szathmari A, Aubriot Lorton MH, et al. (2012). Utility of Ki67 immunostaining in the grading of pineal parenchymal tumours: a multicentre study. Neuropathol Appl Neurobiol. 38(1):87–94. PMID:21696422

703. Figarella-Branger D, Civatte M, Bouvier-Labit C, Gouvernet J, Gambarelli D, Gentet JC, et al. (2000). Prognostic factors in intracranial ependymomas in children. J Neurosurg. 93(4):605–13. PMID:11014538

704. Figarella-Branger D, Gambarelli D, Dollo C, Devictor B, Perez-Castillo AM, Genitori L, et al. (1991). Infratentorial ependymomas of childhood. Correlation between histological features, immunohistological phenotype, silver nucleolar organizer region staining values and post-operative survival in 16 cases. Acta Neuropathol. 82(3):208–16. PMID:1718129

705. Figarella-Branger D, Pellissier JF, Daumas-Duport C, Delisle MB, Pasquier B, Parent M, et al. (1992). Central neurocytomas. Critical evaluation of a small-cell neuronal tumor. Am J Surg Pathol. 16(2):97–109. PMID:1370756

706. Figueroa ME, Abdel-Wahab O, Lu C, Ward PS, Patel J, Shih A, et al. (2010). Leukemic IDH1 and IDH2 mutations result in a hypermethylation phenotype, disrupt TET2 function, and impair hematopoietic differentiation. Cancer Cell. 18(6):553–67. PMID:21130701

707. Fine SW, McClain SA, Li M (2004). Immunohistochemical staining for calretinin is useful for differentiating schwannomas from neurofibromas. Am J Clin Pathol. 122(4):552–9. PMID:15487453

708. Fischer I, Gagner JP, Law M, Newcomb EW, Zagzag D (2005). Angiogenesis in gliomas: biology and molecular pathophysiology. Brain Pathol. 15(4):297–310. PMID:16389942

709. Fisher PG, Breiter SN, Carson BS, Wharam MD, Williams JA, Weingart JD, et al. (2000). A clinicopathologic reappraisal of brain stem tumor classification. Identification of pilocystic astrocytoma and fibrillary astrocytoma as distinct entities. Cancer. 89(7):1569–76. PMID:11013373

710. Fix SE, Nelson J, Schochet SS Jr (1989). Focal leptomeningeal rhabdomyomatosis of the posterior fossa. Arch Pathol Lab Med. 113(8):872–3. PMID:2757487

711. Flament-Durand J, Brion JP (1985). Tanycytes: morphology and functions: a review. Int Rev Cytol. 96:121–55. PMID:2416706

712. Flamme I, Krieg M, Plate KH (1998). Up-regulation of vascular endothelial growth factor in stromal cells of hemangioblastomas is correlated with up-regulation of the transcription factor HRF/HIF-2alpha. Am J Pathol. 153(1):25–9. PMID:9665461

713. Flannery T, Cawley D, Zulfiger A, Alderazi Y, Heffernan J, Brett F, et al. (2008). Familial occurrence of oligodendroglial tumours. Br J Neurosurg. 22(3):436–8. PMID:18568735

713A. Flavahan WA, Drier Y, Liau BB, Gillespie SM, Venteicher AS, Stemmer-Rachamimov AO, et al. (2016). Insulator dysfunction and oncogene activation in IDH mutant gliomas. Nature. 529(7584):110–4. PMID:26700815

714. Fletcher CDM, Bridge JA, Hogendoorn PCW, Mertens F (2013). WHO Classification of Tumours of Soft Tissue and Bone. 4th ed. Lyon: IARC.

715. Fletcher CDM, Unni KK, Mertens F, editors. (2002). World Health Organization Classification of Tumours. Pathology and Genetics of Tumours of Soft Tissue and Bone. 3rd ed. Lyon: IARC Press.

716. Flint-Richter P, Mandelzweig L, Oberman B, Sadetzki S (2011). Possible interaction between ionizing radiation, smoking, and gender in the causation of meningioma. Neuro Oncol. 13(3):345–52. PMID:21339193

717. Flint-Richter P, Sadetzki S (2007). Genetic predisposition for the development of radiation-associated meningioma: an epidemiological study. Lancet Oncol. 8(5):403–10. PMID:17466897

718. Folpe AL (2014). Selected topics in the pathology of epithelioid soft tissue tumors. Mod Pathol. 27 Suppl 1:S64–79. PMID:24384854

719. Folpe AL, Billings SD, McKenney JK, Walsh SV, Nusrat A, Weiss SW (2002). Expression of claudin-1, a recently described tight junction-associated protein, distinguishes soft tissue perineurioma from potential mimics. Am J Surg Pathol. 26(12):1620–6. PMID:12459629

720. Font RL, Truong LD (1984). Melanotic schwannoma of soft tissues. Electron-microscopic observations and review of literature. Am J Surg Pathol. 8(2):129–38. PMID:6703189

721. Fontebasso AM, Papillon-Cavanagh S, Schwartzentruber J, Nikbakht H, Gerges N, Fiset PO, et al. (2014). Recurrent somatic mutations in ACVR1 in pediatric midline high-grade astrocytoma. Nat Genet. 46(5):462–6. PMID:24705250

722. Fontebasso AM, Schwartzentruber J, Khuong-Quang DA, Liu XY, Sturm D, Korshunov A, et al. (2013). Mutations in SETD2 and genes affecting histone H3K36 methylation target hemispheric high-grade gliomas. Acta Neuropathol. 125(5):659–69. PMID:23417712

723. Forest F, David A, Arrufat S, Pierron G, Ranchere-Vince D, Stephan JL, et al. (2012). Conventional chondrosarcoma in a survivor of rhabdoid tumor: enlarging the spectrum of tumors associated with SMARCB1 germline mutations. Am J Surg Pathol. 36(12):1892–6. PMID:23154773

724. Forshew T, Tatevossian RG, Lawson AR, Ma J, Neale G, Ogunkolade BW, et al. (2009). Activation of the ERK/MAPK pathway: a signature genetic defect in posterior fossa pilocytic astrocytomas. J Pathol. 218(2):172–81. PMID:19373855

725. Forsyth PA, Shaw EG, Scheithauer BW, O'Fallon JR, Layton DD Jr, Katzmann JA (1993). Supratentorial pilocytic astrocytomas. A clinicopathologic, prognostic, and flow cytometric study of 51 patients. Cancer. 72(4):1335–42. PMID:8339223

726. Foster RD, Williams ML, Barkovich AJ, Hoffman WY, Mathes SJ, Frieden IJ (2001). Giant congenital melanocytic nevi: the significance of neurocutaneous melanosis in neurologically asymptomatic children. Plast Reconstr Surg. 107(4):933–41. PMID:11252085

727. Fouladi M, Helton K, Dalton J, Gilger E, Gajjar A, Merchant T, et al. (2003). Clear cell ependymoma: a clinicopathologic and radiographic analysis of 10 patients. Cancer. 98(10):2232–44. PMID:14601094

728. Foulkes WD, Clarke BA, Hasselblatt M, Majewski J, Albrecht S, McCluggage WG (2014). No small surprise - small cell carcinoma of the ovary, hypercalcaemic type, is a malignant rhabdoid tumour. J Pathol. 233(3):209–14. PMID:24752781

729. Fountas KN, Karampelas I, Nikolakakos LG, Troup EC, Robinson JS (2005). Primary spinal cord oligodendroglioma: case report and review of the literature. Childs Nerv Syst. 21(2):171–5. PMID:15138790

730. Fowler M, Simpson DA (1962). A malignant melanin-forming tumour of the cerebellum. J Pathol Bacteriol. 84:307–11. PMID:13958991

731. Fox BD, Cheung VJ, Patel AJ, Suki D, Rao G (2011). Epidemiology of metastatic brain tumors. Neurosurg Clin N Am. 22(1):1–6, v. PMID:21109143

732. Francis JM, Zhang CZ, Maire CL, Jung J, Manzo VE, Adalsteinsson VA, et al. (2014). EGFR variant heterogeneity in glioblastoma resolved through single-nucleus sequencing. Cancer Discov. 4(8):956–71. PMID:24893890

732A. Franz DN, Belousova E, Sparagana S, Bebin EM, Frost M, Kuperman R, et al. (2013). Efficacy and safety of everolimus for subependymal giant cell astrocytomas associated with tuberous sclerosis complex (EXIST-1): a multicentre, randomised, placebo-controlled phase 3 trial. Lancet. 381(9861):125–32. PMID:23158522

733. Franz DN, Belousova E, Sparagana S, Bebin EM, Frost M, Kuperman R, et al. (2014). Everolimus for subependymal giant cell astrocytoma in patients with tuberous sclerosis complex: 2-year open-label extension of the randomised EXIST-1 study. Lancet Oncol. 15(13):1513–20. PMID:25456370

734. Frappaz D, Ricci AC, Kohler R, Bret P, Mottolese C (1999). Diffuse brain stem tumor in an adolescent with multiple enchondromatosis (Ollier's disease). Childs Nerv Syst. 15(5):222–5. PMID:10392492

735. Frattini V, Trifonov V, Chan JM, Castano A, Lia M, Abate F, et al. (2013). The integrated landscape of driver genomic alterations in glioblastoma. Nat Genet. 45(10):1141–9. PMID:23917401

736. Frebourg T, Barbier N, Yan YX, Garber JE, Dreyfus M, Fraumeni J Jr, et al. (1995). Germline p53 mutations in 15 families with Li-Fraumeni syndrome. Am J Hum Genet. 56(3):608–15. PMID:7887414

737. Freilich RJ, Thompson SJ, Walker RW, Rosenblum MK (1995). Adenocarcinomatous transformation of intracranial germ cell tumors. Am J Surg Pathol. 19(5):537–44. PMID:7726363

738. Frenk E, Marazzi A (1984). Neurofibromatosis of von Recklinghausen: a quantitative study of the epidermal keratinocyte and melanocyte populations. J Invest Dermatol. 83(1):23–5. PMID:6203987

739. Freudenstein D, Wagner A, Bornemann A, Ernemann U, Bauer T, Duffner F (2004). Primary melanocytic lesions of the CNS: report of five cases. Zentralbl Neurochir. 65(3):146–53. PMID:15306980

739A. Friedman JM. Neurofibromatosis 1. 1998 [Updated 2014 Sep 4]. In: Pagon RA, Adam MP, Ardinger HH, et al., editors. GeneReviews® [Internet]. Seattle (WA): University of Washington, Seattle; 1993–2016. Available from: http://www.ncbi.nlm.nih.gov/books/NBK1109/

740. Friedman JM, Arbiser J, Epstein JA, Gutmann DH, Huot SJ, Lin AE, et al. (2002). Cardiovascular disease in neurofibromatosis 1: report of the NF1 Cardiovascular Task Force. Genet Med. 4(3):105–11. PMID:12180143

741. Friedrich C, Warmuth-Metz M, von Bueren AO, Nowak J, Bison B, von Hoff K, et al. (2015). Primitive neuroectodermal tumors of the brainstem in children treated according to the HIT trials: clinical findings of a rare disease. J Neurosurg Pediatr. 15(3):227–35. PMID:25555122

742. Fritchie KJ, Carver P, Sun Y, Batiouchko G, Billings SD, Rubin BP, et al. (2012). Solitary fibrous tumor: is there a molecular relationship with cellular angiofibroma, spindle cell lipoma, and mammary-type myofibroblastoma? Am J Clin Pathol. 137(6):963–70. PMID:22586056

742A. Fritz A, Percy C, Jack A, Shanmugaratnam K, Sobin L, Parkin DM, et al. (2000). International Classification of Diseases for Oncology (ICD-O). Third edition. World Health Organization: Geneva.

743. Fruehwald-Pallamar J, Puchner SB, Rossi A, Garre ML, Cama A, Koelblinger C, et al. (2011). Magnetic resonance imaging spectrum of medulloblastoma. Neuroradiology. 53(6):387–96. PMID:21279509

744. Fryssira H, Leventopoulos G, Psoni S, Kitsiou-Tzeli S, Stavrianeas N, Kanavakis E (2008). Tumor development in three patients with Noonan syndrome. Eur J Pediatr. 167(9):1025–31. PMID:18057963

745. Fu YJ, Taniguchi Y, Takeuchi S, Shiga A, Okamoto K, Hirato J, et al. (2013). Cerebral astroblastoma in an adult: an immunohistochemical, ultrastructural and genetic study. Neuropathology. 33(3):312–9. PMID:22994361

746. Fu YS, Chen AT, Kay S, Young H (1974). Is subependymoma (subependymal glomerate astrocytoma) an astrocytoma or ependymoma? A comparative ultrastructural and tissue culture study. Cancer. 34(6):1992–2008. PMID:4434329

746A. Fujii K, Miyashita T (2014). Gorlin syndrome (nevoid basal cell carcinoma syndrome): update and literature review. Pediatr Int. 56(5):667–74. PMID:25131638

747. Fujii K, Ohashi H, Suzuki M, Hatsuse H, Shiohama T, Uchikawa H, et al. (2013). Frameshift mutation in the PTCH2 gene can cause nevoid basal cell carcinoma syndrome. Fam Cancer. 12(4):611–4. PMID:23479190

748. Fujimaki T, Matsutani M, Funada N, Kirino T, Takakura K, Nakamura O, et al. (1994). CT and MRI features of intracranial germ cell tumors. J Neurooncol. 19(3):217–26. PMID:7807172

749. Fujimoto K, Ohnishi H, Tsujimoto M, Hoshida T, Nakazato Y (2000). Dysembryoplastic neuroepithelial tumor of the cerebellum and brainstem. Case report. J Neurosurg. 93(3):487–9. PMID:10969950

750. Fujisawa H, Kurrer M, Reis RM, Yonekawa Y, Kleihues P, Ohgaki H (1999). Acquisition of the glioblastoma phenotype during astrocytoma progression is associated with loss of heterozygosity on 10q25-qter. Am J Pathol. 155(2):387–94. PMID:10433932

751. Fujisawa H, Marukawa K, Hasegawa M, Tohma Y, Hayashi Y, Uchiyama N, et al. (2002). Genetic differences between neurocytoma and dysembryoplastic neuroepithelial tumor and oligodendroglial tumors. J Neurosurg. 97(6):1350–5. PMID:12507133

752. Fujisawa H, Reis RM, Nakamura M, Colella S, Yonekawa Y, Kleihues P, et al. (2000). Loss of heterozygosity on chromosome 10 is more extensive in primary (de novo) than in secondary glioblastomas. Lab Invest. 80(1):65–72. PMID:10653004

753. Fujisawa H, Tohma Y, Muramatsu N, Kida S, Kaizaki Y, Tamamura H (2012). Spindle cell oncocytoma of the adenohypophysis with marked hypervascularity. Case report. Neurol Med Chir (Tokyo). 52(8):594–8. PMID:22976144

754. Fukuda T, Akiyama N, Ikegami M, Takahashi H, Sasaki A, Oka H, et al. (2010). Expression of hydroxyindole-O-methyltransferase enzyme in the human central nervous system and in pineal parenchymal cell tumors. J Neuropathol Exp Neurol. 69(5):498–510. PMID:20418777

755. Fukuda T, Yasumichi K, Suzuki T (2008). Immunohistochemistry of gliosarcoma with liposarcomatous differentiation. Pathol Int. 58(6):396–401. PMID:18477220

756. Fukunaga M (2001). Unusual malignant perineurioma of soft tissue. Virchows Arch. 439(2):212–4. PMID:11561764

757. Fukuoka K, Sasaki A, Yanagisawa T, Suzuki T, Wakiya K, Adachi J, et al. (2012). Pineal parenchymal tumor of intermediate differentiation with marked elevation of MIB-1 labeling index. Brain Tumor Pathol. 29(4):229–34. PMID:22362162

758. Fukushima S, Otsuka A, Suzuki T, Yanagisawa T, Mishima K, Mukasa A, et al.; Intracranial Germ Cell Tumor Genome Analysis Consortium (iGCT Consortium) (2014). Mutually exclusive mutations of KIT and RAS are associated with KIT mRNA expression and chromosomal instability in primary intracranial pure germinomas. Acta Neuropathol. 127(6):911–25. PMID:24452629

759. Fukushima S, Yoshida A, Narita Y, Arita H, Ohno M, Miyakita Y, et al. (2015). Multinodular and vacuolating neuronal tumor of the cerebrum. Brain Tumor Pathol. 32(2):131–6.

PMID:25146549
760. Fuld AD, Speck ME, Harris BT, Simmons NE, Corless CL, Tsongalis GJ, et al. (2011). Primary melanoma of the spinal cord: a case report, molecular footprint, and review of the literature. J Clin Oncol. 29(17):e499–502. PMID:21444862
761. Fulham MJ, Melisi JW, Nishimiya J, Dwyer AJ, Di Chiro G (1993). Neuroimaging of juvenile pilocytic astrocytomas: an enigma. Radiology. 189(1):221–5. PMID:8372197
762. Fuller C, Fouladi M, Gajjar A, Dalton J, Sanford RA, Helton KJ (2006). Chromosome 17 abnormalities in pediatric neuroblastic tumor with abundant neuropil and true rosettes. Am J Clin Pathol. 126(2):277–83. PMID:16891204
763. Fuller CE, Perry A (2002). Fluorescence in situ hybridization (FISH) in diagnostic and investigative neuropathology. Brain Pathol. 12(1):67–86. PMID:11770903
764. Fuller GN, Bigner SH (1992). Amplified cellular oncogenes in neoplasms of the human central nervous system. Mutat Res. 276(3):299–306. PMID:1374522
765. Fuller GN, Hess KR, Rhee CH, Yung WK, Sawaya RA, Bruner JM, et al. (2002). Molecular classification of human diffuse gliomas by multidimensional scaling analysis of gene expression profiles parallels morphology-based classification, correlates with survival, and reveals clinically-relevant novel glioma subsets. Brain Pathol. 12(1):108–16. PMID:11771519
766. Fung KM, Fang W, Norton RE, Torres N, Chu A, Langford LA (2003). Cerebellar central liponeurocytoma. Ultrastruct Pathol. 27(2):109–14. PMID:12746202
767. Furnari FB, Huang HJ, Cavenee WK (1998). The phosphoinositol phosphatase activity of PTEN mediates a serum-sensitive G1 growth arrest in glioma cells. Cancer Res. 58(22):5002–8. PMID:9823298
768. Furnari FB, Lin H, Huang HS, Cavenee WK (1997). Growth suppression of glioma cells by PTEN requires a functional phosphatase catalytic domain. Proc Natl Acad Sci U S A. 94(23):12479–84. PMID:9356475
769. Furtado A, Arantes M, Silva R, Romao H, Resende M, Honavar M (2010). Comprehensive review of extraventricular neurocytoma with report of two cases, and comparison with central neurocytoma. Clin Neuropathol. 29(3):134–40. PMID:20423686
770. Furuya K, Takanashi S, Ogawa A, Takahashi Y, Nakagomi T (2014). High-dose methotrexate monotherapy followed by radiation for CD30-positive, anaplastic lymphoma kinase-1-positive anaplastic large-cell lymphoma in the brain of a child. J Neurosurg Pediatr. 14(3):311–5. PMID:25014324
771. Gabeau-Lacet D, Aghi M, Betensky RA, Barker FG, Loeffler JS, Louis DN (2009). Bone involvement predicts poor outcome in atypical meningioma. J Neurosurg. 111(3):464–71. PMID:19267533
772. Gadish T, Tulchinsky H, Deutsch AA, Rabau M (2005). Pinealoblastoma in a patient with familial adenomatous polyposis: variant of Turcot syndrome type 2? Report of a case and review of the literature. Dis Colon Rectum. 48(12):2343–6. PMID:16400511
773. Gaffney EF, Doorly T, Dinn JJ (1986). Aggressive oncocytic neuroendocrine tumour ('oncocytic paraganglioma') of the cauda equina. Histopathology. 10(3):311–9. PMID:2422107
774. Gailani MR, Ståhle-Bäckdahl M, Leffell DJ, Glynn M, Zaphiropoulos PG, Pressman C, et al. (1996). The role of the human homologue of Drosophila patched in sporadic basal cell carcinomas. Nat Genet. 14(1):78–81. PMID:8782823
775. Gajjar A, Bhargava R, Jenkins JJ, Heideman R, Sanford RA, Langston JW, et al. (1995). Low-grade astrocytoma with neuraxis dissemination at diagnosis. J Neurosurg. 83(1):67–71. PMID:7782852
776. Gajjar A, Packer RJ, Foreman NK, Cohen K, Haas-Kogan D, Merchant TE; COG Brain Tumor Committee (2013). Children's Oncology Group's 2013 blueprint for research: central nervous system tumors. Pediatr Blood Cancer. 60(6):1022–6. PMID:23255213
777. Gajjar A, Pfister SM, Taylor MD, Gilbertson RJ (2014). Molecular insights into pediatric brain tumors have the potential to transform therapy. Clin Cancer Res. 20(22):5630–40. PMID:25398846
778. Galan SR, Kann PH (2013). Genetics and molecular pathogenesis of pheochromocytoma and paraganglioma. Clin Endocrinol (Oxf). 78(2):165–75. PMID:23061808
779. Galanis E, Buckner JC, Dinapoli RP, Scheithauer BW, Jenkins RB, Wang CH, et al. (1998). Clinical outcome of gliosarcoma compared with glioblastoma multiforme: North Central Cancer Treatment Group results. J Neurosurg. 89(3):425–30. PMID:9724117
780. Galli R, Binda E, Orfanelli U, Cipelletti B, Gritti A, De Vitis S, et al. (2004). Isolation and characterization of tumorigenic, stem-like neural precursors from human glioblastoma. Cancer Res. 64(19):7011–21. PMID:15466194
781. Gallina P, Buccoliero AM, Mariotti F, Mennonna P, Di Lorenzo N (2006). Oncocytic meningiomas: Cases with benign histopathological features and a favorable clinical course. J Neurosurg. 105(5):736–8. PMID:17121136
782. Gao J, Aksoy BA, Dogrusoz U, Dresdner G, Gross B, Sumer SO, et al. (2013). Integrative analysis of complex cancer genomics and clinical profiles using the cBioPortal. Sci Signal. 6(269):pl1. PMID:23550210
783. Gao X, Zhang Y, Arrazola P, Hino O, Kobayashi T, Yeung RS, et al. (2002). Tsc tumour suppressor proteins antagonize amino-acid-TOR signalling. Nat Cell Biol. 4(9):699–704. PMID:12172555
784. Garcia DM, Fulling KH (1985). Juvenile pilocytic astrocytoma of the cerebrum in adults. A distinctive neoplasm with favorable prognosis. J Neurosurg. 63(3):382–6. PMID:4020465
785. Garcia-Lavandeira M, Saez C, Diaz-Rodriguez E, Perez-Romero S, Senra A, Dieguez C, et al. (2012). Craniopharyngiomas express embryonic stem cell markers (SOX2, OCT4, KLF4, and SOX9) as pituitary stem cells but do not coexpress RET/GFRA3 receptors. J Clin Endocrinol Metab. 97(1):E80–7. PMID:22031517
786. Gardiman MP, Fassan M, Orvieto E, D'Avella D, Denaro L, Calderone M, et al. (2010). Diffuse leptomeningeal glioneuronal tumors: a new entity? Brain Pathol. 20(2):361–6. PMID:19486008
787. Garrè ML, Cama A, Bagnasco F, Morana G, Giangaspero F, Brisigotti M, et al. (2009). Medulloblastoma variants: age-dependent occurrence and relation to Gorlin syndrome–a new clinical perspective. Clin Cancer Res. 15(7):2463–71. PMID:19276247
788. Gasco J, Franklin B, Fuller GN, Salinas P, Prabhu S (2009). Multifocal epithelioid glioblastoma mimicking cerebral metastasis: case report. Neurocirugia (Astur). 20(6):550–4. PMID:19967320
789. Gaspar LE, Mackenzie IR, Gilbert JJ, Kaufmann JC, Fisher BF, Macdonald DR, et al. (1993). Primary cerebral fibrosarcomas. Clinicopathologic study and review of the literature. Cancer. 72(11):3277–81. PMID:8242554
790. Gaston-Massuet C, Andoniadou CL, Signore M, Jayakody SA, Charolidi N, Kyeyune R, et al. (2011). Increased Wingless (Wnt) signaling in pituitary progenitor/stem cells gives rise to pituitary tumors in mice and humans. Proc Natl Acad Sci U S A. 108(28):11482–7. PMID:21636786
791. Gatta G, Botta L, Rossi S, Aareleid T, Bielska-Lasota M, Clavel J, et al.; EUROCARE Working Group (2014). Childhood cancer survival in Europe 1999–2007: results of EUROCARE-5–a population-based study. Lancet Oncol. 15(1):35–47. PMID:24314616
792. Gavrilovic IT, Posner JB (2005). Brain metastases: epidemiology and pathophysiology. J Neurooncol. 75(1):5–14. PMID:16215811
793. Geddes JF, Thom M, Robinson SF, Révész T (1996). Granular cell change in astrocytic tumors. Am J Surg Pathol. 20(1):55–63. PMID:8540609
794. Gelabert-González M (2005). Paragangliomas of the lumbar region. Report of two cases and review of the literature. J Neurosurg Spine. 2(3):354–65. PMID:15796363
795. Gempt J, Baldawa SS, Weirich G, Delbridge C, Hempel M, Lohse P, et al. (2013). Recurrent multiple spinal paragangliomas as a manifestation of a metastatic composite paraganglioma-ganglioneuroblastoma. Acta Neurochir (Wien). 155(7):1241–2. PMID:23532344
796. Gempt J, Ringel F, Oexle K, Delbridge C, Förschler A, Schlegel J, et al. (2012). Familial pineocytoma. Acta Neurochir (Wien). 154(8):1413–6. PMID:22699425
797. George DH, Scheithauer BW, Aker FV, Kurtin PJ, Burger PC, Cameselle-Teijeiro J, et al. (2003). Primary anaplastic large cell lymphoma of the central nervous system: prognostic effect of ALK-1 expression. Am J Surg Pathol. 27(4):487–93. PMID:12657933
798. Gerson SL (2004). MGMT: its role in cancer aetiology and cancer therapeutics. Nat Rev Cancer. 4(4):296–307. PMID:15057289
799. Gerstner ER, Abrey LE, Schiff D, Ferreri AJ, Lister A, Montoto S, et al. (2008). CNS Hodgkin lymphoma. Blood. 112(5):1658–61. PMID:18591379
800. Gessi M, Abdel Moneim Y, Hammes J, Waha A, Pietsch T (2014). FGFR1 N546K mutation in a case of papillary glioneuronal tumor (PGNT). Acta Neuropathol. 127(6):935–6. PMID:24777483
801. Gessi M, Giangaspero F, Lauriola L, Gardiman M, Scheithauer BW, Halliday W, et al. (2009). Embryonal tumors with abundant neuropil and true rosettes: a distinctive CNS primitive neuroectodermal tumor. Am J Surg Pathol. 33(2):211–7. PMID:18987548
802. Gessi M, Giangaspero F, Pietsch T (2003). Atypical teratoid/rhabdoid tumors and choroid plexus tumors: when genetics "surprise" pathology. Brain Pathol. 13(3):409–14. PMID:12946029
803. Gessi M, Lambert SR, Lauriola L, Waha A, Collins VP, Pietsch T (2012). Absence of KIAA1549-BRAF fusion in rosette-forming glioneuronal tumors of the fourth ventricle (RGNT). J Neurooncol. 110(1):21–5. PMID:22814862
804. Gessi M, Moneim YA, Hammes J, Goschzik T, Scholz M, Denkhaus D, et al. (2014). FGFR1 mutations in Rosette-forming glioneuronal tumors of the fourth ventricle. J Neuropathol Exp Neurol. 73(6):580–4. PMID:24806303
805. Gessi M, Setty P, Bisceglia M, zur Muehlen A, Lauriola L, Waha A, et al. (2011). Supratentorial primitive neuroectodermal tumors of the central nervous system in adults: molecular and histopathologic analysis of 12 cases. Am J Surg Pathol. 35(4):573–82. PMID:21378543
806. Gessi M, von Bueren A, Treszl A, zur Mühlen A, Hartmann W, Warmuth-Metz M, et al. (2014). MYCN amplification predicts poor outcome for patients with supratentorial primitive neuroectodermal tumors of the central nervous system. Neuro Oncol. 16(7):924–32. PMID:24470553
807. Gessi M, Waha A, Setty P, Waha A, Pietsch T (2011). Analysis of KIAA1549-BRAF fusion status in a case of rosette-forming glioneuronal tumor of the fourth ventricle (RGNT). Neuropathology. 31(6):654–7. PMID:21518014
808. Gessi M, Zur Mühlen A, Hammes J, Waha A, Denkhaus D, Pietsch T (2013). Genome-wide DNA copy number analysis of desmoplastic infantile astrocytomas and desmoplastic infantile gangliogliomas. J Neuropathol Exp Neurol. 72(9):807–15. PMID:23965740
809. Geyer JR, Sposto R, Jennings M, Boyett JM, Axtell RA, Breiger D, et al.; Children's Cancer Group (2005). Multiagent chemotherapy and deferred radiotherapy in infants with malignant brain tumors: a report from the Children's Cancer Group. J Clin Oncol. 23(30):7621–31. PMID:16234523
810. Geyer JR, Zeltzer PM, Boyett JM, Rorke LB, Stanley P, Albright AL, et al. (1994). Survival of infants with primitive neuroectodermal tumors or malignant ependymomas of the CNS treated with eight drugs in 1 day: a report from the Childrens Cancer Group. J Clin Oncol. 12(8):1607–15. PMID:8040673
811. Gherardi R, Baudrimont M, Nguyen JP, Gaston A, Cesaro P, Degos JD, et al. (1986). Monstrocellular heavily lipidized malignant glioma. Acta Neuropathol. 69(1-2):28–32. PMID:3515829
812. Gheyi V, Hui FK, Doppenberg EM, Todd W, Broaddus WC (2004). Glioblastoma multiforme causing calvarial destruction: an unusual manifestation revisited. AJNR Am J Neuroradiol. 25(9):1533–7. PMID:15502132
813. Ghia AJ, Allen PK, Mahajan A, Penas-Prado M, McCutcheon IE, Brown PD (2013). Intracranial hemangiopericytoma and the role of radiation therapy: a population based analysis. Neurosurgery. 72(2):203–9. PMID:23149953
814. Ghia AJ, Chang EL, Allen PK, Mahajan A, Penas-Prado M, McCutcheon IE, et al. (2013). Intracranial hemangiopericytoma: patterns of failure and the role of radiation therapy. Neurosurgery. 73(4):624–30, discussion 630–1. PMID:23839520
815. Ghose A, Guha G, Kundu R, Tew J, Chaudhary R (2014). CNS Hemangiopericytoma: A Systematic Review of 523 Patients. Am J Clin Oncol. PMID:25350465
816. Giangaspero F, Cenacchi G, Losi L, Cerasoli S, Bisceglia M, Burger PC (1997). Extraventricular neoplasms with neurocytoma features. A clinicopathological study of 11 cases. Am J Surg Pathol. 21(2):206–12. PMID:9042288
817. Giangaspero F, Cenacchi G, Roncaroli F, Rigobello L, Manetto V, Gambacorta M, et al. (1996). Medullocytoma (lipidized medulloblastoma). A cerebellar neoplasm of adults with favorable prognosis. Am J Surg Pathol. 20(6):656–64. PMID:8651344
818. Giangaspero F, Chieco P, Ceccarelli C, Lisignoli G, Pozzuoli R, Gambacorta M, et al. (1991). "Desmoplastic" versus "classic" medulloblastoma: comparison of DNA content, histopathology and differentiation. Virchows Arch A Pathol Anat Histopathol. 418(3):207–14. PMID:1900966
819. Giangaspero F, Guiducci A, Lenz FA, Mastronardi L, Burger PC (1999). Meningioma with meningioangiomatosis: a condition mimicking invasive meningiomas in children and young adults: report of two cases and review of the literature. Am J Surg Pathol. 23(8):872–5. PMID:10435554
820. Giangaspero F, Perilongo G, Fondelli MP, Brisigotti M, Carollo C, Burnelli R, et al. (1999). Medulloblastoma with extensive nodularity: a variant with favorable prognosis. J Neurosurg. 91(6):971–7. PMID:10584843
821. Giangaspero F, Rigobello L, Badiali M, Loda M, Andreini L, Basso G, et al. (1992). Large-cell medulloblastomas. A distinct variant with highly aggressive behavior. Am J Surg Pathol. 16(7):687–93. PMID:1530108
822. Giangaspero F, Wellek S, Masuoka J, Gessi M, Kleihues P, Ohgaki H (2006). Stratification of medulloblastoma on the basis of histopathological grading. Acta Neuropathol. 112(1):5–12. PMID:16685513
823. Giannini C, Fratkin JD, Wyatt-Ashmead J, Aleff PC (2014). Rhabdoid-like meningioma with inclusions consisting of accumulations of complex interdigitating cell processes rather than intermediate filaments. Acta Neuropathol.

127(6):937–9. PMID:24691783
824. Giannini C, Hebrink D, Scheithauer BW, Dei Tos AP, James CD (2001). Analysis of p53 mutation and expression in pleomorphic xanthoastrocytoma. Neurogenetics. 3(3):159–62. PMID:11523567
825. Giannini C, Scheithauer BW, Burger PC, Brat DJ, Wollan PC, Lach B, et al. (1999). Pleomorphic xanthoastrocytoma: what do we really know about it? Cancer. 85(9):2033–45. PMID:10223246
826. Giannini C, Scheithauer BW, Burger PC, Christensen MR, Wollan PC, Sebo TJ, et al. (1999). Cellular proliferation in pilocytic and diffuse astrocytomas. J Neuropathol Exp Neurol. 58(1):46–53. PMID:10068313
827. Giannini C, Scheithauer BW, Jenkins RB, Erlandson RA, Perry A, Borell TJ, et al. (1997). Soft-tissue perineurioma. Evidence for an abnormality of chromosome 22, criteria for diagnosis, and review of the literature. Am J Surg Pathol. 21(2):164–73. PMID:9042282
828. Giannini C, Scheithauer BW, Lopes MB, Hirose T, Kros JM, VandenBerg SR (2002). Immunophenotype of pleomorphic xanthoastrocytoma. Am J Surg Pathol. 26(4):479–85. PMID:11914626
829. Giannini C, Scheithauer BW, Steinberg J, Cosgrove TJ (1998). Intraventricular perineurioma: case report. Neurosurgery. 43(6):1478–81, discussion 1481–2. PMID:9848865
830. Giannini C, Scheithauer BW, Weaver AL, Burger PC, Kros JM, Mork S, et al. (2001). Oligodendrogliomas: reproducibility and prognostic value of histologic diagnosis and grading. J Neuropathol Exp Neurol. 60(3):248–62. PMID:11245209
831. Gibson P, Tong Y, Robinson G, Thompson MC, Currle DS, Eden C, et al. (2010). Subtypes of medulloblastoma have distinct developmental origins. Nature. 468(7327):1095–9. PMID:21150899
832. Gielen GH, Gessi M, Buttarelli FR, Baldi C, Hammes J, zur Muehlen A, et al. (2015). Genetic Analysis of Diffuse High-Grade Astrocytomas in Infancy Defines a Novel Molecular Entity. Brain Pathol. 25(4):409–17 PMID:25231549
833. Gielen GH, Gessi M, Hammes J, Kramm CM, Waha A, Pietsch T (2013). H3F3A K27M mutation in pediatric CNS tumors: a marker for diffuse high-grade astrocytomas. Am J Clin Pathol. 139(3):345–9. PMID:23429371
834. Giese A, Bjerkvig R, Berens ME, Westphal M (2003). Cost of migration: invasion of malignant gliomas and implications for treatment. J Clin Oncol. 21(8):1624–36. PMID:12697889
835. Giese A, Loo MA, Tran N, Haskett D, Coons SW, Berens ME (1996). Dichotomy of astrocytoma migration and proliferation. Int J Cancer. 67(2):275–82. PMID:8760599
836. Gil-Gouveia R, Cristino N, Farias JP, Trindade A, Ruivo NS, Pimentel J (2004). Pleomorphic xanthoastrocytoma of the cerebellum: illustrated review. Acta Neurochir (Wien). 146(11):1241–4. PMID:15455217
837. Gilbert MR, Dignam JJ, Armstrong TS, Wefel JS, Blumenthal DT, Vogelbaum MA, et al. (2014). A randomized trial of bevacizumab for newly diagnosed glioblastoma. N Engl J Med. 370(8):699–708. PMID:24552317
838. Gilbert MR, Wang M, Aldape KD, Stupp R, Hegi ME, Jaeckle KA, et al. (2013). Dose-dense temozolomide for newly diagnosed glioblastoma: a randomized phase III clinical trial. J Clin Oncol. 31(32):4085–91. PMID:24101040
839. Gilbertson RJ, Ellison DW (2008). The origins of medulloblastoma subtypes. Annu Rev Pathol. 3:341–65. PMID:18039127
840. Gill AJ, Benn DE, Chou A, Clarkson A, Muljono A, Meyer-Rochow GY, et al. (2010). Immunohistochemistry for SDHB triages genetic testing of SDHB, SDHC, and SDHD in paraganglioma-pheochromocytoma syndromes. Hum Pathol. 41(6):805–14. PMID:20236688
841. Gill AJ, Hes O, Papathomas T, Šedivcová M, Tan PH, Agaimy A, et al. (2014). Succinate dehydrogenase (SDH)-deficient renal carcinoma: a morphologically distinct entity: a clinicopathologic series of 36 tumors from 27 patients. Am J Surg Pathol. 38(12):1588–602. PMID:25025441
842. Gimm O, Attié-Bitach T, Lees JA, Vekemans M, Eng C (2000). Expression of the PTEN tumour suppressor protein during human development. Hum Mol Genet. 9(11):1633–9. PMID:10861290
843. Giorgianni A, Pellegrino C, De Benedictis A, Mercuri A, Baruzzi F, Minotto R, et al. (2013). Lhermitte-Duclos disease. A case report. Neuroradiol J. 26(6):655–60. PMID:24355184
844. Gire J, Deveze A, Garcia S, Menelli C, Curto CL, Tardivet L, et al. (2008). [Paraganglioma of the cerebellopontine angle: report of two cases]. Rev Laryngol Otol Rhinol (Bord). 129(3):213–6. PMID:19694167
845. Giulioni M, Galassi E, Zucchelli M, Volpi L (2005). Seizure outcome of lesionectomy in glioneuronal tumors associated with epilepsy in children. J Neurosurg. 102(3) Suppl:288–93. PMID:15881752
846. Gjerris F, Agerlin N, Børgesen SE, Buhl L, Haase J, Klinken L, et al. (1998). Epidemiology and prognosis in children treated for intracranial tumours in Denmark 1960–1984. Childs Nerv Syst. 14(7):302–11. PMID:9726580
847. Gjerris F, Klinken L (1978). Long-term prognosis in children with benign cerebellar astrocytoma. J Neurosurg. 49(2):179–84. PMID:671072
848. Gleissner B, Chamberlain MC (2006). Neoplastic meningitis. Lancet Neurol. 5(5):443–52. PMID:16632315
849. Glick R, Baker C, Husain S, Hays A, Hibshoosh H (1997). Primary melanocytomas of the spinal cord: a report of seven cases. Clin Neuropathol. 16(3):127–32. PMID:9197936
850. Gläsker S, Bender BU, Apel TW, Natt E, van Velthoven V, Scheremet R, et al. (1999). The impact of molecular genetic analysis of the VHL gene in patients with haemangioblastomas of the central nervous system. J Neurol Neurosurg Psychiatry. 67(6):758–62. PMID:10567493
851. Gläsker S, Bender BU, Apel TW, van Velthoven V, Mulligan LM, Zentner J, et al. (2001). Reconsideration of biallelic inactivation of the VHL tumour suppressor gene in hemangioblastomas of the central nervous system. J Neurol Neurosurg Psychiatry. 70(5):644–8. PMID:11309459
852. Gläsker S, Berlis A, Pagenstecher A, Vougioukas VI, Van Velthoven V (2005). Characterization of hemangioblastomas of spinal nerves. Neurosurgery. 56(3):503–9, discussion 503–9. PMID:15730575
853. Gläsker S, Krüger MT, Klingler JH, Wlodarski M, Klompen J, Schatlo B, et al. (2013). Hemangioblastomas and neurogenic polyglobulia. Neurosurgery. 72(6):930–5, discussion 935. PMID:23407287
854. Gläsker S, Li J, Xia JB, Okamoto H, Zeng W, Lonser RR, et al. (2006). Hemangioblastomas share protein expression with embryonal hemangioblast progenitor cell. Cancer Res. 66(8):4167–72. PMID:16618738
855. Gläsker S, Van Velthoven V (2005). Risk of hemorrhage in hemangioblastomas of the central nervous system. Neurosurgery. 57(1):71–6, discussion 71–6. PMID:15987542
856. Godfraind C (2009). Classification and controversies in pathology of ependymomas. Childs Nerv Syst. 25(10):1185–93. PMID:19212775
857. Godfraind C, Kaczmarska JM, Kocak M, Dalton J, Wright KD, Sanford RA, et al. (2012). Distinct disease-risk groups in pediatric supratentorial and posterior fossa ependymomas. Acta Neuropathol. 124(2):247–57. PMID:22526017
858. Goebel HH, Cravioto H (1972). Ultrastructure of human and experimental ependymomas. A comparative study. J Neuropathol Exp Neurol. 31(1):54–71. PMID:5060130
859. Goellner JR, Laws ER Jr, Soule EH, Okazaki H (1978). Hemangiopericytoma of the meninges. Mayo Clinic experience. Am J Clin Pathol. 70(3):375–80. PMID:707404
860. Goerig M (1990). [Comments on the paper by J.-P. Jantzen et al. An active charcoal filter for removing volatile anesthetics]. Anaesthesist. 39(12):637–9. PMID:2073047
861. Gold JS, Antonescu CR, Hajdu C, Ferrone CR, Hussain M, Lewis JJ, et al. (2002). Clinicopathologic correlates of solitary fibrous tumors. Cancer. 94(4):1057–68. PMID:11920476
862. Goldman JE, Corbin E (1991). Rosenthal fibers contain ubiquitinated alpha B-crystallin. Am J Pathol. 139(4):933–8. PMID:1656764
863. Gomez MR (1991). Phenotypes of the tuberous sclerosis complex with a revision of diagnostic criteria. Ann N Y Acad Sci. 615:1–7. PMID:2039135
864. Gonzalez KD, Noltner KA, Buzin CH, Gu D, Wen-Fong CY, Nguyen VQ, et al. (2009). Beyond Li Fraumeni Syndrome: clinical characteristics of families with p53 germline mutations. J Clin Oncol. 27(8):1250–6. PMID:19204208
865. Gonzalez-Aguilar A, Idbaih A, Boisselier B, Habbita N, Rossetto M, Laurenge A, et al. (2012). Recurrent mutations of MYD88 and TBL1XR1 in primary central nervous system lymphomas. Clin Cancer Res. 18(19):5203–11. PMID:22837180
866. González-Cámpora R, Weller RO (1998). Lipidized mature neuroectodermal tumour of the cerebellum with myoid differentiation. Neuropathol Appl Neurobiol. 24(5):397–402. PMID:9821171
867. Goodrich LV, Milenković L, Higgins KM, Scott MP (1997). Altered neural cell fates and medulloblastoma in mouse patched mutants. Science. 277(5329):1109–13. PMID:9262482
868. Goodrich LV, Scott MP (1998). Hedgehog and patched in neural development and disease. Neuron. 21(6):1243–57. PMID:9883719
869. Gorlin RJ (1987). Nevoid basal-cell carcinoma syndrome. Medicine (Baltimore). 66(2):98–113. PMID:3547011
870. Gorovets D, Kannan K, Shen R, Kastenhuber ER, Islamdoust N, Campos C, et al. (2012). IDH mutation and neuroglial developmental features define clinically distinct subclasses of lower grade diffuse astrocytic glioma. Clin Cancer Res. 18(9):2490–501. PMID:22415316
871. Górski GK, McMorrow LE, Donaldson MH, Freed M (1992). Multiple chromosomal abnormalities in a case of craniopharyngioma. Cancer Genet Cytogenet. 60(2):212–3. PMID:1606570
872. Goschzik T, Gessi M, Denkhaus D, Pietsch T (2014). PTEN mutations and activation of the PI3K/Akt/mTOR signaling pathway in papillary tumors of the pineal region. J Neuropathol Exp Neurol. 73(8):747–51. PMID:25003235
873. Gossage L, Eisen T, Maher ER (2015). VHL, the story of a tumour suppressor gene. Nat Rev Cancer. 15(1):55–64. PMID:25533676
874. Goto J, Talos DM, Klein P, Qin W, Chekaluk YI, Anderl S, et al. (2011). Regulable neural progenitor-specific Tsc1 loss yields giant cells with organellar dysfunction in a model of tuberous sclerosis complex. Proc Natl Acad Sci U S A. 108(45):E1070–9. PMID:22025691
875. Gould VE, Rorke LB, Jansson DS, Molenaar WM, Trojanowski JQ, Lee VM, et al. (1990). Primitive neuroectodermal tumors of the central nervous system express neuroendocrine markers and may express all classes of intermediate filaments. Hum Pathol. 21(3):245–52. PMID:2155868
876. Goutagny S, Nault JC, Mallet M, Henin D, Rossi JZ, Kalamarides M (2014). High incidence of activating TERT promoter mutations in meningiomas undergoing malignant progression. Brain Pathol. 24(2):184–9. PMID:24261697
877. Goutagny S, Yang HW, Zucman-Rossi J, Chan J, Dreyfuss JM, Park PJ, et al. (2010). Genomic profiling reveals alternative genetic pathways of meningioma malignant progression dependent on the underlying NF2 status. Clin Cancer Res. 16(16):4155–64. PMID:20682713
878. Gozali AE, Britt B, Shane L, Gonzalez I, Gilles F, McComb JG, et al. (2012). Choroid plexus tumors; management, outcome, and association with the Li-Fraumeni syndrome: the Children's Hospital Los Angeles (CHLA) experience, 1991–2010. Pediatr Blood Cancer. 58(6):905–9. PMID:21990040
879. Graadt van Roggen JF, McMenamin ME, Belchis DA, Nielsen GP, Rosenberg AE, Fletcher CD (2001). Reticular perineurioma: a distinctive variant of soft tissue perineurioma. Am J Surg Pathol. 25(4):485–93. PMID:11257623
880. Grabb PA, Albright AL, Pang D (1992). Dissemination of supratentorial malignant gliomas via the cerebrospinal fluid in children. Neurosurgery. 30(1):64–71. PMID:1738457
882. Graham DI, Lantos PL, editors. (2002). Greenfield's Neuropathology. 7th ed. London: Arnold.
883. Grajkowska W, Kotulska K, Jurkiewicz E, Roszkowski M, Daszkiewicz P, Jóźwiak S, et al. (2011). Subependymal giant cell astrocytomas with atypical histological features mimicking malignant gliomas. Folia Neuropathol. 49(1):39–46. PMID:21455842
884. Grammel D, Warmuth-Metz M, von Bueren AO, Kool M, Pietsch T, Kretzschmar HA, et al. (2012). Sonic hedgehog-associated medulloblastoma arising from the cochlear nuclei of the brainstem. Acta Neuropathol. 123(4):601–14. PMID:22349907
885. Grant JW, Steart PV, Aguzzi A, Jones DB, Gallagher PJ (1989). Gliosarcoma: an immunohistochemical study. Acta Neuropathol. 79(3):305–9. PMID:2609937
886. Gravendeel LA, Kouwenhoven MC, Gevaert O, de Rooi JJ, Stubbs AP, Duijm JE, et al. (2009). Intrinsic gene expression profiles of gliomas are a better predictor of survival than histology. Cancer Res. 69(23):9065–72. PMID:19920198
887. Griffin CA, Burger P, Morsberger L, Yonescu R, Swierczynski S, Weingart JD, et al. (2006). Identification of der(1;19)(q10;p10) in five oligodendrogliomas suggests mechanism of concurrent 1p and 19q loss. J Neuropathol Exp Neurol. 65(10):988–94. PMID:17021403
888. Grill J, Avet-Loiseau H, Lellouch-Tubiana A, Sévenet N, Terrier-Lacombe MJ, Vénuat AM, et al. (2002). Comparative genomic hybridization detects specific cytogenetic abnormalities in pediatric ependymomas and choroid plexus papillomas. Cancer Genet Cytogenet. 136(2):121–5. PMID:12237235
888A. Grimm T, Teglund S, Tackels D, Sangiorgi E, Gurrieri F, Schwartz C, et al. (2001). Genomic organization and embryonic expression of Suppressor of Fused, a candidate gene for the split-hand/split-foot malformation type 3. FEBS Lett. 505(1):13–7. PMID:11557033
889. Grois N, Fahrner B, Arceci RJ, Henter JI, McClain K, Lassmann H, Nanduri V, Prosch H, Prayer D, (2010). Central nervous system disease in Langerhans cell histiocytosis . J Pediatr 156: 873-81, 881.e1. PMID:20434166
890. Grosse G, Lindner G, Matthies HJ (1976). [Effect of orotic acid on the in vitro cultured nerve tissue]. Z Mikrosk Anat Forsch. 90(3):499–506. PMID:1088565
891. Filbin MG, Dabral SK, Pazyra-Murphy MF, Ramkissoon S, Kung AL, Pak E, et al. (2013). Coordinate activation of Shh and PI3K signaling in PTEN-deficient glioblastoma: new therapeutic opportunities. Nat Med. 19(11):1518–23. PMID:24076665
892. Gu J, Tamura M, Yamada KM (1998). Tumor suppressor PTEN inhibits integrin- and growth factor-mediated mitogen-activated protein (MAP) kinase signaling pathways. J Cell Biol. 143(5):1375–83. PMID:9832564

893. Guan H, Huang Y, Wen W, Xu M, Zan Q, Zhang Z (2011). Primary central nervous system extranodal NK/T-cell lymphoma, nasal type: case report and review of the literature. J Neurooncol. 103(2):387–91. PMID:20845062
894. Gucer H, Mete O (2014). Endobronchial gangliocytic paraganglioma: not all keratin-positive endobronchial neuroendocrine neoplasms are pulmonary carcinoids. Endocr Pathol. 25(3):356–8. PMID:23912549
895. Guermazi A, De Kerviler E, Zagdanski AM, Frija J (2000). Diagnostic imaging of choroid plexus disease. Clin Radiol. 55(7):503–16. PMID:10924373
896. Guesmi H, Houtteville JP, Courthéoux P, Derlon JM, Chapon F (1999). [Dysembryoplastic neuroepithelial tumors. Report of 8 cases including two with unusual localization]. Neurochirurgie. 45(3):190–200. PMID:10567958
897. Gunny RS, Hayward RD, Phipps KP, Harding BN, Saunders DE (2005). Spontaneous regression of residual low-grade cerebellar pilocytic astrocytomas in children. Pediatr Radiol. 35(11):1086–91. PMID:16047140
898. Guppy KH, Akins PT, Moes GS, Prados MD (2009). Spinal cord oligodendroglioma with 1p and 19q deletions presenting with cerebral oligodendrogliomatosis. J Neurosurg Spine. 10(6):557–63. PMID:19558288
899. Gurney JG, Smith MA, Bunin GR CNS and miscellaneous intracranial and intraspinal neoplasms. In: Ries LAG, Smith MA, Gurney JG, Linet M, Tamra T, Young JL, Bunin GR, editors (1995).Cancer incidence and survival among children and adolescents United States SEER Program 1975-1995. NIH Pub no. 99-4649 Bethesda, MD: National Cancer Institute.
900. Gusella JF, Ramesh V, MacCollin M, Jacoby LB (1996). Neurofibromatosis 2: loss of merlin's protective spell. Curr Opin Genet Dev. 6(1):87–92. PMID:8791482
901. Gusella JF, Ramesh V, MacCollin M, Jacoby LB (1999). Merlin: the neurofibromatosis 2 tumor suppressor. Biochim Biophys Acta. 1423(2):M29–36. PMID:10214350
902. Gutenberg A, Brandis A, Hong B, Gunawan B, Enders C, Schaefer IM, et al. (2011). Common molecular cytogenetic pathway in papillary tumors of the pineal region (PTPR). Brain Pathol. 21(6):672–7. PMID:21470326
903. Guthrie BL, Ebersold MJ, Scheithauer BW, Shaw EG (1989). Meningeal hemangiopericytoma: histopathological features, treatment, and long-term follow-up of 44 cases. Neurosurgery. 25(4):514–22. PMID:2797389
904. Gutman DA, Cooper LA, Hwang SN, Holder CA, Gao J, Aurora TD, et al. (2013). MR imaging predictors of molecular profile and survival: multi-institutional study of the TCGA glioblastoma data set. Radiology. 267(2):560–9. PMID:23392431
905. Gutmann DH, Aylsworth A, Carey JC, Korf B, Marks J, Pyeritz RE, et al. (1997). The diagnostic evaluation and multidisciplinary management of neurofibromatosis 1 and neurofibromatosis 2. JAMA. 278(1):51–7. PMID:9207339
906. Gutmann DH, Collins FS (1993). The neurofibromatosis type 1 gene and its protein product, neurofibromin. Neuron. 10(3):335–43. PMID:8461130
907. Gutmann DH, Donahoe J, Perry A, Lemke N, Gorse K, Kittiniyom K, et al. (2000). Loss of DAL-1, a protein 4.1-related tumor suppressor, is an important early event in the pathogenesis of meningiomas. Hum Mol Genet. 9(10):1495–500. PMID:10888600
908. Gutmann DH, James CD, Poyhonen M, Louis DN, Ferner R, Guha A, et al. (2003). Molecular analysis of astrocytomas presenting after age 10 in individuals with NF1. Neurology. 61(10):1397–400. PMID:14638962
909. Gutmann DH, McLellan MD, Hussain I, Wallis JW, Fulton LL, Fulton RS, et al. (2013). Somatic neurofibromatosis type 1 (NF1) inactivation characterizes NF1-associated pilocytic astrocytoma. Genome Res. 23(3):431–9. PMID:23222849
910. Gutmann DH, Parada LF, Silva AJ, Ratner N (2012). Neurofibromatosis type 1: modeling CNS dysfunction. J Neurosci. 32(41):14087–93. PMID:23055477
911. Gutmann DH, Wood DL, Collins FS (1991). Identification of the neurofibromatosis type 1 gene product. Proc Natl Acad Sci U S A. 88(21):9658–62. PMID:1946382
912. Gyure KA, Morrison AL (2000). Cytokeratin 7 and 20 expression in choroid plexus tumors: utility in differentiating these neoplasms from metastatic carcinomas. Mod Pathol. 13(6):638–43. PMID:10874668
913. Gyure KA, Prayson RA (1997). Subependymal giant cell astrocytoma: a clinicopathologic study with HMB45 and MIB-1 immunohistochemical analysis. Mod Pathol. 10(4):313–7. PMID:9110292
914. Götze S, Wolter M, Reifenberger G, Müller O, Sievers S (2010). Frequent promoter hypermethylation of Wnt pathway inhibitor genes in malignant astrocytic gliomas. Int J Cancer. 126(11):2584–93. PMID:19847810
915. Haapasalo H, Isola J, Sallinen P, Kalimo H, Helin H, Rantala I (1993). Aberrant p53 expression in astrocytic neoplasms of the brain: association with proliferation. Am J Pathol. 142(5):1347–51. PMID:7684193
916. Haas JE, Palmer NF, Weinberg AG, Beckwith JB (1981). Ultrastructure of malignant rhabdoid tumor of the kidney. A distinctive renal tumor of children. Hum Pathol. 12(7):646–57. PMID:7275104
917. Haberler C, Jarius C, Lang S, Rössler K, Gruber A, Hainfellner JA, et al. (2002). Fibrous meningeal tumours with extensive non-calcifying collagenous whorls and glial fibrillary acidic protein expression: the whorling-sclerosing variant of meningioma. Neuropathol Appl Neurobiol. 28(1):42–7. PMID:11849562
918. Haberler C, Laggner U, Slavc I, Czech T, Ambros IM, Ambros PF, et al. (2006). Immunohistochemical analysis of INI1 protein in malignant pediatric CNS tumors: Lack of INI1 in atypical teratoid/rhabdoid tumors and in a fraction of primitive neuroectodermal tumors without rhabdoid phenotype. Am J Surg Pathol. 30(11):1462–8. PMID:17063089
919. Haddad SF, Hitchon PW, Godersky JC (1991). Idiopathic and glucocorticoid-induced spinal epidural lipomatosis. J Neurosurg. 74(1):38–42. PMID:1984504
920. Haddad SF, Moore SA, Schelper RL, Goeken JA (1992). Vascular smooth muscle hyperplasia underlies the formation of glomeruloid vascular structures of glioblastoma multiforme. J Neuropathol Exp Neurol. 51(5):488–92. PMID:1381413
921. Hadfield KD, Newman WG, Bowers NL, Wallace A, Bolger C, Colley A, et al. (2008). Molecular characterisation of SMARCB1 and NF2 in familial and sporadic schwannomatosis. J Med Genet. 45(6):332–9. PMID:18285426
922. Hadfield KD, Smith MJ, Urquhart JE, Wallace AJ, Bowers NL, King AT, et al. (2010). Rates of loss of heterozygosity and mitotic recombination in NF2 schwannomas, sporadic vestibular schwannomas and schwannomatosis schwannomas. Oncogene. 29(47):6216–21. PMID:20729918
923. Hagel C, Stemmer-Rachamimov AO, Bornemann A, Schuhmann M, Nagel C, Huson S, et al. (2012). Clinical presentation, immunohistochemistry and electron microscopy indicate neurofibromatosis type 2-associated gliomas to be spinal ependymomas. Neuropathology. 32(6):611–6. PMID:22394059
924. Hahn H, Wicking C, Zaphiropoulous PG, Gailani MR, Shanley S, Chidambaram A, et al. (1996). Mutations of the human homolog of Drosophila patched in the nevoid basal cell carcinoma syndrome. Cell. 85(6):841–51. PMID:8681379
925. Hainaut P, Olivier M, Wiman K (2013).p53 in the Clinics. New York: Springer.
926. Hair LS, Symmans F, Powers JM, Carmel P (1992). Immunohistochemistry and proliferative activity in Lhermitte-Duclos disease. Acta Neuropathol. 84(5):570–3. PMID:1462769
927. Hajnsek S, Paladino J, Gadze ZP, Nanković S, Mrak G, Lupret V (2013). Clinical and neurophysiological changes in patients with pineal region expansions. Coll Antropol. 37(1):35–40. PMID:23697248
928. Haliloglu G, Jobard F, Oguz KK, Anlar B, Akalan N, Coskun T, et al. (2008). L-2-hydroxyglutaric aciduria and brain tumors in children with mutations in the L2HGDH gene: neuroimaging findings. Neuropediatrics. 39(2):119–22. PMID:18671189
929. Haller F, Bieg M, Moskalev EA, Barthelmeß S, Geddert H, Boltze C, et al. (2015). Recurrent mutations within the amino-terminal region of β-catenin are probable key molecular driver events in sinonasal hemangiopericytoma. Am J Pathol. 185(2):563–71. PMID:25482924
930. Haller F, Moskalev EA, Faucz FR, Barthelmeß S, Wiemann S, Bieg M, et al. (2014). Aberrant DNA hypermethylation of SDHC: a novel mechanism of tumor development in Carney triad. Endocr Relat Cancer. 21(4):567–77. PMID:24859990
931. Halling KC, Scheithauer BW, Halling AC, Nascimento AG, Ziesmer SC, Roche PC, et al. (1996). p53 expression in neurofibroma and malignant peripheral nerve sheath tumor. An immunohistochemical study of sporadic and NF1-associated tumors. Am J Clin Pathol. 106(3):282–8. PMID:8816583
932. Hama S, Arita K, Nishisaka T, Fukuhara T, Tominaga A, Sugiyama K, et al. (2002). Changes in the epithelium of Rathke cleft cyst associated with inflammation. J Neurosurg. 96(2):209–16. PMID:11838792
933. Hamasaki T, Yamada K, Kuratsu J (2013). Seizures as a presenting symptom in neurosurgical patients: a retrospective single-institution analysis. Clin Neurol Neurosurg. 115(11):2336–40. PMID:24011499
934. Hamazaki S, Nakashima H, Matsumoto K, Taguchi K, Okada S (2001). Metastasis of renal cell carcinoma to central nervous system hemangioblastoma in two patients with von Hippel-Lindau disease. Pathol Int. 51(12):948–53. PMID:11844068
935. Hamilton JD, Rapp M, Schneiderhan T, Sabel M, Hayman A, Scherer A, et al. (2014). Glioblastoma multiforme metastasis outside the CNS: three case reports and possible mechanisms of escape. J Clin Oncol. 32(22):e80–4. PMID:24567434
936. Hamilton RL, Pollack IF (1997). The molecular biology of ependymomas. Brain Pathol. 7(2):807–22. PMID:9161731
937. Hamilton SR, Liu B, Parsons RE, Papadopoulos N, Jen J, Powell SM, et al. (1995). The molecular basis of Turcot's syndrome. N Engl J Med. 332(13):839–47. PMID:7661930
938. Han L, Niu H, Wang J, Wan F, Shu K, Ke C, et al. (2013). Extraventricular neurocytoma in pediatric populations: A case report and review of the literature. Oncol Lett. 6(5):1397–405. PMID:24179531
939. Han SJ, Yang I, Otero JJ, Ahn BJ, Tihan T, McDermott MW, et al. (2010). Secondary gliosarcoma after diagnosis of glioblastoma: clinical experience with 30 consecutive patients. J Neurosurg. 112(5):990–6. PMID:19817543
940. Hannan F, Ho I, Tong JJ, Zhu Y, Nurnberg P, Zhong Y (2006). Effect of neurofibromatosis type I mutations on a novel pathway for adenylyl cyclase activation requiring neurofibromin and Ras. Hum Mol Genet. 15(7):1087–98. PMID:16513807
941. Hanssen AM, Fryns JP (1995). Cowden syndrome. J Med Genet. 32(2):117–9. PMID:7760320
942. Hansson CM, Buckley PG, Grigelioniene G, Piotrowski A, Hellström AR, Mantripragada K, et al. (2007). Comprehensive genetic and epigenetic analysis of sporadic meningioma for macro-mutations on 22q and micro-mutations within the NF2 locus. BMC Genomics. 8:16. PMID:17222329
943. Hao C, Beguinot F, Condorelli G, Trencia A, Van Meir EG, Yong VW, et al. (2001). Induction and intracellular regulation of tumor necrosis factor-related apoptosis-inducing ligand (TRAIL) mediated apotosis in human malignant glioma cells. Cancer Res. 61(3):1162–70. PMID:11221847
944. Hardee ME, Zagzag D (2012). Mechanisms of glioma-associated neovascularization. Am J Pathol. 181(4):1126–41. PMID:22858156
945. Harder A, Wesemann M, Hagel C, Schittenhelm J, Fischer S, Tatagiba M, et al. (2012). Hybrid neurofibroma/schwannoma is overrepresented among schwannomatosis and neurofibromatosis patients. Am J Surg Pathol. 36(5):702–9. PMID:22446939
946. Haroche J, Charlotte F, Arnaud L, von Deimling A, Hélias-Rodzewicz Z, Hervier B, et al. (2012). High prevalence of BRAF V600E mutations in Erdheim-Chester disease but not in other non-Langerhans cell histiocytoses. Blood. 120(13):2700–3. PMID:22879539
947. Haroche J, Cohen-Aubart F, Emile JF, Maksud P, Drier A, Tolédano D, et al. (2015). Reproducible and sustained efficacy of targeted therapy with vemurafenib in patients with BRAF(V600E)-mutated Erdheim-Chester disease. J Clin Oncol. 33(5):411–8. PMID:25422482
948. Harris CP, Townsend JJ, Brockmeyer DL, Heilbrun MP (1991). Cerebral granular cell tumor occurring with glioblastoma multiforme: case report. Surg Neurol. 36(3):202–6. PMID:1652163
949. Harter DH, Omeis I, Forman S, Braun A (2006). Endoscopic resection of an intraventricular dysembryoplastic neuroepithelial tumor of the septum pellucidum. Pediatr Neurosurg. 42(2):105–7. PMID:16465080
950. Hartmann C, Hentschel B, Simon M, Westphal M, Schackert G, Tonn JC, et al.; German Glioma Network (2013). Long-term survival in primary glioblastoma with versus without isocitrate dehydrogenase mutations. Clin Cancer Res. 19(18):5146–57. PMID:23918605
951. Hartmann C, Hentschel B, Tatagiba M, Schramm J, Schnell O, Seidel C, et al.; German Glioma Network (2011). Molecular markers in low-grade gliomas: predictive or prognostic? Clin Cancer Res. 17(13):4588–99. PMID:21558404
952. Hartmann C, Hentschel B, Wick W, Capper D, Felsberg J, Simon M, et al. (2010). Patients with IDH1 wild type anaplastic astrocytomas exhibit worse prognosis than IDH1-mutated glioblastomas, and IDH1 mutation status accounts for the unfavorable prognostic effect of higher age: implications for classification of gliomas. Acta Neuropathol. 120(6):707–18. PMID:21088844
953. Hartmann C, Meyer J, Balss J, Capper D, Mueller W, Christians A, et al. (2009). Type and frequency of IDH1 and IDH2 mutations are related to astrocytic and oligodendroglial differentiation and age: a study of 1,010 diffuse gliomas. Acta Neuropathol. 118(4):469–74. PMID:19554337
954. Hartmann C, Sieberns J, Gehlhaar C, Simon M, Paulus W, von Deimling A (2006). NF2 mutations in secretory and other rare variants of meningiomas. Brain Pathol. 16(1):15–9. PMID:16612978
955. Hartmann C, Xu X, Bartels G, Holtkamp N, Gonzales IA, Tallen G, et al. (2004). Pdgfr-alpha in 1p/19q LOH oligodendrogliomas. Int J Cancer. 112(6):1081–2. PMID:15386438
956. Hashimoto T, Sasagawa I, Ishigooka M, Kubota Y, Nakada T, Fujita T, et al. (1995). Down's syndrome associated with intracranial

germinoma and testicular embryonal carcinoma. Urol Int. 55(2):120–2. PMID:8533196
957. Hasselblatt M, Blümcke I, Jeibmann A, Rickert CH, Jouvet A, van de Nes JA, et al. (2006). Immunohistochemical profile and chromosomal imbalances in papillary tumours of the pineal region. Neuropathol Appl Neurobiol. 32(3):278–83. PMID:16640646
958. Hasselblatt M, Böhm C, Tatenhorst L, Dinh V, Newrzella D, Keyvani K, et al. (2006). Identification of novel diagnostic markers for choroid plexus tumors: a microarray-based approach. Am J Surg Pathol. 30(1):66–74. PMID:16330944
959. Hasselblatt M, Gesk S, Oyen F, Rossi S, Viscardi E, Giangaspero F, et al. (2011). Nonsense mutation and inactivation of SMARCA4 (BRG1) in an atypical teratoid/rhabdoid tumor showing retained SMARCB1 (INI1) expression. Am J Surg Pathol. 35(6):933–5. PMID:21566516
960. Hasselblatt M, Jeibmann A, Guerry M, Senner V, Paulus W, McLendon RE (2008). Choroid plexus papilloma with neuropil-like islands. Am J Surg Pathol. 32(1):162–6. PMID:18162784
961. Hasselblatt M, Mühlisch J, Wrede B, Kallinger B, Jeibmann A, Peters O, et al. (2009). Aberrant MGMT (O6-methylguanine-DNA methyltransferase) promoter methylation in choroid plexus tumors. J Neurooncol. 91(2):151–5. PMID:18795231
962. Hasselblatt M, Nagel I, Oyen F, Bartelheim K, Russell RB, Schüller U, et al. (2014). SMARCA4-mutated atypical teratoid/rhabdoid tumors are associated with inherited germline alterations and poor prognosis. Acta Neuropathol. 128(3):453–6. PMID:25060813
963. Hasselblatt M, Nolte KW, Paulus W (2004). Angiomatous meningioma: a clinicopathologic study of 38 cases. Am J Surg Pathol. 28(3):390–3. PMID:15104303
964. Hasselblatt M, Oyen F, Gesk S, Kordes U, Wrede B, Bergmann M, et al. (2009). Cribriform neuroepithelial tumor (CRINET): a nonrhabdoid ventricular tumor with INI1 loss and relatively favorable prognosis. J Neuropathol Exp Neurol. 68(12):1249–55. PMID:19915490
965. Hasselblatt M, Paulus W (2003). Sensitivity and specificity of epithelial membrane antigen staining patterns in ependymomas. Acta Neuropathol. 106(4):385–8. PMID:12898159
965A. Hasselblatt M, Riesmeier B, Lechtape B, Brentrup A, Stummer W, Albert FK, et al. (2011). BRAF-KIAA1549 fusion transcripts are less frequent in pilocytic astrocytomas diagnosed in adults. Neuropathol Appl Neurobiol. 37(7):803–6. PMID:21696415
966. Hasselblatt M, Sepehrnia A, von Falkenhausen M, Paulus W (2003). Intracranial follicular dendritic cell sarcoma. Case report. J Neurosurg. 99(6):1089–90. PMID:14705740
967. Hassoun J, Gambarelli D, Grisoli F, Pellet W, Salamon G, Pellissier JF, et al. (1982). Central neurocytoma. An electron-microscopic study of two cases. Acta Neuropathol. 56(2):151–6. PMID:7064664
968. Hassoun J, Gambarelli D, Peragut JC, Toga M (1983). Specific ultrastructural markers of human pinealomas. A study of four cases. Acta Neuropathol. 62(1-2):31–40. PMID:6318505
969. Hassoun J, Söylemezoglu F, Gambarelli D, Figarella-Branger D, von Ammon K, Kleihues P (1993). Central neurocytoma: a synopsis of clinical and histological features. Brain Pathol. 3(3):297–306. PMID:8293189
970. Hatton BA, Villavicencio EH, Tsuchiya KD, Pritchard JI, Ditzler S, Pullar B, et al. (2008). The Smo/Smo model: hedgehog-induced medulloblastoma with 90% incidence and leptomeningeal spread. Cancer Res. 68(6):1768–76. PMID:18339857
971. Hatva E, Böhling T, Jääskeläinen J, Persico MG, Haltia M, Alitalo K (1996). Vascular growth factors and receptors in capillary hemangioblastomas and hemangiopericytomas. Am J Pathol. 148(3):763–75. PMID:8774132
972. Hayasaka K, Nihashi T, Takebayashi S, Bundoh M (2008). FDG PET in Lhermitte-Duclos disease. Clin Nucl Med. 33(1):52–4. PMID:18097262
973. Hayashi K, Ohara N, Jeon HJ, Akagi S, Takahashi K, Akagi T, et al. (1993). Gliosarcoma with features of chondroblastic osteosarcoma. Cancer. 72(3):850–5. PMID:8334639
974. Hayostek CJ, Shaw EG, Scheithauer B, O'Fallon JR, Weiland TL, Schomberg PJ, et al. (1993). Astrocytomas of the cerebellum. A comparative clinicopathologic study of pilocytic and diffuse astrocytomas. Cancer. 72(3):856–69. PMID:8334640
975. He J, Mokhtari K, Sanson M, Marie Y, Kujas M, Huguet S, et al. (2001). Glioblastomas with an oligodendroglial component: a pathological and molecular study. J Neuropathol Exp Neurol. 60(9):863–71. PMID:11556543
976. He MX, Wang JJ (2011). Rhabdoid glioblastoma: case report and literature review. Neuropathology. 31(4):421–6. PMID:21092062
977. Heaphy CM, de Wilde RF, Jiao Y, Klein AP, Edil BH, Shi C, et al. (2011). Altered telomeres in tumors with ATRX and DAXX mutations. Science. 333(6041):425. PMID:21719641
978. Heath JA, Ng J, Beshay V, Coleman L, Lo P, Amor DJ (2013). Anaplastic oligodendroglioma in an adolescent with Lynch syndrome. Pediatr Blood Cancer. 60(6):E13–5. PMID:23255519
979. Hébert-Blouin MN, Scheithauer BW, Amrami KK, Durham SR, Spinner RJ (2012). Fibromatosis: a potential sequela of neuromuscular choristoma. J Neurosurg. 116(2):399–408. PMID:21819193
980. Heegaard S, Sommer HM, Broholm H, Broendstrup O (1995). Proliferating cell nuclear antigen and Ki-67 immunohistochemistry of oligodendrogliomas with special reference to prognosis. Cancer. 76(10):1809–13. PMID:8625052
981. Heesters M, Molenaar W, Go GK (2003). Radiotherapy in supratentorial gliomas. A study of 821 cases. Strahlenther Onkol. 179(9):606–14. PMID:14628126
982. Hegi ME, Diserens AC, Gorlia T, Hamou MF, de Tribolet N, Weller M, et al. (2005). MGMT gene silencing and benefit from temozolomide in glioblastoma. N Engl J Med. 352(10):997–1003. PMID:15758010
983. Hegi ME, Janzer RC, Lambiv WL, Gorlia T, Kouwenhoven MC, Hartmann C, et al.; European Organisation for Research and Treatment of Cancer Brain Tumour and Radiation Oncology Groups; National Cancer Institute of Canada Clinical Trials Group (2012). Presence of an oligodendroglioma-like component in newly diagnosed glioblastoma identifies a pathogenetically heterogeneous subgroup and lacks prognostic value: central pathology review of the EORTC_26981/NCIC_CE.3 trial. Acta Neuropathol. 123(6):841–52. PMID:22249618
984. Heim S, Beschorner R, Mittelbronn M, Keyvani K, Riemenschneider MJ, Vajtai I, et al. (2014). Increased mitotic and proliferative activity are associated with worse prognosis in papillary tumors of the pineal region. Am J Surg Pathol. 38(1):106–10. PMID:24121176
985. Heim S, Coras R, Ganslandt O, Kufeld M, Blümcke I, Paulus W, et al. (2013). Papillary tumor of the pineal region with anaplastic small cell component. J Neurooncol. 115(1):127–30. PMID:23817812
986. Heim S, Sill M, Jones DT, Vasiljevic A, Jouvet A, Fèvre-Montange M, et al. (2015). Papillary tumor of the pineal region: A distinct molecular entity. Brain Pathol. PMID:26113311
987. Heimdal K, Evensen SA, Fosså SD, Hirscberg H, Langholm R, Brøgger A, et al. (1991). Karyotyping of a hematologic neoplasia developing shortly after treatment for cerebral extragonadal germ cell tumor. Cancer Genet Cytogenet. 57(1):41–6. PMID:1756483
988. Helseth A, Helseth E, Unsgaard G (1989). Primary meningeal melanoma. Acta Oncol. 28(1):103–4. PMID:2706127
989. Hemminki K, Kyyrönen P, Vaittinen P (1999). Parental age as a risk factor of childhood leukemia and brain cancer in offspring. Epidemiology. 10(3):271–5. PMID:10230837
990. Hemminki K, Liu X, Försti A, Ji J, Sundquist J, Sundquist K (2013). Subsequent brain tumors in patients with autoimmune disease. Neuro Oncol. 15(9):1142–50. PMID:23757294
991. Hennessy MJ, Elwes RD, Rabe-Hesketh S, Binnie CD, Polkey CE (2001). Prognostic factors in the surgical treatment of medically intractable epilepsy associated with mesial temporal sclerosis. Acta Neurol Scand. 103(6):344–50. PMID:11421846
992. Henske EP, Wessner LL, Golden J, Scheithauer BW, Vortmeyer AO, Zhuang Z, et al. (1997). Loss of tuberin in both subependymal giant cell astrocytomas and angiomyolipomas supports a two-hit model for the pathogenesis of tuberous sclerosis tumors. Am J Pathol. 151(6):1639–47. PMID:9403714
993. Henson JW, Schnitker BL, Correa KM, von Deimling A, Fassbender F, Xu HJ, et al. (1994). The retinoblastoma gene is involved in malignant progression of astrocytomas. Ann Neurol. 36(5):714–21. PMID:7979217
994. Herpers MJ, Budka H (1984). Glial fibrillary acidic protein (GFAP) in oligodendroglial tumors: gliofibrillary oligodendroglioma and transitional oligoastrocytoma as subtypes of oligodendroglioma. Acta Neuropathol. 64(4):265–72. PMID:6391068
995. Herpers MJ, Ramaekers FC, Aldeweireldt J, Moesker O, Slooff J (1986). Co-expression of glial fibrillary acidic protein- and vimentin-type intermediate filaments in human astrocytomas. Acta Neuropathol. 70(3-4):333–9. PMID:3020864
996. Herregodts P, Vloeberghs M, Schmedding E, Goossens A, Stadnik T, D'Haens J (1991). Solitary dorsal intramedullary schwannoma. Case report. J Neurosurg. 74(5):816–20. PMID:2013780
997. Herrick MK, Rubinstein LJ (1979). The cytological differentiating potential of pineal parenchymal neoplasms (true pinealomas). A clinicopathological study of 28 tumours . Brain 102: 289-320. PMID:88244
998. Hertzler DA 2nd, DePowell JJ, Stevenson CB, Mangano FT (2010). Tethered cord syndrome: a review of the literature from embryology to adult presentation. Neurosurg Focus. 29(1):E1. PMID:20593997
999. Herva R, Serlo W, Laitinen J, Becker LE (1996). Intraventricular rhabdomyosarcoma after resection of hyperplastic choroid plexus. Acta Neuropathol. 92(2):213–6. PMID:8841669
1000. Hewer E, Beck J, Murek M, Kappeler A, Vassella E, Vajtai I (2014). Polymorphous oligodendroglioma of Zülch revisited: a genetically heterogeneous group of anaplastic gliomas including tumors of bona fide oligodendroglial differentiation. Neuropathology. 34(4):323–32. PMID:24444336
1001. Hijiya N, Hudson MM, Lensing S, Zacher M, Onciu M, Behm FG, et al. (2007). Cumulative incidence of secondary neoplasms as a first event after childhood acute lymphoblastic leukemia. JAMA. 297(11):1207–15. PMID:17374815
1002. Hilden JM, Meerbaum S, Burger P, Finlay J, Janss A, Scheithauer BW, et al. (2004). Central nervous system atypical teratoid/rhabdoid tumor: results of therapy in children enrolled in a registry. J Clin Oncol. 22(14):2877–84. PMID:15254056
1003. Hill RM, Kuijper S, Lindsey JC, Petrie K, Schwalbe EC, Barker K, et al. (2015). Combined MYC and P53 defects emerge at medulloblastoma relapse and define rapidly progressive, therapeutically targetable disease. Cancer Cell. 27(1):72–84. PMID:25533335
1004. Hiniker A, Hagenkord JM, Powers MP, Aghi MK, Prados MD, Perry A (2013). Gliosarcoma arising from an oligodendroglioma (oligosarcoma). Clin Neuropathol. 32(3):165–70. PMID:23254140
1005. Hinkes BG, von Hoff K, Deinlein F, Warmuth-Metz M, Soerensen N, Timmermann B, et al. (2007). Childhood pineoblastoma: experiences from the prospective multicenter trials HIT-SKK87, HIT-SKK92 and HIT91. J Neurooncol. 81(2):217–23. PMID:16941074
1006. Hirbe AC, Gutmann DH (2014). Neurofibromatosis type 1: a multidisciplinary approach to care. Lancet Neurol. 13(8):834–43. PMID:25030515
1007. Hirose T, Giannini C, Scheithauer BW (2001). Ultrastructural features of pleomorphic xanthoastrocytoma: a comparative study with glioblastoma multiforme. Ultrastruct Pathol. 25(6):469–78. PMID:11783911
1008. Hirose T, Scheithauer BW (1998). Mixed dysembryoplastic neuroepithelial tumor and ganglioglioma. Acta Neuropathol. 95(6):649–54. PMID:9650758
1009. Hirose T, Scheithauer BW, Lopes MB, Gerber HA, Altermatt HJ, Hukee MJ, et al. (1995). Tuber and subependymal giant cell astrocytoma associated with tuberous sclerosis: an immunohistochemical, ultrastructural, and immunoelectron and microscopic study. Acta Neuropathol. 90(4):387–99. PMID:8546029
1010. Hirose T, Scheithauer BW, Lopes MB, Gerber HA, Altermatt HJ, VandenBerg SR (1997). Ganglioglioma: an ultrastructural and immunohistochemical study. Cancer. 79(5):989–1003. PMID:9041162
1011. Hirose T, Scheithauer BW, Sano T (1998). Perineurial malignant peripheral nerve sheath tumor (MPNST): a clinicopathologic, immunohistochemical, and ultrastructural study of seven cases. Am J Surg Pathol. 22(11):1368–78. PMID:9808129
1012. Hirose T, Tani T, Shimada T, Ishizawa K, Shimada S, Sano T (2003). Immunohistochemical demonstration of EMA/Glut1-positive perineurial cells and CD34-positive fibroblastic cells in peripheral nerve sheath tumors. Mod Pathol. 16(4):293–8. PMID:12692193
1013. Hiroyuki M, Ogino J, Takahashi A, Hasegawa T, Wakabayashi T (2015). Rhabdoid glioblastoma: an aggressive variaty of astrocytic tumor. Nagoya J Med Sci. 77(1-2):321–8. PMID:25797998
1014. Hitotsumatsu T, Iwaki T, Kitamoto T, Mizoguchi M, Suzuki SO, Hamada Y, et al. (1997). Expression of neurofibromatosis 2 protein in human brain tumors: an immunohistochemical study. Acta Neuropathol. 93(3):225–32. PMID:9083553
1015. Hjalmars U, Kulldorff M, Wahlqvist Y, Lannering B (1999). Increased incidence rates but no space-time clustering of childhood astrocytoma in Sweden, 1973–1992: a population-based study of pediatric brain tumors. Cancer. 85(9):2077–90. PMID:10223251
1016. Ho DM, Hsu CY, Wong TT, Ting LT, Chiang H (2000). Atypical teratoid/rhabdoid tumor of the central nervous system: a comparative study with primitive neuroectodermal tumor/medulloblastoma. Acta Neuropathol. 99(5):482–8. PMID:10805090
1017. Ho DM, Liu HC (1992). Primary intracranial germ cell tumor. Pathologic study of 51 patients. Cancer. 70(6):1577–84. PMID:1325276
1018. Ho KL (1990). Intercellular septate-like junction of neoplastic cells in myxopapillary ependymoma of the filum terminale. Acta Neuropathol. 79(4):432–7. PMID:2339595
1019. Ho KL (1990). Microtubular aggregates within rough endoplasmic reticulum in myxopapillary ependymoma of the filum terminale. Arch Pathol Lab Med. 114(9):956–60. PMID:2390011
1020. Ho YS, Wei CH, Tsai MD, Wai YY (1992).

Intracerebral malignant fibrous histiocytoma: case report and review of the literature. Neurosurgery. 31(3):567–71. PMID:1328926
1021. Hoang MP, Amirkhan RH (2003). Inhibin alpha distinguishes hemangioblastoma from clear cell renal cell carcinoma. Am J Surg Pathol. 27(8):1152–6. PMID:12883249
1022. Hoang-Xuan K, Capelle L, Kujas M, Taillibert S, Duffau H, Lejeune J, et al. (2004). Temozolomide as initial treatment for adults with low-grade oligodendrogliomas or oligoastrocytomas and correlation with chromosome 1p deletions. J Clin Oncol. 22(15):3133–8. PMID:15284265
1023. Hobbs J, Nikiforova MN, Fardo DW, Bortoluzzi S, Cieply K, Hamilton RL, et al. (2012). Paradoxical relationship between the degree of EGFR amplification and outcome in glioblastomas. Am J Surg Pathol. 36(8):1186–93. PMID:22472960
1024. Hoefnagel LD, van der Groep P, van de Vijver MJ, Boers JE, Wesseling P, Wesseling J, et al.; Dutch Distant Breast Cancer Metastases Consortium (2013). Discordance in ERα, PR and HER2 receptor status across different distant breast cancer metastases within the same patient. Ann Oncol. 24(12):3017–23. PMID:24114857
1025. Hoffman HJ, Otsubo H, Hendrick EB, Humphreys RP, Drake JM, Becker LE, et al. (1991). Intracranial germ-cell tumors in children. J Neurosurg. 74(4):545–51. PMID:1848284
1026. Hoffman LM, Donson AM, Nakachi I, Griesinger AM, Birks DK, Amani V, et al. (2014). Molecular sub-group-specific immunophenotypic changes are associated with outcome in recurrent posterior fossa ependymoma. Acta Neuropathol. 127(5):731–45. PMID:24240813
1027. Hofman S, Heeg M, Klein JP, Krikke AP (1998). Simultaneous occurrence of a supra- and an infratentorial glioma in a patient with Ollier's disease: more evidence for non-mesodermal tumor predisposition in multiple enchondromatosis. Skeletal Radiol. 27(12):688–91. PMID:9921931
1028. Hofmann BM, Kreutzer J, Saeger W, Buchfelder M, Blümcke I, Fahlbusch R, et al. (2006). Nuclear beta-catenin accumulation as reliable marker for the differentiation between cystic craniopharyngiomas and rathke cleft cysts: a clinico-pathologic approach. Am J Surg Pathol. 30(12):1595–603. PMID:17122517
1029. Hoischen A, Ehrler M, Fassunke J, Simon M, Baudis M, Landwehr C, et al. (2008). Comprehensive characterization of genomic aberrations in gangliogliomas by CGH, array-based CGH and interphase FISH. Brain Pathol. 18(3):326–37. PMID:18371186
1030. Holash J, Maisonpierre PC, Compton D, Boland P, Alexander CR, Zagzag D, et al. (1999). Vessel cooption, regression, and growth in tumors mediated by angiopoietins and VEGF. Science. 284(5422):1994–8. PMID:10373119
1031. Homma T, Fukushima T, Vaccarella S, Yonekawa Y, Di Patre PL, Franceschi S, et al. (2006). Correlation among pathology, genotype, and patient outcomes in glioblastoma. J Neuropathol Exp Neurol. 65(9):846–54. PMID:16957578
1032. Honan WP, Anderson M, Carey MP, Williams B (1987). Familial subependymomas. Br J Neurosurg. 1(3):317–21. PMID:3268127
1033. Honavar M, Janota I (1994). 73 cases of dysembryoplastic neuroepithelial tumour: the range of histological appearances. Brain Pathol. 4:428.
1034. Horbinski C (2013). To BRAF or not to BRAF: is that even a question anymore? J Neuropathol Exp Neurol. 72(1):2–7. PMID:23242278
1035. Horbinski C, Dacic S, McLendon RE, Cieply K, Datto M, Brat DJ, et al. (2009). Chordoid glioma: a case report and molecular characterization of five cases. Brain Pathol. 19(3):439–48. PMID:18652591
1036. Horbinski C, Hobbs J, Cieply K, Dacic S, Hamilton RL (2011). EGFR expression stratifies oligodendroglioma behavior. Am J Pathol. 179(4):1638–44. PMID:21839716
1037. Horbinski C, Kofler J, Yeaney G, Camelo-Piragua S, Venneti S, Louis DN, et al. (2011). Isocitrate dehydrogenase 1 analysis differentiates gangliogliomas from infiltrative gliomas. Brain Pathol. 21(5):564–74. PMID:21314850
1038. Horiguchi H, Hirose T, Kannuki S, Nagahiro S, Sano T (1998). Gliosarcoma: an immunohistochemical, ultrastructural and fluorescence in situ hybridization study. Pathol Int. 48(8):595–602. PMID:9736406
1039. Horiguchi H, Hirose T, Sano T, Nagahiro S, Seki K, Fujimoto N, et al. (2000). Meningioma with granulofilamentous inclusions. Ultrastruct Pathol. 24(4):267–71. PMID:11013967
1040. Hornick JL, Bundock EA, Fletcher CD (2009). Hybrid schwannoma/perineurioma: clinicopathologic analysis of 42 distinctive benign nerve sheath tumors. Am J Surg Pathol. 33(10):1554–61. PMID:19623031
1041. Hornick JL, Fletcher CD (2005). Intestinal perineuriomas: clinicopathologic definition of a new anatomic subset in a series of 10 cases. Am J Surg Pathol. 29(7):859–65. PMID:15958849
1042. Hornick JL, Fletcher CD (2005). Soft tissue perineurioma: clinicopathologic analysis of 81 cases including those with atypical histologic features. Am J Surg Pathol. 29(7):845–58. PMID:15958848
1043. Hornick JL, Jaffe ES, Fletcher CD (2004). Extranodal histiocytic sarcoma: clinicopathologic analysis of 14 cases of a rare epithelioid malignancy. Am J Surg Pathol. 28(9):1133–44. PMID:15316312
1044. Horstmann S, Perry A, Reifenberger G, Giangaspero F, Huang H, Hara A, et al. (2004). Genetic and expression profiles of cerebellar liponeurocytomas. Brain Pathol. 14(3):281–9. PMID:15446583
1045. Horten BC, Rubinstein LJ (1976). Primary cerebral neuroblastoma. A clinicopathological study of 35 cases. Brain. 99(4):735–56. PMID:1030655
1046. Hoshino T, Wilson BC, Ellis WG (1975). Gemistocytic astrocytes in gliomas. An autoradiographic study. J Neuropathol Exp Neurol. 34(3):263–81. PMID:167133
1047. Hosokawa Y, Tsuchihashi Y, Okabe H, Toyama M, Namura K, Kuga M, et al. (1991). Pleomorphic xanthoastrocytoma. Ultrastructural, immunohistochemical, and DNA cytofluorometric study of a case. Cancer. 68(4):853–9. PMID:1855184
1048. Hou Z, Wu Z, Zhang J, Zhang L, Tian R, Liu B, et al. (2013). Clinical features and management of intracranial subependymomas in children. J Clin Neurosci. 20(1):84–8. PMID:23117139
1049. Hovestadt V, Remke M, Kool M, Pietsch T, Northcott PA, Fischer R, et al. (2013). Robust molecular subgrouping and copy-number profiling of medulloblastoma from small amounts of archival tumour material using high-density DNA methylation arrays. Acta Neuropathol. 125(6):913–6. PMID:23670100
1050. Howard BM, Hofstetter C, Wagner PL, Muskin ET, Lavi E, Boockvar JA (2009). Transformation of a low-grade pineal parenchymal tumour to secondary pineoblastoma. Neuropathol Appl Neurobiol. 35(2):214–7. PMID:19284482
1051. Howard JE, Dwivedi RC, Masterson L, Jani P (2015). Langerhans cell sarcoma: a systematic review. Cancer Treat Rev. 41(4):320–31. PMID:25805533
1052. Howe JR, Ringold JC, Summers RW, Mitros FA, Nishimura DY, Stone EM (1998). A gene for familial juvenile polyposis maps to chromosome 18q21.1. Am J Hum Genet. 62(5):1129–36. PMID:9545410
1053. Howe JR, Roth S, Ringold JC, Summers RW, Järvinen HJ, Sistonen P, et al. (1998). Mutations in the SMAD4/DPC4 gene in juvenile polyposis. Science. 280(5366):1086–8. PMID:9582123
1054. Hoyt WF, Baghdassarian SA (1969). Optic glioma of childhood. Natural history and rationale for conservative management. Br J Ophthalmol. 53(12):793–8. PMID:5386369
1055. Hruban RH, Shiu MH, Senie RT, Woodruff JM (1990). Malignant peripheral nerve sheath tumors of the buttock and lower extremity. A study of 43 cases. Cancer. 66(6):1253–65. PMID:2119249
1056. Hsu DW, Louis DN, Efird JT, Hedley-Whyte ET (1997). Use of MIB-1 (Ki-67) immunoreactivity in differentiating grade II and grade III gliomas. J Neuropathol Exp Neurol. 56(8):857–65. PMID:9258255
1057. Huang H, Mahler-Araujo BM, Sankila A, Chimelli L, Yonekawa Y, Kleihues P, et al. (2000). APC mutations in sporadic medulloblastomas. Am J Pathol. 156(2):433–7. PMID:10666372
1058. Huang H, Reis R, Yonekawa Y, Lopes JM, Kleihues P, Ohgaki H (1999). Identification in human brain tumors of DNA sequences specific for SV40 large T antigen. Brain Pathol. 9(1):33–42. PMID:9989448
1058A. Huang J, Grotzer MA, Watanabe T, Hewer E, Pietsch T, Rutkowski S, et al. (2008). Mutations in the Nijmegen breakage syndrome gene in medulloblastomas. Clin Cancer Res. 14(13):4053–8. PMID:18593981
1059. Huang JG, Kavar B, Smith PD (2007). Intradural extramedullary spinal spread of oligoastrocytoma. J Clin Neurosci. 14(9):879–82. PMID:17582770
1060. Huang MC, Kubo O, Tajika Y, Takakura K (1996). A clinico-immunohistochemical study of giant cell glioblastoma. Noshuyo Byori. 13(1):11–6. PMID:8916121
1061. Hufnagel TJ, Kim JH, True LD, Manuelidis EE (1989). Immunohistochemistry of capillary hemangioblastoma. Immunoperoxidase-labeled antibody staining resolves the differential diagnosis with metastatic renal cell carcinoma, but does not explain the histogenesis of the capillary hemangioblastoma. Am J Surg Pathol. 13(3):207–16. PMID:2465700
1062. Hulsebos TJ, Kenter S, Siebers-Renelt U, Hans V, Wesseling P, Flucke U (2014). SMARCB1 involvement in the development of leiomyoma in a patient with schwannomatosis. Am J Surg Pathol. 38(3):421–5. PMID:24525513
1063. Hulsebos TJ, Kenter S, Verhagen WI, Baas F, Flucke U, Wesseling P (2014). Premature termination of SMARCB1 translation may be followed by reinitiation in schwannomatosis-associated schwannomas, but results in absence of SMARCB1 expression in rhabdoid tumors. Acta Neuropathol. 128(3):439–48. PMID:24740647
1064. Hulsebos TJ, Plomp AS, Wolterman RA, Robanus-Maandag EC, Baas F, Wesseling P (2007). Germline mutation of INI1/SMARCB1 in familial schwannomatosis. Am J Hum Genet. 80(4):805–10. PMID:17357086
1065. Hung KL, Wu CM, Huang JS, How SW (1990). Familial medulloblastoma in siblings: report in one family and review of the literature. Surg Neurol. 33(5):341–6. PMID:2184531
1066. Husain AN, Leestma JE (1986). Cerebral astroblastoma: immunohistochemical and ultrastructural features. Case report. J Neurosurg. 64(4):657–61. PMID:3950749
1067. Huse JT, Diamond EL, Wang L, Rosenblum MK (2015). Mixed glioma with molecular features of composite oligodendroglioma and astrocytoma: a true "oligoastrocytoma"? Acta Neuropathol. 129(1):151–3. PMID:25359109
1068. Huse JT, Edgar M, Halliday J, Mikolaenko I, Lavi E, Rosenblum MK (2013). Multinodular and vacuolating neuronal tumors of the cerebrum: 10 cases of a distinctive seizure-associated lesion. Brain Pathol. 23(5):515–24. PMID:23324039
1069. Husemann K, Wolter M, Büschges R, Boström J, Sabel M, Reifenberger G (1999). Identification of two distinct deleted regions on the short arm of chromosome 1 and rare mutation of the CDKN2C gene from 1p32 in oligodendroglial tumors. J Neuropathol Exp Neurol. 58(10):1041–50. PMID:10515227
1070. Hussain N, Curran A, Pilling D, Malluci CL, Ladusans EJ, Alfirevic Z, et al. (2006). Congenital subependymal giant cell astrocytoma diagnosed on fetal MRI. Arch Dis Child. 91(6):520. PMID:16714726
1071. Husseini L, Saleh A, Reifenberger G, Hartung HP, Kieseier BC (2012). Inflammatory demyelinating brain lesions heralding primary CNS lymphoma. Can J Neurol Sci. 39(1):6–10. PMID:22384490
1072. Huttenlocher PR, Heydemann PT (1984). Fine structure of cortical tubers in tuberous sclerosis: a Golgi study. Ann Neurol. 16(5):595–602. PMID:6508241
1073. Hutter S, Piro RM, Reuss DE, Hovestadt V, Sahm F, Farschtschi S, et al. (2014). Whole exome sequencing reveals that the majority of schwannomatosis cases remain unexplained after excluding SMARCB1 and LZTR1 germline variants. Acta Neuropathol. 128(3):449–52. PMID:25008767
1074. Huynh DP, Mautner V, Baser ME, Stavrou D, Pulst SM (1997). Immunohistochemical detection of schwannomin and neurofibromin in vestibular schwannomas, ependymomas and meningiomas. J Neuropathol Exp Neurol. 56(4):382–90. PMID:9100669
1075. Hyman SL, Arthur Shores E, North KN (2006). Learning disabilities in children with neurofibromatosis type 1: subtypes, cognitive profile, and attention-deficit-hyperactivity disorder. Dev Med Child Neurol. 48(12):973–7. PMID:17109785
1076. Hütt-Cabezas M, Karajannis MA, Zagzag D, Shah S, Horkayne-Szakaly I, Rushing EJ, et al. (2013). Activation of mTORC1/mTORC2 signaling in pediatric low-grade glioma and pilocytic astrocytoma reveals mTOR as a therapeutic target. Neuro Oncol. 15(12):1604–14. PMID:24203892
1077. Hölsken A, Kreutzer J, Hofmann BM, Hans V, Oppel F, Buchfelder M, et al. (2009). Target gene activation of the Wnt signaling pathway in nuclear beta-catenin accumulating cells of adamantinomatous craniopharyngiomas. Brain Pathol. 19(3):357–64. PMID:18540944
1078. Ichimura K, Pearson DM, Kocialkowski S, Bäcklund LM, Chan R, Jones DT, et al. (2009). IDH1 mutations are present in the majority of common adult gliomas but rare in primary glioblastomas. Neuro Oncol. 11(4):341–7. PMID:19435942
1079. Ichimura K, Schmidt EE, Miyakawa A, Goike HM, Collins VP (1998). Distinct patterns of deletion on 10p and 10q suggest involvement of multiple tumor suppressor genes in the development of astrocytic gliomas of different malignancy grades. Genes Chromosomes Cancer. 22(1):9–15. PMID:9591629
1080. Iczkowski KA, Butler SL, Shanks JH, Hossain D, Schall A, Meiers I, et al. (2008). Trials of new germ cell immunohistochemical stains in 93 extragonadal and metastatic germ cell tumors. Hum Pathol. 39(2):275–81. PMID:18045648
1081. Ida CM, Rodriguez FJ, Burger PC, Caron AA, Jenkins SM, Spears GM, et al. (2015). Pleomorphic Xanthoastrocytoma: Natural History and Long-Term Follow-Up. Brain Pathol. 25(5):575–86 PMID:25318587
1082. Ida CM, Vrana JA, Rodriguez FJ, Jentoft ME, Caron AA, Jenkins SM, et al. (2013). Immunohistochemistry is highly sensitive and specific for detection of BRAF V600E mutation in pleomorphic xanthoastrocytoma. Acta Neuropathol Commun. 1:20. PMID:24252190
1083. Idbaih A, Crinière E, Marie Y, Rousseau A, Mokhtari K, Kujas M, et al. (2008). Gene

amplification is a poor prognostic factor in anaplastic oligodendrogliomas. Neuro Oncol. 10(4):540–7. PMID:18544654
1084. Idbaih A, Ducray F, Dehais C, Courdy C, Carpentier C, de Bernard S, et al.; POLA Network (2012). SNP array analysis reveals novel genomic abnormalities including copy neutral loss of heterozygosity in anaplastic oligodendrogliomas. PLoS One. 7(10):e45950. PMID:23071531
1085. Idbaih A, Mokhtari K, Emile JF, Galanaud D, Belaid H, de Bernard S, et al. (2014). Dramatic response of a BRAF V600E-mutated primary CNS histiocytic sarcoma to vemurafenib. Neurology. 83(16):1478–80. PMID:25209580
1086. Ikeda J, Sawamura Y, van Meir EG (1998). Pineoblastoma presenting in familial adenomatous polyposis (FAP): random association, FAP variant or Turcot syndrome? Br J Neurosurg. 12(6):576–8. PMID:10070471
1087. Ikezaki K, Matsushima T, Inoue T, Yokoyama N, Kaneko Y, Fukui M (1993). Correlation of microanatomical localization with postoperative survival in posterior fossa ependymomas. Neurosurgery. 32(1):38–44. PMID:8421555
1088. Ikota H, Tanaka Y, Yokoo H, Nakazato Y (2011). Clinicopathological and immunohistochemical study of 20 choroid plexus tumors: their histological diversity and the expression of markers useful for differentiation from metastatic cancer. Brain Tumor Pathol. 28(3):215–21. PMID:21394517
1089. Ilhan I, Berberoglu S, Kutluay L, Maden HA (1998). Subcutaneous sacrococcygeal myxopapillary ependymoma. Med Pediatr Oncol. 30(2):81–4. PMID:9403014
1090. Imperiale A, Moussallieh FM, Roche P, Battini S, Cicek AE, Sebag F, et al. (2015). Metabolome profiling by HRMAS NMR spectroscopy of pheochromocytomas and paragangliomas detects SDH deficiency: clinical and pathophysiological implications. Neoplasia. 17(1):55–65. PMID:25622899
1091. Inatomi Y, Ito T, Nagae K, Yamada Y, Kiyomatsu M, Nakano-Nakamura M, et al. (2014). Hybrid perineurioma-neurofibroma in a patient with neurofibromatosis type 1, clinically mimicking malignant peripheral nerve sheath tumor. Eur J Dermatol. 24(3):412–3. PMID:24751814
1092. Ingham PW (1998). The patched gene in development and cancer. Curr Opin Genet Dev. 8(1):88–94. PMID:9529611
1093. Ingold B, Wild PJ, Nocito A, Amin MB, Storz M, Heppner FL, et al. (2008). Renal cell carcinoma marker reliably discriminates central nervous system haemangioblastoma from brain metastases of renal cell carcinoma. Histopathology. 52(6):674–81. PMID:18393979
1094. Inoue Y, Nemoto Y, Murata R, Tashiro T, Shakudo M, Kohno K, et al. (1998). CT and MR imaging of cerebral tuberous sclerosis. Brain Dev. 20(4):209–21. PMID:9661965
1095. Cairncross G, Berkey B, Shaw E, Jenkins R, Scheithauer B, Brachman D, et al.; Intergroup Radiation Therapy Oncology Group Trial 9402 (2006). Phase III trial of chemotherapy plus radiotherapy compared with radiotherapy alone for pure and mixed anaplastic oligodendroglioma: Intergroup Radiation Therapy Oncology Group Trial 9402. J Clin Oncol. 24(18):2707–14. PMID:16782910
1096. Ironside JW, Jefferson AA, Royds JA, Taylor CB, Timperley WR (1984). Carcinoid tumour arising in a recurrent intradural spinal teratoma. Neuropathol Appl Neurobiol. 10(6):479–89. PMID:6084821
1097. Ishida M, Hotta M, Tsukamura A, Taga T, Kato H, Ohta S, et al. (2010). Malignant transformation in craniopharyngioma after radiation therapy: a case report and review of the literature. Clin Neuropathol. 29(1):2–8. PMID:20040326
1098. Ishii N, Sawamura Y, Tada M, Daub DM, Janzer RC, Meagher-Villemure M, et al. (1998). Absence of p53 gene mutations in a tumor panel representative of pilocytic astrocytoma diversity using a p53 functional assay. Int J Cancer. 76(6):797–800. PMID:9626343
1099. Ishizawa K, Kan-nuki S, Kumagai H, Komori T, Hirose T (2002). Lipomatous primitive neuroectodermal tumor with a glioblastoma component: a case report. Acta Neuropathol. 103(2):193–8. PMID:11810187
1100. Ishizawa K, Komori T, Hirose T (2005). Stromal cells in hemangioblastoma: neuroectodermal differentiation and morphological similarities to ependymoma. Pathol Int. 55(7):377–85. PMID:15982211
1101. Ishizawa K, Komori T, Shimada S, Hirose T (2008). Olig2 and CD99 are useful negative markers for the diagnosis of brain tumors. Clin Neuropathol. 27(3):118–28. PMID:18552083
1102. Ishizawa T, Komori T, Shibahara J, Ishizawa K, Adachi J, Nishikawa R, et al. (2006). Papillary glioneuronal tumor with minigemistocytic components and increased proliferative activity. Hum Pathol. 37(5):627–30. PMID:16647962
1103. Ismat FA, Xu J, Lu MM, Epstein JA (2006). The neurofibromin GAP-related domain rescues endothelial but not neural crest development in Nf1 mice. J Clin Invest. 116(9):2378–84. PMID:16906226
1104. Italiano A, Sung YS, Zhang L, Singer S, Maki RG, Coindre JM, et al. (2012). High prevalence of CIC fusion with double-homeobox (DUX4) transcription factors in EWSR1-negative undifferentiated small blue round cell sarcomas. Genes Chromosomes Cancer. 51(3):207–18. PMID:22072439
1105. Ito T, Kanno H, Sato K, Oikawa M, Ozaki Y, Nakamura H, et al. (2014). Clinicopathologic study of pineal parenchymal tumors of intermediate differentiation. World Neurosurg. 81(5-6):783–9. PMID:23396072
1106. Iwaki T, Fukui M, Kondo A, Matsushima T, Takeshita I (1987). Epithelial properties of pleomorphic xanthoastrocytomas determined in ultrastructural and immunohistochemical studies. Acta Neuropathol. 74(2):142–50. PMID:3673505
1107. Iwamoto FM, DeAngelis LM, Abrey LE (2006). Primary dural lymphomas: a clinicopathologic study of treatment and outcome in eight patients. Neurology. 66(11):1763–5. PMID:16769960
1108. Iwashita T, Enjoji M (1987). Plexiform neurilemmoma: a clinicopathological and immunohistochemical analysis of 23 tumours from 20 patients. Virchows Arch A Pathol Anat Histopathol. 411(4):305–9. PMID:3114942
1109. Iwata H, Mori Y, Takagi H, Shirahashi K, Shinoda J, Shimokawa K, et al. (2004). Mediastinal growing teratoma syndrome after cisplatin-based chemotherapy and radiotherapy for intracranial germinoma. J Thorac Cardiovasc Surg. 127(1):291–3. PMID:14752454
1110. Jacks T, Shih TS, Schmitt EM, Bronson RT, Bernards A, Weinberg RA (1994). Tumour predisposition in mice heterozygous for a targeted mutation in Nf1. Nat Genet. 7(3):353–61. PMID:7920653
1111. Jackson CG (2001). Glomus tympanicum and glomus jugulare tumors . Otolaryngol Clin North Am 34: 941-70, vii. PMID:11557448
1112. Jackson M, Hassiotou F, Nowak A (2015). Glioblastoma stem-like cells: at the root of tumor recurrence and a therapeutic target. Carcinogenesis. 36(2):177–85. PMID:25504149
1113. Jacob K, Albrecht S, Sollier C, Faury D, Sader E, Montpetit A, et al. (2009). Duplication of 7q34 is specific to juvenile pilocytic astrocytomas and a hallmark of cerebellar and optic pathway tumours. Br J Cancer. 101(4):722–33. PMID:19603027
1114. Jacobs JJ, Rosenberg AE (1989). Extracranial skeletal metastasis from a pinealoblastoma. A case report and review of the literature. Clin Orthop Relat Res. (247):256–60. PMID:2676297
1115. Jacoby LB, Jones D, Davis K, Kronn D, Short MP, Gusella J, et al. (1997). Molecular analysis of the NF2 tumor-suppressor gene in schwannomatosis. Am J Hum Genet. 61(6):1293–302. PMID:9399891
1116. Jacoby LB, MacCollin M, Barone R, Ramesh V, Gusella JF (1996). Frequency and distribution of NF2 mutations in schwannomas. Genes Chromosomes Cancer. 17(1):45–55. PMID:8889506
1117. Jacoby LB, MacCollin M, Louis DN, Mohney T, Rubio MP, Pulaski K, et al. (1994). Exon scanning for mutation of the NF2 gene in schwannomas. Hum Mol Genet. 3(3):413–9. PMID:8012353
1118. Jacoby LB, Pulaski K, Rouleau GA, Martuza RL (1990). Clonal analysis of human meningiomas and schwannomas. Cancer Res. 50(21):6783–6. PMID:2208143
1119. Jacques TS, Eldridge C, Patel A, Saleem NM, Powell M, Kitchen ND, et al. (2006). Mixed glioneuronal tumour of the fourth ventricle with prominent rosette formation. Neuropathol Appl Neurobiol. 32(2):217–20. PMID:16599951
1120. Jacques TS, Valentine A, Bradford R, McLaughlin JE (2004). December 2003: a 70-year-old woman with a recurrent meningeal mass. Recurrent meningioma with rhabdomyosarcomatous differentiation. Brain Pathol. 14(2):229–30. PMID:15193039
1121. Jaeckle KA, Decker PA, Ballman KV, Flynn PJ, Giannini C, Scheithauer BW, et al. (2011). Transformation of low grade glioma and correlation with outcome: an NCCTG database analysis. J Neurooncol. 104(1):253–9. PMID:21153680
1122. Jaffe ES, Harris NL, Vardiman JW, Campo E, Arber DA, editors. (2010). Hematopathology. 1st Philadelphia. Saunders/ Elsevier.
1123. Jahnke K, Korfel A, Komm J, Bechrakis NE, Stein H, Thiel E, et al. (2006). Intraocular lymphoma 2000–2005: results of a retrospective multicentre trial. Graefes Arch Clin Exp Ophthalmol. 244(6):663–9. PMID:16228920
1124. Jahnke K, Thiel E, Martus P, Herrlinger U, Weller M, Fischer L, et al.; German Primary Central Nervous System Lymphoma Study Group (2006). Relapse of primary central nervous system lymphoma: clinical features, outcome and prognostic factors. J Neurooncol. 80(2):159–65. PMID:16699873
1125. Jahnke K, Thiel E, Schilling A, Herrlinger U, Weller M, Coupland SE, et al. (2005). Low-grade primary central nervous system lymphoma in immunocompetent patients. Br J Haematol. 128(5):616–24. PMID:15725082
1126. Jain A, Amin AG, Jain P, Burger P, Jallo GI, Lim M, et al. (2012). Subependymoma: clinical features and surgical outcomes. Neurol Res. 34(7):677–84. PMID:22747714
1127. Jain RK, Carmeliet P (2012). SnapShot: Tumor angiogenesis. Cell. 149(6):1408–1408.e1. PMID:22682256
1128. Jakacki RI, Burger PC, Kocak M, Boyett JM, Goldwein J, Mehta M, et al. (2015). Outcome and prognostic factors for children with supratentorial primitive neuroectodermal tumors treated with carboplatin during radiotherapy: a report from the Children's Oncology Group. Pediatr Blood Cancer. 62(5):776–83. PMID:25704363
1129. Jakobiec FA, Kool M, Stagner AM, Pfister SM, Eagle RC, Proia AD, et al. (2015). Intraocular Medulloepitheliomas and Embryonal Tumors With Multilayered Rosettes of the Brain: Comparative Roles of LIN28A and C19MC. Am J Ophthalmol. 159(6):1065–1074.e1. PMID:25748578
1130. Jallo GI, Zagzag D, Epstein F (1996). Intramedullary subependymoma of the spinal cord. Neurosurgery. 38(2):251–7. PMID:8869051
1131. Jamal SE, Li S, Bajaj R, Wang Z, Kenyon L, Glass J, et al. (2014). Primary central nervous system Epstein-Barr virus-positive diffuse large B-cell lymphoma of the elderly: a clinicopathologic study of five cases. Brain Tumor Pathol. 31(4):265–73. PMID:24399201
1132. Jansen M, Mohapatra G, Betensky RA, Keohane C, Louis DN (2012). Gain of chromosome arm 1q in atypical meningioma correlates with shorter progression-free survival. Neuropathol Appl Neurobiol. 38(2):213–9. PMID:21988727
1133. Janson K, Nedzi LA, David O, Schorin M, Walsh JW, Bhattacharjee M, et al. (2006). Predisposition to atypical teratoid/rhabdoid tumor due to an inherited INI1 mutation. Pediatr Blood Cancer. 47(3):279–84. PMID:16261613
1134. Janssen D, Harms D (2005). Juvenile xanthogranuloma in childhood and adolescence: a clinicopathologic study of 129 patients from the kiel pediatric tumor registry. Am J Surg Pathol. 29(1):21–8. PMID:15613853
1135. Janz C, Buhl R (2014). Astroblastoma: report of two cases with unexpected clinical behavior and review of the literature. Clin Neurol Neurosurg. 125:114–24. PMID:25108699
1136. Japp AS, Gessi M, Messing-Jünger M, Denkhaus D, Zur Mühlen A, Wolff JE, et al. (2015). High-resolution genomic analysis does not qualify atypical plexus papilloma as a separate entity among choroid plexus tumors. J Neuropathol Exp Neurol. 74(2):110–20. PMID:25575132
1137. Jaros E, Perry RH, Adam L, Kelly PJ, Crawford PJ, Kalbag RM, et al. (1992). Prognostic implications of p53 protein, epidermal growth factor receptor, and Ki-67 labelling in brain tumours. Br J Cancer. 66(2):373–85. PMID:1503912
1138. Jarrell ST, Vortmeyer AO, Linehan WM, Oldfield EH, Lonser RR (2006). Metastases to hemangioblastomas in von Hippel-Lindau disease. J Neurosurg. 105(2):256–63. PMID:17219831
1139. Javahery RJ, Davidson L, Fangusaro J, Finlay JL, Gonzalez-Gomez I, McComb JG (2009). Aggressive variant of a papillary glioneuronal tumor. Report of 2 cases. J Neurosurg Pediatr. 3(1):46–52. PMID:19119904
1140. Jay V, Edwards V, Squire J, Rutka J (1993). Astroblastoma: report of a case with ultrastructural, cell kinetic, and cytogenetic analysis. Pediatr Pathol. 13(3):323–32. PMID:8516227
1141. Jay V, Squire J, Becker LE, Humphreys R (1994). Malignant transformation in a ganglioglioma with anaplastic neuronal and astrocytic components. Report of a case with flow cytometric and cytogenetic analysis. Cancer. 73(11):2862–8. PMID:8194028
1142. Jay V, Squire J, Blaser S, Hoffman HJ, Hwang P (1997). Intracranial and spinal metastases from a ganglioglioma with unusual cytogenetic abnormalities in a patient with complex partial seizures. Childs Nerv Syst. 13(10):550–5. PMID:9403205
1143. Jeffs GJ, Lee GY, Wong GT (2003). Functioning paraganglioma of the thoracic spine: case report. Neurosurgery. 53(4):992–4, discussion 994–5. PMID:14519233
1144. Jehi L, Yardi R, Chagin K, Tassi L, Russo GL, Worrell G, et al. (2015). Development and validation of nomograms to provide individualised predictions of seizure outcomes after epilepsy surgery: a retrospective analysis. Lancet Neurol. 14(3):283–90. PMID:25638640
1145. Jeibmann A, Eikmeier K, Linge A, Kool M, Koos B, Schulz J, et al. (2014). Identification of genes involved in the biology of atypical teratoid/rhabdoid tumours using Drosophila melanogaster. Nat Commun. 5:4005. PMID:24892285
1146. Jeibmann A, Hasselblatt M, Gerss J, Wrede B, Egensperger R, Beschorner R, et al. (2006). Prognostic implications of atypical histologic features in choroid plexus papilloma. J Neuropathol Exp Neurol. 65(11):1069–73. PMID:17086103

1147. Jeibmann A, Wrede B, Peters O, Wolff JE, Paulus W, Hasselblatt M (2007). Malignant progression in choroid plexus papillomas. J Neurosurg. 107(3) Suppl:199–202. PMID:17918524
1148. Jellinger K (2009). Metastatic oligodendrogliomas: a review of the literature and case report. Acta Neurochir (Wien). 151(8):987. PMID:19424658
1149. Jellinger K, Böck F, Brenner H (1988). Meningeal melanocytoma. Report of a case and review of the literature. Acta Neurochir (Wien). 94(1-2):78–87. PMID:3051898
1150. Jenevein EP (1964). A neurohypophyseal tumor originating from pituicytes. Am J Clin Pathol. 41:522–6. PMID:14165459
1151. Jenkins RB, Blair H, Ballman KV, Giannini C, Arusell RM, Law M, et al. (2006). A t(1;19)(q10;p10) mediates the combined deletions of 1p and 19q and predicts a better prognosis of patients with oligodendroglioma. Cancer Res. 66(20):9852–61. PMID:17047046
1152. Jenkins RB, Xiao Y, Sicotte H, Decker PA, Kollmeyer TM, Hansen HM, et al. (2012). A low-frequency variant at 8q24.21 is strongly associated with risk of oligodendroglial tumors and astrocytomas with IDH1 or IDH2 mutation. Nat Genet. 44(10):1122–5. PMID:22922872
1153. Jenkinson MD, Bosma JJ, Du Plessis D, Ohgaki H, Kleihues P, Warnke P, et al. (2003). Cerebellar liponeurocytoma with an unusually aggressive clinical course: case report. Neurosurgery. 53(6):1425–7, discussion 1428. PMID:14633310
1154. Jennings MT, Gelman R, Hochberg F (1985). Intracranial germ-cell tumors: natural history and pathogenesis. J Neurosurg. 63(2):155–67. PMID:2991485
1155. Jensen RL, Caamano E, Jensen EM, Couldwell WT (2006). Development of contrast enhancement after long-term observation of a dysembryoplastic neuroepithelial tumor. J Neurooncol. 78(1):59–62. PMID:16314940
1156. Jentoft M, Giannini C, Rossi S, Mota R, Jenkins RB, Rodriguez FJ (2011). Oligodendroglial tumors with marked desmoplasia: clinicopathologic and molecular features of 7 cases. Am J Surg Pathol. 35(6):845–52. PMID:21552114
1157. Jeong JY, Suh YL, Hong SW (2014). Atypical teratoid/rhabdoid tumor arising in pleomorphic xanthoastrocytoma: a case report. Neuropathology. 34(4):398–405. PMID:25268025
1159. Jeuken JW, Sprenger SH, Gilhuis J, Teepen HL, Grotenhuis AJ, Wesseling P (2002). Correlation between localization, age, and chromosomal imbalances in ependymal tumours as detected by CGH. J Pathol. 197(2):238–44. PMID:12015749
1159A. Jhawar BS, Fuchs CS, Colditz GA, Stampfer MJ (2003). Sex steroid hormone exposures and risk for meningioma. J Neurosurg. 99(5):848–53. PMID:14609164
1160. Jiao Y, Killela PJ, Reitman ZJ, Rasheed AB, Heaphy CM, de Wilde RF, et al. (2012). Frequent ATRX, CIC, FUBP1 and IDH1 mutations refine the classification of malignant gliomas. Oncotarget. 3(7):709–22. PMID:22869205
1161. Jimsheleishvili S, Alshareef AT, Papadimitriou K, Bregy A, Shah AH, Graham RM, et al. (2014). Extracranial glioblastoma in transplant recipients. J Cancer Res Clin Oncol. 140(5):801–7. PMID:24595597
1162. Jo VY, Fletcher CD (2015). Epithelioid malignant peripheral nerve sheath tumor: clinicopathologic analysis of 63 cases. Am J Surg Pathol. 39(5):673–82. PMID:25602794
1163. Jóźwiak S, Kwiatkowski D, Kotulska K, Larysz-Brysz M, Lewin-Kowalik J, Grajkowska W, et al. (2004). Tuberin and hamartin expression is reduced in the majority of subependymal giant cell astrocytomas in tuberous sclerosis complex consistent with a two-hit model of pathogenesis. J Child Neurol. 19(2):102–6. PMID:15072102
1164. Joachim T, Ram Z, Rappaport ZH, Simon M, Schramm J, Wiestler OD, et al. (2001). Comparative analysis of the NF2, TP53, PTEN, KRAS, NRAS and HRAS genes in sporadic and radiation-induced human meningiomas. Int J Cancer. 94(2):218–21. PMID:11668501
1165. Johannsson O, Ostermeyer EA, Håkansson S, Friedman LS, Johansson U, Sellberg G, et al. (1996). Founding BRCA1 mutations in hereditary breast and ovarian cancer in southern Sweden. Am J Hum Genet. 58(3):441–50. PMID:8644702
1166. Goldblum JR, Weiss SW, Folpe AL (2013). Enzinger and Weiss's Soft Tissue Tumors. 6th ed. Philadephia: Elsevier Saunders.
1167. Johnson BE, Mazor T, Hong C, Barnes M, Aihara K, McLean CY, et al. (2014). Mutational analysis reveals the origin and therapy-driven evolution of recurrent glioma. Science. 343(6167):189–93. PMID:24336570
1168. Johnson MW, Eberhart CG, Perry A, Tihan T, Cohen KJ, Rosenblum MK, et al. (2010). Spectrum of pilomyxoid astrocytomas: intermediate pilomyxoid tumors. Am J Surg Pathol. 34(12):1783–91. PMID:21107083
1169. Johnson MW, Emelin JK, Park SH, Vinters HV (1999). Co-localization of TSC1 and TSC2 gene products in tubers of patients with tuberous sclerosis. Brain Pathol. 9(1):45–54. PMID:9989450
1170. Johnson MW, Kerfoot C, Bushnell T, Li M, Vinters HV (2001). Hamartin and tuberin expression in human tissues. Mod Pathol. 14(3):202–10. PMID:11266527
1171. Johnson RA, Wright KD, Poppleton H, Mohankumar KM, Finkelstein D, Pounds SB, et al. (2010). Cross-species genomics matches driver mutations and cell compartments to model ependymoma. Nature. 466(7306):632–6. PMID:20639864
1172. Johnson RL, Rothman AL, Xie J, Goodrich LV, Bare JW, Bonifas JM, et al. (1996). Human homolog of patched, a candidate gene for the basal cell nevus syndrome. Science. 272(5268):1668–71. PMID:8658145
1173. Johnston DL, Keene DL, Lafay-Cousin L, Steinbok P, Sung L, Carret AS, et al. (2008). Supratentorial primitive neuroectodermal tumors: a Canadian pediatric brain tumor consortium report. J Neurooncol. 86(1):101–8. PMID:17619825
1174. Jones AC, Shyamsundar MM, Thomas MW, Maynard J, Idziaszczyk S, Tomkins S, et al. (1999). Comprehensive mutation analysis of TSC1 and TSC2-and phenotypic correlations in 150 families with tuberous sclerosis. Am J Hum Genet. 64(5):1305–15. PMID:10205261
1175. Jones C, Baker SJ (2014). Unique genetic and epigenetic mechanisms driving paediatric diffuse high-grade glioma. Nat Rev Cancer. 14(10):14. PMID:25230881
1176. Jones DT, Hutter B, Jäger N, Korshunov A, Kool M, Warnatz HJ, et al.; International Cancer Genome Consortium PedBrain Tumor Project (2013). Recurrent somatic alterations of FGFR1 and NTRK2 in pilocytic astrocytoma. Nat Genet. 45(8):927–32. PMID:23817572
1177. Jones DT, Ichimura K, Liu L, Pearson DM, Plant K, Collins VP (2006). Genomic analysis of pilocytic astrocytomas at 0.97 Mb resolution shows an increasing tendency toward chromosomal copy number change with age. J Neuropathol Exp Neurol. 65(11):1049–58. PMID:17086101
1178. Jones DT, Kocialkowski S, Liu L, Pearson DM, Bäcklund LM, Ichimura K, et al. (2008). Tandem duplication producing a novel oncogenic BRAF fusion gene defines the majority of pilocytic astrocytomas. Cancer Res. 68(21):8673–7. PMID:18974108
1179. Jones H, Steart PV, Weller RO (1991). Spindle-cell glioblastoma or gliosarcoma? Neuropathol Appl Neurobiol. 17(3):177–87. PMID:1653908
1180. Jones RT, Abedalthagafi MS, Brahmandam M, Greenfield EA, Hoang MP, Louis DN, et al. (2015). Cross-reactivity of the BRAF VE1 antibody with epitopes in axonemal dyneins leads to staining of cilia. Mod Pathol. 28(4):596–606. PMID:25412847
1181. Jordanova ES, Riemersma SA, Philippo K, Giphart-Gassler M, Schuuring E, Kluin PM (2002). Hemizygous deletions in the HLA region account for loss of heterozygosity in the majority of diffuse large B-cell lymphomas of the testis and the central nervous system. Genes Chromosomes Cancer. 35(1):38–48. PMID:12203788
1182. Joseph NM, Mosher JT, Buchstaller J, Snider P, McKeever PE, Lim M, et al. (2008). The loss of Nf1 transiently promotes self-renewal but not tumorigenesis by neural crest stem cells. Cancer Cell. 13(2):129–40. PMID:18242513
1183. Joseph NM, Phillips J, Dahiya S, M Felicella M, Tihan T, Brat DJ, et al. (2013). Diagnostic implications of IDH1-R132H and OLIG2 expression patterns in rare and challenging glioblastoma variants. Mod Pathol. 26(3):315–26. PMID:23041832
1184. Jouvet A, Fauchon F, Liberski P, Saint-Pierre G, Didier-Bazes M, Heitzmann A, et al. (2003). Papillary tumor of the pineal region. Am J Surg Pathol. 27(4):505–12. PMID:12657936
1185. Jouvet A, Fèvre-Montange M, Besançon R, Derrington E, Saint-Pierre G, Belin MF, et al. (1994). Structural and ultrastructural characteristics of human pineal gland, and pineal parenchymal tumors. Acta Neuropathol. 88(4):334–48. PMID:7839826
1186. Jouvet A, Lellouch-Tubiana A, Boddaert N, Zerah M, Champier J, Fèvre-Montange M (2005). Fourth ventricle neurocytoma with lipomatous and ependymal differentiation. Acta Neuropathol. 109(3):346–51. PMID:15627205
1187. Jouvet A, Saint-Pierre G, Fauchon F, Privat K, Bouffet E, Ruchoux MM, et al. (2000). Pineal parenchymal tumors: a correlation of histological features with prognosis in 66 cases. Brain Pathol. 10(1):49–60. PMID:10668895
1188. Jozwiak J, Jozwiak S, Skopinski P (2005). Immunohistochemical and microscopic studies on giant cells in tuberous sclerosis. Histol Histopathol. 20(4):1321–6. PMID:16136513
1189. Juco J, Horvath E, Smyth H, Rotondo F, Kovacs K (2007). Hemangiopericytoma of the sella mimicking pituitary adenoma: case report and review of the literature. Clin Neuropathol. 26(6):288–93. PMID:18232595
1190. Judkins AR, Burger PC, Hamilton RL, Kleinschmidt-DeMasters B, Perry A, Pomeroy SL, et al. (2005). INI1 protein expression distinguishes atypical teratoid/rhabdoid tumor from choroid plexus carcinoma. J Neuropathol Exp Neurol. 64(5):391–7. PMID:15892296
1191. Judkins AR, Ellison DW (2010). Ependymoblastoma: dear, damned, distracting diagnosis, farewell!*. Brain Pathol. 20(1):133–9. PMID:19120373
1192. Judkins AR, Mauger J, Ht A, Rorke LB, Biegel JA (2004). Immunohistochemical analysis of hSNF5/INI1 in pediatric CNS neoplasms. Am J Surg Pathol. 28(5):644–50. PMID:15105654
1192A. Jung KW, Ha J, Lee SH, Won YJ, Yoo H (2013). An updated nationwide epidemiology of primary brain tumors in republic of Korea. Brain Tumor Res Treat. 1(1):16–23. PMID:24904884
1193. Jung SM, Kuo TT (2005). Immunoreactivity of CD10 and inhibin alpha in differentiating hemangioblastoma of central nervous system from metastatic clear cell renal cell carcinoma. Mod Pathol. 18(6):788–94. PMID:15578072
1194. Jurco S 3rd, Nadji M, Harvey DG, Parker JC Jr, Font RL, Morales AR (1982). Hemangioblastomas: histogenesis of the stromal cell studied by immunocytochemistry. Hum Pathol. 13(1):13–8. PMID:6176519
1195. Jänisch W, Janda J, Link I (1994). [Primary diffuse leptomeningeal leiomyomatosis]. Zentralbl Pathol. 140(2):195–200. PMID:7947627
1196. Jänisch W, Staneczek W (1989). [Primary tumors of the choroid plexus. Frequency, localization and age]. Zentralbl Allg Pathol. 135(3):235–40. PMID:2773602
1197. Jääskeläinen J (1986). Seemingly complete removal of histologically benign intracranial meningioma: late recurrence rate and factors predicting recurrence in 657 patients. A multivariate analysis. Surg Neurol. 26(5):461–9. PMID:3764651
1198. Jääskeläinen J, Paetau A, Pyykkö I, Blomstedt G, Palva T, Troupp H (1994). Interface between the facial nerve and large acoustic neurinomas. Immunohistochemical study of the cleavage plane in NF2 and non-NF2 cases. J Neurosurg. 80(3):541–7. PMID:8113868
1199. Kacerovska D, Michal M, Kuroda N, Tanaka A, Sima R, Denisjuk N, et al. (2013). Hybrid peripheral nerve sheath tumors, including a malignant variant in type 1 neurofibromatosis. Am J Dermatopathol. 35(6):641–9. PMID:23676318
1200. Kachhara R, Bhattacharya RN, Nair S, Radhakrishnan VV (2003). Liponeurocytoma of the cerebellum–a case report. Neurol India. 51(2):274–6. PMID:14571027
1201. Kadonaga JN, Frieden IJ (1991). Neurocutaneous melanosis: definition and review of the literature. J Am Acad Dermatol. 24(5 Pt 1):747–55. PMID:1869648
1202. Kaido T, Sasaoka Y, Hashimoto H, Taira K (2003). De novo germinoma in the brain in association with Klinefelter's syndrome: case report and review of the literature. Surg Neurol. 60(6):553–8, discussion 559. PMID:14670679
1203. Kakita A, Inenaga C, Kameyama S, Masuda H, Ueno T, Honma J, et al. (2005). Cerebral lipoma and the underlying cortex of the temporal lobe: pathological features associated with the malformation. Acta Neuropathol. 109(3):339–45. PMID:15622498
1204. Kalamarides M, Niwa-Kawakita M, Leblois H, Abramowski V, Perricaudet M, Janin A, et al. (2002). Nf2 gene inactivation in arachnoidal cells is rate-limiting for meningioma development in the mouse. Genes Dev. 16(9):1060–5. PMID:12000789
1205. Kalamarides M, Stemmer-Rachamimov AO, Niwa-Kawakita M, Chareyre F, Taranchon E, Han ZY, et al. (2011). Identification of a progenitor cell of origin capable of generating diverse meningioma histological subtypes. Oncogene. 30(20):2333–44. PMID:21242963
1206. Kaloshi G, Alikaj V, Rroji A, Vreto G, Petrela M (2013). Visual and auditory hallucinations revealing cerebellar extraventricular neurocytoma: uncommon presentation for uncommon tumor in uncommon location. Gen Hosp Psychiatry. 35(6):680.e1–3. PMID:24199787
1207. Kalyan-Raman UP, Olivero WC (1987). Ganglioglioma: a correlative clinicopathological and radiological study of ten surgically treated cases with follow-up. Neurosurgery. 20(3):428–33. PMID:3574619
1208. Kambham N, Chang Y, Matsushima AY (1998). Primary low-grade B-cell lymphoma of mucosa-associated lymphoid tissue (MALT) arising in dura. Clin Neuropathol. 17(6):311–7. PMID:9832258
1209. Kamoshima Y, Sawamura Y, Sugiyama T, Yamaguchi S, Houkin K, Kubota K (2011). Primary central nervous system mucosa-associated lymphoid tissue lymphoma–case report. Neurol Med Chir (Tokyo). 51(7):527–30. PMID:21785250
1210. Kanamori M, Kumabe T, Saito R, Yamashita Y, Sonoda Y, Ariga H, et al. (2009). Optimal treatment strategy for intracranial germ cell tumors: a single institution analysis. J Neurosurg Pediatr. 4(6):506–14. PMID:19951035
1211. Kandenwein JA, Bostroem A, Feuss M, Pietsch T, Simon M (2011). Surgical management of intracranial subependymomas.

Acta Neurochir (Wien). 153(7):1469–75. PMID:21499782
1212. Kandt RS, Haines JL, Smith M, Northrup H, Gardner RJ, Short MP, et al. (1992). Linkage of an important gene locus for tuberous sclerosis to a chromosome 16 marker for polycystic kidney disease. Nat Genet. 2(1):37–41. PMID:1303246
1213. Kane AJ, Sughrue ME, Rutkowski MJ, Aranda D, Mills SA, Lehil M, et al. (2012). Atypia predicting prognosis for intracranial extraventricular neurocytomas. J Neurosurg. 116(2):349–54. PMID:22054208
1214. Kane AJ, Sughrue ME, Rutkowski MJ, Shangari G, Fang S, McDermott MW, et al. (2011). Anatomic location is a risk factor for atypical and malignant meningiomas. Cancer. 117(6):1272–8. PMID:21381014
1215. Kannan K, Inagaki A, Silber J, Gorovets D, Zhang J, Kastenhuber ER, et al. (2012). Whole-exome sequencing identifies ATRX mutation as a key molecular determinant in lower-grade glioma. Oncotarget. 3(10):1194–203. PMID:23104868
1216. Kanner AA, Staugaitis SM, Castilla EA, Chernova O, Prayson RA, Vogelbaum MA, et al. (2006). The impact of genotype on outcome in oligodendroglioma: validation of the loss of chromosome arm 1p as an important factor in clinical decision making. J Neurosurg. 104(4):542–50. PMID:16619658
1217. Kanno H, Nishihara H, Oikawa M, Ozaki Y, Murata J, Sawamura Y, et al. (2012). Expression of O^6-methylguanine DNA methyltransferase (MGMT) and immunohistochemical analysis of 12 pineal parenchymal tumors. Neuropathology. 32(6):647–53. PMID:22458700
1218. Kannuki S, Bando K, Soga T, Matsumoto K, Hirose T (1996). [A case report of dysembryoplastic neuroepithelial tumor associated with neurofibromatosis type 1]. No Shinkei Geka. 24(2):183–8. PMID:8849480
1219. Kapadia SB, Frisman DM, Hitchcock CL, Ellis GL, Popek EJ (1993). Melanotic neuroectodermal tumor of infancy. Clinicopathological, immunohistochemical, and flow cytometric study. Am J Surg Pathol. 17(6):566–73. PMID:8392815
1220. Karafin M, Jallo GI, Ayars M, Eberhart CG, Rodriguez FJ (2011). Rosette forming glioneuronal tumor in association with Noonan syndrome: pathobiological implications. Clin Neuropathol. 30(6):297–300. PMID:22011734
1221. Karaki S, Mochida J, Lee YH, Nishimura K, Tsutsumi Y (1999). Low-grade malignant perineurioma of the paravertebral column, transforming into a high-grade malignancy. Pathol Int. 49(9):820–5. PMID:10504555
1222. Karamchandani JR, Nielsen TO, van de Rijn M, West RB (2012). Sox10 and S100 in the diagnosis of soft-tissue neoplasms. Appl Immunohistochem Mol Morphol. 20(5):445–50. PMID:22495377
1223. Karamitopoulou E, Perentes E, Diamantis I, Maraziotis T (1994). Ki-67 immunoreactivity in human central nervous system tumors: a study with MIB 1 monoclonal antibody on archival material. Acta Neuropathol. 87(1):47–54. PMID:7511316
1224. Karnes PS, Tran TN, Cui MY, Raffel C, Gilles FH, Barranger JA, et al. (1992). Cytogenetic analysis of 39 pediatric central nervous system tumors. Cancer Genet Cytogenet. 59(1):12–9. PMID:1313329
1225. Karpinski NC, Yaghmai R, Barba D, Hansen LA (1999). Case of the month: March 1999–A 26 year old HIV positive male with dura based masses. Brain Pathol. 9(3):609–10. PMID:10416997
1226. Karremann M, Butenhoff S, Rausche U, Pietsch T, Wolff JE, Kramm CM (2009). Pediatric giant cell glioblastoma: New insights into a rare tumor entity. Neuro Oncol. 11(3):323–9. PMID:19050301
1227. Karremann M, Pietsch T, Janssen G, Kramm CM, Wolff JE (2009). Anaplastic ganglioglioma in children. J Neurooncol. 92(2):157–63. PMID:19043777
1228. Karremann M, Rausche U, Fleischhack G, Nathrath M, Pietsch T, Kramm CM, et al. (2010). Clinical and epidemiological characteristics of pediatric gliosarcomas. J Neurooncol. 97(2):257–65. PMID:19806321
1229. Karremann M, Rausche U, Roth D, Kühn A, Pietsch T, Gielen GH, et al. (2013). Cerebellar location may predict an unfavourable prognosis in paediatric high-grade glioma. Br J Cancer. 109(4):844–51. PMID:23868007
1230. Kasashima S, Oda Y, Nozaki J, Shirasaki M, Nakanishi I (2000). A case of atypical granular cell tumor of the neurohypophysis. Pathol Int. 50(7):568–73. PMID:10886742
1231. Kato K, Nakatani Y, Kanno H, Inayama Y, Ijiri R, Nagahara N, et al. (2004). Possible linkage between specific histological structures and aberrant reactivation of the Wnt pathway in adamantinomatous craniopharyngioma. J Pathol. 203(3):814–21. PMID:15221941
1232. Kato S, Han SY, Liu W, Otsuka K, Shibata H, Kanamaru R, et al. (2003). Understanding the function-structure and function-mutation relationships of p53 tumor suppressor protein by high-resolution missense mutation analysis. Proc Natl Acad Sci U S A. 100(14):8424–9. PMID:12826609
1233. Katoh M, Aida T, Sugimoto S, Suwamura Y, Abe H, Isu T, et al. (1995). Immunohistochemical analysis of giant cell glioblastoma. Pathol Int. 45(4):275–82. PMID:7550996
1234. Katsetos CD, Herman MM, Frankfurter A, Gass P, Collins VP, Walker CC, et al. (1989). Cerebellar desmoplastic medulloblastomas. A further immunohistochemical characterization of the reticulin-free pale islands. Arch Pathol Lab Med. 113(9):1019–29. PMID:2505732
1235. Katsetos CD, Herman MM, Krishna L, Vender JR, Vinores SA, Agamanolis DP, et al. (1995). Calbindin-D28k in subsets of medulloblastomas and in the human medulloblastoma cell line D283 Med. Arch Pathol Lab Med. 119(8):734–43. PMID:7646332
1236. Katsetos CD, Krishna L, Friedberg E, Reidy J, Karkavelas G, Savory J (1994). Lobar pilocytic astrocytomas of the cerebral hemispheres: II. Pathobiology–morphogenesis of the eosinophilic granular bodies. Clin Neuropathol. 13(6):306–14. PMID:7851045
1237. Kaufman DL, Heinrich BS, Willett C, Perry A, Finseth F, Sobel RA, et al. (2003). Somatic instability of the NF2 gene in schwannomatosis. Arch Neurol. 60(9):1317–20. PMID:12975302
1238. Kaulich K, Blaschke B, Nümann A, von Deimling A, Wiestler OD, Weber RG, et al. (2002). Genetic alterations commonly found in diffusely infiltrating cerebral gliomas are rare or absent in pleomorphic xanthoastrocytomas. J Neuropathol Exp Neurol. 61(12):1092–9. PMID:12484572
1239. Kaur B, Khwaja FW, Severson EA, Matheny SL, Brat DJ, Van Meir EG (2005). Hypoxia and the hypoxia-inducible-factor pathway in glioma growth and angiogenesis. Neuro Oncol. 7(2):134–53. PMID:15831232
1240. Kaur K, Kakkar A, Kumar A, Mallick S, Julka PK, Gupta D, et al. (2015). Integrating molecular subclassification of medulloblastomas into routine clinical practice: A simplified approach. Brain Pathol. PMID:26222673
1241. Kawano N, Yasui Y, Utsuki S, Oka H, Fujii K, Yamashina S (2004). Light microscopic demonstration of the microlumen of ependymoma: a study of the usefulness of antigen retrieval for epithelial membrane antigen (EMA) immunostaining. Brain Tumor Pathol. 21(1):17–21. PMID:15696964
1242. Kehrer-Sawatzki H, Cooper DN (2008). Mosaicism in sporadic neurofibromatosis type 1: variations on a theme common to other hereditary cancer syndromes? J Med Genet. 45(10):622–31. PMID:18511569
1243. Keith J, Lownie S, Ang LC (2006). Co-existence of paraganglioma and myxopapillary ependymoma of the cauda equina. Acta Neuropathol. 111(6):617–8. PMID:16718356
1244. Kelleher T, Aquilina K, Keohane C, O'Sullivan MG (2005). Intramedullary capillary haemangioma. Br J Neurosurg. 19(4):345–8. PMID:16455542
1245. Kelsey KT, Wrensch M, Zuo ZF, Miike R, Wiencke JK (1997). A population-based case-control study of the CYP2D6 and GSTT1 polymorphisms and malignant brain tumors. Pharmacogenetics. 7(6):463–8. PMID:9429231
1246. Kepes JJ (1978). Transitional cell tumor of the pituitary gland developing from a Rathke's cleft cyst. Cancer. 41(1):337–43. PMID:626939
1247. Kepes JJ (1987). Astrocytomas: old and newly recognized variants, their spectrum of morphology and antigen expression. Can J Neurol Sci. 14(2):109–21. PMID:3607613
1248. Kepes JJ (1993). Pleomorphic xanthoastrocytoma: the birth of a diagnosis and a concept. Brain Pathol. 3(3):269–74. PMID:8293186
1249. Kepes JJ, Chen WY, Connors MH, Vogel FS (1988). "Chordoid" meningeal tumors in young individuals with peritumoral lymphoplasmacellular infiltrates causing systemic manifestations of the Castleman syndrome. A report of seven cases. Cancer. 62(2):391–406. PMID:3383139
1250. Kepes JJ, Fulling KH, Garcia JH (1982). The clinical significance of "adenoid" formations of neoplastic astrocytes, imitating metastatic carcinoma, in gliosarcomas. A review of five cases. Clin Neuropathol. 1(4):139–50. PMID:6188569
1251. Kepes JJ, Lewis RC, Vergara GG (1980). Cerebellar astrocytoma invading the musculature and soft tissues of the neck. Case report. J Neurosurg. 52(3):414–8. PMID:7359199
1252. Kepes JJ, Moral LA, Wilkinson SB, Abdullah A, Llena JF (1998). Rhabdoid transformation of tumor cells in meningiomas: a histologic indication of increased proliferative activity: report of four cases. Am J Surg Pathol. 22(2):231–8. PMID:9500225
1253. Kepes JJ, Rubinstein LJ (1981). Malignant gliomas with heavily lipidized (foamy) tumor cells: a report of three cases with immunoperoxidase study. Cancer. 47(10):2451–9. PMID:7023643
1254. Kepes JJ, Rubinstein LJ, Eng LF (1979). Pleomorphic xanthoastrocytoma: a distinctive meningocerebral glioma of young subjects with relatively favorable prognosis. A study of 12 cases. Cancer. 44(5):1839–52. PMID:498051
1255. Kerfoot C, Wienecke R, Menchine M, Emelin J, Maize JC Jr, Welsh CT, et al. (1996). Localization of tuberous sclerosis 2 mRNA and its protein product tuberin in normal human brain and in cerebral lesions of patients with tuberous sclerosis. Brain Pathol. 6(4):367–75. PMID:8944308
1256. Kesari S, Schiff D, Drappatz J, LaFrankie D, Doherty L, Macklin EA, et al. (2009). Phase II study of protracted daily temozolomide for low-grade gliomas in adults. Clin Cancer Res. 15(1):330–7. PMID:19118062
1257. Keser H, Barnes M, Moes G, Lee HS, Tıhan T (2014). Well-differentiated pediatric glial neoplasms with features of oligodendroglioma, angiocentric glioma and dysembryoplastic neuroepithelial tumors: a morphological diagnostic challenge. Turk Patoloji Derg. 30(1):23–9. PMID:24448703
1258. Kessler BA, Bookhout C, Jaikumar S, Hipps J, Lee YZ (2015). Disseminated oligodendroglial-like leptomeningeal tumor with anaplastic progression and presumed extraneural disease: case report. Clin Imaging. 39(2):300–4. PMID:25518979
1259. Khalatbari MR, Hamidi M, Moharamzad Y (2013). Primary alveolar rhabdomyosarcoma of the brain with long-term survival. J Neurooncol. 115(1):131–3. PMID:23857335
1260. Khalid L, Carone M, Dumrongpisutikul N, Intrapiromkul J, Bonekamp D, Barker PB, et al. (2012). Imaging characteristics of oligodendrogliomas that predict grade. AJNR Am J Neuroradiol. 33(5):852–7. PMID:22268087
1261. Khanani MF, Hawkins C, Shroff M, Dirks P, Capra M, Burger PC, et al. (2006). Pilomyxoid astrocytoma in a patient with neurofibromatosis. Pediatr Blood Cancer. 46(3):377–80. PMID:15800886
1262. Khanna M, Siraj F, Chopra P, Bhalla S, Roy S (2011). Gliosarcoma with prominent smooth muscle component (gliomyosarcoma): a report of 10 cases. Indian J Pathol Microbiol. 54(1):51–4. PMID:21393877
1263. Khuong-Quang DA, Buczkowicz P, Rakopoulos P, Liu XY, Fontebasso AM, Bouffet E, et al. (2012). K27M mutation in histone H3.3 defines clinically and biologically distinct subgroups of pediatric diffuse intrinsic pontine gliomas. Acta Neuropathol. 124(3):439–47. PMID:22661320
1264. Kienast Y, von Baumgarten L, Fuhrmann M, Klinkert WE, Goldbrunner R, Herms J, et al. (2010). Real-time imaging reveals the single steps of brain metastasis formation. Nat Med. 16(1):116–22. PMID:20023634
1265. Kijima C, Miyashita T, Suzuki M, Oka H, Fujii K (2012). Two cases of nevoid basal cell carcinoma syndrome associated with meningioma caused by a PTCH1 or SUFU germline mutation. Fam Cancer. 11(4):565–70. PMID:22829011
1266. Kilday JP, Mitra B, Domerg C, Ward J, Andreiuolo F, Osteso-Ibanez T, et al. (2012). Copy number gain of 1q25 predicts poor progression-free survival for pediatric intracranial ependymomas and enables patient risk stratification: a prospective European clinical trial cohort analysis on behalf of the Children's Cancer Leukaemia Group (CCLG), Societe Francaise d'Oncologie Pediatrique (SFOP), and International Society for Pediatric Oncology (SIOP). Clin Cancer Res. 18(7):2001–11. PMID:22338015
1267. Kilday JP, Rahman R, Dyer S, Ridley L, Lowe J, Coyle B, et al. (2009). Pediatric ependymoma: biological perspectives. Mol Cancer Res. 7(6):765–86. PMID:19531565
1268. Killela PJ, Pirozzi CJ, Healy P, Reitman ZJ, Lipp E, Rasheed BA, et al. (2014). Mutations in IDH1, IDH2, and in the TERT promoter define clinically distinct subgroups of adult malignant gliomas. Oncotarget. 5(6):1515–25. PMID:24722048
1269. Killela PJ, Pirozzi CJ, Reitman ZJ, Jones S, Rasheed BA, Lipp E, et al. (2014). The genetic landscape of anaplastic astrocytoma. Oncotarget. 5(6):1452–7. PMID:24140581
1270. Killela PJ, Reitman ZJ, Jiao Y, Bettegowda C, Agrawal N, Diaz LA Jr, et al. (2013). TERT promoter mutations occur frequently in gliomas and a subset of tumors derived from cells with low rates of self-renewal. Proc Natl Acad Sci U S A. 110(15):6021–6. PMID:23530248
1271. Kim B, Chung CK, Myung JK, Park SH (2009). Pleomorphic xanthoastrocytoma associated with long-standing Taylor-type IIB-focal cortical dysplasia in an adult. Pathol Res Pract. 205(2):113–7. PMID:18657915
1272. Kim BS, Kim DK, Park SH (2009). Pineal parenchymal tumor of intermediate differentiation showing malignant progression at relapse. Neuropathology. 29(5):602–8. PMID:19170892
1273. Kim DG, Lee DY, Paek SH, Chi JG, Choe G, Jung HW (2002). Supratentorial primitive neuroectodermal tumors in adults. J Neurooncol. 60(1):43–52. PMID:12416545
1274. Kim DH, Suh YL (1997). Pseudopapillary neurocytoma of temporal lobe with glial differentiation. Acta Neuropathol. 94(2):187–91. PMID:9255395
1275. Kim ES, Kwon MJ, Song JH, Kim DH, Park HR (2015). Adenocarcinoma arising from intracranial recurrent mature teratoma and featuring mutated KRAS and wild-type

BRAF genes. Neuropathology. 35(1):44–9. PMID:25039399
1276. Kim KH, Roberts CW (2014). Mechanisms by which SMARCB1 loss drives rhabdoid tumor growth. Cancer Genet. 207(9):365–72. PMID:24853101
1277. Kim MS, Kim YS, Lee HK, Lee GJ, Choi CY, Lee CH (2014). Primary intracranial ectopic craniopharyngioma in a patient with probable Gardner's syndrome. J Neurosurg. 120(2):337–41. PMID:24266539
1278. Kim SD, Nakagawa H, Mizuno J, Inoue T (2005). Thoracic subpial intramedullary schwannoma involving a ventral nerve root: a case report and review of the literature. Surg Neurol. 63(4):389–93, discussion 393. PMID:15808734
1279. Kim Y, Lee SY, Yi KS, Cha SH, Gang MH, Cho BS, et al. (2014). Infratentorial and intraparenchymal subependymoma in the cerebellum: case report. Korean J Radiol. 15(1):151–5. PMID:24497806
1280. Kim YH, Kim JW, Park CK, Kim DG, Sohn CH, Chang KH, et al. (2010). Papillary tumor of pineal region presenting with leptomeningeal seeding. Neuropathology. 30(6):654–60. PMID:20374498
1281. Kim YH, Nobusawa S, Mittelbronn M, Paulus W, Brokinkel B, Keyvani K, et al. (2010). Molecular classification of low-grade diffuse gliomas. Am J Pathol. 177(6):2708–14. PMID:21075857
1282. Kim YH, Nonoguchi N, Paulus W, Brokinkel B, Keyvani K, Sure U, et al. (2012). Frequent BRAF gain in low-grade diffuse gliomas with 1p/19q loss. Brain Pathol. 22(6):834–40. PMID:22568401
1283. Kim YH, Ohta T, Oh JE, Le Calvez-Kelm F, McKay J, Voegele C, et al. (2014). TP53, MSH4, and LATS1 germline mutations in a family with clustering of nervous system tumors. Am J Pathol. 184(9):2374–81. PMID:25041856
1284. Kimonis VE, Goldstein AM, Pastakia B, Yang ML, Kase R, DiGiovanna JJ, et al. (1997). Clinical manifestations in 105 persons with nevoid basal cell carcinoma syndrome. Am J Med Genet. 69(3):299–308. PMID:9096761
1285. Kimura T, Budka H, Soler-Federsppiel S (1986). An immunocytochemical comparison of the glia-associated proteins glial fibrillary acidic protein (GFAP) and S-100 protein (S100P) in human brain tumors. Clin Neuropathol. 5(1):21–7. PMID:3512139
1286. Kinsler VA, Thomas AC, Ishida M, Bulstrode NW, Loughlin S, Hing S, et al. (2013). Multiple congenital melanocytic nevi and neurocutaneous melanosis are caused by postzygotic mutations in codon 61 of NRAS. J Invest Dermatol. 133(9):2229–36. PMID:23392294
1287. Kirkpatrick PJ, Honavar M, Janota I, Polkey CE (1993). Control of temporal lobe epilepsy following en bloc resection of low-grade tumors. J Neurosurg. 78(1):19–25. PMID:8416237
1288. Kissil JL, Wilker EW, Johnson KC, Eckman MS, Yaffe MB, Jacks T (2003). Merlin, the product of the Nf2 tumor suppressor gene, is an inhibitor of the p21-activated kinase, Pak1. Mol Cell. 12(4):841–9. PMID:14580336
1288A. Kita D, Yonekawa Y, Weller M, Ohgaki H (2007). PIK3CA alterations in primary (de novo) and secondary glioblastomas. Acta Neuropathol. 113(3):295–302. PMID:17235514
1289. Kleihues P, Burger PC, Scheithauer BW (1993). The new WHO classification of brain tumours. Brain Pathol. 3(3):255–68. PMID:8293185
1290. Kleihues P, Burger PC, Scheithauer BW, editors. (1993). Histological Typing of Tumours of the Central Nervous System. World Health Organization International Histological Classification of Tumours. 2nd ed. Berlin, Heidelberg: Springer Verlag.
1291. Kleihues P, Cavenee WK, editors. (2000). World Health Organization Classification of Tumours. Pathology and Genetics of Tumours of the Nervous System. 3rd ed. Lyon: IARC Press.
1292. Kleihues P, Kiessling M, Janzer RC (1987). Morphological markers in neuro-oncology. Curr Top Pathol. 77:307–38. PMID:2827963
1293. Kleihues P, Louis DN, Scheithauer BW, Rorke LB, Reifenberger G, Burger PC, et al. (2002). The WHO classification of tumors of the nervous system. J Neuropathol Exp Neurol. 61(3):215–25, discussion 226–9. PMID:11895036
1294. Kleihues P, Schäuble B, zur Hausen A, Estève J, Ohgaki H (1997). Tumors associated with p53 germline mutations: a synopsis of 91 families. Am J Pathol. 150(1):1–13. PMID:9006316
1295. Kleinman CL, Gerges N, Papillon-Cavanagh S, Sin-Chan P, Pramatarova A, Quang DA, et al. (2014). Fusion of TTYH1 with the C19MC microRNA cluster drives expression of a brain-specific DNMT3B isoform in the embryonal brain tumor ETMR. Nat Genet. 46(1):39–44. PMID:24316981
1296. Kleinman GM, Schoene WC, Walshe TM 3rd, Richardson EP Jr (1978). Malignant transformation in benign cerebellar astrocytoma. Case report. J Neurosurg. 49(1):111–8. PMID:660255
1297. Kleinschmidt-DeMasters BK, Aisner DL, Birks DK, Foreman NK (2013). Epithelioid GBMs show a high percentage of BRAF V600E mutation. Am J Surg Pathol. 37(5):685–98. PMID:23552385
1298. Kleinschmidt-DeMasters BK, Aisner DL, Foreman NK (2015). BRAF VE1 immunoreactivity patterns in epithelioid glioblastomas positive for BRAF V600E mutation. Am J Surg Pathol. 39(4):528–40. PMID:25581727
1299. Kleinschmidt-DeMasters BK, Alassiri AH, Birks DK, Newell KL, Moore W, Lillehei KO (2010). Epithelioid versus rhabdoid glioblastomas are distinguished by monosomy 22 and immunohistochemical expression of INI-1 but not claudin 6. Am J Surg Pathol. 34(3):341–54. PMID:20118769
1300. Kleinschmidt-DeMasters BK, Boylan A, Capocelli K, Boyer PJ, Foreman NK (2011). Multinodular leptomeningeal metastases from ETANTR contain both small blue cell and maturing neuropil elements. Acta Neuropathol. 122(6):783–5. PMID:22033877
1301. Kleinschmidt-DeMasters BK, Lopes MB (2013). Update on hypophysitis and TTF-1 expressing sellar region masses. Brain Pathol. 23(5):495–514. PMID:23701182
1302. Kleinschmidt-DeMasters BK, Meltesen L, McGavran L, Lillehei KO (2006). Characterization of glioblastomas in young adults. Brain Pathol. 16(4):273–86. PMID:17107596
1303. Kliewer KE, Cochran AJ (1989). A review of the histology, ultrastructure, immunohistology, and molecular biology of extra-adrenal paragangliomas. Arch Pathol Lab Med. 113(11):1209–18. PMID:2684087
1304. Klintworth GK, Garner A, editors. (2008). Garner and Klintworth's Pathobiology of ocular disease. 3rd Boca Raton. CRC Press.
1305. Kloub O, Perry A, Tu PH, Lipper M, Lopes MB (2005). Spindle cell oncocytoma of the adenohypophysis: report of two recurrent cases. Am J Surg Pathol. 29(2):247–53. PMID:15644783
1306. Kluwe L, MacCollin M, Tatagiba M, Thomas S, Hazim W, Haase W, et al. (1998). Phenotypic variability associated with 14 splice-site mutations in the NF2 gene. Am J Med Genet. 77(3):228–33. PMID:9605590
1307. Kluwe L, Mautner V, Heinrich B, Dezube R, Jacoby LB, Friedrich RE, et al. (2003). Molecular study of frequency of mosaicism in neurofibromatosis 2 patients with bilateral vestibular schwannomas. J Med Genet. 40(2):109–14. PMID:12566519
1308. Kluwe L, Mautner VF (1998). Mosaicism in sporadic neurofibromatosis 2 patients. Hum Mol Genet. 7(13):2051–5. PMID:9817921
1309. Knobbe CB, Trampe-Kieslich A, Reifenberger G (2005). Genetic alteration and expression of the phosphoinositol-3-kinase/Akt pathway genes PIK3CA and PIKE in human glioblastomas. Neuropathol Appl Neurobiol. 31(5):486–90. PMID:16150119
1310. Knowles DM (1999). Immunodeficiency-associated lymphoproliferative disorders. Mod Pathol. 12(2):200–17. PMID:10071343
1311. Ko LJ, Prives C (1996). p53: puzzle and paradigm. Genes Dev. 10(9):1054–72. PMID:8654922
1312. Kochi N, Budka H (1987). Contribution of histiocytic cells to sarcomatous development of the gliosarcoma. An immunohistochemical study. Acta Neuropathol. 73(2):124–30. PMID:3111162
1313. Koelsche C, Hovestadt V, Jones DT, Capper D, Sturm D, Sahm F, et al. (2015). Melanotic tumors of the nervous system are characterized by distinct mutational, chromosomal and epigenomic profiles. Brain Pathol. 25(2):202–8. PMID:25399693
1314. Koelsche C, Sahm F, Capper D, Reuss D, Sturm D, Jones DT, et al. (2013). Distribution of TERT promoter mutations in pediatric and adult tumors of the nervous system. Acta Neuropathol. 126(6):907–15. PMID:24154961
1315. Koelsche C, Sahm F, Paulus W, Mittelbronn M, Giangaspero F, Antonelli M, et al. (2014). BRAF V600E expression and distribution in desmoplastic infantile astrocytoma/ganglioglioma. Neuropathol Appl Neurobiol. 40(3):337–44. PMID:23822828
1316. Koelsche C, Sahm F, Wöhrer A, Jeibmann A, Schittenhelm J, Kohlhof P, et al. (2014). BRAF-mutated pleomorphic xanthoastrocytoma is associated with temporal location, reticulin fiber deposition and CD34 expression. Brain Pathol. 24(3):221–9. PMID:24345274
1317. Koelsche C, Schweizer L, Renner M, Warth A, Jones DT, Sahm F, et al. (2014). Nuclear relocation of STAT6 reliably predicts NAB2-STAT6 fusion for the diagnosis of solitary fibrous tumour. Histopathology. 65(5):613–22. PMID:24702701
1318. Koelsche C, Wöhrer A, Jeibmann A, Schittenhelm J, Schindler G, Preusser M, et al. (2013). Mutant BRAF V600E protein in ganglioglioma is predominantly expressed by neuronal tumor cells. Acta Neuropathol. 125(6):891–900. PMID:23435618
1319. Koen JL, McLendon RE, George TM (1998). Intradural spinal teratoma: evidence for a dysembryogenic origin. Report of four cases. J Neurosurg. 89(5):844–51. PMID:9817426
1320. Koga T, Iwasaki H, Ishiguro M, Matsuzaki A, Kikuchi M (2002). Losses in chromosomes 17, 19, and 22q in neurofibromatosis type 1 and sporadic neurofibromas: a comparative genomic hybridization analysis. Cancer Genet Cytogenet. 136(2):113–20. PMID:12237234
1320A. Kogerman P, Grimm T, Kogerman L, Krause D, Undén AB, Sandstedt B, et al. (1999). Mammalian suppressor-of-fused modulates nuclear-cytoplasmic shuttling of Gli-1. Nat Cell Biol. 1(5):312–9. PMID:10559945
1321. Komakula S, Warmuth-Metz M, Hildenbrand P, Loevner L, Hewlett R, Salzman K, et al. (2011). Pineal parenchymal tumor of intermediate differentiation: imaging spectrum of an unusual tumor in 11 cases. Neuroradiology. 53(8):577–84. PMID:21080159
1322. Komakula ST, Fenton LZ, Kleinschmidt-DeMasters BK, Foreman NK (2007). Pilomyxoid astrocytoma: neuroimaging with clinicopathologic correlates in 4 cases followed over time. J Pediatr Hematol Oncol. 29(7):465–70. PMID:17609624
1323. Komori T, Arai N (2013). Dysembryoplastic neuroepithelial tumor, a pure glial tumor? Immunohistochemical and morphometric studies. Neuropathology. 33(4):459–68. PMID:23530928
1324. Komori T, Scheithauer BW, Anthony DC, Rosenblum MK, McLendon RE, Scott RM, et al. (1998). Papillary glioneuronal tumor: a new variant of mixed neuronal-glial neoplasm. Am J Surg Pathol. 22(10):1171–83. PMID:9777979
1325. Komori T, Scheithauer BW, Hirose T (2002). A rosette-forming glioneuronal tumor of the fourth ventricle: infratentorial form of dysembryoplastic neuroepithelial tumor? Am J Surg Pathol. 26(5):582–91. PMID:11979088
1326. Komotar RJ, Burger PC, Carson BS, Brem H, Olivi A, Goldthwaite PT, et al. (2004). Pilocytic and pilomyxoid hypothalamic/chiasmatic astrocytomas. Neurosurgery. 54(1):72–9, discussion 79–80. PMID:14683543
1327. Komuro Y, Mikami M, Sakaiya N, Kurahashi T, Komiyama S, Tei C, et al. (2001). Tumor imprint cytology of ovarian ependymoma. A case report. Cancer. 92(12):3165–9. PMID:11753996
1328. Kondziolka D, Parry PV, Lunsford LD, Kano H, Flickinger JC, Rakfal S, et al. (2014). The accuracy of predicting survival in individual patients with cancer. J Neurosurg. 120(1):24–30. PMID:24160479
1329. Kong LY, Wei J, Haider AS, Liebelt BD, Ling X, Conrad CA, et al. (2014). Therapeutic targets in subependymoma. J Neuroimmunol. 277(1-2):168–75. PMID:25465288
1330. Konishi E, Ibayashi N, Yamamoto S, Scheithauer BW (2003). Isolated intracranial Rosai-Dorfman disease (sinus histiocytosis with massive lymphadenopathy). AJNR Am J Neuroradiol. 24(3):515–8. PMID:12637307
1331. Konno S, Oka H, Utsuki S, Kondou K, Tanaka S, Fujii K, et al. (2002). Germinoma with a granulomatous reaction. Problems of differential diagnosis. Clin Neuropathol. 21(6):248–51. PMID:12489672
1332. Konovalov AN, Pitskhelauri DI (2003). Principles of treatment of the pineal region tumors. Surg Neurol. 59(4):250–68. PMID:12748006
1333. Kool M, Jones DT, Jäger N, Northcott PA, Pugh TJ, Hovestadt V, et al.; ICGC PedBrain Tumor Project (2014). Genome sequencing of SHH medulloblastoma predicts genotype-related response to smoothened inhibition. Cancer Cell. 25(3):393–405. PMID:24651015
1334. Kool M, Korshunov A, Remke M, Jones DT, Schlanstein M, Northcott PA, et al. (2012). Molecular subgroups of medulloblastoma: an international meta-analysis of transcriptome, genetic aberrations, and clinical data of WNT, SHH, Group 3, and Group 4 medulloblastomas. Acta Neuropathol. 123(4):473–84. PMID:22358457
1335. Kool M, Koster J, Bunt J, Hasselt NE, Lakeman A, van Sluis P, et al. (2008). Integrated genomics identifies five medulloblastoma subtypes with distinct genetic profiles, pathway signatures and clinicopathological features. PLoS One. 3(8):e3088. PMID:18769486
1336. Koperek O, Gelpi E, Birner P, Haberler C, Budka H, Hainfellner JA (2004). Value and limits of immunohistochemistry in differential diagnosis of clear cell primary brain tumors. Acta Neuropathol. 108(1):24–30. PMID:15108012
1337. Koral K, Koral KM, Sklar F (2012). Angiocentric glioma in a 4-year-old boy: imaging characteristics and review of the literature. Clin Imaging. 36(1):61–4. PMID:22226445
1338. Koral K, Weprin B, Rollins NK (2006). Sphenoid sinus craniopharyngioma simulating mucocele. Acta Radiol. 47(5):494–6. PMID:16796313
1339. Kordek R, Biernat W, Sapieja W, Alwasiak J, Liberski PP (1995). Pleomorphic xanthoastrocytoma with a gangliomatous component: an immunohistochemical and ultrastructural study. Acta Neuropathol. 89(2):194–7. PMID:7732793
1340. Korfel A, Schlegel U (2013). Diagnosis and treatment of primary CNS lymphoma. Nat Rev Neurol. 9(6):317–27. PMID:23670107

1341. Korfel A, Weller M, Martus P, Roth P, Klasen HA, Roeth A, et al. (2012). Prognostic impact of meningeal dissemination in primary CNS lymphoma (PCNSL): experience from the G-PCNSL-SG1 trial. Ann Oncol. 23(9):2374–80. PMID:22396446
1342. Kornreich L, Blaser S, Schwarz M, Shuper A, Vishne TH, Cohen IJ, et al. (2001). Optic pathway glioma: correlation of imaging findings with the presence of neurofibromatosis. AJNR Am J Neuroradiol. 22(10):1963–9. PMID:11733333
1343. Korogi Y, Takahashi M, Ushio Y (2001). MRI of pineal region tumors. J Neurooncol. 54(3):251–61. PMID:11767291
1344. Korshunov A, Golanov A (2001). The prognostic significance of DNA topoisomerase II-alpha (Ki-S1), p21/Cip-1, and p27/Kip-1 protein immunoexpression in oligodendrogliomas. Arch Pathol Lab Med. 125(7):892–8. PMID:11419973
1345. Korshunov A, Golanov A, Sycheva R, Timirgaz V (2004). The histologic grade is a main prognostic factor for patients with intracranial ependymomas treated in the microneurosurgical era: an analysis of 258 patients. Cancer. 100(6):1230–7. PMID:15022291
1345A. Korshunov A, Jakobiec FA, Eberhart CG, Hovestadt V, Capper D, Jones DT, et al. (2015). Comparative integrated molecular analysis of intraocular medulloepitheliomas and central nervous system embryonal tumors with multilayered rosettes confirms that they are distinct nosologic entities. Neuropathology. 35(6):538–44. PMID:26183384
1346. Korshunov A, Remke M, Gessi M, Ryzhova M, Hielscher T, Witt H, et al. (2010). Focal genomic amplification at 19q13.42 comprises a powerful diagnostic marker for embryonal tumors with ependymoblastic rosettes. Acta Neuropathol. 120(2):253–60. PMID:20407781
1347. Korshunov A, Remke M, Werft W, Benner A, Ryzhova M, Witt H, et al. (2010). Adult and pediatric medulloblastomas are genetically distinct and require different algorithms for molecular risk stratification. J Clin Oncol. 28(18):3054–60. PMID:20479417
1348. Korshunov A, Ryzhova M, Jones DT, Northcott PA, van Sluis P, Volckmann R, et al. (2012). LIN28A immunoreactivity is a potent diagnostic marker of embryonal tumor with multilayered rosettes (ETMR). Acta Neuropathol. 124(6):875–81. PMID:23161096
1349. Korshunov A, Sturm D, Ryzhova M, Hovestadt V, Gessi M, Jones DT, et al. (2014). Embryonal tumor with abundant neuropil and true rosettes (ETANTR), ependymoblastoma, and medulloepithelioma share molecular similarity and comprise a single clinicopathological entity. Acta Neuropathol. 128(2):279–89. PMID:24337497
1350. Korshunov A, Sycheva R, Golanov A (2007). Recurrent cytogenetic aberrations in central neurocytomas and their biological relevance. Acta Neuropathol. 113(3):303–12. PMID:17123091
1351. Korshunov A, Witt H, Hielscher T, Benner A, Remke M, Ryzhova M, et al. (2010). Molecular staging of intracranial ependymoma in children and adults. J Clin Oncol. 28(19):3182–90. PMID:20516456
1352. Korten AG, ter Berg HJ, Spincemaille GH, van der Laan RT, Van de Wel AM (1998). Intracranial chondrosarcoma: review of the literature and report of 15 cases. J Neurol Neurosurg Psychiatry. 65(1):88–92. PMID:9667567
1353. Koschny R, Holland H, Koschny T, Vitzthum HE (2006). Comparative genomic hybridization pattern of non-anaplastic and anaplastic oligodendrogliomas–a meta-analysis. Pathol Res Pract. 202(1):23–30. PMID:16356658
1354. Koutourousiou M, Georgakoulias N, Kontogeorgos G, Seretis A (2009). Subependymomas of the lateral ventricle: tumor recurrence correlated with increased Ki-67 labeling index. Neurol India. 57(2):191–3. PMID:19439853
1355. Kowalski RJ, Prayson RA, Mayberg MR (2004). Pituicytoma. Ann Diagn Pathol. 8(5):290–4. PMID:15494936
1356. Kozak KR, Moody JS (2009). Giant cell glioblastoma: a glioblastoma subtype with distinct epidemiology and superior prognosis. Neuro Oncol. 11(6):833–41. PMID:19332771
1357. Kraan W, Horlings HM, van Keimpema M, Schilder-Tol EJ, Oud ME, Scheepstra C, et al. (2013). High prevalence of oncogenic MYD88 and CD79B mutations in diffuse large B-cell lymphomas presenting at immune-privileged sites. Blood Cancer J. 3:e139. PMID:24013661
1358. Kramm CM, Butenhoff S, Rausche U, Warmuth-Metz M, Kortmann RD, Pietsch T, et al. (2011). Thalamic high-grade gliomas in children: a distinct clinical subset? Neuro Oncol. 13(6):680–9. PMID:21636712
1359. Kraus JA, Koopmann J, Kaskel P, Maintz D, Brandner S, Schramm J, et al. (1995). Shared allelic losses on chromosomes 1p and 19q suggest a common origin of oligodendroglioma and oligoastrocytoma. J Neuropathol Exp Neurol. 54(1):91–5. PMID:7815084
1360. Kraus JA, Lamszus K, Glesmann N, Beck M, Wolter M, Sabel M, et al. (2001). Molecular genetic alterations in glioblastomas with oligodendroglial component. Acta Neuropathol. 101(4):311–20. PMID:11355302
1361. Kreiger PA, Okada Y, Simon S, Rorke LB, Louis DN, Golden JA (2005). Losses of chromosomes 1p and 19q are rare in pediatric oligodendrogliomas. Acta Neuropathol. 109(4):387–92. PMID:15739101
1362. Kresse SH, Skårn M, Ohnstad HO, Namløs HM, Bjerkehagen B, Myklebost O, et al. (2008). DNA copy number changes in high-grade malignant peripheral nerve sheath tumors by array CGH. Mol Cancer. 7:48. PMID:18522746
1363. Krieg M, Marti HH, Plate KH (1998). Coexpression of erythropoietin and vascular endothelial growth factor in nervous system tumors associated with von Hippel-Lindau tumor suppressor gene loss of function. Blood. 92(9):3388–93. PMID:9787178
1364. Krieger MD, Gonzalez-Gomez I, Levy ML, McComb JG (1997). Recurrence patterns and anaplastic change in a long-term study of pilocytic astrocytomas. Pediatr Neurosurg. 27(1):1–11. PMID:9486830
1365. Krishnan S, Brown PD, Scheithauer BW, Ebersold MJ, Hammack JE, Buckner JC (2004). Choroid plexus papillomas: a single institutional experience. J Neurooncol. 68(1):49–55. PMID:15174521
1366. Kristof RA, Van Roost D, Wolf HK, Schramm J (1997). Intravascular papillary endothelial hyperplasia of the sellar region. Report of three cases and review of the literature. J Neurosurg. 86(3):558–63. PMID:9046317
1367. Kros J, de Greve K, van Tilborg A, Hop W, Pieterman H, Avezaat C, et al. (2001). NF2 status of meningiomas is associated with tumour localization and histology. J Pathol. 194(3):367–72. PMID:11439370
1368. Kros JM, Cella F, Bakker SL, Paz Y Geuze D, Egeler RM, Egeler RM (2000). Papillary meningioma with pleural metastasis: case report and literature review. Acta Neurol Scand. 102(3):200–2. PMID:10987382
1369. Kros JM, Delwel EJ, de Jong TH, Tanghe HL, van Run PR, Vissers K, et al. (2002). Desmoplastic infantile astrocytoma and ganglioglioma: a search for genomic characteristics. Acta Neuropathol. 104(2):144–8. PMID:12111357
1370. Kros JM, Gorlia T, Kouwenhoven MC, Zheng PP, Collins VP, Figarella-Branger D, et al. (2007). Panel review of anaplastic oligodendroglioma from European Organization For Research and Treatment of Cancer Trial 26951: assessment of consensus in diagnosis, influence of 1p/19q loss, and correlations with outcome. J Neuropathol Exp Neurol. 66(6):545–51. PMID:17549014
1371. Kros JM, Hop WC, Godschalk JJ, Krishnadath KK (1996). Prognostic value of the proliferation-related antigen Ki-67 in oligodendrogliomas. Cancer. 78(5):1107–13. PMID:8780550
1372. Kros JM, Schouten WC, Janssen PJ, van der Kwast TH (1996). Proliferation of gemistocytic cells and glial fibrillary acidic protein (GFAP)-positive oligodendroglial cells in gliomas: a MIB-1/GFAP double labeling study. Acta Neuropathol. 91(1):99–103. PMID:8773153
1373. Kros JM, van den Brink WA, van Loon-van Luyt JJ, Stefanko SZ (1997). Signet-ring cell oligodendroglioma–report of two cases and discussion of the differential diagnosis. Acta Neuropathol. 93(6):638–43. PMID:9194905
1374. Kros JM, Van Eden CG, Stefanko SZ, Waayer-Van Batenburg M, van der Kwast TH (1990). Prognostic implications of glial fibrillary acidic protein containing cell types in oligodendrogliomas. Cancer. 66(6):1204–12. PMID:2205356
1375. Kros JM, Vecht CJ, Stefanko SZ (1991). The pleomorphic xanthoastrocytoma and its differential diagnosis: a study of five cases. Hum Pathol. 22(11):1128–35. PMID:1743696
1376. Krossnes BK, Wester K, Moen G, Mørk SJ (2005). Multifocal dysembryoplastic neuroepithelial tumour in a male with the XYY syndrome. Neuropathol Appl Neurobiol. 31(5):556–60. PMID:16150126
1377. Krouwer HG, Davis RL, Silver P, Prados M (1991). Gemistocytic astrocytomas: a reappraisal. J Neurosurg. 74(3):399–406. PMID:1993905
1378. Krueger DA, Northrup H; International Tuberous Sclerosis Complex Consensus Group (2013). Tuberous sclerosis complex surveillance and management: recommendations of the 2012 International Tuberous Sclerosis Complex Consensus Conference. Pediatr Neurol. 49(4):255–65. PMID:24053983
1379. Krutilkova V, Trkova M, Fleitz J, Gregor V, Novotna K, Krepelova A, et al. (2005). Identification of five new families strengthens the link between childhood choroid plexus carcinoma and germline TP53 mutations. Eur J Cancer. 41(11):1597–603. PMID:15925506
1380. Kubo O, Sasahara A, Tajika Y, Kawamura H, Kawabatake H, Takakura K (1996). Pleomorphic xanthoastrocytoma with neurofibromatosis type 1: case report. Noshuyo Byori. 13(1):79–83. PMID:8916131
1381. Kubota T, Sato K, Arishima H, Takeuchi H, Kitai R, Nakagawa T (2006). Astroblastoma: immunohistochemical and ultrastructural study of distinctive epithelial and probable tanycytic differentiation. Neuropathology. 26(1):72–81. PMID:16521483
1382. Kuchelmeister K, Demirel T, Schlörer E, Bergmann M, Gullotta F (1995). Dysembryoplastic neuroepithelial tumour of the cerebellum. Acta Neuropathol. 89(4):385–90. PMID:7610772
1383. Kuchelmeister K, Hügens-Penzel M, Jödicke A, Schachenmayr W (2006). Papillary tumour of the pineal region: histodiagnostic considerations. Neuropathol Appl Neurobiol. 32(2):203–8. PMID:16599948
1384. Kuchelmeister K, von Borcke IM, Klein H, Bergmann M, Gullotta F (1994). Pleomorphic pineocytoma with extensive neuronal differentiation: report of two cases. Acta Neuropathol. 88(5):448–53. PMID:7847074
1385. Kudo H, Oi S, Tamaki N, Nishida Y, Matsumoto S (1990). Ependymoma diagnosed in the first year of life in Japan in collaboration with the International Society for Pediatric Neurosurgery. Childs Nerv Syst. 6(7):375–8. PMID:1669244
1386. Kuhlmann T, Lassmann H, Brück W (2008). Diagnosis of inflammatory demyelination in biopsy specimens: a practical approach. Acta Neuropathol. 115(3):275–87. PMID:18175128
1387. Kujas M, Faillot T, Lalam T, Roncier B, Catala M, Poirier J (2000). Astroblastomas revisited. Report of two cases with immunocytochemical and electron microscopic study. Histogenetic considerations. Neuropathol Appl Neurobiol. 26(3):295–8. PMID:10886687
1388. Kukreja S, Ambekar S, Sharma M, Sin AH, Nanda A (2015). Outcome predictors in the management of spinal myxopapillary ependymoma: an integrative survival analysis. World Neurosurg. 83(5):852–9 PMID:25108296
1389. Kukreja S, Ambekar S, Sin AH, Nanda A (2014). Cumulative survival analysis of patients with spinal myxopapillary ependymomas in the first 2 decades of life. J Neurosurg Pediatr. 13(4):400–7. PMID:24527863
1390. Kulkarni AV, Pierre-Kahn A, Zerah M (2004). Spontaneous regression of congenital spinal lipomas of the conus medullaris. Report of two cases. J Neurosurg. 101(2) Suppl:226–7. PMID:15835113
1391. Kumar A, Pathak P, Purkait S, Faruq M, Jha P, Mallick S, et al. (2015). Oncogenic KIAA1549-BRAF fusion with activation of the MAPK/ERK pathway in pediatric oligodendrogliomas. Cancer Genet. 208(3):91–5. PMID:25794445
1392. Kumar S, Kumar D, Kaldjian EP, Bauserman S, Raffeld M, Jaffe ES (1997). Primary low-grade B-cell lymphoma of the dura: a mucosa associated lymphoid tissue-type lymphoma. Am J Surg Pathol. 21(1):81–7. PMID:8990144
1393. Kuratsu J, Matsukado Y, Sonoda H (1983). Pseudopsammoma bodies in meningotheliomatous meningioma. A histochemical and ultrastructural study. Acta Neurochir (Wien). 68(1-2):55–62. PMID:6858731
1394. Kurian KM, Summers DM, Statham PF, Smith C, Bell JE, Ironside JW (2005). Third ventricular chordoid glioma: clinicopathological study of two cases with evidence for a poor clinical outcome despite low grade histological features. Neuropathol Appl Neurobiol. 31(4):354–61. PMID:16008819
1395. Kuroiwa T, Bergey GK, Rothman MI, Zoarski GH, Wolf A, Zagardo MT, et al. (1995). Radiologic appearance of the dysembryoplastic neuroepithelial tumor. Radiology. 197(1):233–8. PMID:7568829
1396. Kurose K, Araki T, Matsunaka T, Takada Y, Emi M (1999). Variant manifestation of Cowden disease in Japan: hamartomatous polyposis of the digestive tract with mutation of the PTEN gene. Am J Hum Genet. 64(1):308–10. PMID:9915974
1397. Kurt E, Beute GN, Sluzewski M, van Rooij WJ, Teepen JL (1996). Giant chondroma of the falx. Case report and review of the literature. J Neurosurg. 85(6):1161–4. PMID:8929512
1398. Kurt E, Zheng PP, Hop WC, van der Weiden M, Bol M, van den Bent MJ, et al. (2006). Identification of relevant prognostic histopathologic features in 69 intracranial ependymomas, excluding myxopapillary ependymomas and subependymomas. Cancer. 106(2):388–95. PMID:16342252
1399. Kurtkaya-Yapicier O, Elmaci I, Boran B, Kiliç T, Sav A, Pamir MN (2002). Dysembryoplastic neuroepithelial tumor of the midbrain tectum: a case report. Brain Tumor Pathol. 19(2):97–100. PMID:12622140
1400. Kurzwelly D, Glas M, Roth P, Weimann E, Lohner H, Waha A, et al. (2010). Primary CNS lymphoma in the elderly: temozolomide therapy and MGMT status. J Neurooncol. 97(3):389–92. PMID:19841864
1401. Kwon CH, Zhu X, Zhang J, Knoop LL, Tharp R, Smeyne RJ, et al. (2001). Pten regulates neuronal soma size: a mouse model of Lhermitte-Duclos disease. Nat Genet. 29(4):404–11. PMID:11726927
1402. Küchler J, Hartmann W, Waha A, Koch A, Endl E, Wurst P, et al. (2011). p75(NTR) induces apoptosis in medulloblastoma cells. Int J Cancer. 128(8):1804–12. PMID:20549701

1403. Küker W, Nägele T, Korfel A, Heckl S, Thiel E, Bamberg M, et al. (2005). Primary central nervous system lymphomas (PCNSL): MRI features at presentation in 100 patients. J Neurooncol. 72(2):169–77. PMID:15925998
1403A. Küsters-Vandevelde HV, Creytens D, Grunsven AC, Jeunink M, Winnepenninckx V, Groenen PJ, et al. (2016). SF3B1 and EIF1AX mutations occur in primary leptomeningeal melanocytic neoplasms; yet another similarity to uveal melanomas. Acta Neuropathol Commun. 4(1):5. PMID:26769193
1404. Küsters-Vandevelde HV, Klaasen A, Küsters B, Groenen PJ, van Engen-van Grunsven IA, van Dijk MR, et al. (2010). Activating mutations of the GNAQ gene: a frequent event in primary melanocytic neoplasms of the central nervous system. Acta Neuropathol. 119(3):317–23. PMID:19936769
1405. Küsters-Vandevelde HV, Küsters B, van Engen-van Grunsven AC, Groenen PJ, Wesseling P, Blokx WA (2015). Primary melanocytic tumors of the central nervous system: a review with focus on molecular aspects. Brain Pathol. 25(2):209–26. PMID:25534128
1406. Küsters-Vandevelde HV, van Engen-van Grunsven IA, Küsters B, van Dijk MR, Groenen PJ, Wesseling P, et al. (2010). Improved discrimination of melanotic schwannoma from melanocytic lesions by combined morphological and GNAQ mutational analysis. Acta Neuropathol. 120(6):755–64. PMID:20865267
1407. Labreche K, Simeonova I, Kamoun A, Gleize V, Chubb D, Letouzé E, et al.; POLA Network (2015). TCF12 is mutated in anaplastic oligodendroglioma. Nat Commun. 6:7207. PMID:26068201
1408. Labussière M, Di Stefano AL, Gleize V, Boisselier B, Giry M, Mangesius S, et al. (2014). TERT promoter mutations in gliomas, genetic associations and clinico-pathological correlations. Br J Cancer. 111(10):2024–32. PMID:25314060
1409. Lach B, Duggal N, DaSilva VF, Benoit BG (1996). Association of pleomorphic xanthoastrocytoma with cortical dysplasia and neuronal tumors. A report of three cases. Cancer. 78(12):2551–63. PMID:8952564
1410. Lach B, Duncan E, Rippstein P, Benoit BG (1994). Primary intracranial pleomorphic angioleiomyoma–a new morphologic variant. An immunohistochemical and electron microscopic study. Cancer. 74(7):1915–20. PMID:8082097
1411. Lachenal F, Cotton F, Desmurs-Clavel H, Haroche J, Taillia H, Magy N, et al. (2006). Neurological manifestations and neuroradiological presentation of Erdheim-Chester disease: report of 6 cases and systematic review of the literature. J Neurol. 253(10):1267–77. PMID:17063320
1412. Lack EE (1994). Paragangliomas. In: Sternberg SS, editor. Diagnostic Surgical Pathology. New York: Raven Press; pp. 559–621.
1413. Lafay-Cousin L, Hader W, Wei XC, Nordal R, Strother D, Hawkins C, et al. (2014). Post-chemotherapy maturation in supratentorial primitive neuroectodermal tumors. Brain Pathol. 24(2):166–72. PMID:24033491
1414. Lafay-Cousin L, Hawkins C, Carret AS, Johnston D, Zelcer S, Wilson B, et al. (2012). Central nervous system atypical teratoid rhabdoid tumours: the Canadian Paediatric Brain Tumour Consortium experience. Eur J Cancer. 48(3):353–9. PMID:22023887
1415. Lafay-Cousin L, Keene D, Carret AS, Fryer C, Brossard J, Crooks B, et al. (2011). Choroid plexus tumors in children less than 36 months: the Canadian Pediatric Brain Tumor Consortium (CPBTC) experience. Childs Nerv Syst. 27(2):259–64. PMID:20809071
1416. LaFemina J, Qin LX, Moraco NH, Antonescu CR, Fields RC, Crago AM, et al. (2013). Oncologic outcomes of sporadic, neurofibromatosis-associated, and radiation-induced malignant peripheral nerve sheath tumors. Ann Surg Oncol. 20(1):66–72. PMID:22878618
1417. Lai A, Kharbanda S, Pope WB, Tran A, Solis OE, Peale F, et al. (2011). Evidence for sequenced molecular evolution of IDH1 mutant glioblastoma from a distinct cell of origin. J Clin Oncol. 29(34):4482–90. PMID:22025148
1418. Laigle-Donadey F, Martin-Duverneuil N, Lejeune J, Crinière E, Capelle L, Duffau H, et al. (2004). Correlations between molecular profile and radiologic pattern in oligodendroglial tumors. Neurology. 63(12):2360–2. PMID:15623700
1419. Laigle-Donadey F, Taillibert S, Mokhtari K, Hildebrand J, Delattre JY (2005). Dural metastases. J Neurooncol. 75(1):57–61. PMID:16215816
1420. Lakings DR, Gehrke CW, Waalkes TP (1976). Determination of trimethylsilyl methylated nucleic acid bases in urine by gas-liquid chromatography . J Chromatogr 116: 69-81. PMID:1411
1421. Lal A, Dahiya S, Gonzales M, Hiniker A, Prayson R, Kleinschmidt-DeMasters BK, et al. (2014). IgG4 overexpression is rare in meningiomas with a prominent inflammatory component: a review of 16 cases. Brain Pathol. 24(4):352–9. PMID:24467316
1422. Lam CW, Xie J, To KF, Ng HK, Lee KC, Yuen NW, et al. (1999). A frequent activated smoothened mutation in sporadic basal cell carcinomas. Oncogene. 18(3):833–6. PMID:9989836
1423. Lamb RF, Roy C, Diefenbach TJ, Vinters HV, Johnson MW, Jay DG, et al. (2000). The TSC1 tumour suppressor hamartin regulates cell adhesion through ERM proteins and the GTPase Rho. Nat Cell Biol. 2(5):281–7. PMID:10806479
1424. Lambert SR, Witt H, Hovestadt V, Zucknick M, Kool M, Pearson DM, et al. (2013). Differential expression and methylation of brain developmental genes define location-specific subsets of pilocytic astrocytoma. Acta Neuropathol. 126(2):291–301. PMID:23660940
1425. Lambiv WL, Vassallo I, Delorenzi M, Shay T, Diserens AC, Misra A, et al. (2011). The Wnt inhibitory factor 1 (WIF1) is targeted in glioblastoma and has a tumor suppressing function potentially by induction of senescence. Neuro Oncol. 13(7):736–47. PMID:21642372
1426. Lamont JM, McManamy CS, Pearson AD, Clifford SC, Ellison DW (2004). Combined histopathological and molecular cytogenetic stratification of medulloblastoma patients. Clin Cancer Res. 10(16):5482–93. PMID:15328187
1427. Lamzabi I, Arvanitis LD, Reddy VB, Bitterman P, Gattuso P (2013). Immunophenotype of myxopapillary ependymomas. Appl Immunohistochem Mol Morphol. 21(6):485–9. PMID:23455181
1428. Lang FF, Epstein FJ, Ransohoff J, Allen JC, Wisoff J, Abbott IR, et al. (1993). Central nervous system gangliogliomas. Part 2: Clinical outcome. J Neurosurg. 79(6):867–73. PMID:8246055
1429. Langford LA (1986). The ultrastructure of the ependymoblastoma. Acta Neuropathol. 71(1-2):136–41. PMID:3776467
1430. Langford LA, Camel MH (1987). Palisading pattern in cerebral neuroblastoma mimicking the primitive polar spongioblastoma. An ultrastructural study. Acta Neuropathol. 73(2):153–9. PMID:3604582
1431. Lannering B, Rutkowski S, Doz F, Pizer B, Gustafsson G, Navajas A, et al. (2012). Hyperfractionated versus conventional radiotherapy followed by chemotherapy in standard-risk medulloblastoma: results from the randomized multicenter HIT-SIOP PNET 4 trial. J Clin Oncol. 30(26):3187–93. PMID:22851561
1432. Larkin SJ, Preda V, Karavitaki N, Grossman A, Ansorge O (2014). BRAF V600E mutations are characteristic for papillary craniopharyngioma and may coexist with CTNNB1-mutated adamantinomatous craniopharyngioma. Acta Neuropathol. 127(6):927–9. PMID:24715106
1433. Larson JJ, Tew JM Jr, Simon M, Menon AG (1995). Evidence for clonal spread in the development of multiple meningiomas. J Neurosurg. 83(4):705–9. PMID:7674021
1434. Lashner BA, Riddell RH, Winans CS (1986). Ganglioneuromatosis of the colon and extensive glycogenic acanthosis in Cowden's disease. Dig Dis Sci. 31(2):213–6. PMID:3943449
1435. Laskin WB, Weiss SW, Bratthauer GL (1991). Epithelioid variant of malignant peripheral nerve sheath tumor (malignant epithelioid schwannoma). Am J Surg Pathol. 15(12):1136–45. PMID:1746681
1436. Lassman AB, Iwamoto FM, Cloughesy TF, Aldape KD, Rivera AL, Eichler AF, et al. (2011). International retrospective study of over 1000 adults with anaplastic oligodendroglial tumors. Neuro Oncol. 13(6):649–59. PMID:21636710
1437. Lau D, La Marca F, Camelo-Piragua S, Park P (2013). Metastatic paraganglioma of the spine: case report and review of the literature. Clin Neurol Neurosurg. 115(9):1571–4. PMID:23398849
1438. Lauer DH, Enzinger FM (1980). Cranial fasciitis of childhood. Cancer. 45(2):401–6. PMID:7351023
1439. Lavrnic S, Macvanski M, Ristic-Balos D, Gavrilov M, Damjanovic D, Gavrilovic S, et al. (2012). Papillary glioneuronal tumor: unexplored entity. J Neurol Surg A Cent Eur Neurosurg. 73(4):224–9. PMID:21842459
1440. Laws ER Jr, Goldberg WJ, Bernstein JJ (1993). Migration of human malignant astrocytoma cells in the mammalian brain: Scherer revisited. Int J Dev Neurosci. 11(5):691–7. PMID:8116480
1441. Le DT, Uram JN, Wang H, Bartlett BR, Kemberling H, Eyring AD, et al. (2015). PD-1 Blockade in Tumors with Mismatch-Repair Deficiency. N Engl J Med. 372(26):2509–20. PMID:26028255
1442. Le LQ, Shipman T, Burns DK, Parada LF (2009). Cell of origin and microenvironment contribution for NF1-associated dermal neurofibromas. Cell Stem Cell. 4(5):453–63. PMID:19427294
1443. Le Mercier M, Hastir D, Moles Lopez X, De Nève N, Maris C, Trepant AL, et al. (2012). A simplified approach for the molecular classification of glioblastomas. PLoS One. 7(9):e45475. PMID:23029035
1445. LeBoit PE, Burg G, Weedon D, Sarasin A, editors. (2005). World Health Organization Classification of Tumours. Pathology and Genetics of Skin Tumours. 3rd ed. Lyon: IARC Press.1157.
1446. Lebrun C, Fontaine D, Ramaioli A, Vandenbos F, Chanalet S, Lonjon M, et al.; Nice Brain Tumor Study Group (2004). Long-term outcome of oligodendrogliomas. Neurology. 62(10):1783–7. PMID:15159478
1447. Lechapt-Zalcman E, Chapon F, Guillamo JS, Khouri S, Menegalli-Boggelli D, Loussouarn D, et al. (2011). Long-term clinicopathological observations on a papillary tumour of the pineal region. Neuropathol Appl Neurobiol. 37(4):431–5. PMID:20942871
1448. Lee D, Cho YH, Kang SY, Yoon N, Sung CO, Suh YL (2015). BRAF V600E mutations are frequent in dysembryoplastic neuroepithelial tumors and subependymal giant cell astrocytomas. J Surg Oncol. 111(3):359–64. PMID:25346165
1449. Lee D, Suh YL (2010). Histologically confirmed intracranial germ cell tumors; an analysis of 62 patients in a single institute. Virchows Arch. 457(3):347–57. PMID:20652714
1450. Lee DK, Jung HW, Kim DG, Paek SH, Gwak HS, Choe G (2001). Postoperative spinal seeding of craniopharyngioma. Case report. J Neurosurg. 94(4):617–20. PMID:11302661
1451. Lee DY, Chung CK, Hwang YS, Choe G, Chi JG, Kim HJ, et al. (2000). Dysembryoplastic neuroepithelial tumor: radiological findings (including PET, SPECT, and MRS) and surgical strategy. J Neurooncol. 47(2):167–74. PMID:10982159
1452. Lee EB, Tihan T, Scheithauer BW, Zhang PJ, Gonatas NK (2009). Thyroid transcription factor 1 expression in sellar tumors: a histogenetic marker? J Neuropathol Exp Neurol. 68(5):482–8. PMID:19525896
1453. Lee EQ (2015). Nervous system metastases from systemic cancer. Continuum (Minneap Minn). 21 2 Neuro-oncology:415–28. PMID:25837904
1454. Lee HY, Yoon CS, Sevenet N, Rajalingam V, Delattre O, Walford NQ (2002). Rhabdoid tumor of the kidney is a component of the rhabdoid predisposition syndrome. Pediatr Dev Pathol. 5(4):395–9. PMID:12016529
1455. Lee JH, Sundaram V, Stein DJ, Kinney SE, Stacey DW, Golubić M (1997). Reduced expression of schwannomin/merlin in human sporadic meningiomas. Neurosurgery. 40(3):578–87. PMID:9055299
1456. Lee JY, Dong SM, Park WS, Yoo NJ, Kim CS, Jang JJ, et al. (1998). Loss of heterozygosity and somatic mutations of the VHL tumor suppressor gene in sporadic cerebellar hemangioblastomas. Cancer Res. 58(3):504–8. PMID:9458097
1457. Lee JY, Wakabayashi T, Yoshida J (2005). Management and survival of pineoblastoma: an analysis of 34 adults from the brain tumor registry of Japan. Neurol Med Chir (Tokyo). 45(3):132–41, discussion 141–2. PMID:15782004
1458. Lee S, Cimica V, Ramachandra N, Zagzag D, Kalpana GV (2011). Aurora A is a repressed effector target of the chromatin remodeling protein INI1/hSNF5 required for rhabdoid tumor cell survival. Cancer Res. 71(9):3225–35. PMID:21521802
1459. Lee SH, Appleby V, Jeyapalan JN, Palmer RD, Nicholson JC, Sottile V, et al. (2011). Variable methylation of the imprinted gene, SNRPN, supports a relationship between intracranial germ cell tumours and neural stem cells. J Neurooncol. 101(3):419–28. PMID:20582452
1460. Lee W, Teckie S, Wiesner T, Ran L, Prieto Granada CN, Lin M, et al. (2014). PRC2 is recurrently inactivated through EED or SUZ12 loss in malignant peripheral nerve sheath tumors. Nat Genet. 46(11):1227–32. PMID:25240281
1461. Leeds NE, Lang FF, Ribalta T, Sawaya R, Fuller GN (2006). Origin of chordoid glioma of the third ventricle. Arch Pathol Lab Med. 130(4):460–4. PMID:16594739
1462. Leenstra JL, Rodriguez FJ, Frechette CM, Giannini C, Stafford SL, Pollock BE, et al. (2007). Central neurocytoma: management recommendations based on a 35-year experience. Int J Radiat Oncol Biol Phys. 67(4):1145–54. PMID:17187939
1463. Lehman NL (2008). Patterns of brain infiltration and secondary structure formation in supratentorial ependymal tumors. J Neuropathol Exp Neurol. 67(9):900–10. PMID:18716554
1464. Lehman NL, Horoupian DS, Warnke RA, Sundram UN, Peterson K, Harsh GR 4th (2002). Dural marginal zone lymphoma with massive amyloid deposition: rare low-grade primary central nervous system B-cell lymphoma. Case report. J Neurosurg. 96(2):368–72. PMID:11838814
1465. Lehman NL, Jorden MA, Huhn SL, Barnes PD, Nelson GB, Fisher PG, et al. (2003). Cortical ependymoma. A case report and review. Pediatr Neurosurg. 39(1):50–4. PMID:12784079
1466. Lekanne Deprez RH, Bianchi AB, Groen NA, Seizinger BR, Hagemeijer A, van Drunen E, et al. (1994). Frequent NF2 gene transcript mutations in sporadic meningiomas and vestibular schwannomas. Am J Hum Genet.

54(6):1022–9. PMID:7911002
1467. Lellouch-Tubiana A, Boddaert N, Bourgeois M, Fohlen M, Jouvet A, Delalande O, et al. (2005). Angiocentric neuroepithelial tumor (ANET): a new epilepsy-related clinicopathological entity with distinctive MRI. Brain Pathol. 15(4):281–6. PMID:16389940
1468. Lellouch-Tubiana A, Bourgeois M, Vekemans M, Robain O (1995). Dysembryoplastic neuroepithelial tumors in two children with neurofibromatosis type 1. Acta Neuropathol. 90(3):319–22. PMID:8525807
1469. Lemke D, Pfenning PN, Sahm F, Klein AC, Kempf T, Warnken U, et al. (2012). Costimulatory protein 4IgB7H3 drives the malignant phenotype of glioblastoma by mediating immune escape and invasiveness. Clin Cancer Res. 18(1):105–17. PMID:22080438
1470. Leonard JR, Perry A, Rubin JB, King AA, Chicoine MR, Gutmann DH (2006). The role of surgical biopsy in the diagnosis of glioma in individuals with neurofibromatosis-1. Neurology. 67(8):1509–12. PMID:17060590
1471. Leone PE, Bello MJ, Mendiola M, Kusak ME, De Campos JM, Vaquero J, et al. (1998). Allelic status of 1p, 14q, and 22q and NF2 gene mutations in sporadic schwannomas. Int J Mol Med. 1(5):889–92. PMID:9852312
1472. Leoz ML, Carballal S, Moreira L, Ocaña T, Balaguer F (2015). The genetic basis of familial adenomatous polyposis and its implications for clinical practice and risk management. Appl Clin Genet. 8:95–107. PMID:25931827
1473. Lermen O, Frank S, Hassler W (2010). Postoperative spinal recurrence of craniopharyngioma. Acta Neurochir (Wien). 152(2):309–11, discussion 311. PMID:19838829
1474. Lester RA, Brown LC, Eckel LJ, Foote RT, NageswaraRao AA, Buckner JC, et al. (2014). Clinical outcomes of children and adults with central nervous system primitive neuroectodermal tumor. J Neurooncol. 120(2):371–9. PMID:25115737
1475. Letouzé E, Martinelli C, Loriot C, Burnichon N, Abermil N, Ottolenghi C, et al. (2013). SDH mutations establish a hypermethylator phenotype in paraganglioma. Cancer Cell. 23(6):739–52. PMID:23707781
1476. Levin N, Lavon I, Zelikovitsh B, Fuchs D, Bokstein F, Fellig Y, et al. (2006). Progressive low-grade oligodendrogliomas: response to temozolomide and correlation between genetic profile and O6-methylguanine DNA methyltransferase protein expression. Cancer. 106(8):1759–65. PMID:16541434
1477. Levine AJ (1997). p53, the cellular gatekeeper for growth and division. Cell. 88(3):323–31. PMID:9039259
1478. Levy RA (1993). Paraganglioma of the filum terminale: MR findings. AJR Am J Roentgenol. 160(4):851–2. PMID:8456679
1479. Lewis JJ, Brennan MF (1996). Soft tissue sarcomas. Curr Probl Surg. 33(10):817–72. PMID:8885853
1480. Lewis PW, Müller MM, Koletsky MS, Cordero F, Lin S, Banaszynski LA, et al. (2013). Inhibition of PRC2 activity by a gain-of-function H3 mutation found in pediatric glioblastoma. Science. 340(6134):857–61. PMID:23539183
1481. Lewis RA, Gerson LP, Axelson KA, Riccardi VM, Whitford RP (1984). von Recklinghausen neurofibromatosis. II. Incidence of optic gliomata. Ophthalmology. 91(8):929–35. PMID:6436764
1482. Lhermitte J, Duclos P (1920). Sur un ganglioneurome diffus du coertex du cervelet. Bull Assoc Fr Etud Cancer. 9:99–107.
1483. Li D, Schauble B, Moll C, Fisch U (1996). Intratemporal facial nerve perineurioma. Laryngoscope. 106(3 Pt 1):328–33. PMID:8614198
1484. Li D, Wang JM, Li GL, Hao SY, Yang Y, Wu Z, et al. (2014). Clinical, radiological, and pathological features of 16 papillary glioneuronal tumors. Acta Neurochir (Wien). 156(4):627–39. PMID:24553727
1485. Li DM, Sun H (1997). TEP1, encoded by a candidate tumor suppressor locus, is a novel protein tyrosine phosphatase regulated by transforming growth factor beta. Cancer Res. 57(11):2124–9. PMID:9187108
1486. Li FP, Fraumeni JF Jr, Mulvihill JJ, Blattner WA, Dreyfus MG, Tucker MA, et al. (1988). A cancer family syndrome in twenty-four kindreds. Cancer Res. 48(18):5358–62. PMID:3409256
1487. Li G, Mitra S, Karamchandani J, Edwards MS, Wong AJ (2010). Pineal parenchymal tumor of intermediate differentiation: clinicopathological report and analysis of epidermal growth factor receptor variant III expression. Neurosurgery. 66(5):963–8, discussion 968. PMID:20404701
1488. Li J, Simpson L, Takahashi M, Miliaresis C, Myers MP, Tonks N, et al. (1998). The PTEN/MMAC1 tumor suppressor induces cell death that is rescued by the AKT/protein kinase B oncogene. Cancer Res. 58(24):5667–72. PMID:9865719
1489. Li J, Yen C, Liaw D, Podsypanina K, Bose S, Wang SI, et al. (1997). PTEN, a putative protein tyrosine phosphatase gene mutated in human brain, breast, and prostate cancer. Science. 275(5308):1943–7. PMID:9072974
1490. Li JY, Langford LA, Adesina A, Bodhireddy SR, Wang M, Fuller GN (2012). The high mitotic count detected by phospho-histone H3 immunostain does not alter the benign behavior of angiocentric glioma. Brain Tumor Pathol. 29(1):68–72. PMID:21892765
1491. Li M, Lee KF, Lu Y, Clarke I, Shih D, Eberhart C, et al. (2009). Frequent amplification of a chr19q13.41 microRNA polycistron in aggressive primitive neuroectodermal brain tumors. Cancer Cell. 16(6):533–46. PMID:19962671
1492. Li P, James SL, Evans N, Davies AM, Herron B, Sumathi VP (2007). Paraganglioma of the cauda equina with subarachnoid haemorrhage. Clin Radiol. 62(3):277–80. PMID:17293223
1493. Li W, Cooper J, Zhou L, Yang C, Erdjument-Bromage H, Zagzag D, et al. (2014). Merlin/NF2 loss-driven tumorigenesis linked to CRL4(DCAF1)-mediated inhibition of the hippo pathway kinases Lats1 and 2 in the nucleus. Cancer Cell. 26(1):48–60. PMID:25026211
1494. Li W, Graeber MB (2012). The molecular profile of microglia under the influence of glioma. Neuro Oncol. 14(8):958–78. PMID:22573310
1495. Li YS, Ramsay DA, Fan YS, Armstrong RF, Del Maestro RF (1995). Cytogenetic evidence that a tumor suppressor gene in the long arm of chromosome 1 contributes to glioma growth. Cancer Genet Cytogenet. 84(1):46–50. PMID:7497442
1496. Li ZJ, Lan XL, Hao FY, Yao WC, Wang MY, Chen XD, et al. (2014). Primary cerebellar paraganglioma: a pediatric case report and review of the literature. Pediatr Neurol. 50(4):303–6. PMID:24485927
1497. Liang L, Korogi Y, Sugahara T, Ikushima I, Shigematsu Y, Okuda T, et al. (2002). MRI of intracranial germ-cell tumours. Neuroradiology. 44(5):382–8. PMID:12012121
1498. Liang X, Shen D, Huang Y, Yin C, Bojanowski CM, Zhuang Z, et al. (2007). Molecular pathology and CXCR4 expression in surgically excised retinal hemangioblastomas associated with von Hippel-Lindau disease. Ophthalmology. 114(1):147–56. PMID:17070589
1499. Liaw D, Marsh DJ, Li J, Dahia PL, Wang SI, Zheng Z, et al. (1997). Germline mutations of the PTEN gene in Cowden disease, an inherited breast and thyroid cancer syndrome. Nat Genet. 16(1):64–7. PMID:9140396
1500. Ligon KL, Alberta JA, Kho AT, Weiss J, Kwaan MR, Nutt CL, et al. (2004). The oligodendroglial lineage marker OLIG2 is universally expressed in diffuse gliomas. J Neuropathol Exp Neurol. 63(5):499–509. PMID:15198128
1501. Lillehei KO, Donson AM, Kleinschmidt-DeMasters BK (2008). Radiation-induced meningiomas: clinical, cytogenetic, and microarray features. Acta Neuropathol. 116(3):289–301. PMID:18604545
1502. Lim SC, Jang SJ (2006). Myxopapillary ependymoma of the fourth ventricle. Clin Neurol Neurosurg. 108(2):211–4. PMID:16412846
1503. Lim T, Kim SJ, Kim K, Lee JI, Lim H, Lee DJ, et al. (2011). Primary CNS lymphoma other than DLBCL: a descriptive analysis of clinical features and treatment outcomes. Ann Hematol. 90(12):1391–8. PMID:21479535
1504. Lin AL, Liu J, Evans J, Leuthardt EC, Rich KM, Dacey RG, et al. (2014). Codeletions at 1p and 19q predict a lower risk of pseudoprogression in oligodendrogliomas and mixed oligoastrocytomas. Neuro Oncol. 16(1):123–30. PMID:24285548
1505. Lin NU, Amiri-Kordestani L, Palmieri D, Liewehr DJ, Steeg PS (2013). CNS metastases in breast cancer: old challenge, new frontiers. Clin Cancer Res. 19(23):6404–18. PMID:24298071
1506. Lin SL, Wang JS, Huang CS, Tseng HH (1996). Primary intracerebral leiomyoma: a case with eosinophilic inclusions of actin filaments. Histopathology. 28(4):365–9. PMID:8732347
1507. Lin YJ, Yang QX, Tian XY, Li B, Li Z (2013). Unusual primary intracranial dural-based poorly differentiated synovial sarcoma with t(X; 18)(p11; q11). Neuropathology. 33(1):75–82. PMID:22537253
1508. Lindberg N, Jiang Y, Xie Y, Bolouri H, Kastemar M, Olofsson T, et al. (2014). Oncogenic signaling is dominant to cell of origin and dictates astrocytic or oligodendroglial tumor development from oligodendrocyte precursor cells. J Neurosci. 34(44):14644–51. PMID:25355217
1509. Lindstrom KM, Cousar JB, Lopes MB (2010). IgG4-related meningeal disease: clinico-pathological features and proposal for diagnostic criteria. Acta Neuropathol. 120(6):765–76. PMID:20844883
1510. Lindström E, Shimokawa T, Toftgård R, Zaphiropoulos PG (2006). PTCH mutations: distribution and analyses. Hum Mutat. 27(3):215–9. PMID:16419085
1511. Linnebank M, Moskau S, Kowoll A, Semmler A, Bangard C, Vogt-Schaden M, et al. (2012). Association of transcobalamin c. 776C>G with overall survival in patients with primary central nervous system lymphoma. Br J Cancer. 107(11):1840–3. PMID:23099805
1512. Linnebank M, Schmidt S, Kölsch H, Linnebank A, Heun R, Schmidt-Wolf IG, et al. (2004). The methionine synthase polymorphism D919G alters susceptibility to primary central nervous system lymphoma. Br J Cancer. 90(10):1969–71. PMID:15138479
1513. Lipper S, Decker RE (1984). Paraganglioma of the cauda equina. A histologic, immunohistochemical, and ultrastructural study and review of the literature. Surg Neurol. 22(4):415–20. PMID:6474349
1514. Liss L, Kahn EA (1958). Pituicytoma, tumor of the sella turcica; a clinicopathological study. J Neurosurg. 15(5):481–8. PMID:13576191
1515. Listernick R, Charrow J, Greenwald M, Mets M (1994). Natural history of optic pathway tumors in children with neurofibromatosis type 1: a longitudinal study. J Pediatr. 125(1):63–6. PMID:8021787
1516. Listernick R, Ferner RE, Liu GT, Gutmann DH (2007). Optic pathway gliomas in neurofibromatosis-1: controversies and recommendations. Ann Neurol. 61(3):189–98. PMID:17387725
1517. Listernick R, Mancini AJ, Charrow J (2003). Segmental neurofibromatosis in childhood. Am J Med Genet A. 121A(2):132–5. PMID:12910491
1518. Liu K, Wen G, Lv XF, Deng YJ, Deng YJ, Hou GQ, et al. (2013). MR imaging of cerebral extraventricular neurocytoma: a report of 9 cases. AJNR Am J Neuroradiol. 34(3):541–6. PMID:23042917
1519. Liu XY, Gerges N, Korshunov A, Sabha N, Khuong-Quang DA, Fontebasso AM, et al. (2012). Frequent ATRX mutations and loss of expression in adult diffuse astrocytic tumors carrying IDH1/IDH2 and TP53 mutations. Acta Neuropathol. 124(5):615–25. PMID:22886134
1520. Liverman C, Mafra M, Chuang SS, Shivane A, Chakrabarty A, Highley R, et al. (2015). A clinicopathologic study of 11 rosette-forming meningiomas: a rare and potentially confusing pattern. Acta Neuropathol. 130(2):311–3. PMID:26106026
1521. Lloyd KM 2nd, Dennis M (1963). Cowden's disease. A possible new symptom complex with multiple system involvement. Ann Intern Med. 58:136–42. PMID:13931122
1522. Lodding P, Kindblom LG, Angervall L, Stenman G (1990). Cellular schwannoma. A clinicopathologic study of 29 cases. Virchows Arch A Pathol Anat Histopathol. 416(3):237–48. PMID:2105560
1523. Loh JK, Lieu AS, Chai CY, Howng SL (2011). Malignant transformation of a desmoplastic infantile ganglioglioma. Pediatr Neurol. 45(2):135–7. PMID:21763958
1524. Longatti P, Basaldella L, Orvieto E, Dei Tos AP, Martinuzzi A (2006). Aquaporin 1 expression in cystic hemangioblastomas. Neurosci Lett. 392(3):178–80. PMID:16300893
1525. Longy M, Lacombe D (1996). Cowden disease. Report of a family and review. Ann Genet. 39(1):35–42. PMID:9297442
1526. Lopes MB, Altermatt HJ, Scheithauer BW, Shepherd CW, VandenBerg SR (1996). Immunohistochemical characterization of subependymal giant cell astrocytomas. Acta Neuropathol. 91(4):368–75. PMID:8928613
1526A. Los M, Jansen GH, Kaelin WG, Lips CJ, Blijham GH, Voest EE (1996). Expression pattern of the von Hippel-Lindau protein in human tissues. Lab Invest. 75(2):231–8. PMID:8765323
1527. Losa M, Saeger W, Mortini P, Pandolfi C, Terreni MR, Taccagni G, et al. (2000). Acromegaly associated with a granular cell tumor of the neurohypophysis: a clinical and histological study. Case report. J Neurosurg. 93(1):121–6. PMID:10883914
1528. Lossos C, Bayraktar S, Weinzierl E, Younes SF, Hosein PJ, Tibshirani RJ, et al. (2014). LMO2 and BCL6 are associated with improved survival in primary central nervous system lymphoma. Br J Haematol. 165(5):640–8. PMID:24571259
1529. Lotan I, Khlebtovsky A, Inbar E, Strenov J, Djaldetti R, Steiner I (2012). Primary brain T-cell lymphoma in an HTLV-1 serologically positive male. J Neurol Sci. 314(1-2):163–5. PMID:22118868
1530. Louis DN (1994). The p53 gene and protein in human brain tumors. J Neuropathol Exp Neurol. 53(1):11–21. PMID:8301315
1531. Louis DN, Hamilton AJ, Sobel RA, Ojemann RG (1991). Pseudopsammomatous meningioma with elevated serum carcinoembryonic antigen: a true secretory meningioma. Case report. J Neurosurg. 74(1):129–32. PMID:1984492
1532. Louis DN, Hedley-Whyte ET, Martuza RL (1990). Sarcomatous proliferation of the vasculature in a subependymoma: a follow-up study of sarcomatous dedifferentiation. Acta Neuropathol. 80(5):573–4. PMID:2251917
1533. Louis DN, Ohgaki H, Wiestler OD, Cavenee WK, editors. (2007). WHO Classification of Tumours of the Central Nervous System. 4th ed. Lyon: International Agency for Research on Cancer.
1534. Louis DN, Ohgaki H, Wiestler OD, Cavenee WK, Burger PC, Jouvet A, et al. (2007). The 2007 WHO classification of tumours of

the central nervous system. Acta Neuropathol. 114(2):97–109. PMID:17618441
1535. Louis DN, Perry A, Burger P, Ellison DW, Reifenberger G, von Deimling A, et al.; International Society Of Neuropathology--Haarlem (2014). International Society Of Neuropathology–Haarlem consensus guidelines for nervous system tumor classification and grading. Brain Pathol. 24(5):429–35. PMID:24990071
1536. Louis DN, Ramesh V, Gusella JF (1995). Neuropathology and molecular genetics of neurofibromatosis 2 and related tumors. Brain Pathol. 5(2):163–72. PMID:7670657
1537. Louis DN, Richardson EP Jr, Dickersin GR, Petrucci DA, Rosenberg AE, Ojemann RG (1989). Primary intracranial leiomyosarcoma. Case report. J Neurosurg. 71(2):279–82. PMID:2746352
1538. Louis DN, von Deimling A, Dickersin GR, Dooling EC, Seizinger BR (1992). Desmoplastic cerebral astrocytomas of infancy: a histopathologic, immunohistochemical, ultrastructural, and molecular genetic study. Hum Pathol. 23(12):1402–9. PMID:1468778
1539. Lovly CM, Gupta A, Lipson D, Otto G, Brennan T, Chung CT, et al. (2014). Inflammatory myofibroblastic tumors harbor multiple potentially actionable kinase fusions. Cancer Discov. 4(8):889–95. PMID:24875859
1540. Lu C, Ward PS, Kapoor GS, Rohle D, Turcan S, Abdel-Wahab O, et al. (2012). IDH mutation impairs histone demethylation and results in a block to cell differentiation. Nature. 483(7390):474–8. PMID:22343901
1541. Lu JQ, Patel S, Wilson BA, Pugh J, Mehta V (2013). Malignant glioma with angiocentric features. J Neurosurg Pediatr. 11(3):350–5. PMID:23240849
1542. Lu L, Dai Z, Zhong Y, Lv G (2013). Cervical intradural paraganglioma presenting as progressive cervicodynia: case report and literature review. Clin Neurol Neurosurg. 115(3):359–61. PMID:22721774
1543. Lu-Emerson C, Duda DG, Emblem KE, Taylor JW, Gerstner ER, Loeffler JS, et al. (2015). Lessons from anti-vascular endothelial growth factor and anti-vascular endothelial growth factor receptor trials in patients with glioblastoma. J Clin Oncol. 33(10):1197–213. PMID:25713439
1544. Lubs ML, Bauer MS, Formas ME, Djokic B (1991). Lisch nodules in neurofibromatosis type 1. N Engl J Med. 324(18):1264–6. PMID:1901624
1545. Ludwin SK, Rubinstein LJ, Russell DS (1975). Papillary meningioma: a malignant variant of meningioma. Cancer. 36(4):1363–73. PMID:1175134
1546. Lun M, Lok E, Gautam S, Wu E, Wong ET (2011). The natural history of extracranial metastasis from glioblastoma multiforme. J Neurooncol. 105(2):261–73. PMID:21512826
1547. Luse SA, Kernohan JW (1955). Granular-cell tumors of the stalk and posterior lobe of the pituitary gland. Cancer. 8(3):616–22. PMID:14379151
1548. Lusis EA, Watson MA, Chicoine MR, Lyman M, Roerig P, Reifenberger G, et al. (2005). Integrative genomic analysis identifies NDRG2 as a candidate tumor suppressor gene frequently inactivated in clinically aggressive meningioma. Cancer Res. 65(16):7121–6. PMID:16103061
1549. Lutterbach J, Fauchon F, Schild SE, Chang SM, Pagenstecher A, Volk B, et al. (2002). Malignant pineal parenchymal tumors in adult patients: patterns of care and prognostic factors. Neurosurgery. 51(1):44–55, discussion 55–6. PMID:12182434
1550. Lutterbach J, Liegibel J, Koch D, Madlinger A, Frommhold H, Pagenstecher A (2001). Atypical teratoid/rhabdoid tumors in adult patients: case report and review of the literature. J Neurooncol. 52(1):49–56. PMID:11451202
1551. Luyken C, Blümcke I, Fimmers R, Urbach H, Elger CE, Wiestler OD, et al. (2003). The spectrum of long-term epilepsy-associated tumors: long-term seizure and tumor outcome and neurosurgical aspects. Epilepsia. 44(6):822–30. PMID:12790896
1552. Luyken C, Blümcke I, Fimmers R, Urbach H, Wiestler OD, Schramm J (2004). Supratentorial gangliogliomas: histopathologic grading and tumor recurrence in 184 patients with a median follow-up of 8 years. Cancer. 101(1):146–55. PMID:15222000
1553. Lübbe J, von Ammon K, Watanabe K, Hegi ME, Kleihues P (1995). Familial brain tumour syndrome associated with a p53 germline deletion of codon 236. Brain Pathol. 5(1):15–23. PMID:7767487
1554. Lynch ED, Ostermeyer EA, Lee MK, Arena JF, Ji H, Dann J, et al. (1997). Inherited mutations in PTEN that are associated with breast cancer, cowden disease, and juvenile polyposis. Am J Hum Genet. 61(6):1254–60. PMID:9399897
1555. MacCollin M, Chiocca EA, Evans DG, Friedman JM, Horvitz R, Jaramillo D, et al. (2005). Diagnostic criteria for schwannomatosis. Neurology. 64(11):1838–45. PMID:15955931
1556. MacCollin M, Ramesh V, Jacoby LB, Louis DN, Rubio MP, Pulaski K, et al. (1994). Mutational analysis of patients with neurofibromatosis 2. Am J Hum Genet. 55(2):314–20. PMID:7913580
1557. MacCollin M, Willett C, Heinrich B, Jacoby LB, Acierno JS Jr, Perry A, et al. (2003). Familial schwannomatosis: exclusion of the NF2 locus as the germline event. Neurology. 60(12):1968–74. PMID:12821741
1558. MacCollin M, Woodfin W, Kronn D, Short MP (1996). Schwannomatosis: a clinical and pathologic study. Neurology. 46(4):1072–9. PMID:8780094
1559. Machein MR, Plate KH (2004). Role of VEGF in developmental angiogenesis and in tumor angiogenesis in the brain. Cancer Treat Res. 117:191–218. PMID:15015562
1560. Mack SC, Witt H, Piro RM, Gu L, Zuyderduyn S, Stütz AM, et al. (2014). Epigenomic alterations define lethal CIMP-positive ependymomas of infancy. Nature. 506(7489):445–50. PMID:24553142
1561. Mackenzie IR (1999). Central neurocytoma: histologic atypia, proliferation potential, and clinical outcome. Cancer. 85(7):1606–10. PMID:10193953
1562. Mader I, Stock KW, Radue EW, Steinbrich W (1996). Langerhans cell histiocytosis in monocygote twins: case reports. Neuroradiology. 38(2):163–5. PMID:8692432
1563. Maehama T, Dixon JE (1998). The tumor suppressor, PTEN/MMAC1, dephosphorylates the lipid second messenger, phosphatidylinositol 3,4,5-trisphosphate. J Biol Chem. 273(22):13375–8. PMID:9593664
1564. Maertens O, Brems H, Vandesompele J, De Raedt T, Heyns I, Rosenbaum T, et al. (2006). Comprehensive NF1 screening on cultured Schwann cells from neurofibromas. Hum Mutat. 27(10):1030–40. PMID:16941471
1565. Maesawa C, Tamura G, Iwaya T, Ogasawara S, Ishida K, Sato N, et al. (1998). Mutations in the human homologue of the Drosophila patched gene in esophageal squamous cell carcinoma. Genes Chromosomes Cancer. 21(3):276–9. PMID:9523206
1566. Magri L, Cambiaghi M, Cominelli M, Alfaro-Cervello C, Cursi M, Pala M, et al. (2011). Sustained activation of mTOR pathway in embryonic neural stem cells leads to development of tuberous sclerosis complex-associated lesions. Cell Stem Cell. 9(5):447–62. PMID:22056141
1567. Maher ER, Yates JR, Ferguson-Smith MA (1990). Statistical analysis of the two stage mutation model in von Hippel-Lindau disease, and in sporadic cerebellar haemangioblastoma and renal cell carcinoma. J Med Genet. 27(5):311–4. PMID:2352258
1568. Mahzoni P, Zavareh MH, Bagheri M, Hani N, Moqtader B (2012). Intracranial ROSAI-DORFMAN Disease. J Res Med Sci. 17(3):304–7. PMID:23267385
1569. Maier H, Ofner D, Hittmair A, Kitz K, Budka H (1992). Classic, atypical, and anaplastic meningioma: three histopathological subtypes of clinical relevance. J Neurosurg. 77(4):616–23. PMID:1527622
1570. Majores M, von Lehe M, Fassunke J, Schramm J, Becker AJ, Simon M (2008). Tumor recurrence and malignant progression of gangliogliomas. Cancer. 113(12):3355–63. PMID:18988291
1571. Majós C, Aguilera C, Cos M, Camins A, Candiota AP, Delgado-Goñi T, et al. (2009). In vivo proton magnetic resonance spectroscopy of intraventricular tumours of the brain. Eur Radiol. 19(8):2049–59. PMID:19277673
1572. Makino K, Nakamura H, Yano S, Kuratsu J; Kumamoto Brain Tumor Group (2010). Population-based epidemiological study of primary intracranial tumors in childhood. Childs Nerv Syst. 26(8):1029–34. PMID:20349186
1573. Makino K, Nakamura H, Yano S, Kuratsu J; Kumamoto Brain Tumor Research Group (2013). Incidence of primary central nervous system germ cell tumors in childhood: a regional survey in Kumamoto prefecture in southern Japan. Pediatr Neurosurg. 49(3):155–8. PMID:24751890
1574. Makkar HS, Frieden IJ (2002). Congenital melanocytic nevi: an update for the pediatrician. Curr Opin Pediatr. 14(4):397–403. PMID:12130901
1575. Malkin D, Li FP, Strong LC, Fraumeni JF Jr, Nelson CE, Kim DH, et al. (1990). Germ line p53 mutations in a familial syndrome of breast cancer, sarcomas, and other neoplasms. Science. 250(4985):1233–8. PMID:1978757
1576. Mallory SB (1995). Cowden syndrome (multiple hamartoma syndrome). Dermatol Clin. 13(1):27–31. PMID:7712647
1577. Malmström A, Grønberg BH, Marosi C, Stupp R, Frappaz D, Schultz H, et al.; Nordic Clinical Brain Tumour Study Group (NCBTSG) (2012). Temozolomide versus standard 6-week radiotherapy versus hypofractionated radiotherapy in patients older than 60 years with glioblastoma: the Nordic randomised, phase 3 trial. Lancet Oncol. 13(9):916–26. PMID:22877848
1578. Manjila S, Ray A, Hu Y, Cai DX, Cohen ML, Cohen AR (2011). Embryonal tumors with abundant neuropil and true rosettes: 2 illustrative cases and a review of the literature. Neurosurg Focus. 30(1):E2. PMID:21194275
1579. Mantripragada KK, Spurlock G, Kluwe L, Chuzhanova N, Ferner RE, Frayling IM, et al. (2008). High-resolution DNA copy number profiling of malignant peripheral nerve sheath tumors using targeted microarray-based comparative genomic hybridization. Clin Cancer Res. 14(4):1015–24. PMID:18281533
1580. Marano SR, Johnson PC, Spetzler RF (1988). Recurrent Lhermitte-Duclos disease in a child. Case report. J Neurosurg. 69(4):599–603. PMID:3418394
1581. Marcel V, Dichtel-Danjoy ML, Sagne C, Hafsi H, Ma D, Ortiz-Cuaran S, et al. (2011). Biological functions of p53 isoforms through evolution: lessons from animal and cellular models. Cell Death Differ. 18(12):1815–24. PMID:21941372
1581A. Marciscano AE, Stemmer-Rachamimov AO, Niemierko A, Larvie M, Curry WT, Barker FG 2nd, et al. (2016). Benign meningiomas (WHO Grade I) with atypical histological features: correlation of histopathological features with clinical outcomes. J Neurosurg. 124(1):106–14. PMID:26274991
1582. Marcotte L, Aronica E, Baybis M, Crino PB (2012). Cytoarchitectural alterations are widespread in cerebral cortex in tuberous sclerosis complex. Acta Neuropathol. 123(5):685–93. PMID:22327361
1583. Marden FA, Wippold FJ 2nd, Perry A (2003). Fast magnetic resonance imaging in steady-state precession (true FISP) in the prenatal diagnosis of a congenital brain teratoma. J Comput Assist Tomogr. 27(3):427–30. PMID:12794611
1584. Margetts JC, Kalyan-Raman UP (1989). Giant-celled glioblastoma of brain. A clinico-pathological and radiological study of ten cases (including immunohistochemistry and ultrastructure). Cancer. 63(3):524–31. PMID:2912529
1585. Marigo V, Davey RA, Zuo Y, Cunningham JM, Tabin CJ (1996). Biochemical evidence that patched is the Hedgehog receptor. Nature. 384(6605):176–9. PMID:8906794
1586. Markesbery WR, Duffy PE, Cowen D (1973). Granular cell tumors of the central nervous system. J Neuropathol Exp Neurol. 32(1):92–109. PMID:4346659
1587. Markesbery WR, Haugh RM, Young AB (1981). Ultrastructure of pineal parenchymal neoplasms. Acta Neuropathol. 55(2):143–9. PMID:7315200
1588. Marsh A, Wicking C, Wainwright B, Chenevix-Trench G (2005). DHPLC analysis of patients with Nevoid Basal Cell Carcinoma Syndrome reveals novel PTCH missense mutations in the sterol-sensing domain. Hum Mutat. 26(3):283. PMID:16088933
1589. Marsh DJ, Coulon V, Lunetta KL, Rocca-Serra P, Dahia PL, Zheng Z, et al. (1998). Mutation spectrum and genotype-phenotype analyses in Cowden disease and Bannayan-Zonana syndrome, two hamartoma syndromes with germline PTEN mutation. Hum Mol Genet. 7(3):507–15. PMID:9467011
1590. Marsh DJ, Dahia PL, Caron S, Kum JB, Frayling IM, Tomlinson IP, et al. (1998). Germline PTEN mutations in Cowden syndrome-like families. J Med Genet. 35(11):881–5. PMID:9832031
1591. Marsh DJ, Dahia PL, Zheng Z, Liaw D, Parsons R, Gorlin RJ, et al. (1997). Germline mutations in PTEN are present in Bannayan-Zonana syndrome. Nat Genet. 16(4):333–4. PMID:9241266
1592. Marsh DJ, Kum JB, Lunetta KL, Bennett MJ, Gorlin RJ, Ahmed SF, et al. (1999). PTEN mutation spectrum and genotype-phenotype correlations in Bannayan-Riley-Ruvalcaba syndrome suggest a single entity with Cowden syndrome. Hum Mol Genet. 8(8):1461–72. PMID:10400993
1593. Marsh DJ, Roth S, Lunetta KL, Hemminki A, Dahia PL, Sistonen P, et al. (1997). Exclusion of PTEN and 10q22–24 as the susceptibility locus for juvenile polyposis syndrome. Cancer Res. 57(22):5017–21. PMID:9371495
1594. Marsh DJ, Trahair TN, Martin JL, Chee WY, Walker J, Kirk EP, et al. (2008). Rapamycin treatment for a child with germline PTEN mutation. Nat Clin Pract Oncol. 5(6):357–61. PMID:18431376
1595. Marshman LA, Pollock JR, King A, Chawda SJ (2005). Primary extradural epithelioid leiomyosarcoma of the cervical spine: case report and literature review. Neurosurgery. 57(2):E372, discussion E372. PMID:16094142
1596. Martinez R, Roggendorf W, Baretton G, Klein R, Toedt G, Lichter P, et al. (2007). Cytogenetic and molecular genetic analyses of giant cell glioblastoma multiforme reveal distinct profiles in giant cell and non-giant cell subpopulations. Cancer Genet Cytogenet. 175(1):26–34. PMID:17498554
1597. Martinez-Diaz H, Kleinschmidt-DeMasters BK, Powell SZ, Yachnis AT (2003). Giant cell glioblastoma and pleomorphic xanthoastrocytoma show different immunohistochemical profiles for neuronal antigens and p53 but share reactivity for class III beta-tubulin. Arch Pathol Lab Med. 127(9):1187–91. PMID:12946225

1598. Martinez-Salazar A, Supler M, Rojiani AM (1997). Primary intracerebral malignant fibrous histiocytoma: immunohistochemical findings and etiopathogenetic considerations. Mod Pathol. 10(2):149–54. PMID:9127321
1599. Martuza RL, Eldridge R (1988). Neurofibromatosis 2 (bilateral acoustic neurofibromatosis). N Engl J Med. 318(11):684–8. PMID:3125435
1600. Marucci G, Di Oto E, Farnedi A, Panzacchi R, Ligorio C, Foschini MP (2012). Nogo-A: a useful marker for the diagnosis of oligodendroglioma and for identifying 1p19q codeletion. Hum Pathol. 43(3):374–80. PMID:21835431
1601. Maruoka R, Takenouchi T, Torii C, Shimizu A, Misu K, Higasa K, et al. (2014). The use of next-generation sequencing in molecular diagnosis of neurofibromatosis type 1: a validation study. Genet Test Mol Biomarkers. 18(11):722–35. PMID:25325900
1602. Maruya J, Seki Y, Morita K, Nishimaki K, Minakawa T (2006). Meningeal hemangiopericytoma manifesting as massive intracranial hemorrhage–two case reports. Neurol Med Chir (Tokyo). 46(2):92–7. PMID:16498220
1603. Massimino M, Antonelli M, Gandola L, Miceli R, Pollo B, Biassoni V, et al. (2013). Histological variants of medulloblastoma are the most powerful clinical prognostic indicators. Pediatr Blood Cancer. 60(2):210–6. PMID:22693015
1604. Massimino M, Solero CL, Garrè ML, Biassoni V, Cama A, Genitori L, et al. (2011). Second-look surgery for ependymoma: the Italian experience. J Neurosurg Pediatr. 8(3):246–50. PMID:21882914
1605. Masuoka J, Brandner S, Paulus W, Soffer D, Vital A, Chimelli L, et al. (2001). Germline SDHD mutation in paraganglioma of the spinal cord. Oncogene. 20(36):5084–6. PMID:11526495
1606. Mathew RK, O'Kane R, Parslow R, Stiller C, Kenny T, Picton S, et al. (2014). Comparison of survival between the UK and US after surgery for most common pediatric CNS tumors. Neuro Oncol. 16(8):1137–45. PMID:24799454
1607. Mathews JD, Forsythe AV, Brady Z, Butler MW, Goergen SK, Byrnes GB, et al. (2013). Cancer risk in 680,000 people exposed to computed tomography scans in childhood or adolescence: data linkage study of 11 million Australians. BMJ. 346:f2360. PMID:23694687
1608. Mathews T, Moossy J (1974). Gliomas containing bone and cartilage. J Neuropathol Exp Neurol. 33(3):456–71. PMID:4365915
1609. Mathon B, Carpentier A, Clemenceau S, Boch AL, Bitar A, Mokhtari K, et al. (2012). [Paraganglioma of the cauda equina region: Report of six cases and review of the literature]. Neurochirurgie. 58(6):341–5. PMID:22770767
1610. Matsushima T, Inoue T, Takeshita I, Fukui M, Iwaki T, Kitamoto T (1988). Choroid plexus papillomas: an immunohistochemical study with particular reference to the coexpression of prealbumin. Neurosurgery. 23(3):384–9. PMID:3226520
1611. Matsutani M; Japanese Pediatric Brain Tumor Study Group (2001). Combined chemotherapy and radiation therapy for CNS germ cell tumors–the Japanese experience. J Neurooncol. 54(3):311–6. PMID:11767296
1612. Matsutani M, Sano K, Takakura K, Fujimaki T, Nakamura O, Funata N, et al. (1997). Primary intracranial germ cell tumors: a clinical analysis of 153 histologically verified cases. J Neurosurg. 86(3):446–55. PMID:9046301
1613. Matthies C, Samii M (1997). Management of 1000 vestibular schwannomas (acoustic neuromas): clinical presentation. Neurosurgery. 40(1):1–9, discussion 9–10. PMID:8971818
1614. Matyakhina L, Bei TA, McWhinney SR, Pasini B, Cameron S, Gunawan B, et al. (2007). Genetics of carney triad: recurrent losses at chromosome 1 but lack of germline mutations in genes associated with paragangliomas and gastrointestinal stromal tumors. J Clin Endocrinol Metab. 92(8):2938–43. PMID:17535989
1615. Mawrin C, Perry A (2010). Pathological classification and molecular genetics of meningiomas. J Neurooncol. 99(3):379–91. PMID:20809251
1616. Mayer-Proschel M, Kalyani AJ, Mujtaba T, Rao MS (1997). Isolation of lineage-restricted neuronal precursors from multipotent neuroepithelial stem cells. Neuron. 19(4):773–85. PMID:9354325
1617. Mazur MA, Gururangan S, Bridge JA, Cummings TJ, Mukundan S, Fuchs H, et al. (2005). Intracranial Ewing sarcoma. Pediatr Blood Cancer. 45(6):850–6. PMID:15929128
1618. McCabe MG, Ichimura K, Liu L, Plant K, Bäcklund LM, Pearson DM, et al. (2006). High-resolution array-based comparative genomic hybridization of medulloblastomas and supratentorial primitive neuroectodermal tumors. J Neuropathol Exp Neurol. 65(6):549–61. PMID:16783165
1619. McClatchey AI, Giovannini M (2005). Membrane organization and tumorigenesis–the NF2 tumor suppressor, Merlin. Genes Dev. 19(19):2265–77. PMID:16204178
1620. McCubrey JA, Steelman LS, Abrams SL, Lee JT, Chang F, Bertrand FE, et al. (2006). Roles of the RAF/MEK/ERK and PI3K/PTEN/AKT pathways in malignant transformation and drug resistance. Adv Enzyme Regul. 46:249–79. PMID:16854453
1621. McGarvey TW, Maruta Y, Tomaszewski JE, Linnenbach AJ, Malkowicz SB (1998). PTCH gene mutations in invasive transitional cell carcinoma of the bladder. Oncogene. 17(9):1167–72. PMID:9764827
1622. McGirr SJ, Kelly PJ, Scheithauer BW (1987). Stereotactic resection of juvenile pilocytic astrocytomas of the thalamus and basal ganglia. Neurosurgery. 20(3):447–52. PMID:3553982
1623. McHugh BJ, Baranoski JF, Malhotra A, Vortmeyer AO, Sze G, Duncan CC (2014). Intracranial infantile hemangiopericytoma. J Neurosurg Pediatr. 14(2):149–54. PMID:24905842
1624. McKusick VA. Online Mendelian Inheritance in Man [www.omim.org]
1625. McLendon RE, Bentley RC, Parisi JE, Tien RD, Harrison JC, Tarbell NJ, et al. (1997). Malignant supratentorial glial-neuronal neoplasms: report of two cases and review of the literature. Arch Pathol Lab Med. 121(5):485–92. PMID:9167602
1626. McManamy CS, Lamont JM, Taylor RE, Cole M, Pearson AD, Clifford SC, et al.; United Kingdom Children's Cancer Study Group (2003). Morphophenotypic variation predicts clinical behavior in childhood non-desmoplastic medulloblastomas. J Neuropathol Exp Neurol. 62(6):627–32. PMID:12834107
1627. McManamy CS, Pears J, Weston CL, Hanzely Z, Ironside JW, Taylor RE, et al.; Clinical Brain Tumour Group (2007). Nodule formation and desmoplasia in medulloblastomas-defining the nodular/desmoplastic variant and its biological behavior. Brain Pathol. 17(2):151–64. PMID:17388946
1628. McMenamin ME, Fletcher CD (2001). Expanding the spectrum of malignant change in schwannomas: epithelioid malignant change, epithelioid malignant peripheral nerve sheath tumor, and epithelioid angiosarcoma: a study of 17 cases. Am J Surg Pathol. 25(1):13–25. PMID:11145248
1629. McNatt SA, Gonzalez-Gomez I, Nelson MD, McComb JG (2005). Synchronous multicentric pleomorphic xanthoastrocytoma: case report. Neurosurgery. 57(1):E191, discussion E191. PMID:15987556
1630. Medhkour A, Traul D, Husain M (2002). Neonatal subependymal giant cell astrocytoma. Pediatr Neurosurg. 36(5):271–4. PMID:12053047
1631. Mei K, Liu A, Allan RW, Wang P, Lane Z, Abel TW, et al. (2009). Diagnostic utility of SALL4 in primary germ cell tumors of the central nervous system: a study of 77 cases. Mod Pathol. 22(12):1628–36. PMID:19820689
1632. Meijer-Jorna LB, Aronica E, van der Loos CM, Troost D, van der Wal AC (2012). Congenital vascular malformations–cerebral lesions differ from extracranial lesions by their immune expression of the glucose transporter protein GLUT1. Clin Neuropathol. 31(3):135–41. PMID:22551917
1633. Meis JM, Ho KL, Nelson JS (1990). Gliosarcoma: a histologic and immunohistochemical reaffirmation. Mod Pathol. 3(1):19–24. PMID:2155418
1634. Mellinghoff IK, Wang MY, Vivanco I, Haas-Kogan DA, Zhu S, Dia EQ, et al. (2005). Molecular determinants of the response of glioblastomas to EGFR kinase inhibitors. N Engl J Med. 353(19):2012–24. PMID:16282176
1635. Memoli VA, Brown EF, Gould VE (1984). Glial fibrillary acidic protein (GFAP) immunoreactivity in peripheral nerve sheath tumors. Ultrastruct Pathol. 7(4):269–75. PMID:6543600
1636. Mena H, Ribas JL, Enzinger FM, Parisi JE (1991). Primary angiosarcoma of the central nervous system. Study of eight cases and review of the literature. J Neurosurg. 75(1):73–6. PMID:2045922
1637. Mena H, Ribas JL, Pezeshkpour GH, Cowan DN, Parisi JE (1991). Hemangiopericytoma of the central nervous system: a review of 94 cases. Hum Pathol. 22(1):84–91. PMID:1985083
1638. Mena H, Rushing EJ, Ribas JL, Delahunt B, McCarthy WF (1995). Tumors of pineal parenchymal cells: a correlation of histological features, including nucleolar organizer regions, with survival in 35 cases. Hum Pathol. 26(1):20–30. PMID:7821912
1639. Mendrzyk F, Korshunov A, Benner A, Toedt G, Pfister S, Radlwimmer B, et al. (2006). Identification of gains on 1q and epidermal growth factor receptor overexpression as independent prognostic markers in intracranial ependymoma. Clin Cancer Res. 12(7 Pt 1):2070–9. PMID:16609018
1640. Mendrzyk F, Radlwimmer B, Joos S, Kokocinski F, Benner A, Stange DE, et al. (2005). Genomic and protein expression profiling identifies CDK6 as novel independent prognostic marker in medulloblastoma. J Clin Oncol. 23(34):8853–62. PMID:16314645
1641. Menke JR, Raleigh DR, Gown AM, Thomas S, Perry A, Tihan T (2015). Somatostatin receptor 2a is a more sensitive diagnostic marker of meningioma than epithelial membrane antigen. Acta Neuropathol. 130(3):441–3. PMID:26195322
1642. Menko FH, Kaspers GL, Meijer GA, Claes K, van Hagen JM, Gille JJ (2004). A homozygous MSH6 mutation in a child with café-au-lait spots, oligodendroglioma and rectal cancer. Fam Cancer. 3(2):123–7. PMID:15340263
1643. Merchant TE, Jenkins JJ, Burger PC, Sanford RA, Sherwood SH, Jones-Wallace D, et al. (2002). Influence of tumor grade on time to progression after irradiation for localized ependymoma in children. Int J Radiat Oncol Biol Phys. 53(1):52–7. PMID:12007941
1644. Merchant TE, Li C, Xiong X, Kun LE, Boop FA, Sanford RA (2009). Conformal radiotherapy after surgery for paediatric ependymoma: a prospective study. Lancet Oncol. 10(3):258–66. PMID:19274783
1645. Merchant TE, Pollack IF, Loeffler JS (2010). Brain tumors across the age spectrum: biology, therapy, and late effects. Semin Radiat Oncol. 20(1):58–66. PMID:19959032
1646. Mercuri S, Gazzeri R, Galarza M, Esposito S, Giordano M (2005). Primary meningeal pheochromocytoma: case report. J Neurooncol. 73(2):169–72. PMID:15981108
1647. Mérel P, Hoang-Xuan K, Sanson M, Bijlsma E, Rouleau G, Laurent-Puig P, et al. (1995). Screening for germ-line mutations in the NF2 gene. Genes Chromosomes Cancer. 12(2):117–27. PMID:7535084
1648. Merino DM, Shlien A, Villani A, Pienkowska M, Mack S, Ramaswamy V, et al. (2015). Molecular characterization of choroid plexus tumors reveals novel clinically relevant subgroups. Clin Cancer Res. 21(1):184–92. PMID:25336695
1649. Merker VL, Esparza S, Smith MJ, Stemmer-Rachamimov A, Plotkin SR (2012). Clinical features of schwannomatosis: a retrospective analysis of 87 patients. Oncologist. 17(10):1317–22. PMID:22927469
1650. Merlin E, Chabrier S, Verkarre V, Cramer E, Delabesse E, Stéphan JL (2008). Primary leptomeningeal ALK+ lymphoma in a 13-year-old child. J Pediatr Hematol Oncol. 30(12):963–7. PMID:19131793
1651. Merrell R, Nabors LB, Perry A, Palmer CA (2006). 1p/19q chromosome deletions in metastatic oligodendroglioma. J Neurooncol. 80(2):203–7. PMID:16710746
1652. Messiaen LM, Callens T, Mortier G, Beysen D, Vandenbroucke I, Van Roy N, et al. (2000). Exhaustive mutation analysis of the NF1 gene allows identification of 95% of mutations and reveals a high frequency of unusual splicing defects. Hum Mutat. 15(6):541–55. PMID:10862084
1653. Mester J, Eng C (2012). Estimate of de novo mutation frequency in probands with PTEN hamartoma tumor syndrome. Genet Med. 14(9):819–22. PMID:22595938
1654. Mete O, Lopes MB, Asa SL (2013). Spindle cell oncocytomas and granular cell tumors of the pituitary are variants of pituicytoma. Am J Surg Pathol. 37(11):1694–9. PMID:23887161
1655. Mete O, Tischler AS, de Krijger R, McNicol AM, Eisenhofer G, Pacak K, et al. (2014). Protocol for the examination of specimens from patients with pheochromocytomas and extra-adrenal paragangliomas. Arch Pathol Lab Med. 138(2):182–8. PMID:24476517
1656. Metellus P, Bouvier C, Guyotat J, Fuentes S, Jouvet A, Vasiljevic A, et al. (2007). Solitary fibrous tumors of the central nervous system: clinicopathological and therapeutic considerations of 18 cases. Neurosurgery. 60(4):715–22, discussion 722. PMID:17415209
1657. Meyer P, Eberle MM, Probst A, Tolnay M (2000). [Ganglioglioma of optic nerve in neurofibromatosis type 1. Case report and review of the literature]. Klin Monbl Augenheilkd. 217(1):55–8. PMID:10949818
1658. Meyer-Puttlitz B, Hayashi Y, Waha A, Rollbrocker B, Boström J, Wiestler OD, et al. (1997). Molecular genetic analysis of giant cell glioblastomas. Am J Pathol. 151(3):853–7. PMID:9284834
1659. Meyers SP, Khademian ZP, Biegel JA, Chuang SH, Korones DN, Zimmerman RA (2006). Primary intracranial atypical teratoid/rhabdoid tumors of infancy and childhood: MRI features and patient outcomes. AJNR Am J Neuroradiol. 27(5):962–71. PMID:16687525
1660. Meyers SP, Khademian ZP, Chuang SH, Pollack IF, Korones DN, Zimmerman RA (2004). Choroid plexus carcinomas in children: MRI features and patient outcomes. Neuroradiology. 46(9):770–80. PMID:15309348
1661. Michal M, Kazakov DV, Belousova I, Bisceglia M, Zamecnik M, Mukensnabl P (2004). A benign neoplasm with histopathological features of both schwannoma and retiform perineurioma (benign schwannoma-perineurioma): a report of six cases of a distinctive soft tissue tumor with a predilection for the fingers. Virchows Arch. 445(4):347–53. PMID:15322875
1662. Miettinen M, Shekitka KM, Sobin LH (2001). Schwannomas in the colon and rectum: a clinicopathologic and immunohistochemical study of 20 cases. Am J Surg Pathol. 25(7):846–55. PMID:11420455
1663. Migheli A, Cavalla P, Marino S, Schiffer

D (1994). A study of apoptosis in normal and pathologic nervous tissue after in situ end-labeling of DNA strand breaks. J Neuropathol Exp Neurol. 53(6):606–16. PMID:7525880
1664. Milbouw G, Born JD, Martin D, Collignon J, Hans P, Reznik M, et al. (1988). Clinical and radiological aspects of dysplastic gangliocytoma (Lhermitte-Duclos disease): a report of two cases with review of the literature. Neurosurgery. 22(1 Pt 1):124–8. PMID:3278250
1665. Millard NE, Dunkel IJ (2014). Advances in the management of central nervous system germ cell tumors. Curr Oncol Rep. 16(7):393. PMID:24838613
1666. Miller CA, Torack RM (1970). Secretory ependymoma of the filum terminale. Acta Neuropathol. 15(3):240–50. PMID:4193811
1667. Miller CR, Dunham CP, Scheithauer BW, Perry A (2006). Significance of necrosis in grading of oligodendroglial neoplasms: a clinicopathologic and genetic study of newly diagnosed high-grade gliomas. J Clin Oncol. 24(34):5419–26. PMID:17135643
1668. Miller S, Rogers HA, Lyon P, Rand V, Adamowicz-Brice M, Clifford SC, et al. (2011). Genome-wide molecular characterization of central nervous system primitive neuroectodermal tumor and pineoblastoma. Neuro Oncol. 13(8):866–79. PMID:21798848
1669. Miller S, Ward JH, Rogers HA, Lowe J, Grundy RG (2013). Loss of INI1 protein expression defines a subgroup of aggressive central nervous system primitive neuroectodermal tumors. Brain Pathol. 23(1):19–27. PMID:22672440
1670. Min HS, Lee JY, Kim SK, Park SH (2013). Genetic grouping of medulloblastomas by representative markers in pathologic diagnosis. Transl Oncol. 6(3):265–72. PMID:23730405
1671. Min HS, Lee YJ, Park K, Cho BK, Park SH (2006). Medulloblastoma: histopathologic and molecular markers of anaplasia and biologic behavior. Acta Neuropathol. 112(1):13–20. PMID:16691420
1672. Min KW, Scheithauer BW (1990). Pineal germinomas and testicular seminoma: a comparative ultrastructural study with special references to early carcinomatous transformation. Ultrastruct Pathol. 14(6):483–96. PMID:2281547
1673. Min KW, Scheithauer BW (1997). Clear cell ependymoma: a mimic of oligodendroglioma: clinicopathologic and ultrastructural considerations. Am J Surg Pathol. 21(7):820–6. PMID:9236838
1674. Min KW, Scheithauer BW, Bauserman SC (1994). Pineal parenchymal tumors: an ultrastructural study with prognostic implications. Ultrastruct Pathol. 18(1-2):69–85. PMID:8191649
1675. Min KW, Seo IS, Song J (1987). Postnatal evolution of the human pineal gland. An immunohistochemical study. Lab Invest. 57(6):724–8. PMID:3695415
1676. Minaguchi T, Waite KA, Eng C (2006). Nuclear localization of PTEN is regulated by Ca(2+) through a tyrosil phosphorylation-independent conformational modification in major vault protein. Cancer Res. 66(24):11677–82. PMID:17178862
1677. Minehan KJ, Brown PD, Scheithauer BW, Krauss WE, Wright MP (2009). Prognosis and treatment of spinal cord astrocytoma. Int J Radiat Oncol Biol Phys. 73(3):727–33. PMID:18687533
1678. Minehan KJ, Shaw EG, Scheithauer BW, Davis DL, Onofrio BM (1995). Spinal cord astrocytoma: pathological and treatment considerations. J Neurosurg. 83(4):590–5. PMID:7674006
1678A. Ming JE, Kaupas ME, Roessler E, Brunner HG, Golabi M, Tekin M, et al. (2002). Mutations in PATCHED-1, the receptor for SONIC HEDGEHOG, are associated with holoprosencephaly. Hum Genet. 110(4):297–301. PMID:11941477
1679. Ming JE, Kaupas ME, Roessler E, Brunner HG, Nance WE, Stratton RF, et al. (1998). Mutations of PATCHED in holoprosencephaly. Am J Hum Genet. 63:A140–140.
1680. Mirsattari SM, Chong JJ, Hammond RR, Megyesi JF, Macdonald DR, Lee DH, et al. (2011). Do epileptic seizures predict outcome in patients with oligodendroglioma? Epilepsy Res. 94(1-2):39–44. PMID:21315558
1681. Mishima K, Nakamura M, Nakamura H, Nakamura O, Funata N, Shitara N (1992). Leptomeningeal dissemination of cerebellar pilocytic astrocytoma. Case report. J Neurosurg. 77(5):788–91. PMID:1403124
1682. Mishra T, Goel NA, Goel AH (2014). Primary paraganglioma of the spine: A clinicopathological study of eight cases. J Craniovertebr Junction Spine. 5(1):20–4. PMID:25013343
1683. Mistry M, Zhukova N, Merico D, Rakopoulos P, Krishnatry R, Shago M, et al. (2015). BRAF mutation and CDKN2A deletion define a clinically distinct subgroup of childhood secondary high-grade glioma. J Clin Oncol. 33(9):1015–22. PMID:25667294
1684. Mitchell A, Scheithauer BW, Ebersold MJ, Forbes GS (1991). Intracranial fibromatosis. Neurosurgery. 29(1):123–6. PMID:1870673
1685. Mitchell A, Scheithauer BW, Unni KK, Forsyth PJ, Wold LE, McGivney DJ (1993). Chordoma and chondroid neoplasms of the spheno-occiput. An immunohistochemical study of 41 cases with prognostic and nosologic implications. Cancer. 72(10):2943–9. PMID:7693324
1686. Mittal P, Gupta K, Saggar K, Kaur S (2009). Adult medulloblastoma mimicking Lhermitte-Duclos disease: can diffusion weighted imaging help? Neurol India. 57(2):203–5. PMID:19439857
1687. Miyagami M, Katayama Y, Nakamura S (2000). Clinicopathological study of vascular endothelial growth factor (VEGF), p53, and proliferative potential in familial von Hippel-Lindau disease and sporadic hemangioblastomas. Brain Tumor Pathol. 17(3):111–20. PMID:11310918
1688. Miyagi Y, Suzuki SO, Iwaki T, Shima F, Ishido K, Araki T, et al. (2001). Pleomorphic xanthoastrocytoma with predominantly exophytic growth: case report. Surg Neurol. 56(5):330–2. PMID:11750009
1689. Miyamori T, Mizukoshi H, Yamano K, Takayanagi N, Sugino M, Hayase H, et al. (1990). Intracranial chondrosarcoma–case report. Neurol Med Chir (Tokyo). 30(4):263–7. PMID:1696697
1690. Miyata H, Chiang AC, Vinters HV (2004). Insulin signaling pathways in cortical dysplasia and TSC-tubers: tissue microarray analysis. Ann Neurol. 56(4):510–9. PMID:15455398
1691. Miyata H, Ryufuku M, Kubota Y, Ochiai T, Niimura K, Hori T (2012). Adult-onset angiocentric glioma of epithelioid cell-predominant type of the mesial temporal lobe suggestive of a rare but distinct clinicopathological subset within a spectrum of angiocentric cortical ependymal tumors. Neuropathology. 32(5):479–91. PMID:22151480
1692. Mizoguchi M, Nutt CL, Mohapatra G, Louis DN (2004). Genetic alterations of phosphoinositide 3-kinase subunit genes in human glioblastomas. Brain Pathol. 14(4):372–7. PMID:15605984
1693. Mizuguchi M, Ikeda K, Takashima S (2000). Simultaneous loss of hamartin and tuberin from the cerebrum, kidney and heart with tuberous sclerosis. Acta Neuropathol. 99(5):503–10. PMID:10805093
1694. Mizuguchi M, Kato M, Yamanouchi H, Ikeda K, Takashima S (1996). Loss of tuberin from cerebral tissues with tuberous sclerosis and astrocytoma. Ann Neurol. 40(6):941–4. PMID:9007104
1695. Mizuno J, Iwata K, Takei Y (1993). Immunohistochemical study of hemangioblastoma with special reference to its cytogenesis. Neurol Med Chir (Tokyo). 33(7):420–4. PMID:7692317
1696. Mobley BC, Roulston D, Shah GV, Bijwaard KE, McKeever PE (2006). Peripheral primitive neuroectodermal tumor/Ewing's sarcoma of the craniospinal vault: case reports and review. Hum Pathol. 37(7):845–53. PMID:16784984
1697. Modena P, Lualdi E, Facchinetti F, Galli L, Teixeira MR, Pilotti S, et al. (2005). SMARCB1/INI1 tumor suppressor gene is frequently inactivated in epithelioid sarcomas. Cancer Res. 65(10):4012–9. PMID:15899790
1698. Moles KJ, Gowans GC, Gedela S, Beversdorf D, Yu A, Seaver LH, et al. (2012). NF1 microduplications: identification of seven nonrelated individuals provides further characterization of the phenotype. Genet Med. 14(5):508–14. PMID:22241097
1699. Momota H, Iwami K, Fujii M, Motomura K, Natsume A, Ogino J, et al. (2011). Rhabdoid glioblastoma in a child: case report and literature review. Brain Tumor Pathol. 28(1):65–70. PMID:21213124
1700. Momota H, Narita Y, Maeshima AM, Miyakita Y, Shinomiya A, Maruyama T, et al. (2010). Prognostic value of immunohistochemical profile and response to high-dose methotrexate therapy in primary CNS lymphoma. J Neurooncol. 98(3):341–8. PMID:20012911
1701. Monje M, Mitra SS, Freret ME, Raveh TB, Kim J, Masek M, et al. (2011). Hedgehog-responsive candidate cell of origin for diffuse intrinsic pontine glioma. Proc Natl Acad Sci U S A. 108(11):4453–8. PMID:21368213
1702. Montesinos-Rongen M, Besleaga R, Heinsohn S, Siebert R, Kabisch H, Wiestler OD, et al. (2004). Absence of simian virus 40 DNA sequences in primary central nervous system lymphoma in HIV-negative patients. Virchows Arch. 444(5):436–8. PMID:15042369
1703. Montesinos-Rongen M, Godlewska E, Brunn A, Wiestler OD, Siebert R, Deckert M (2011). Activating L265P mutations of the MYD88 gene are common in primary central nervous system lymphoma. Acta Neuropathol. 122(6):791–2. PMID:22020631
1704. Montesinos-Rongen M, Hans VH, Eis-Hübinger AM, Prinz M, Schaller C, Van Roost D, et al. (2001). Human herpes virus-8 is not associated with primary central nervous system lymphoma in HIV-negative patients. Acta Neuropathol. 102(5):489–95. PMID:11699563
1705. Montesinos-Rongen M, Küppers R, Schlüter D, Spieker T, Van Roost D, Schaller C, et al. (1999). Primary central nervous system lymphomas are derived from germinal-center B cells and show a preferential usage of the V4-34 gene segment. Am J Pathol. 155(6):2077–86. PMID:10595937
1706. Montesinos-Rongen M, Schmitz R, Brunn A, Gesk S, Richter J, Hong K, et al. (2010). Mutations of CARD11 but not TNFAIP3 may activate the NF-kappaB pathway in primary CNS lymphoma. Acta Neuropathol. 120(4):529–35. PMID:20544211
1707. Montesinos-Rongen M, Schmitz R, Courts C, Stenzel W, Bechtel D, Niedobitek G, et al. (2005). Absence of immunoglobulin class switch in primary lymphomas of the central nervous system. Am J Pathol. 166(6):1773–9. PMID:15920162
1708. Montesinos-Rongen M, Schäfer E, Siebert R, Deckert M (2012). Genes regulating the B cell receptor pathway are recurrently mutated in primary central nervous system lymphoma. Acta Neuropathol. 124(6):905–6. PMID:23138649
1709. Montesinos-Rongen M, Van Roost D, Schaller C, Wiestler OD, Deckert M (2004). Primary diffuse large B-cell lymphomas of the central nervous system are targeted by aberrant somatic hypermutation. Blood. 103(5):1869–75. PMID:14592832
1710. Montesinos-Rongen M, Zühlke-Jenisch R, Gesk S, Martín-Subero JI, Schaller C, Van Roost D, et al. (2002). Interphase cytogenetic analysis of lymphoma-associated chromosomal breakpoints in primary diffuse large B-cell lymphomas of the central nervous system. J Neuropathol Exp Neurol. 61(10):926–33. PMID:12387458
1711. Moody P, Murtagh K, Piduru S, Brem S, Murtagh R, Rojiani AM (2012). Tumor-to-tumor metastasis: pathology and neuroimaging considerations. Int J Clin Exp Pathol. 5(4):367–73. PMID:22670183
1712. Moran CA, Rush W, Mena H (1997). Primary spinal paragangliomas: a clinicopathological and immunohistochemical study of 30 cases. Histopathology. 31(2):167–73. PMID:9279569
1713. Morantz RA, Feigin I, Ransohoff J 3rd (1976). Clinical and pathological study of 24 cases of gliosarcoma. J Neurosurg. 45(4):398–408. PMID:956876
1714. Moriguchi S, Yamashita A, Marutsuka K, Yoneyama T, Nakano S, Wakisaka S, et al. (2006). Atypical extraventricular neurocytoma. Pathol Int. 56(1):25–9. PMID:16398676
1715. Moskowitz SI, Jin T, Prayson RA (2006). Role of MIB1 in predicting survival in patients with glioblastomas. J Neurooncol. 76(2):193–200. PMID:16234986
1716. Moss TH (1984). Observations on the nature of subependymoma: an electron microscopic study. Neuropathol Appl Neurobiol. 10(1):63–75. PMID:6738805
1717. Mott RT, Goodman BK, Burchette JL, Cummings TJ (2005). Loss of chromosome 13 in a case of soft tissue perineurioma. Clin Neuropathol. 24(2):69–76. PMID:15803806
1718. Mrak RE, Yasargil MG, Mohapatra G, Earel J Jr, Louis DN (2004). Atypical extraventricular neurocytoma with oligodendroglioma-like spread and an unusual pattern of chromosome 1p and 19q loss. Hum Pathol. 35(9):1156–9. PMID:15343519
1719. Mu Q, Yu J, Qu L, Hu X, Gao H, Liu P, et al. (2015). Spindle cell oncocytoma of the adenohypophysis: two case reports and a review of the literature. Mol Med Rep. 12(1):871–6. PMID:25777996
1720. Mueller W, Mizoguchi M, Silen E, D'Amore K, Nutt CL, Louis DN (2005). Mutations of the PIK3CA gene are rare in human glioblastoma. Acta Neuropathol. 109(6):654–5. PMID:15924252
1721. Muller C, Adroos N, Lockhat Z, Slavik T, Kruger H (2011). Toothy craniopharyngioma: a literature review and case report of craniopharyngioma with extensive odontogenic differentiation and tooth formation. Childs Nerv Syst. 27(2):323–6. PMID:20922394
1722. Mullins KJ, Rubio A, Myers SP, Korones DN, Pilcher WH (1998). Malignant ependymomas in a patient with Turcot's syndrome: case report and management guidelines. Surg Neurol. 49(3):290–4. PMID:9508117
1723. Mur P, Mollejo M, Ruano Y, de Lope ÁR, Fiaño C, García JF, et al. (2013). Codeletion of 1p and 19q determines distinct gene methylation and expression profiles in IDH-mutated oligodendroglial tumors. Acta Neuropathol. 126(2):277–89. PMID:23689617
1724. Murali R, Wiesner T, Rosenblum MK, Bastian BC (2012). GNAQ and GNA11 mutations in melanocytomas of the central nervous system. Acta Neuropathol. 123(3):457–9. PMID:22307269
1725. Murray JM, Morgello S (2004). Polyomaviruses and primary central nervous system lymphomas. Neurology. 63(7):1299–301. PMID:15477558
1726. Murthy A, Gonzalez-Agosti C, Cordero E, Pinney D, Candia C, Solomon F, et al. (1998). NHE-RF, a regulatory cofactor for Na(+)-H+ exchange, is a common interactor for merlin and ERM (MERM) proteins. J Biol Chem. 273(3):1273–6. PMID:9430655

1727. Mustafa D, Swagemakers S, French P, Luider TM, van der Spek P, Kremer A, et al. (2013). Structural and expression differences between the vasculature of pilocytic astrocytomas and glioblastomas. J Neuropathol Exp Neurol. 72(12):1171–81. PMID:24226271
1728. Mut M, Schiff D, Shaffrey ME (2005). Metastasis to nervous system: spinal epidural and intramedullary metastases. J Neurooncol. 75(1):43–56. PMID:16215815
1729. Myers MP, Stolarov JP, Eng C, Li J, Wang SI, Wigler MH, et al. (1997). P-TEN, the tumor suppressor from human chromosome 10q23, is a dual-specificity phosphatase. Proc Natl Acad Sci U S A. 94(17):9052–7. PMID:9256433
1730. Müller HL, Gebhardt U, Teske C, Faldum A, Zwiener I, Warmuth-Metz M, et al.; Study Committee of KRANIOPHARYNGEOM 2000 (2011). Post-operative hypothalamic lesions and obesity in childhood craniopharyngioma: results of the multinational prospective trial KRANIOPHARYNGEOM 2000 after 3-year follow-up. Eur J Endocrinol. 165(1):17–24. PMID:21490122
1731. Myung JK, Byeon SJ, Kim B, Suh J, Kim SK, Park CK, et al. (2011). Papillary glioneuronal tumors: a review of clinicopathologic and molecular genetic studies. Am J Surg Pathol. 35(12):1794–805. PMID:22020040
1732. Myung JK, Cho HJ, Park CK, Chung CK, Choi SH, Kim SK, et al. (2013). Clinicopathological and genetic characteristics of extraventricular neurocytomas. Neuropathology. 33(2):111–21. PMID:22672632
1733. Möllemann M, Wolter M, Felsberg J, Collins VP, Reifenberger G (2005). Frequent promoter hypermethylation and low expression of the MGMT gene in oligodendroglial tumors. Int J Cancer. 113(3):379–85. PMID:15455350
1734. Mørk SJ, Rubinstein LJ, Kepes JJ, Perentes E, Uphoff DF (1988). Patterns of epithelial metaplasia in malignant gliomas. II. Squamous differentiation of epithelial-like formations in gliosarcomas and glioblastomas. J Neuropathol Exp Neurol. 47(2):101–18. PMID:3339369
1735. Nagai S, Kurimoto M, Ishizawa S, Hayashi N, Hamada H, Kamiyama H, et al. (2009). A rare astrocytic tumor with rhabdoid features. Brain Tumor Pathol. 26(1):19–24. PMID:19408093
1736. Nagaishi M, Kim YH, Mittelbronn M, Giangaspero F, Paulus W, Brokinkel B, et al. (2012). Amplification of the STOML3, FREM2, and LHFP genes is associated with mesenchymal differentiation in gliosarcoma. Am J Pathol. 180(5):1816–23. PMID:22538188
1737. Nagaishi M, Paulus W, Brokinkel B, Vital A, Tanaka Y, Nakazato Y, et al. (2012). Transcriptional factors for epithelial-mesenchymal transition are associated with mesenchymal differentiation in gliosarcoma. Brain Pathol. 22(5):670–6. PMID:22288519
1738. Nagaishi M, Yokoo H, Nobusawa S, Fujii Y, Sugiura Y, Suzuki R, et al. (2015). Localized overexpression of alpha-internexin within nodules in multinodular and vacuolating neuronal tumors. Neuropathology. PMID:26073706
1739. Nagao K, Togawa N, Fujii K, Uchikawa H, Kohno Y, Yamada M, et al. (2005). Detecting tissue-specific alternative splicing and disease-associated aberrant splicing of the PTCH gene with exon junction microarrays. Hum Mol Genet. 14(22):3379–88. PMID:16203740
1740. Nagao K, Toyoda M, Takeuchi-Inoue K, Fujii K, Yamada M, Miyashita T (2005). Identification and characterization of multiple isoforms of a murine and human tumor suppressor, patched, having distinct first exons. Genomics. 85(4):462–71. PMID:15780749
1741. Nagashima T, Hoshino T, Cho KG (1987). Proliferative potential of vascular components in human glioblastoma multiforme. Acta Neuropathol. 73(3):301–5. PMID:3039783
1742. Naggara O, Varlet P, Page P, Oppenheim C, Meder JF (2005). Suprasellar paraganglioma: a case report and review of the literature. Neuroradiology. 47(10):753–7. PMID:16047139
1743. Nair S, Fort JA, Yachnis AT, Williams CA (2015). Optic nerve pilomyxoid astrocytoma in a patient with Noonan syndrome. Pediatr Blood Cancer. 62(6):1084–6. PMID:25585602
1744. Naitoh Y, Sasajima T, Kinouchi H, Mikawa S, Mizoi K (2002). Medulloblastoma with extensive nodularity: single photon emission CT study with iodine-123 metaiodobenzylguanidine. AJNR Am J Neuroradiol. 23(9):1564–7. PMID:12372749
1745. Najm I, Jehi L, Palmini A, Gonzalez-Martinez J, Paglioli E, Bingaman W (2013). Temporal patterns and mechanisms of epilepsy surgery failure. Epilepsia. 54(5):772–82. PMID:23586531
1746. Nakagawa Y, Perentes E, Rubinstein LJ (1986). Immunohistochemical characterization of oligodendrogliomas: an analysis of multiple markers. Acta Neuropathol. 72(1):15–22. PMID:2435103
1747. Nakagawa Y, Perentes E, Rubinstein LJ (1987). Non-specificity of anti-carbonic anhydrase C antibody as a marker in human neurooncology. J Neuropathol Exp Neurol. 46(4):451–60. PMID:3110380
1748. Nakama S, Higashi T, Kimura A, Yamamuro K, Kikkawa I, Hoshino Y (2005). Double myxopapillary ependymoma of the cauda equina. J Orthop Sci. 10(5):543–5. PMID:16193371
1749. Nakamura M, Chiba K, Matsumoto M, Ikeda E, Toyama Y (2006). Pleomorphic xanthoastrocytoma of the spinal cord. Case report. J Neurosurg Spine. 5(1):72–5. PMID:16850961
1751. Nakamura M, Saeki N, Iwadate Y, Sunami K, Osato K, Yamaura A (2000). Neuroradiological characteristics of pineocytoma and pineoblastoma. Neuroradiology. 42(7):509–14. PMID:10952183
1752. Nakamura M, Watanabe T, Klangby U, Asker C, Wiman K, Yonekawa Y, et al. (2001). p14ARF deletion and methylation in genetic pathways to glioblastomas. Brain Pathol. 11(2):159–68. PMID:11303791
1753. Nakamura M, Watanabe T, Yonekawa Y, Kleihues P, Ohgaki H (2001). Promoter methylation of the DNA repair gene MGMT in astrocytomas is frequently associated with G:C -> A:T mutations of the TP53 tumor suppressor gene. Carcinogenesis. 22(10):1715–9. PMID:11577014
1754. Nakamura M, Yang F, Fujisawa H, Yonekawa Y, Kleihues P, Ohgaki H (2000). Loss of heterozygosity on chromosome 19 in secondary glioblastomas. J Neuropathol Exp Neurol. 59(6):539–43. PMID:10850866
1755. Nakamura M, Yonekawa Y, Kleihues P, Ohgaki H (2001). Promoter hypermethylation of the RB1 gene in glioblastomas. Lab Invest. 81(1):77–82. PMID:11204276
1756. Nakano I (2015). Stem cell signature in glioblastoma: therapeutic development for a moving target. J Neurosurg. 122(2):324–30. PMID:25397368
1757. Narod SA, Parry DM, Parboosingh J, Lenoir GM, Ruttledge M, Fischer G, et al. (1992). Neurofibromatosis type 2 appears to be a genetically homogeneous disease. Am J Hum Genet. 51(3):486–96. PMID:1496982
1758. National Institutes of Health Consensus Development Conference (1988). Neurofibromatosis. Conference statement. Arch Neurol. 45(5):575–8. PMID:3128965
1759. Nauen D, Haley L, Lin MT, Perry A, Giannini C, Burger PC, et al. (2015). Molecular Analysis of Pediatric Oligodendrogliomas Highlights Genetic Differences with Adult Counterparts and Other Pediatric Gliomas. Brain Pathol. PMID:26206478
1760. Nayak L, Abrey LE, Iwamoto FM (2009). Intracranial dural metastases. Cancer. 115(9):1947–53. PMID:19241421
1761. Neal MT, Ellis TL, Stanton CA (2012). Pleomorphic xanthoastrocytoma in two siblings with neurofibromatosis type 1 (NF-1). Clin Neuropathol. 31(1):54–6. PMID:22192706
1762. Neelima R, Easwer HV, Kapilamoorthy TR, Hingwala DR, Radhakrishnan VV (2012). Embryonal tumor with multilayered rosettes: Two case reports with a review of the literature. Neurol India. 60(1):96–9. PMID:22406791
1763. Neff BA, Willcox TO Jr, Sataloff RT (2003). Intralabyrinthine schwannomas. Otol Neurotol. 24(2):299–307. PMID:12621348
1764. Nelen MR, Kremer H, Konings IB, Schoute F, van Essen AJ, Koch R, et al. (1999). Novel PTEN mutations in patients with Cowden disease: absence of clear genotype-phenotype correlations. Eur J Hum Genet. 7(3):267–73. PMID:10234502
1765. Nelen MR, Padberg GW, Peeters EA, Lin AY, van den Helm B, Frants RR, et al. (1996). Localization of the gene for Cowden disease to chromosome 10q22–23. Nat Genet. 13(1):114–6. PMID:8673088
1766. Nelen MR, van Staveren WC, Peeters EA, Hassel MB, Gorlin RJ, Hamm H, et al. (1997). Germline mutations in the PTEN/MMAC1 gene in patients with Cowden disease. Hum Mol Genet. 6(8):1383–7. PMID:9259288
1767. Nemes Z (1992). Fibrohistiocytic differentiation in capillary hemangioblastoma. Hum Pathol. 23(7):805–10. PMID:1351864
1768. Nestor SL, Perry A, Kurtkaya O, Abell-Aleff P, Rosemblat AM, Burger PC, et al. (2003). Melanocytic colonization of a meningothelial meningioma: histopathological and ultrastructural findings with immunohistochemical and genetic correlation: case report. Neurosurgery. 53(1):211–4, discussion 214–5. PMID:12823892
1769. Neumann HP, Eggert HR, Weigel K, Friedburg H, Wiestler OD, Schollmeyer P (1989). Hemangioblastomas of the central nervous system. A 10-year study with special reference to von Hippel-Lindau syndrome. J Neurosurg. 70(1):24–30. PMID:2909683
1770. Neves S, Mazal PR, Wanschitz J, Rudnay AC, Drlicek M, Czech T, et al. (2001). Pseudogliomatous growth pattern of anaplastic small cell carcinomas metastatic to the brain. Clin Neuropathol. 20(1):38–42. PMID:11220694
1771. Newcomb EW, Madonia WJ, Pisharody S, Lang FF, Koslow M, Miller DC (1993). A correlative study of p53 protein alteration and p53 gene mutation in glioblastoma multiforme. Brain Pathol. 3(3):229–35. PMID:8293182
1772. Newton HB, Dalton J, Ray-Chaudhury A, Gahbauer R, McGregor J (2008). Aggressive papillary glioneuronal tumor: case report and literature review. Clin Neuropathol. 27(5):317–24. PMID:18808063
1773. Ng HK, Lo ST (1989). Cytokeratin immunoreactivity in gliomas. Histopathology. 14(4):359–68. PMID:2472343
1774. Ng HK, Poon WS (1990). Gliosarcoma of the posterior fossa with features of a malignant fibrous histiocytoma. Cancer. 65(5):1161–6. PMID:2154322
1775. Ng HK, Poon WS (1999). Diffuse leptomeningeal gliomatosis with oligodendroglioma. Pathology. 31(1):59–63. PMID:10212927
1776. Ng TH, Fung CF, Ma LT (1990). The pathological spectrum of desmoplastic infantile gangliogliomas. Histopathology. 16(3):235–41. PMID:2332209
1777. Ngeow J, Mester J, Rybicki LA, Ni Y, Milas M, Eng C (2011). Incidence and clinical characteristics of thyroid cancer in prospective series of individuals with Cowden and Cowden-like syndrome characterized by germline PTEN, SDH, or KLLN alterations. J Clin Endocrinol Metab. 96(12):E2063–71. PMID:21956414
1778. Nguyen R, Dombi E, Akshintala S, Baldwin A, Widemann BC (2015). Characterization of spinal findings in children and adults with neurofibromatosis type 1 enrolled in a natural history study using magnetic resonance imaging. J Neurooncol. 121(1):209–15. PMID:25293439
1779. Nguyen SA, Stechishin OD, Luchman HA, Lun XQ, Senger DL, Robbins SM, et al. (2014). Novel MSH6 mutations in treatment-naïve glioblastoma and anaplastic oligodendroglioma contribute to temozolomide resistance independently of MGMT promoter methylation. Clin Cancer Res. 20(18):4894–903. PMID:25078279
1780. Ni HC, Chen SY, Chen L, Lu DH, Fu YJ, Piao YS (2015). Angiocentric glioma: a report of nine new cases, including four with atypical histological features. Neuropathol Appl Neurobiol. 41(3):333–46. PMID:24861831
1781. Ni Y, He X, Chen J, Moline J, Mester J, Orloff MS, et al. (2012). Germline SDHx variants modify breast and thyroid cancer risks in Cowden and Cowden-like syndrome via FAD/NAD-dependant destabilization of p53. Hum Mol Genet. 21(2):300–10. PMID:21979946
1782. Ni Y, Zbuk KM, Sadler T, Patocs A, Lobo G, Edelman E, et al. (2008). Germline mutations and variants in the succinate dehydrogenase genes in Cowden and Cowden-like syndromes. Am J Hum Genet. 83(2):261–8. PMID:18678321
1783. Nieder C, Spanne O, Mehta MP, Grosu AL, Geinitz H (2011). Presentation, patterns of care, and survival in patients with brain metastases: what has changed in the last 20 years? Cancer. 117(11):2505–12. PMID:24048799
1784. Nielsen EH, Feldt-Rasmussen U, Poulsgaard L, Kristensen LO, Astrup J, Jørgensen JO, et al. (2011). Incidence of craniopharyngioma in Denmark (n = 189) and estimated world incidence of craniopharyngioma in children and adults. J Neurooncol. 104(3):755–63. PMID:21336771
1785. Nielsen GP, Stemmer-Rachamimov AO, Ino Y, Moller MB, Rosenberg AE, Louis DN (1999). Malignant transformation of neurofibromas in neurofibromatosis 1 is associated with CDKN2A/p16 inactivation. Am J Pathol. 155(6):1879–84. PMID:10595918
1786. Nieuwenhuis MH, Kets CM, Murphy-Ryan M, Yntema HG, Evans DG, Colas C, et al. (2014). Cancer risk and genotype-phenotype correlations in PTEN hamartoma tumor syndrome. Fam Cancer. 13(1):57–63. PMID:23934601
1787. Niida Y, Stemmer-Rachamimov AO, Logrip M, Tapon D, Perez R, Kwiatkowski DJ, et al. (2001). Survey of somatic mutations in tuberous sclerosis complex (TSC) hamartomas suggests different genetic mechanisms for pathogenesis of TSC lesions. Am J Hum Genet. 69(3):493–503. PMID:11468687
1788. Niiro T, Tokimura H, Hanaya R, Hirano H, Fukukura Y, Sugiyma K, et al. (2012). MRI findings in patients with central neurocytomas with special reference to differential diagnosis from other ventricular tumours near the foramen of Monro. J Clin Neurosci. 19(5):681–6. PMID:22410173
1789. Nishikawa R, Furnari FB, Lin H, Arap W, Berger MS, Cavenee WK, et al. (1995). Loss of P16INK4 expression is frequent in high grade gliomas. Cancer Res. 55(9):1941–5. PMID:7728764
1790. Nishimoto T, Kaya B (2012). Cerebellar liponeurocytoma. Arch Pathol Lab Med. 136(8):965–9. PMID:22849747
1791. Nishio S, Morioka T, Inamura T, Takeshita I, Fukui M, Sasaki M, et al. (1998). Radiation-induced brain tumours: potential late complications of radiation therapy for brain tumours. Acta Neurochir (Wien). 140(8):763–70. PMID:9810442
1792. Nishio S, Takeshita I, Kaneko Y, Fukui M (1992). Cerebral neurocytoma. A new subset of benign neuronal tumors of the cerebrum. Cancer. 70(2):529–37. PMID:1617603
1793. Nitta H, Hayase H, Moriyama Y, Yamashima T, Yamashita J (1993). Gliosarcoma of the posterior cranial fossa: MRI findings.

Neuroradiology. 35(4):279–80. PMID:8492894
1794. Noble M, Wren D, Wolswijk G (1992). The O-2A(adult) progenitor cell: a glial stem cell of the adult central nervous system. Semin Cell Biol. 3(6):413–22. PMID:1489973
1795. Nobusawa S, Hirato J, Kurihara H, Ogawa A, Okura N, Nagaishi M, et al. (2014). Intratumoral heterogeneity of genomic imbalance in a case of epithelioid glioblastoma with BRAF V600E mutation. Brain Pathol. 24(3):239–46. PMID:24354918
1796. Nobusawa S, Orimo K, Horiguchi K, Ikota H, Yokoo H, Hirato J, et al. (2014). Embryonal tumor with abundant neuropil and true rosettes with only one structure suggestive of an ependymoblastic rosette. Pathol Int. 64(9):472–7. PMID:25186165
1797. Nobusawa S, Watanabe T, Kleihues P, Ohgaki H (2009). IDH1 mutations as molecular signature and predictive factor of secondary glioblastomas. Clin Cancer Res. 15(19):6002–7. PMID:19755387
1798. Nobusawa S, Yokoo H, Hirato J, Kakita A, Takahashi H, Sugino T, et al. (2012). Analysis of chromosome 19q13.42 amplification in embryonal brain tumors with ependymoblastic multilayered rosettes. Brain Pathol. 22(5):689–97. PMID:22324795
1799. Noell S, Beschorner R, Bisdas S, Beyer U, Weber RG, Fallier-Becker P, et al. (2014). Simultaneous subependymomas in monozygotic female twins: further evidence for a common genetic or developmental disorder background. J Neurosurg. 121(3):570–5. PMID:24655099
1800. Nolan MA, Sakuta R, Chuang N, Otsubo H, Rutka JT, Snead OC 3rd, et al. (2004). Dysembryoplastic neuroepithelial tumors in childhood: long-term outcome and prognostic features. Neurology. 62(12):2270–6. PMID:15210893
1801. Nonoguchi N, Ohta T, Oh JE, Kim YH, Kleihues P, Ohgaki H (2013). TERT promoter mutations in primary and secondary glioblastomas. Acta Neuropathol. 126(6):931–7. PMID:23955565
1802. Nora FE, Scheithauer BW (1996). Primary epithelioid hemangioendothelioma of the brain. Am J Surg Pathol. 20(6):707–14. PMID:8651350
1803. Norman MG, Harrison KJ, Poskitt KJ, Kalousek DK (1995). Duplication of 9P and hyperplasia of the choroid plexus: a pathologic, radiologic, and molecular cytogenetics study. Pediatr Pathol Lab Med. 15(1):109–20. PMID:8736601
1804. Northcott PA, Jones DT, Kool M, Robinson GW, Gilbertson RJ, Cho YJ, et al. (2012). Medulloblastomics: the end of the beginning. Nat Rev Cancer. 12(12):818–34. PMID:23175120
1805. Northcott PA, Korshunov A, Witt H, Hielscher T, Eberhart CG, Mack S, et al. (2011). Medulloblastoma comprises four distinct molecular variants. J Clin Oncol. 29(11):1408–14 PMID:20823417
1806. Northcott PA, Lee C, Zichner T, Stütz AM, Erkek S, Kawauchi D, et al. (2014). Enhancer hijacking activates GFI1 family oncogenes in medulloblastoma. Nature. 511(7510):428–34. PMID:25043047
1807. Northcott PA, Shih DJ, Peacock J, Garzia L, Morrissy AS, Zichner T, et al. (2012). Subgroup-specific structural variation across 1,000 medulloblastoma genomes. Nature. 488(7409):49–56. PMID:22832581
1808. Northcott PA, Shih DJ, Remke M, Cho YJ, Kool M, Hawkins C, et al. (2012). Rapid, reliable, and reproducible molecular sub-grouping of clinical medulloblastoma samples. Acta Neuropathol. 123(4):615–26. PMID:22057785
1809. Northrup H, Krueger DA; International Tuberous Sclerosis Complex Consensus Group (2013). Tuberous sclerosis complex diagnostic criteria update: recommendations of the 2012 Iinternational Tuberous Sclerosis Complex Consensus Conference. Pediatr Neurol. 49(4):243–54. PMID:24053982
1810. Noushmehr H, Weisenberger DJ, Diefes K, Phillips HS, Pujara K, Berman BP, et al.; Cancer Genome Atlas Research Network (2010). Identification of a CpG island methylator phenotype that defines a distinct subgroup of glioma. Cancer Cell. 17(5):510–22. PMID:20399149
1811. Numoto RT (1994). Pineal parenchymal tumors: cell differentiation and prognosis. J Cancer Res Clin Oncol. 120(11):683–90. PMID:7525594
1812. Nutt CL, Mani DR, Betensky RA, Tamayo P, Cairncross JG, Ladd C, et al. (2003). Gene expression-based classification of malignant gliomas correlates better with survival than histological classification. Cancer Res. 63(7):1602–7. PMID:12670911
1813. O'Malley S, Weitman D, Olding M, Sekhar L (1997). Multiple neoplasms following craniospinal irradiation for medulloblastoma in a patient with nevoid basal cell carcinoma syndrome. Case report. J Neurosurg. 86(2):286–8. PMID:9010431
1814. O'Marcaigh AS, Ledger GA, Roche PC, Parisi JE, Zimmerman D (1995). Aromatase expression in human germinomas with possible biological effects. J Clin Endocrinol Metab. 80(12):3763–6. PMID:8530631
1815. Oderich GS, Sullivan TM, Bower TC, Gloviczki P, Miller DV, Babovic-Vuksanovic D, et al. (2007). Vascular abnormalities in patients with neurofibromatosis syndrome type I: clinical spectrum, management, and results. J Vasc Surg. 46(3):475–84. PMID:17681709
1816. Ogiwara H, Dubner S, Shafizadeh S, Raizer J, Chandler JP (2011). Spindle cell oncocytoma of the pituitary and pituicytoma: Two tumors mimicking pituitary adenoma. Surg Neurol Int. 2:116. PMID:21886889
1817. Ogura R, Aoki H, Natsumeda M, Shimizu H, Kobayashi T, Saito T, et al. (2013). Epstein-Barr virus-associated primary central nervous system cytotoxic T-cell lymphoma. Neuropathology. 33(4):436–41. PMID:23279449
1818. Oh D, Prayson RA (1999). Evaluation of epithelial and keratin markers in glioblastoma multiforme: an immunohistochemical study. Arch Pathol Lab Med. 123(10):917–20. PMID:10506444
1819. Oh JE, Ohta T, Nonoguchi N, Satomi K, Capper D, Pierscianek D, et al. (2015). Genetic alterations in gliosarcoma and giant cell glioblastoma. Brain Pathol. PMID:26443480
1820. Oh T, Rutkowski MJ, Safaee M, Sun MZ, Sayegh ET, Bloch O, et al. (2014). Survival outcomes of giant cell glioblastoma: institutional experience in the management of 20 patients. J Clin Neurosci. 21(12):2129–34. PMID:25037316
1821. Ohba Y, Mochizuki N, Yamashita S, Chan AM, Schrader JW, Hattori S, et al. (2000). Regulatory proteins of R-Ras, TC21/R-Ras2, and M-Ras/R-Ras3. J Biol Chem. 275(26):20020–6. PMID:10777492
1822. Ohgaki H, Burger P, Kleihues P (2014). Definition of primary and secondary glioblastoma–response. Clin Cancer Res. 20(7):2013. PMID:24557936
1823. Ohgaki H, Dessen P, Jourde B, Horstmann S, Nishikawa T, Di Patre PL, et al. (2004). Genetic pathways to glioblastoma: a population-based study. Cancer Res. 64(19):6892–9. PMID:15466178
1824. Ohgaki H, Eibl RH, Schwab M, Reichel MB, Mariani L, Gehring M, et al. (1993). Mutations of the p53 tumor suppressor gene in neoplasms of the human nervous system. Mol Carcinog. 8(2):74–80. PMID:8397797
1825. Ohgaki H, Kleihues P (2005). Epidemiology and etiology of gliomas. Acta Neuropathol. 109(1):93–108. PMID:15685439
1826. Ohgaki H, Kleihues P (2005). Population-based studies on incidence, survival rates, and genetic alterations in astrocytic and oligodendroglial gliomas. J Neuropathol Exp Neurol. 64(6):479–89. PMID:15977639
1827. Ohgaki H, Kleihues P (2007). Genetic pathways to primary and secondary glioblastoma. Am J Pathol. 170(5):1445–53. PMID:17456751
1828. Ohgaki H, Kleihues P (2009). Genetic alterations and signaling pathways in the evolution of gliomas. Cancer Sci. 100(12):2235–41. PMID:19737147
1829. Ohgaki H, Kleihues P (2011). Genetic profile of astrocytic and oligodendroglial gliomas. Brain Tumor Pathol. 28(3):177–83. PMID:21442241
1830. Ohgaki H, Kleihues P (2013). The definition of primary and secondary glioblastoma. Clin Cancer Res. 19(4):764–72. PMID:23209033
1831. Ojha BK, Sharma MC, Rastogi M, Chandra A, Husain M, Husain N (2007). Dumbbell-shaped paraganglioma of the cervical spine in a child. Pediatr Neurosurg. 43(1):60–4. PMID:17190992
1832. Okada M, Yano H, Hirose Y, Nakayama N, Ohe N, Shinoda J, et al. (2011). Olig2 is useful in the differential diagnosis of oligodendrogliomas and extraventricular neurocytomas. Brain Tumor Pathol. 28(2):157–61. PMID:21312066
1833. Okada Y, Nishikawa R, Matsutani M, Louis DN (2002). Hypomethylated X chromosome gain and rare isochromosome 12p in diverse intracranial germ cell tumors. J Neuropathol Exp Neurol. 61(6):531–8. PMID:12071636
1834. Okamoto Y, Di Patre PL, Burkhard C, Horstmann S, Jourde B, Fahey M, et al. (2004). Population-based study on incidence, survival rates, and genetic alterations of low-grade diffuse astrocytomas and oligodendrogliomas. Acta Neuropathol. 108(1):49–56. PMID:15118874
1835. Okita Y, Narita Y, Miyakita Y, Ohno M, Matsushita Y, Fukushima S, et al. (2012). IDH1/2 mutation is a prognostic marker for survival and predicts response to chemotherapy for grade II gliomas concomitantly treated with radiation therapy. Int J Oncol. 41(4):1325–36. PMID:22825915
1836. Olar A, Wani KM, Alfaro-Munoz KD, Heathcock LE, van Thuijl HF, Gilbert MR, et al. (2015). IDH mutation status and role of WHO grade and mitotic index in overall survival in grade II-III diffuse gliomas. Acta Neuropathol. 129(4):585–96. PMID:25701198
1837. Olar A, Wani KM, Sulman EP, Mansouri A, Zadeh G, Wilson CD, et al. (2015). Mitotic Index is an Independent Predictor of Recurrence-Free Survival in Meningioma. Brain Pathol. 25(3):266–75 PMID:25040885
1838. Oliveira AM, Scheithauer BW, Salomao DR, Parisi JE, Burger PC, Nascimento AG (2002). Primary sarcomas of the brain and spinal cord: a study of 18 cases. Am J Surg Pathol. 26(8):1056–63. PMID:12170093
1839. Oliver TG, Grasfeder LL, Carroll AL, Kaiser C, Gillingham CL, Lin SM, et al. (2003). Transcriptional profiling of the Sonic hedgehog response: a critical role for N-myc in proliferation of neuronal precursors. Proc Natl Acad Sci U S A. 100(12):7331–6. PMID:12777630
1840. Oliver TG, Read TA, Kessler JD, Mehmeti A, Wells JF, Huynh TT, et al. (2005). Loss of patched and disruption of granule cell development in a pre-neoplastic stage of medulloblastoma. Development. 132(10):2425–39. PMID:15843415
1841. Olivier M, Goldgar DE, Sodha N, Ohgaki H, Kleihues P, Hainaut P, et al. (2003). Li-Fraumeni and related syndromes: correlation between tumor type, family structure, and TP53 genotype. Cancer Res. 63(20):6643–50. PMID:14583457
1842. Olivier M, Hollstein M, Hainaut P (2010). TP53 mutations in human cancers: origins, consequences, and clinical use. Cold Spring Harb Perspect Biol. 2(1):a001008. PMID:20182602
1843. Olivier M, Hussain SP, Caron de Fromentel C, Hainaut P, Harris CC (2004). TP53 mutation spectra and load: a tool for generating hypotheses on the etiology of cancer. IARC Sci Publ. 157:247–70. PMID:15055300
1844. Olschwang S, Serova-Sinilnikova OM, Lenoir GM, Thomas G (1998). PTEN germ-line mutations in juvenile polyposis coli. Nat Genet. 18(1):12–4. PMID:9425889
1845. Olson JD, Riedel E, DeAngelis LM (2000). Long-term outcome of low-grade oligodendroglioma and mixed glioma. Neurology. 54(7):1442–8. PMID:10751254
1846. Olson JM, Breslow NE, Barce J (1993). Cancer in twins of Wilms tumor patients. Am J Med Genet. 47(1):91–4. PMID:8396323
1847. Onda K, Davis RL, Wilson CB, Hoshino T (1994). Regional differences in bromodeoxyuridine uptake, expression of Ki-67 protein, and nucleolar organizer region counts in glioblastoma multiforme. Acta Neuropathol. 87(6):586–93. PMID:8091951
1848. Ongürü O, Deveci S, Sirin S, Timurkaynak E, Günhan O (2003). Dysembryoplastic neuroepithelial tumor in the left lateral ventricle. Minim Invasive Neurosurg. 46(5):306–9. PMID:14628248
1849. Onilude OE, Lusher ME, Lindsey JC, Pearson AD, Ellison DW, Clifford SC (2006). APC and CTNNB1 mutations are rare in sporadic ependymomas. Cancer Genet Cytogenet. 168(2):158–61. PMID:16843107
1850. Oosterhuis JW, Stoop H, Honecker F, Looijenga LH (2007). Why human extragonadal germ cell tumours occur in the midline of the body: old concepts, new perspectives. Int J Androl. 30(4):256–63, discussion 263–4. PMID:17705807
1851. Orloff MS, Eng C (2008). Genetic and phenotypic heterogeneity in the PTEN hamartoma tumour syndrome. Oncogene. 27(41):5387–97. PMID:18794875
1852. Orloff MS, He X, Peterson C, Chen F, Chen JL, Mester JL, et al. (2013). Germline PIK3CA and AKT1 mutations in Cowden and Cowden-like syndromes. Am J Hum Genet. 92(1):76–80. PMID:23246288
1853. Ortega A, Nuño M, Walia S, Mukherjee D, Black KL, Patil CG (2014). Treatment and survival of patients harboring histological variants of glioblastoma. J Clin Neurosci. 21(10):1709–13. PMID:24980627
1854. Ortega-Aznar A, Romero-Vidal FJ, de la Torre J, Castellvi J, Nogues P (2001). Neonatal tumors of the CNS: a report of 9 cases and a review. Clin Neuropathol. 20(5):181–9. PMID:11594502
1855. Oruckaptan HH, Berker M, Soylemezoglu F, Ozcan OE (2001). Parafalcine chondrosarcoma: an unusual localization for a classical variant. Case report and review of the literature. Surg Neurol. 55(3):174–9. PMID:11311919
1856. Osawa T, Tosaka M, Nagaishi M, Yoshimoto Y (2013). Factors affecting peritumoral brain edema in meningioma: special histological subtypes with prominently extensive edema. J Neurooncol. 111(1):49–57. PMID:23104516
1857. Osborn AG, et al. (2004). Diagnostic Imaging Brain. first Salt Lake City. Utah: Amirsys.
1858. Osorio JA, Hervey-Jumper SL, Walsh KM, Clarke JL, Butowski NA, Prados MD, et al. (2015). Familial gliomas: cases in two pairs of brothers. J Neurooncol. 121(1):135–40. PMID:25208478
1859. Ostendorf AP, Gutmann DH, Weisenberg JL (2013). Epilepsy in individuals with neurofibromatosis type 1. Epilepsia. 54(10):1810–4. PMID:24032542
1860. Ostertun B, Wolf HK, Campos MG, Matus C, Solymosi L, Elger CE, et al. (1996). Dysembryoplastic neuroepithelial tumors: MR and CT evaluation. AJNR Am J Neuroradiol. 17(3):419–30. PMID:8881234
1861. Ostrom QT, Bauchet L, Davis FG, Deltour I, Fisher JL, Langer CE, et al. (2014). The epidemiology of glioma in adults: a "state of the science" review. Neuro Oncol. 16(7):896–913. PMID:24842956

1862. Ostrom QT, de Blank PM, Kruchko C, Petersen CM, Liao P, Finlay JL, et al. (2015). Alex's Lemonade Stand Foundation Infant and Childhood Primary Brain and Central Nervous System Tumors Diagnosed in the United States in 2007–2011. Neuro Oncol. 16 Suppl 10:x1–36. PMID:25542864
1862A. Ostrom QT, Gittleman H, Farah P, Ondracek A, Chen Y, Wolinsky Y, et al. (2013). CBTRUS statistical report: Primary brain and central nervous system tumors diagnosed in the United States in 2006-2010. Neuro Oncol. 15 Suppl 2:ii1–56. PMID:24137015
1863. Ostrom QT, Gittleman H, Liao P, Rouse C, Chen Y, Dowling J, et al. (2014). CBTRUS statistical report: primary brain and central nervous system tumors diagnosed in the United States in 2007–2011. Neuro Oncol. 16 Suppl 4:iv1–63. PMID:25304271
1864. Ota S, Crabbe DC, Tran TN, Triche TJ, Shimada H (1993). Malignant rhabdoid tumor. A study with two established cell lines. Cancer. 71(9):2862–72. PMID:8385567
1865. Otero JJ, Rowitch D, Vandenberg S (2011). OLIG2 is differentially expressed in pediatric astrocytic and in ependymal neoplasms. J Neurooncol. 104(2):423–38. PMID:21193945
1866. Ouladan S, Trautmann M, Orouji E, Hartmann W, Huss S, Büttner R, et al. (2015). Differential diagnosis of solitary fibrous tumors: A study of 454 soft tissue tumors indicating the diagnostic value of nuclear STAT6 relocation and ALDH1 expression combined with in situ proximity ligation assay. Int J Oncol. 46(6):2595–605. PMID:25901508
1867. Owler BK, Makeham JM, Shingde M, Besser M (2005). Cerebellar liponeurocytoma. J Clin Neurosci. 12(3):326–9. PMID:15851097
1868. Owonikoko TK, Arbiser J, Zelnak A, Shu HK, Shim H, Robin AM, et al. (2014). Current approaches to the treatment of metastatic brain tumours. Nat Rev Clin Oncol. 11(4):203–22. PMID:24569448
1869. Ozawa T, Brennan CW, Wang L, Squatrito M, Sasayama T, Nakada M, et al. (2010). PDGFRA gene rearrangements are frequent genetic events in PDGFRA-amplified glioblastomas. Genes Dev. 24(19):2205–18. PMID:20889717
1870. Ozek MM, Sav A, Pamir MN, Ozer AF, Ozek E, Erzen C (1993). Pleomorphic xanthoastrocytoma associated with von Recklinghausen neurofibromatosis. Childs Nerv Syst. 9(1):39–42. PMID:8481944
1871. Ozolek JA, Finkelstein SD, Couce ME (2004). Gliosarcoma with epithelial differentiation: immunohistochemical and molecular characterization. A case report and review of the literature. Mod Pathol. 17(6):739–45. PMID:15148503
1872. Ozören N, El-Deiry WS (2003). Cell surface Death Receptor signaling in normal and cancer cells. Semin Cancer Biol. 13(2):135–47. PMID:12654257
1873. Padberg GW, Schot JD, Vielvoye GJ, Bots GT, de Beer FC (1991). Lhermitte-Duclos disease and Cowden disease: a single phakomatosis. Ann Neurol. 29(5):517–23. PMID:1859181
1874. Padovani L, Colin C, Fernandez C, Maues de Paula A, Mercurio S, Scavarda D, et al. (2012). Search for distinctive markers in DNT and cortical grade II glioma in children: same clinicopathological and molecular entities? Curr Top Med Chem. 12(15):1683–92. PMID:22978341
1875. Paek SH, Kim SH, Chang KH, Park CK, Kim JE, Kim DG, et al. (2005). Microcystic meningiomas: radiological characteristics of 16 cases. Acta Neurochir (Wien). 147(9):965–72, discussion 972. PMID:16028111
1876. Paek SH, Shin HY, Kim JW, Park SH, Son JH, Kim DG (2010). Primary culture of central neurocytoma: a case report. J Korean Med Sci. 25(5):798–803. PMID:20436722
1877. Paganini I, Chang VY, Capone GL, Vitte J, Benelli M, Barbetti L, et al. (2015). Expanding the mutational spectrum of LZTR1 in schwannomatosis. Eur J Hum Genet. 23(7):963–8 PMID:25335493
1878. Pagni CA, Giordana MT, Canavero S (1991). Benign recurrence of a pilocytic cerebellar astrocytoma 36 years after radical removal: case report. Neurosurgery. 28(4):606–9. PMID:2034360
1879. Pagon RA, Adam MP, Ardinger HH, et al. (1993-2015).GeneReviews® [Internet]. [Updated 2014 Mar 27]. Seattle: University of Washington.
1880. Pajtler KW, Witt H, Sill M, Jones DT, Hovestadt V, Kratochwil F, et al. (2015). Molecular Classification of Ependymal Tumors across All CNS Compartments, Histopathological Grades, and Age Groups. Cancer Cell. 27(5):728–43. PMID:25965575
1881. Pakos EE, Goussia AC, Zina VP, Pitouli EJ, Tsekeris PG (2005). Multi-focal gliosarcoma: a case report and review of the literature. J Neurooncol. 74(3):301–4. PMID:16086111
1882. Palma L, Russo A, Celli P (1984). Prognosis of the so-called "diffuse" cerebellar astrocytoma. Neurosurgery. 15(3):315–7. PMID:6483145
1883. Palmero EI, Achatz MI, Ashton-Prolla P, Olivier M, Hainaut P (2010). Tumor protein 53 mutations and inherited cancer: beyond Li-Fraumeni syndrome. Curr Opin Oncol. 22(1):64–9. PMID:19952748
1884. Panageas KS, Reiner AS, Iwamoto FM, Cloughesy TF, Aldape KD, Rivera AL, et al. (2014). Recursive partitioning analysis of prognostic variables in newly diagnosed anaplastic oligodendroglial tumors. Neuro Oncol. 16(11):1541–6. PMID:24997140
1885. Pantazis G, Harter PN, Capper D, Kohlhof P, Mittelbronn M, Schittenhelm J (2014). The embryonic stem cell factor UTF1 serves as a reliable diagnostic marker for germinomas. Pathology. 46(3):225–9. PMID:24614704
1886. Papanicolau-Sengos A, Wang-Rodriguez J, Wang HY, Lee RR, Wong A, Hansen LA, et al. (2012). Rare case of a primary non-dural central nervous system low grade B-cell lymphoma and literature review. Int J Clin Exp Pathol. 5(1):89–95. PMID:22295152
1886A. Paraf F, Jothy S, Van Meir EG (1997). Brain tumor-polyposis syndrome: two genetic diseases? J Clin Oncol. 15(7):2744–58. PMID:9215849
1887. Parham DM, Weeks DA, Beckwith JB (1994). The clinicopathologic spectrum of putative extrarenal rhabdoid tumors. An analysis of 42 cases studied with immunohistochemistry or electron microscopy. Am J Surg Pathol. 18(10):1010–29. PMID:8092393
1888. Park CK, Phi JH, Park SH (2015). Glial tumors with neuronal differentiation. Neurosurg Clin N Am. 26(1):117–38. PMID:25432191
1889. Park DH, Park YK, Oh JI, Kwon TH, Chung HS, Cho HD, et al. (2002). Oncocytic paraganglioma of the cauda equina in a child. Case report and review of the literature. Pediatr Neurosurg. 36(5):260–5. PMID:12053045
1890. Park JS, Park H, Park S, Kim SJ, Seol HJ, Ko YH (2013). Primary central nervous system ALK positive anaplastic large cell lymphoma with predominantly leptomeningeal involvement in an adult. Yonsei Med J. 54(3):791–6. PMID:23549832
1891. Parker M, Mohankumar KM, Punchihewa C, Weinlich R, Dalton JD, Li Y, et al. (2014). C11orf95-RELA fusions drive oncogenic NF-κB signalling in ependymoma. Nature. 506(7489):451–5. PMID:24553141
1892. Parkin DM, Whelan SL, Ferlay J, Teppo L, Thomas DB (2003). Cancer Incidence in Five Continents. IARC Scientific Publications. Volume 155. Lyon: IARC Press.
1893. Parry DM, Eldridge R, Kaiser-Kupfer MI, Bouzas EA, Pikus A, Patronas N (1994). Neurofibromatosis 2 (NF2): clinical characteristics of 63 affected individuals and clinical evidence for heterogeneity. Am J Med Genet. 52(4):450–61. PMID:7747758
1894. Parsa CF, Hoyt CS, Lesser RL, Weinstein JM, Strother CM, Muci-Mendoza R, et al. (2001). Spontaneous regression of optic gliomas: thirteen cases documented by serial neuroimaging. Arch Ophthalmol. 119(4):516–29. PMID:11296017
1895. Parsons DW, Jones S, Zhang X, Lin JC, Leary RJ, Angenendt P, et al. (2008). An integrated genomic analysis of human glioblastoma multiforme. Science. 321(5897):1807–12. PMID:18772396
1896. Partap S, Curran EK, Propp JM, Le GM, Sainani KL, Fisher PG (2009). Medulloblastoma incidence has not changed over time: a CBTRUS study. J Pediatr Hematol Oncol. 31(12):970–1. PMID:19887963
1897. Pascual-Castroviejo I, Pascual-Pascual SI, Viaño J, Velazquez-Fragua R, López-Gutierrez JC (2012). Bilateral spinal neurofibromas in patients with neurofibromatosis 1. Brain Dev. 34(7):563–9. PMID:21999966
1898. Pasini B, McWhinney SR, Bei T, Matyakhina L, Stergiopoulos S, Muchow M, et al. (2008). Clinical and molecular genetics of patients with the Carney-Stratakis syndrome and germline mutations of the genes coding for the succinate dehydrogenase subunits SDHB, SDHC, and SDHD. Eur J Hum Genet. 16(1):79–88. PMID:17667967
1899. Pasmant E, Masliah-Planchon J, Lévy P, Laurendeau I, Ortonne N, Parfait B, et al. (2011). Identification of genes potentially involved in the increased risk of malignancy in NF1-microdeleted patients. Mol Med. 17(1-2):79–87. PMID:20844836
1900. Pasquale G, Maria BA, Vania P, Gastone P, Nicola DL (2009). Cerebellar liponeurocytoma: an updated follow-up of a case presenting histopathological and clinically aggressive features. Neurol India. 57(2):194–6. PMID:19439854
1901. Pasquier B, Gasnier F, Pasquier D, Keddari E, Morens A, Couderc P (1986). Papillary meningioma. Clinicopathologic study of seven cases and review of the literature. Cancer. 58(2):299–305. PMID:3719522
1902. Pasquier B, Pasquier D, N'Golet A, Panh MH, Couderc P (1980). Extraneural metastases of astrocytomas and glioblastomas: clinicopathological study of two cases and review of literature. Cancer. 45(1):112–25. PMID:6985826
1903. Pasquier B, Péoc'H M, Fabre-Bocquentin B, Bensaadi L, Pasquier D, Hoffmann D, et al. (2002). Surgical pathology of drug-resistant partial epilepsy. A 10-year-experience with a series of 327 consecutive resections. Epileptic Disord. 4(2):99–119. PMID:12105073
1904. Pasquier B, Péoc'h M, Morrison AL, Gay E, Pasquier D, Grand S, et al. (2002). Chordoid glioma of the third ventricle: a report of two new cases, with further evidence supporting an ependymal differentiation, and review of the literature. Am J Surg Pathol. 26(10):1330–42. PMID:12360048
1905. Passone E, Pizzolitto S, D'Agostini S, Skrap M, Gardiman MP, Nocerino A, et al. (2006). Non-anaplastic pleomorphic xanthoastrocytoma with neuroradiological evidences of leptomeningeal dissemination. Childs Nerv Syst. 22(6):614–8. PMID:16369851
1905A. Pastorino L, Ghiorzo P, Nasti S, Battistuzzi L, Cusano R, Marzocchi C, et al. (2009). Identification of a SUFU germline mutation in a family with Gorlin syndrome. Am J Med Genet A. 149A(7):1539–43. PMID:19533801
1906. Patel AP, Tirosh I, Trombetta JJ, Shalek AK, Gillespie SM, Wakimoto H, et al. (2014). Single-cell RNA-seq highlights intratumoral heterogeneity in primary glioblastoma. Science. 344(6190):1396–401. PMID:24925914
1907. Patel DM, Schmidt RF, Liu JK (2013). Update on the diagnosis, pathogenesis, and treatment strategies for central neurocytoma. J Clin Neurosci. 20(9):1193–9. PMID:23810386
1908. Patel N, Fallah A, Provias J, Jha NK (2009). Cerebellar liponeurocytoma. Can J Surg. 52(4):E117–9. PMID:19680499
1909. Patil S, Perry A, Maccollin M, Dong S, Betensky RA, Yeh TH, et al. (2008). Immunohistochemical analysis supports a role for INI1/SMARCB1 in hereditary forms of schwannomas, but not in solitary, sporadic schwannomas. Brain Pathol. 18(4):517–9. PMID:18422762
1910. Patil S, Scheithauer BW, Strom RG, Mafra M, Chicoine MR, Perry A (2011). Malignant meningiomas with epithelial (adenocarcinoma-like) metaplasia: a study of 3 cases. Neurosurgery. 69(4):884–92. PMID:21558975
1911. Patsalides AD, Atac G, Hedge U, Janik J, Grant N, Jaffe ES, et al. (2005). Lymphomatoid granulomatosis: abnormalities of the brain at MR imaging. Radiology. 237(1):265–73. PMID:16100084
1912. Paulli M, Bergamaschi G, Tonon L, Viglio A, Rosso R, Facchetti F, et al. (1995). Evidence for a polyclonal nature of the cell infiltrate in sinus histiocytosis with massive lymphadenopathy (Rosai-Dorfman disease). Br J Haematol. 91(2):415–8. PMID:8547085
1913. Paulus W, Bayas A, Ott G, Roggendorf W (1994). Interphase cytogenetics of glioblastoma and gliosarcoma. Acta Neuropathol. 88(5):420–5. PMID:7847070
1914. Paulus W, Honegger J, Keyvani K, Fahlbusch R (1999). Xanthogranuloma of the sellar region: a clinicopathological entity different from adamantinomatous craniopharyngioma. Acta Neuropathol. 97(4):377–82. PMID:10208277
1915. Paulus W, Jellinger K, Hallas C, Ott G, Müller-Hermelink HK (1993). Human herpesvirus-6 and Epstein-Barr virus genome in primary cerebral lymphomas. Neurology. 43(8):1591–3. PMID:8394522
1916. Paulus W, Jänisch W (1990). Clinicopathologic correlations in epithelial choroid plexus neoplasms: a study of 52 cases. Acta Neuropathol. 80(6):635–41. PMID:1703384
1917. Paulus W, Lisle DK, Tonn JC, Wolf HK, Roggendorf W, Reeves SA, et al. (1996). Molecular genetic alterations in pleomorphic xanthoastrocytoma. Acta Neuropathol. 91(3):293–7. PMID:8834542
1918. Paulus W, Schlote W, Perentes E, Jacobi G, Warmuth-Metz M, Roggendorf W (1992). Desmoplastic supratentorial neuroepithelial tumours of infancy. Histopathology. 21(1):43–9. PMID:1634201
1919. Paulus W, Slowik F, Jellinger K (1991). Primary intracranial sarcomas: histopathological features of 19 cases. Histopathology. 18(5):395–402. PMID:1715839
1920. Pearce MS, Salotti JA, Little MP, McHugh K, Lee C, Kim KP, et al. (2012). Radiation exposure from CT scans in childhood and subsequent risk of leukaemia and brain tumours: a retrospective cohort study. Lancet. 380(9840):499–505. PMID:22681860
1921. Pedersen M, Küsters-Vandevelde HV, Viros A, Groenen PJ, Sanchez-Laorden B, Gilhuis JH, et al. (2013). Primary melanoma of the CNS in children is driven by congenital expression of oncogenic NRAS in melanocytes. Cancer Discov. 3(4):458–69. PMID:23303902
1922. Pekmezci M, Louie J, Gupta N, Bloomer MM, Tihan T (2010). Clinicopathological characteristics of adamantinomatous and papillary craniopharyngiomas: University of California, San Francisco experience 1985–2005. Neurosurgery. 67(5):1341–9, discussion 1349. PMID:20871436
1923. Pekmezci M, Perry A (2013). Neuropathology of brain metastases. Surg Neurol Int. 4 Suppl 4:S245–55. PMID:23717796
1924. Pekmezci M, Reuss DE, Hirbe AC, Dahiya S, Gutmann DH, von Deimling A, et al. (2015). Morphologic and immunohistochemical features of malignant peripheral nerve sheath

tumors and cellular schwannomas. Mod Pathol. 28(2):187–200. PMID:25189642
1925. Pels H, Montesinos-Rongen M, Schaller C, Schlegel U, Schmidt-Wolf IG, Wiestler OD, et al. (2005). VH gene analysis of primary CNS lymphomas. J Neurol Sci. 228(2):143–7. PMID:15694195
1926. Pels H, Schlegel U (2006). Primary central nervous system lymphoma. Curr Treat Options Neurol. 8(4):346–57. PMID:16942677
1927. Pencalet P, Maixner W, Sainte-Rose C, Lellouch-Tubiana A, Cinalli G, Zerah M, et al. (1999). Benign cerebellar astrocytomas in children. J Neurosurg. 90(2):265–73. PMID:9950497
1928. Per H, Kontaş O, Kumandaş S, Kurtsoy A (2009). A report of a desmoplastic non-infantile ganglioglioma in a 6-year-old boy with review of the literature. Neurosurg Rev. 32(3):369–74, discussion 374. PMID:19280238
1929. Peraud A, Ansari H, Bise K, Reulen HJ (1998). Clinical outcome of supratentorial astrocytoma WHO grade II. Acta Neurochir (Wien). 140(12):1213–22. PMID:9932120
1930. Peraud A, Kreth FW, Wiestler OD, Kleihues P, Reulen HJ (2002). Prognostic impact of TP53 mutations and P53 protein overexpression in supratentorial WHO grade II astrocytomas and oligoastrocytomas. Clin Cancer Res. 8(5):1117–24. PMID:12006527
1931. Peraud A, Watanabe K, Plate KH, Yonekawa Y, Kleihues P, Ohgaki H (1997). p53 mutations versus EGF receptor expression in giant cell glioblastomas. J Neuropathol Exp Neurol. 56(11):1236–41. PMID:9370234
1932. Peraud A, Watanabe K, Schwechheimer K, Yonekawa Y, Kleihues P, Ohgaki H (1999). Genetic profile of the giant cell glioblastoma. Lab Invest. 79(2):123–9. PMID:10068201
1933. Perentes E, Rubinstein LJ, Herman MM, Donoso LA (1986). S-antigen immunoreactivity in human pineal glands and pineal parenchymal tumors. A monoclonal antibody study. Acta Neuropathol. 71(3-4):224–7. PMID:3541480
1934. Perilongo G, Carollo C, Salviati L, Murgia A, Pillon M, Basso G, et al. (1997). Diencephalic syndrome and disseminated juvenile pilocytic astrocytomas of the hypothalamic-optic chiasm region. Cancer. 80(1):142–6. PMID:9210720
1935. Perkins SM, Mitra N, Fei W, Shinohara ET (2012). Patterns of care and outcomes of patients with pleomorphic xanthoastrocytoma: a SEER analysis. J Neurooncol. 110(1):99–104. PMID:22843450
1936. Perreault S, Ramaswamy V, Achrol AS, Chao K, Liu TT, Shih D, et al. (2014). MRI surrogates for molecular subgroups of medulloblastoma. AJNR Am J Neuroradiol. 35(7):1263–9. PMID:24831600
1937. Perry A, Aldape KD, George DH, Burger PC (2004). Small cell astrocytoma: an aggressive variant that is clinicopathologically and genetically distinct from anaplastic oligodendroglioma. Cancer. 101(10):2318–26. PMID:15470710
1938. Perry A, Banerjee R, Lohse CM, Kleinschmidt-DeMasters BK, Scheithauer BW (2002). A role for chromosome 9p21 deletions in the malignant progression of meningiomas and the prognosis of anaplastic meningiomas. Brain Pathol. 12(2):183–90. PMID:11958372
1939. Perry A, Burton SS, Fuller GN, Robinson CA, Palmer CA, Resch L, et al. (2010). Oligodendroglial neoplasms with ganglioglioma-like maturation: a diagnostic pitfall. Acta Neuropathol. 120(2):237–52. PMID:20464403
1940. Perry A, Cai DX, Scheithauer BW, Swanson PE, Lohse CM, Newsham IF, et al. (2000). Merlin, DAL-1, and progesterone receptor expression in clinicopathologic subsets of meningioma: a correlative immunohistochemical study of 175 cases. J Neuropathol Exp Neurol. 59(10):872–9. PMID:11079777
1941. Perry A, Fuller CE, Judkins AR, Dehner LP, Biegel JA (2005). INI1 expression is retained in composite rhabdoid tumors, including rhabdoid meningiomas. Mod Pathol. 18(7):951–8. PMID:15761491
1942. Perry A, Giannini C, Raghavan R, Scheithauer BW, Banerjee R, Margraf L, et al. (2001). Aggressive phenotypic and genotypic features in pediatric and NF2-associated meningiomas: a clinicopathologic study of 53 cases. J Neuropathol Exp Neurol. 60(10):994–1003. PMID:11589430
1943. Perry A, Giannini C, Scheithauer BW, Rojiani AM, Yachnis AT, Seo IS, et al. (1997). Composite pleomorphic xanthoastrocytoma and ganglioglioma: report of four cases and review of the literature. Am J Surg Pathol. 21(7):763–71. PMID:9236832
1944. Perry A, Kurtkaya-Yapicier O, Scheithauer BW, Robinson S, Prayson RA, Kleinschmidt-DeMasters BK, et al. (2005). Insights into meningioangiomatosis with and without meningioma: a clinicopathologic and genetic series of 24 cases with review of the literature. Brain Pathol. 15(1):55–65. PMID:15779237
1945. Perry A, Lusis EA, Gutmann DH (2005). Meningothelial hyperplasia: a detailed clinicopathologic, immunohistochemical and genetic study of 11 cases. Brain Pathol. 15(2):109–15. PMID:15912882
1946. Perry A, Miller CR, Gujrati M, Scheithauer BW, Zambrano SC, Jost SC, et al. (2009). Malignant gliomas with primitive neuroectodermal tumor-like components: a clinicopathologic and genetic study of 53 cases. Brain Pathol. 19(1):81–90. PMID:18452568
1947. Perry A, Roth KA, Banerjee R, Fuller CE, Gutmann DH (2001). NF1 deletions in S-100 protein-positive and negative cells of sporadic and neurofibromatosis 1 (NF1)-associated plexiform neurofibromas and malignant peripheral nerve sheath tumors. Am J Pathol. 159(1):57–61. PMID:11438454
1948. Perry A, Scheithauer BW, Macaulay RJ, Raffel C, Roth KA, Kros JM (2002). Oligodendrogliomas with neurocytic differentiation. A report of 4 cases with diagnostic and histogenetic implications. J Neuropathol Exp Neurol. 61(11):947–55. PMID:12430711
1949. Perry A, Scheithauer BW, Nascimento AG (1997). The immunophenotypic spectrum of meningeal hemangiopericytoma: a comparison with fibrous meningioma and solitary fibrous tumor of meninges. Am J Surg Pathol. 21(11):1354–60. PMID:9351573
1950. Perry A, Scheithauer BW, Stafford SL, Abell-Aleff PC, Meyer FB (1998). "Rhabdoid" meningioma: an aggressive variant. Am J Surg Pathol. 22(12):1482–90. PMID:9850174
1951. Perry A, Scheithauer BW, Stafford SL, Lohse CM, Wollan PC (1999). "Malignancy" in meningiomas: a clinicopathologic study of 116 patients, with grading implications. Cancer. 85(9):2046–56. PMID:10223247
1952. Perry A, Stafford SL, Scheithauer BW, Suman VJ, Lohse CM (1997). Meningioma grading: an analysis of histologic parameters. Am J Surg Pathol. 21(12):1455–65. PMID:9414189
1953. Perry A, Stafford SL, Scheithauer BW, Suman VJ, Lohse CM (1998). The prognostic significance of MIB-1, p53, and DNA flow cytometry in completely resected primary meningiomas. Cancer. 82(11):2262–9. PMID:9610708
1954. Persson AI, Petritsch C, Swartling FJ, Itsara M, Sim FJ, Auvergne R, et al. (2010). Non-stem cell origin for oligodendroglioma. Cancer Cell. 18(6):669–82. PMID:21156288
1955. Persu A, Hamoir M, Grégoire V, Garin P, Duvivier E, Reychler H, et al. (2008). High prevalence of SDHB mutations in head and neck paraganglioma in Belgium. J Hypertens. 26(7):1395–401. PMID:18551016
1956. Burger PC (2009). Smears and Frozen Sections in Surgical Neuropathology. Baltimore (MD): PB Medical Publishing.
1957. Peters KB, Cummings TJ, Gururangan S (2011). Transformation of juvenile pilocytic astrocytoma to anaplastic pilocytic astrocytoma in patients with neurofibromatosis type I. J Pediatr Hematol Oncol. 33(5):e198–201. PMID:21572348
1958. Petitjean A, Mathe E, Kato S, Ishioka C, Tavtigian SV, Hainaut P, et al. (2007). Impact of mutant p53 functional properties on TP53 mutation patterns and tumor phenotype: lessons from recent developments in the IARC TP53 database. Hum Mutat. 28(6):622–9. PMID:17311302
1959. Peyre M, Bah A, Kalamarides M (2012). Multifocal choroid plexus papillomas: case report. Acta Neurochir (Wien). 154(2):295–9. PMID:21953479
1960. Peyre M, Stemmer-Rachamimov A, Clermont-Taranchon E, Quentin S, El-Taraya N, Walczak C, et al. (2013). Meningioma progression in mice triggered by Nf2 and Cdkn2ab inactivation. Oncogene. 32(36):4264–72. PMID:23045274
1961. Pfister S, Janzarik WG, Remke M, Ernst A, Werft W, Becker N, et al. (2008). BRAF gene duplication constitutes a mechanism of MAPK pathway activation in low-grade astrocytomas. J Clin Invest. 118(5):1739–49. PMID:18398503
1962. Pfister S, Remke M, Castoldi M, Bai AH, Muckenthaler MU, Kulozik A, et al. (2009). Novel genomic amplification targeting the microRNA cluster at 19q13.42 in a pediatric embryonal tumor with abundant neuropil and true rosettes. Acta Neuropathol. 117(4):457–64. PMID:19057917
1963. Phi JH, Koh EJ, Kim SK, Park SH, Cho BK, Wang KC (2011). Desmoplastic infantile astrocytoma: recurrence with malignant transformation into glioblastoma: a case report. Childs Nerv Syst. 27(12):2177–81. PMID:21947035
1964. Phi JH, Park SH, Chae JH, Hong KH, Park SS, Kang JH, et al. (2008). Congenital subependymal giant cell astrocytoma: clinical considerations and expression of radial glial cell markers in giant cells. Childs Nerv Syst. 24(12):1499–503. PMID:18629509
1965. Phillips CL, Miles L, Jones BV, Sutton M, Crone K, Fouladi M (2011). Medulloblastoma with melanotic differentiation: case report and review of the literature. J Neurooncol. 103(3):759–64. PMID:20953660
1966. Phillips JJ, Misra A, Feuerstein BG, Kunwar S, Tihan T (2010). Pituicytoma: characterization of a unique neoplasm by histology, immunohistochemistry, ultrastructure, and array-based comparative genomic hybridization. Arch Pathol Lab Med. 134(7):1063–9. PMID:20586639
1967. Picard D, Miller S, Hawkins CE, Bouffet E, Rogers HA, Chan TS, et al. (2012). Markers of survival and metastatic potential in childhood CNS primitive neuro-ectodermal brain tumours: an integrative genomic analysis. Lancet Oncol. 13(8):838–48. PMID:22691720
1968. Pickuth D, Leutloff U (1996). Computed tomography and magnetic resonance imaging findings in primitive neuroectodermal tumours in adults. Br J Radiol. 69(817):1–5. PMID:8785615
1969. Pierallini A, Bonamini M, Pantano P, Palmeggiani F, Raguso M, Osti MF, et al. (1998). Radiological assessment of necrosis in glioblastoma: variability and prognostic value. Neuroradiology. 40(3):150–3. PMID:9561517
1970. Piercecchi-Marti MD, Mohamed H, Liprandi A, Gambarelli D, Grisoli F, Pellissier JF (2002). Intracranial meningeal melanocytoma associated with ipsilateral nevus of Ota. Case report. J Neurosurg. 96(3):619–23. PMID:11883852
1971. Pierron G, Tirode F, Lucchesi C, Reynaud S, Ballet S, Cohen-Gogo S, et al. (2012). A new subtype of bone sarcoma defined by BCOR-CCNB3 gene fusion. Nat Genet. 44(4):461–6. PMID:22387997
1972. Pietsch T, Schmidt R, Remke M, Korshunov A, Hovestadt V, Jones DT, et al. (2014). Prognostic significance of clinical, histopathological, and molecular characteristics of medulloblastomas in the prospective HIT2000 multicenter clinical trial cohort. Acta Neuropathol. 128(1):137–49. PMID:24791927
1973. Pietsch T, Waha A, Koch A, Kraus J, Albrecht S, Tonn J, et al. (1997). Medulloblastomas of the desmoplastic variant carry mutations of the human homologue of Drosophila patched. Cancer Res. 57(11):2085–8. PMID:9187099
1974. Pietsch T, Wohlers I, Goschzik T, Dreschmann V, Denkhaus D, Dörner E, et al. (2014). Supratentorial ependymomas of childhood carry C11orf95-RELA fusions leading to pathological activation of the NF-κB signaling pathway. Acta Neuropathol. 127(4):609–11. PMID:24562983
1975. Pignatti F, van den Bent M, Curran D, Debruyne C, Sylvester R, Therasse P, et al.; European Organization for Research and Treatment of Cancer Brain Tumor Cooperative Group; European Organization for Research and Treatment of Cancer Radiotherapy Cooperative Group (2002). Prognostic factors for survival in adult patients with cerebral low-grade glioma. J Clin Oncol. 20(8):2076–84. PMID:11956268
1976. Pimentel J, Barroso C, Miguéns J, Firmo C, Antunes JL (2009). Papillary glioneuronal tumor–prognostic value of the extension of surgical resection. Clin Neuropathol. 28(4):287–94. PMID:19642508
1977. Pimentel J, Silva R, Pimentel T (2003). Primary malignant rhabdoid tumors of the central nervous system: considerations about two cases of adulthood presentation. J Neurooncol. 61(2):121–6. PMID:12622450
1978. Pinna V, Lanari V, Daniele P, Consoli F, Agolini E, Margiotti K, et al. (2015). p.Arg1809Cys substitution in neurofibromin is associated with a distinctive NF1 phenotype without neurofibromas. Eur J Hum Genet. 23(8):1068–71. PMID:25370043
1979. Pinto Gama HP, da Rocha AJ, Braga FT, da Silva CJ, Maia AC Jr, de Campos Meirelles RG, et al. (2006). Comparative analysis of MR sequences to detect structural brain lesions in tuberous sclerosis. Pediatr Radiol. 36(2):119–25. PMID:16283285
1980. Piotrowski A, Xie J, Liu YF, Poplawski AB, Gomes AR, Madanecki P, et al. (2014). Germline loss-of-function mutations in LZTR1 predispose to an inherited disorder of multiple schwannomas. Nat Genet. 46(2):182–7. PMID:24362817
1981. Pirini MG, Mascalchi M, Salvi F, Tassinari CA, Zanella L, Bacchini P, et al. (2003). Primary diffuse meningeal melanomatosis: radiologic-pathologic correlation. AJNR Am J Neuroradiol. 24(1):115–8. PMID:12533338
1982. Pirotte B, Krischek B, Levivier M, Bolyn S, Brucher JM, Brotchi J (1998). Diagnostic and microsurgical presentation of intracranial angiolipomas. Case report and review of the literature. J Neurosurg. 88(1):129–32. PMID:9420085
1983. Pitche P, Ategbo S, Gbadoe A, Bassuka-Parent A, Mouzou B, Tchangaï-Walla K (1997). [Bullous toxidermatosis and HIV infection in hospital environment in Lome (Togo)]. Bull Soc Pathol Exot. 90(3):186–8. PMID:9410257
1984. Pizer BL, Moss T, Oakhill A, Webb D, Coakham HB (1995). Congenital astroblastoma: an immunohistochemical study. Case report. J Neurosurg. 83(3):550–5. PMID:7545227
1985. Pizzuti A, Bottillo I, Inzana F, Lanari V, Buttarelli F, Torrente I, et al. (2011). Familial spinal neurofibromatosis due to a multiexonic NF1 gene deletion. Neurogenetics. 12(3):233–40. PMID:21365283
1986. Plank TL, Logginidou H, Klein-Szanto A, Henske EP (1999). The expression of hamartin, the product of the TSC1 gene, in normal human tissues and in TSC1- and TSC2-linked angiomyolipomas. Mod Pathol. 12(5):539–45. PMID:10349994
1987. Plank TL, Yeung RS, Henske EP (1998).

Hamartin, the product of the tuberous sclerosis 1 (TSC1) gene, interacts with tuberin and appears to be localized to cytoplasmic vesicles. Cancer Res. 58(21):4766–70. PMID:9809973
1988. Plate KH, Breier G, Weich HA, Risau W (1992). Vascular endothelial growth factor is a potential tumour angiogenesis factor in human gliomas in vivo. Nature. 359(6398):845–8. PMID:1279432
1989. Plate KH, Scholz A, Dumont DJ (2012). Tumor angiogenesis and anti-angiogenic therapy in malignant gliomas revisited. Acta Neuropathol. 124(6):763–75. PMID:23143192
1990. Plotkin SR, Blakeley JO, Evans DG, Hanemann CO, Hulsebos TJ, Hunter-Schaedle K, et al. (2013). Update from the 2011 International Schwannomatosis Workshop: From genetics to diagnostic criteria. Am J Med Genet A. 161A(3):405–16. PMID:23401320
1991. Plowman PN, Pizer B, Kingston JE (2004). Pineal parenchymal tumours: II. On the aggressive behaviour of pineoblastoma in patients with an inherited mutation of the RB1 gene. Clin Oncol (R Coll Radiol). 16(4):244–7. PMID:15214647
1992. Podsypanina K, Ellenson LH, Nemes A, Gu J, Tamura M, Yamada KM, et al. (1999). Mutation of Pten/Mmac1 in mice causes neoplasia in multiple organ systems. Proc Natl Acad Sci U S A. 96(4):1563–8. PMID:9990064
1993. Pohl U, Cairncross JG, Louis DN (1999). Homozygous deletions of the CDKN2C/p18INK4C gene on the short arm of chromosome 1 in anaplastic oligodendrogliomas. Brain Pathol. 9(4):639–43. PMID:10517502
1994. Pollack IF, Claassen D, al-Shboul Q, Janosky JE, Deutsch M (1995). Low-grade gliomas of the cerebral hemispheres in children: an analysis of 71 cases. J Neurosurg. 82(4):536–47. PMID:7897512
1995. Pollack IF, Hoffman HJ, Humphreys RP, Becker L (1993). The long-term outcome after surgical treatment of dorsally exophytic brainstem gliomas. J Neurosurg. 78(6):859–63. PMID:8487066
1996. Pollack IF, Hurtt M, Pang D, Albright AL (1994). Dissemination of low grade intracranial astrocytomas in children. Cancer. 73(11):2869–78. PMID:8194029
1997. Pollak A, Friede RL (1977). Fine structure of medulloepithelioma. J Neuropathol Exp Neurol. 36(4):712–25. PMID:886367
1998. Pollock E, Ford-Jones EL, Corey M, Barker G, Mindorff CM, Gold R, et al. (1991). Use of the Pediatric Risk of Mortality score to predict nosocomial infection in a pediatric intensive care unit. Crit Care Med. 19(2):160–5. PMID:1989753
1999. Polydorides AD, Rosenblum MK, Edgar MA (2007). Metastatic renal cell carcinoma to hemangioblastoma in von Hippel-Lindau disease. Arch Pathol Lab Med. 131(4):641–5. PMID:17425399
2000. Pomeroy SL, Tamayo P, Gaasenbeek M, Sturla LM, Angelo M, McLaughlin ME, et al. (2002). Prediction of central nervous system embryonal tumour outcome based on gene expression. Nature. 415(6870):436–42. PMID:11807556
2001. Pomper MG, Passe TJ, Burger PC, Scheithauer BW, Brat DJ (2001). Chordoid glioma: a neoplasm unique to the hypothalamus and anterior third ventricle. AJNR Am J Neuroradiol. 22(3):464–9. PMID:11237967
2002. Pompili A, Calvosa F, Caroli F, Mastrostefano R, Occhipinti E, Raus L, et al. (1993). The transdural extension of gliomas. J Neurooncol. 15(1):67–74. PMID:8455064
2003. Ponzoni M, Arrigoni G, Gould VE, Del Curto B, Maggioni M, Scapinello A, et al. (2000). Lack of CD 29 (beta1 integrin) and CD 54 (ICAM-1) adhesion molecules in intravascular lymphomatosis. Hum Pathol. 31(2):220–6. PMID:10685637
2004. Ponzoni M, Berger F, Chassagne-Clement C, Tinguely M, Jouvet A, Ferreri AJ, et al.; International Extranodal Lymphoma Study Group (2007). Reactive perivascular T-cell infiltrate predicts survival in primary central nervous system B-cell lymphomas. Br J Haematol. 138(3):316–23. PMID:17555470
2005. Ponzoni M, Bonetti F, Poliani PL, Vermi W, Bottelli C, Dolcetti R, et al. (2011). Central nervous system marginal zone B-cell lymphoma associated with Chlamydophila psittaci infection. Hum Pathol. 42(5):738–42. PMID:21239044
2006. Ponzoni M, Ferreri AJ, Campo E, Facchetti F, Mazzucchelli L, Yoshino T, et al. (2007). Definition, diagnosis, and management of intravascular large B-cell lymphoma: proposals and perspectives from an international consensus meeting. J Clin Oncol. 25(21):3168–73. PMID:17577023
2007. Popova SN, Bergqvist M, Dimberg A, Edqvist PH, Ekman S, Hesselager G, et al. (2014). Subtyping of gliomas of various WHO grades by the application of immunohistochemistry. Histopathology. 64(3):365–79. PMID:24410805
2008. Poppleton H, Gilbertson RJ (2007). Stem cells of ependymoma. Br J Cancer. 96(1):6–10. PMID:17179988
2009. Poremba C, Dockhorn-Dworniczak B, Merritt V, Li CY, Heidl G, Tauber PF, et al. (1993). Immature teratomas of different origin carried by a pregnant mother and her fetus. Diagn Mol Pathol. 2(2):131–6. PMID:8269278
2010. Portela A, Esteller M (2010). Epigenetic modifications and human disease. Nat Biotechnol. 28(10):1057–68. PMID:20944598
2011. Portela-Oliveira E, Torres US, Lancellotti CL, Souza AS, Ferraz-Filho JR (2014). Solid intraventricular papillary glioneuronal tumor: magnetic resonance imaging findings with histopathological correlation. Pediatr Neurol. 50(2):199–200. PMID:24314675
2012. Poulgrain K, Gurgo R, Winter C, Ong B, Lau Q (2011). Papillary tumour of the pineal region. J Clin Neurosci. 18(8):1007–17. PMID:21658955
2013. Powell SZ, Yachnis AT, Rorke LB, Rojiani AM, Eskin TA (1996). Divergent differentiation in pleomorphic xanthoastrocytoma. Evidence for a neuronal element and possible relationship to ganglion cell tumors. Am J Surg Pathol. 20(1):80–5. PMID:8540612
2014. Prabhu VC, Brown HG (2005). The pathogenesis of craniopharyngiomas. Childs Nerv Syst. 21(8-9):622–7. PMID:15965669
2015. Prabowo AS, Iyer AM, Veersema TJ, Anink JJ, Schouten-van Meeteren AY, Spliet WG, et al. (2014). BRAF V600E mutation is associated with mTOR signaling activation in glioneuronal tumors. Brain Pathol. 24(1):52–66. PMID:23941441
2016. Prabowo AS, van Thuijl HF, Scheinin I, Sie D, van Essen HF, Iyer AM, et al. (2015). Landscape of chromosomal copy number aberrations in gangliogliomas and dysembryoplastic neuroepithelial tumours. Neuropathol Appl Neurobiol. 41(6):743–55. PMID:25764012
2017. Prajapati HJ, Vincentelli C, Hwang SN, Voloschin A, Crocker I, Dehkharghani S (2014). Primary CNS natural killer/T-cell lymphoma of the nasal type presenting in a woman: case report and review of the literature. J Clin Oncol. 32(8):e26–9. PMID:24419127
2018. Prayer D, Grois N, Prosch H, Gadner H, Barkovich AJ (2004). MR imaging presentation of intracranial disease associated with Langerhans cell histiocytosis. AJNR Am J Neuroradiol. 25(5):880–91. PMID:15140741
2019. Prayson RA (1997). Myxopapillary ependymomas: a clinicopathologic study of 14 cases including MIB-1 and p53 immunoreactivity. Mod Pathol. 10(4):304–10. PMID:9110291
2020. Prayson RA (1999). Clinicopathologic study of 61 patients with ependymoma including MIB-1 immunohistochemistry. Ann Diagn Pathol. 3(1):11–8. PMID:9990108
2021. Prayson RA (1999). Composite ganglioglioma and dysembryoplastic neuroepithelial tumor. Arch Pathol Lab Med. 123(3):247–50. PMID:10086515
2022. Prayson RA (2000). Papillary glioneuronal tumor. Arch Pathol Lab Med. 124(12):1820–3. PMID:11100065
2023. Prayson RA (2012). Pleomorphic xanthoastrocytoma arising in neurofibromatosis Type 1. Clin Neuropathol. 31(3):152–4. PMID:22551920
2024. Prayson RA, Castilla EA, Hembury TA, Liu W, Noga CM, Prok AL (2003). Interobserver variability in determining MIB-1 labeling indices in oligodendrogliomas. Ann Diagn Pathol. 7(1):9–13. PMID:12616468
2025. Prayson RA, Chahlavi A, Luciano M (2004). Cerebellar paraganglioma. Ann Diagn Pathol. 8(4):219–23. PMID:15290673
2026. Prayson RA, Estes ML (1992). Dysembryoplastic neuroepithelial tumor. Am J Clin Pathol. 97(3):398–401. PMID:1543164
2027. Prayson RA, Khajavi K, Comair YG (1995). Cortical architectural abnormalities and MIB1 immunoreactivity in gangliogliomas: a study of 60 patients with intracranial tumors. J Neuropathol Exp Neurol. 54(4):513–20. PMID:7541447
2028. Prayson RA, Suh JH (1999). Subependymomas: clinicopathologic study of 14 tumors, including comparative MIB-1 immunohistochemical analysis with other ependymal neoplasms. Arch Pathol Lab Med. 123(4):306–9. PMID:10320142
2029. Preston DL, Ron E, Yonehara S, Kobuke T, Fujii H, Kishikawa M, et al. (2002). Tumors of the nervous system and pituitary gland associated with atomic bomb radiation exposure. J Natl Cancer Inst. 94(20):1555–63. PMID:12381708
2030. Preuss M, Christiansen H, Merkenschlager A, Hirsch FW, Kiess W, Müller W, et al. (2015). Disseminated oligodendroglial cell-like leptomeningeal tumors: preliminary diagnostic and therapeutic results for a novel tumor entity. J Neurooncol.
2031. Preusser M, Budka H, Rössler K, Hainfellner JA (2007). OLIG2 is a useful immunohistochemical marker in differential diagnosis of clear cell primary CNS neoplasms. Histopathology. 50(3):365–70. PMID:17257132
2032. Preusser M, Capper D, Ilhan-Mutlu A, Berghoff AS, Birner P, Bartsch R, et al. (2012). Brain metastases: pathobiology and emerging targeted therapies. Acta Neuropathol. 123(2):205–22. PMID:22212630
2033. Preusser M, Dietrich W, Czech T, Prayer D, Budka H, Hainfellner JA (2003). Rosette-forming glioneuronal tumor of the fourth ventricle. Acta Neuropathol. 106(5):506–8. PMID:12915951
2034. Preusser M, Hoeftberger R, Woehrer A, Gelpi E, Kouwenhoven M, Kros JM, et al. (2012). Prognostic value of Ki67 index in anaplastic oligodendroglial tumours–a translational study of the European Organization for Research and Treatment of Cancer Brain Tumor Group. Histopathology. 60(6):885–94. PMID:22335622
2035. Preusser M, Hoischen A, Novak K, Czech T, Prayer D, Hainfellner JA, et al. (2007). Angiocentric glioma: report of clinico-pathologic and genetic findings in 8 cases. Am J Surg Pathol. 31(11):1709–18. PMID:18059228
2036. Preusser M, Laggner U, Haberler C, Heinzl H, Budka H, Hainfellner JA (2006). Comparative analysis of NeuN immunoreactivity in primary brain tumours: conclusions for rational use in diagnostic histopathology. Histopathology. 48(4):438–44. PMID:16487366
2037. Preusser M, Woehrer A, Koperek O, Rottenfusser A, Dieckmann K, Gatterbauer B, et al. (2010). Primary central nervous system lymphoma: a clinicopathological study of 75 cases. Pathology. 42(6):547–52. PMID:20854073
2038. Prévot S, Bienvenu L, Vaillant JC, de Saint-Maur PP (1999). Benign schwannoma of the digestive tract: a clinicopathologic and immunohistochemical study of five cases, including a case of esophageal tumor. Am J Surg Pathol. 23(4):431–6. PMID:10199472
2038A. Prieto-Granada CN, Wiesner T, Messina JL, Jungbluth AA, Chi P, Antonescu CR (2015). Loss of H3K27me3 Expression Is a Highly Sensitive Marker for Sporadic and Radiation-induced MPNST. Am J Surg Pathol. [Epub ahead of print] PMID:26645727
2039. Probst-Cousin S, Bergmann M, Schröder R, Kuchelmeister K, Schmid KW, Ernestus RJ, et al. (1996). Ki-67 and biological behaviour in meningeal haemangiopericytomas. Histopathology. 29(1):57–61. PMID:8818695
2040. Proescholdt MA, Mayer C, Kubitza M, Schubert T, Liao SY, Stanbridge EJ, et al. (2005). Expression of hypoxia-inducible carbonic anhydrases in brain tumors. Neuro Oncol. 7(4):465–75. PMID:16212811
2041. Pruchon E, Chauveinc L, Sabatier L, Dutrillaux AM, Ricoul M, Delattre JY, et al. (1994). A cytogenetic study of 19 recurrent gliomas. Cancer Genet Cytogenet. 76(2):85–92. PMID:7923073
2042. Pugh TJ, Weeraratne SD, Archer TC, Pomeranz Krummel DA, Auclair D, Bochicchio J, et al. (2012). Medulloblastoma exome sequencing uncovers subtype-specific somatic mutations. Nature. 488(7409):106–10. PMID:22820256
2043. Pulido R, Baker SJ, Barata JT, Carracedo A, Cid VJ, Chin-Sang ID, et al. (2014). A unified nomenclature and amino acid numbering for human PTEN. Sci Signal. 7(332):pe15. PMID:24985344
2044. Pummi KP, Aho HJ, Laato MK, Peltonen JT, Peltonen SA (2006). Tight junction proteins and perineurial cells in neurofibromas. J Histochem Cytochem. 54(1):53–61. PMID:16087703
2045. Purav P, Ganapathy K, Mallikarjuna VS, Annapurneswari S, Kalyanaraman S, Reginald J, et al. (2005). Rosai-Dorfman disease of the central nervous system. J Clin Neurosci. 12(6):656–9. PMID:16099162
2046. Purdy E, Johnston DL, Bartels U, Fryer C, Carret AS, Crooks B, et al. (2014). Ependymoma in children under the age of 3 years: a report from the Canadian Pediatric Brain Tumour Consortium. J Neurooncol. 117(2):359–64. PMID:24532240
2047. Qian H, Lin S, Zhang M, Cao Y (2012). Surgical management of intraventricular central neurocytoma: 92 cases. Acta Neurochir (Wien). 154(11):1951–60. PMID:22941394
2048. Qin W, Chan JA, Vinters HV, Mathern GW, Franz DN, Taillon BE, et al. (2010). Analysis of TSC cortical tubers by deep sequencing of TSC1, TSC2 and KRAS demonstrates that small second-hit mutations in these genes are rare events. Brain Pathol. 20(6):1096–105. PMID:20633017
2049. Qin Y, Yao L, King EE, Buddavarapu K, Lenci RE, Chocron ES, et al. (2010). Germline mutations in TMEM127 confer susceptibility to pheochromocytoma. Nat Genet. 42(3):229–33. PMID:20154675
2050. Qu M, Olofsson T, Sigurdardottir S, You C, Kalimo H, Nistér M, et al. (2007). Genetically distinct astrocytic and oligodendroglial components in oligoastrocytomas. Acta Neuropathol. 113(2):129–36. PMID:17031656
2051. Quillien V, Lavenu A, Karayan-Tapon L, Carpentier C, Labussière M, Lesimple T, et al. (2012). Comparative assessment of 5 methods (methylation-specific polymerase chain reaction, MethyLight, pyrosequencing, methylation-sensitive high-resolution melting, and immunohistochemistry) to analyze O6-methylguanine-DNA-methyltranferase in a series of 100 glioblastoma patients. Cancer. 118(17):4201–11. PMID:22294349
2052. Rades D, Fehlauer F, Lamszus K, Schild SE, Hagel C, Westphal M, et al. (2005).

Well-differentiated neurocytoma: what is the best available treatment? Neuro Oncol. 7(1):77–83. PMID:15701284
2053. Rades D, Schild SE, Fehlauer F (2004). Prognostic value of the MIB-1 labeling index for central neurocytomas. Neurology. 62(6):987–9. PMID:15037708
2054. Radke J, Gehlhaar C, Lenze D, Capper D, Bock A, Heppner FL, et al. (2015). The evolution of the anaplastic cerebellar liponeurocytoma: case report and review of the literature. Clin Neuropathol. 34(1):19–25. PMID:25250652
2055. Raffel C, Jenkins RB, Frederick L, Hebrink D, Alderete B, Fults DW, et al. (1997). Sporadic medulloblastomas contain PTCH mutations. Cancer Res. 57(5):842–5. PMID:9041183
2056. Ragel BT, Osborn AG, Whang K, Townsend JJ, Jensen RL, Couldwell WT (2006). Subependymomas: an analysis of clinical and imaging features. Neurosurgery. 58(5):881–90, discussion 881–90. PMID:16639322
2057. Raghavan R, Balani J, Perry A, Margraf L, Vono MB, Cai DX, et al. (2003). Pediatric oligodendrogliomas: a study of molecular alterations on 1p and 19q using fluorescence in situ hybridization. J Neuropathol Exp Neurol. 62(5):530–7. PMID:12769192
2058. Raghavan R, Dickey WT Jr, Margraf LR, White CL 3rd, Coimbra C, Hynan LS, et al. (2000). Proliferative activity in craniopharyngiomas: clinicopathological correlations in adults and children. Surg Neurol. 54(3):241–7, discussion 248. PMID:11118571
2059. Raghavan R, Steart PV, Weller RO (1990). Cell proliferation patterns in the diagnosis of astrocytomas, anaplastic astrocytomas and glioblastoma multiforme: a Ki-67 study. Neuropathol Appl Neurobiol. 16(2):123–33. PMID:2161084
2060. Raghunathan A, Wani K, Armstrong TS, Vera-Bolanos E, Fouladi M, Gilbertson R, et al.; Collaborative Ependymoma Research Network (2013). Histological predictors of outcome in ependymoma are dependent on anatomic site within the central nervous system. Brain Pathol. 23(5):584–94. PMID:23452038
2061. Rainho CA, Rogatto SR, de Moraes LC, Barbieri-Neto J (1992). Cytogenetic study of a pineocytoma. Cancer Genet Cytogenet. 64(2):127–32. PMID:1486561
2062. Rainov NG, Lübbe J, Renshaw J, Pritchard-Jones K, Lüthy AR, Aguzzi A (1995). Association of Wilms' tumor with primary brain tumor in siblings. J Neuropathol Exp Neurol. 54(2):214–23. PMID:7876889
2063. Raisanen J, Biegel JA, Hatanpaa KJ, Judkins A, White CL, Perry A (2005). Chromosome 22q deletions in atypical teratoid/rhabdoid tumors in adults. Brain Pathol. 15(1):23–8. PMID:15779233
2064. Raja AI, Yeaney GA, Jakacki RI, Hamilton RL, Pollack IF (2008). Extraventricular neurocytoma in neurofibromatosis Type 1: case report. J Neurosurg Pediatr. 2(1):63–7. PMID:18590398
2065. Rajan B, Ashley S, Gorman C, Jose CC, Horwich A, Bloom HJ, et al. (1993). Craniopharyngioma–a long-term results following limited surgery and radiotherapy. Radiother Oncol. 26(1):1–10. PMID:8438080
2066. Rajaram V, Brat DJ, Perry A (2004). Anaplastic meningioma versus meningeal hemangiopericytoma: immunohistochemical and genetic markers. Hum Pathol. 35(11):1413–8. PMID:15668900
2067. Raju GP, Urion DK, Sahin M (2007). Neonatal subependymal giant cell astrocytoma: new case and review of literature. Pediatr Neurol. 36(2):128–31. PMID:17275668
2068. Ramkissoon LA, Horowitz PM, Craig JM, Ramkissoon SH, Rich BE, Schumacher SE, et al. (2013). Genomic analysis of diffuse pediatric low-grade gliomas identifies recurrent oncogenic truncating rearrangements in the transcription factor MYBL1. Proc Natl Acad Sci U S A. 110(20):8188–93. PMID:23633565
2069. Raney RB, Ater JL, Herman-Liu A, Leeds NE, Cleary KR, Womer RB, et al. (1994). Primary intraspinal soft-tissue sarcoma in childhood: report of two cases with a review of the literature. Med Pediatr Oncol. 23(4):359–64. PMID:8058008
2070. Rankine AJ, Filion PR, Platten MA, Spagnolo DV (2004). Perineurioma: a clinicopathological study of eight cases. Pathology. 36(4):309–15. PMID:15370128
2071. Raoux D, Duband S, Forest F, Trombert B, Chambonnière ML, Dumollard JM, et al. (2010). Primary central nervous system lymphoma: immunohistochemical profile and prognostic significance. Neuropathology. 30(3):232–40. PMID:19925562
2072. Rasheed BK, McLendon RE, Friedman HS, Friedman AH, Fuchs HE, Bigner DD, et al. (1995). Chromosome 10 deletion mapping in human gliomas: a common deletion region in 10q25. Oncogene. 10(11):2243–6. PMID:7784070
2073. Rauen KA (2013). The RASopathies. Annu Rev Genomics Hum Genet. 14:355–69. PMID:23875798
2074. Rauhut F, Reinhardt V, Budach V, Wiedemayer H, Nau HE (1989). Intramedullary pilocytic astrocytomas–a clinical and morphological study after combined surgical and photon or neutron therapy. Neurosurg Rev. 12(4):309–13. PMID:2594208
2075. Rausch T, Jones DT, Zapatka M, Stütz AM, Zichner T, Weischenfeldt J, et al. (2012). Genome sequencing of pediatric medulloblastoma links catastrophic DNA rearrangements with TP53 mutations. Cell. 148(1-2):59–71. PMID:22265402
2076. Rawlinson DG, Herman MM, Rubinstein LJ (1973). The fine structure of a myxopapillary ependymoma of the filum terminale. Acta Neuropathol. 25(1):1–13. PMID:4727729
2077. Ray WZ, Blackburn SL, Casavilca-Zambrano S, Barrionuevo C, Orrego JE, Heinicke H, et al. (2009). Clinicopathologic features of recurrent dysembryoplastic neuroepithelial tumor and rare malignant transformation: a report of 5 cases and review of the literature. J Neurooncol. 94(2):283–92. PMID:19267228
2078. Raymond AA, Halpin SF, Alsanjari N, Cook MJ, Kitchen ND, Fish DR, et al. (1994). Dysembryoplastic neuroepithelial tumor. Features in 16 patients. Brain. 117(Pt 3):461–75. PMID:8032857
2079. Raza SM, Lang FF, Aggarwal BB, Fuller GN, Wildrick DM, Sawaya R (2002). Necrosis and glioblastoma: a friend or a foe? A review and a hypothesis. Neurosurgery. 51(1):2–12, discussion 12–3. PMID:12182418
2080. Read TA, Fogarty MP, Markant SL, McLendon RE, Wei Z, Ellison DW, et al. (2009). Identification of CD15 as a marker for tumor-propagating cells in a mouse model of medulloblastoma. Cancer Cell. 15(2):135–47. PMID:19185848
2081. Reardon W, Zhou XP, Eng C (2001). A novel germline mutation of the PTEN gene in a patient with macrocephaly, ventricular dilatation, and features of VATER association. J Med Genet. 38(12):820–3. PMID:11748304
2082. Reddy AT, Janss AJ, Phillips PC, Weiss HL, Packer RJ (2000). Outcome for children with supratentorial primitive neuroectodermal tumors treated with surgery, radiation, and chemotherapy. Cancer. 88(9):2189–93. PMID:10813733
2083. Reifenberger G, Kaulich K, Wiestler OD, Blümcke I (2003). Expression of the CD34 antigen in pleomorphic xanthoastrocytomas. Acta Neuropathol. 105(4):358–64. PMID:12624789
2084. Reifenberger G, Liu L, Ichimura K, Schmidt EE, Collins VP (1993). Amplification and overexpression of the MDM2 gene in a subset of human malignant gliomas without p53 mutations. Cancer Res. 53(12):2736–9. PMID:8504413
2085. Reifenberger G, Louis DN (2003). Oligodendroglioma: toward molecular definitions in diagnostic neuro-oncology. J Neuropathol Exp Neurol. 62(2):111–26. PMID:12578221
2086. Reifenberger G, Reifenberger J, Ichimura K, Meltzer PS, Collins VP (1994). Amplification of multiple genes from chromosomal region 12q13–14 in human malignant gliomas: preliminary mapping of the amplicons shows preferential involvement of CDK4, SAS, and MDM2. Cancer Res. 54(16):4299–303. PMID:8044775
2087. Reifenberger G, Szymas J, Wechsler W (1987). Differential expression of glial- and neuronal-associated antigens in human tumors of the central and peripheral nervous system. Acta Neuropathol. 74(2):105–23. PMID:3314309
2088. Reifenberger G, Weber RG, Riehmer V, Kaulich K, Willscher E, Wirth H, et al.; German Glioma Network (2014). Molecular characterization of long-term survivors of glioblastoma using genome- and transcriptome-wide profiling. Int J Cancer. 135(8):1822–31. PMID:24615357
2089. Reifenberger G, Weber T, Weber RG, Wolter M, Brandis A, Kuchelmeister K, et al. (1999). Chordoid glioma of the third ventricle: immunohistochemical and molecular genetic characterization of a novel tumor entity. Brain Pathol. 9(4):617–26. PMID:10517500
2090. Reifenberger J, Reifenberger G, Ichimura K, Schmidt EE, Wechsler W, Collins VP (1996). Epidermal growth factor receptor expression in oligodendroglial tumors. Am J Pathol. 149(1):29–35. PMID:8686753
2091. Reifenberger J, Reifenberger G, Liu L, James CD, Wechsler W, Collins VP (1994). Molecular genetic analysis of oligodendroglial tumors shows preferential allelic deletions on 19q and 1p. Am J Pathol. 145(5):1175–90. PMID:7977648
2092. Reifenberger J, Ring GU, Gies U, Cobbers L, Oberstrass J, An HX, et al. (1996). Analysis of p53 mutation and epidermal growth factor receptor amplification in recurrent gliomas with malignant progression. J Neuropathol Exp Neurol. 55(7):822–31. PMID:8965097
2093. Reis F, Faria AV, Zanardi VA, Menezes JR, Cendes F, Queiroz LS (2006). Neuroimaging in pineal tumors. J Neuroimaging. 16(1):52–8. PMID:16483277
2094. Reis RM, Hara A, Kleihues P, Ohgaki H (2001). Genetic evidence of the neoplastic nature of gemistocytes in astrocytomas. Acta Neuropathol. 102(5):422–5. PMID:11699553
2095. Reis RM, Könü-Lebleblicioglu D, Lopes JM, Kleihues P, Ohgaki H (2000). Genetic profile of gliosarcomas. Am J Pathol. 156(2):425–32. PMID:10666371
2096. Reis-Filho JS, Faoro LN, Carrilho C, Bleggi-Torres LF, Schmitt FC (2000). Evaluation of cell proliferation, epidermal growth factor receptor, and bcl-2 immunoexpression as prognostic factors for patients with World Health Organization grade 2 oligodendroglioma. Cancer. 88(4):862–9. PMID:10679656
2097. Reithmeier T, Gumprecht H, Stölzle A, Lumenta CB (2000). Intracerebral paraganglioma. Acta Neurochir (Wien). 142(9):1063–6. PMID:11086818
2098. Remke M, Ramaswamy V, Peacock J, Shih DJ, Koelsche C, Northcott PA, et al. (2013). TERT promoter mutations are highly recurrent in SHH subgroup medulloblastoma. Acta Neuropathol. 126(6):917–29. PMID:24174164
2099. Rencic A, Gordon J, Otte J, Curtis M, Kovatich A, Zoltick P, et al. (1996). Detection of JC virus DNA sequence and expression of the viral oncoprotein, tumor antigen, in brain of immunocompetent patient with oligoastrocytoma. Proc Natl Acad Sci U S A. 93(14):7352–7. PMID:8692997
2100. Reni M, Ferreri AJ, Zoldan MC, Villa E (1997). Primary brain lymphomas in patients with a prior or concomitant malignancy. J Neurooncol. 32(2):135–42. PMID:9120542
2101. Resta N, Lauriola L, Puca A, Susca FC, Albanese A, Sabatino G, et al. (2006). Ganglioglioma arising in a Peutz-Jeghers patient: a case report with molecular implications. Acta Neuropathol. 112(1):106–11. PMID:16733653
2102. Reuss DE, Habel A, Hagenlocher C, Mucha J, Ackermann U, Tessmer C, et al. (2014). Neurofibromin specific antibody differentiates malignant peripheral nerve sheath tumors (MPNST) from other spindle cell neoplasms. Acta Neuropathol. 127(4):565–72. PMID:24464231
2103. Reuss DE, Mamatjan Y, Schrimpf D, Capper D, Hovestadt V, Kratz A, et al. (2015). IDH mutant diffuse and anaplastic astrocytomas have similar age at presentation and little difference in survival: a grading problem for WHO. Acta Neuropathol. 129(6):867–73. PMID:25962792
2104. Reuss DE, Piro RM, Jones DT, Simon M, Ketter R, Kool M, et al. (2013). Secretory meningiomas are defined by combined KLF4 K409Q and TRAF7 mutations. Acta Neuropathol. 125(3):351–8. PMID:23404370
2105. Reuss DE, Sahm F, Schrimpf D, Wiestler B, Capper D, Koelsche C, et al. (2015). ATRX and IDH1-R132H immunohistochemistry with subsequent copy number analysis and IDH sequencing as a basis for an "integrated" diagnostic approach for adult astrocytoma, oligodendroglioma and glioblastoma. Acta Neuropathol. 129(1):133–46. PMID:25427834
2106. Reyes-Mugica M, Chou P, Byrd S, Ray V, Castelli M, Gattuso P, et al. (1993). Nevomelanocytic proliferations in the central nervous system of children. Cancer. 72(7):2277–85. PMID:8374887
2108. Rezai AR, Woo HH, Lee M, Cohen H, Zagzag D, Epstein FJ (1996). Disseminated ependymomas of the central nervous system. J Neurosurg. 85(4):618–24. PMID:8814165
2109. Rhiew RB, Manjila S, Lozen A, Guthikonda M, Sood S, Kupsky WJ (2010). Leptomeningeal dissemination of a pediatric neoplasm with 1p19q deletion showing mixed immunohistochemical features of an oligodendroglioma and neurocytoma. Acta Neurochir (Wien). 152(8):1425–9. PMID:20446099
2110. Rhodes RH, Cole M, Takaoka Y, Roessmann U, Cotes EE, Simon J (1994). Intraventricular cerebral neuroblastoma. Analysis of subtypes and comparison with hemispheric neuroblastoma. Arch Pathol Lab Med. 118(9):897–911. PMID:8080360
2111. Ribeiro RC, Sandrini F, Figueiredo B, Zambetti GP, Michalkiewicz E, Lafferty AR, et al. (2001). An inherited p53 mutation that contributes in a tissue-specific manner to pediatric adrenal cortical carcinoma. Proc Natl Acad Sci U S A. 98(16):9330–5. PMID:11481490
2112. Ribeiro S, Napoli I, White IJ, Parrinello S, Flanagan AM, Suter U, et al. (2013). Injury signals cooperate with Nf1 loss to relieve the tumor-suppressive environment of adult peripheral nerve. Cell Rep. 5(1):126–36. PMID:24075988
2113. Ricci A Jr, Parham DM, Woodruff JM, Callihan T, Green A, Erlandson RA (1984). Malignant peripheral nerve sheath tumors arising from ganglioneuromas. Am J Surg Pathol. 8(1):19–29. PMID:6696163
2114. Rickard KA, Parker JR, Vitaz TW, Plaga AR, Wagner S, Parker JC Jr (2011). Papillary tumor of the pineal region: two case studies and a review of the literature. Ann Clin Lab Sci. 41(2):174–81. PMID:21844577
2115. Rickert CH, Hasselblatt M (2006). Cytogenetic features of ependymoblastomas. Acta Neuropathol. 111(6):559–62. PMID:16718352
2116. Rickert CH, Paulus W (2001). Epidemiology of central nervous system tumors in childhood and adolescence based on the new WHO classification. Childs Nerv Syst. 17(9):503–11. PMID:11585322
2117. Rickert CH, Paulus W (2001). Tumors

of the choroid plexus. Microsc Res Tech. 52(1):104–11. PMID:11135453
2118. Rickert CH, Paulus W (2002). Genetic characterisation of granular cell tumours. Acta Neuropathol. 103(4):309–12. PMID:11904749
2119. Rickert CH, Paulus W (2002). No chromosomal imbalances detected by comparative genomic hybridisation in a case of fetal immature teratoma. Childs Nerv Syst. 18(11):639–43. PMID:12420126
2120. Rickert CH, Paulus W (2004). Comparative genomic hybridization in central and peripheral nervous system tumors of childhood and adolescence. J Neuropathol Exp Neurol. 63(5):399–417. PMID:15198120
2121. Rickert CH, Simon R, Bergmann M, Dockhorn-Dworniczak B, Paulus W (2000). Comparative genomic hybridization in pineal germ cell tumors. J Neuropathol Exp Neurol. 59(9):815–21. PMID:11005262
2122. Rickert CH, Simon R, Bergmann M, Dockhorn-Dworniczak B, Paulus W (2001). Comparative genomic hybridization in pineal parenchymal tumors. Genes Chromosomes Cancer. 30(1):99–104. PMID:11107183
2123. Rickert CH, Wiestler OD, Paulus W (2002). Chromosomal imbalances in choroid plexus tumors. Am J Pathol. 160(3):1105–13. PMID:11891207
2124. Rickman DS, Bobek MP, Misek DE, Kuick R, Blaivas M, Kurnit DM, et al. (2001). Distinctive molecular profiles of high-grade and low-grade gliomas based on oligonucleotide microarray analysis. Cancer Res. 61(18):6885–91. PMID:11559565
2125. Riegert-Johnson DL, Gleeson FC, Roberts M, Tholen K, Youngborg L, Bullock M, et al. (2010). Cancer and Lhermitte-Duclos disease are common in Cowden syndrome patients. Hered Cancer Clin Pract. 8(1):6. PMID:20565722
2126. Riemenschneider MJ, Reifenberger G (2009). Molecular neuropathology of gliomas. Int J Mol Sci. 10(1):184–212. PMID:19333441
2127. Riemersma SA, Jordanova ES, Schop RF, Philippo K, Looijenga LH, Schuuring E, et al. (2000). Extensive genetic alterations of the HLA region, including homozygous deletions of HLA class II genes in B-cell lymphomas arising in immune-privileged sites. Blood. 96(10):3569–77. PMID:11071656
2128. Riemersma SA, Oudejans JJ, Vonk MJ, Dreef EJ, Prins FA, Jansen PM, et al. (2005). High numbers of tumour-infiltrating activated cytotoxic T lymphocytes, and frequent loss of HLA class I and II expression, are features of aggressive B cell lymphomas of the brain and testis. J Pathol. 206(3):328–36. PMID:15887291
2129. Rienstein S, Adams EF, Pilzer D, Goldring AA, Goldman B, Friedman E (2003). Comparative genomic hybridization analysis of craniopharyngiomas. J Neurosurg. 98(1):162–4. PMID:12546365
2130. Ringertz N (1950). Grading of gliomas. Acta Pathol Microbiol Scand. 27(1):51–64. PMID:15406242
2131. Ritter JH, Mills SE, Nappi O, Wick MR (1995). Angiosarcoma-like neoplasms of epithelial organs: true endothelial tumors or variants of carcinoma? Semin Diagn Pathol. 12(3):270–82. PMID:8545593
2132. Rivera AL, Takei H, Zhai J, Shen SS, Ro JY, Powell SZ (2010). Useful immunohistochemical markers in differentiating hemangioblastoma versus metastatic renal cell carcinoma. Neuropathology. 30(6):580–5. PMID:20374497
2133. Roach ES, Sparagana SP (2010). Diagnostic criteria for tuberous sclerosis complex. In: Tuberous sclerosis complex. Genes, clinical features, and therapeutics. Kwiatkowski DJ, Whittemore VH, Thiele EA, eds. Wiley-Blackwell: Weinheim, Germany, pp. 21-25.
2134. Robbins P, Segal A, Narula S, Stokes B, Lee M, Thomas W, et al. (1995). Central neurocytoma. A clinicopathological, immunohistochemical and ultrastructural study of 7 cases. Pathol Res Pract. 191(2):100–11. PMID:7567679
2135. Roberts AE, Allanson JE, Tartaglia M, Gelb BD (2013). Noonan syndrome. Lancet. 381(9863):333–42. PMID:23312968
2136. Roberts CW, Biegel JA (2009). The role of SMARCB1/INI1 in development of rhabdoid tumor. Cancer Biol Ther. 8(5):412–6. PMID:19305156
2137. Roberts CW, Orkin SH (2004). The SWI/SNF complex–chromatin and cancer. Nat Rev Cancer. 4(2):133–42. PMID:14964309
2138. Roberts RO, Lynch CF, Jones MP, Hart MN (1991). Medulloblastoma: a population-based study of 532 cases. J Neuropathol Exp Neurol. 50(2):134–44. PMID:2010773
2139. Robertson RP (2011).Translational Endocrinology & Metabolism. Neoplasia Update Chevy Chase, Maryland 20815: The Endocrine Society.
2140. Robin YM, Guillou L, Michels JJ, Coindre JM (2004). Human herpesvirus 8 immunostaining: a sensitive and specific method for diagnosing Kaposi sarcoma in paraffin-embedded sections. Am J Clin Pathol. 121(3):330–4. PMID:15023036
2141. Robinson DR, Wu YM, Kalyana-Sundaram S, Cao X, Lonigro RJ, Sung YS, et al. (2013). Identification of recurrent NAB2-STAT6 gene fusions in solitary fibrous tumor by integrative sequencing. Nat Genet. 45(2):180–5. PMID:23313952
2142. Robinson G, Parker M, Kranenburg TA, Lu C, Chen X, Ding L, et al. (2012). Novel mutations target distinct subgroups of medulloblastoma. Nature. 488(7409):43–8. PMID:22722829
2143. Robinson GW, Orr BA, Wu G, Gururangan S, Lin T, Qaddoumi I, et al. (2015). Vismodegib Exerts Targeted Efficacy Against Recurrent Sonic Hedgehog-Subgroup Medulloblastoma: Results From Phase II Pediatric Brain Tumor Consortium Studies PBTC-025B and PBTC-032. J Clin Oncol. 33(24):2646–54. PMID:26169613
2144. Roche PH, Figarella-Branger D, Regis J, Peragut JC (1996). Cauda equina paraganglioma with subsequent intracranial and intraspinal metastases. Acta Neurochir (Wien). 138(4):475–9. PMID:8738400
2145. Rodriguez EF, Scheithauer BW, Giannini C, Rynearson A, Cen L, Hoesley B, et al. (2011). PI3K/AKT pathway alterations are associated with clinically aggressive and histologically anaplastic subsets of pilocytic astrocytoma. Acta Neuropathol. 121(3):407–20. PMID:21113787
2146. Rodriguez FJ, Folpe AL, Giannini C, Perry A (2012). Pathology of peripheral nerve sheath tumors: diagnostic overview and update on selected diagnostic problems. Acta Neuropathol. 123(3):295–319. PMID:22327363
2147. Rodriguez FJ, Mota RA, Scheithauer BW, Giannini C, Blair H, New KC, et al. (2009). Interphase cytogenetics for 1p19q and t(1;19)(q10;p10) may distinguish prognostically relevant subgroups in extraventricular neurocytoma. Brain Pathol. 19(4):623–9. PMID:18710393
2148. Rodriguez FJ, Perry A, Gutmann DH, O'Neill BP, Leonard J, Bryant S, et al. (2008). Gliomas in neurofibromatosis type 1: a clinicopathologic study of 100 patients. J Neuropathol Exp Neurol. 67(3):240–9. PMID:18344915
2149. Rodriguez FJ, Perry A, Rosenblum MK, Krawitz S, Cohen KJ, Lin D, et al. (2012). Disseminated oligodendroglial-like leptomeningeal tumor of childhood: a distinctive clinicopathologic entity. Acta Neuropathol. 124(5):627–41. PMID:22941225
2150. Rodriguez FJ, Scheithauer BW, Burger PC, Jenkins S, Giannini C (2010). Anaplasia in pilocytic astrocytoma predicts aggressive behavior. Am J Surg Pathol. 34(2):147–60. PMID:20061938
2151. Rodriguez FJ, Scheithauer BW, Giannini C, Bryant SC, Jenkins RB (2008). Epithelial and pseudoepithelial differentiation in glioblastoma and gliosarcoma: a comparative morphologic and molecular genetic study. Cancer. 113(10):2779–89. PMID:18816605
2152. Rodriguez FJ, Scheithauer BW, Jenkins R, Burger PC, Rudzinskiy P, Vlodavsky E, et al. (2007). Gliosarcoma arising in oligodendroglial tumors ("oligosarcoma"): a clinicopathologic study. Am J Surg Pathol. 31(3):351–62. PMID:17325476
2153. Rodriguez FJ, Scheithauer BW, Perry A, Oliveira AM, Jenkins RB, Oviedo A, et al. (2008). Ependymal tumors with sarcomatous change ("ependymosarcoma"): a clinicopathologic and molecular cytogenetic study. Am J Surg Pathol. 32(5):699–709. PMID:18347506
2154. Rodriguez FJ, Scheithauer BW, Robbins PD, Burger PC, Hessler RB, Perry A, et al. (2007). Ependymomas with neuronal differentiation: a morphologic and immunohistochemical spectrum. Acta Neuropathol. 113(3):313–24. PMID:17061076
2155. Rodriguez FJ, Scheithauer BW, Tsunoda S, Kovacs K, Vidal S, Piepgras DG (2007). The spectrum of malignancy in craniopharyngioma. Am J Surg Pathol. 31(7):1020–8. PMID:17592268
2156. Rodriguez FJ, Schniederjan MJ, Nicolaides T, Tihan T, Burger PC, Perry A (2015). High rate of concurrent BRAF-KIAA1549 gene fusion and 1p deletion in disseminated oligodendroglioma-like leptomeningeal neoplasms (DOLN). Acta Neuropathol. 129(4):609–10. PMID:25720745
2157. Rodriguez FJ, Tihan T, Lin D, McDonald W, Nigro J, Feuerstein B, et al. (2014). Clinicopathologic features of pediatric oligodendrogliomas: a series of 50 patients. Am J Surg Pathol. 38(8):1058–70. PMID:24805856
2158. Rodriguez HA, Berthrong M (1966). Multiple primary intracranial tumors in von Recklinghausen's neurofibromatosis. Arch Neurol. 14(5):467–75. PMID:4957904
2159. Rodriguez LA, Edwards MS, Levin VA (1990). Management of hypothalamic gliomas in children: an analysis of 33 cases. Neurosurgery. 26(2):242–6, discussion 246–7. PMID:2308672
2160. Roerig P, Nessling M, Radlwimmer B, Joos S, Wrobel G, Schwaenen C, et al. (2005). Molecular classification of human gliomas using matrix-based comparative genomic hybridization. Int J Cancer. 117(1):95–103. PMID:15880582
2161. Roessler E, Belloni E, Gaudenz K, Jay P, Berta P, Scherer SW, et al. (1996). Mutations in the human Sonic Hedgehog gene cause holoprosencephaly. Nat Genet. 14(3):357–60. PMID:8896572
2162. Roggendorf W, Strupp S, Paulus W (1996). Distribution and characterization of microglia/macrophages in human brain tumors. Acta Neuropathol. 92(3):288–93. PMID:8870831
2163. Roldán G, Chan J, Eliasziw M, Cairncross JG, Forsyth PA (2011). Leptomeningeal disease in oligodendroglial tumors: a population-based study. J Neurooncol. 104(3):811–5. PMID:21373968
2164. Rollison DE, Utaipat U, Ryschkewitsch C, Hou J, Goldthwaite P, Daniel R, et al. (2005). Investigation of human brain tumors for the presence of polyomavirus genome sequences by two independent laboratories. Int J Cancer. 113(5):769–74. PMID:15499616
2165. Romani R, Niemelä M, Celik O, Isarakul P, Paetau A, Hernesniemi J (2010). Ectopic recurrence of craniopharyngioma along the surgical route: case report and literature review. Acta Neurochir (Wien). 152(2):297–302, discussion 302. PMID:19499168
2166. Romero-Rojas AE, Diaz-Perez JA, Ariza-Serrano LM, Amaro D, Lozano-Castillo A (2013). Primary gliosarcoma of the brain: radiologic and histopathologic features. Neuroradiol J. 26(6):639–48. PMID:24355182
2167. Romero-Rojas AE, Melo-Uribe MA, Barajas-Solano PA, Chinchilla-Olaya SI, Escobar LI, Hernandez-Walteros DM (2011). Spindle cell oncocytoma of the adenohypophysis. Brain Tumor Pathol. 28(4):359–64. PMID:21833579
2168. Roncaroli F, Riccioni L, Cerati M, Capella C, Calbucci F, Trevisan C, et al. (1997). Oncocytic meningioma. Am J Surg Pathol. 21(4):375–82. PMID:9130983
2169. Roncaroli F, Scheithauer BW, Cenacchi G, Horvath E, Kovacs K, Lloyd RV, et al. (2002). 'Spindle cell oncocytoma' of the adenohypophysis: a tumor of folliculostellate cells? Am J Surg Pathol. 26(8):1048–55. PMID:12170092
2170. Rong Y, Durden DL, Van Meir EG, Brat DJ (2006). 'Pseudopalisading' necrosis in glioblastoma: a familiar morphologic feature that links vascular pathology, hypoxia, and angiogenesis. J Neuropathol Exp Neurol. 65(6):529–39. PMID:16783163
2171. Rorke LB (1983). The cerebellar medulloblastoma and its relationship to primitive neuroectodermal tumors. J Neuropathol Exp Neurol. 42(1):1–15. PMID:6296325
2172. Rorke LB, Packer RJ, Biegel JA (1996). Central nervous system atypical teratoid/rhabdoid tumors of infancy and childhood: definition of an entity. J Neurosurg. 85(1):56–65. PMID:8683283
2173. Rosai J, Parkash V, Reuter V (1994). Invited Review: The Origin of Mediastinal Germ Cell Tumors. Int J Surg Pathol. 2:73–8.
2174. Rosemberg S, Fujiwara D (2005). Epidemiology of pediatric tumors of the nervous system according to the WHO 2000 classification: a report of 1,195 cases from a single institution. Childs Nerv Syst. 21(11):940–4. PMID:16044344
2175. Rosemberg S, Vieira GS (1998). [Dysembryoplastic neuroepithelial tumor. An epidemiological study from a single institution]. Arq Neuropsiquiatr. 56(2):232–6. PMID:9698733
2176. Rosenberg AS, Langee CL, Stevens GL, Morgan MB (2002). Malignant peripheral nerve sheath tumor with perineurial differentiation: "malignant perineurioma". J Cutan Pathol. 29(6):362–7. PMID:12135468
2177. Rosenberg DS, Demarquay G, Jouvet A, Le Bars D, Streichenberger N, Sindou M, et al. (2005). [11C]-Methionine PET: dysembryoplastic neuroepithelial tumours compared with other epileptogenic brain neoplasms. J Neurol Neurosurg Psychiatry. 76(12):1686–92. PMID:16291894
2178. Rosenblum MK (1998). Ependymal tumors: A review of their diagnostic surgical pathology. Pediatr Neurosurg. 28(3):160–5. PMID:9705595
2179. Rosenblum MK, Erlandson RA, Aleksic SN, Budzilovich GN (1990). Melanotic ependymoma and subependymoma. Am J Surg Pathol. 14(8):729–36. PMID:2378394
2180. Rosenblum MK, Erlandson RA, Budzilovich GN (1991). The lipid-rich epithelioid glioblastoma. Am J Surg Pathol. 15(10):925–34. PMID:1718177
2181. Roser F, Nakamura M, Bellinzona M, Rosahl SK, Ostertag H, Samii M (2004). The prognostic value of progesterone receptor status in meningiomas. J Clin Pathol. 57(10):1033–7. PMID:15452155
2182. Roser F, Nakamura M, Brandis A, Hans V, Vorkapic P, Samii M (2004). Transition from meningeal melanocytoma to primary cerebral melanoma. Case report. J Neurosurg. 101(3):528–31. PMID:15352613
2183. Rossi A, Cama A, Consales A, Gandolfo C, Garrè ML, Milanaccio C, et al. (2006). Neuroimaging of pediatric craniopharyngiomas: a pictorial essay. J Pediatr Endocrinol Metab. 19 Suppl 1:299–319. PMID:16700305
2184. Rossi ML, Jones NR, Candy E, Nicoll JA, Compton JS, Hughes JT, et al. (1989). The

mononuclear cell infiltrate compared with survival in high-grade astrocytomas. Acta Neuropathol. 78(2):189–93. PMID:2750489
2185. Rossi S, Rodriguez FJ, Mota RA, Dei Tos AP, Di Paola F, Bendini M, et al. (2009). Primary leptomeningeal oligodendroglioma with documented progression to anaplasia and t(1;19)(q10;p10) in a child. Acta Neuropathol. 118(4):575–7. PMID:19562354
2186. Rossitch E Jr, Zeidman SM, Burger PC, Curnes JT, Harsh C, Anscher M, et al. (1990). Clinical and pathological analysis of spinal cord astrocytomas in children. Neurosurgery. 27(2):193–6. PMID:2385335
2187. Rostomily RC, Bermingham-McDonogh O, Berger MS, Tapscott SJ, Reh TA, Olson JM (1997). Expression of neurogenic basic helix-loop-helix genes in primitive neuroectodermal tumors. Cancer Res. 57(16):3526–31. PMID:9270024
2188. Roth J, Roach ES, Bartels U, Jóźwiak S, Koenig MK, Weiner HL, et al. (2013). Subependymal giant cell astrocytoma: diagnosis, screening, and treatment. Recommendations from the International Tuberous Sclerosis Complex Consensus Conference 2012. Pediatr Neurol. 49(6):439–44. PMID:24138953
2189. Rotman JA, Kucharczyk W, Zadeh G, Kiehl TR, Al-Ahmadi H (2014). Spindle cell oncocytoma of the adenohypophysis: a case report illustrating its natural history with 8-year observation and a review of the literature. Clin Imaging. 38(4):499–504. PMID:24721021
2190. Rouleau GA, Merel P, Lutchman M, Sanson M, Zucman J, Marineau C, et al. (1993). Alteration in a new gene encoding a putative membrane-organizing protein causes neuro-fibromatosis type 2. Nature. 363(6429):515–21. PMID:8379998
2191. Rousseau G, Noguchi T, Bourdon V, Sobol H, Olschwang S (2011). SMARCB1/INI1 germline mutations contribute to 10% of sporadic schwannomatosis. BMC Neurol. 11:9. PMID:21255467
2192. Roussel MF, Robinson GW (2013). Role of MYC in Medulloblastoma. Cold Spring Harb Perspect Med. 3(11):3. PMID:24186490
2193. Roy S, Chu A, Trojanowski JQ, Zhang PJ (2005). D2-40, a novel monoclonal antibody against the M2A antigen as a marker to distinguish hemangioblastomas from renal cell carcinomas. Acta Neuropathol. 109(5):497–502. PMID:15864611
2194. Rubin JB, Gutmann DH (2005). Neurofibromatosis type 1 - a model for nervous system tumour formation? Nat Rev Cancer. 5(7):557–64. PMID:16069817
2195. Rubinstein LJ (1986). The malformative central nervous system lesions in the central and peripheral forms of neurofibromatosis. A neuropathological study of 22 cases. Ann N Y Acad Sci. 486:14–29. PMID:3105387
2196. Rueda-Pedraza ME, Heifetz SA, Sesterhenn IA, Clark GB (1987). Primary intracranial germ cell tumors in the first two decades of life. A clinical, light-microscopic, and immunohistochemical analysis of 54 cases. Perspect Pediatr Pathol. 10:160–207. PMID:3588245
2197. Ruggieri M, Polizzi A, Spalice A, Salpietro V, Caltabiano R, D'Orazi V, et al. (2015). The natural history of spinal neurofibromatosis: a critical review of clinical and genetic features. Clin Genet. 87(5):401–10 PMID:25211147
2198. Ruland V, Hartung S, Kordes U, Wolff JE, Paulus W, Hasselblatt M (2014). Choroid plexus carcinomas are characterized by complex chromosomal alterations related to patient age and prognosis. Genes Chromosomes Cancer. 53(5):373–80. PMID:24478045
2199. Rupani A, Modi C, Desai S, Rege J (2005). Primary anaplastic large cell lymphoma of central nervous system–a case report. J Postgrad Med. 51(4):326–7. PMID:16388180
2200. Rushing EJ, Armonda RA, Ansari Q, Mena H (1996). Mesenchymal chondrosarcoma: a clinicopathologic and flow cytometric study of 13 cases presenting in the central nervous system. Cancer. 77(9):1884–91. PMID:8646689
2201. Rushing EJ, Cooper PB, Quezado M, Begnami M, Crespo A, Smirniotopoulos JG, et al. (2007). Subependymoma revisited: clinicopathological evaluation of 83 cases. J Neurooncol. 85(3):297–305. PMID:17569000
2202. Rushing EJ, Olsen C, Mena H, Rueda ME, Lee YS, Keating RF, et al. (2005). Central nervous system meningiomas in the first two decades of life: a clinicopathological analysis of 87 patients. J Neurosurg. 103(6) Suppl:489–95. PMID:16383246
2203. Rushing EJ, Thompson LD, Mena H (2003). Malignant transformation of a dysembryoplastic neuroepithelial tumor after radiation and chemotherapy. Ann Diagn Pathol. 7(4):240–4. PMID:12913847
2204. Russell DS, Rubinstein LJ (1989). Pathology of Tumours of the Nervous System. London: Edward Arnold.
2205. Russell, DS and Rubinstein, LJ ().Pathology of tumours of the nervous system. 5th London: Edward Arnold.
2206. Russo C, Pellarin M, Tingby O, Bollen AW, Lamborn KR, Mohapatra G, et al. (1999). Comparative genomic hybridization in patients with supratentorial and infratentorial primitive neuroectodermal tumors. Cancer. 86(2):331–9. PMID:10421270
2207. Rutkowski S, Bode U, Deinlein F, Ottensmeier H, Warmuth-Metz M, Soerensen N, et al. (2005). Treatment of early childhood medulloblastoma by postoperative chemotherapy alone. N Engl J Med. 352(10):978–86. PMID:15758008
2208. Rutkowski S, von Hoff K, Emser A, Zwiener I, Pietsch T, Figarella-Branger D, et al. (2010). Survival and prognostic factors of early childhood medulloblastoma: an international meta-analysis. J Clin Oncol. 28(33):4961–8. PMID:20940197
2209. Ryken TC, Robinson RA, VanGilder JC (1994). Familial occurrence of subependymoma. Report of two cases. J Neurosurg. 80(6):1108–11. PMID:8189269
2210. Sabbaghian N, Hamel N, Srivastava A, Albrecht S, Priest JR, Foulkes WD (2012). Germline DICER1 mutation and associated loss of heterozygosity in a pineoblastoma. J Med Genet. 49(7):417–9. PMID:22717647
2211. Sachdeva MU, Vankalakunti M, Rangan A, Radotra BD, Chhabra R, Vasishta RK (2008). The role of immunohistochemistry in medullomyoblastoma–a case series highlighting divergent differentiation. Diagn Pathol. 3:18. PMID:18439235
2212. Sadetzki S, Bruchim R, Oberman B, Armstrong GN, Lau CC, Claus EB, et al.; Gliogene Consortium (2013). Description of selected characteristics of familial glioma patients - results from the Gliogene Consortium. Eur J Cancer. 49(6):1335–45. PMID:23290425
2213. Sadetzki S, Chetrit A, Freedman L, Stovall M, Modan B, Novikov I (2005). Long-term follow-up for brain tumor development after childhood exposure to ionizing radiation for tinea capitis. Radiat Res. 163(4):424–32. PMID:15799699
2214. Saesue P, Chankaew E, Chawalparit O, Na Ayudhya NS, Muangsomboon S, Sangruchi T (2004). Primary extraskeletal osteosarcoma in the pineal region. Case report. J Neurosurg. 101(6):1061–4. PMID:15597771
2215. Safaee M, Oh MC, Bloch O, Sun MZ, Kaur G, Auguste KI, et al. (2013). Choroid plexus papillomas: advances in molecular biology and understanding of tumorigenesis. Neuro Oncol. 15(3):255–67. PMID:23172371
2216. Safaee M, Oh MC, Mummaneni PV, Weinstein PR, Ames CP, Chou D, et al. (2014). Surgical outcomes in spinal cord ependymomas and the importance of extent of resection in children and young adults. J Neurosurg Pediatr. 13(4):393–9. PMID:24506340
2217. Sahm F, Bissel J, Koelsche C, Schweizer L, Capper D, Reuss D, et al. (2013). AKT1E17K mutations cluster with meningothelial and transitional meningiomas and can be detected by SFRP1 immunohistochemistry. Acta Neuropathol. 126(5):757–62. PMID:24096618
2218. Sahm F, Capper D, Preusser M, Meyer J, Stenzinger A, Lasitschka F, et al. (2012). BRAF-V600E mutant protein is expressed in cells of variable maturation in Langerhans cell histiocytosis. Blood. 120(12):e28–34. PMID:22859608
2219. Sahm F, Koelsche C, Meyer J, Pusch S, Lindenberg K, Mueller W, et al. (2012). CIC and FUBP1 mutations in oligodendrogliomas, oligoastrocytomas and astrocytomas. Acta Neuropathol. 123(6):853–60. PMID:22588899
2220. Sahm F, Reuss D, Koelsche C, Capper D, Schittenhelm J, Heim S, et al. (2014). Farewell to oligoastrocytoma: in situ molecular genetics favor classification as either oligodendroglioma or astrocytoma. Acta Neuropathol. 128(4):551–9. PMID:25143301
2220A. Sahm F, Schrimpf D, Olar A, Koelsche C, Reuss D, Bissel J, et al. (2015). TERT Promoter Mutations and Risk of Recurrence in Meningioma. J Natl Cancer Inst. 108(5). PMID:26668184
2221. Sainz J, Figueroa K, Baser ME, Mautner VF, Pulst SM (1995). High frequency of nonsense mutations in the NF2 gene caused by C to T transitions in five CGA codons. Hum Mol Genet. 4(1):137–9. PMID:7711726
2222. Sainz J, Huynh DP, Figueroa K, Ragge NK, Baser ME, Pulst SM (1994). Mutations of the neurofibromatosis type 2 gene and lack of the gene product in vestibular schwannomas. Hum Mol Genet. 3(6):885–91. PMID:7951231
2223. Sakaguchi N, Sano K, Ito M, Baba T, Fukuzawa M, Hotchi M (1996). A case of von Recklinghausen's disease with bilateral pheochromocytoma-malignant peripheral nerve sheath tumors of the adrenal and gastrointestinal autonomic nerve tumors. Am J Surg Pathol. 20(7):889–97. PMID:8669538
2224. Sakuta R, Otsubo H, Nolan MA, Weiss SK, Hawkins C, Rutka JT, et al. (2005). Recurrent intractable seizures in children with cortical dysplasia adjacent to dysembryoplastic neuroepithelial tumor. J Child Neurol. 20(4):377–84. PMID:15921242
2225. Salgado CM, Basu D, Nikiforova M, Bauer BS, Johnson D, Rundell V, et al. (2015). BRAF mutations are also associated with neurocutaneous melanocytosis and large/giant congenital melanocytic nevi. Pediatr Dev Pathol. 18(1):1–9. PMID:25490715
2226. Salunke PS, Gupta K, Srinivasa R, Sura S (2011). Functional? Paraganglioma of the cerebellum. Acta Neurochir (Wien). 153(7):1527–8. PMID:21491190
2227. Salvati M, Ciappetta P, Raco A (1993). Osteosarcomas of the skull. Clinical remarks on 19 cases. Cancer. 71(7):2210–6. PMID:8453540
2228. Salvati M, Oppido PA, Artizzu S, Fiorenza F, Puzzilli F, Orlando ER (1991). Multicentric gliomas. Report of seven cases. Tumori. 77(6):518–22. PMID:1666470
2229. Sampson JR, Maheshwar MM, Aspinwall R, Thompson P, Cheadle JP, Ravine D, et al. (1997). Renal cystic disease in tuberous sclerosis: role of the polycystic kidney disease 1 gene. Am J Hum Genet. 61(4):843–51. PMID:9382094
2229A. Sampson JR, Scahill SJ, Stephenson JB, Mann L, Connor JM (1989). Genetic aspects of tuberous sclerosis in the west of Scotland. J Med Genet. 26(1):28–31. PMID:2918523
2230. Sanai N, Alvarez-Buylla A, Berger MS (2005). Neural stem cells and the origin of gliomas. N Engl J Med. 353(8):811–22. PMID:16120861
2231. Sancak O, Nellist M, Goedbloed M, Elfferich P, Wouters C, Maat-Kievit A, et al. (2005). Mutational analysis of the TSC1 and TSC2 genes in a diagnostic setting: genotype–phenotype correlations and comparison of diagnostic DNA techniques in Tuberous Sclerosis Complex. Eur J Hum Genet. 13(6):731–41. PMID:15798777
2232. Sandberg DI, Ragheb J, Dunoyer C, Bhatia S, Olavarria G, Morrison G (2005). Surgical outcomes and seizure control rates after resection of dysembryoplastic neuroepithelial tumors. Neurosurg Focus. 18 6A:E5. PMID:16048291
2233. Sanford RA, Bowman R, Tomita T, De Leon G, Palka P (1999). A 16-year-old male with Noonan's syndrome develops progressive scoliosis and deteriorating gait. Pediatr Neurosurg. 30(1):47–52. PMID:10202309
2234. Sanford RA, Gajjar A (1997). Ependymomas. Clin Neurosurg. 44:559–70. PMID:10080027
2235. Sangoi AR, Dulai MS, Beck AH, Brat DJ, Vogel H (2009). Distinguishing chordoid meningiomas from their histologic mimics: an immunohistochemical evaluation. Am J Surg Pathol. 33(5):669–81. PMID:19194275
2236. Sankhla S, Khan GM (2004). Cauda equina paraganglioma presenting with intracranial hypertension: case report and review of the literature. Neurol India. 52(2):243–4. PMID:15269482
2237. Sanoudou D, Tingby O, Ferguson-Smith MA, Collins VP, Coleman N (2000). Analysis of pilocytic astrocytoma by comparative genomic hybridization. Br J Cancer. 82(6):1218–22. PMID:10735509
2238. Sanson M, Marie Y, Paris S, Idbaih A, Laffaire J, Ducray F, et al. (2009). Isocitrate dehydrogenase 1 codon 132 mutation is an important prognostic biomarker in gliomas. J Clin Oncol. 27(25):4150–4. PMID:19636000
2239. Santagata S, Hornick JL, Ligon KL (2006). Comparative analysis of germ cell transcription factors in CNS germinoma reveals diagnostic utility of NANOG. Am J Surg Pathol. 30(12):1613–8. PMID:17122519
2240. Santagata S, Ligon KL, Hornick JL (2007). Embryonic stem cell transcription factor signatures in the diagnosis of primary and metastatic germ cell tumors. Am J Surg Pathol. 31(6):836–45. PMID:17527070
2241. Santagata S, Maire CL, Idbaih A, Geffers L, Correll M, Holton K, et al. (2009). CRX is a diagnostic marker of retinal and pineal lineage tumors. PLoS One. 4(11):e7932. PMID:19936203
2242. Sarkar C, Sharma MC, Sudha K, Gaikwad S, Varma A (1997). A clinico-pathological study of 29 cases of gliosarcoma with special reference to two unique variants. Indian J Med Res. 106:229–35. PMID:9378529
2243. Sarkar H, K S, Ghosh S (2013). Pure intraventricular origin of gliosarcoma - a rare entity. Turk Neurosurg. 23(3):392–4. PMID:23756982
2244. Sarkaria JN, Kitange GJ, James CD, Plummer R, Calvert H, Weller M, et al. (2008). Mechanisms of chemoresistance to alkylating agents in malignant glioma. Clin Cancer Res. 14(10):2900–8. PMID:18483356
2245. Sartoretti-Schefer S, Wichmann W, Aguzzi A, Valavanis A (1997). MR differentiation of adamantinous and squamous-papillary craniopharyngiomas. AJNR Am J Neuroradiol. 18(1):77–87. PMID:9010523
2246. Sasaki H, Zlatescu MC, Betensky RA, Ino Y, Cairncross JG, Louis DN (2001). PTEN is a target of chromosome 10q loss in anaplastic oligodendrogliomas and PTEN alterations are associated with poor prognosis. Am J Pathol. 159(1):359–67. PMID:11438483
2247. Sato H, Ohmura K, Mizushima M, Ito J, Kuyama H (1983). Myxopapillary ependymoma of the lateral ventricle. A study on the mechanism of its stromal myxoid change. Acta Pathol Jpn. 33(5):1017–25. PMID:6359815
2248. Sato TS, Kirby PA, Buatti JM, Moritani T (2009). Papillary tumor of the pineal region: report of a rapidly progressive tumor with possible

multicentric origin. Pediatr Radiol. 39(2):188–90. PMID:19037636
2249. Satoh T, Smith A, Sarde A, Lu HC, Mian S, Trouillet C, et al. (2012). B-RAF mutant alleles associated with Langerhans cell histiocytosis, a granulomatous pediatric disease. PLoS One. 7(4):e33891. PMID:22506009
2250. Sawamura Y, Hamou MF, Kuppner MC, de Tribolet N (1989). Immunohistochemical and in vitro functional analysis of pineal-germinoma infiltrating lymphocytes: report of a case. Neurosurgery. 25(3):454–7, discussion 457–8. PMID:2671789
2251. Sawamura Y, Ikeda J, Shirato H, Tada M, Abe H (1998). Germ cell tumours of the central nervous system: treatment consideration based on 111 cases and their long-term clinical outcomes. Eur J Cancer. 34(1):104–10. PMID:9624246
2252. Sawin PD, Theodore N, Rekate HL (1999). Spinal cord ganglioglioma in a child with neurofibromatosis type 2. Case report and literature review. J Neurosurg. 90(2) Suppl:231–3. PMID:10199253
2253. Sawyer JR, Roloson GJ, Chadduck WM, Boop FA (1991). Cytogenetic findings in a pleomorphic xanthoastrocytoma. Cancer Genet Cytogenet. 55(2):225–30. PMID:1933824
2254. Sawyer JR, Thomas EL, Roloson GJ, Chadduck WM, Boop FA (1992). Telomeric associations evolving to ring chromosomes in a recurrent pleomorphic xanthoastrocytoma. Cancer Genet Cytogenet. 60(2):152–7. PMID:1606558
2254A. Schaefer IM, Fletcher CD, Hornick JL (2016). Loss of H3K27 trimethylation distinguishes malignant peripheral nerve sheath tumors from histologic mimics. Mod Pathol.29(1):4–13. PMID:26585554
2256. Scheie D, Meling TR, Cvancarova M, Skullerud K, Mørk S, Lote K, et al. (2011). Prognostic variables in oligodendroglial tumors: a single-institution study of 95 cases. Neuro Oncol. 13(11):1225–33. PMID:21856683
2257. Scheithauer BW (1978). Symptomatic subependymoma. Report of 21 cases with review of the literature. J Neurosurg. 49(5):689–96. PMID:712391
2258. Scheithauer BW (1999). Pathobiology of the pineal gland with emphasis on parenchymal tumors. Brain Tumor Pathol. 16(1):1–9. PMID:10532417
2259. Scheithauer BW, Amrami KK, Folpe AL, Silva AI, Edgar MA, Woodruff JM, et al. (2011). Synovial sarcoma of nerve. Hum Pathol. 42(4):568–77. PMID:21295819
2260. Scheithauer BW, Erdogan S, Rodriguez FJ, Burger PC, Woodruff JM, Kros JM, et al. (2009). Malignant peripheral nerve sheath tumors of cranial nerves and intracranial contents: a clinicopathologic study of 17 cases. Am J Surg Pathol. 33(3):325–38. PMID:19065105
2261. Scheithauer BW, Horvath E, Kovacs K (1992). Ultrastructure of the neurohypophysis. Microsc Res Tech. 20(2):177–86. PMID:1547358
2262. Scheithauer BW, Rubinstein LJ (1978). Meningeal mesenchymal chondrosarcoma: report of 8 cases with review of the literature. Cancer. 42(6):2744–52. PMID:365318
2263. Scheithauer BW, Silva AI, Ketterling RP, Pula JH, Lininger JF, Krinock MJ (2009). Rosette-forming glioneuronal tumor: report of a chiasmal-optic nerve example in neurofibromatosis type 1: special pathology report. Neurosurgery. 64(4):E771–2, discussion E772. PMID:193498062264
2264. Schenk PW, Van Es S, Kesbeke F, Snaar-Jagalska BE (1991). Involvement of cyclic AMP cell surface receptors and G-proteins in signal transduction during slug migration of Dictyostelium discoideum. Dev Biol. 145(1):110–8. PMID:1850366
2265. Scherer H-J (1940). Cerebral astrocytomas and their derivatives. Am J Cancer. 40:159–98.
2266. Scherer HJ (1938). Structural development in gliomas. Am J Cancer. 34:333–51.
2267. Scherer HJ (1940). The forms of growth in gliomas and their practical significance. Brain. 63:1–35.
2268. Scheurlen WG, Schwabe GC, Joos S, Mollenhauer J, Sörensen N, Kühl J (1998). Molecular analysis of childhood primitive neuroectodermal tumors defines markers associated with poor outcome. J Clin Oncol. 16(7):2478–85. PMID:9667267
2269. Schiariti M, Goetz P, El-Maghraby H, Tailor J, Kitchen N (2011). Hemangiopericytoma: long-term outcome revisited. Clinical article. J Neurosurg. 114(3):747–55. PMID:20672899
2270. Schiefer AI, Vastagh I, Molnar MJ, Bereczki D, Varallyay G, Deak B, et al. (2012). Extranodal marginal zone lymphoma of the CNS arising after a long-standing history of atypical white matter disease. Leuk Res. 36(7):e155–7. PMID:22520340
2271. Schiff D, O'Neill B, Wijdicks E, Antin JH, Wen PY (2001). Gliomas arising in organ transplant recipients: an unrecognized complication of transplantation? Neurology. 57(8):1486–8. PMID:11673595
2272. Schiffer D, Cavalla P, Migheli A, Chiò A, Giordana MT, Marino S, et al. (1995). Apoptosis and cell proliferation in human neuroepithelial tumors. Neurosci Lett. 195(2):81–4. PMID:7478273
2273. Schiffer D, Chiò A, Giordana MT, Leone M, Soffietti R (1988). Prognostic value of histologic factors in adult cerebral astrocytoma. Cancer. 61(7):1386–93. PMID:3345492
2274. Schiffer D, Chiò A, Giordana MT, Migheli A, Palma L, Pollo B, et al. (1991). Histologic prognostic factors in ependymoma. Childs Nerv Syst. 7(4):177–82. PMID:1933913
2275. Schiffer D, Giordana MT (1998). Prognosis of ependymoma. Childs Nerv Syst. 14(8):357–61. PMID:9753400
2276. Schiffer D, Giordana MT, Mauro A, Migheli A (1984). GFAP, F VIII/RAg, laminin, and fibronectin in gliosarcomas: an immunohistochemical study. Acta Neuropathol. 63(2):108–16. PMID:6428154
2277. Schiffman JD, Hodgson JG, VandenBerg SR, Flaherty P, Polley MY, Yu M, et al. (2010). Oncogenic BRAF mutation with CDKN2A inactivation is characteristic of a subset of pediatric malignant astrocytomas. Cancer Res. 70(2):512–9. PMID:20068183
2278. Schild SE, Scheithauer BW, Haddock MG, Wong WW, Lyons MK, Marks LB, et al. (1996). Histologically confirmed pineal tumors and other germ cell tumors of the brain. Cancer. 78(12):2564–71. PMID:8952565
2279. Schild SE, Scheithauer BW, Schomberg PJ, Hook CC, Kelly PJ, Frick L, et al. (1993). Pineal parenchymal tumors. Clinical, pathologic, and therapeutic aspects. Cancer. 72(3):870–80. PMID:8334641
2280. Schindler G, Capper D, Meyer J, Janzarik W, Omran H, Herold-Mende C, et al. (2011). Analysis of BRAF V600E mutation in 1,320 nervous system tumors reveals high mutation frequencies in pleomorphic xanthoastrocytoma, ganglioglioma and extra-cerebellar pilocytic astrocytoma. Acta Neuropathol. 121(3):397–405. PMID:21274720
2281. Schittenhelm J, Mittelbronn M, Nguyen TD, Meyermann R, Beschorner R (2008). WT1 expression distinguishes astrocytic tumor cells from normal and reactive astrocytes. Brain Pathol. 18(3):344–53. PMID:18371184
2282. Schittenhelm J, Mittelbronn M, Wolff M, Truebenbach J, Will BE, Meyermann R, et al. (2007). Multifocal dysembryoplastic neuroepithelial tumor with signs of atypia after regrowth. Neuropathology. 27(4):383–9. PMID:17899694
2283. Schittenhelm J, Psaras T (2010). Glioblastoma with granular cell astrocytoma features: a case report and literature review. Clin Neuropathol. 29(5):323–9. PMID:20860896
2284. Schittenhelm J, Roser F, Tatagiba M, Beschorner R (2012). Diagnostic value of EAAT-1 and Kir7.1 for distinguishing endolymphatic sac tumors from choroid plexus tumors. Am J Clin Pathol. 138(1):85–9. PMID:22706862
2285. Schlamann A, von Bueren AO, Hagel C, Zwiener I, Seidel C, Kortmann RD, et al. (2014). An individual patient data meta-analysis on characteristics and outcome of patients with papillary glioneuronal tumor, rosette glioneuronal tumor with neuropil-like islands and rosette forming glioneuronal tumor of the fourth ventricle. PLoS One. 9(7):e101211. PMID:24991807
2286. Schlegel U (2009). Primary CNS lymphoma. Ther Adv Neurol Disord. 2(2):93–104. PMID:21180644
2287. Schmalisch K, Beschorner R, Psaras T, Honegger J (2010). Postoperative intracranial seeding of craniopharyngiomas–report of three cases and review of the literature. Acta Neurochir (Wien). 152(2):313–9, discussion 319. PMID:19859655
2288. Schmidbauer M, Budka H, Pilz P (1989). Neuroepithelial and ectomesenchymal differentiation in a primitive pineal tumor ("pineal anlage tumor"). Clin Neuropathol. 8(1):7–10. PMID:2650944
2289. Schmidt MC, Antweiler S, Urban N, Mueller W, Kuklik A, Meyer-Puttlitz B, et al. (2002). Impact of genotype and morphology on the prognosis of glioblastoma. J Neuropathol Exp Neurol. 61(4):321–8. PMID:11939587
2290. Schmidt Y, Kleinschmidt-DeMasters BK, Aisner DL, Lillehei KO, Damek D (2013). Anaplastic PXA in adults: case series with clinicopathologic and molecular features. J Neurooncol. 111(1):59–69. PMID:23096133
2291. Schmitz U, Mueller W, Weber M, Sévenet N, Delattre O, von Deimling A (2001). INI1 mutations in meningiomas at a potential hotspot in exon 9. Br J Cancer. 84(2):199–201. PMID:11161377
2292. Schneider DT, Zahn S, Sievers S, Alemazkour K, Reifenberger G, Wiestler OD, et al. (2006). Molecular genetic analysis of central nervous system germ cell tumors with comparative genomic hybridization. Mod Pathol. 19(6):864–73. PMID:16607373
2293. Schneppenheim R, Frühwald MC, Gesk S, Hasselblatt M, Jeibmann A, Kordes U, et al. (2010). Germline nonsense mutation and somatic inactivation of SMARCA4/BRG1 in a family with rhabdoid tumor predisposition syndrome. Am J Hum Genet. 86(2):279–84. PMID:20137775
2294. Schniederjan MJ, Alghamdi S, Castellano-Sanchez A, Mazewski C, Brahma B, Brat DJ, et al. (2013). Diffuse leptomeningeal neuroepithelial tumor: 9 pediatric cases with chromosome 1p/19q deletion status and IDH1 (R132H) immunohistochemistry. Am J Surg Pathol. 37(5):763–71. PMID:23588371
2294A. Schoemaker MJ, Swerdlow AJ, Hepworth SJ, van Tongeren M, Muir KR, McKinney PA (2007). History of allergic disease and risk of meningioma. Am J Epidemiol. 165(5):477–85. PMID:17182979
2295. Schoenberg BS, Schoenberg DG, Christine BW, Gomez MR (1976). The epidemiology of primary intracranial neoplasms of childhood. A population study. Mayo Clin Proc. 51(1):51–6. PMID:1249998
2296. Schofield D, West DC, Anthony DC, Marshal R, Sklar J (1995). Correlation of loss of heterozygosity at chromosome 9q with histological subtype in medulloblastomas. Am J Pathol. 146(2):472–80. PMID:7856756
2297. Schouten LJ, Rutten J, Huveneers HA, Twijnstra A (2002). Incidence of brain metastases in a cohort of patients with carcinoma of the breast, colon, kidney, and lung and melanoma. Cancer. 94(10):2698–705. PMID:12173339
2298. Schrager CA, Schneider D, Gruener AC, Tsou HC, Peacocke M (1998). Clinical and pathological features of breast disease in Cowden's syndrome: an underrecognized syndrome with an increased risk of breast cancer. Hum Pathol. 29(1):47–53. PMID:9445133
2299. Schroers R, Baraniskin A, Heute C, Vorgerd M, Brunn A, Kuhnhenn J, et al. (2010). Diagnosis of leptomeningeal disease in diffuse large B-cell lymphomas of the central nervous system by flow cytometry and cytopathology. Eur J Haematol. 85(6):520–8. PMID:20727005
2300. Schuettpelz LG, McDonald S, Whitesell K, Desruisseau DM, Grange DK, Gurnett CA, et al. (2009). Pilocytic astrocytoma in a child with Noonan syndrome. Pediatr Blood Cancer. 53(6):1147–9. PMID:19621452
2301. Schumacher T, Bunse L, Pusch S, Sahm F, Wiestler B, Quandt J, et al. (2014). A vaccine targeting mutant IDH1 induces antitumour immunity. Nature. 512(7514):324–7. PMID:25043048
2302. Schuss P, Ulrich CT, Harter PN, Tews DS, Seifert V, Franz K (2011). Gliosarcoma with bone infiltration and extracranial growth: case report and review of literature. J Neurooncol. 103(3):765–70. PMID:20957407
2303. Schwartz AM, Ghatak NR (1990). Malignant transformation of benign cerebellar astrocytoma. Cancer. 65(2):333–6. PMID:2403835
2304. Schwartzentruber J, Korshunov A, Liu XY, Jones DT, Pfaff E, Jacob K, et al. (2012). Driver mutations in histone H3.3 and chromatin remodelling genes in paediatric glioblastoma. Nature. 482(7384):226–31. PMID:22286061
2305. Schwartzkroin PA, Wenzel HJ (2012). Are developmental dysplastic lesions epileptogenic? Epilepsia. 53 Suppl 1:35–44. PMID:22612807
2306. Schwechheimer K, Huang S, Cavenee WK (1995). EGFR gene amplification–rearrangement in human glioblastomas. Int J Cancer. 62(2):145–8. PMID:7622287
2307. Schweizer L, Capper D, Hölsken A, Fahlbusch R, Flitsch J, Buchfelder M, et al. (2015). BRAF V600E analysis for the differentiation of papillary craniopharyngiomas and Rathke's cleft cysts. Neuropathol Appl Neurobiol. 41(6):733–42 PMID:25442675
2308. Schweizer L, Koelsche C, Sahm F, Piro RM, Capper D, Reuss DE, et al. (2013). Meningeal hemangiopericytoma and solitary fibrous tumors carry the NAB2-STAT6 fusion and can be diagnosed by nuclear expression of STAT6 protein. Acta Neuropathol. 125(5):651–8. PMID:23575898
2309. Schwindt H, Vater I, Kreuz M, Montesinos-Rongen M, Brunn A, Richter J, et al. (2009). Chromosomal imbalances and partial uniparental disomies in primary central nervous system lymphoma. Leukemia. 23(10):1875–84. PMID:19494841
2310. Schüller U, Heine VM, Mao J, Kho AT, Dillon AK, Han YG, et al. (2008). Acquisition of granule neuron precursor identity is a critical determinant of progenitor cell competence to form Shh-induced medulloblastoma. Cancer Cell. 14(2):123–34. PMID:18691547
2311. Sciot R, Dal Cin P, Hagemeijer A, De Smet L, Van Damme B, Van den Berghe H (1999). Cutaneous sclerosing perineurioma with cryptic NF2 gene deletion. Am J Surg Pathol. 23(7):849–53. PMID:10403310
2312. Scott RM, Ballantine HT Jr (1973). Cerebellar astrocytoma: malignant recurrence after prolonged postoperative survival. Case report. J Neurosurg. 39(6):777–9. PMID:4759666
2313. Seiz M, Tuettenberg J, Meyer J, Essig M, Schmieder K, Mawrin C, et al. (2010). Detection of IDH1 mutations in gliomatosis cerebri, but only in tumors with additional solid component: evidence for molecular subtypes. Acta Neuropathol. 120(2):261–7. PMID:20514489
2314. Seizinger BR, Martuza RL, Gusella JF (1986). Loss of genes on chromosome 22 in tumorigenesis of human acoustic neuroma. Nature. 322(6080):644–7. PMID:3092103

2315. Seizinger BR, Rouleau GA, Ozelius LJ, Lane AH, Faryniarz AG, Chao MV, et al. (1987). Genetic linkage of von Recklinghausen neurofibromatosis to the nerve growth factor receptor gene. Cell. 49(5):589–94. PMID:2884037
2316. Sekine S, Shibata T, Kokubu A, Morishita Y, Noguchi M, Nakanishi Y, et al. (2002). Craniopharyngiomas of adamantinomatous type harbor beta-catenin gene mutations. Am J Pathol. 161(6):1997–2001. PMID:12466115
2317. Sekine S, Takata T, Shibata T, Mori M, Morishita Y, Noguchi M, et al. (2004). Expression of enamel proteins and LEF1 in adamantinomatous craniopharyngioma: evidence for its odontogenic epithelial differentiation. Histopathology. 45(6):573–9. PMID:15569047
2318. Sener RN (2002). Astroblastoma: diffusion MRI, and proton MR spectroscopy. Comput Med Imaging Graph. 26(3):187–91. PMID:11918982
2319. Senft C, Raabe A, Hattingen E, Sommerlad D, Seifert V, Franz K (2008). Pineal parenchymal tumor of intermediate differentiation: diagnostic pitfalls and discussion of treatment options of a rare tumor entity. Neurosurg Rev. 31(2):231–6. PMID:18266015
2320. SenGupta SK, Webb S, Cooke RA, Igo JD (1992). Breast filariasis diagnosed by needle aspiration cytology. Diagn Cytopathol. 8(4):392–3. PMID:1638940
2321. Seol HJ, Hwang SK, Choi YL, Chi JG, Jung HW (2003). A case of recurrent subependymoma with subependymal seeding: case report. J Neurooncol. 62(3):315–20. PMID:12777084
2322. Seppälä MT, Sainio MA, Haltia MJ, Kinnunen JJ, Setälä KH, Jääskeläinen JE (1998). Multiple schwannomas: schwannomatosis or neurofibromatosis type 2? J Neurosurg. 89(1):36–41. PMID:9647170
2323. Serracino HS, Kleinschmidt-Demasters BK (2013). Skull invaders: when surgical pathology and neuropathology worlds collide. J Neuropathol Exp Neurol. 72(7):600–13. PMID:23771219
2324. Serrano M, Lin AW, McCurrach ME, Beach D, Lowe SW (1997). Oncogenic ras provokes premature cell senescence associated with accumulation of p53 and p16INK4a. Cell. 88(5):593–602. PMID:9054499
2325. Sestini R, Bacci C, Provenzano A, Genuardi M, Papi L (2008). Evidence of a four-hit mechanism involving SMARCB1 and NF2 in schwannomatosis-associated schwannomas. Hum Mutat. 29(2):227–31. PMID:18072270
2326. Setzer M, Lang J, Turowski B, Marquardt G (2002). Primary meningeal osteosarcoma: case report and review of the literature. Neurosurgery. 51(2):488–92, discussion 492. PMID:12182789
2327. Sévenet N, Sheridan E, Amram D, Schneider P, Handgretinger R, Delattre O (1999). Constitutional mutations of the hSNF5/INI1 gene predispose to a variety of cancers. Am J Hum Genet. 65(5):1342–8. PMID:10521299
2328. Shankar GM, Chen L, Kim AH, Ross GL, Folkerth RD, Friedlander RM (2010). Composite ganglioneuroma-paraganglioma of the filum terminale. J Neurosurg Spine. 12(6):709–13. PMID:20515359
2329. Shankar GM, Taylor-Weiner A, Lelic N, Jones RT, Kim JC, Francis JM, et al. (2014). Sporadic hemangioblastomas are characterized by cryptic VHL inactivation. Acta Neuropathol Commun. 2:167. PMID:25589003
2330. Shanklin WM (1953). The origin, histology and senescence of tumorettes in the human neurohypophysis. Acta Anat (Basel). 18(1):1–20. PMID:13064969
2331. Shanley S, Ratcliffe J, Hockey A, Haan E, Oley C, Ravine D, et al. (1994). Nevoid basal cell carcinoma syndrome: review of 118 affected individuals. Am J Med Genet. 50(3):282–90. PMID:8042673
2332. Sharif S, Upadhyaya M, Ferner R, Majounie E, Shenton A, Baser M, et al. (2011). A molecular analysis of individuals with neurofibromatosis type 1 (NF1) and optic pathway gliomas (OPGs), and an assessment of genotype-phenotype correlations. J Med Genet. 48(4):256–60. PMID:21278392
2333. Sharma M, Ralte A, Arora R, Santosh V, Shankar SK, Sarkar C (2004). Subependymal giant cell astrocytoma: a clinicopathological study of 23 cases with special emphasis on proliferative markers and expression of p53 and retinoblastoma gene proteins. Pathology. 36(2):139–44. PMID:15203749
2334. Sharma MC, Ralte AM, Gaekwad S, Santosh V, Shankar SK, Sarkar C (2004). Subependymal giant cell astrocytoma–a clinicopathological study of 23 cases with special emphasis on histogenesis. Pathol Oncol Res. 10(4):219–24. PMID:15619643
2335. Sharma MK, Mansur DB, Reifenberger G, Perry A, Leonard JR, Aldape KD, et al. (2007). Distinct genetic signatures among pilocytic astrocytomas relate to their brain region origin. Cancer Res. 67(3):890–900. PMID:17283119
2336. Sharpless NE, Bardeesy N, Lee KH, Carrasco D, Castrillon DH, Aguirre AJ, et al. (2001). Loss of p16Ink4a with retention of p19Arf predisposes mice to tumorigenesis. Nature. 413(6851):86–91. PMID:11544531
2337. Shaw EG, Scheithauer BW, O'Fallon JR, Tazelaar HD, Davis DH (1992). Oligodendrogliomas: the Mayo Clinic experience. J Neurosurg. 76(3):428–34. PMID:1738022
2338. Shaw EG, Wang M, Coons SW, Brachman DG, Buckner JC, Stelzer KJ, et al. (2012). Randomized trial of radiation therapy plus procarbazine, lomustine, and vincristine chemotherapy for supratentorial adult low-grade glioma: initial results of RTOG 9802. J Clin Oncol. 30(25):3065–70. PMID:22851558
2339. Shaw RJ, Paez JG, Curto M, Yaktine A, Pruitt WM, Saotome I, et al. (2001). The Nf2 tumor suppressor, merlin, functions in Rac-dependent signaling. Dev Cell. 1(1):63–72. PMID:11703924
2340. Shen WH, Balajee AS, Wang J, Wu H, Eng C, Pandolfi PP, et al. (2007). Essential role for nuclear PTEN in maintaining chromosomal integrity. Cell. 128(1):157–70. PMID:17218262
2341. Shenkier TN, Blay JY, O'Neill BP, Poortmans P, Thiel E, Jahnke K, et al. (2005). Primary CNS lymphoma of T-cell origin: a descriptive analysis from the international primary CNS lymphoma collaborative group. J Clin Oncol. 23(10):2233–9. PMID:15800313
2342. Shepherd CW, Houser OW, Gomez MR (1995). MR findings in tuberous sclerosis complex and correlation with seizure development and mental impairment. AJNR Am J Neuroradiol. 16(1):149–55. PMID:7900584
2343. Shibahara J, Fukayama M (2005). Secondary glioblastoma with advanced neuronal immunophenotype. Virchows Arch. 447(3):665–8. PMID:15968544
2344. Shibahara J, Todo T, Morita A, Mori H, Aoki S, Fukayama M (2004). Papillary neuroepithelial tumor of the pineal region. A case report. Acta Neuropathol. 108(4):337–40. PMID:15221340
2345. Shih DJ, Northcott PA, Remke M, Korshunov A, Ramaswamy V, Kool M, et al. (2014). Cytogenetic prognostication within medulloblastoma subgroups. J Clin Oncol. 32(9):886–96. PMID:24493713
2346. Shimbo Y, Takahashi H, Hayano M, Kumagai T, Kameyama S (1997). Temporal lobe lesion demonstrating features of dysembryoplastic neuroepithelial tumor and ganglioglioma: a transitional form? Clin Neuropathol. 16(2):65–8. PMID:9101106
2347. Shinojima N, Kochi M, Hamada J, Nakamura H, Yano S, Makino K, et al. (2004). The influence of sex and the presence of giant cells on postoperative long-term survival in adult patients with supratentorial glioblastoma multiforme. J Neurosurg. 101(2):219–26. PMID:15309911
2348. Shinojima N, Ohta K, Yano S, Nakamura H, Kochi M, Ishimaru Y, et al. (2002). Myofibroblastoma in the suprasellar region. Case report. J Neurosurg. 97(5):1203–7. PMID:12450045
2349. Shintaku M, Yoneda H, Hirato J, Nagaishi M, Okabe H (2013). Gliosarcoma with ependymal and PNET-like differentiation. Clin Neuropathol. 32(6):508–14. PMID:23863343
2350. Shishiba T, Niimura M, Ohtsuka F, Tsuru N (1984). Multiple cutaneous neurilemmomas as a skin manifestation of neurilemmomatosis. J Am Acad Dermatol. 10(5 Pt 1):744–54. PMID:6427303
2351. Shiurba RA, Buffinger NS, Spencer EM, Urich H (1991). Basic fibroblast growth factor and somatomedin C in human medulloepithelioma. Cancer. 68(4):798–808. PMID:1855180
2352. Shively SB, Falke EA, Li J, Tran MG, Thompson ER, Maxwell PH, et al. (2011). Developmentally arrested structures preceding cerebellar tumors in von Hippel-Lindau disease. Mod Pathol. 24(8):1023–30. PMID:21499240
2353. Shlien A, Campbell BB, de Borja R, Alexandrov LB, Merico D, Wedge D, et al.; Biallelic Mismatch Repair Deficiency Consortium (2015). Combined hereditary and somatic mutations of replication error repair genes result in rapid onset of ultra-hypermutated cancers. Nat Genet. 47(3):257–62. PMID:25642631
2354. Short MP, Richardson EP Jr, Haines JL, Kwiatkowski DJ (1995). Clinical, neuropathological and genetic aspects of the tuberous sclerosis complex. Brain Pathol. 5(2):173–9. PMID:7670658
2355. Shou Y, Robinson DM, Amakye DD, Rose KL, Cho YJ, Ligon KL, et al. (2015). A five-gene hedgehog signature developed as a patient preselection tool for hedgehog inhibitor therapy in medulloblastoma. Clin Cancer Res. 21(3):585–93. PMID:25473003
2356. Shuangshoti S, Rushing EJ, Mena H, Olsen C, Sandberg GD (2005). Supratentorial extraventricular ependymal neoplasms: a clinicopathologic study of 32 patients. Cancer. 103(12):2598–605. PMID:15861411
2357. Shweiki D, Itin A, Soffer D, Keshet E (1992). Vascular endothelial growth factor induced by hypoxia may mediate hypoxia-initiated angiogenesis. Nature. 359(6398):843–5. PMID:1279431
2358. Siami-Namini K, Shuey-Drake R, Wilson D, Francel P, Perry A, Fung KM (2005). A 15-year-old female with progressive myelopathy. Brain Pathol. 15(3):265–7. PMID:16196395
2359. Sievers S, Alemazkour K, Zahn S, Perlman EJ, Gillis AJ, Looijenga LH, et al. (2005). IGF2/H19 imprinting analysis of human germ cell tumors (GCTs) using the methylation-sensitive single-nucleotide primer extension method reflects the origin of GCTs in different stages of primordial germ cell development. Genes Chromosomes Cancer. 44(3):256–64. PMID:16001432
2360. Sievert AJ, Jackson EM, Gai X, Hakonarson H, Judkins AR, Resnick AC, et al. (2009). Duplication of 7q34 in pediatric low-grade astrocytomas detected by high-density single-nucleotide polymorphism-based genotype arrays results in a novel BRAF fusion gene. Brain Pathol. 19(3):449–58. PMID:19016743
2361. Simon SL, Moonis G, Judkins AR, Scobie J, Burnett MG, Riina HA, et al. (2005). Intracranial capillary hemangioma: case report and review of the literature. Surg Neurol. 64(2):154–9. PMID:16051010
2362. Simoneau-Roy J, O'Gorman C, Pencharz P, Adeli K, Daneman D, Hamilton J (2010). Insulin sensitivity and secretion in children and adolescents with hypothalamic obesity following treatment for craniopharyngioma. Clin Endocrinol (Oxf). 72(3):364–70. PMID:19486023
2363. Simpson LN, Hughes BD, Karikari IO, Mehta AI, Hodges TR, Cummings TJ, et al. (2012). Catecholamine-secreting paraganglioma of the thoracic spinal column: report of an unusual case and review of the literature. Neurosurgery. 70(4):E1049–52, discussion E1052. PMID:21788916
2364. Singh D, Chan JM, Zoppoli P, Niola F, Sullivan R, Castano A, et al. (2012). Transforming fusions of FGFR and TACC genes in human glioblastoma. Science. 337(6099):1231–5. PMID:22837387
2365. Singh SK, Hawkins C, Clarke ID, Squire JA, Bayani J, Hide T, et al. (2004). Identification of human brain tumour initiating cells. Nature. 432(7015):396–401. PMID:15549107
2366. Sinicrope FA, Sargent DJ (2012). Molecular pathways: microsatellite instability in colorectal cancer: prognostic, predictive, and therapeutic implications. Clin Cancer Res. 18(6):1506–12. PMID:22302899
2367. Sinson G, Gennarelli TA, Wells GB (1998). Suprasellar osteolipoma: case report. Surg Neurol. 50(5):457–60. PMID:9842872
2368. Skardelly M, Pantazis G, Bisdas S, Feigl GC, Schuhmann MU, Tatagiba MS, et al. (2013). Primary cerebral low-grade B-cell lymphoma, monoclonal immunoglobulin deposition disease, cerebral light chain deposition disease and "aggregoma": an update on classification and diagnosis. BMC Neurol. 13:107. PMID:23947787
2369. Skullerud K, Stenwig AE, Brandtzaeg P, Nesland JM, Kerty E, Langmoen I, et al. (1995). Intracranial primary leiomyosarcoma arising in a teratoma of the pineal area. Clin Neuropathol. 14(4):245–8. PMID:8521631
2370. Slowik F, Jellinger K, Gaszó L, Fischer J (1985). Gliosarcomas: histological, immunohistochemical, ultrastructural, and tissue culture studies. Acta Neuropathol. 67(3-4):201–10. PMID:4050334
2371. Smedby KE, Brandt L, Bäcklund ML, Blomqvist P (2009). Brain metastases admissions in Sweden between 1987 and 2006. Br J Cancer. 101(11):1919–24. PMID:19826419
2372. Smith AB, Rushing EJ, Smirniotopoulos JG (2009). Pigmented lesions of the central nervous system: radiologic-pathologic correlation. Radiographics. 29(5):1503–24. PMID:19755608
2373. Smith AB, Rushing EJ, Smirniotopoulos JG (2010). From the archives of the AFIP: lesions of the pineal region: radiologic-pathologic correlation. Radiographics. 30(7):2001–20. PMID:21057132
2374. Smith JS, Tachibana I, Passe SM, Huntley BK, Borell TJ, Iturria N, et al. (2001). PTEN mutation, EGFR amplification, and outcome in patients with anaplastic astrocytoma and glioblastoma multiforme. J Natl Cancer Inst. 93(16):1246–56. PMID:11504770
2375. Smith MJ (2015). Germline and somatic mutations in meningiomas. Cancer Genet. 208(4):107–14. PMID:25857641
2376. Smith MJ, Beetz C, Williams SG, Bhaskar SS, O'Sullivan J, Anderson B, et al. (2014). Germline mutations in SUFU cause Gorlin syndrome-associated childhood medulloblastoma and redefine the risk associated with PTCH1 mutations. J Clin Oncol. 32(36):4155–61. PMID:25403219
2377. Smith MJ, Isidor B, Beetz C, Williams SG, Bhaskar SS, Richer W, et al. (2015). Mutations in LZTR1 add to the complex heterogeneity of schwannomatosis. Neurology. 84(2):141–7. PMID:25480913
2378. Smith MJ, Kulkarni A, Rustad C, Bowers NL, Wallace AJ, Holder SE, et al. (2012). Vestibular schwannomas occur in schwannomatosis and should not be considered an exclusion criterion for clinical diagnosis. Am J Med Genet A. 158A(1):215–9. PMID:22105938
2379. Smith MJ, Wallace AJ, Bennett C, Hasselblatt M, Elert-Dobkowska E, Evans LT, et al. (2014). Germline SMARCE1 mutations predispose to both spinal and cranial clear

cell meningiomas. J Pathol. 234(4):436–40. PMID:25143307
2380. Smith MJ, Wallace AJ, Bowers NL, Eaton H, Evans DG (2014). SMARCB1 mutations in schwannomatosis and genotype correlations with rhabdoid tumors. Cancer Genet. 207(9):373–8. PMID:24933152
2381. Smith MJ, Wallace AJ, Bowers NL, Rustad CF, Woods CG, Leschziner GD, et al. (2012). Frequency of SMARCB1 mutations in familial and sporadic schwannomatosis. Neurogenetics. 13(2):141–5. PMID:22434358
2382. Smoll NR, Drummond KJ (2012). The incidence of medulloblastomas and primitive neurectodermal tumours in adults and children. J Clin Neurosci. 19(11):1541–4. PMID:22981874
2383. Smolle E, Al-Qubati S, Stefanits H, Haberler C, Kleinert R, Haybaeck J (2012). Medullomyoblastoma: a case report and literature review of a rare tumor entity. Anticancer Res. 32(11):4939–44. PMID:23155263
2384. Smyth I, Narang MA, Evans T, Heimann C, Nakamura Y, Chenevix-Trench G, et al. (1999). Isolation and characterization of human patched 2 (PTCH2), a putative tumour suppressor gene inbasal cell carcinoma and medulloblastoma on chromosome 1p32. Hum Mol Genet. 8(2):291–7. PMID:9931336
2385. Snuderl M, Fazlollahi L, Le LP, Nitta M, Zhelyazkova BH, Davidson CJ, et al. (2011). Mosaic amplification of multiple receptor tyrosine kinase genes in glioblastoma. Cancer Cell. 20(6):810–7. PMID:22137795
2386. Snyder LA, Wolf AB, Oppenlander ME, Bina R, Wilson JR, Ashby L, et al. (2014). The impact of extent of resection on malignant transformation of pure oligodendrogliomas. J Neurosurg. 120(2):309–14. PMID:24313617
2387. Sobel RA (1993). Vestibular (acoustic) schwannomas: histologic features in neurofibromatosis 2 and in unilateral cases. J Neuropathol Exp Neurol. 52(2):106–13. PMID:8440992
2388. Sofela AA, Hettige S, Curran O, Bassi S (2014). Malignant transformation in craniopharyngiomas. Neurosurgery. 75(3):306–14, discussion 314. PMID:24978859
2389. Soffer D, Pittaluga S, Caine Y, Feinsod M (1983). Paraganglioma of cauda equina. A report of a case and review of the literature. Cancer. 51(10):1907–10. PMID:6831356
2390. Soffietti R, Baumert BG, Bello L, von Deimling A, Duffau H, Frénay M, et al.; European Federation of Neurological Societies (2010). Guidelines on management of low-grade gliomas: report of an EFNS-EANO Task Force. Eur J Neurol. 17(9):1124–33. PMID:20718851
2391. Sohda T, Yun K (1996). Insulin-like growth factor II expression in primary meningeal hemangiopericytoma and its metastasis to the liver accompanied by hypoglycemia. Hum Pathol. 27(8):858–61. PMID:8760024
2392. Solis OE, Mehta RI, Lai A, Mehta RI, Farchoukh LO, Green RM, et al. (2011). Rosette-forming glioneuronal tumor: a pineal region case with IDH1 and IDH2 mutation analyses and literature review of 43 cases. J Neurooncol. 102(3):477–84. PMID:20872044
2392A. Solomon DA, Wood MD, Tihan T, Bollen AW, Gupta N, Phillips JJ, et al. (2015). Diffuse Midline Gliomas with Histone H3-K27M Mutation: A Series of 47 Cases Assessing the Spectrum of Morphologic Variation and Associated Genetic Alterations. Brain Pathol. doi: 10.1111/bpa.12336. [Epub ahead of print]
2393. Song MK, Chung JS, Joo YD, Lee SM, Oh SY, Shin DH, et al. (2011). Clinical importance of Bcl-6-positive non-deep-site involvement in non-HIV-related primary central nervous system diffuse large B-cell lymphoma. J Neurooncol. 104(3):825–31. PMID:21380743
2394. Song X, Andrew Allen R, Terence Dunn S, Fung KM, Farmer P, Gandhi S, et al. (2011). Glioblastoma with PNET-like components has a higher frequency of isocitrate dehydrogenase 1 (IDH1) mutation and likely a better prognosis than primary glioblastoma. Int J Clin Exp Pathol. 4(7):651–60. PMID:22076165
2395. Sonneland PR, Scheithauer BW, LeChago J, Crawford BG, Onofrio BM (1986). Paraganglioma of the cauda equina region. Clinicopathologic study of 31 cases with special reference to immunocytology and ultrastructure. Cancer. 58(8):1720–35. PMID:2875784
2396. Sonneland PR, Scheithauer BW, Onofrio BM (1985). Myxopapillary ependymoma. A clinicopathologic and immunocytochemical study of 77 cases. Cancer. 56(4):883–93. PMID:4016681
2397. Sonoda Y, Yoshimoto T, Sekiya T (1995). Homozygous deletion of the MTS1/p16 and MTS2/p15 genes and amplification of the CDK4 gene in glioma. Oncogene. 11(10):2145–9. PMID:7478535
2398. Sorensen AG, Emblem KE, Polaskova P, Jennings D, Kim H, Ancukiewicz M, et al. (2012). Increased survival of glioblastoma patients who respond to antiangiogenic therapy with elevated blood perfusion. Cancer Res. 72(2):402–7. PMID:22127927
2399. Soylemezoglu F, Onder S, Tezel GG, Berker M (2003). Neuronal nuclear antigen (NeuN): a new tool in the diagnosis of central neurocytoma. Pathol Res Pract. 199(7):463–8. PMID:14521262
2400. Soylemezoglu F, Soffer D, Onol B, Schwechheimer K, Kleihues P (1996). Lipomatous medulloblastoma in adults. A distinct clinicopathological entity. Am J Surg Pathol. 20(4):413–8. PMID:8604807
2401. Spanberger T, Berghoff AS, Dinhof C, Ilhan-Mutlu A, Magerle M, Hutterer M, et al. (2013). Extent of peritumoral brain edema correlates with prognosis, tumoral growth pattern, HIF1a expression and angiogenic activity in patients with single brain metastases. Clin Exp Metastasis. 30(4):357–68. PMID:23076770
2402. Specht CS, Smith TW, DeGirolami U, Price JM (1986). Myxopapillary ependymoma of the filum terminale. A light and electron microscopic study. Cancer. 58(2):310–7. PMID:3521831
2403. Spence T, Sin-Chan P, Picard D, Barszczyk M, Hoss K, Lu M, et al. (2014). CNS-PNETs with C19MC amplification and/or LIN28 expression comprise a distinct histogenetic diagnostic and therapeutic entity. Acta Neuropathol. 128(2):291–303. PMID:24839957
2404. Sperduto PW, Chao ST, Sneed PK, Luo X, Suh J, Roberge D, et al. (2010). Diagnosis-specific prognostic factors, indexes, and treatment outcomes for patients with newly diagnosed brain metastases: a multi-institutional analysis of 4,259 patients. Int J Radiat Oncol Biol Phys. 77(3):655–61. PMID:19942357
2405. Sperfeld AD, Hein C, Schröder JM, Ludolph AC, Hanemann CO (2002). Occurrence and characterization of peripheral nerve involvement in neurofibromatosis type 2. Brain. 125(Pt 5):996–1004. PMID:11960890
2406. Spiegel E (1920). Hyperplasie des Kleinhirns. Beitr Pathol Anat. 67:539–48.
2407. Squarize CH, Castilho RM, Gutkind JS (2008). Chemoprevention and treatment of experimental Cowden's disease by mTOR inhibition with rapamycin. Cancer Res. 68(17):7066–72. PMID:18757421
2408. Squire JA, Arab S, Marrano P, Bayani J, Karaskova J, Taylor M, et al. (2001). Molecular cytogenetic analysis of glial tumors using spectral karyotyping and comparative genomic hybridization. Mol Diagn. 6(2):93–108. PMID:11468694
2409. Sredni ST, Tomita T (2015). Rhabdoid tumor predisposition syndrome. Pediatr Dev Pathol. 18(1):49–58. PMID:25494491
2410. Stache C, Hölsken A, Fahlbusch R, Flitsch J, Schlaffer SM, Buchfelder M, et al. (2014). Tight junction protein claudin-1 is differentially expressed in craniopharyngioma subtypes and indicates invasive tumor growth. Neuro Oncol. 16(2):256–64. PMID:24305709
2411. Stambolic V, Suzuki A, de la Pompa JL, Brothers GM, Mirtsos C, Sasaki T, et al. (1998). Negative regulation of PKB/Akt-dependent cell survival by the tumor suppressor PTEN. Cell. 95(1):29–39. PMID:9778245
2412. Stanescu Cosson R, Varlet P, Beuvon F, Daumas Duport C, Devaux B, Chassoux F, et al. (2001). Dysembryoplastic neuroepithelial tumors: CT, MR findings and imaging follow-up: a study of 53 cases. J Neuroradiol. 28(4):230–40. PMID:11924137
2413. Stangl AP, Wellenreuther R, Lenartz D, Kraus JA, Menon AG, Schramm J, et al. (1997). Clonality of multiple meningiomas. J Neurosurg. 86(5):853–8. PMID:9126902
2414. Starink TM, van der Veen JP, Arwert F, de Waal LP, de Lange GG, Gille JJ, et al. (1986). The Cowden syndrome: a clinical and genetic study in 21 patients. Clin Genet. 29(3):222–33. PMID:3698331
2415. Starzyk J, Starzyk B, Bartnik-Mikuta A, Urbanowicz W, Dziatkowiak H (2001). Gonadotropin releasing hormone-independent precocious puberty in a 5 year-old girl with suprasellar germ cell tumor secreting beta-hCG and alpha-fetoprotein. J Pediatr Endocrinol Metab. 14(6):789–96. PMID:11453531
2416. Stavrou T, Bromley CM, Nicholson HS, Byrne J, Packer RJ, Goldstein AM, et al. (2001). Prognostic factors and secondary malignancies in childhood medulloblastoma. J Pediatr Hematol Oncol. 23(7):431–6. PMID:11878577
2417. Stüer C, Vilz B, Majores M, Becker A, Schramm J, Simon M (2007). Frequent recurrence and progression in pilocytic astrocytoma in adults. Cancer. 110(12):2799–808. PMID:17973253
2418. Steck PA, Pershouse MA, Jasser SA, Yung WK, Lin H, Ligon AH, et al. (1997). Identification of a candidate tumour suppressor gene, MMAC1, at chromosome 10q23.3 that is mutated in multiple advanced cancers. Nat Genet. 15(4):356–62. PMID:9090379
2419. Steel TR, Botterill P, Sheehy JP (1994). Paraganglioma of the cauda equina with associated syringomyelia: case report. Surg Neurol. 42(6):489–93. PMID:7825103
2420. Steinberg GK, Shuer LM, Conley FK, Hanbery JW (1985). Evolution and outcome in malignant astroglial neoplasms of the cerebellum. J Neurosurg. 62(1):9–17. PMID:3964859
2421. Steinbok P, Poskitt K, Hendson G (2006). Spontaneous regression of cerebellar astrocytoma after subtotal resection. Childs Nerv Syst. 22(6):572–6. PMID:16552566
2422. Stemmer-Rachamimov AO, Gonzalez-Agosti C, Xu L, Burwick JA, Beauchamp R, Pinney D, et al. (1997). Expression of NF2-encoded merlin and related ERM family proteins in the human central nervous system. J Neuropathol Exp Neurol. 56(6):735–42. PMID:9184664
2423. Stemmer-Rachamimov AO, Horgan MA, Taratuto AL, Munoz DG, Smith TW, Frosch MP, et al. (1997). Meningioangiomatosis is associated with neurofibromatosis 2 but not with somatic alterations of the NF2 gene. J Neuropathol Exp Neurol. 56(5):485–9. PMID:9143261
2424. Stemmer-Rachamimov AO, Ino Y, Lim ZY, Jacoby LB, MacCollin M, Gusella JF, et al. (1998). Loss of the NF2 gene and merlin occur by the tumorlet stage of schwannoma development in neurofibromatosis 2. J Neuropathol Exp Neurol. 57(12):1164–7. PMID:9862639
2425. Stenzel W, Pels H, Staib P, Impekoven P, Bektas N, Deckert M (2004). Concomitant manifestation of primary CNS lymphoma and Toxoplasma encephalitis in a patient with AIDS. J Neurol. 251(6):764–6. PMID:15311360
2426. Stephen JH, Sievert AJ, Madsen PJ, Judkins AR, Resnick AC, Storm PB, et al. (2012). Spinal cord ependymomas and myxopapillary ependymomas in the first 2 decades of life: a clinicopathological and immunohistochemical characterization of 19 cases. J Neurosurg Pediatr. 9(6):646–53. PMID:22656257
2427. Stern J, Jakobiec FA, Housepian EM (1980). The architecture of optic nerve gliomas with and without neurofibromatosis. Arch Ophthalmol. 98(3):505–11. PMID:6767467
2428. Stockhammer F, Misch M, Helms HJ, Lengler U, Prall F, von Deimling A, et al. (2012). IDH1/2 mutations in WHO grade II astrocytomas associated with localization and seizure as the initial symptom. Seizure. 21(3):194–7. PMID:22217666
2429. Stoffel EM, Mangu PB, Gruber SB, Hamilton SR, Kalady MF, Lau MW, et al.; American Society of Clinical Oncology; European Society of Clinical Oncology (2015). Hereditary colorectal cancer syndromes: American Society of Clinical Oncology Clinical Practice Guideline endorsement of the familial risk-colorectal cancer: European Society for Medical Oncology Clinical Practice Guidelines. J Clin Oncol. 33(2):209–17. PMID:25452455
2430. Stojanova A, Penn LZ (2009). The role of INI1/hSNF5 in gene regulation and cancer. Biochem Cell Biol. 87(1):163–77. PMID:19234532
2431. Stokland T, Liu JF, Ironside JW, Ellison DW, Taylor R, Robinson KJ, et al. (2010). A multivariate analysis of factors determining tumor progression in childhood low-grade glioma: a population-based cohort study (CCLG CNS9702). Neuro Oncol. 12(12):1257–68. PMID:20861086
2432. Stommel JM, Kimmelman AC, Ying H, Nabioullin R, Ponugoti AH, Wiedemeyer R, et al. (2007). Coactivation of receptor tyrosine kinases affects the response of tumor cells to targeted therapies. Science. 318(5848):287–90. PMID:17872411
2433. Stone DM, Hynes M, Armanini M, Swanson TA, Gu Q, Johnson RL, et al. (1996). The tumour-suppressor gene patched encodes a candidate receptor for Sonic hedgehog. Nature. 384(6605):129–34. PMID:8906787
2433A. Stone DM, Murone M, Luoh S, Ye W, Armanini MP, Gurney A, et al. (1999). Characterization of the human suppressor of fused, a negative regulator of the zinc-finger transcription factor Gli. J Cell Sci. 112(Pt 23):4437–48. PMID:10564661
2434. Storlazzi CT, Von Steyern FV, Domanski HA, Mandahl N, Mertens F (2005). Biallelic somatic inactivation of the NF1 gene through chromosomal translocations in a sporadic neurofibroma. Int J Cancer. 117(6):1055–7. PMID:15986446
2435. Stratakis CA (2002). Mutations of the gene encoding the protein kinase A type I-alpha regulatory subunit (PRKAR1A) in patients with the "complex of spotty skin pigmentation, myxomas, endocrine overactivity, and schwannomas" (Carney complex). Ann N Y Acad Sci. 968:3–21. PMID:12119264
2436. Stratakis CA, Carney JA (2009). The triad of paragangliomas, gastric stromal tumours and pulmonary chondromas (Carney triad), and the dyad of paragangliomas and gastric stromal sarcomas (Carney-Stratakis syndrome): molecular genetics and clinical implications. J Intern Med. 266(1):43–52. PMID:19522824
2437. Stratmann R, Krieg M, Haas R, Plate KH (1997). Putative control of angiogenesis in hemangioblastomas by the von Hippel-Lindau tumor suppressor gene. J Neuropathol Exp Neurol. 56(11):1242–52. PMID:9370235
2438. Strommer KN, Brandner S, Sarioglu AC, Sure U, Yonekawa Y (1995). Symptomatic cerebellar metastasis and late local recurrence of a cauda equina paraganglioma. Case report. J Neurosurg. 83(1):166–9. PMID:7782837
2439. Stucky CC, Johnson KN, Gray RJ, Pockaj BA, Ocal IT, Rose PS, et al. (2012). Malignant peripheral nerve sheath tumors (MPNST): the Mayo Clinic experience. Ann Surg Oncol. 19(3):878–85. PMID:21861229
2440. Stuivenvolt M, Mandl E, Verheul J, Fleischeuer R, Tijssen CC (2012). Atypical

transformation in sacral drop metastasis from posterior fossa choroid plexus papilloma. BMJ Case Rep. 2012:2012. PMID:22922909
2441. Stupp R, Hegi ME, Gorlia T, Erridge SC, Perry J, Hong YK, et al.; European Organisation for Research and Treatment of Cancer (EORTC); Canadian Brain Tumor Consortium; CENTRIC study team (2014). Cilengitide combined with standard treatment for patients with newly diagnosed glioblastoma with methylated MGMT promoter (CENTRIC EORTC 26071–22072 study): a multicentre, randomised, open-label, phase 3 trial. Lancet Oncol. 15(10):1100–8. PMID:25163906
2442. Stupp R, Hegi ME, Mason WP, van den Bent MJ, Taphoorn MJ, Janzer RC, et al.; European Organisation for Research and Treatment of Cancer Brain Tumour and Radiation Oncology Groups; National Cancer Institute of Canada Clinical Trials Group (2009). Effects of radiotherapy with concomitant and adjuvant temozolomide versus radiotherapy alone on survival in glioblastoma in a randomised phase III study: 5-year analysis of the EORTC-NCIC trial. Lancet Oncol. 10(5):459–66. PMID:19269895
2443. Sturm D, Bender S, Jones DT, Lichter P, Grill J, Becher O, et al. (2014). Paediatric and adult glioblastoma: multiform (epi)genomic culprits emerge. Nat Rev Cancer. 14(2):92–107. PMID:24457416
2444. Sturm D, Witt H, Hovestadt V, Khuong-Quang DA, Jones DT, Konermann C, et al. (2012). Hotspot mutations in H3F3A and IDH1 define distinct epigenetic and biological subgroups of glioblastoma. Cancer Cell. 22(4):425–37. PMID:23079654
2445. Stödberg T, Deniz Y, Esteitie N, Jacobsson B, Mousavi-Jazi M, Dahl H, et al. (2002). A case of diffuse leptomeningeal oligodendrogliomatosis associated with HHV-6 variant A. Neuropediatrics. 33(5):266–70. PMID:12536370
2446. Sugawa N, Ekstrand AJ, James CD, Collins VP (1990). Identical splicing of aberrant epidermal growth factor receptor transcripts from amplified rearranged genes in human glioblastomas. Proc Natl Acad Sci U S A. 87(21):8602–6. PMID:2236070
2447. Sughrue ME, Choi J, Rutkowski MJ, Aranda D, Kane AJ, Barani IJ, et al. (2011). Clinical features and post-surgical outcome of patients with astroblastoma. J Clin Neurosci. 18(6):750–4. PMID:21507653
2448. Sughrue ME, Sanai N, Shangari G, Parsa AT, Berger MS, McDermott MW (2010). Outcome and survival following primary and repeat surgery for World Health Organization Grade III meningiomas. J Neurosurg. 113(2):202–9. PMID:20225922
2449. Sugiarto S, Persson AI, Munoz EG, Waldhuber M, Lamagna C, Andor N, et al. (2011). Asymmetry-defective oligodendrocyte progenitors are glioma precursors. Cancer Cell. 20(3):328–40. PMID:21907924
2450. Sugino T, Mikami T, Akiyama Y, Wanibuchi M, Hasegawa T, Mikuni N (2013). Primary central nervous system anaplastic large-cell lymphoma mimicking lymphomatosis cerebri. Brain Tumor Pathol. 30(1):61–5. PMID:22426596
2451. Sugiyama K, Arita K, Shima T, Nakaoka M, Matsuoka T, Taniguchi E, et al. (2002). Good clinical course in infants with desmoplastic cerebral neuroepithelial tumor treated by surgery alone. J Neurooncol. 59(1):63–9. PMID:12222839
2452. Suh YL, Koo H, Kim TS, Chi JG, Park SH, Khang SK, et al.; Neuropathology Study Group of the Korean Society of Pathologists (2002). Tumors of the central nervous system in Korea: a multicenter study of 3221 cases. J Neurooncol. 56(3):251–9. PMID:12061732
2453. Sukov WR, Cheville JC, Giannini C, Carlson AW, Shearer BM, Sinnwell JP, et al. (2010). Isochromosome 12p and polysomy 12 in primary central nervous system germ cell tumors: frequency and association with clinicopathologic features. Hum Pathol. 41(2):232–8. PMID:19801160
2454. Sullivan JP, Nahed BV, Madden MW, Oliveira SM, Springer S, Bhere D, et al. (2014). Brain tumor cells in circulation are enriched for mesenchymal gene expression. Cancer Discov. 4(11):1299–309. PMID:25139148
2455. Sulman EP, Guerrero M, Aldape K (2009). Beyond grade: molecular pathology of malignant gliomas. Semin Radiat Oncol. 19(3):142–9. PMID:19464628
2456. Sundgren P, Annertz M, Englund E, Strömblad LG, Holtås S (1999). Paragangliomas of the spinal canal. Neuroradiology. 41(10):788–94. PMID:10552032
2457. Sung CC, Collins R, Li J, Pearl DK, Coons SW, Scheithauer BW, et al. (1996). Glycolipids and myelin proteins in human oligodendrogliomas. Glycoconj J. 13(3):433–43. PMID:8781974
2458. Surawicz TS, McCarthy BJ, Kupelian V, Jukich PJ, Bruner JM, Davis FG (1999). Descriptive epidemiology of primary brain and CNS tumors: results from the Central Brain Tumor Registry of the United States, 1990–1994. Neuro Oncol. 1(1):14–25. PMID:11554386
2459. Suresh TN, Santosh V, Yasha TC, Anandh B, Mohanty A, Indiradevi B, et al. (2004). Medulloblastoma with extensive nodularity: a variant occurring in the very young-clinicopathological and immunohistochemical study of four cases. Childs Nerv Syst. 20(1):55–60. PMID:14657995
2460. Suster D, Plaza JA, Shen R (2005). Low-grade malignant perineurioma (perineurial sarcoma) of soft tissue: a potential diagnostic pitfall on fine needle aspiration. Ann Diagn Pathol. 9(4):197–201. PMID:16084452
2461. Suvà ML, Rheinbay E, Gillespie SM, Patel AP, Wakimoto H, Rabkin SD, et al. (2014). Reconstructing and reprogramming the tumor-propagating potential of glioblastoma stem-like cells. Cell. 157(3):580–94. PMID:24726434
2462. Suvà ML, Riggi N, Bernstein BE (2013). Epigenetic reprogramming in cancer. Science. 339(6127):1567–70. PMID:23539597
2463. Suzuki A, de la Pompa JL, Stambolic V, Elia AJ, Sasaki T, del Barco Barrantes I, et al. (1998). High cancer susceptibility and embryonic lethality associated with mutation of the PTEN tumor suppressor gene in mice. Curr Biol. 8(21):1169–78. PMID:9799734
2464. Suzuki H, Aoki K, Chiba K, Sato Y, Shiozawa Y, Shiraishi Y, et al. (2015). Mutational landscape and clonal architecture in grade II and III gliomas. Nat Genet. 47(5):458–68. PMID:25848751
2465. Svajdler M Jr, Rychlý B, Gajdoš M, Pataky F, Fröhlichová L, Perry A (2012). Gliosarcoma with alveolar rhabdomyosarcoma-like component: report of a case with a hitherto undescribed sarcomatous component. Cesk Patol. 48(4):210–4. PMID:23121030
2466. Swaidan MY, Hussaini M, Sultan I, Mansour A (2012). Radiological findings in gliosarcoma. A single institution experience. Neuroradiol J. 25(2):173–80. PMID:24028910
2467. Swanson KR, Bridge C, Murray JD, Alvord EC Jr (2003). Virtual and real brain tumors: using mathematical modeling to quantify glioma growth and invasion. J Neurol Sci. 216(1):1–10. PMID:14607296
2468. Swartling FJ, Savov V, Persson AI, Chen J, Hackett CS, Northcott PA, et al. (2012). Distinct neural stem cell populations give rise to disparate brain tumors in response to N-MYC. Cancer Cell. 21(5):601–13. PMID:22624711
2469. Sweet K, Willis J, Zhou XP, Gallione C, Sawada T, Alhopuro P, et al. (2005). Molecular classification of patients with unexplained hamartomatous and hyperplastic polyposis. JAMA. 294(19):2465–73. PMID:16287957
2470. Sweiss FB, Lee M, Sherman JH (2015). Extraventricular neurocytomas. Neurosurg Clin N Am. 26(1):99–104. PMID:25432188
2471. Swensen AR, Bushhouse SA (1998). Childhood cancer incidence and trends in Minnesota, 1988–1994. Minn Med. 81(12):27–32. PMID:9866372
2472. Swensen JJ, Keyser J, Coffin CM, Biegel JA, Viskochil DH, Williams MS (2009). Familial occurrence of schwannomas and malignant rhabdoid tumour associated with a duplication in SMARCB1. J Med Genet. 46(1):68–72. PMID:19124645
2473. Swerdlow SH, Campo E, Harris NL, Jaffe ES, Pileri SA, Stein H, et al., editors. (2008). WHO Classification of Tumours of Haematopoietic and Lymphoid Tissues. 4th ed. Lyon: International Agency for Research on Cancer.
2474. Szathmari A, Champier J, Ghersi-Egea JF, Jouvet A, Watrin C, Wierinckx A, et al. (2013). Molecular characterization of circumventricular organs and third ventricle ependyma in the rat: potential markers for periventricular tumors. Neuropathology. 33(1):17–29. PMID:22537279
2475. Szeifert GT, Pásztor E (1993). Could craniopharyngiomas produce pituitary hormones? Neurol Res. 15(1):68–9. PMID:8098858
2476. Szudek J, Birch P, Riccardi VM, Evans DG, Friedman JM (2000). Associations of clinical features in neurofibromatosis 1 (NF1). Genet Epidemiol. 19(4):429–39. PMID:11108651
2477. Szudek J, Joe H, Friedman JM (2002). Analysis of intrafamilial phenotypic variation in neurofibromatosis 1 (NF1). Genet Epidemiol. 23(2):150–64. PMID:12214308
2478. Söylemezoglu F, Scheithauer BW, Esteve J, Kleihues P (1997). Atypical central neurocytoma. J Neuropathol Exp Neurol. 56(5):551–6. PMID:9143268
2479. Söylemezoglu F, Tezel GG, Köybaşoglu F, Er U, Akalan N (2001). Cranial infantile myofibromatosis: report of three cases. Childs Nerv Syst. 17(9):524–7. PMID:11585325
2480. Taal W, Oosterkamp HM, Walenkamp AM, Dubbink HJ, Beerepoot LV, Hanse MC, et al. (2014). Single-agent bevacizumab or lomustine versus a combination of bevacizumab plus lomustine in patients with recurrent glioblastoma (BELOB trial): a randomised controlled phase 2 trial. Lancet Oncol. 15(9):943–53. PMID:25035291
2481. Taal W, van der Rijt CC, Dinjens WN, Sillevis Smitt PA, Wertenbroek AA, Bromberg JE, et al. (2015). Treatment of large low-grade oligodendroglial tumors with upfront procarbazine, lomustine, and vincristine chemotherapy with long follow-up: a retrospective cohort study with growth kinetics. J Neurooncol. 121(2):365–72. PMID:25344884
2482. Tabori U, Baskin B, Shago M, Alon N, Taylor MD, Ray PN, et al. (2010). Universal poor survival in children with medulloblastoma harboring somatic TP53 mutations. J Clin Oncol. 28(8):1345–50. PMID:20142599
2483. Tabori U, Shlien A, Baskin B, Levitt S, Ray P, Alon N, et al. (2010). TP53 alterations determine clinical subgroups and survival of patients with choroid plexus tumors. J Clin Oncol. 28(12):1995–2001. PMID:20308654
2484. Tabouret E, Chinot O, Metellus P, Tallet A, Viens P, Gonçalves A (2012). Recent trends in epidemiology of brain metastases: an overview. Anticancer Res. 32(11):4655–62. PMID:23155227
2485. Tachibana O, Nakazawa H, Lampe J, Watanabe K, Kleihues P, Ohgaki H (1995). Expression of Fas/APO-1 during the progression of astrocytomas. Cancer Res. 55(23):5528–30. PMID:7585627
2486. Tachibana O, Yamashima T, Yamashita J, Takabatake Y (1994). Immunohistochemical expression of human chorionic gonadotropin and P-glycoprotein in human pituitary glands and craniopharyngiomas. J Neurosurg. 80(1):79–84. PMID:7903692
2487. Tada T, Katsuyama T, Aoki T, Kobayashi S, Shigematsu H (1987). Mixed glioblastoma and sarcoma with osteoid-chondral tissue. Clin Neuropathol. 6(4):160–3. PMID:3115659
2488. Taggard DA, Menezes AH (2000). Three choroid plexus papillomas in a patient with Aicardi syndrome. A case report. Pediatr Neurosurg. 33(4):219–23. PMID:11124640
2489. Taillibert S, Chodkiewicz C, Laigle-Donadey F, Napolitano M, Cartalat-Carel S, Sanson M (2006). Gliomatosis cerebri: a review of 296 cases from the ANOCEF database and the literature. J Neurooncol. 76(2):201–5. PMID:16200347
2490. Taillibert S, Laigle-Donadey F, Chodkiewicz C, Sanson M, Hoang-Xuan K, Delattre JY (2005). Leptomeningeal metastases from solid malignancy: a review. J Neurooncol. 75(1):85–99. PMID:16215819
2491. Taipale J, Cooper MK, Maiti T, Beachy PA (2002). Patched acts catalytically to suppress the activity of Smoothened. Nature. 418(6900):892–7. PMID:12192414
2492. Takahashi E, Kajimoto K, Fukatsu T, Yoshida M, Eimoto T, Nakamura S (2005). Intravascular large T-cell lymphoma: a case report of CD30-positive and ALK-negative anaplastic type with cytotoxic molecule expression. Virchows Arch. 447(6):1000–6. PMID:16189700
2493. Takahashi E, Nakamura S (2013). Histiocytic sarcoma : an updated literature review based on the 2008 WHO classification. J Clin Exp Hematop. 53(1):1–8. PMID:23801128
2494. Takahashi M, Yamamoto J, Aoyama Y, Soejima Y, Akiba D, Nishizawa S (2009). Efficacy of multi-staged surgery and adjuvant chemotherapy for successful treatment of atypical choroid plexus papilloma in an infant: case report. Neurol Med Chir (Tokyo). 49(10):484–7. PMID:19855149
2495. Takami H, Fukushima S, Fukuoka K, Suzuki T, Yanagisawa T, Matsushita Y, et al. (2015). Human chorionic gonadotropin is expressed virtually in all intracranial germ cell tumors. J Neurooncol. 124(1):23–32. PMID:25994796
2496. Takami H, Yoshida A, Fukushima S, Arita H, Matsushita Y, Nakamura T, et al. (2015). Revisiting TP53 Mutations and Immunohistochemistry–A Comparative Study in 157 Diffuse Gliomas. Brain Pathol. 25(3):256–65 PMID:25040820
2497. Takei H, Adesina AM, Mehta V, Powell SZ, Langford LA (2010). Atypical teratoid/rhabdoid tumor of the pineal region in an adult. J Neurosurg. 113(2):374–9. PMID:19911885
2498. Takei Y, Mirra SS, Miles ML (1976). Eosinophilic granular ceels in oligodendrogliomas. An ultrastructural study. Cancer. 38(5):1968–76. PMID:991110
2499. Takei Y, Seyama S, Pearl GS, Tindall GT (1980). Ultrastructural study of the human neurohypophysis. II. Cellular elements of neural parenchyma, the pituicytes. Cell Tissue Res. 205(2):273–87. PMID:7188885
2500. Takeshima H, Kawahara Y, Hirano H, Obara S, Niiro M, Kuratsu J (2003). Postoperative regression of desmoplastic infantile gangliogliomas: report of two cases. Neurosurgery. 53(4):979–83, discussion 983–4. PMID:14519230
2501. Tamura M, Gu J, Matsumoto K, Aota S, Parsons R, Yamada KM (1998). Inhibition of cell migration, spreading, and focal adhesions by tumor suppressor PTEN. Science. 280(5369):1614–7. PMID:9616126
2502. Tan C, Scotting PJ (2013). Stem cell research points the way to the cell of origin for intracranial germ cell tumours. J Pathol. 229(1):4–11. PMID:22926997
2503. Tan MH, Mester J, Peterson C, Yang Y, Chen JL, Rybicki LA, et al. (2011). A clinical scoring system for selection of patients for PTEN mutation testing is proposed on the basis of a prospective study of 3042 probands. Am J Hum Genet. 88(1):42–56. PMID:21194675

2504. Tan MH, Mester JL, Ngeow J, Rybicki LA, Orloff MS, Eng C (2012). Lifetime cancer risks in individuals with germline PTEN mutations. Clin Cancer Res. 18(2):400–7. PMID:22252256
2505. Tan W, Huang W, Xiong J, Pan J, Geng D, Jun Z (2014). Neuroradiological features of papillary glioneuronal tumor: a study of 8 cases. J Comput Assist Tomogr. 38(5):634–8. PMID:24879457
2506. Tanaka K, Waga S, Itho H, Shimizu DM, Namiki H (1989). Superficial location of malignant glioma with heavily lipidized (foamy) tumor cells: a case report. J Neurooncol. 7(3):293–7. PMID:2795123
2507. Tanaka M, Suda M, Ishikawa Y, Fujitake J, Fujii H, Tatsuoka Y (1996). Idiopathic hypertrophic cranial pachymeningitis associated with hydrocephalus and myocarditis: remarkable steriod-induced remission of hypertrophic dura mater. Neurology. 46(2):554–6. PMID:8614532
2508. Tanaka S, Nakada M, Nobusawa S, Suzuki SO, Sabit H, Miyashita K, et al. (2014). Epithelioid glioblastoma arising from pleomorphic xanthoastrocytoma with the BRAF V600E mutation. Brain Tumor Pathol. 31(3):172–6. PMID:24894018
2509. Tanaka Y, Yokoo H, Komori T, Makita Y, Ishizawa T, Hirose T, et al. (2005). A distinct pattern of Olig2-positive cellular distribution in papillary glioneuronal tumors: a manifestation of the oligodendroglial phenotype? Acta Neuropathol. 110(1):39–47. PMID:15906048
2510. Tanas MR, Sboner A, Oliveira AM, Erickson-Johnson MR, Hespelt J, Hanwright PJ, et al. (2011). Identification of a disease-defining gene fusion in epithelioid hemangioendothelioma. Sci Transl Med. 3(98):98ra82. PMID:21885404
2510A. Tanboon J, Williams EA, Louis DN (2015). The Diagnostic Use of Immunohistochemical Surrogates for Signature Molecular Genetic Alterations in Gliomas. J Neuropathol Exp Neurol. [Epub ahead of print] PMID:26671986
2511. Tandon A, Schiff D (2014). Therapeutic decision making in patients with newly diagnosed low grade glioma. Curr Treat Options Oncol. 15(4):529–38. PMID:25139406
2512. Tanimura A, Nakamura Y, Hachisuka H, Tanimura Y, Fukumura A (1984). Hemangioblastoma of the central nervous system: nature of the stromal cells as studied by the immunoperoxidase technique. Hum Pathol. 15(9):866–9. PMID:6432675
2513. Taratuto AL, Molina HA, Diez B, Zúccaro G, Monges J (1985). Primary rhabdomyosarcoma of brain and cerebellum. Report of four cases in infants: an immunohistochemical study. Acta Neuropathol. 66(2):98–104. PMID:4013672
2514. Taratuto AL, Monges J, Lylyk P, Leiguarda R (1984). Superficial cerebral astrocytoma attached to dura. Report of six cases in infants. Cancer. 54(11):2505–12. PMID:6498740
2515. Taratuto AL, Pomata H, Sevlever G, Gallo G, Monges J (1995). Dysembryoplastic neuroepithelial tumor: morphological, immunocytochemical, and deoxyribonucleic acid analyses in a pediatric series. Neurosurgery. 36(3):474–81. PMID:7753346
2516. Tashjian VS, Khanlou N, Vinters HV, Canalis RF, Becker DP (2009). Hemangiopericytoma of the cerebellopontine angle: a case report and review of the literature. Surg Neurol. 72(3):290–5. PMID:18786704
2517. Tate M, Sughrue ME, Rutkowski MJ, Kane AJ, Aranda D, McClinton L, et al. (2012). The long-term postsurgical prognosis of patients with pineoblastoma. Cancer. 118(1):173–9. PMID:21717450
2518. Tatevossian RG, Tang B, Dalton J, Forshew T, Lawson AR, Ma J, et al. (2010). MYB upregulation and genetic aberrations in a subset of pediatric low-grade gliomas. Acta Neuropathol. 120(6):731–43. PMID:21046410
2519. Tatter SB, Borges LF, Louis DN (1994). Central neurocytomas of the cervical spinal cord. Report of two cases. J Neurosurg. 81(2):288–93. PMID:8027814
2520. Tavangar SM, Larijani B, Mahta A, Hosseini SM, Mehrazine M, Bandarian F (2004). Craniopharyngioma: a clinicopathological study of 141 cases. Endocr Pathol. 15(4):339–44. PMID:15681858
2521. Taylor KR, Mackay A, Truffaux N, Butterfield YS, Morozova O, Philippe C, et al. (2014). Recurrent activating ACVR1 mutations in diffuse intrinsic pontine glioma. Nat Genet. 46(5):457–61. PMID:24705252
2522. Taylor MD, Gokgoz N, Andrulis IL, Mainprize TG, Drake JM, Rutka JT (2000). Familial posterior fossa brain tumors of infancy secondary to germline mutation of the hSNF5 gene. Am J Hum Genet. 66(4):1403–6. PMID:10739763
2523. Taylor MD, Liu L, Raffel C, Hui CC, Mainprize TG, Zhang X, et al. (2002). Mutations in SUFU predispose to medulloblastoma. Nat Genet. 31(3):306–10. PMID:12068298
2524. Taylor MD, Northcott PA, Korshunov A, Remke M, Cho YJ, Clifford SC, et al. (2012). Molecular subgroups of medulloblastoma: the current consensus. Acta Neuropathol. 123(4):465–72. PMID:22134537
2525. Taylor MD, Perry J, Zlatescu MC, Stemmer-Rachamimov AO, Ang LC, Ino Y, et al. (1999). The hPMS2 exon 5 mutation and malignant glioma. Case report. J Neurosurg. 90(5):946–50. PMID:10223463
2526. Taylor MD, Poppleton H, Fuller C, Su X, Liu Y, Jensen P, et al. (2005). Radial glia cells are candidate stem cells of ependymoma. Cancer Cell. 8(4):323–35. PMID:16226707
2526A. Taylor TE, Furnari FB, Cavenee WK (2012). Targeting EGFR for treatment of glioblastoma: molecular basis to overcome resistance. Curr Cancer Drug Targets. 12(3):197–209. PMID:22268382
2527. Tchoghandjian A, Fernandez C, Colin C, El Ayachi I, Voutsinos-Porche B, Fina F, et al. (2009). Pilocytic astrocytoma of the optic pathway: a tumour deriving from radial glia cells with a specific gene signature. Brain. 132(Pt 6):1523–35. PMID:19336457
2528. Tee AR, Fingar DC, Manning BD, Kwiatkowski DJ, Cantley LC, Blenis J (2002). Tuberous sclerosis complex-1 and -2 gene products function together to inhibit mammalian target of rapamycin (mTOR)-mediated downstream signaling. Proc Natl Acad Sci U S A. 99(21):13571–6. PMID:12271141
2529. Tehrani M, Friedman TM, Olson JJ, Brat DJ (2008). Intravascular thrombosis in central nervous system malignancies: a potential role in astrocytoma progression to glioblastoma. Brain Pathol. 18(2):164–71. PMID:18093251
2530. Tekautz TM, Fuller CE, Blaney S, Fouladi M, Broniscer A, Merchant TE, et al. (2005). Atypical teratoid/rhabdoid tumors (ATRT): improved survival in children 3 years of age and older with radiation therapy and high-dose alkylator-based chemotherapy. J Clin Oncol. 23(7):1491–9. PMID:15735125
2531. Telera S, Carosi M, Cerasoli V, Facciolo F, Occhipinti E, Vidiri A, et al. (2006). Hemothorax presenting as a primitive thoracic paraganglioma. Case illustration. J Neurosurg Spine. 4(6):515. PMID:16776367
2532. Telfeian AE, Judkins A, Younkin D, Pollock AN, Crino P (2004). Subependymal giant cell astrocytoma with cranial and spinal metastases in a patient with tuberous sclerosis. Case report. J Neurosurg. 100(5) Suppl Pediatrics:498–500. PMID:15287462
2533. Temme A, Geiger KD, Wiedemuth R, Conseur K, Pietsch T, Felsberg J, et al. (2010). Giant cell glioblastoma is associated with altered aurora b expression and concomitant p53 mutation. J Neuropathol Exp Neurol. 69(6):632–42. PMID:20467329
2534. Teo WY, Shen J, Su JM, Yu A, Wang J, Chow WY, et al. (2013). Implications of tumor location on subtypes of medulloblastoma. Pediatr Blood Cancer. 60(9):1408–10. PMID:23512859
2535. Terada T (2015). Expression of cytokeratins in glioblastoma multiforme. Pathol Oncol Res. 21(3):817–9. PMID:25633990
2536. Terashima K, Yu A, Chow WY, Hsu WC, Chen P, Wong S, et al. (2014). Genome-wide analysis of DNA copy number alterations and loss of heterozygosity in intracranial germ cell tumors. Pediatr Blood Cancer. 61(4):593–600. PMID:24249158
2537. Thiel G, Losanowa T, Kintzel D, Nisch G, Martin H, Vorpahl K, et al. (1992). Karyotypes in 90 human gliomas. Cancer Genet Cytogenet. 58(2):109–20. PMID:1551072
2538. Thiele EA (2010). Managing and understanding epilepsy in tuberous sclerosis complex. Epilepsia. 51 Suppl 1:90–1. PMID:20331728
2539. Thiessen B, Finlay J, Kulkarni R, Rosenblum MK (1998). Astroblastoma: does histology predict biologic behavior? J Neurooncol. 40(1):59–65. PMID:9874187
2540. Thines L, Lejeune JP, Ruchoux MM, Assaker R (2006). Management of delayed intracranial and intraspinal metastases of intradural spinal paragangliomas. Acta Neurochir (Wien). 148(1):63–6, discussion 66. PMID:16283104
2541. Thom M, Blümcke I, Aronica E (2012). Long-term epilepsy-associated tumors. Brain Pathol. 22(3):350–79. PMID:22497610
2542. Thom M, Gomez-Anson B, Revesz T, Harkness W, O'Brien CJ, Kett-White R, et al. (1999). Spontaneous intralesional haemorrhage in dysembryoplastic neuroepithelial tumours: a series of five cases. J Neurol Neurosurg Psychiatry. 67(1):97–101. PMID:10369831
2543. Thom M, Toma A, An S, Martinian L, Hadjivassiliou G, Ratilal B, et al. (2011). One hundred and one dysembryoplastic neuroepithelial tumors: an adult epilepsy series with immunohistochemical, molecular genetic, and clinical correlations and a review of the literature. J Neuropathol Exp Neurol. 70(10):859–78. PMID:21937911
2544. Thomas C, Ruland V, Kordes U, Hartung S, Capper D, Pietsch T, et al. (2015). Pediatric atypical choroid plexus papilloma reconsidered: increased mitotic activity is prognostic only in older children. Acta Neuropathol. 129(6):925–7. PMID:25935663
2545. Thomas L, Spurlock G, Eudall C, Thomas NS, Mort M, Hamby SE, et al. (2012). Exploring the somatic NF1 mutational spectrum associated with NF1 cutaneous neurofibromas. Eur J Hum Genet. 20(4):411–9. PMID:22108604
2546. Thomas PK, King RH, Chiang TR, Scaravilli F, Sharma AK, Downie AW (1990). Neurofibromatous neuropathy. Muscle Nerve. 13(2):93–101. PMID:2156160
2547. Thommen F, Hewer E, Schäfer SC, Vassella E, Kappeler A, Vajtai I (2013). Rosette-forming glioneuronal tumor of the cerebellum in statu nascendi: an incidentally detected diminutive example indicates derivation from the internal granule cell layer. Clin Neuropathol. 32(5):370–6. PMID:23547894
2548. Thompsett AR, Ellison DW, Stevenson FK, Zhu D (1999). V(H) gene sequences from primary central nervous system lymphomas indicate derivation from highly mutated germinal center B cells with ongoing mutational activity. Blood. 94(5):1738–46. PMID:10477699
2549. Thompson MC, Fuller C, Hogg TL, Dalton J, Finkelstein D, Lau CC, et al. (2006). Genomics identifies medulloblastoma subgroups that are enriched for specific genetic alterations. J Clin Oncol. 24(12):1924–31. PMID:16567768
2550. Tian R, Hao S, Hou Z, Bian L, Zhang Y, Wu W, et al. (2013). Clinical characteristics and prognostic analysis of recurrent hemangiopericytoma in the central nervous system: a review of 46 cases. J Neurooncol. 115(1):53–9. PMID:23824534
2551. Tian Y, Wang J, Ge Jz, Ma Z, Ge M (2015). Intracranial Rosai-Dorfman disease mimicking multiple meningiomas in a child: a case report and review of the literature. Childs Nerv Syst. 31(2):317–23. PMID:25183389
2552. Tibbetts KM, Emnett RJ, Gao F, Perry A, Gutmann DH, Leonard JR (2009). Histopathologic predictors of pilocytic astrocytoma event-free survival. Acta Neuropathol. 117(6):657–65. PMID:19271226
2553. Tien RD, Barkovich AJ, Edwards MS (1990). MR imaging of pineal tumors. AJR Am J Roentgenol. 155(1):143–51. PMID:2162137
2554. Tien RD, Brasch RC, Jackson DE, Dillon WP (1989). Cerebral Erdheim-Chester disease: persistent enhancement with Gd-DTPA on MR images. Radiology. 172(3):791–2. PMID:2772189
2555. Tihan T, Fisher PG, Kepner JL, Godfraind C, McComb RD, Goldthwaite PT, et al. (1999). Pediatric astrocytomas with monomorphous pilomyxoid features and a less favorable outcome. J Neuropathol Exp Neurol. 58(10):1061–8. PMID:10515229
2556. Tihan T, Vohra P, Berger MS, Keles GE (2006). Definition and diagnostic implications of gemistocytic astrocytomas: a pathological perspective. J Neurooncol. 76(2):175–83. PMID:16132490
2557. Tihan T, Zhou T, Holmes E, Burger PC, Ozuysal S, Rushing EJ (2008). The prognostic value of histological grading of posterior fossa ependymomas in children: a Children's Oncology Group study and a review of prognostic factors. Mod Pathol. 21(2):165–77. PMID:18084249
2558. Timmermann B, Kortmann RD, Kühl J, Rutkowski S, Meisner C, Pietsch T, et al. (2006). Role of radiotherapy in supratentorial primitive neuroectodermal tumor in young children: results of the German HIT-SKK87 and HIT-SKK92 trials. J Clin Oncol. 24(10):1554–60. PMID:16575007
2559. Tinat J, Bougeard G, Baert-Desurmont S, Vasseur S, Martin C, Bouvignies E, et al. (2009). 2009 version of the Chompret criteria for Li Fraumeni syndrome. J Clin Oncol. 27(26):e108–9, author reply e110. PMID:19652052
2560. Tirakotai W, Mennel HD, Celik I, Hellwig D, Bertalanffy H, Riegel T (2006). Secretory meningioma: immunohistochemical findings and evaluation of mast cell infiltration. Neurosurg Rev. 29(1):41–8. PMID:16010579
2561. Toedt G, Barbus S, Wolter M, Felsberg J, Tews B, Blond F, et al. (2011). Molecular signatures classify astrocytic gliomas by IDH1 mutation status. Int J Cancer. 128(5):1095–103. PMID:20473936
2562. Tohma Y, Gratas C, Biernat W, Peraud A, Fukuda M, Yonekawa Y, et al. (1998). PTEN (MMAC1) mutations are frequent in primary glioblastomas (de novo) but not in secondary glioblastomas. J Neuropathol Exp Neurol. 57(7):684–9. PMID:9690672
2563. Tohma Y, Gratas C, Van Meir EG, Desbaillets I, Tenan M, Tachibana O, et al. (1998). Necrogenesis and Fas/APO-1 (CD95) expression in primary (de novo) and secondary glioblastomas. J Neuropathol Exp Neurol. 57(3):239–45. PMID:9600216
2564. Tomita T, Gates E (1999). Pituitary adenomas and granular cell tumors. Incidence, cell type, and location of tumor in 100 pituitary glands at autopsy. Am J Clin Pathol. 111(6):817–25. PMID:10361519
2565. Tomlinson FH, Scheithauer BW, Hayostek CJ, Parisi JE, Meyer FB, Shaw EG, et al. (1994). The significance of atypia and histologic malignancy in pilocytic astrocytoma of the cerebellum: a clinicopathologic and flow cytometric study. J Child Neurol. 9(3):301–10. PMID:7930411

2566. Tomlinson FH, Scheithauer BW, Kelly PJ, Forbes GS (1991). Subependymoma with rhabdomyosarcomatous differentiation: report of a case and literature review. Neurosurgery. 28(5):761–8. PMID:1876259
2567. Tomura N, Hirano H, Watanabe O, Watarai J, Itoh Y, Mineura K, et al. (1997). Central neurocytoma with clinically malignant behavior. AJNR Am J Neuroradiol. 18(6):1175–8. PMID:9194446
2568. Tong J, Hannan F, Zhu Y, Bernards A, Zhong Y (2002). Neurofibromin regulates G protein-stimulated adenylyl cyclase activity. Nat Neurosci. 5(2):95–6. PMID:11788835
2569. Torchia J, Picard D, Lafay-Cousin L, Hawkins CE, Kim SK, Letourneau L, et al. (2015). Molecular subgroups of atypical teratoid rhabdoid tumours in children: an integrated genomic and clinicopathological analysis. Lancet Oncol. 16(5):569–82. PMID:25882982
2570. Torres CF, Korones DN, Pilcher W (1997). Multiple ependymomas in a patient with Turcot's syndrome. Med Pediatr Oncol. 28(1):59–61. PMID:8950338
2571. Trehan G, Bruge H, Vinchon M, Khalil C, Ruchoux MM, Dhellemmes P, et al. (2004). MR imaging in the diagnosis of desmoplastic infantile tumor: retrospective study of six cases. AJNR Am J Neuroradiol. 25(6):1028–33. PMID:15205142
2572. Tresser N, Parveen T, Roessmann U (1993). Intracranial lipomas with teratomatous elements. Arch Pathol Lab Med. 117(9):918–20. PMID:8368905
2573. Trifanescu R, Ansorge O, Wass JA, Grossman AB, Karavitaki N (2012). Rathke's cleft cysts. Clin Endocrinol (Oxf). 76(2):151–60. PMID:21951110
2574. Trimbath JD, Petersen GM, Erdman SH, Ferre M, Luce MC, Giardiello FM (2001). Café-au-lait spots and early onset colorectal neoplasia: a variant of HNPCC? Fam Cancer. 1(2):101–5. PMID:14574005
2575. Trofatter JA, MacCollin MM, Rutter JL, Murrell JR, Duyao MP, Parry DM, et al. (1993). A novel moesin-, ezrin-, radixin-like gene is a candidate for the neurofibromatosis 2 tumor suppressor. Cell. 72(5):791–800. PMID:8453669
2576. Troost D, Jansen GH, Dingemans KP (1990). Cerebral medulloepithelioma–electron microscopy and immunohistochemistry. Acta Neuropathol. 80(1):103–7. PMID:2360414
2577. Trost D, Ehrler M, Fimmers R, Felsberg J, Sabel MC, Kirsch L, et al. (2007). Identification of genomic aberrations associated with shorter overall survival in patients with oligodendroglial tumors. Int J Cancer. 120(11):2368–76. PMID:17285580
2578. Tsai CJ, Wang Y, Allen PK, Mahajan A, McCutcheon IE, Rao G, et al. (2014). Outcomes after surgery and radiotherapy for spinal myxopapillary ependymoma: update of the MD Anderson Cancer Center experience. Neurosurgery. 75(3):205–14, discussion 213–4. PMID:24818785
2579. Tsikitis M, Zhang Z, Edelman W, Zagzag D, Kalpana GV (2005). Genetic ablation of Cyclin D1 abrogates genesis of rhabdoid tumors resulting from Ini1 loss. Proc Natl Acad Sci U S A. 102(34):12129–34. PMID:16099835
2580. Tso CL, Freije WA, Day A, Chen Z, Merriman B, Perlina A, et al. (2006). Distinct transcription profiles of primary and secondary glioblastoma subgroups. Cancer Res. 66(1):159–67. PMID:16397228
2581. Tsou HC, Teng DH, Ping XL, Brancolini V, Davis T, Hu R, et al. (1997). The role of MMAC1 mutations in early-onset breast cancer: causative in association with Cowden syndrome and excluded in BRCA1-negative cases. Am J Hum Genet. 61(5):1036–43. PMID:9345101
2582. Tsuchida T, Matsumoto M, Shirayama Y, Imahori T, Kasai H, Kawamoto K (1996). Neuronal and glial characteristics of central neurocytoma: electron microscopical analysis of two cases. Acta Neuropathol. 91(6):573–7. PMID:8781655
2583. Tsukayama C, Arakawa Y (2002). A papillary glioneuronal tumor arising in an elderly woman: a case report. Brain Tumor Pathol. 19(1):35–9. PMID:12455887
2584. Tsumanuma I, Sato M, Okazaki H, Tanaka R, Washiyama K, Kawasaki T, et al. (1995). The analysis of p53 tumor suppressor gene in pineal parenchymal tumors. Noshuyo Byori. 12(1):39–43. PMID:7795728
2585. Tsumanuma I, Tanaka R, Abe S, Kawasaki T, Washiyama K, Kumanishi T (1997). Infrequent mutation of Waf1/p21 gene, a CDK inhibitor gene, in brain tumors. Neurol Med Chir (Tokyo). 37(2):150–6, discussion 156–7. PMID:9059037
2586. Tsumanuma I, Tanaka R, Washiyama K (1999). Clinicopathological study of pineal parenchymal tumors: correlation between histopathological features, proliferative potential, and prognosis. Brain Tumor Pathol. 16(2):61–8. PMID:10746962
2587. Tu PH, Giannini C, Judkins AR, Schwalb JM, Burack R, O'Neill BP, et al. (2005). Clinicopathologic and genetic profile of intracranial marginal zone lymphoma: a primary low-grade CNS lymphoma that mimics meningioma. J Clin Oncol. 23(24):5718–27. PMID:16009945
2588. Tucker T, Wolkenstein P, Revuz J, Zeller J, Friedman JM (2005). Association between benign and malignant peripheral nerve sheath tumors in NF1. Neurology. 65(2):205–11. PMID:16043787
2589. Turcan S, Rohle D, Goenka A, Walsh LA, Fang F, Yilmaz E, et al. (2012). IDH1 mutation is sufficient to establish the glioma hypermethylator phenotype. Nature. 483(7390):479–83. PMID:22343889
2590. Turcot J, Despres JP, St Pierre F (1959). Malignant tumors of the central nervous system associated with familial polyposis of the colon: report of two cases. Dis Colon Rectum. 2:465–8. PMID:13839882
2591. Uchikawa H, Toyoda M, Nagao K, Miyauchi H, Nishikawa R, Fujii K, et al. (2006). Brain- and heart-specific Patched-1 containing exon 12b is a dominant negative isoform and is expressed in medulloblastomas. Biochem Biophys Res Commun. 349(1):277–83. PMID:16934747
2592. Ud Din N, Memon A, Aftab K, Ahmad Z, Ahmed R, Hassan S (2012). Oligodendroglioma arising in the glial component of ovarian teratomas: a series of six cases and review of literature. J Clin Pathol. 65(7):631–4. PMID:22496515
2593. Ueba T, Okawa M, Abe H, Inoue T, Takano K, Hayashi H, et al. (2013). Central nervous system marginal zone B-cell lymphoma of mucosa-associated lymphoid tissue type involving the brain and spinal cord parenchyma. Neuropathology. 33(3):306–11. PMID:22994302
2594. Ueki K, Ono Y, Henson JW, Efird JT, von Deimling A, Louis DN (1996). CDKN2/p16 or RB alterations occur in the majority of glioblastomas and are inversely correlated. Cancer Res. 56(1):150–3. PMID:8548755
2595. Ulbright TM, Hattab EM, Zhang S, Ehrlich Y, Foster RS, Einhorn LH, et al. (2010). Primitive neuroectodermal tumors in patients with testicular germ cell tumors usually resemble pediatric-type central nervous system embryonal neoplasms and lack chromosome 22 rearrangements. Mod Pathol. 23(7):972–80. PMID:20348883
2596. Ulm AJ, Yachnis AT, Brat DJ, Rhoton AL Jr (2004). Pituicytoma: report of two cases and clues regarding histogenesis. Neurosurgery. 54(3):753–7, discussion 757–8. PMID:15028154
2597. Ulrich J, Heitz PU, Fischer T, Obrist E, Gullotta F (1987). Granular cell tumors: evidence for heterogeneous tumor cell differentiation. An immunocytochemical study. Virchows Arch B Cell Pathol Incl Mol Pathol. 53(1):52–7. PMID:2885972
2598. Uluc K, Arsava EM, Ozkan B, Cila A, Zorlu F, Tan E (2004). Primary leptomeningeal sarcomatosis; a pathology proven case with challenging MRI and clinical findings. J Neurooncol. 66(3):307–12. PMID:15015662
2599. Uno K, Takita J, Yokomori K, Tanaka Y, Ohta S, Shimada H, et al. (2002). Aberrations of the hSNF5/INI1 gene are restricted to malignant rhabdoid tumors or atypical teratoid/rhabdoid tumors in pediatric solid tumors. Genes Chromosomes Cancer. 34(1):33–41. PMID:11921280
2600. Upadhyaya M, Huson SM, Davies M, Thomas N, Chuzhanova N, Giovannini S, et al. (2007). An absence of cutaneous neurofibromas associated with a 3-bp inframe deletion in exon 17 of the NF1 gene (c.2970–2972 delAAT): evidence of a clinically significant NF1 genotype-phenotype correlation. Am J Hum Genet. 80(1):140–51. PMID:17160901
2601. Upadhyaya M, Spurlock G, Kluwe L, Chuzhanova N, Bennett E, Thomas N, et al. (2009). The spectrum of somatic and germline NF1 mutations in NF1 patients with spinal neurofibromas. Neurogenetics. 10(3):251–63. PMID:19221814
2602. Urbach H (2012). High-field magnetic resonance imaging for epilepsy. Neuroimaging Clin N Am. 22(2):173–89, ix–x. [ix-x.] PMID:22548927
2603. Ushio Y, Arita N, Yoshimine T, Ikeda T, Mogami H (1987). Malignant recurrence of childhood cerebellar astrocytoma: case report. Neurosurgery. 21(2):251–5. PMID:3309714
2604. Usul H, Kuzeyli K, Cakir E, Caylan R, Sayin OC, Peksoylu B, et al. (2005). Giant cranial extradural primary fibroxanthoma: a case report. Surg Neurol. 63(3):281–4. PMID:15734528
2605. Vajtai I, Beck J, Kappeler A, Hewer E (2011). Spindle cell oncocytoma of the pituitary gland with follicle-like component: organotypic differentiation to support its origin from folliculo-stellate cells. Acta Neuropathol. 122(2):253–8. PMID:21590491
2606. Vajtai I, Kappeler A, Lukes A, Arnold M, Lüthy AR, Leibundgut K (2006). Papillary glioneuronal tumor. Pathol Res Pract. 202(2):107–12. PMID:16413693
2607. Vajtai I, Varga Z, Aguzzi A (1996). MIB-1 immunoreactivity reveals different labelling in low-grade and in malignant epithelial neoplasms of the choroid plexus. Histopathology. 29(2):147–51. PMID:8872148
2608. Val-Bernal JF, Hernando M, Garijo MF, Villa P (1997). Renal perineurioma in childhood. Gen Diagn Pathol. 143(1):75–81. PMID:9269912
2609. Valdez R, McKeever P, Finn WG, Gebarski S, Schnitzer B (2002). Composite germ cell tumor and B-cell non-Hodgkin's lymphoma arising in the sella turcica. Hum Pathol. 33(10):1044–7. PMID:12395379
2610. Valenti MP, Froelich S, Armspach JP, Chenard MP, Dietemann JL, Kerhli P, et al. (2002). Contribution of SISCOM imaging in the presurgical evaluation of temporal lobe epilepsy related to dysembryoplastic neuroepithelial tumors. Epilepsia. 43(3):270–6. PMID:11906512
2611. van den Bent MJ (2010). Interobserver variation of the histopathological diagnosis in clinical trials on glioma: a clinician's perspective. Acta Neuropathol. 120(3):297–304. PMID:20644945
2612. van den Bent MJ (2014). Practice changing mature results of RTOG study 9802: another positive PCV trial makes adjuvant chemotherapy part of standard of care in low-grade glioma. Neuro Oncol. 16(12):1570–4. PMID:25355680
2613. van den Bent MJ, Afra D, de Witte O, Ben Hassel M, Schraub S, Hoang-Xuan K, et al.; EORTC Radiotherapy and Brain Tumor Groups and the UK Medical Research Council (2005). Long-term efficacy of early versus delayed radiotherapy for low-grade astrocytoma and oligodendroglioma in adults: the EORTC 22845 randomised trial. Lancet. 366(9490):985–90. PMID:16168780
2614. van den Bent MJ, Brandes AA, Rampling R, Kouwenhoven MC, Kros JM, Carpentier AF, et al. (2009). Randomized phase II trial of erlotinib versus temozolomide or carmustine in recurrent glioblastoma: EORTC brain tumor group study 26034. J Clin Oncol. 27(8):1268–74. PMID:19204207
2615. van den Bent MJ, Brandes AA, Taphoorn MJ, Kros JM, Kouwenhoven MC, Delattre JY, et al. (2013). Adjuvant procarbazine, lomustine, and vincristine chemotherapy in newly diagnosed anaplastic oligodendroglioma: long-term follow-up of EORTC brain tumor group study 26951. J Clin Oncol. 31(3):344–50. PMID:23071237
2616. van den Bent MJ, Bromberg JE (2012). Anaplastic oligodendroglial tumors. Handb Clin Neurol. 105:467–84. PMID:22230513
2617. van den Bent MJ, Carpentier AF, Brandes AA, Sanson M, Taphoorn MJ, Bernsen HJ, et al. (2006). Adjuvant procarbazine, lomustine, and vincristine improves progression-free survival but not overall survival in newly diagnosed anaplastic oligodendrogliomas and oligoastrocytomas: a randomized European Organisation for Research and Treatment of Cancer phase III trial. J Clin Oncol. 24(18):2715–22. PMID:16782911
2618. van den Bent MJ, Dubbink HJ, Marie Y, Brandes AA, Taphoorn MJ, Wesseling P, et al. (2010). IDH1 and IDH2 mutations are prognostic but not predictive for outcome in anaplastic oligodendroglial tumors: a report of the European Organization for Research and Treatment of Cancer Brain Tumor Group. Clin Cancer Res. 16(5):1597–604. PMID:20160062
2619. van den Bent MJ, Dubbink HJ, Sanson M, van der Lee-Haarloo CR, Hegi M, Jeuken JW, et al. (2009). MGMT promoter methylation is prognostic but not predictive for outcome to adjuvant PCV chemotherapy in anaplastic oligodendroglial tumors: a report from EORTC Brain Tumor Group Study 26951. J Clin Oncol. 27(35):5881–6. PMID:19901104
2620. van den Bent MJ, Gravendeel LA, Gorlia T, Kros JM, Lapre L, Wesseling P, et al. (2011). A hypermethylated phenotype is a better predictor of survival than MGMT methylation in anaplastic oligodendroglial brain tumors: a report from EORTC study 26951. Clin Cancer Res. 17(22):7148–55. PMID:21914791
2621. Van den Bent MJ, Reni M, Gatta G, Vecht C (2008). Oligodendroglioma. Crit Rev Oncol Hematol. 66(3):262–72. PMID:18272388
2622. van den Munckhof P, Christiaans I, Kenter SB, Baas F, Hulsebos TJ (2012). Germline SMARCB1 mutation predisposes to multiple meningiomas and schwannomas with preferential location of cranial meningiomas at the falx cerebri. Neurogenetics. 13(1):1–7. PMID:22038540
2623. Van Gompel JJ, Koeller KK, Meyer FB, Marsh WR, Burger PC, Roncaroli F, et al. (2011). Cortical ependymoma: an unusual epileptogenic lesion. J Neurosurg. 114(4):1187–94. PMID:21235315
2624. Van Meir EG (1998). "Turcot's syndrome": phenotype of brain tumors, survival and mode of inheritance. Int J Cancer. 75(1):162–4. PMID:9426707
2625. van Slegtenhorst M, de Hoogt R, Hermans C, Nellist M, Janssen B, Verhoef S, et al. (1997). Identification of the tuberous sclerosis gene TSC1 on chromosome 9q34. Science. 277(5327):805–8. PMID:9242607
2626. van Slegtenhorst M, Verhoef S, Tempelaars A, Bakker L, Wang Q, Wessels M, et al. (1999). Mutational spectrum of the TSC1 gene in a cohort of 225 tuberous sclerosis complex

patients: no evidence for genotype-phenotype correlation. J Med Genet. 36(4):285–9. PMID:10227394

2627. van Thuijl HF, Mazor T, Johnson BE, Fouse SD, Aihara K, Hong C, et al. (2015). Evolution of DNA repair defects during malignant progression of low-grade gliomas after temozolomide treatment. Acta Neuropathol. 129(4):597–607. PMID:25724300

2628. VandenBerg SR (1993). Desmoplastic infantile ganglioglioma and desmoplastic cerebral astrocytoma of infancy. Brain Pathol. 3(3):275–81. PMID:8293187

2629. VandenBerg SR, May EE, Rubinstein LJ, Herman MM, Perentes E, Vinores SA, et al. (1987). Desmoplastic supratentorial neuroepithelial tumors of infancy with divergent differentiation potential ("desmoplastic infantile gangliogliomas"). Report on 11 cases of a distinctive embryonal tumor with favorable prognosis. J Neurosurg. 66(1):58–71. PMID:3097276

2630. Vandewalle G, Brucher JM, Michotte A (1995). Intracranial facial nerve rhabdomyoma. Case report. J Neurosurg. 83(5):919–22. PMID:7472566

2631. Vang R, Heck K, Fuller GN, Medeiros LJ (2000). Granular cell tumor of intracranial meninges. Clin Neuropathol. 19(1):41–4. PMID:10774952

2632. Varga Z, Vajtai I, Aguzzi A (1996). The standard isoform of CD44 is preferentially expressed in atypical papillomas and carcinomas of the choroid plexus. Pathol Res Pract. 192(12):1225–31. PMID:9182293

2633. Varikatt W, Dexter M, Mahajan H, Murali R, Ng T (2009). Usefulness of smears in intra-operative diagnosis of newly described entities of CNS. Neuropathology. 29(6):641–8. PMID:19563508

2634. Varley JM, McGown G, Thorncroft M, Santibanez-Koref MF, Kelsey AM, Tricker KJ, et al. (1997). Germ-line mutations of TP53 in Li-Fraumeni families: an extended study of 39 families. Cancer Res. 57(15):3245–52. PMID:9242456

2635. Vasen HF, Ghorbanoghli Z, Bourdeaut F, Cabaret O, Caron O, Duval A, et al.; EU-Consortium Care for CMMR-D (C4CMMR-D) (2014). Guidelines for surveillance of individuals with constitutional mismatch repair-deficiency proposed by the European Consortium "Care for CMMR-D" (C4CMMR-D). J Med Genet. 51(5):283–93. PMID:24556086

2636. Vasen HF, Tomlinson I, Castells A (2015). Clinical management of hereditary colorectal cancer syndromes. Nat Rev Gastroenterol Hepatol. 12(2):88–97. PMID:25582351

2637. Vasiljevic A, Champier J, Figarella-Branger D, Wierinckx A, Jouvet A, Fèvre-Montange M (2013). Molecular characterization of central neurocytomas: potential markers for tumor typing and progression. Neuropathology. 33(2):149–61. PMID:22816789

2638. Vasiljevic A, François P, Loundou A, Fèvre-Montange M, Jouvet A, Roche PH, et al. (2012). Prognostic factors in central neurocytomas: a multicenter study of 71 cases. Am J Surg Pathol. 36(2):220–7. PMID:22251941

2639. Vater I, Montesinos-Rongen M, Schlesner M, Haake A, Purschke F, Sprute R, et al. (2015). The mutational pattern of primary lymphoma of the central nervous system determined by whole-exome sequencing. Leukemia. 29(3):677–85. PMID:25189415

2639A. Vaubel RA, Chen SG, Raleigh DR, Link MJ, Chicoine MR, Barani I, et al. (2016). Meningiomas With Rhabdoid Features Lacking Other Histologic Features of Malignancy: A Study of 44 Cases and Review of the Literature. J Neuropathol Exp Neurol. 75(1):44–52. PMID:26705409

2640. Vecht CJ, Kerkhof M, Duran-Pena A (2014). Seizure prognosis in brain tumors: new insights and evidence-based management. Oncologist. 19(7):751–9. PMID:24899645

2641. Vege KD, Giannini C, Scheithauer BW (2000). The immunophenotype of ependymomas. Appl Immunohistochem Mol Morphol. 8(1):25–31. PMID:10937045

2642. Venkataraman G, Rizzo KA, Chavez JJ, Streubel B, Raffeld M, Jaffe ES, et al. (2011). Marginal zone lymphomas involving meningeal dura: possible link to IgG4-related diseases. Mod Pathol. 24(3):355–66. PMID:21102421

2643. Venkataraman S, Pandian C, Kumar SA (2013). Primary spinal primitive neuroectodermal tumour - a case report. Ann Neurosci. 20(2):80–2. PMID:25206019

2644. Venneti S, Santi M, Felicella MM, Yarilin D, Phillips JJ, Sullivan LM, et al. (2014). A sensitive and specific histopathologic prognostic marker for H3F3A K27M mutant pediatric glioblastomas. Acta Neuropathol. 128(5):743–53. PMID:25200322

2645. Verhaak RG, Hoadley KA, Purdom E, Wang V, Qi Y, Wilkerson MD, et al.; Cancer Genome Atlas Research Network (2010). Integrated genomic analysis identifies clinically relevant subtypes of glioblastoma characterized by abnormalities in PDGFRA, IDH1, EGFR, and NF1. Cancer Cell. 17(1):98–110. PMID:20129251

2646. Verhoef S, Bakker L, Tempelaars AM, Hesseling-Janssen AL, Mazurczak T, Jozwiak S, et al. (1999). High rate of mosaicism in tuberous sclerosis complex. Am J Hum Genet. 64(6):1632–7. PMID:10330349

2647. Verma A, Zhou H, Chin S, Bruggers C, Kestle J, Khatua S (2012). EGFR as a predictor of relapse in myxopapillary ependymoma. Pediatr Blood Cancer. 59(4):746–8. PMID:22190537

2648. Versteege I, Medjkane S, Rouillard D, Delattre O (2002). A key role of the hSNF5/INI1 tumour suppressor in the control of the G1-S transition of the cell cycle. Oncogene. 21(42):6403–12. PMID:12226744

2649. Versteege I, Sévenet N, Lange J, Rousseau-Merck MF, Ambros P, Handgretinger R, et al. (1998). Truncating mutations of hSNF5/INI1 in aggressive paediatric cancer. Nature. 394(6689):203–6. PMID:9671307

2650. Vescovi AL, Galli R, Reynolds BA (2006). Brain tumour stem cells. Nat Rev Cancer. 6(6):425–36. PMID:16723989

2651. Villà S, Miller RC, Krengli M, Abusaris H, Baumert BG, Servagi-Vernat S, et al. (2012). Primary pineal tumors: outcome and prognostic factors–a study from the Rare Cancer Network (RCN). Clin Transl Oncol. 14(11):827–34. PMID:22914906

2652. Villano JL, Koshy M, Shaikh H, Dolecek TA, McCarthy BJ (2011). Age, gender, and racial differences in incidence and survival in primary CNS lymphoma. Br J Cancer. 105(9):1414–8. PMID:21915121

2653. Villano JL, Parker CK, Dolecek TA (2013). Descriptive epidemiology of ependymal tumours in the United States. Br J Cancer. 108(11):2367–71. PMID:23660944

2654. Vinchon M, Blond S, Lejeune JP, Krivosik I, Fossati P, Assaker R, et al. (1994). Association of Lhermitte-Duclos and Cowden disease: report of a new case and review of the literature. J Neurol Neurosurg Psychiatry. 57(6):699–704. PMID:8006650

2655. Vinters HV, Park SH, Johnson MW, Mischel PS, Catania M, Kerfoot C (1999). Cortical dysplasia, genetic abnormalities and neurocutaneous syndromes. Dev Neurosci. 21(3-5):248–59. PMID:10575248

2656. Vital A, Vital C, Martin-Negrier ML, McGrogan G, Bioulac P, Trojani M, et al. (1994). Lhermitte-Duclos type cerebellum hamartoma and Cowden disease. Clin Neuropathol. 13(4):229–31. PMID:7955671

2657. Vivekanandan S, Dickinson P, Bessell E, O'Connor S (2011). An unusual case of primary anaplastic large cell central nervous system lymphoma: an 8-year success story. BMJ Case Rep. 2011:2011. PMID:22707580

2658. Vogazianou AP, Chan R, Bäcklund LM, Pearson DM, Liu L, Langford CF, et al. (2010). Distinct patterns of 1p and 19q alterations identify subtypes of human gliomas that have different prognoses. Neuro Oncol. 12(7):664–78. PMID:20164239

2659. Vogelgesang S, Junge MH, Pahnke J, Gaab MR, Warzok RW (2002). August 2001: Sellar/suprasellar mass in a 59-year-old woman. Brain Pathol. 12(1):135–6, 139. PMID:11770897

2660. von Deimling A, Fimmers R, Schmidt MC, Bender B, Fassbender F, Nagel J, et al. (2000). Comprehensive allelotype and genetic anaysis of 466 human nervous system tumors. J Neuropathol Exp Neurol. 59(6):544–58. PMID:10850867

2661. von Deimling A, Janzer R, Kleihues P, Wiestler OD (1990). Patterns of differentiation in central neurocytoma. An immunohistochemical study of eleven biopsies. Acta Neuropathol. 79(5):473–9. PMID:2109481

2662. von Deimling A, Kleihues P, Saremaslani P, Yasargil MG, Spoerri O, Südhof TC, et al. (1991). Histogenesis and differentiation potential of central neurocytomas. Lab Invest. 64(4):585–91. PMID:1901927

2663. von Deimling A, Larson J, Wellenreuther R, Stangl AP, van Velthoven V, Warnick R, et al. (1999). Clonal origin of recurrent meningiomas. Brain Pathol. 9(4):645–50. PMID:10517503

2664. von Hoff K, Hartmann W, von Bueren AO, Gerber NU, Grotzer MA, Pietsch T, et al. (2010). Large cell/anaplastic medulloblastoma: outcome according to myc status, histopathological, and clinical risk factors. Pediatr Blood Cancer. 54(3):369–76. PMID:19908297

2665. von Hoff K, Hinkes B, Dannenmann-Stern E, von Bueren AO, Warmuth-Metz M, Soerensen N, et al. (2011). Frequency, risk-factors and survival of children with atypical teratoid rhabdoid tumors (AT/RT) of the CNS diagnosed between 1988 and 2004, and registered to the German HIT database. Pediatr Blood Cancer. 57(6):978–85. PMID:21796761

2666. von Koch CS, Gulati M, Aldape K, Berger MS (2002). Familial medulloblastoma: case report of one family and review of the literature. Neurosurgery. 51(1):227–33, discussion 233. PMID:12182422

2667. Vorechovský I, Tingby O, Hartman M, Strömberg B, Nister M, Collins VP, et al. (1997). Somatic mutations in the human homologue of Drosophila patched in primitive neuroectodermal tumours. Oncogene. 15(3):361–6. PMID:9233770

2668. Vorechovský I, Undén AB, Sandstedt B, Toftgård R, Ståhle-Bäckdahl M (1997). Trichoepitheliomas contain somatic mutations in the overexpressed PTCH gene: support for a gatekeeper mechanism in skin tumorigenesis. Cancer Res. 57(21):4677–81. PMID:9354420

2669. Vortmeyer AO, Frank S, Jeong SY, Yuan K, Ikejiri B, Lee YS, et al. (2003). Developmental arrest of angioblastic lineage initiates tumorigenesis in von Hippel-Lindau disease. Cancer Res. 63(21):7051–5. PMID:14612494

2670. Vortmeyer AO, Gnarra JR, Emmert-Buck MR, Katz D, Linehan WM, Oldfield EH, et al. (1997). von Hippel-Lindau gene deletion detected in the stromal cell component of a cerebellar hemangioblastoma associated with von Hippel-Lindau disease. Hum Pathol. 28(5):540–3. PMID:9158701

2671. Vredenburgh JJ, Desjardins A, Herndon JE 2nd, Dowell JM, Reardon DA, Quinn JA, et al. (2007). Phase II trial of bevacizumab and irinotecan in recurrent malignant glioma. Clin Cancer Res. 13(4):1253–9. PMID:17317837

2672. Vujovic S, Henderson S, Presneau N, Odell E, Jacques TS, Tirabosco R, et al. (2006). Brachyury, a crucial regulator of notochordal development, is a novel biomarker for chordomas. J Pathol. 209(2):157–65. PMID:16538613

2673. Vuorinen V, Sallinen P, Haapasalo H, Visakorpi T, Kallio M, Jääskeläinen J (1996). Outcome of 31 intracranial haemangiopericytomas: poor predictive value of cell proliferation indices. Acta Neurochir (Wien). 138(12):1399–408. PMID:9030346

2674. Wacker MR, Cogen PH, Etzell JE, Daneshvar L, Davis RL, Prados MD (1992). Diffuse leptomeningeal involvement by a ganglioglioma in a child. Case report. J Neurosurg. 77(2):302–6. PMID:1625019

2675. Wakai S, Segawa H, Kitahara S, Asano T, Sano K, Ogihara R, et al. (1980). Teratoma in the pineal region in two brothers. Case reports. J Neurosurg. 53(2):239–43. PMID:7431063

2676. Wakamatsu T, Matsuo T, Kawano S, Teramoto S, Matsumura H (1971). Glioblastoma with extracranial metastasis through ventriculopleural shunt. Case report. J Neurosurg. 34(5):697–701. PMID:4326303

2677. Waldron JS, Tihan T (2003). Epidemiology and pathology of intraventricular tumors. Neurosurg Clin N Am. 14(4):469–82. PMID:15024796

2678. Walker C, Baborie A, Crooks D, Wilkins S, Jenkinson MD (2011). Biology, genetics and imaging of glial cell tumours. Br J Radiol. 84(Spec No 2):S90–106. PMID:22433833

2679. Walker C, Joyce KA, Thompson-Hehir J, Davies MP, Gibbs FE, Halliwell N, et al. (2001). Characterisation of molecular alterations in microdissected archival gliomas. Acta Neuropathol. 101(4):321–33. PMID:11355303

2680. Walker L, Thompson D, Easton D, Ponder B, Ponder M, Frayling I, et al. (2006). A prospective study of neurofibromatosis type 1 cancer incidence in the UK. Br J Cancer. 95(2):233–8. PMID:16786042

2681. Walker LS, Sansom DM (2011). The emerging role of CTLA4 as a cell-extrinsic regulator of T cell responses. Nat Rev Immunol. 11(12):852–63. PMID:22116087

2682. Wallner KE, Gonzales MF, Edwards MS, Wara WM, Sheline GE (1988). Treatment results of juvenile pilocytic astrocytoma. J Neurosurg. 69(2):171–6. PMID:3392563

2683. Wanebo JE, Lonser RR, Glenn GM, Oldfield EH (2003). The natural history of hemangioblastomas of the central nervous system in patients with von Hippel-Lindau disease. J Neurosurg. 98(1):82–94. PMID:12546356

2684. Wang CC, Turner J, Steel T (2013). Spontaneous pineal apoplexy in a pineal parenchymal tumor of intermediate differentiation. Cancer Biol Med. 10(1):43–6. PMID:23691444

2685. Wang F, Travins J, DeLaBarre B, Penard-Lacronique V, Schalm S, Hansen E, et al. (2013). Targeted inhibition of mutant IDH2 in leukemia cells induces cellular differentiation. Science. 340(6132):622–6. PMID:23558173

2686. Wang H, Zhang S, Rehman SK, Zhang Z, Li W, Makki MS, et al. (2014). Clinicopathological features of myxopapillary ependymoma. J Clin Neurosci. 21(4):569–73. PMID:24332590

2687. Wang H, Zhang S, Wu C, Zhang Z, Qin T (2013). Melanocytomas of the central nervous system: a clinicopathological and molecular study. Eur J Clin Invest. 43(8):809–15. PMID:23683178

2688. Wang L, Motoi T, Khanin R, Olshen A, Mertens F, Bridge J, et al. (2012). Identification of a novel, recurrent HEY1-NCOA2 fusion in mesenchymal chondrosarcoma based on a genome-wide screen of exon-level expression data. Genes Chromosomes Cancer. 51(2):127–39. PMID:22034177

2689. Wang L, Yamaguchi S, Burstein MD, Terashima K, Chang K, Ng HK, et al. (2014). Novel somatic and germline mutations in intracranial germ cell tumours. Nature. 511(7508):241–5. PMID:24896186

2690. Wang M, Jia D, Shen J, Zhang J, Li G (2013). Clinical and imaging features of central neurocytomas. J Clin Neurosci. 20(5):679–85. PMID:23522930

2691. Wang M, Tihan T, Rojiani AM, Bodhireddy

SR, Prayson RA, Iacuone JJ, et al. (2005). Monomorphous angiocentric glioma: a distinctive epileptogenic neoplasm with features of infiltrating astrocytoma and ependymoma. J Neuropathol Exp Neurol. 64(10):875–81. PMID:16215459
2692. Wang X, Dubuc AM, Ramaswamy V, Mack S, Gendoo DM, Remke M, et al. (2015). Medulloblastoma subgroups remain stable across primary and metastatic compartments. Acta Neuropathol. 129(3):449–57. PMID:25689980
2693. Wang XQ, Zhou Q, Li ST, Liao CL, Zhang H, Zhang BY (2013). Solitary fibrous tumors of the central nervous system: clinical features and imaging findings in 22 patients. J Comput Assist Tomogr. 37(5):658–65. PMID:24045237
2694. Wang Y, Xiong J, Chu SG, Liu Y, Cheng HX, Wang YF, et al. (2009). Rosette-forming glioneuronal tumor: report of an unusual case with intraventricular dissemination. Acta Neuropathol. 118(6):813–9. PMID:19585134
2695. Wanggou S, Jiang X, Li Q, Zhang L, Liu D, Li G, et al. (2012). HESRG: a novel biomarker for intracranial germinoma and embryonal carcinoma. J Neurooncol. 106(2):251–9. PMID:21861197
2696. Wani K, Armstrong TS, Vera-Bolanos E, Raghunathan A, Ellison D, Gilbertson R, et al.; Collaborative Ependymoma Research Network (2012). A prognostic gene expression signature in infratentorial ependymoma. Acta Neuropathol. 123(5):727–38. PMID:22322993
2697. Warmuth-Metz M, Bison B, Gerber NU, Pietsch T, Hasselblatt M, Frühwald MC (2013). Bone involvement in atypical teratoid/rhabdoid tumors of the CNS. AJNR Am J Neuroradiol. 34(10):2039–42. PMID:23681355
2698. Warnick RE, Raisanen J, Adornato BT, Prados MD, Davis RL, Larson DA, et al. (1993). Intracranial myxopapillary ependymoma: case report. J Neurooncol. 15(3):251–6. PMID:8360710
2699. Warren C, James LA, Ramsden RT, Wallace A, Baser ME, Varley JM, et al. (2003). Identification of recurrent regions of chromosome loss and gain in vestibular schwannomas using comparative genomic hybridisation. J Med Genet. 40(11):802–6. PMID:14627667
2700. Warren KE (2012). Diffuse intrinsic pontine glioma: poised for progress. Front Oncol. 2:205. PMID:23293772
2701. Wasdahl DA, Scheithauer BW, Andrews BT, Jeffrey RA Jr (1994). Cerebellar pleomorphic xanthoastrocytoma: case report. Neurosurgery. 35(5):947–50, discussion 950–1. PMID:7838347
2702. Watanabe K, Ogata N, von Ammon K, Yonekawa Y, Nagai M, Ohgaki H, et al. (1996). Immunohistochemical assessments of p53 protein accumulation and tumor growth fraction during the progression of astrocytomas. In: Brain Tumour Research and Therapy. Nagai
2702A. Watanabe T, Nakamura M, Yonekawa Y, Kleihues P, Ohgaki H (2001). Promoter hypermethylation and homozygous deletion of the p14ARF and p16INK4a genes in oligodendrogliomas. Acta Neuropathol. 101(3):185–9. PMID:11307615
2703. Watanabe K, Peraud A, Gratas C, Wakai S, Kleihues P, Ohgaki H (1998). p53 and PTEN gene mutations in gemistocytic astrocytomas. Acta Neuropathol. 95(6):559–64. PMID:9650746
2704. Watanabe K, Sato K, Biernat W, Tachibana O, von Ammon K, Ogata N, et al. (1997). Incidence and timing of p53 mutations during astrocytoma progression in patients with multiple biopsies. Clin Cancer Res. 3(4):523–30. PMID:9815715
2705. Watanabe K, Tachibana O, Sata K, Yonekawa Y, Kleihues P, Ohgaki H (1996). Overexpression of the EGF receptor and p53 mutations are mutually exclusive in the evolution of primary and secondary glioblastomas. Brain Pathol. 6(3):217–23, discussion 23–4. PMID:8864278
2706. Watanabe K, Tachibana O, Yonekawa Y, Kleihues P, Ohgaki H (1997). Role of gemistocytes in astrocytoma progression. Lab Invest. 76(2):277–84. PMID:9042164
2707. Watanabe T, Makiyama Y, Nishimoto H, Matsumoto M, Kikuchi A, Tsubokawa T (1995). Metachronous ovarian dysgerminoma after a suprasellar germ-cell tumor treated by radiation therapy. Case report. J Neurosurg. 83(1):149–53. PMID:7782834
2708. Watanabe T, Mizowaki T, Arakawa Y, Iizuka Y, Ogura K, Sakanaka K, et al. (2014). Pineal parenchymal tumor of intermediate differentiation: Treatment outcomes of five cases. Mol Clin Oncol. 2(2):197–202. PMID:24649332
2709. Watanabe T, Nobusawa S, Kleihues P, Ohgaki H (2009). IDH1 mutations are early events in the development of astrocytomas and oligodendrogliomas. Am J Pathol. 174(4):1149–53. PMID:19246647
2710. Watanabe T, Vital A, Nobusawa S, Kleihues P, Ohgaki H (2009). Selective acquisition of IDH1 R132C mutations in astrocytomas associated with Li-Fraumeni syndrome. Acta Neuropathol. 117(6):653–6. PMID:19340432
2711. Weber DC, Wang Y, Miller R, Villà S, Zaucha R, Pica A, et al. (2015). Long-term outcome of patients with spinal myxopapillary ependymoma: treatment results from the MD Anderson Cancer Center and institutions from the Rare Cancer Network. Neuro Oncol. 17(4):588–95 PMID:25301811
2712. Weber HC, Marsh DJ, Lubensky IA, Lin AY, Eng C (1998). Germline PTEN/MMAC1/TEP1 mutations and association with gastrointestinal manifestations in Cowden disease. Gastroenterology. 114S:G2902.
2713. Weber RG, Hoischen A, Ehrler M, Zipper P, Kaulich K, Blaschke B, et al. (2007). Frequent loss of chromosome 9, homozygous CDKN2A/p14(ARF)/CDKN2B deletion and low TSC1 mRNA expression in pleomorphic xanthoastrocytomas. Oncogene. 26(7):1088–97. PMID:16909113
2714. Wechsler J, Lantieri L, Zeller J, Voisin MC, Martin-Garcia N, Wolkenstein P (2003). Aberrant axon neurofilaments in schwannomas associated with phacomatoses. Virchows Arch. 443(6):768–73. PMID:14508685
2715. Wechsler-Reya RJ, Scott MP (1999). Control of neuronal precursor proliferation in the cerebellum by Sonic Hedgehog. Neuron. 22(1):103–14. PMID:10027293
2716. Wefers AK, Warmuth-Metz M, Pöschl J, von Bueren AO, Monoranu CM, Seelos K, et al. (2014). Subgroup-specific localization of human medulloblastoma based on pre-operative MRI. Acta Neuropathol. 127(6):931–3. PMID:24699697
2717. Wei D, Rich P, Bridges L, Martin AJ, Chau I, Bodi I, et al. (2013). Rare case of cerebral MALToma presenting with stroke-like symptoms and seizures. BMJ Case Rep. 2013:2013. PMID:23608841
2718. Wei G, Zhang W, Li Q, Kang X, Zhao H, Liu X, et al. (2014). Magnetic resonance characteristics of adult-onset Lhermitte-Duclos disease: An indicator for active cancer surveillance? Mol Clin Oncol. 2(3):415–20. PMID:24772310
2719. Wei YQ, Hang ZB, Liu KF (1992). In situ observation of inflammatory cell-tumor cell interaction in human seminomas (germinomas): light, electron microscopic, and immunohistochemical study. Hum Pathol. 23(4):421–8. PMID:1563744
2720. Weinbreck N, Marie B, Bressenot A, Montagne K, Joud A, Baumann C, et al. (2008). Immunohistochemical markers to distinguish between hemangioblastoma and metastatic clear-cell renal cell carcinoma in the brain: utility of aquaporin1 combined with cytokeratin AE1/AE3 immunostaining. Am J Surg Pathol. 32(7):1051–9. PMID:18496143
2721. Weiner HL, Wisoff JH, Rosenberg ME, Kupersmith MJ, Cohen H, Zagzag D, et al. (1994). Craniopharyngiomas: a clinicopathological analysis of factors predictive of recurrence and functional outcome. Neurosurgery. 35(6):1001–10, discussion 1010–1. PMID:7885544
2722. Weiner HL, Zagzag D, Babu R, Weinreb HJ, Ransohoff J (1993). Schwannoma of the fourth ventricle presenting with hemifacial spasm. A report of two cases. J Neurooncol. 15(1):37–43. PMID:8455061
2723. Weingart MF, Roth JJ, Hutt-Cabezas M, Busse TM, Kaur H, Price A, et al. (2015). Disrupting LIN28 in atypical teratoid rhabdoid tumors reveals the importance of the mitogen activated protein kinase pathway as a therapeutic target. Oncotarget. 6(5):3165–77. PMID:25638158
2724. Weiss SW, Langloss JM, Enzinger FM (1983). Value of S-100 protein in the diagnosis of soft tissue tumors with particular reference to benign and malignant Schwann cell tumors. Lab Invest. 49(3):299–308. PMID:6310227
2725. Weiss WA, Burns MJ, Hackett C, Aldape K, Hill JR, Kuriyama H, et al. (2003). Genetic determinants of malignancy in a mouse model for oligodendroglioma. Cancer Res. 63(7):1589–95. PMID:12670909
2726. Welander J, Larsson C, Bäckdahl M, Hareni N, Sivlér T, Brauckhoff M, et al. (2012). Integrative genomics reveals frequent somatic NF1 mutations in sporadic pheochromocytomas. Hum Mol Genet. 21(26):5406–16. PMID:23010473
2727. Wellenreuther R, Kraus JA, Lenartz D, Menon AG, Schramm J, Louis DN, et al. (1995). Analysis of the neurofibromatosis 2 gene reveals molecular variants of meningioma. Am J Pathol. 146(4):827–32. PMID:7717450
2728. Weller M, Felsberg J, Hartmann C, Berger H, Steinbach JP, Schramm J, et al. (2009). Molecular predictors of progression-free and overall survival in patients with newly diagnosed glioblastoma: a prospective translational study of the German Glioma Network. J Clin Oncol. 27(34):5743–50. PMID:19805672
2729. Weller M, Tabatabai G, Kästner B, Felsberg J, Steinbach JP, Wick A, et al.; DIRECTOR Study Group (2015). MGMT promoter methylation is a strong prognostic biomarker for benefit from dose-intensified temozolomide rechallenge in progressive glioblastoma: the DIRECTOR trial. Clin Cancer Res. 21(9):2057–64. PMID:25655102
2730. Weller M, van den Bent M, Hopkins K, Tonn JC, Stupp R, Falini A, et al.; European Association for Neuro-Oncology (EANO) Task Force on Malignant Glioma (2014). EANO guideline for the diagnosis and treatment of anaplastic gliomas and glioblastoma. Lancet Oncol. 15(9):e395–403. PMID:25079102
2731. Weller M, Weber RG, Willscher E, Riehmer V, Hentschel B, Kreuz M, et al. (2015). Molecular classification of diffuse cerebral WHO grade II/III gliomas using genome- and transcriptome-wide profiling improves stratification of prognostically distinct patient groups. Acta Neuropathol. 129(5):679–93. PMID:25783747
2732. Wellons JC 3rd, Reddy AT, Tubbs RS, Abdullatif H, Oakes WJ, Blount JP, et al. (2004). Neuroendoscopic findings in patients with intracranial germinomas correlating with diabetes insipidus. J Neurosurg. 100(5) Suppl Pediatrics:430–6. PMID:15287450
2733. Wen PY, Kesari S (2008). Malignant gliomas in adults. N Engl J Med. 359(5):492–507. PMID:18669428
2734. Wesseling P, Schlingemann RO, Rietveld FJ, Link M, Burger PC, Ruiter DJ (1995). Early and extensive contribution of pericytes/vascular smooth muscle cells to microvascular proliferation in glioblastoma multiforme: an immuno-light and immuno-electron microscopic study. J Neuropathol Exp Neurol. 54(3):304–10. PMID:7745429
2735. Wester DJ, Falcone S, Green BA, Camp A, Quencer RM (1993). Paraganglioma of the filum: MR appearance. J Comput Assist Tomogr. 17(6):967–9. PMID:8227586
2736. Wharton SB, Chan KK, Anderson JR, Stoeber K, Williams GH (2001). Replicative Mcm2 protein as a novel proliferation marker in oligodendrogliomas and its relationship to Ki67 labelling index, histological grade and prognosis. Neuropathol Appl Neurobiol. 27(4):305–13. PMID:11532161
2737. White FV, Dehner LP, Belchis DA, Conard K, Davis MM, Stocker JT, et al. (1999). Congenital disseminated malignant rhabdoid tumor: a distinct clinicopathologic entity demonstrating abnormalities of chromosome 22q11. Am J Surg Pathol. 23(3):249–56. PMID:10078913
2738. White W, Shiu MH, Rosenblum MK, Erlandson RA, Woodruff JM (1990). Cellular schwannoma. A clinicopathologic study of 57 patients and 58 tumors. Cancer. 66(6):1266–75. PMID:2400975
2739. Whittle IR, Dow GR, Lammie GA, Wardlaw J (1999). Dsyembryoplastic neuroepithelial tumour with discrete bilateral multifocality: further evidence for a germinal origin. Br J Neurosurg. 13(5):508–11. PMID:10627786
2740. Wick W, Hartmann C, Engel C, Stoffels M, Felsberg J, Stockhammer F, et al. (2009). NOA-04 randomized phase III trial of sequential radiochemotherapy of anaplastic glioma with procarbazine, lomustine, and vincristine or temozolomide. J Clin Oncol. 27(35):5874–80. PMID:19901110
2741. Wick W, Meisner C, Hentschel B, Platten M, Schilling A, Wiestler B, et al. (2013). Prognostic or predictive value of MGMT promoter methylation in gliomas depends on IDH1 mutation. Neurology. 81(17):1515–22. PMID:24068788
2742. Wick W, Platten M, Meisner C, Felsberg J, Tabatabai G, Simon M, et al.; NOA-08 Study Group of Neuro-oncology Working Group (NOA) of German Cancer Society (2012). Temozolomide chemotherapy alone versus radiotherapy alone for malignant astrocytoma in the elderly: the NOA-08 randomised, phase 3 trial. Lancet Oncol. 13(7):707–15. PMID:22578793
2743. Wick W, Weller M, van den Bent M, Sanson M, Weiler M, von Deimling A, et al. (2014). MGMT testing–the challenges for biomarker-based glioma treatment. Nat Rev Neurol. 10(7):372–85. PMID:24912512
2744. Wicking C, Gillies S, Smyth I, Shanley S, Fowles L, Ratcliffe J, et al. (1997). De novo mutations of the Patched gene in nevoid basal cell carcinoma syndrome help to define the clinical phenotype. Am J Med Genet. 73(3):304–7. PMID:9415689
2745. Wicking C, Shanley S, Smyth I, Gillies S, Negus K, Graham S, et al. (1997). Most germline mutations in the nevoid basal cell carcinoma syndrome lead to a premature termination of the PATCHED protein, and no genotype-phenotype correlations are evident. Am J Hum Genet. 60(1):21–6. PMID:8981943
2746. Wiemels J, Wrensch M, Claus EB (2010). Epidemiology and etiology of meningioma. J Neurooncol. 99(3):307–14. PMID:20821343
2747. Wiemels JL, Wrensch M, Sison JD, Zhou M, Bondy M, Calvocoressi L, et al. (2011). Reduced allergy and immunoglobulin E among adults with intracranial meningioma compared to controls. Int J Cancer. 129(8):1932–9. PMID:21520030
2748. Wiens AL, Cheng L, Bertsch EC, Johnson KA, Zhang S, Hattab EM (2012). Polysomy of chromosomes 1 and/or 19 is common and associated with less favorable clinical outcome in oligodendrogliomas: fluorescent in situ hybridization analysis of 84 consecutive cases. J Neuropathol Exp Neurol. 71(7):618–24. PMID:22710961
2749. Wiens AL, Hattab EM (2014). The

pathological spectrum of solid CNS metastases in the pediatric population. J Neurosurg Pediatr. 14(2):129–35. PMID:24926970
2750. Wiestler B, Capper D, Holland-Letz T, Korshunov A, von Deimling A, Pfister SM, et al. (2013). ATRX loss refines the classification of anaplastic gliomas and identifies a subgroup of IDH mutant astrocytic tumors with better prognosis. Acta Neuropathol. 126(3):443–51. PMID:23904111
2751. Wiestler B, Capper D, Sill M, Jones DT, Hovestadt V, Sturm D, et al. (2014). Integrated DNA methylation and copy-number profiling identify three clinically and biologically relevant groups of anaplastic glioma. Acta Neuropathol. 128(4):561–71. PMID:25008768
2752. Wiestler OD, von Siebenthal K, Schmitt HP, Feiden W, Kleihues P (1989). Distribution and immunoreactivity of cerebral micro-hamartomas in bilateral acoustic neurofibromatosis (neurofibromatosis 2). Acta Neuropathol. 79(2):137–43. PMID:2596263
2752A. Wigertz A, Lönn S, Hall P, Auvinen A, Christensen HC, Johansen C, et al. (2008). Reproductive factors and risk of meningioma and glioma. Cancer Epidemiol Biomarkers Prev. 17(10):2663–70. PMID:18843008
2752B. Wigertz A, Lönn S, Schwartzbaum J, Hall P, Auvinen A, Christensen HC, et al. (2007). Allergic conditions and brain tumor risk. Am J Epidemiol. 166(8):941–50. PMID:17646205
2753. Wikstrand CJ, Reist CJ, Archer GE, Zalutsky MR, Bigner DD (1998). The class III variant of the epidermal growth factor receptor (EGFRvIII): characterization and utilization as an immunotherapeutic target. J Neurovirol. 4(2):148–58. PMID:9584952
2754. Wilcox P, Li CC, Lee M, Shivalingam B, Brennan J, Suter CM, et al. (2015). Oligoastrocytomas: throwing the baby out with the bathwater? Acta Neuropathol. 129(1):147–9. PMID:25304041
2755. Willard N, Kleinschmidt-DeMasters BK (2015). Massive dissemination of adult glioblastomas. Clin Neuropathol. 34(6):330–42. PMID:26308254
2756. Williams D, Mori T, Reiter A, Woessman W, Rosolen A, Wrobel G, et al.; European Intergroup for Childhood Non-Hodgkin Lymphoma, the Japanese Pediatric Leukemia/Lymphoma Study Group (2013). Central nervous system involvement in anaplastic large cell lymphoma in childhood: results from a multicentre European and Japanese study. Pediatr Blood Cancer. 60(10):E118–21. PMID:23720354
2757. Williams SR, Joos BW, Parker JC, Parker JR (2008). Papillary glioneuronal tumor: a case report and review of the literature. Ann Clin Lab Sci. 38(3):287–92. PMID:18715860
2758. Willis B, Ablin A, Weinberg V, Zoger S, Wara WM, Matthay KK (1996). Disease course and late sequelae of Langerhans' cell histiocytosis: 25-year experience at the University of California, San Francisco. J Clin Oncol. 14(7):2073–82. PMID:8683239
2759. Willis SN, Mallozzi SS, Rodig SJ, Cronk KM, McArdel SL, Caron T, et al. (2009). The microenvironment of germ cell tumors harbors a prominent antigen-driven humoral response. J Immunol. 182(5):3310–7. PMID:19234230
2760. Wilson BG, Roberts CW (2011). SWI/SNF nucleosome remodellers and cancer. Nat Rev Cancer. 11(7):481–92. PMID:21654818
2761. Wilson BG, Wang X, Shen X, McKenna ES, Lemieux ME, Cho YJ, et al. (2010). Epigenetic antagonism between polycomb and SWI/SNF complexes during oncogenic transformation. Cancer Cell. 18(4):316–28. PMID:20951942
2762. Wilson C, Bonnet C, Guy C, Idziaszczyk S, Colley J, Humphreys V, et al. (2006). Tsc1 haploinsufficiency without mammalian target of rapamycin activation is sufficient for renal cyst formation in Tsc1+/- mice. Cancer Res. 66(16):7934–8. PMID:16912167
2763. Wimmer K, Kratz CP, Vasen HF, Caron O, Colas C, Entz-Werle N, et al.; EU-Consortium Care for CMMRD (C4CMMRD) (2014). Diagnostic criteria for constitutional mismatch repair deficiency syndrome: suggestions of the European consortium 'care for CMMRD' (C4CMMRD). J Med Genet. 51(6):355–65. PMID:24737826
2764. Winek RR, Scheithauer BW, Wick MR (1989). Meningioma, meningeal hemangiopericytoma (angioblastic meningioma), peripheral hemangiopericytoma, and acoustic schwannoma. A comparative immunohistochemical study. Am J Surg Pathol. 13(4):251–61. PMID:2648875
2765. Wippold FJ 2nd, Smirniotopoulos JG, Pilgram TK (1997). Lesions of the cauda equina: a clinical and pathology review from the Armed Forces Institute of Pathology. Clin Neurol Neurosurg. 99(4):229–34. PMID:9491294
2766. Witkowski L, Lalonde E, Zhang J, Albrecht S, Hamel N, Cavallone L, et al. (2013). Familial rhabdoid tumour 'avant la lettre'–from pathology review to exome sequencing and back again. J Pathol. 231(1):35–43. PMID:23775540
2767. Witt H, Mack SC, Ryzhova M, Bender S, Sill M, Isserlin R, et al. (2011). Delineation of two clinically and molecularly distinct subgroups of posterior fossa ependymoma. Cancer Cell. 20(2):143–57. PMID:21840481
2768. Wizigmann-Voos S, Breier G, Risau W, Plate KH (1995). Up-regulation of vascular endothelial growth factor and its receptors in von Hippel-Lindau disease-associated and sporadic hemangioblastomas. Cancer Res. 55(6):1358–64. PMID:7533661
2769. Wizigmann-Voos S, Plate KH (1996). Pathology, genetics and cell biology of hemangioblastomas. Histol Histopathol. 11(4):1049–61. PMID:8930647
2770. Woehrer A, Hackl M, Waldhör T, Weis S, Pichler J, Olschowski A, et al.; Austrian Brain Tumour Registry (2014). Relative survival of patients with non-malignant central nervous system tumours: a descriptive study by the Austrian Brain Tumour Registry. Br J Cancer. 110(2):286–96. PMID:24253501
2771. Woehrer A, Slavc I, Peyrl A, Czech T, Dorfer C, Prayer D, et al. (2011). Embryonal tumor with abundant neuropil and true rosettes (ETANTR) with loss of morphological but retained genetic key features during progression. Acta Neuropathol. 122(6):787–90. PMID:22057788
2772. Wolf HK, Buslei R, Blümcke I, Wiestler OD, Pietsch T (1997). Neural antigens in oligodendrogliomas and dysembryoplastic neuroepithelial tumors. Acta Neuropathol. 94(5):436–43. PMID:9386775
2773. Wolf HK, Buslei R, Schmidt-Kastner R, Schmidt-Kastner PK, Pietsch T, Wiestler OD, et al. (1996). NeuN: a useful neuronal marker for diagnostic histopathology. J Histochem Cytochem. 44(10):1167–71. PMID:8813082
2774. Wolf HK, Müller MB, Spänle M, Zentner J, Schramm J, Wiestler OD (1994). Ganglioglioma: a detailed histopathological and immunohistochemical analysis of 61 cases. Acta Neuropathol. 88(2):166–73. PMID:7985497
2775. Wolf HK, Normann S, Green AJ, von Bakel I, Blümcke I, Pietsch T, et al. (1997). Tuberous sclerosis-like lesions in epileptogenic human neocortex lack allelic loss at the TSC1 and TSC2 regions. Acta Neuropathol. 93(1):93–6. PMID:9006662
2776. Wolff B, Ng A, Roth D, Parthey K, Warmuth-Metz M, Eyrich M, et al. (2012). Pediatric high grade glioma of the spinal cord: results of the HIT-GBM database. J Neurooncol. 107(1):139–46. PMID:21964697
2777. Wolff JE, Sajedi M, Brant R, Coppes MJ, Egeler RM (2002). Choroid plexus tumours. Br J Cancer. 87(10):1086–91. PMID:12402146
2778. Wolfsberger S, Fischer I, Höftberger R, Birner P, Slavc I, Dieckmann K, et al. (2004). Ki-67 immunolabeling index is an accurate predictor of outcome in patients with intracranial ependymoma. Am J Surg Pathol. 28(7):914–20. PMID:15223962
2779. Wolter M, Reifenberger J, Blaschke B, Ichimura K, Schmidt EE, Collins VP, et al. (2001). Oligodendroglial tumors frequently demonstrate hypermethylation of the CDKN2A (MTS1, p16INK4a), p14ARF, and CDKN2B (MTS2, p15INK4b) tumor suppressor genes. J Neuropathol Exp Neurol. 60(12):1170–80. PMID:11764089
2780. Wong AJ, Bigner SH, Bigner DD, Kinzler KW, Hamilton SR, Vogelstein B (1987). Increased expression of the epidermal growth factor receptor gene in malignant gliomas is invariably associated with gene amplification. Proc Natl Acad Sci U S A. 84(19):6899–903. PMID:3477813
2781. Wong K, Gyure KA, Prayson RA, Morrison AL, Le TQ, Armstrong RC (1999). Dysembryoplastic neuroepithelial tumor: in situ hybridization of proteolipid protein (PLP) messenger ribonucleic acid (mRNA). J Neuropathol Exp Neurol. 58:542–542.
2782. Wong KK, Tsang YT, Chang YM, Su J, Di Francesco AM, Meco D, et al. (2006). Genome-wide allelic imbalance analysis of pediatric gliomas by single nucleotide polymorphic allele array. Cancer Res. 66(23):11172–8. PMID:17145861
2783. Wong TT, Ho DM, Chang KP, Yen SH, Guo WY, Chang FC, et al. (2005). Primary pediatric brain tumors: statistics of Taipei VGH, Taiwan (1975–2004). Cancer. 104(10):2156–67. PMID:16220552
2784. Wong TT, Ho DM, Chang TK, Yang DD, Lee LS (1995). Familial neurofibromatosis 1 with germinoma involving the basal ganglion and thalamus. Childs Nerv Syst. 11(8):456–8. PMID:7585682
2785. Woodruff JM, Christensen WN (1993). Glandular peripheral nerve sheath tumors. Cancer. 72(12):3618–28. PMID:8252477
2786. Woodruff JM, Godwin TA, Erlandson RA, Susin M, Martini N (1981). Cellular schwannoma: a variety of schwannoma sometimes mistaken for a malignant tumor. Am J Surg Pathol. 5(8):733–44. PMID:7337161
2787. Woodruff JM, Marshall ML, Godwin TA, Funkhouser JW, Thompson NJ, Erlandson RA (1983). Plexiform (multinodular) schwannoma. A tumor simulating the plexiform neurofibroma. Am J Surg Pathol. 7(7):691–7. PMID:6638259
2788. Woodruff JM, Scheithauer BW, Kurtkaya-Yapicier O, Raffel C, Amr SS, LaQuaglia MP, et al. (2003). Congenital and childhood plexiform (multinodular) cellular schwannoma: a troublesome mimic of malignant peripheral nerve sheath tumor. Am J Surg Pathol. 27(10):1321–9. PMID:14508393
2789. Woodruff JM, Selig AM, Crowley K, Allen PW (1994). Schwannoma (neurilemoma) with malignant transformation. A rare, distinctive peripheral nerve tumor. Am J Surg Pathol. 18(9):882–95. PMID:8067509
2790. Wrede B, Hasselblatt M, Peters O, Thall PF, Kutluk T, Moghrabi A, et al. (2009). Atypical choroid plexus papilloma: clinical experience in the CPT-SIOP-2000 study. J Neurooncol. 95(3):383–92. PMID:19543851
2791. Wu G, Broniscer A, McEachron TA, Lu C, Paugh BS, Becksfort J, et al.; St. Jude Children's Research Hospital–Washington University Pediatric Cancer Genome Project (2012). Somatic histone H3 alterations in pediatric diffuse intrinsic pontine gliomas and non-brainstem glioblastomas. Nat Genet. 44(3):251–3. PMID:22286216
2792. Wu G, Diaz AK, Paugh BS, Rankin SL, Ju B, Li Y, et al.; St. Jude Children's Research Hospital–Washington University Pediatric Cancer Genome Project (2014). The genomic landscape of diffuse intrinsic pontine glioma and pediatric non-brainstem high-grade glioma. Nat Genet. 46(5):444–50. PMID:24705251
2793. Wu J, Williams JP, Rizvi TA, Kordich JJ, Witte D, Meijer D, et al. (2008). Plexiform and dermal neurofibromas and pigmentation are caused by Nf1 loss in desert hedgehog-expressing cells. Cancer Cell. 13(2):105–16. PMID:18242511
2794. Wu L, Yang T, Deng X, Yang C, Zhao L, Fang J, et al. (2014). Surgical outcomes in spinal cord subependymomas: an institutional experience. J Neurooncol. 116(1):99–106. PMID:24062139
2795. Wu W, Tanrivermis Sayit A, Vinters HV, Pope W, Mirsadraei L, Said J (2013). Primary central nervous system histiocytic sarcoma presenting as a postradiation sarcoma: case report and literature review. Hum Pathol. 44(6):1177–83. PMID:23356953
2796. Wu YT, Ho JT, Lin YJ, Lin JW (2011). Rhabdoid papillary meningioma: a clinicopathologic case series study. Neuropathology. 31(6):599–605. PMID:21382093
2797. Wöhrer A, Waldhör T, Heinzl H, Hackl M, Feichtinger J, Gruber-Mösenbacher U, et al. (2009). The Austrian Brain Tumour Registry: a cooperative way to establish a population-based brain tumour registry. J Neurooncol. 95(3):401–11. PMID:19562257
2798. Xekouki P, Stratakis CA (2012). Succinate dehydrogenase (SDHx) mutations in pituitary tumors: could this be a new role for mitochondrial complex II and/or Krebs cycle defects? Endocr Relat Cancer. 19(6):C33–40. PMID:22889736
2799. Xiao GH, Jin F, Yeung RS (1995). Identification of tuberous sclerosis 2 messenger RNA splice variants that are conserved and differentially expressed in rat and human tissues. Cell Growth Differ. 6(9):1185–91. PMID:8519695
2800. Xiong J, Liu Y, Chu SG, Chen H, Chen HX, Mao Y, et al. (2012). Dysembryoplastic neuroepithelial tumor-like neoplasm of the septum pellucidum: review of 2 cases with chromosome 1p/19q and IDH1 analysis. Clin Neuropathol. 31(1):31–8. PMID:22192702
2801. Xiong J, Liu Y, Chu SG, Chen H, Chen HX, Mao Y, et al. (2012). Rosette-forming glioneuronal tumor of the septum pellucidum with extension to the supratentorial ventricles: rare case with genetic analysis. Neuropathology. 32(3):301–5. PMID:22017246
2802. Xu HM, Gutmann DH (1998). Merlin differentially associates with the microtubule and actin cytoskeleton. J Neurosci Res. 51(3):403–15. PMID:9486775
2803. Xu J, Yang Y, Liu Y, Wei M, Ren J, Chang Y, et al. (2012). Rosette-forming glioneuronal tumor in the pineal gland and the third ventricle: a case with radiological and clinical implications. Quant Imaging Med Surg. 2(3):227–31. PMID:23256084
2804. Xu W, Yang H, Liu Y, Yang Y, Wang P, Kim SH, et al. (2011). Oncometabolite 2-hydroxyglutarate is a competitive inhibitor of α-ketoglutarate-dependent dioxygenases. Cancer Cell. 19(1):17–30. PMID:21251613
2805. Xu X, Zhao J, Xu Z, Peng B, Huang Q, Arnold E, et al. (2004). Structures of human cytosolic NADP-dependent isocitrate dehydrogenase reveal a novel self-regulatory mechanism of activity. J Biol Chem. 279(32):33946–57. PMID:15173171
2806. Yaşargil MG, Curcic M, Kis M, Siegenthaler G, Teddy PJ, Roth P (1990). Total removal of craniopharyngiomas. Approaches and long-term results in 144 patients. J Neurosurg. 73(1):3–11. PMID:2352020
2807. Yamada H, Haratake J, Narasaki T, Oda T (1995). Embryonal craniopharyngioma. Case report of the morphogenesis of a craniopharyngioma. Cancer. 75(12):2971–7. PMID:7773950
2808. Yamamoto K, Yamada K, Nakahara T, Ishihara A, Takaki S, Kochi M, et al. (2002). Rapid regrowth of solitary subependymal giant cell astrocytoma–case report. Neurol Med Chir (Tokyo). 42(5):224–7. PMID:12064158
2809. Yamane Y, Mena H, Nakazato Y (2002).

Immunohistochemical characterization of pineal parenchymal tumors using novel monoclonal antibodies to the pineal body. Neuropathology. 22(2):66–76. PMID:12075938
2810. Yan H, Parsons DW, Jin G, McLendon R, Rasheed BA, Yuan W, et al. (2009). IDH1 and IDH2 mutations in gliomas. N Engl J Med. 360(8):765–73. PMID:19228619
2811. Yang C, Li G, Fang J, Wu L, Yang T, Deng X, et al. (2015). Clinical characteristics and surgical outcomes of primary spinal paragangliomas. J Neurooncol. 122(3):539–47. PMID:25720695
2812. Yang HJ, Kim JE, Paek SH, Chi JG, Jung HW, Kim DG (2003). The significance of gemistocytes in astrocytoma. Acta Neurochir (Wien). 145(12):1097–103, discussion 1103. PMID:14663567
2813. Yang I, Tihan T, Han SJ, Wrensch MR, Wiencke J, Sughrue ME, et al. (2010). CD8+ T-cell infiltrate in newly diagnosed glioblastoma is associated with long-term survival. J Clin Neurosci. 17(11):1381–5. PMID:20727764
2814. Yang P, Kollmeyer TM, Buckner K, Bamlet W, Ballman KV, Jenkins RB (2005). Polymorphisms in GLTSCR1 and ERCC2 are associated with the development of oligodendrogliomas. Cancer. 103(11):2363–72. PMID:15834925
2815. Yang SY, Jin YJ, Park SH, Jahng TA, Kim HJ, Chung CK (2005). Paragangliomas in the cauda equina region: clinicopathoradiologic findings in four cases. J Neurooncol. 72(1):49–55. PMID:15803375
2816. Yang X, Zeng Y, Wang J (2013). Hybrid schwannoma/perineurioma: report of 10 Chinese cases supporting a distinctive entity. Int J Surg Pathol. 21(1):22–8. PMID:22832113
2817. Yang ZJ, Ellis T, Markant SL, Read TA, Kessler JD, Bourboulas M, et al. (2008). Medulloblastoma can be initiated by deletion of Patched in lineage-restricted progenitors or stem cells. Cancer Cell. 14(2):135–45. PMID:18691548
2818. Yasargil MG, von Ammon K, von Deimling A, Valavanis A, Wichmann W, Wiestler OD (1992). Central neurocytoma: histopathological variants and therapeutic approaches. J Neurosurg. 76(1):32–7. PMID:1727166
2819. Yasha TC, Mohanty A, Radhesh S, Santosh V, Das S, Shankar SK (1998). Infratentorial dysembryoplastic neuroepithelial tumor (DNT) associated with Arnold-Chiari malformation. Clin Neuropathol. 17(6):305–10. PMID:9832257
2820. Yassa M, Bahary JP, Bourguoin P, Bélair M, Berthelet F, Bouthillier A (2005). Intra-parenchymal mesenchymal chondrosarcoma of the cerebellum: case report and review of the literature. J Neurooncol. 74(3):329–31. PMID:16187026
2821. Yeh-Nayre LA, Malicki DM, Vinocur DN, Crawford JR (2012). Medulloblastoma with excessive nodularity: radiographic features and pathologic correlate. Case Rep Radiol. 2012:310359. PMID:23133782
2822. Yi KS, Sohn CH, Yun TJ, Choi SH, Kim JH, Han MH, et al. (2012). MR imaging findings of extraventricular neurocytoma: a series of ten patients confirmed by immunohistochemistry of IDH1 gene mutation. Acta Neurochir (Wien). 154(11):1973–9, discussion 1980. PMID:22945896
2823. Yildiz H, Hakyemez B, Koroglu M, Yesildag A, Baykal B (2006). Intracranial lipomas: importance of localization. Neuroradiology. 48(1):1–7. PMID:16237548
2824. Yin XL, Hui AB, Pang JC, Poon WS, Ng HK (2002). Genome-wide survey for chromosomal imbalances in ganglioglioma using comparative genomic hybridization. Cancer Genet Cytogenet. 134(1):71–6. PMID:11996800
2825. Yip S, Butterfield YS, Morozova O, Chittaranjan S, Blough MD, An J, et al. (2012). Concurrent CIC mutations, IDH mutations, and 1p/19q loss distinguish oligodendrogliomas from other cancers. J Pathol. 226(1):7–16. PMID:22072542
2826. Yip S, Miao J, Cahill DP, Iafrate AJ, Aldape K, Nutt CL, et al. (2009). MSH6 mutations arise in glioblastomas during temozolomide therapy and mediate temozolomide resistance. Clin Cancer Res. 15(14):4622–9. PMID:19584161
2827. Yokota T, Tachizawa T, Fukino K, Teramoto A, Kouno J, Matsumoto K, et al. (2003). A family with spinal anaplastic ependymoma: evidence of loss of chromosome 22q in tumor. J Hum Genet. 48(11):598–602. PMID:14566482
2828. Yoo JH, Rivera A, Naeini RM, Yedururi S, Bayindir P, Megahead H, et al. (2008). Melanotic paraganglioma arising in the temporal horn following Langerhans cell histiocytosis. Pediatr Radiol. 38(5):571–4. PMID:18196230
2829. Yoshimoto M, de Toledo SR, da Silva NS, Bayani J, Bertozzi AP, Stavale JN, et al. (2004). Comparative genomic hybridization analysis of pediatric adamantinomatous craniopharyngiomas and a review of the literature. J Neurosurg. 101(1) Suppl:85–90. PMID:16206977
2830. Yoshimoto T, Takahashi-Fujigasaki J, Inoshita N, Fukuhara N, Nishioka H, Yamada S (2015). TTF-1-positive oncocytic sellar tumor with follicle formation/ependymal differentiation: non-adenomatous tumor capable of two different interpretations as a pituicytoma or a spindle cell oncocytoma. Brain Tumor Pathol. 32(3):221–7. PMID:25893822
2831. Yoshimura J, Onda K, Tanaka R, Takahashi H (2003). Clinicopathological study of diffuse type brainstem gliomas: analysis of 40 autopsy cases. Neurol Med Chir (Tokyo). 43(8):375–82, discussion 382. PMID:12968803
2832. You H, Kim YI, Im SY, Suh-Kim H, Paek SH, Park SH, et al. (2005). Immunohistochemical study of central neurocytoma, subependymoma, and subependymal giant cell astrocytoma. J Neurooncol. 74(1):1–8. PMID:16078101
2833. Young RJ, Sills AK, Brem S, Knopp EA (2005). Neuroimaging of metastatic brain disease. Neurosurgery. 57(5) Suppl:S10–23, S1–4. PMID:16237282
2834. Yu J, Deshmukh H, Payton JE, Dunham C, Scheithauer BW, Tihan T, et al. (2011). Array-based comparative genomic hybridization identifies CDK4 and FOXM1 alterations as independent predictors of survival in malignant peripheral nerve sheath tumor. Clin Cancer Res. 17(7):1924–34. PMID:21325289
2835. Yu T, Sun X, Wang J, Ren X, Lin N, Lin S (2015). Twenty-seven cases of pineal parenchymal tumours of intermediate differentiation: mitotic count, Ki-67 labelling index and extent of resection predict prognosis. J Neurol Neurosurg Psychiatry. PMID:25911570
2836. Zacharia BE, Bruce SS, Goldstein H, Malone HR, Neugut AI, Bruce JN (2012). Incidence, treatment and survival of patients with craniopharyngioma in the surveillance, epidemiology and end results program. Neuro Oncol. 14(8):1070–8. PMID:22735773
2837. Zada G, Lin N, Ojerholm E, Ramkissoon S, Laws ER (2010). Craniopharyngioma and other cystic epithelial lesions of the sellar region: a review of clinical, imaging, and histopathological relationships. Neurosurg Focus. 28(4):E4. PMID:20367361
2838. Zagzag D, Esencay M, Mendez O, Yee H, Smirnova I, Huang Y, et al. (2008). Hypoxia- and vascular endothelial growth factor-induced stromal cell-derived factor-1alpha/CXCR4 expression in glioblastomas: one plausible explanation of Scherer's structures. Am J Pathol. 173(2):545–60. PMID:18599607
2839. Zagzag D, Krishnamachary B, Yee H, Okuyama H, Chiriboga L, Ali MA, et al. (2005). Stromal cell-derived factor-1alpha and CXCR4 expression in hemangioblastoma and clear cell-renal cell carcinoma: von Hippel-Lindau loss-of-function induces expression of a ligand and its receptor. Cancer Res. 65(14):6178–88. PMID:16024619
2840. Zagzag D, Lukyanov Y, Lan L, Ali MA, Esencay M, Mendez O, et al. (2006). Hypoxia-inducible factor 1 and VEGF upregulate CXCR4 in glioblastoma: implications for angiogenesis and glioma cell invasion. Lab Invest. 86(12):1221–32. PMID:17075581
2841. Zagzag D, Zhong H, Scalzitti JM, Laughner E, Simons JW, Semenza GL (2000). Expression of hypoxia-inducible factor 1alpha in brain tumors: association with angiogenesis, invasion, and progression. Cancer. 88(11):2606–18. PMID:10861440
2842. Zajac V, Kirchhoff T, Levy ER, Horsley SW, Miller A, Steichen-Gersdorf E, et al. (1997). Characterisation of X;17(q12;p13) translocation breakpoints in a female patient with hypomelanosis of Ito and choroid plexus papilloma. Eur J Hum Genet. 5(2):61–8. PMID:9195154
2843. Zakrzewska M, Wojcik I, Zakrzewski K, Polis L, Grajkowska W, Roszkowski M, et al. (2005). Mutational analysis of hSNF5/INI1 and TP53 genes in choroid plexus carcinomas. Cancer Genet Cytogenet. 156(2):179–82. PMID:15642401
2844. Zaky W, Dhall G, Khatua S, Brown RJ, Ginn KF, Gardner SL, et al. (2015). Choroid plexus carcinoma in children: the Head Start experience. Pediatr Blood Cancer. 62(5):784–9. PMID:25662896
2845. Zamecnik M, Michal M (2001). Perineurial cell differentiation in neurofibromas. Report of eight cases including a case with composite perineurioma-neurofibroma features. Pathol Res Pract. 197(8):537–44. PMID:11518046
2846. Zang KD (2001). Meningioma: a cytogenetic model of a complex benign human tumor, including data on 394 karyotyped cases. Cytogenet Cell Genet. 93(3-4):207–20. PMID:11528114
2847. Zarate JO, Sampaolesi R (1999). Pleomorphic xanthoastrocytoma of the retina. Am J Surg Pathol. 23(1):79–81. PMID:9888706
2848. Zaveri J, La Q, Yarmish G, Neuman J (2014). More than just Langerhans cell histiocytosis: a radiologic review of histiocytic disorders. Radiographics. 34(7):2008–24. PMID:25384298
2848A. Zawlik I, Kita D, Vaccarella S, Mittelbronn M, Franceschi S, Ohgaki H (2009). Common polymorphisms in the MDM2 and TP53 genes and the relationship between TP53 mutations and patient outcomes in glioblastomas. Brain Pathol. 19(2):188–94. PMID:18462472
2849. Zbuk KM, Eng C (2007). Cancer phenomics: RET and PTEN as illustrative models. Nat Rev Cancer. 7(1):35–45. PMID:17167516
2850. Zbuk KM, Eng C (2007). Hamartomatous polyposis syndromes. Nat Clin Pract Gastroenterol Hepatol. 4(9):492–502. PMID:17768394
2851. Zevallos-Giampietri EA, Yañes HH, Orrego Puelles J, Barrionuevo C (2004). Primary meningeal Epstein-Barr virus-related leiomyosarcoma in a man infected with human immunodeficiency virus: review of literature, emphasizing the differential diagnosis and pathogenesis. Appl Immunohistochem Mol Morphol. 12(4):387–91. PMID:15536343
2852. Zhang CZ, Leibowitz ML, Pellman D (2013). Chromothripsis and beyond: rapid genome evolution from complex chromosomal rearrangements. Genes Dev. 27(23):2513–30. PMID:24298051
2853. Zhang F, Tan L, Wainwright LM, Bartolomei MS, Biegel JA (2002). No evidence for hypermethylation of the hSNF5/INI1 promoter in pediatric rhabdoid tumors. Genes Chromosomes Cancer. 34(4):398–405. PMID:12112529
2854. Zhang J, Cheng H, Qiao Q, Zhang JS, Wang YM, Fu X, et al. (2010). Malignant solitary fibrous tumor arising from the pineal region: case study and literature review. Neuropathology. 30(3):294–8. PMID:19845865
2855. Zhang J, Wu G, Miller CP, Tatevossian RG, Dalton JD, Tang B, et al.; St. Jude Children's Research Hospital–Washington University Pediatric Cancer Genome Project (2013). Whole-genome sequencing identifies genetic alterations in pediatric low-grade gliomas. Nat Genet. 45(6):602–12. PMID:23583981
2856. Zhang K, Lin JW, Wang J, Wu X, Gao H, Hsieh YC, et al. (2014). A germline missense mutation in COQ6 is associated with susceptibility to familial schwannomatosis. Genet Med. 16(10):787–92. PMID:24763291
2857. Zhang M, Wang Y, Jones S, Sausen M, McMahon K, Sharma R, et al. (2014). Somatic mutations of SUZ12 in malignant peripheral nerve sheath tumors. Nat Genet. 46(11):1170–2. PMID:25305755
2858. Zhang ZK, Davies KP, Allen J, Zhu L, Pestell RG, Zagzag D, et al. (2002). Cell cycle arrest and repression of cyclin D1 transcription by INI1/hSNF5. Mol Cell Biol. 22(16):5975–88. PMID:12138206
2859. Zheng H, Chang L, Patel N, Yang J, Lowe L, Burns DK, et al. (2008). Induction of abnormal proliferation by nonmyelinating schwann cells triggers neurofibroma formation. Cancer Cell. 13(2):117–28. PMID:18242512
2860. Zheng PP, Pang JC, Hui AB, Ng HK (2000). Comparative genomic hybridization detects losses of chromosomes 22 and 16 as the most common recurrent genetic alterations in primary ependymomas. Cancer Genet Cytogenet. 122(1):18–25. PMID:11104027
2861. Zhong H, De Marzo AM, Laughner E, Lim M, Hilton DA, Zagzag D, et al. (1999). Overexpression of hypoxia-inducible factor 1alpha in common human cancers and their metastases. Cancer Res. 59(22):5830–5. PMID:10582706
2862. Zhou H, Coffin CM, Perkins SL, Tripp SR, Liew M, Viskochil DH (2003). Malignant peripheral nerve sheath tumor: a comparison of grade, immunophenotype, and cell cycle/growth activation marker expression in sporadic and neurofibromatosis 1-related lesions. Am J Surg Pathol. 27(10):1337–45. PMID:14508395
2862A. Zhou J, Shrikhande G, Xu J, McKay RM, Burns DK, Johnson JE, Parada LF (2011). Tsc1 mutant neural stem/progenitor cells exhibit migration deficits and give rise to subependymal lesions in the lateral ventricle. Genes Dev. 25(15):1595–600. PMID:21828270
2863. Zhou X, Hampel H, Thiele H, Gorlin RJ, Hennekam RC, Parisi M, et al. (2001). Association of germline mutation in the PTEN tumour suppressor gene and Proteus and Proteus-like syndromes. Lancet. 358(9277):210–1. PMID:11476841
2864. Zhou XP, Marsh DJ, Morrison CD, Chaudhury AR, Maxwell M, Reifenberger G, et al. (2003). Germline inactivation of PTEN and dysregulation of the phosphoinositol-3-kinase/Akt pathway cause human Lhermitte-Duclos disease in adults. Am J Hum Genet. 73(5):1191–8. PMID:14566704
2865. Zhou XP, Waite KA, Pilarski R, Hampel H, Fernandez MJ, Bos C, et al. (2003). Germline PTEN promoter mutations and deletions in Cowden/Bannayan-Riley-Ruvalcaba syndrome result in aberrant PTEN protein and dysregulation of the phosphoinositol-3-kinase/Akt pathway. Am J Hum Genet. 73(2):404–11. PMID:12844284
2866. Zhu HD, Xie Q, Gong Y, Mao Y, Zhong P, Hang FP, et al. (2013). Lymphoplasmacyte-rich meningioma: our experience with 19 cases and a systematic literature review. Int J Clin Exp Med. 6(7):504–15. PMID:23936588
2867. Zhu J, Frosch MP, Busque L, Beggs AH, Dashner K, Gilliland DG, et al. (1995). Analysis of meningiomas by methylation- and transcription-based clonality assays. Cancer Res. 55(17):3865–72. PMID:7641206
2868. Zhu L, Ren G, Li K, Liang ZH, Tang WJ, Ji YM, et al. (2011). Pineal parenchymal tumours: minimum apparent diffusion coefficient in prediction of tumour grading. J Int Med Res. 39(4):1456–63. PMID:21986148

2869. Zhu Y, Ghosh P, Charnay P, Burns DK, Parada LF (2002). Neurofibromas in NF1: Schwann cell origin and role of tumor environment. Science. 296(5569):920–2. PMID:11988578

2870. Zhukova N, Ramaswamy V, Remke M, Pfaff E, Shih DJ, Martin DC, et al. (2013). Subgroup-specific prognostic implications of TP53 mutation in medulloblastoma. J Clin Oncol. 31(23):2927–35. PMID:23835706

2871. Zlatescu MC, TehraniYazdi A, Sasaki H, Megyesi JF, Betensky RA, Louis DN, et al. (2001). Tumor location and growth pattern correlate with genetic signature in oligodendroglial neoplasms. Cancer Res. 61(18):6713–5. PMID:11559541

2872. Zong H, Parada LF, Baker SJ (2015). Cell of origin for malignant gliomas and its implication in therapeutic development. Cold Spring Harb Perspect Biol. 7(5) PMID:25635044

2873. Zorludemir S, Scheithauer BW, Hirose T, Van Houten C, Miller G, Meyer FB (1995). Clear cell meningioma. A clinicopathologic study of a potentially aggressive variant of meningioma. Am J Surg Pathol. 19(5):493–505. PMID:7726360

2874. Zou C, Smith KD, Liu J, Lahat G, Myers S, Wang WL, et al. (2009). Clinical, pathological, and molecular variables predictive of malignant peripheral nerve sheath tumor outcome. Ann Surg. 249(6):1014–22. PMID:19474676

2875. Zuccaro G, Taratuto AL, Monges J (1986). Intracranial neoplasms during the first year of life. Surg Neurol. 26(1):29–36. PMID:3715697

2876. Zulch KJ (1957). Brain Tumours. Their Biology and Pathology. New York: Springer-Verlag.

2877. Zygourakis CC, Rolston JD, Lee HS, Partow C, Kunwar S, Aghi MK (2015). Pituicytomas and spindle cell oncocytomas: modern case series from the University of California, San Francisco. Pituitary. 18(1):150–8. PMID:24823438

2878. Zülch KJ, editor (1979). Histological typing of tumours of the central nervous system. 1st Edition Geneva: World Health Organization.

2879. Zöller ME, Rembeck B, Odén A, Samuelsson M, Angervall L (1997). Malignant and benign tumors in patients with neurofibromatosis type 1 in a defined Swedish population. Cancer. 79(11):2125–31. PMID:9179058

Subject index

L

L1 antigen 282
L1CAM 108, 112, 206
L2HGDH 43
L-2-hydroxyglutaric aciduria 42
Lactate dehydrogenase 37, 64
Laminin 84, 217, 218, 223
Langerhans cell histiocytosis **280**, 281
Langerin 280, 282
LARGE 235
Large cell / anaplastic medulloblastoma 184, **200**
LATS1 313
LDB1 197
LDB2 141
Leiomyoma **262**
Leiomyosarcoma **262**
Leptomyelolipomas 260
LEU4 143
LEU7 64, 217, 256
LFL-B 310
LFL-E2 310
LFS See Li–Fraumeni syndrome
Lhermitte–Duclos disease 136, **142**, 143, 314
Li–Fraumeni syndrome 21, 42, 43, 54, 56, 59, 128, 188, 191, 192, 197, **310**, 317
LIN28A 202, 204, 206, 207, 289, 290
Lipidized glioblastoma 35
Lipidized mature neuroectodermal tumour of the cerebellum 161
Lipoma 240, **260**
Lipomatous glioneurocytoma 161
Liposarcoma 260
Lisch nodules 294, 295
LMO2 275
Low-grade B-cell lymphomas **276**
LRP1B 50, 193
LSAMP 50
Lupus erythematosus 275
Lymphomatoid granulomatosis **276**
Lymphomatosis cerebri 272
Lymphoplasmacyte-rich meningioma **240**
Lymphoplasmacytic lymphoma 276
Lynch syndrome 67, 317, 318
Lys656 mutation 151
Lysozyme 280, 282, 283
LZTR1 218, 301–303

M

MAC387 282, 283
MACF1 86, 140
Maffucci syndrome 249
Malignant ectomesenchymoma 262
Malignant fibrous histiocytoma See Undifferentiated pleomorphic sarcoma / malignant fibrous histiocytoma
Malignant perineurioma See MPNST with perineurial differentiation
Malignant peripheral nerve sheath tumour **226**, 228, 294
Malignant peripheral nerve sheath tumour with divergent differentiation **227**
Malignant pineocytoma 173
Malignant triton tumour 227
MALT1 274
MALT lymphoma See Extranodal marginal zone lymphoma of mucosa-associated lymphoid tissue of the dura

MAP2K1 137, 280
Mature teratoma **291**
MAX 167
MBEN See Medulloblastoma with extensive nodularity
MDM2 39, 40, 49, 96, 103, 118, 129, 146
MDM4 39, 191
Medulloblastoma, classic 184, **194**
Medulloblastoma, group 3 184, **193**
Medulloblastoma, group 4 184, **193**
Medulloblastoma, non-WNT/non-SHH 184, **193**
Medulloblastoma, NOS 184, **186**
Medulloblastoma, SHH-activated and TP53-mutant 184, **190**
Medulloblastoma, SHH-activated and TP53-wildtype 184, **190**, 191
Medulloblastoma with extensive nodularity 184, **198**, 199, 319
Medulloblastoma, WNT-activated 184,**188**, 189, 318
Medullocytoma 161
Medulloepithelioma 201, **202**–204, 206, **207**
MEG3 235
Melan-A 51, 187, 228, 266, 341
Melanotic neuroectodermal tumour of infancy (retinal anlage tumour) 266
Melanotic schwannoma 218
Meningeal melanocytoma 268
Meningeal melanocytosis 266, **267**
Meningeal melanoma 269
Meningeal melanomatosis 266, **267**, 269
Meningioangiomatosis 299
Meningioma **232**
Meningioma with oncocytic features 245
Meningothelial meningioma 233, **237**
Merlin 117, 214, 217, 235, 299, 300
Mesenchymal chondrosarcoma 253, 263
MET 39, 51, 59, 146, 151, 229
Metaplastic meningioma 233, **240**
Metastatic tumours of the CNS 338
MGMT promoter methylation 21, 28, 41–44, 68, 69, 74, 125
Microcystic meningioma 233, **239**
Microtubule-associated protein tau 171
Microvascular proliferation 17, 32, 36, 37, 46, 98, 114, 148, 157, 180
Minigemistocytes 23, 62, 64, 68, 72, 148, 149
Mismatch repair cancer syndrome 188, 317, 318
MITF 266, 341
Mixed germ cell tumour **291**
Mixed pineocytoma–pineoblastoma 173, 177
MKRN1 86
MLH1 43, 317, 318
MLL 41, 59
MLLT10 236
MMP2 31, 49
MMP9 31, 49
MN1 235
Moesin 299, 308
Monomorphous angiocentric glioma 119
Monosomy 22 42, 238
Mosaicism 92, 296, 308
MPNST See Malignant peripheral nerve sheath tumour
MPNST with perineurial differentiation (malignant perineurioma) **228**

MRAS 295
MSH2 43, 317, 318
MSH3 43, 317
MSH4 313
MSH6 43, 69, 317, 318
mTOR1 93
mTORC1 300
MUC4 224
Multifocal glioblastoma 31
Multinodular and vacuolating neuronal tumour of the cerebrum **137**
Multiple endocrine neoplasia type 2 167
Multiple germline mutations 313
Multiple neurilemmomas 301
MUM1/IRF4 273
MYB 23, 60, 68, 120
MYC 21, 34, 59, 185, 193, 200, 273
MYCL 190, 191
MYCN 34, 59, 158, 185, 190–193, 197, 200
MYC-PVT1 fusion 193
MYD88 274
Myelin-associated glycoprotein 64
Myelin basic protein 64
Myofibroblastoma **260**
Myogenin 187, 262
Myxopapillary ependymoma 104, 105, 109, 167

N

N546K mutation 86, 149
NAB2 249, 250, 253, 254
NAB2-STAT6 fusion 249, 250, 253, 254
NADP+ 55
Naevoid basal cell carcinoma syndrome 188, 191, 192, 195, 197–199, 236, **319**–321
NANOG 289
Napsin-A 341
NCAM1 58, 103, 105, 122, 181, 194, 256, 341
NCOA2 264
NDRG2 235
Nerve growth factor 67
Nestin 38
Neurilemmomatosis 301
Neurilemoma 214
Neurinoma 214
Neuroendocrine islet cell tumour 304
Neurofibroma **219**, 221, 294, 295, 298
Neurofibromatosis type 1 42, 43, 59, 80, 89, 94, 97, 135, 141, 151, 167, 219, 222, 224, 226, 274, 287, **294**–297, 301, 317
Neurofibromatosis type 2 109, **297**, 301
Neurolipocytoma 161
Neuromuscular choristoma 262
Neuron-specific enolase 256
Nf1–/– 295
NF1 See Neurofibromatosis type 1
NF2 See Neurofibromatosis type 2
NF-kappaB 112, 274
NFKB1A deletion 39
NGN1 163
Nijmegen breakage syndrome 188
NOGO-A 65, 69, 134
Non-polyposis colorectal carcinoma 42
Non-WNT/non-SHH medulloblastoma 193
Noonan syndrome 87–89, 151
NOTCH1 66, 72, 73
NPM1 277

Rubinstein–Taybi syndrome 188

List of abbreviations

AIDS	Acquired immunodeficiency syndrome
ATP	Adenosine triphosphate
cAMP	Cyclic adenosine monophosphate
cDNA	Complementary deoxyribonucleic acid
CI	Confidence interval
CNS	Central nervous system
CT	Computed tomography
DNA	Deoxyribonucleic acid
EBV	Epstein–Barr virus
EGFR	Epidermal growth factor receptor
EMA	Epithelial membrane antigen
FDG-PET	18F-fluorodeoxyglucose positron emission tomography
FISH	Fluorescence in situ hybridization
G-CIMP	Glioma CpG island methylator phenotype
GDP	Guanosine diphosphate
GFAP	Glial fibrillary acidic protein
GTP	Guanosine-5′-triphosphate
H&E	Haematoxylin and eosin
HAART	Highly active antiretroviral therapy
HHV6	Human herpesvirus 6
HHV8	Human herpesvirus 8
HIV	Human immunodeficiency virus
ICD-O	International Classification of Diseases for Oncology
LOH	Loss of heterozygosity
MIM number	Mendelian Inheritance in Man number
MR angiography	Magnetic resonance angiography
MR spectroscopy	Magnetic resonance spectroscopy
MRI	Magnetic resonance imaging
mRNA	Messenger ribonucleic acid
NFP	Neurofilament protein
NOS	Not otherwise specified
OR	Odds ratio
PCR	Polymerase chain reaction
PCV	Procarbazine, lomustine, and vincristine
RNA	Ribonucleic acid
RT-PCR	Reverse transcriptase polymerase chain reaction
SEER	Surveillance, Epidemiology, and End Results
SNP	Sngle nucleotide polymorphism
SV40	Simian virus 40
TNM	Tumour, node, metastasis